R 728.8 .S275   Saunders manual of medical assisting practice / [edited by] Karen Lane.

DATE DUE

8/2/96			
10/8/96			
GAYLORD			PRINTED IN U.S.A.

SAUNDERS MANUAL OF MEDICAL ASSISTING PRACTICE

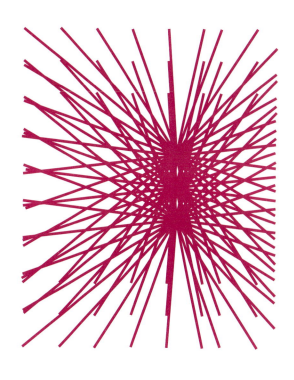

Section Editors

JEAN ERWIN KEENON, BS, MA, CMA-A
Professor and Program Director,
Medical Assistant,
Multiple Competency Clinical Technician
and Medical Transcription Programs
School of Health Related Professions
The University of Alabama at Birmingham
Birmingham, Alabama

1990–1991 President
American Association of Medical Assistants

CRYSTAL COLEMAN, CMA-AC
Currently Serving as:
Member, Board of Trustees
Manager, Annual Convention Strategy Team
Member, Task Force to Study Feasibility of a Managers' Section
Member, Speakers Bureau Strategy Team
Chairman, Resolutions Committee
Speakers Bureau Representative:
1992 — Iowa, Montana, Virginia
1991 — New Jersey, Virginia

Division Administrator, Northridge Internal Medicine,
University of Virginia Health Sciences Center,
Charlottesville, Virginia

Formerly:
Chairman, Continuing Education Board
Member, Continuing Education Board Task Force
Chairman, National Convention
Member, Resolutions Committee
Member, Public Relations Committee

SAUNDERS MANUAL OF MEDICAL ASSISTING PRACTICE

Karen Lane, CMA-AC
Former Program Director, Medical Assisting Program
Instructor, Medical Assisting Program
Medix School, Baltimore, Maryland

Former Chairman, Curriculum Review Board of the
American Association of Medical Assistants Endowment

Former Consultant, Certification Test Construction
Task Force, American Association of Medical Assistants

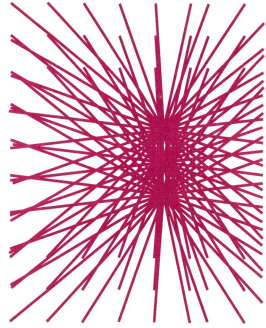

W. B. SAUNDERS COMPANY
Harcourt Brace Jovanovich, Inc.
Philadelphia London Montreal Toronto Sydney Tokyo

W. B. Saunders Company
Harcourt Brace Jovanovich, Inc.

The Curtis Center
Independence Square West
Philadelphia, Pennsylvania 19106

Library of Congress Cataloging-in-Publication Data

Saunders manual of medical assisting practice / [edited by] Karen
  Lane.
     p.   cm.
     Includes index.
     ISBN 0-7216-3063-4
     1. Medical assistants.   I. Lane, Karen
     [DNLM: 1. Allied Health Personnel. 2. Practice Management. W 80
S257]
R728.8.S275   1993
610.73'7—dc20
DNLM/DLC   92-49703

Saunders Manual of Medical Assisting Practice   ISBN 0-7216-3063-4

Copyright © 1993 by W. B. Saunders Company

All rights reserved. No part of this publication may be reproduced or transmitted in any form or by any means, electronic or mechanical, including photocopy, recording, or any information storage and retrieval system, without permission in writing from the publisher.

Printed in the United States of America.

Last digit is the print number.   9   8   7   6   5   4   3   2   1

To Shirley Kuhn, the best quarterback any team of writers could have.

CONTRIBUTORS

Carolyn C. Avery, CMA-A, is founder and president of her own medical malpractice consulting firm and has over 25 years' experience as a medical assistant. She teaches medical assistants at Trevecca Nazarene College in Nashville, Tennessee, and coordinates insurance workshops for the Tennessee Medical Association. She lectures and has published numerous booklets in the areas of medical malpractice and office management.

Jeannette R. Bell, CLS(NCA), MT(ASCP), is Associate Professor, Clinical Laboratory Sciences Division, at The University of Alabama at Birmingham. She has written for the *American Journal of Medical Technology* and has assisted in developing the CLS and CLT examinations for the National Certification Agency for Clinical Laboratory Personnel.

Juanita N. Blocker, LPN, CMA-AC, has been a practicing medical assistant for more than 25 years. She was President of the American Association of Medical Assistants from 1989 to 1990 and has been a part-time instructor at Enterprise State Junior College in Enterprise, Alabama. She is an author and editor of numerous medical assisting journal articles and publications.

Nancy Vines Campbell, CMA, is an administrative medical assistant specializing in insurance and billing, Department of Family Medicine, at the University of Alabama at Birmingham. She teaches practice management to family medicine residents and is a management consultant to private practices in the Birmingham area.

Carol S. Champagne, RMA, CMA-C, ICEA, CCE, is a respected leader in continuing education. She resides in Hayesville, Kansas, where she runs her own business publishing continuing education books for medical assistants. She has authored countless study guides and articles that appear regularly in *AMT Events*. She has five times been the recipient of national American Medical Technologists achievement awards for her work in post-graduate medical assistant education.

Crystal Coleman, CMA-AC, Section Editor, is the Division Administrator of the Northridge Internal Medicine Center at the University of Virginia Health Sciences Center in Charlottesville, Virginia. She is active on the national level and served as Chairman of the Continuing Education Board of the American Association of Medical Assistants. She currently is serving on a national task force to research the feasibility of an advanced medical assistant management program.

Joan B. Conrad, CMA-A, has been the practice administrator of a professional corporation for internal medicine specialists for over 20 years. In addition, she has taught the administrative portions of medical assisting in a proprietary setting on a part-time basis. Her special areas of interest and study are employment law and handwriting analysis. She has written articles and lectured on both topics. Her articles have appeared in the *Professional Medical Assistant* magazine.

Dale Davis, RCT, is a partner in Cardiac Educational Resources—an organization dedicated to providing educational programs for the allied health professional in the cardiac field. She is the author of three books: *How to Quickly and Accurately Master ECG Interpretation* (Lippincott, 1985); *How to Quickly and Accurately Master Arrhythmia Interpretation* (Lippincott, 1989); and *Differential Diagnosis of Arrhythmias,* released in 1991 by W.B. Saunders. She is a past assistant director and instructor for the Morristown Memorial Hospital School of Cardiovascular Technology. She currently resides in Hawaii.

Julianna S. Drumheller, CMA, manages a busy family practice in Charlottesville, Virginia. She is a member of the Curriculum Review Board of the American Association of Medical Assistants and additionally participates at both the local and state society levels. She is a medical assisting program consultant and surveyor.

June M. Francis, RN, CMA, has been managing the practices of general surgeons for the past 15 years in Silverdale, Washington. She divides her time and abilities between her management and clinical duties and has managed medical assisting student externs in association with the local community college, with signal successes at each.

Walter R. Frank, III, BS, RT(R), is President and CEO of Medical Diagnostics Limited in Baltimore, Maryland. He is a past chief technologist and has taught radiology to medical assisting students.

Margaret Giddens Fritsma, MA, MT(ASCP)SBB, is Associate Professor, Clinical Laboratory Sciences Division, Applied Health Sciences, School of Health Related Professions, at the University of Alabama at Birmingham. She has presented courses, seminars, and workshops in immunohematology, hemostasis, and immunology, and serves as an inspector for accreditation of blood banks and hospital transfusion services by the American Association of Blood Banks.

Ann M. Gray, BS, CMA-AC, lives in Essex Junction, Vermont, with her four cats. She has worked in a vascular surgery practice for 26 years. She has been a guest lecturer to the Medical Assisting Department at Champlain College in Burlington, Vermont, and edits a monthly newsletter for the local chamber of commerce. She has contributed numerous journal articles to the *Professional Medical Assistant* and *Medical Economics*.

Loretta Hatlestad, CMA, is an office manager in an urology practice in Bozeman, Montana, where she divides her time between management and patient care. She teaches certification examination preparation classes for the local medical assisting society.

Nanette L. Hoffman combines her degree in health policy and administration with a career in a privately owned computer company in Charlottesville, Virginia. She performs installations of both computer hardware and software and provides computerized practice management services to physicians and other health care providers.

Patricia S. Hurlbut, BS, CLS(NCA), MT(ASCP), CMA, is Program Director of Medical Assisting at Stratton College in Milwaukee, Wisconsin. She spends her time outside of Stratton leading courses in Christian bioethics and bilingual first-aid and CPR. She has served in most of the offices and committees of the local medical assisting society.

Linda Jeff, MA, MT(ASCP), is Associate Professor, Clinical Laboratory Sciences Division, Applied Health Sciences, School of Health Related Professions, at the University of Alabama at Birmingham. She has made presentations and written publications and self-instructional units in microbiology, immunology, and laboratory medicine instruction.

Jean Erwin Keenon, BS, MA, CMA-A, Section Editor, is a Professor and Program Director for the Medical Assisting, Multiple Competency Clinical Technician, and Medical Transcriptionist Programs at the School of Health Related Professions, University of Alabama at Birmingham. She was Chairman of the AAMA Certifying Board for four years and 1990–1991 President of the AAMA.

Mary A. Klinge, RRA, CMA-A, is Manager of Patient Planning Services at a large medical center in Great Bend, Kansas. Her responsibilities include utilization review, quality assurance, risk management, credentialing, and safety and social services. She has taught numerous *ICD-9* coding workshops across the United States and writes for the *Professional Medical Assistant* in the areas of medical records and coding.

Karen Lane, CMA-AC, Editor, is the author of *Medications: A Guide for the Health Professions* (F.A. Davis Company, 1992) and *The Medical Assisting Examination Guide* (F.A. Davis Company, 1990), and has provided special editorial assistance to the sixth edition of *The Medical Assistant: Administrative and Clinical* (W.B. Saunders, 1988). During her 20 years as a medical assisting educator, she has served on numerous national accreditation and certification committees. She is co-authoring a medical assisting student textbook revision soon to be published.

Marcia "Marti" Lewis, RN, EdD, CMA-AC, writes in the areas of law and ethics. Her approach to the patient with understanding, sensitivity, and compassion is highly regarded by educators and practitioners alike. She is an administrator who teaches at Olymic College in Bremerton, Washington. She is co-author of *Law and Ethics in the Medical Office Including Bioethical Issues* (2nd ed., F.A. Davis Company, 1988) and *Diseases of the Human Body* (F.A. Davis Company, 1989). Her textbooks are widely used at colleges everywhere.

Lisa C. McCollum, BS, CMA-AC, is the Director of Operations of the American Association of Medical Assistants at its headquarters in Chicago. She has served on the Association's Curriculum Review Board and was a medical assisting practitioner in Washington State. She has taught behavior modification courses and medical assisting students at Olympic Community College in Seattle, Washington.

Gary M. Munson, BS, is a radiographer with Medical Diagnostics Limited in Baltimore, Maryland. He is currently pursuing graduate study in molecular biology. He is a military-trained radiographer and was formerly a health services technician in the United States Coast Guard.

Linda T. Powell, RN, CMA, is Associate Faculty for the Medical Assistant and Multiple Competency Clinical Technician Programs at The University of Alabama at Birmingham. In addition to her teaching responsibilities, she is a staff nurse at the University of Alabama Hospital in Birmingham.

Midge Noel Ray, MSN, CMA-C, is Associate Professor, Division of Health Information Management, School of Health Related Professions, at the University of Alabama at Birmingham. She divides her time between teaching and working in the newborn intensive care unit at the University of Alabama Hospital.

Vicki S. Sanders, MA, CMA, teaches courses in administrative medical assisting and is coordinator of the Medical Transcriptionist Program, School of Health Related Professions at the University of Alabama at Birmingham. Before accepting her teaching position, she worked as an office manager for a family practice clinic and an after-hour emergency care center. Other professional activities have included editing and consulting for numerous publications and continuing education workshops.

Jane B. Seelig, CMA-A, is a practice management consultant and seminar speaker specializing in practice organization and personnel management. She currently is the hospital billing coordinator for the Departments of Pathology and Anesthesiology. She has managed the office and business for a multiphysician specialty practice with multiple satellite offices and taught part-time as a medical assisting instructor at the Indiana Vocational Technical College, in Columbus, Indiana.

Deborah A. Standefer, CMA, is an administrative medical assistant of 17 years in Soldotna, Alaska. Her experience includes group and solo practices and responsibilities for managing the start-up of two practices. Her special interests include medical practice finance and accounting.

Betty Bates Tempkin, BA, RTR, RDMS, is the previous Clinical Director of the Sonography Program at Hillsborough Community College in Tampa, Florida. She is currently writing three sonography textbooks from her home and is a free-lance consultant for various hospitals and radiology offices in the Tampa Bay area. Prior to her sonography career, Betty taught medical assistants at Webster College in Bradenton, Florida.

Lois E. Wolfgang, MHS, BSN, CMA, is an associate professor at Trevecca Nazarene College in Nashville, Tennessee, and has served as its Medical Assistant Program Director for the last 14 years. For 30 years as a baccalaureate nurse, she has been active in general duty, administration, and nursing education at several different levels.

Rachel K. Younger, BA, C(ASCP), RMA, CMA-ACP, is retired as Assistant Professor of Surgery, Vanderbilt University Medical Center, Nashville, Tennessee. She has served as a medical assistant lecturer and is a past Chairman of the Education Committee and Continuing Education Board of the American Association of Medical Assistants. Her contributions to the medical assisting profession on a national level span a period of more than 20 years, testimony to her enduring quality.

PREFACE

The Saunders Manual of Medical Assisting Practice is designed for both the practitioner and the student. As a procedure and reference manual, its purpose is to help medical assistants keep up to date on diagnostic and treatment procedures, on office management responsibilities, and on the recent outpouring of legislation that has been designed to regulate the delivery of health care. In these times of such rapid change, it is important that medical assistants be knowledgeable about their increasing role and function to enhance administrative and clinical judgment and high-quality patient care in the ambulatory setting.

A key feature of this manual is that the procedures are designed in the competency-based format. The format of each procedure includes *Universal Precaution symbols;* the purpose of the procedure; a list of necessary equipment and materials; the step-by-step order for performing the procedure; and rationales for steps, when further explanations are necessary. The Universal Precaution symbols are presented in an instantly recognizable format that designates when and which Universal Precautions apply.

Another key feature of this manual is the use of the *Medical Assisting Alert* and *Special Hints*. The *Medical Assisting Alert* focuses the medical assistant's attention on potential complications or dangers in patient care. The *Special Hints* are invaluable because they provide information beyond the usual entry-level material contained in textbooks.

Numerous illustrations and tables are included to enhance the reader's understanding of the procedures and processes contained in the book. There are four appendices: Appendix A, General Information Resources; Appendix B, Administrative Information; Appendix C, Clinical Information; and Appendix D, Standards and Regulations. The appendices include actual texts of the government standards and regulations requiring compliance in physician offices and laboratories.

The Saunders Manual of Medical Assisting Practice contains chapters on material not usually included in entry-level texts or in procedure manuals designed for hospital-based physicians and nurses. This manual is the first definitive single source to contain not only the tasks required of the entry-level medical assistant but also advanced tasks in the areas of office management, finance, laboratory and diagnostic tests, and caring for the pediatric and OB-GYN patient. The topical format of the chapters and the cross-referencing approach both within the chapters and in the indexing should ensure quick and easy retrieval of the procedures.

The manual was developed by more than 30 educators and practitioners across the United States. It is our hope that it reflects not only the DACUM

(*Developing A CurriculUM*) process (developed by the American Association of Medical Assistants to define the scope of instruction for a medical assisting curriculum) but also the daily scope of practice as it is performed on the job everywhere. We also hope that this manual answers once and for all what medical assistants can do in the ambulatory setting. It is our belief that the *Saunders Manual of Medical Assisting Practice* will be an invaluable quick reference for all levels of personnel working in the physician's office or other outpatient setting.

We thank the contributors who have shared their knowledge and clinical expertise and express our gratitude for their professonalism and desire to share with the reader their excellence in high-quality patient care. While realizing that nothing is ever constant in health care, this manual reflects the degree of our participation in the kind and quality of health care being delivered into the community.

KAREN LANE
CRYSTAL COLEMAN
JEAN ERWIN KEENON

ACKNOWLEDGMENTS

We wish to extend our gratitude to the wide variety of friends and co-workers and to the W.B. Saunders Company staff who have contributed their time and expertise in the development of this text. Thanks also to our families, who willingly supported the time we spent from them researching and creating the manuscripts.

We would also like to recognize Lisa C. McCollum, for her advice on the organization of the material; and Danyka Wolfkill-Hoffman, for reviewing portions of the manuscript.

A special expression of gratitude is extended to Linda R. Garber, Production Manager, who helped immeasurably to keep the project moving; and to Tom Stringer, for his superb copy editing skills. We thank Charles Keenan, former assistant to Margaret Biblis, for coordinating the mounds of correspondence to and from the contributors in the early phases of this effort.

Much of the original artwork in this book can be attributed to the highly skilled professionals assigned to our project: Cecilia Roberts, our illustration specialist who coordinated the entire art program; Bill Donnelly, who designed the interior of the book; and Ellen Bodner-Zanolle, who designed the cover. The processing of many of the illustrations was the computerized genius of Beach Studios. We also wish to thank all those outside contributors who so generously supplied us with existing illustrations.

Finally, we thank our developmental editor, Shirley Kuhn, who used her outstanding management skills to cajole, support, kindly nag, and guide us to the end; and our acquisitions editor, Margaret Biblis, who believed in our abilities and the importance of this project from the start.

KAREN LANE
CRYSTAL COLEMAN
JEAN ERWIN KEENON

CONTENTS

Section One
ADMINISTRATIVE PRACTICES   1

Chapter 1
APPOINTMENTS AND TELECOMMUNICATIONS   3
    CAROLYN C. AVERY and RACHEL K. YOUNGER

SCHEDULING APPOINTMENTS IN THE OFFICE   3
Mission Statement   3
Decisions to Be Made   4
Setting up a Manual Appointment System in a Primary Care Setting   4
Setting up a Manual Appointment System in a Specialist's Office   9
Making Appointments   9
Ethical/Legal Considerations Involving the Appointment Book   13
Computerized Appointment Systems   13
APPOINTMENT SCHEDULING OUTSIDE THE OFFICE   13
Referrals for Consultations and Clinical Tests   13
Referral to Outpatient Surgery Center and Hospitals   13
TELEPHONE MANAGEMENT   15
Screening Telephone Calls   15
What to Tell the Caller   16
Answering the Telephone   16
Getting the Message to the Physician   16
Getting the Message to the Client   16
Taking Messages after Hours   17

Chapter 2
MEDICAL RECORDS AND CORRESPONDENCE   19
    ANN M. GRAY

MEDICAL RECORDS   19
Filing and Identification Systems   19
Source-Oriented Medical Records   25
Problem-Oriented Medical Records   26
Patient Data Collection   27
Authorization to Release Records   31
MEDICAL CORRESPONDENCE   34
Mail Processing   34
Letter-Writing Formats   38
Attending Physician Statement   40
Medical Reports   41
Manuscript Preparation   42

Chapter 3
FACILITIES MANAGEMENT 45
JULIANNA S. DRUMHELLER

OPENING A PRACTICE 45
Suggested Time Frame for Opening a Practice 45
Renting Versus Owning 46
Site Selection 46
Space Planning 46
Construction and Building Negotiation 46
Supplies and Furniture 47
OBTAINING NEW OR ADDITIONAL SPACE 47
CLOSING A PRACTICE 48
LANDLORD RELATIONS 49
COMMUNITY RELATIONS 53

Chapter 4
OFFICE EQUIPMENT AND SERVICES 55
JANE B. SEELIG

LEASE AND PURCHASE AGREEMENTS 55
Financial And Tax Advantages 56
Depreciation 56
Policy and Procedure Development 56
Policy/Procedure Manuals and Updating Procedures 58
Maintenance Agreements 58
SECURITY 58
Access and Activation 59
Sensor Placement 59
Options 59
GROUNDS AND PARKING SYSTEMS 59
Waste Disposal 60
Custodial and Housekeeping Services 60
Security Violation, Incident Handling, Reporting, and Follow-up 60
PURCHASING AND INVENTORY CONTROL 61
Purchasing Control 61
Storage and Inventory 62
Inventory Control 63
OFFICE EQUIPMENT AND MAINTENANCE 64
Telephone Systems and Services 64
Photocopy Machines and Services 64
Facsimile (Fax) Machines and Services 65
Computers 65
SALES REPRESENTATIVES 65
Sample Handling 65
Recourse from Suppliers 65

Chapter 5
QUALITY ASSURANCE 67
LOIS E. WOLFGANG

QUALITY ASSURANCE 67
Purpose of Quality Assurance 68
Quality Assurance Process 68
QUALITY OF CARE 70
Qualifications of Allied Health Personnel 70
Continuing Education 70
Job Performance 71

MEDICAL RECORDS   72
RISK MANAGEMENT   72
Incident Report and Follow-up   74
QUALITY CONTROL   74
Safety Management   74
Laboratory and Radiology   75
Infection Control   75

Chapter 6
BOOKKEEPING, CREDIT, AND COLLECTIONS   77
VICKI S. SANDERS

BOOKKEEPING SYSTEMS   77
Starting a System   77
Bookkeeping Methods   78
Double-Entry Accounting   78
Bookkeeping Systems   79
Maintaining an Accounts Receivable Bookkeeping System   82
Posting Special Accounting Entries   87
Completing an Accounts Receivable Trial Balance   92
Maintaining an Accounts Payable Bookkeeping System   93
Completing a Disbursements Journal Trial Balance   94
Completing a Year-to-Date Cash Disbursements Summary   97
Maintaining Petty Cash Records   97
BANKING   98
Opening a Checking Account   98
Selecting Checks   100
Writing Checks   100
Accepting Checks for Payment   101
Endorsing Checks   101
Making Bank Deposits   101
Reconciling a Bank Statement   104
CREDIT AND COLLECTIONS   108
Establishing a Credit and Collection System   108
Billing Patients   112
Collecting Past Due Accounts   114
Collection Ratio   122
Preparing an Accounts Receivable Aging Record   122
Preparing a Monthly Accounts Receivable Analysis   122

Chapter 7
ACCOUNTING AND TAXES   123
DEBORAH A. STANDEFER

ACCOUNTING   123
Accounting Methods   123
Chart of Accounts   124
Revenue   124
Expenditures   131
Balance Sheet   142
Income Statement   143
Analysis of Profit and Loss   144
Cost Analysis of Services and Procedures   144
Budget   144
TAXES   146
Property Tax   146
State Tax   146
Federal Taxes   146

Chapter 8
INSURANCE AND CODING 157
  NANCY VINES CAMPBELL and MARY KLINGE

COVERAGE AND POLICIES 157
Types of Health Insurance Coverage 157
Types of Health Insurance Policies 158
CLAIMS PROCESSING 170
Information from the Medical Record/Patient 170
Assignments 170
Claim Forms 173
Claim Filing Deadline 179
Insurance Log 179
PAYMENTS AND REJECTIONS 179
Methods of Payments 179
Explanation of Benefit 181
Rejections 183
Refiles 183
HEALTH MAINTENANCE ORGANIZATIONS 186
Types of HMOs 186
ICD-9-CM CODING 187
History 187
Impact of the *ICD-9-CM* on Physicians' Offices 187
Prerequisites for Accurate Coding 189
The *ICD-9-CM* Coding Books 189
Remembering the Basics: Some Guidelines 193
The Employee's Role in Coding 195
Physician Education 196
Validation of the Diagnosis in the Medical Record 197
Guidelines for Coding Specific Conditions 197
Additional Coding Information 203
Diagnosis-Related Groups 203
The Future of the ICD 204

Chapter 9
COMPUTERIZATION AND PRACTICE MANAGEMENT FOR THE HEALTH CARE PROVIDER 205
  NANETTE HOFFMAN

BENEFITS OF COMPUTERIZING A MEDICAL PRACTICE 205
Efficient Patient Billing 205
Efficient Third-Party Reimbursement 206
Efficient Patient Recall and Scheduling 206
Evaluation of the Practice 206
Better Patient Care 206
More Efficient Office Staff 206
Flexibility of the Software to Grow with the Practice and Handle Changes in the Health Care Industry 206
HARDWARE CONSIDERATIONS 207
SOFTWARE CONSIDERATIONS 207
Flow of the Program 207
Keeping Additional Records 221
Preparing Practice Management Reports 221
Security 222
Summary of Software 222
CHOOSING THE VENDOR 222
TRAINING AND SUPPORT 222
UPGRADES 223

Chapter 10
EMPLOYMENT PRACTICES   225
JOAN B. CONRAD

RECRUITMENT AND HIRING   225
The Planning Process   225
Job Descriptions   226
Sources of Job Candidates   227
Interviewing Process   230
Selection of Candidates   234
WAGES AND SALARIES   234
Determining and Evaluating Pay Scales   234
Federal Wage and Hour Regulations   235
BENEFIT PACKAGES   239
Required Programs   239
Retirement Programs   239
Health Insurance Programs   239
Life Insurance Programs   240
Disability Insurance Programs   241
Sick Leave and Personal Leave Programs   241
Other Benefits   242
Legal Requirements   242

Chapter 11
PERSONNEL AND OFFICE POLICIES   245
JOAN B. CONRAD

POLICY MANUAL   245
The Outline   245
Contents of the Manual   246
Writing the Manual   247
Updating the Manual   247
EMPLOYMENT AND LABOR LAWS   248
Worker's Compensation   248
Issues in the Workplace   250
SELECTION OF ANCILLARY SERVICES   258
Criteria for Selection of Attorneys, Accountants, and Consultants   258
SEPARATION FROM EMPLOYMENT   260
Warnings   260
Suspensions   260
Discharges   260
Exit Interviews   261

Chapter 12
ETHICS   263
MARCIA LEWIS

INTRODUCTION   263
What Are Ethics?   263
Why Ethics?   264
Ethical Conflicts   264
Moral Principles   265
ETHICS AND PROFESSIONALISM FOR MEDICAL PERSONNEL   267
Code of Ethics   267
Ethics Related to the Analysis of the Profession   268
THE ETHICS OF CONFIDENTIALITY   269
THE ETHICS OF CONSENT   269
BIOETHICAL ISSUES IN AMBULATORY CARE   270
Patients' Right to Health Care   270

Patients' Right to Live or to Die 271
Patients' Right to Procreate or to Abort 271
PRACTICAL IMPLICATIONS OF ETHICS AND BIOETHICS FOR MEDICAL PERSONNEL IN AMBULATORY CARE 272
The "Ethics Check" Questions 272
What to Do When You Don't Know What to Do 272
Ethical Dos and Don'ts 272

Chapter 13
MEDICAL LAW 275
LISA McCOLLUM

REGULATION OF MEDICAL OFFICES 275
Sources of Information Regarding Federal and State Laws 276
Branches of Law 277
CREDENTIALING OF HEALTH CARE PERSONNEL 278
Licensure 278
Certification 279
Registration 279
MEDICAL ASSISTING PRACTICE 279
Laboratory Testing 279
Venipuncture and Injections 280
Radiography 280
MEDICAL PROFESSIONAL LIABILITY 280
Contracts 280
Standard of Care 281
Statute of Limitations 282
Insurance 286
PATIENT CARE 286
Emergency Aid 286
Appointments 287
Consent 287
Minors 288
MEDICAL RECORDS 290
Ownership and Access 290
Retention 290
Confidentiality 291
Disposal 291
PUBLIC HEALTH REPORTING REQUIREMENTS 291
COMPREHENSIVE DRUG ABUSE PREVENTION AND CONTROL ACT OF 1970 291
Registration 291
Record Keeping 293
Inventory 293
Prescriptions 293
DRUG SCREENING 293
UNIFORM ANATOMICAL GIFT ACT OF 1968 294
DEATH AND DYING 294
Living Wills 294
Durable Power of Attorney for Health Care 297
Withdrawal of Life Support 297
MONITORING LEGISLATION 298

Section Two
CLINICAL PRACTICES — 299

Chapter 14
GENERAL PATIENT CARE — 301
CAROL S. CHAMPAGNE and KAREN LANE

MEDICAL ASEPSIS 301
CDC Universal Blood and Body Fluid Precautions 301
Sanitization 303
Sterilization and Disinfection 304
PATIENT INTERVIEWING 306
Skills for Successful Patient Interviewing 306
The New Patient Interview 307
VITAL SIGNS 309
Height 309
Weight 310
Pulse 312
Respiration 313
Temperature 313
Blood Pressure 316
MEDICAL EXAMINATIONS 320
Positions for Examination 320
Preparing for a Complete Physical Examination 322
Preparing for a Proctological Examination 322
The Eye and Ear Examinations 324
The Neurological Examination 330
Employment, School, and Insurance Examinations 333
Patient Self-Examination 333

Chapter 15
MEDICATION ADMINISTRATION — 335
KAREN LANE

RESPONSIBILITIES IN DRUG THERAPY 335
READING AND UNDERSTANDING WRITTEN AND ORAL ORDERS 336
Abbreviations 336
Systems of Measurement 336
MEASURING AND CALCULATING DRUG DOSAGE 340
Measuring Medications 340
Drugs that Require Reconstitution 341
UNDERSTANDING HOW DRUGS ARE ABSORBED, DISTRIBUTED, AND EXCRETED BY THE BODY 345
Drug Delivery and Absorption 345
Factors that Influence the Effects of Drugs 345
ASSESSING THE PATIENT, THE DRUG, AND THE ENVIRONMENT 345
Patient Assessment 345
Drug Assessment 346
The Environment 346
CHOOSING THE CORRECT ROUTE AND SITE 347
Oral Medications 347
Mucous Membrane Medications 347
Topical Medications 348
Parenteral (By Injection) Medications 348
USING CORRECT TECHNIQUES AND EQUIPMENT FOR INJECTIONS 352
Advantages of Injections 352
Routes of Administration 352
Landmarks 356

USING SPECIAL SYRINGE TECHNIQUES 361
Using Syringe Dead Space and Air Bubbles 361
Admixing Two Drugs in a Single Syringe 361
ADMINISTERING PARENTERAL MEDICATIONS 363
Assessing the Patient Prior to Injection 363
Using the Z-tract Technique 365
Steps to Reducing Injection Pain 366
TUBERCULIN TESTING 366
RECOGNIZING POTENTIAL ADVERSE EFFECTS 370
Emotional Complications of Injections 370
Physical Complications of Injections 370
Managing Drug Emergencies 370

Chapter 16
SURGICAL AND REHABILITATIVE PROCEDURES 371
JUNE M. FRANCIS

SURGICAL PROCEDURES 371
Surgical Instruments 371
Procedures 378
REHABILITATIVE PROCEDURES 397

Chapter 17
PEDIATRIC PROCEDURES 403
JUANITA BLOCKER

NEWBORN EVALUATION AND CARE 403
Instructing Parents on the Care of the Newborn 403
Assessment of Problems by Telephone 406
Common Problems of Newborns 407
GROWTH AND DEVELOPMENT 409
Head and Chest Circumferences 409
Weight 410
Height (Length) 412
Growth Charts 413
IMMUNIZATION SCHEDULES 424
WELL-BABY EXAMINATIONS 427
Vital Signs 427
COMMON CHILDHOOD PROBLEMS AND COMMUNICABLE DISEASES 429
Immunity- and Allergy-Related Conditions 429
Viral Conditions 429
Bacterial Conditions 432
Other Conditions 435
Parasitic Conditions 436
BATTERED CHILD SYNDROME 438

Chapter 18
GYNECOLOGICAL AND OBSTETRICAL PROCEDURES 441
MIDGE NOEL RAY

GYNECOLOGY 441
Terminology 441
Gynecological History 441
Routine Gynecological Examination 441
Physician's Implementation of Pelvic Examination 444
Medical Conditions 445
Contraception 457
OBSTETRICS 466
Terminology 466
Presumptive Evidence of Pregnancy 467

Confirmation of Pregnancy 467
Routine Prenatal Care 467
Obstetrical Disorders 469
Obstetrical Diagnostic Procedures 472
Postpartum Care 473
Infertility 473

Chapter 19
DIAGNOSTIC PROCEDURES 475
WALTER R. FRANK, III, GARY M. MUNSON, DALE DAVIS, and BETTY BATES TEMPKIN

RADIOGRAPHY 476
Safety 476
Radiography Procedures 477
ELECTROCARDIOGRAM AND ARRHYTHMIA INTERPRETATION 499
Electrocardiography 499
Arrhythmias 509
Cardiac Diagnostic Tests 517
SONOGRAPHY 518
How Sonography is Performed 518
Sonography Examinations 518

Chapter 20
SPECIMEN COLLECTION AND PROCESSING 525
PATRICIA S. HURLBUT

TERMINOLOGY 525
LABORATORY REQUEST FORMS 526
CATEGORIES OF LABORATORY TESTS 529
PANELS AND PROFILES 529
PATIENT INSTRUCTION TECHNIQUES 530
Fasting 530
Medications 530
Patient Instructions 530
COLLECTION EQUIPMENT AND SUPPLIES 530
Appropriate Containers 530
Correct Preservatives 531
Collection Time Factors 531
Labeling 532
Centers for Disease Control Universal Precautions for Blood and Body Fluids 532
TYPES AND METHODS OF SPECIMEN COLLECTION 533
Blood 533
Urine 541
Stool 541
Sputum 542
Semen 542
Throat Specimens 543
Genital Tract Specimens 544
SPECIMEN PREPARATION 545
Preservation Techniques 545
METHODS OF DELIVERY OF SPECIMENS 547
In Person 547
Mail Service 547
Pick-Up Service 547
Chain of Custody 547
PROCEDURES FOR DISPOSAL 548
Labeling of Waste 548
Occupational Safety and Health Act Regulations 548
Health and Safety of the Community 549

QUALITY CONTROL 550
Reagent Management 550
Control Requirements 550
Instrument Calibration 550
Instrument and Testing Logbooks/Worksheets 551
Preventive Maintenance of Equipment 551

Chapter 21
URINALYSIS 553
LORETTA HATLESTAD

CLINICAL CONSIDERATIONS 553
Quality Control 553
Safety 554
Recording the Urinalysis 554
Mailing 554
COLLECTION METHODS 554
Fundamentals 554
Catheterized Specimen 556
Specimen for Drug Screening 558
First Morning Specimen 560
Infant Specimen 560
Random, Clean-Catch Specimen 560
Timed (24-Hour) Specimen 561
Two-Glass Specimen 563
URINE TESTS 564
Physical Examination 564
Chemical Examination 567
Microscopic Examination 570

Chapter 22
HEMATOLOGY AND BLOOD CHEMISTRY 577
JEANNETTE R. BELL and PATRICIA S. HURLBUT

HEMATOLOGY 577
Guidelines for Performing a Hematocrit 578
Guidelines for Performing a Hemoglobin Concentration 582
Guidelines for Performing an Erythrocyte Sedimentation Rate 584
Guidelines for Performing a Manual Leukocyte Count 585
Guidelines for Performing a Peripheral Blood Smear Examination 588
Guidelines for Electronic Blood Cell Counting 592
Guidelines for Performing a Prothrombin Time 594
BLOOD CHEMISTRY 597
Purpose and Significance of Routine Blood Chemistries 597
Specimen Integrity 597
Use and Care of Laboratory Equipment 601
Quality Control 601
Accurate Reporting Procedures 601
Testing and Reporting Cholesterol Levels 606

Chapter 23
MICROBIOLOGY, SEROLOGY, AND IMMUNOLOGY 609
LINDA JEFF and MARGARET GIDDENS FRITSMA

MICROBIOLOGY 609
Special Hints for Equipment and Supplies 609
Safety in the Work Area 614
Specimen Collection and Handling 615
Urine Specimens 615
Microscopic Procedures 616
Screening Procedures 623

Culture Techniques 631
SEROLOGY 639
General Guidelines 639
C-Reactive Protein Tests 640
Human Immunodeficiency Virus Antibody Tests 642
Infectious Mononucleosis Antibody Tests 643
Pregnancy Tests 646
Rheumatoid Factor Tests 648
Rapid Plasma Reagin Tests for Syphilis 650
Rubella Antibody Tests 652
Streptococcal Antibody Tests 655

Chapter 24
EMERGENCY PROCEDURES 659
LINDA T. POWELL

SCHEDULING—KEEPING THE OFFICE FUNCTIONAL 659
Assessment of Office 659
Steps to Effective Schedule Management 659
OUTPATIENT EMERGENCY PROCEDURES 661
Developing an Office Emergency Procedures Guide 661
Documentation 661
HANDLING OFFICE EMERGENCIES 661
General Guide for Handling Office Emergencies 661
TRIAGE 663
The Office Triage System 663
Communications Triage 663
General Steps of Triage 664
Patient Assessment Process 664
CARDIOPULMONARY RESUSCITATION 664
EMERGENCY TREATMENTS 667
Medical Emergencies Due to Disease, Illness, or Trauma 667

APPENDIX A: General Information Resources 677

A-1. AIDS Information and Resources 678
A-2. Sources for Patient Education Materials 679
A-3. Directory of Pharmaceutical Manufacturers 682
A-4. Poison Control Centers 686
A-5. Public Health Service Agencies 689
A-6. Voluntary Health and Welfare Agencies and Associations 690
A-7. 1-800 Telephone Numbers for Health Care Information, Products, and Services 693

APPENDIX B: Administrative Information 695

B-1. Abbreviations Commonly Used by Hospitals 696
B-2. Acronyms for Selected Health Care Organizations, Associations, and Agencies 699
B-3. Alphabet Soup of Health Care 702
B-4. Combining Forms in Medical Terminology 703
B-5. Medicare Physician Payment Reform (PPR) 713
B-6. Medicare PPR Procedure Codes Subject to the Outpatient Limit 718
B-7. Medicare PPR Facility-Based Procedures for which Additional Amount for Supplies May Be Payable if Performed in a Physician's Office 720
B-8. Medicare PPR Evaluation and Management Codes 721
B-9. Professional Designations for Health Care Providers 726
B-10. Specialized Terms Used in Medical Records 730
B-11. Symbols Commonly Used in Clinical Practice 731
B-12. Words and Phrases Commonly Misinterpreted 732

APPENDIX C: Clinical Information 737

- C-1. Poisoning by Common Chemicals 738
- C-2. Drugs for Treating Poisoning 741
- C-3. Uses and Effects of Controlled Substances 742
- C-4. Selected Skin Tests 745
- C-5. Tables of Weights and Measures 746
- C-6. Approximate Household Equivalents 751
- C-7. Desirable Weights for Men and Women, According to Height and Frame, Ages 25 to 29 751
- C-8. Ideal Weights for Boys and Girls, According to Height and Age 752
- C-9. Recommended Daily Dietary Allowances (RDAs) 753
- C-10. The Principal Micronutrients (Vitamins and Minerals) 754
- C-11. Laboratory Values of Clinical Importance 757

APPENDIX D: Standards and Regulations 767

- D-1. CDC Recommendations for Prevention of HIV Transmission in Health-Care Settings 768
- D-2. CDC Update: Universal Precautions for Prevention of Transmission of Human Immunodeficiency Virus, Hepatitis B Virus, and Other Bloodborne Pathogens in Health-Care Settings 784
- D-3. CLIA (Clinical Laboratory Improvement Amendments): 1988 Regulations and Requirements 791
- D-4. DACUM (Developing a Curriculum): 1990 Guidelines 797
- D-5. Diagnosis-Related Groups (DRGs) 800
- D-6. OSHA Bloodborne Pathogens Final Standard: Summary of Key Provisions 809
- D-7. OSHA Joint Advisory Notice of the Department of Labor and the Department of Health and Human Services for the Protection Against Occupational Exposure to Hepatitis B Virus (HBV) and Human Immunodeficiency Virus (HIV) 811
- D-8. OSHA Guidelines to Developing a Facility Bloodborne Pathogens Exposure Control Plan 825
- D-9. OSHA Hepatitis B Vaccination Protection 832
- D-10. States with OSHA-Approved Plans 833

Index 835

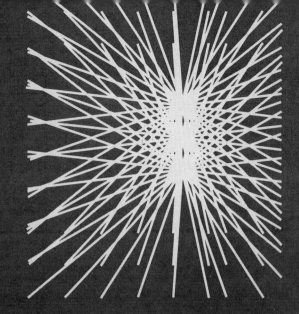

Section One

ADMINISTRATIVE PRACTICES

Chapter 1

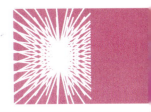

APPOINTMENTS AND TELECOMMUNICATIONS

CAROLYN C. AVERY
RACHEL K. YOUNGER

SCHEDULING APPOINTMENTS IN THE OFFICE
Mission Statement
Decisions to Be Made
Setting Up a Manual Appointment System in a Primary Care Setting
Setting Up a Manual Appointment System in a Specialist's Office
Making Appointments
Ethical/Legal Considerations Involving the Appointment Book
Computerized Appointment Systems

APPOINTMENT SCHEDULING OUTSIDE THE OFFICE
Referrals for Consultations and Clinical Tests
Referral to Outpatient Surgery Center and Hospitals
TELEPHONE MANAGEMENT
Screening Telephone Calls
What to Tell the Caller
Answering the Telephone
Getting the Message to the Physician
Getting the Message to the Patient
Taking Messages after Hours

SCHEDULING APPOINTMENTS IN THE OFFICE

There are no hard and fast rules for scheduling patients for office visits. The scheduling system must be adapted to the goals of the specific practice and the preferences and habits of the physician. The scheduling system should be flexible enough to handle emergencies, walk-ins, and telephone calls without completely disrupting the day. The appointment scheduling system that works for the office in the beginning of practice probably will not be the same one that works best in future years. When patients are consistently waiting more than 30 minutes and/or staff frustration is high, it is time to reassess the appointment scheduling policy and procedures.

Mission Statement

Development of a mission statement might be a beginning point to determine the scheduling system for the practice. The mission (or philosophy) of the practice might be "Our goal is to be the primary care physician for persons in our community from the age of 18 months on. We want to focus on preventive health care through regular office visits and patient education. We want to be available for patients in the community with emergencies, injuries, and acute illnesses. No one will be denied care because of race, creed, color, or ability to pay."

Decisions to Be Made

From the decision regarding the philosophy of the practice comes the framework of whether the office will see patients of all ages, be available 5 days a week, work only by appointments, see Medicaid patients, see patients only on referral, etc. The purpose of an appointment scheduling system is to maximize use of space and personnel while keeping waiting time for the patients to the minimum. Questions to be answered include

- What type of practice?
- How many practitioners?
- What days will patients be seen in office?
- What will the office hours be?
- What about special meetings, lunch hours, etc.?
- What procedures will be done by each practitioner?
- How long will each procedure normally take?
- How many examination rooms?
- How large is the staff?
- Will most appointments be scheduled ahead or on the day seen?
- What about emergencies/walk-ins?
- How many patients do we want to see from a financial point of view?
- When will phone calls be returned?

Usually the type of practice, days to be open, hours to be available, special meetings, and lunch times can be calculated with some sense of accuracy. A primary care practice with a high percentage of walk-in or work-in patients functions much differently from the practice of psychiatry, where most appointments are scheduled ahead and perhaps anticipated at the same time each week for several weeks or even months. A heavily booked office practice, however, may have difficulty finding the slot to accommodate the urgent patient or to respond to the request for an appointment from a valued physician who refers a number of patients each month.

When developing and refining an appointment system, all of the following factors need to be considered:

- The need to provide quality care to each patient
- The need to have a smooth flow of patients from the waiting room to the examination room
- The need to balance the physician's time so that phone calls can be returned
- The need to accommodate the requests for appointments from the medical community

Setting Up a Manual Appointment System in a Primary Care Setting

Determining the time frame for different procedures with different patients is not an accurate science; however, there are ways to begin to allot time frames. One method is to keep a log for 2 or 3 weeks of the amount of time each procedure and/or type of visit usually requires. This could be accomplished by noting on the route sheet or worksheet for each patient the time the medical assistant calls the patient into the examining room and the time the medical assistant leaves the examining room. The patient's time with the physician could be tracked similarly. For example, for the chief complaint of sore throat with the resulting diagnosis of pharyngitis, the medical assistant's time might be 5 minutes (history and vital signs) and the physician's time 5 minutes.

Another way to determine the time frame might be to track an average of how many patients are seen in an hour, in a half day, or in a whole day. If one physician sees an average of six patients per hour and another one four or five with similar complaints, the schedule would be adjusted to the particular physician's method of practice. The office schedule should be able to adjust always to the individual physician's preference and style. In addition, examining room use may be monitored and the clinical staff asked for suggestions on how to improve the patient and/or procedure flow. There may be duties that could be done by the front office staff to allow the clinical process to run more efficiently, such as typing labels for

TABLE 1-1

ESTIMATED TIME REQUIREMENTS FOR COMMON OFFICE PROCEDURES

Procedure	Time in Minutes
Cast change	20–30
Complete physical examination (CPX)	30–60
with electrocardiogram	+15
with sigmoidoscopy	+15
Desensitization injections	20–30
Dressing change	10–20
Hypertension follow-up	10–15
Minor surgery	30–60
Office visit	
Brief	5–10
Intermediate	15–20
Extended	30–45
Pediatric examination and conference	15–30
Pelvic examination and Papanicolaou smear	15–30
Prenatal examination	15–30
Suture removal	10–20
X-ray	10–15

Chapter 1: APPOINTMENTS AND TELECOMMUNICATIONS

TUESDAY, SEPTEMBER 27

HOUR				
8 00				
8 15				
8 30				
8 45				
9 00				
9 15				
9 30				
9 45				
10 00				
10 15				
10 30				
10 45				
11 00				
11 15				
11 30				
11 45				
12 00				
12 15				
12 30				
12 45				
1 00				
1 15				
1 30				
1 45				
2 00				
2 15				
2 30				
2 45				
3 00				
3 15				
3 30				
3 45				
4 00				
4 15				
4 30				
4 45				
5 00				
5 15				
5 30				
5 45				
6 00				
6 15				
6 30				
6 45				
7 00				
NOTES				

FIGURE 1-1

Standard appointment schedule.

Chapter 1: APPOINTMENTS AND TELECOMMUNICATIONS

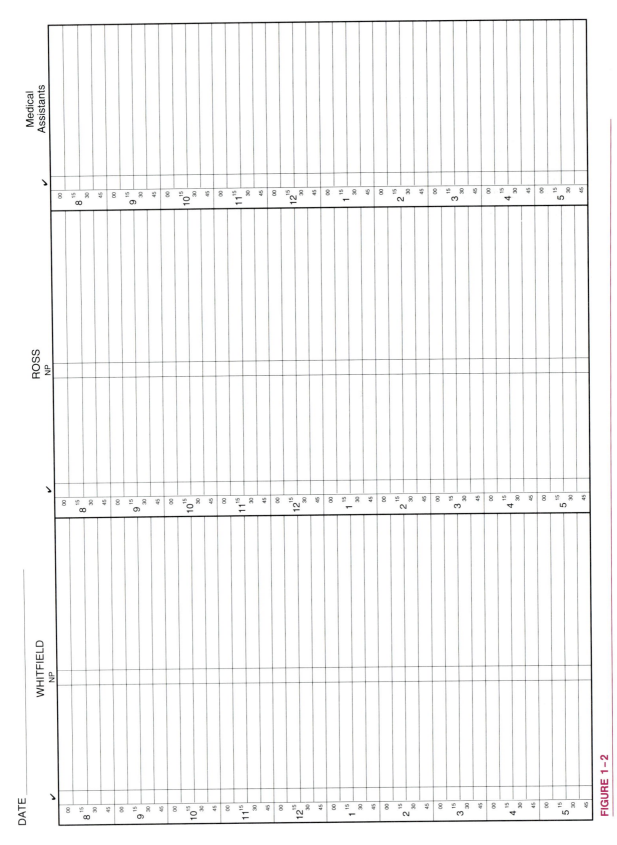

FIGURE 1-2 Specially designed appointment schedule.

Chapter 1: APPOINTMENTS AND TELECOMMUNICATIONS **7**

specimens or biopsy collections and laboratory requisition forms.

Once procedure time requirements are determined (Table 1–1), the appointment book can be designed. Most appointment books, purchased or designed by the medical assistant, have 15-minute time intervals (Figure 1–1).

> **SPECIAL HINT**
>
> The scheduling book needs to work for the practice, *not* the practice for the book. Therefore some offices have only the hours labeled and six to eight lines under each hour for entering times. This allows for more flexibility in time allotment.

Designing an Individualized Appointment Book

Although there are many types of appointment or scheduling books on the market, designing an appointment book for the practice might be important. In a notebook of looseleaf pages, create headings, allowing space for the information needed for each physician (Figure 1–2). The time intervals listed can be limited to only the hours patients are actually seen. Lunch hours and hours when the physician is not in the office need not be included (Figure 1–3). Columns might be made for

- Appointment times
- Patient's name and daytime phone number

	Monday	Tuesday	Wednesday	Thursday	Friday	Saturday
Admit Surgery						
	9:45			2:00		
	10:00	10:00		2:15		
	10:15	10:15		2:30		
	10:30	10:30		2:45		
	10:45	10:45		3:00		Sunday
	11:00	11:00		3:15		
	11:15	11:15		3:30		
	11:30	11:30		3:45		
	11:45	11:45		4:00		
	12:00	12:00		4:15		
	12:15	12:15		4:30		

Month _____ Year _____ Day _____

FIGURE 1–3
Appointment schedule designed with slots for times in the office only.

- Patient's complaint
- Name of referring physician, if any
- New patient notation
- Walk-in or emergency notation (if appropriate)
- Clinical staff tasks

Next, mark out the hours each physician or other practitioner is not available. Remember to mark out time for lunch, business meetings, and speaking engagements. Remember to allow time for phone calls, emergencies, house calls, injuries, etc. The open space left over is when appointments can be scheduled. Determine time segments (15 minutes, 10 minutes, or 5 minutes). There can be a separate page (even a different color) for each physician in the practice. A page or column for nurse scheduling also is helpful, for blood work, allergy shots, and other procedures that can be done without the physician in the room. Scheduling these procedures will prevent overcommitting the nurse's time. Take time to think about some of the peculiarities of the practice:

- Are there more emergencies on Monday?
- Are there more patients between 8:00 and 10:00 in the morning and 3:00 and 5:00 in the afternoon every day?
- Are there slow times in March or May and busy times in January and February?
- Is the schedule heavier on the Monday after the physician has had weekend on-call duty?

Even what seem like unpredictable problems will be able to be predicted after a period of study.

Methods of Scheduling

There are several ways to schedule appointments: stream or time-allotted slots, wave or modified wave, groupings, and open slots.

Stream or Time-Allotted Slots. Scheduling patients in a steady flow or "stream" is the traditional way in which most appointments are scheduled. In theory this would seem to work well, because there would be a consistent flow of patients from waiting room to examining room and gone again. The only drawback is when a patient is late, cancels, or fails to show; the physician is detained; or the patient has multiple problems instead of the one scheduled for. In the time-allotted framework, there can be idle time for the doctor waiting for the next patient. From the drawbacks of this system has evolved what some offices use, called the modified wave.

Wave or Modified Wave. The wave in the true sense would have the number of patients who could been seen in the morning (say 16) all come in at 8:00, and by noon the physician could have seen them all. Patients would certainly not accept this, although it would be efficient use of the physician's time. It usually works out that the physician, day in and day out, averages seeing the same number of patients per day.

With that goal — efficient use of the physician's time — in mind, one method, known as the modified wave, allows for the scheduling of certain blocks of time that can be predicted such as complete physical examinations, insurance examinations, health surveys, well-baby care, and maybe evaluating the effectiveness of a treatment (follow-up). On the appointment schedule, at the same time a physical examination is listed for one examining room, three or four other patients for follow-ups or minor illnesses could be listed for other rooms. This usually averages one long appointment mixed with two shorter ones.

It is not always necessary to see the patients exactly in the same order in which they arrive. If the examination rooms are filled with the first wave of patients when the physician arrives in the office, one needing a physical examination, another needing a follow-up, and another with perhaps a sore throat, the physician might talk with the patient scheduled for the physical examination in his or her office, while the clinical staff obtain vital signs on the other two patients. While the patient for the physical examination undresses, the physician could see the two other patients. The disadvantage of the modified wave system is that patients may object when they realize that several of them have the same appointment time. In the wave system, all examination rooms should be filled when the physician arrives and again when the physician returns from lunch, with a consistent flow in between.

Groupings or Category Scheduling. Some physicians prefer to see the same types of patients grouped together, such as all patients for complete physical examinations in the early morning, all prenatal checks on Tuesday and Wednesday mornings, and rechecks in the early afternoon. The practice might have a pattern of seeing patients for complete physical examinations in the early morning or late afternoon, with some short visits grouped with longer procedures such as breast examinations in midmorning, short visits right after lunch with some longer procedures in midafternoon, and finally, school children after school hours.

Open Slots. Some offices continue to function well with a first-come, first-served schedule. With this type of schedule, patients need to know when the office opens, when the physician is available, and when the office closes. This is not an ideal for the physicians because of the difficulty in using their time efficiently. If the community is accustomed to this practice, it should work well. Remember to allow the physician time to see all patients who arrive to be seen that day. It is difficult to limit the day without the risk of turning away the sickest patient of the day.

> **SPECIAL HINT**
>
> Whatever system works best is the right one for that particular practice. As the practice changes, so should the appointment book.

Double Booking. Scheduling patients for the same appointment is called double booking, which is quite similar to the wave system mentioned earlier. As long as patients do not get the feeling they are being herded through, this method is a useful one. However, if the double-booked patients are walk-ins or work-ins, there needs to be a system to indicate the patients with scheduled appointments to reduce the chance of a patient who has a scheduled appointment having to wait while a walk-in is seen.

Setting Up a Manual Appointment System in a Specialist's Office

The appointment book for a specialist might be quite different from that for the primary care physician (see Figure 1–3). The surgeon who sees only follow-up and referral patients in the office would have a more predictable allotment of examining rooms than would the proceduralist (for example, a gastroenterologist) who is doing procedures and seeing patients in the same suite. It is important to identify on the appointment book or log all the room types so that patient procedures are not scheduled when there is no personnel available because of other types of appointments.

Another type of scheduling involves the practice with a facility, such as an outpatient surgery center, attached. The same staff may be scheduled at both places as well as perhaps assisting with surgeries at the hospital. The appointment logs need to track the available time frames for each type of scheduling situation.

Making Appointments

When making an appointment, which is often done on the telephone, it is necessary to obtain certain information.

Appointments for New Patients

The office policy and procedure manual outlines the basic information needed from the patient who is new to the practice. Issues on which the medical assistant may need to be informed include

- Are patients seen on referral only?
- Is the practice accepting new patients?
- Are there restrictions because of contracted health care plans?
- When does the physician prefer to see new patients?

Normally for a new patient the following information is necessary.

Who. Record the name of the patient. Enter "NP" or some other symbol to designate that the patient is new. Also obtain and record the name of the person who is making the appointment if that person is not the patient.

Phone Number. Both home and work phone numbers are needed. These are necessary in case the schedule needs to be changed or the patient fails to show. A phone number may also be used as an identifying tool, if, for example, the practice has two patients by the name of Jane E. Smith.

The Name of the Referring Physician. This assists in welcoming the patient to your practice, aids the physician with the consultation, and provides information in the event the patient does not show for the appointment.

Why. Record the purpose of the appointment. The reason for the visit, as mentioned before, determines not only the time required, but also what instructions might need to be given to a new patient. If the office policy states that all new patients, unless acutely ill, must have a complete physical examination, this needs to be explained to the patient and the proper amount of

TABLE 1-2
ABBREVIATIONS OF REASONS FOR VISIT

CPE or CPX	Complete physical examination
B/P	Blood pressure check
I&D	Incision and drainage
PAP	Pap smear
P&P	Pap smear and pelvic examination
S/R	Suture removal
N&V	Nausea and vomiting
NP	New patient
ROV or reck	Return office visit/recheck

time allotted. Some common abbreviations for reasons for visits are included in Table 1-2.

When. Determine the time for the office visit. Assist the patient in choosing a convenient time by directing the patient to options, such as morning or afternoon or the beginning or end of the week. Give the patient two choices if possible. Listen carefully to what patients say and ask questions to make sure that the right amount of time is being scheduled. By not having times already written in, the medical assistant can work forward or backward from previously scheduled examinations to fill in the allotted time frame.

Additional Information. Insurance instructions, completion of forms, list of medications, and names of other physicians the new patient is currently seeing may be obtained.

NOTE: A new patient needs directions to the office as well as instructions on where to park, what to bring (insurance cards and list of medications), and an estimate of charges if payment is expected at time of service.

Appointments for Established Patients

As in the case of the new patient, it is important to have an office policy regarding established patients. What is the "established" patient? According to the 1992 American Medical Association CPT coding system, an "established" patient is any patient who has been seen within the past 3 years by the physician or by another physician in the same practice group. Although the patient might be "new" to one physician in the group, the patient would be considered an established patient if seen by any physician in the group. An established patient normally is a patient with an ongoing medical plan, whether it be preventive medical care or follow-up care for a chronic condition or because of family history of illness.

The time frame for an established patient might be more predictable than one for a new patient. Even the individual pattern for the patient might be more predictable. As time goes on in a practice, each patient becomes more of an individual whose own methods can be better planned for. In the modified wave system, the established patient is considered a less time-intensive appointment than the new patient.

The following information is needed at the time of making the appointment:

Who. Record the name of the patient and of the caller (if different). If the patient is not known to the scheduler, it is appropriate to ask when the patient was in last. The reason for this is to explain any policy changes since the patient's last visit.

Phone Number. As for a new patient, obtain both the home and work phone numbers of the patient.

Why. Record the reason for the appointment.

When. Again, give the patient two appointment options, if possible. If the appointment is more than 2-3 weeks away, it is appropriate to ask the patient if he or she would be interested in filling an earlier cancellation if one becomes available. If so, obtain the times when the patient could not make use of a canceled time and phone numbers at which the patient might be reached. Add the patient's name to the list of patients willing to fill cancellations.

Additional Information. It is the policy of some offices to call to remind patients of appointments.

Physician-Referred Appointments

Many practices are "referral only," meaning that all patients scheduled have been sent by some other physician or agency. The promptness and efficiency of these appointments are of upmost importance to the patient and the referring physician or agency. If referrals are a large part of the practice, the office policy might state, "It is the policy of this office to see physician referrals within 24 hours of the request and make a report to the referring physician within 24 hours of the appointment." In this type of practice, slots must be available to accomplish this goal.

The information obtained from the referring office or patient is similar to that obtained for other patients and includes the patient's name and phone number, the reason for the appointment, the name and address of the referring physician, and any pertinent medical information. The appointment slots available are noted. If precertification is necessary, obtain the information regarding the insurance carrier.

If appropriate, a call to the patient might be of benefit to answer any questions about office location and expectations. If the patient cancels the appointment or fails to show for the appointment, it is important to notify the referring party and document the cancellation in the appointment book or other place, such as "consultation file."

Contract or Industrial Appointments

Some practices have contracts or agreements with companies to see all new applicants for pre-employment physicals, drug screens, on-the-job injuries, counseling, and other services. The contract or agreement might define what the arrangements will be: the examination requirements, time restrictions, and specific times of day the physician must be available for appointments. If these agreements are part of the practice, appropriate slots should be available, in keeping with the agreements. Many times the blood tests for a company or insurance examination can take more of the clinical staff's time than a similar examination for a regularly scheduled complete physical examination. At times the physician will go to the site on a regular basis, and at other times the employees will come to the office.

Appointments for Worker's Compensation Patients

In the primary care practice, the Worker's Compensation patient usually initially has an on-the-job injury or illness that needs immediate attention. The office needs to become familiar with the requirements of Worker's Compensation claims. If the proper procedures are not followed, then reimbursement for the physician might be difficult. Necessary information includes the following:

- Who is making the appointment?
- If it is not the employer, who is giving authorization?
- Is this an established patient of the practice?

These questions should be asked in addition to the usual ones eliciting the patient's name, address, and phone number.

Nonroutine Appointments

Again, office policy needs to be established. The development of definitions for the various types of nonroutine appointments could be discussed and decisions made before the situation arises. A screening form might be developed to be used in triaging these calls. Appointment slots should be available for these nonroutine appointments.

Even nonroutine appointments such as emergencies, acute illnesses, consultations, second opinions, and job injuries can be predicted. By tracking or logging appointments over a period of 6 weeks or so, a pattern might develop. There might be an average of eight or more emergencies on Mondays or Fridays. For example, there may be more work injuries on Tuesdays or more surgical problems on Thursday. Any appointment system needs to have slots available for such unplanned but predictable requests for appointments.

Appointments for the Problem Patient

The problem patient might be described as anyone who changes or disregards the plans the practice has made for the appointment. Among these are no-shows, late cancellations, late arrivals, early arrivals, and those who present with one problem but state "By the way . . ." as the appointment ends.

To eliminate no-showing, it might be important to determine the reason. Calling the night or day before might be helpful, especially if the appointment was scheduled originally for some time in the future.

MEDICAL ASSISTING ALERT

All no-shows should be called and the medical record documented according to your office policy. If a charge is to be made for no-show appointments, the patient must be informed of this at the time the appointment is made.

The late cancellation should be rescheduled if possible and the patient reminded that the time had been set aside for that patient. The medical record should be documented as to the cancellation and action taken, for example, "6/1/91—pt cancelled this A.M. 'Forgot.' Rescheduled for 6/2/91 7:30 A.M."

The patient who is late is worked in or rescheduled, depending on the schedule and the patient's condition. However, it is difficult to enforce rules if the office itself is not adhering to the schedule. The early patient could be welcomed and given an estimate of time to be seen. Some patients must depend on others for transportation and must come when the ride is available. Other patients hope to be seen sooner, and some enjoy the social aspects of the waiting room. If space permits, allow the patient to remain.

Perhaps the most difficult patient is the one who says, "Oh, by the way . . ." at the end of the appointment. For example, a patient may say, "Oh, by the way, I was hoping that you might also look at my arm" or "Oh, by the way, I was hoping to stop smoking." If possible, the physician should at that point reply with a remark such as, "Yes, Ms. Jones, we do need to see you about your arm. Ms. Smith will schedule you for that."

The physician's personal and business appointments can take time away from patient appointments, resulting in a late schedule. This might indicate the need for evaluation and discussion during staff meeting. Business and personal appointments should be scheduled in appointment slots. In addition, reminding the person with the business appointment of the time frame in a courteous manner on arrival might be of assistance.

Another problem is the patient whose account has been turned over for collection or who has been discharged from the practice because of noncompliance with medical treatment. Patients who have outstanding accounts cannot be denied an appointment, but the physician may decide to see them on a cash basis. Patients who have been discharged must be referred to another physician or health care facility. Phone conversations with these types of patients should be noted on the patients' records and reported to the physician. It is important to develop office policy and procedure for these incidents to avoid charges of neglect or abandonment.

Miscellaneous Problems in Appointment Scheduling

The physician who insists that appointments must begin at 9:00 A.M. and arrives at 10:00 A.M. consistently creates an appointment scheduling nightmare. It is unlikely that the physician's method of seeing patients can be changed. To reduce patient dissatisfaction and staff frustration, a staff meeting might be useful in planning the appointment scheduling.

SPECIAL HINT

Each physician has a method of seeing patients, which might change over the years. The appointment schedule needs to reflect these changes or preferences.

SPECIAL HINT

Another area of appointment scheduling that creates staff concern and frustration is the practice that is not accepting any new patients.

It would be helpful to have available the names, addresses, and phone numbers of other physicians to whom to refer these requests for appointments.

Some physicians still see selected, usually elderly, patients, for home visits. The physician usually makes these appointments on the way to the office in the morning or on the way home in the afternoon. As with all appointments, documentation needs to be on the appointment book and in the medical record.

Occasionally, it is necessary for the physician to rearrange the schedule and cancel appointments. If it is the day of the appointment, nonurgent patients may be called and rescheduled. If the patient is unable to be contacted and shows up at the office, politely explain the reason for cancellation. If the patients are urgent, it is important to make other arrangements and document the chart. When the change is known in advance, such as for a meeting or speaking engagement, the medical assistant should call to reschedule the patient or send a letter by registered mail with return receipt. The mail receipt should be placed in the patient's chart.

How to Know That the Appointment System Is Not Working

The appointment system needs modification if patients are waiting more than 30 minutes either in the reception area or in the examining room when there are no emergencies. If the physician is not happy with the pace of appointments and if the examining rooms are not being used to the fullest, the scheduling system needs review.

SPECIAL HINT

If the staff is running around with their tongues

hanging out and if the clinical staff is yelling at the front office staff, evaluate the flow of patients.

Ethical/Legal Considerations Involving the Appointment Book

In scheduling appointments, the medical assistant should listen carefully and determine the reason for the appointment. Appointments should be scheduled on the basis of office procedure and office policy, not friendship or other personal attachment.

The appointment book serves as the legal document reflecting the physician's time and contact with the patient. In addition, the documentation of cancelled appointments and of chronic no-shows will serve as a record of the patient's compliance or non-compliance in the treatment plan.

SPECIAL HINT

The appointment schedule should never come between the physician and the patient. When concerned about a slot for an acutely ill or troubled patient, the physician should be consulted as to advisability of appointment time. If the patient thinks the illness is urgent or an emergency, the office must assume the same urgency.

Appointment books should be retained for 7–10 years or at least for the time period in which a lawsuit can be initiated (depending on state statutes of limitations).

Computerized Appointment Systems

Both small and large practices enjoy appointment scheduling by computer software program (see Chapter 9 for additional information).

The same questions and guidelines used in setting up a manual system are used to determine the type of computerized system for the practice. The system should be programmed with the time frames of the practice and physician preferences (Figure 1–4). The system should be able to schedule for individual physicians, special procedures, and space and staff limitations. The system needs to have straightforward commands, such as "F1D" for "forward one day" and be able to move backward and forward among schedules with ease, find future appointments for patients with a minimum of steps, and print copies for other office uses.

SPECIAL HINT

The computer system needs to be able to track cancellations and no-shows and maintain the permanent records needed for medical/legal reasons.

APPOINTMENT SCHEDULING OUTSIDE THE OFFICE

Referrals for Consultations and Clinical Tests

Often the physician will request further appointments for a patient while the patient is in the office. The medical assistant should have available the lists of physicians to whom the practice usually refers, with phone numbers and addresses. The information needed to accomplish this task is

- The procedure(s) requested and its urgency
- Patient and physician preferences
- Any insurance or reimbursement restrictions
- Patient's name, address, and phone numbers

After the appointment is scheduled, it is helpful to have available for the patient a brochure, card, map, or other similar information about the doctor or facility where the appointment will be.

Write the appointment name on the information card and give to the patient.

SPECIAL HINT

If there are any special instructions for the patient in preparation for the appointment, these should be written down for the patient. The patient is not likely to remember everything said at the time.

Referral to Outpatient Surgery Center and Hospitals

For more involved procedures and surgery, the physician may request appointments scheduled in an outpatient surgical center or hospital. These procedures might include magnetic resonance

Chapter 1: APPOINTMENTS AND TELECOMMUNICATIONS

HALIFAX Appointment Scheduling				DOCTOR NUMBER 20		SCHEDULE 05/15/90
BK#	TIME	TYPE	RM	PATIENT ##	PATIENT NAME	HOME PHONE
20	8:00	NE	1	0		0
20	8:00	NE	2	0		0
20	8:00	R	3	0		0
20	8:00	R	4	0		0
20	8:00	R	5	0		0
20	8:00	R	6	0		0
20	8:15	N	1	0		0
20	8:15	R	2	0		0
20	8:30	N	1	0		0
20	8:30	R	2	0		0
20	8:30	K	3	0		0
20	8:45	S	1	0		0
20	8:45	R	2	0		0
20	9:00	NE	1	0		0
20	9:00	R	2	0		0
20	9:00	R	3	0		0
20	9:00	WI	4	0		0
20	9:15	N	1	0		0
20	9:15	R	2	0		0
20	9:30	NE	1	0		0
20	9:30	R	2	0		0
20	9:30	R	3	0		0
20	9:30	WI	4	0		0
20	9:45	N	1	0		0
20	9:45	R	2	0		0
20	10:00	NE	1	0		0
20	10:00	R	2	0		0
20	10:00	R	3	0		0
20	10:00	WI	4	0		0
20	10:15	N	1	0		0
20	10:15	R	2	0		0
20	10:30	R	1	0		0
20	10:30	R	2	0		0
20	10:45	R	1	0		0
20	10:45	R	2	0		0
20	11:00	R	1	0		0
20	11:00	R	2	0		0
20	1:00	HOSP	1	0		0
20	1:15	HOSP	1	0		0
20	1:30	HOSP	1	0		0
20	1:45	HOSP	1	0		0
20	2:00	HOSP	1	0		0
20	2:15	HOSP	1	0		0
20	2:30	HOSP	1	0		0
20	2:45	HOSP	1	0		0
20	3:00	HOSP	1	0		0
20	3:15	HOSP	1	0		0
20	3:30	HOSP	1	0		0
20	3:45	HOSP	1	0		0
20	4:00	HOSP	1	0		0

FIGURE 1-4

Computerized appointment schedule.

imaging, same-day surgeries, and major surgeries and illnesses. Information needed by the facility includes

- The name of the person calling
- The name of the physician and office
- The phone number of caller
- The patient's name and date of birth
- The patient's social security number
- Admitting diagnosis and medical or surgical problem (Medical information needed includes diagnosis, signs and/or symptoms, any abnormal laboratory data pertinent to the diagnosis, and x-ray findings pertinent to the diagnosis. Surgical information needed includes procedure planned, by whom it is to be done, anesthesia type, and severity and intensity of illness.)
- When needed: emergency, urgent, or nonurgent
- Insurance information about patient
- Other hospital or outpatient admissions

Usually the patient will need instructions regarding pre-admission requirements, both medical and administrative. A pre-admission registration form might need to be completed. Blood work and other laboratory procedures might be required before surgical procedures.

Patients scheduled for diagnostic procedures or surgery should know what to expect. Although preparations vary, there are certain expectations, including chest x-rays and an electrocardiogram, a visit with the person administering the anesthesia, and fasting and dietary preparations.

Appointment Scheduling Guidelines

Design manual or computer appointment scheduling system to suit the physician's preference.

Review appointment procedures at least once a year to determine effectiveness, more often if patients are waiting more than 30 minutes past scheduled time.

Listen to patient's complaint and schedule accordingly while being flexible if necessary.

Review appointment time if it is made over the phone. Give patient an appointment card if scheduled in the office. Send office brochure if patient is new.

Apologize for delays in appointment schedules and reschedule if necessary.

Follow up and document all no-shows and cancellations.

Assist patients with referral appointments and provide written instructions as to location, procedures, and preparations.

Plan for the unexpected.

TELEPHONE MANAGEMENT

The telephone is the introductory connection between the patient and the physician most of the time and remains the chief connection over the course of the doctor–patient relationship. The telephone voice and style create expectations and images. It is the vital link in doctor–patient relationships.

Telephones can be a source of frustration. Callers get busy signals and cannot reach the office on the first or second attempt. The staff often views the phone as an interruption of work. Both the physician and staff feel an overall lack of control. The office staff can overcome this sense of frustration by the tone of voice, choice of words, and telephone manners.

SPECIAL HINT

When on the phone, staff members need to use clear speech, project positive attitudes, and maintain control of the conversation.

Screening Telephone Calls

The receptionist should have clear written guidelines to categorize calls. Calls may be categorized as follows:

- Calls to put through to the physician immediately (such as emergencies, other physicians, or family)
- Calls to be directed by message or transfer to the clinical personnel (such as prescription refills, laboratory reports, and status reports)
- Calls to be handled by the receptionist (such as appointments, office hours, cancellations, qualifications of physicians, and business calls)

- Calls to be handled by insurance and billing personnel

The receptionist should ask questions to assess the patient's need.

- What are the symptoms?
- When did the symptoms begin?
- How severe are the symptoms?
- Is there abdominal pain? Excessive bleeding? High fever for more than 2 days? Vomiting? Chest pain?
- Have you been on any medications? What medication? How long? Reaction to medication?

SPECIAL HINT

When unsure of the urgency, the medical office staff should consult the physician. If the patient thinks it is an emergency, it probably should be treated as such.

What to Tell the Caller

With the physician's help, the staff should establish written policies and procedures outlining information that may be released and under what circumstances. When an elderly or acutely ill patient is in the office, the physician could ask him or her to whom in the family information can be released. The information given by the patient is privileged, and the office should have mechanisms to protect the confidentiality of the doctor–patient relationship.

Answering the Telephone

Because the telephone is the vital link between the patient and the physician, the phone should be answered promptly, usually within two to three rings. Adequate phone service should be maintained. Additional phone lines should be added when there are complaints about continual busy signals.

Guidelines for Answering the Telephone

Identify the office by name—slowly and clearly.

Identify yourself and project willingness to help with statements such as "How may I help you?"

Other greetings such as "Happy Holidays" or "Good morning" can be added if appropriate.

Obtain the caller's name and write it down. If other lines begin ringing, place the first caller on hold and answer the second line. Ask the second caller for permission to place him or her on hold and wait for the answer.

Be patient and respectful of the caller.

Maintain control of the conversation by asking questions if the caller appears to not have clarified the reason for the call.

Summarize the conversation for the patient to clarify action taken.

Record the message in a message log. The minimum information should include time, date, name of caller, name of patient, caller's and patient's phone numbers, and message.

Getting the Message to the Physician

The phone message pad should be near the phone at all times so it can be easily used. The office procedures should outline the message flow. The medical record for each medically related call should be attached to the message, and the record should be documented with the action taken. The flow of office duties will be improved if the patients know that phone calls will be returned at certain intervals during the day, such as lunch time, and again later in the afternoon.

SPECIAL HINT

At the end of the day, the phone messages should be checked against the log to make sure that all calls have been taken care of.

Getting the Message to the Patient

- Each telephone message needs a documented action.
- Each outpatient procedure needs a follow-up call from the nurse or the physician the day after discharge from the hospital or the outpatient facility.
- Significant illnesses need follow-up. These include high fevers, new medications, and pain. There needs to be a system for following up laboratory results and documentation of the phone calls relaying laboratory results to patients.

Taking Messages after Hours

The office staff should be aware of the after-hour arrangements for patient care. There are several methods used by physicians:

- An answering service that automatically picks up the office or home phone after a certain number of rings. The phone is answered by a person who will contact the physician for the patient.
- An answering machine that simply tells the patient what the arrangements for emergency care are, when the office will open, etc.
- An answering "mail-box" that automatically answers the phone after hours, relays messages, and beeps the doctor on call until the message is retrieved from the machine.

Whatever the system, it is imperative that it be monitored by the office staff to assess its effectiveness. An answering service should answer the phones with a phrase such as "Dr. Smith's answering service" so patients will know to whom they are talking. The practice brochure should also inform the patient as to after-hour procedures.

The office staff must never be a barrier between the doctor and the patient. The office staff must be sympathetic and understanding and provide answers that are informative and complete.

Bibliography

Frew MA, Frew DR: *Comprehensive Medical Assisting: Administrative and Clinical Procedures,* 2nd ed. Philadelphia: F. A. Davis, 1988.

Kinn ME, Derge EF: *The Medical Assistant: Administrative and Clinical,* 6th ed. Philadelphia: W. B. Saunders, 1988.

Leebov W, Vergare M, Scott G: *Patient Satisfaction.* Oradell, NJ: Medical Economics, 1990.

Chapter 2

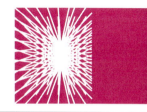

MEDICAL RECORDS AND CORRESPONDENCE

ANN M. GRAY

MEDICAL RECORDS
Filing and Identification Systems
Source-Oriented Medical Records
Problem-Oriented Medical Records
Patient Data Collection
Authorization to Release Records

MEDICAL CORRESPONDENCE
Mail Processing
Letter-Writing Formats
Attending Physician Statements
Medical Reports
Manuscript Preparation

MEDICAL RECORDS

Filing and Identification Systems

Color Coding

Color-coded filing allows for quick storage and retrieval, because recognizing color is faster than reading numbers or names. Color bars of individual folders combine into clearly defined blocks of color (Figure 2–1).

These color bars also make it easy to spot records that have been misfiled. Records of a different color stand out when one is simply scanning the file cabinet because they cause a break in the block of color.

Prepackaged color coding systems are available from manufacturers or can be custom designed by manufacturers or in house. The uses of color coding systems are endless. Filing systems can be color coded by number or by subject. Additional internal codes using colored stickers can further differentiate charts.

Numeric color-coded charts can be filed and retrieved extremely quickly. A numeric color coding system assigns each number a different color. Color-coded folders with preprinted numbers can be purchased, or stickers can be purchased and placed on the folders as needed.

An alphabetic color-coded system assigns each letter of the alphabet a different color. The first letter of the last name of the patient is identified by its color.

To use color coding for subject files, each individual subject would be assigned a different-colored sticker. For example, all files having to do with a particular hospital could have one color.

SPECIAL HINT

Use colored stickers to

- Identify charts of patients with past-due accounts
- Identify patients with specific types of allergic reactions
- Facilitate purging of records by placing color-coded numbers on charts to indicate the last year seen
- Assign each specialty or physician a different-colored sticker

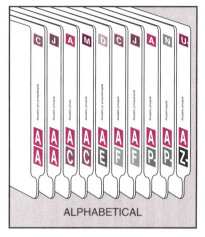
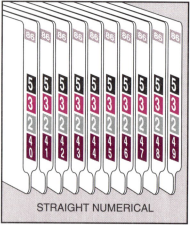
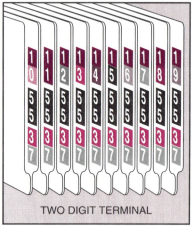
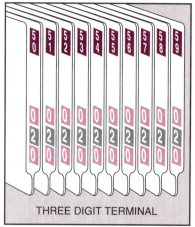

FIGURE 2-1

Examples of color coding.

Alphabetic Coding

Filing alphabetically by name is the most common method of filing because it is so simple to use. No card index cross-referencing is required.

There are many commercial alphabetic filing systems on the market. These systems include preprinted guides and folders. Captions are added to create the files.

Guides and folders can be purchased without preprinting for special office needs. These guides have tabs with inserts that can be prepared according to individual needs.

Filing alphabetically by subject is advisable when

- Records do not refer to the name of a person or organization.
- It is likely that all records will be called for by subject.
- All records about one product or activity are likely to be needed at one time.
- Records might otherwise become minutely subdivided.

Subject files can be difficult to use because it is sometimes impossible to remember exactly where to file information. Considerable thought needs to go into the creation of a subject file so that each subject can be logically remembered in the future.

Medical offices with two or more locations and a centralized business office might consider filing information first by location of satellite office and then alphabetically by name of the patient.

Presorting material to be filed saves much time.

Numeric Coding

Numeric filing is an indirect filing system that requires consulting an alphabetic index to file or retrieve a folder. This cross-reference file can be a listing alphabetized by name or subject.

Numeric files provide a means of quick, accurate identification. Names can be written in different ways, for example, *Rogers* and *Rodgers*. Numbers can be written in only one way.

Numeric filing is arranged consecutively by file number. Because it is not necessary to stop and consider rules of alphabetizing before filing a record, numeric filing can be accomplished in a shorter time period than alphabetic filing.

Numeric files provide for unlimited expansion because numbers are limitless, whereas the alphabet is limited to only 26 letters.

A disadvantage of numeric filing is the necessity of looking up a record in an alphabetic card index before locating the actual record.

Terminal Digit Coding

Filing by terminal digits is easy because numbers are easier to remember than names. Records located by terminal digit are rapidly filed and are retrieved with greater accuracy.

Terminal digit systems have the advantage of an even distribution of records in files at all times. Filing by name causes uneven distribution, because more names begin with certain letters. Permanent numbering of cabinets and guides is possible because the numbers remain the same after files have been transferred.

Terminal digit numeric systems are used most effectively in organizations that have a large number of records, such as hospitals or insurance companies.

In terminal digit filing, the numbers are read from right to left. The last, or terminal, two numbers on the right are primary. The third and fourth numbers from the right are secondary. All the remaining numbers are third in order.

The terminal digits indicate drawer number,

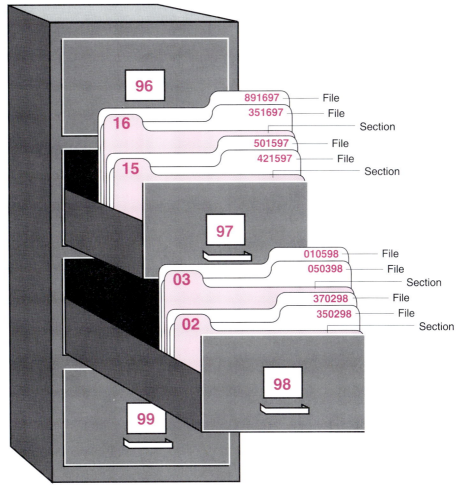

FIGURE 2–2
Example of terminal digit filing.

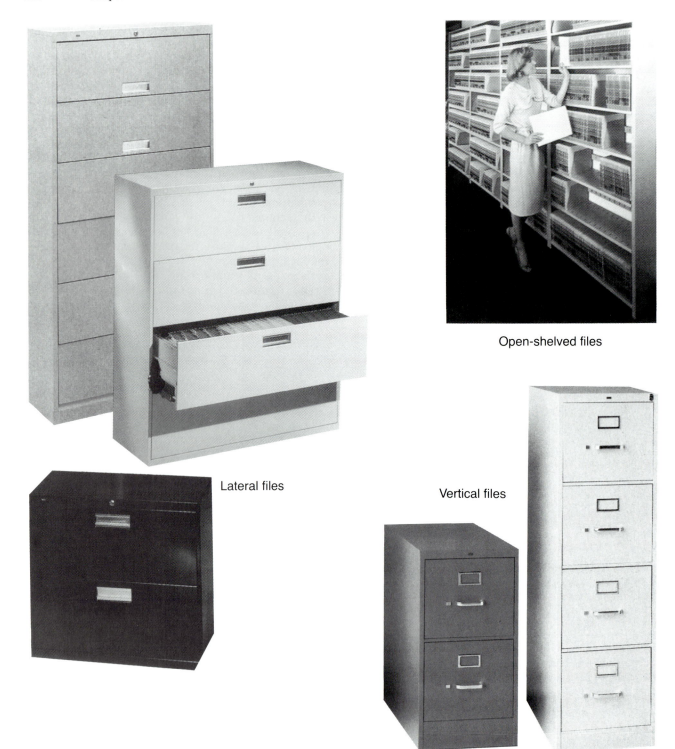

FIGURE 2-3
Examples of file cabinets.

secondary digits indicate folder or section numbers, and remaining numbers indicate sequence within folder or section.

For example, to file a record with the number 421597, the record would be stored in the drawer labeled 97, in the folder or section labeled 15, and would be 42nd within the folder or section (Figure 2-2).

Types of Filing Cabinets

There are four types of filing cabinets (illustrated in Figure 2-3): vertical, lateral, visible, and open-shelved. Each is described below.

Vertical
  Have two to five drawers.
  Are the least efficient type of cabinet because:
    Half of filing time goes into opening and closing drawers.
    Bending or squatting is required to access bottom drawers.
    Stretching is needed to reach folders in back of drawer.

Lateral Filing Cabinets
  Take up less room because they are flush against the wall.
  May be drawer type or open-shelved.
  Are more accessible, making file storage and retrieval faster.

Visible Filing Cabinets
  Are used when information needs to be found rapidly.
  Provide key information on projected edge, which can be seen without handling the stored record.
  Come in many varieties—horizontal trays, vertical racks, open bins or tubs, rotary wheels, or loose-leaf visible books.

Open Shelves
  Take up 50% less space.
  Permit quick access because there are no drawers to open or close.
  Have the disadvantage of collecting dust, particularly in offices without filtration or air conditioning.

Cross-Indexing

Material should be cross-indexed when it might be looked for under more than one caption. File the record under the caption considered to be primary. Cross-index the record under any other captions where material might be filed, indicating correct location of record.

The names of patients in which it is difficult to determine the surname, such as Frank Henry or Charles James, should be filed under proper surname and cross-indexed under the alternative.

Cross-indexing of subject files should include a list of all subjects filed together with major subject classifications under which they are filed.

Converting from One System to Another

Determine how records are requested most frequently and choose a filing system accordingly. Records requested by name should be filed using an alphabetic filing system. Records requested by subject or location should be filed using a subject or geographic filing system. Other considerations in choosing a filing system are expansion needs and the number of records to be filed. Numeric systems, which offer unlimited expansion and fast, accurate filing, are best for handling a large number of records.

Sort out inactive records when converting from one system to another and store them in a separate file using the same system. Conversion of inactive files to a new system should be done when they again become active.

Convert active records to a new system one by one, starting with the first record in the file and continuing until all records are converted.

Because records will be located under two different systems until the conversion is complete, it is best to schedule a file system conversion at a time when records are least likely to be requested. For example, a conversion should be done when the physician is away from the office or over a weekend.

Preserving Records

Microfilm. There is a cost involved in microfilming, and referring to microfilmed files is not as easy as referring to paper. The volume of records and amount of reference made to them after microfilming should be considered before selecting records to transfer to microfilm.

Precautions need to be taken to ensure the safety of microfilmed records and to be sure they are not altered. They should be stored in a locked file and in an area where changes in temperatures cannot damage the microfilm.

> **Guidelines for Microfilming**
>
> - Microfilm records immediately if they are valuable and irreplaceable. Store them in a safe location away from the office, keeping the original in the office for easy reference.
> - Transfer records to storage area rather than to microfilm if records are to be retained less than 7 years.
> - Weigh the cost of microfilming against the cost of storage of original material if records are to be retained from 7 to 12 years.
> - Microfilm records if they are to be retained longer than 12 years.

Microfilm comes in three different formats:

- Roll film (usual format when not specified)
- Strips (stored in special plastic jackets) or
- Microfiche (duplicated sheets in plastic jackets)

Microfilm can be used for transfer of computer data (this is called computer output microfilm—COM). Microfilm uses 2% of the space occupied by original material, comes in either color or black and white film, and is 16 mm or 35 mm.

Computers. All information on a computer's hard disc can be transferred to a computer tape as a means of backing up and preserving records in case any problem occurs. Two or more tapes should be used and rotated when transfers are made. When only one tape is used, the problem can be transferred to the tape, and there will be no way of restoring information to the computer disc without also restoring the problem. Rotation of several tapes provides at least one tape without the problem to use when restoring correct data.

Fire Protection. A fire in an office may not completely destroy the building and its contents, but there is usually considerable water damage. This water can destroy paper files as well as computer systems. It is important to make duplicates of important paper records or backups of computer files and store out of office to prevent loss from fire or water.

Litigation Protection. Duplicate copies of records should be made for any file where there is a chance of litigation. This would include professional liability, insurance claims, or Worker's Compensation claims. It is vital to have the record available for a proper legal defense. The chance of losing the records due to a fire, theft, or other hazards should not be taken. Duplicate records should be stored off the office premises. Alternate locations include the home of the physician or office personnel, an attorney's office, or a bank safe deposit box.

Out Guide for Pulled Records. Recording where a pulled record can be found is of particular importance in multiphysician or multistaff offices where records are used by different physicians or for different administrative functions (billing, dictation, etc.). An *out guide* should be substituted for the record when it is removed, indicating the name of the person who removed the record, the date it was removed, and where it can be found.

SPECIAL HINT

Consideration should be given to having one staff member responsible for retrieving records and inserting an out guide to eliminate problem of misplaced records that occurs when several people have access to file cabinets.

Transfer of Records

Transfer of inactive records can be performed at certain times (such as every 6 months or once a year) or on a continuous basis. This method of transfer creates space in the file cabinet more frequently.

The first transfer of records can be to a less accessible bottom or top file drawer. Records can also be transferred to another file cabinet in a different location (back room, basement, etc.) or to transfer boxes. Filing guides and out guides are not transferred.

Disposal of Records

A *record retention schedule* that lists the time schedule for retention and methods of transfer and/or destruction should be maintained. Destruction of records should be done by paper shredder and the shredded papers disposed of in the wastebasket.

SPECIAL HINT

- State statutes indicate the minimum length of time medical records have to be retained. This length of time runs from last entry.

- Obtain legal advice regarding length of time to retain records, because new statutes are enacted constantly.
- There may be conflicting statutes; the courts must decide which applies to the particular case.

Records should be kept longer than statutes indicate because statutes also provide for bringing suit for professional liability cases for a certain number of years after the *discovery* of the injury. In some cases, an extensive period of time elapses before the discovery of the injury, such as in past prescription of diethylstilbestrol or exposure to toxic or hazardous substances (such as asbestos). Because surviving relatives can bring suit, consider keeping records for a patient until the statute of limitations runs out after the patient's death.

Statutes of limitation in the case of minors do not begin until the minor has reached his or her 18th birthday. Children's records need to be kept for at least the time period specified by the statutes of limitation after their 18th birthday.

Special Indexing

Cross-referencing patients according to treatment, procedure, surgery, or diagnosis allows quick access to this information. Treatment cross-reference is particularly important when experimental drugs are being used. If a patient has an adverse reaction to the drug, names of all patients on the drug are readily available, facilitating the monitoring of other patients for the same reaction. Procedure or surgery cross-reference is useful when a physician is publishing results of cases. Diagnosis cross-reference provides quick notification of patients when new or discontinued treatment of a condition is warranted.

Treatment
List patients undergoing specific treatment.
File card alphabetically by treatment.

Procedure/Surgery
List surgery/procedure.
File alphabetically by surgery/procedure.
List patients chronologically by date of surgery/procedure.
Include complications, special technique or equipment, results, and diagnoses (Figure 2–4).

Diagnosis
File alphabetically by diagnosis.
List current treatment and date it was instituted.
List patient's telephone number, address, and birth date.

Source-Oriented Medical Records

Source-oriented medical records are arranged by section according to the source of each entry. In a source-oriented medical record, all records of like types are kept together: x-ray reports, laboratory reports, etc. Within each section, reports are arranged in chronological order. Office policy

PROCEDURE: CHOLECYSTECTOMY		
DATE	PATIENT	COMPLICATIONS
5/4/85	Patient No. 1	
5/9/85	Patient No. 2	Wound infection
5/20/85	Patient No. 3 (with cholangiogram)	
7/4/85	Patient No. 4 (exploration of common bile duct)	
9/10/85	Patient No. 5	

FIGURE 2–4
Special indexing by surgical procedure.

determines if the most recent is on top or on the bottom, but it is usually more efficient to have the most recent report on the top.

Initial Visit/Progress Notes

Information is arranged according to source. The chief complaint, present illness, past illnesses, and family history provided by the patient are included at the beginning of the record. Results of laboratory and x-ray testing are summarized under separate headings of the record (Figure 2–5).

> **SPECIAL HINT**
>
> A signature, either handwritten or typed, is required on all notes by audit agencies as proof of service rendered. If a signature is absent, repayment to the insurance company of any funds reimbursed for service provided may be necessary.

Problem-Oriented Medical Records

Problem-oriented medical records are arranged according to problems and consist of four essen-

---

PROGRESS NOTE

Name: M.C.G.
Age: 36
Married: 14 years (3 children, ages 13, 10, 8)
Occupation: Housewife

Chief Complaint: Upper abdominal pain, heartburn

Present Illness: About three weeks ago, patient had severe attack of upper abdominal pain.

Past History: Measles and several attacks of sore throat; otherwise healthy childhood. At age 16, had a good deal of heartburn. Medication improved. While at college, heartburn recurred but always responded to medication. Symptoms have recurred at intervals since but have again responded to medication as well as diet. Never had nausea or vomiting.

Habits: Alcohol—at most two cocktails a week. Coffee—two or three cups daily. Meals regular. Does not smoke.

Family History: Father, 68, is well and active. Mother, 60, has had stomach trouble since age 20. One sister, age, 40, has had similar stomach complaints. Two brothers are alive and well.

Physical Examination: Tenderness in the epigastric region.

Laboratory Examination: Blood positive in gastric contents; hemoglobin 11; differential count normal; white count normal.

X-rays: Show an irregular erosion of gastric mucosa 5 cm from the pylorus on the greater curvature.

Diagnosis: Gastric ulcer.

Treatment Prescribed: Special bland diet, no alcohol. Antacid medication. Patient to return in one week.

Physician's Name and Signature

FIGURE 2–5

Example of source-oriented medical record.

```
                          PROBLEM LIST

        PATIENT: D.M.T.

        DATE ONSET:      ACTIVE PROBLEMS:         DATE RESOLVED:

        9/7/86           1. Cholelithiasis        9/14/86 Cholecystectomy

        10/1/87          2. Coronary artery disease

        4/3/89           3. Duodenal ulcer




        TEMPORARY PROBLEMS:

        A. Upper respiratory infection 12/3/88

        B. Rash                         4/8/90
```

FIGURE 2-6
Problem list for problem-oriented medical record.

tial components: (a) the database (chief complaint, present illness, profile, history, physical examination, and diagnostic procedures), (b) the numeric problem list, (c) the initial plans, and (d) progress notes. The problems are numbered in the order the patient presents them to office personnel. Thereafter, the problem is referred to by this number. A problem may be defined as anything that concerns the patient or the physician.

Problem List

A complete problem list is a separate sheet at the front of a patient's chart. This lists all problems the patient has, including resolved problems. The date of onset is indicated. If the problem has resolved, the date of resolution and treatment are indicated (Figure 2-6). For each problem, progress notes are structured according to the SOAP format:

- S: Subjective symptoms — This is the information the patient provides about the problem: date of onset of symptoms, the symptoms, and family history.
- O: Objective findings — This information includes results of the physical examination and testing.
- A: Assessment — This is the physician's diagnosis.
- P: Plan — This includes recommendations for further testing, follow-up, treatment (Figure 2-7).

Patient Data Collection

Creation of registration forms specific to the needs of a particular practice is easy, particularly with a word processor. The form can elicit demographic information and also authorization for release of information to insurance companies and physicians. Photocopies of the master form can be used until it is felt no changes are necessary. The form can then be commercially printed (Figure 2-8).

New Patients

Demographic information obtained from new patients includes

- Patient's name
- Patient's address

```
Name: J.H.

Date: 6/5/90

Problem No. 1: Fractured calcaneus with probable involvement of calcaneal cuboid joint as well as
                anterior process of calcaneus, 3/21/90.

S:  The patient is returning for follow-up for a fracture secondary to a fall down her stairs.
    Treatment has included a short-leg cast and placement in a 3-D brace. She's been attending
    physical therapy sessions three mornings per week for active range of motion and, according to
    the patient, is doing well.

O:  Examination reveals restricted range of motion in the subtalar joint. She has no peroneal
    spasticity. She has a small degree of inversion/eversion. Not tender. Has good dorsiflexion and
    plantar flexion. Walks with a toed opposition of her foot. New x-rays reveal consolidated
    fracture.

A:  Fractured calcaneus, with an articular involvement of the calcaneal cuboid joint with some loss
    of talar motion.

P:  1. Observation
    2. Return in three months to see if she is satisfied with her progress. If there is any worsening,
       then maybe consider further x-rays to see if something could be done.

                                                        Physician's Name and Signature
```

FIGURE 2-7

Example of problem-oriented medical record.

- Patient's phone numbers (both work and home)
- Patient's place of employment
- Patient's next of kin
- Patient's sex
- Patient's marital status
- Patient's date of birth

Insurance information obtained from new patients include

- Name and address of the insurance company
- Patient's group and certificate number
- Name of certificate holder
- Effective date of policy
- Waiting period for coverage

SPECIAL HINT

- Recent effective date of insurance policy should trigger office personnel to advise the patient to review his or her insurance policy or contact his or her agent to make sure that treatment will be covered.
- Obtain signatures authorizing (a) release of information to an insurance company and (b) direct billing of insurance claims at the time of initial visit.

If a new patient has been referred by another physician, the *referral information* obtained includes

- Name, address, phone number, and specialty of the referring physician
- Name, address, and phone number of family physician

Tact should be used in determining whether the patient wants the family physician to know of his or her visit to another physician's office. A

REGISTRATION FORM

PATIENT INFORMATION

Name _____ Home Phone _____ Work Phone _____

Address _____
    Street, Town/City, State, Zip Code

Date of Birth _____ Marital Status _____ Spouse's Name _____

Social Security No. _____ Occupation _____ Employer _____

Family Physician _____ Referring Physician _____

INSURANCE INFORMATION

_____ Blue Cross/Blue Shield Group No. _____ Certificate No. _____

    Certificate Holder _____

_____ Medicare No. _____

_____ Medicaid No. _____ Effective Date _____

_____ MediComp Group No. _____ Certificate No. _____

_____ Other Company _____ No. _____

    Certificate Holder _____

AUTHORIZATION FOR RELEASE OF INFORMATION

I authorize release of medical information to my referring physician and/or family physician. I also authorize release of information to my insurance company.

Signed: _____

On occasion, family members will call inquiring about a patient's treatment and/or medical condition. These members usually include spouse, parents, children, brothers, sisters. If there is any member of your family that you would not want to have your care discussed with, please list below.

I authorize release of medical information to my family except for the following members:

_____

Signed: _____

FOR WORKER'S COMPENSATION CASES

I authorize release of medical information to my employers and/or their insurance company.

Signed: _____

FIGURE 2-8

Custom-designed registration form.

patient may be questioning the care provided by his or her family physician or internist but does not want that physician to know this. Under these circumstances, the patient's wishes should be honored and information should not be sent to the family physician.

Clinical information obtained from new patients includes the following.

- The date of onset of symptoms is helpful to the physician. Insurance companies request this information on claim forms. Verify the date of onset of symptoms with the effective date of the insurance policy. If symptoms occur before expiration of the waiting period, the patient needs to be informed that the cost of treatment may not be covered.
- A patient's medical history can be obtained in several different ways. An oral history can be obtained by office personnel in a private area where there is no chance of other people overhearing. An alternative to an oral history is a written history obtained either at the time of the initial visit or by mailing a history form to the patient, in which case the patient completes the form at home and brings it to the office. Commercial forms are available for purchase, or history forms can be developed for individual office needs.
- Information obtained about a patient's medical history will vary according to the physician's specialty. For example, a pediatrician needs to know what childhood diseases a patient has had. A surgeon needs to know previous surgery, and an obstetrician needs to know about previous pregnancy and any complications. A detailed and complete medical history is needed in an internist's or family physician's office because these specialists treat patients for a wider variety of diseases.
- The amount of family history requested from a patient also depends on the specialty and the condition being treated. A family history is not necessary if a patient is being treated for a fracture. A family history regarding carcinoma of the breast should be obtained if a patient is being treated for a breast mass.
- Allow patients to explain in their own words why they are seeking medical attention. Office personnel should be careful not to put words in a patient's mouth because a clearer understanding of the problem is possible when patients describe their illness themselves. This also creates an atmosphere wherein patients feel they are respected.

Return Visits

1. Verify demographic information.
2. Verify insurance information.
3. Update family and medical history.

Discharge

1. Make sure the proper referring physician and/or family physician are indicated in the records.
2. Make sure the patient has signed all necessary insurance forms.
3. Make sure the patient has authorized release of information to other health care providers.

Research Registry

Agencies that grant money for research have established protocols that the researcher must follow. Information in these protocols includes hypotheses and research methods used. Most protocols have established criteria that patients must meet to be entered into a study.

Hospitals have committees that review research protocols and decide whether the experiment can be conducted on patients in their hospital.

Protection of patients' confidentiality in research studies is accomplished by keeping identifying information separate from research files. Patients are identified only by a number in the research files. Cross-reference by identification number indicating the name of the patient. Keep an alphabetic file by patient name indicating patients' identification numbers.

In double-blind studies, identification numbers are assigned to patients by the agency (for example, the National Institutes of Health) granting the money for research. In this case neither the researcher nor the patient knows who is receiving the experimental drug and who is receiving the placebo.

It is imperative that patients are aware that the treatment they are receiving is experimental. They must sign a consent form stating that the treatment is experimental and they are willing to participate in the study.

Document in research notes that studies are conducted in a humane, moral, and ethical manner. Research notes also include results, adverse reactions, controls, and end point (time when the experiment will stop.)

Authorization to Release Records

Steps in Developing Policies and Procedures for Release of Records

1. Categorize common requests for records (for example, by attorneys, spouses, and health maintenance organizations).
2. Identify the applicable rule of law applying to each.
3. Formalize the procedure for responding to the request, including any fees for preparing the records and how records or parts of records will be reproduced for release.
4. Delegate authority for release to specific personnel.
5. Have these personnel become familiar with laws regarding information release.
6. Document all requests and maintain a record of where information was sent.
7. Review procedures periodically to determine whether laws have changed and modify procedures if indicated.

Releasing Records

Medical records belong to the practitioner, but information in medical records belongs to the patient. The physician is only the custodian of information and needs proper authorization to release it. This confidentiality rule applies to not just the written record but any information that may be in the head of the provider, provider meaning any person working at the health care facility who has access to the information.

Under certain circumstances, the physician has a duty to release this confidential information. This presents a conflict between the physician's duty to keep records confidential and the duty to release the information. Improperly released information can cause the patient to seek legal remedy against the health care provider. Procedures must be established for dealing with requests for release of medical information.

The date the patient signed authorization for release of information must be verified. If it is more than 6 months previous, the authorization should not be accepted and a new one should be obtained from the patient.

Faxing Medical Records. Faxing medical records requires assurance that the person receiving faxed records has the authority to receive confidential medical information. Care needs to be taken to prevent dialing the wrong fax number and faxing records to the wrong office. It is a good policy to ask the requesting office to call and acknowledge their receipt. This provides assurance the records were received by the proper party. Caution must be exercised when using outside agencies to fax records. Consideration should be given to faxing records by identification number and providing the corresponding patient name by phone to the receiving office.

Handling Phone Requests for Medical Records. If a person requests medical information by phone, it must be verified that this person is properly authorized to receive this information, because anyone can call and say he or she is from the office of a physician who needs information on a patient. Information should not be released if there is any question regarding the authority of the person to receive confidential information. Ask for the person's phone number and call back with the information. The phone number can be verified with the phone number of the office for which they were requesting information.

In nonemergent situations, if there is any doubt the patient would want medical information passed on to the other provider, phone requests should not be honored. The other provider should be told written authorization is needed before any information can be released.

Handling Mailed Requests for Medical Records. There is always the possibility that the signature on such a mail request is fake. If there is any question about the authenticity of the signature, a copy of the authorization along with a cover letter requesting confirmation of the signature should be sent to the patient. The patient should sign the cover letter to confirm and return it and the original authorization to the physician.

Releasing Information Generated from Another Health Care Facility. Office staff do not have the right to release information generated from another health care facility. They only have the right to release information generated in their own office. Some health care facilities stamp records they release with the notation "For the use of the receiving facility only, cannot be passed on." Records dictated by a physician but generated by a hospital, such as discharge summaries or operative notes, are probably considered to be part of a physician's records and can be released by that physician. If there is any question, a legal opinion should be obtained prior to release.

Releasing Information without Authorization. Certain types of medical information must be reported to appropriate authorities without authorization from the patient. These include data for some communicable diseases reportable to the state health department or information about the commission of a crime to the police department.

Medical information needed to treat a patient for an emergency condition, when the patient is unable to give proper authorization, may be released under a "need to know" basis to the medical personnel treating the patient. The reason for releasing the information without authorization should be immediately documented in writing.

Requests from Insurance Companies. Third-party payers have provisions in their contracts with patients authorizing release of information required to pay for care provided. If there is any doubt regarding proper authority, or if the health care provider is unwilling to take the risk that such authority exists, a written consent signed by the patient should be obtained.

Insurance companies are contracting with agencies to review the necessity for hospitalization and surgery. Care needs to be taken to make sure that (a) the patient is aware that information is being requested by these fourth parties and (b) the patient authorizes release of this information.

Requests from Employers. The general rule is that employers do not have the right to see an employee's medical records without the employee's consent. The exception to this rule is when a physician provides a pre-employment physical examination requested and paid for by the employer. In this instance, it is presumed there is an absence of a physician–patient relationship and the existence of a legal duty on the part of the physician to the employer. Since this exception is ambiguous, the best policy is to obtain written consent from the person being examined to release the results of the examination to the employer.

A request for information on an employee from a company that is self-insured must be verified to be in the context of claim information. If it is, the rules for third-party payers apply.

A court-appointed guardian for an incompetent individual should have full authority to consent to disclosure of the medical records of the incompetent individual. Verify the extent of the guardian's authority. A guardian of the incompetent person's property may not have the same authority to act as the guardian of the person. The actual text of the appointment document may have to be reviewed to confirm the scope of a guardian's authority before acceptance of an authorization to release records.

Requests from Spouses. In a nonemergency, the spouse of a patient has very little legal authority to act for the patient. It could be argued that the spouse has implied authority to act for the patient because the spouse's consent is usually obtained by the patient before he or she submits to medical care. In nonemergency situations, it is best to obtain the patient's consent before releasing information to a spouse. Although it is common practice to discuss a patient with his or her spouse, legally and ethically this should not be done. Care should be taken to ensure that a couple has not separated or divorced before releasing information to a spouse.

Requests from Attorneys. In a nonlitigation context, a patient's attorney has no special authority to receive information on his or her client. Patients must consent in writing before records can be released to their attorney. If a patient files a lawsuit against a physician, the patient's attorney has the authority to discover all non-privileged information that may lead to evidence. Discovery techniques include written interrogatories or a request for the production of documents. Time limits to respond to a discovery request are short, and there may be severe penalties for non-compliance. An attorney should be consulted immediately when a discovery request is received.

Requests from Other Health Care Providers. In emergency situations, other health care providers providing care to the patient can obtain medical information regarding the patient without a signed consent. In these instances, it can be argued there was implied consent on the part of the patient.

In nonemergency situations, the best approach is to obtain written consent from the patient before releasing records to other health care providers. However, many providers routinely provide information to other providers without consent. Because there is a risk the patient will sue for nonauthorized disclosure, caution should be taken when releasing information to anyone without proper authorization.

If a patient does sue, an available defense to the provider is that the person receiving the information was privileged to receive it; that is, there is a physician–patient privilege between the second provider and the patient just as there is between the first provider and the patient.

Requests from the Government. The federal government generally has the power to override conflicting state rules regarding the release of medical records. States cannot override conflicting federal regulations.

Government entities keep vital statistics, investigate possible child or elder abuse, and monitor communicable diseases. There is a mandatory duty to report these items to the proper government agencies.

Medicare and Medicaid agencies have the right under the law to obtain the medical records of a patient without his or her formal consent. This right has been tested in the court system on many occasions and it still stands.

Requests from Research Agencies. When information is requested for research projects, it should be confirmed there is a legitimate need for the information for the particular project. Information released to research projects should not identify a specific patient. Patients should be assigned a number, and the key identifying the patient with the number should be kept separate from the medical information.

Releasing Records Pertaining to Alcohol and Drug Abuse. Patient records pertaining to alcohol and drug abuse are protected by specific federal statutes and regulations enacted by the Department of Health and Human Services under the authority of the Federal Drug Abuse Prevention, Treatment, and Rehabilitation Act (42 U.S.C. Section 290ee-8) and the Comprehensive Alcohol Abuse and Alcoholism Prevention, Treatment, and Rehabilitation Act (42 U.S.C. Section 290dd-3). These regulations prohibit the disclosure of any information identifying a patient as an alcohol or drug abuser or information regarding the treatment of these patients unless (a) the patient consents in writing; (b) the disclosure is allowed by a court order; or (c) release of records is to other medical personnel in a medical emergency or for research, audit, or program evaluation purposes. These regulations apply to any program that is federally assisted.

SPECIAL HINT

Every physician who receives funds from Medicare or Medicaid programs is considered federally assisted.

Subpoenas for drug and alcohol abuse records should not be acknowledged. Simple acknowledgment of a subpoena can indicate records are available. The response to such a subpoena should be "Your request has been received, but a court judge needs to be contacted because this type of record is federally protected."

The Duty-to-Warn Rule. An exception to the patient privilege rule regarding confidentiality of records is the duty-to-warn rule. When a health care provider has reason to believe a patient will do physical harm to another individual, the provider has a duty to take action to prevent this harm, even though it means release of confidential medical information.

Releasing Records of Minors

Proper authorization is made by the legal guardian of the minor patient, usually the parents. If the parents are separated or divorced, only the parent who has legal custody can authorize release of information. If the minor is in a foster care home, the foster parents or a court-appointed guardian may have legal custody; therefore, it is these parties rather than the natural parents who can authorize release of information.

When a minor has the legal right to consent to treatment, he or she has the right to control release of that information. In many states, minors can consent to drug or alcohol treatment, birth control treatment, or abortions without the consent of their parents. In these instances, written consent of the minor needs to be obtained before release of information.

Medicolegal Forms

Informed Consent. Courts usually accept a signed consent form as proof of informed consent unless the plaintiff can prove there are special circumstances indicating that the form should be ignored. Some attorneys are advising physicians to write a note in the patient's chart specifying what was discussed with the patient or the patient's representative at the time the consent was obtained.

Providing patients with informational material such as pamphlets or videos to supplement explanation of a procedure is a method now being used to further ensure informed consent.

Videotaping the session in which the patient gives consent is a technique to prove that procedures were fully explained to the patient.

Obtaining informed consent for outpatient surgery may be the function of office personnel. They should call to the attention of the physician any patient who seems confused about the surgery or has changed his or her mind about consenting.

Subpoenas. In most states, litigation attorneys have unlimited access to state court subpoenas and can issue them without prior judicial review. Federal subpoenas are issued by the clerk of the federal district court in which the records are located; however, even though issued by a court, in most cases, there is no judicial review. Subpoenas are usually issued after all other attempts to obtain medical records have failed. Caution should be used in responding to subpoenas.

> ### Guidelines for Responding to Subpoenas
>
> 1. Advise the patient in all cases, except when a prior judicial order restricting disclosure has been served with the subpoena.
> 2. Obtain written authorization from the patient to release records.
> 3. Contact an attorney to take legal action to resist the subpoena if written authorization is denied by the patient. Time to respond is short, and there are severe penalties for not responding.
> 4. Verify jurisdiction of the subpoena. State subpoenas have legal force only within the state. There is no duty to respond to out-of-state subpoenas.
> 5. Confirm a case is pending before a court by calling the court clerk. Subpoenas are only valid if they are issued in connection with a pending matter.
> 6. Evaluate the nature of the information being requested. Drug or alcohol abuse records are protected by federal legislation, which supercedes state subpoenas.
> 7. Make a list of records released under a subpoena and have the party issuing the subpoena sign this list to prevent later accusations disclosure was made outside the scope of the authorization.

Search Warrants. Search warrants are limited to criminal proceedings and are issued to obtain evidence against a defendant in a criminal violation. Search warrants are only issued after probable cause and are executed immediately. There is no time to question the legal validity of the warrant. The physician should notify an attorney immediately upon being served with a search warrant. Challenges to search warrants can be made after the warrant has been executed and before the documents or objects taken in the search are introduced as evidence.

MEDICAL CORRESPONDENCE

Mail Processing

Incoming Mail

Incoming mail is processed in the following manner:

1. Sort mail before opening it into first, second, third, and fourth class. Place priority mail on top of first class mail.
2. Check letters for an "enclosure" notation. If the mentioned enclosures were not included, note this on the letter itself.
3. Verify that sender's address is on the letter before throwing away the envelope.
4. Identify personal or confidential mail and distribute to the person to whom it is addressed, unless special authority is given for you to open it.
5. Stamp or handwrite the date of receipt on correspondence (not the envelope) to prove when the mail was received as a defense in a professional liability suit.
6. After you have opened the mail, arrange it by priority or type.
7. Recognize junk mail by the following:
   a. The notation "confidential" or "personal" may be printed on the envelope.
   b. Envelope may not have a return address.
   c. Address may be a computer-printed label or printed by an addressograph machine.
   d. The envelope itself usually is of low-quality paper.
8. Flag laboratory reports with abnormal findings for immediate attention of the physician.

Outgoing Mail

In sending mail, it is helpful to do the following:

1. Verify the address on the envelope to make sure it is the same as on the letter.
2. Verify that all mailing notations ("special han-

dling," "confidential," or "personal") in the letter are also typed on the envelope.
3. Verify that a letter is properly signed by the person writing the letter.
4. Verify "enclosure" (encl) notations to make sure all correspondence indicated as being enclosed has been enclosed.
5. Copy letters for individuals listed in "carbon copy" (cc) notations.
6. Sort and bind mail into local and out-of-town bundles with all addresses facing same direction for faster processing by the postal service.
7. Place special classes of mail (for example, special delivery, special handling, or priority mail) on top of the other mail.
8. Sort by zip code with lowest number first and highest last.
9. If there are more than 10 envelopes to the same zip code, bundle them together.

Use the two-letter abbreviations for states and Canadian provinces. These are listed in the table.

The *National Five-Digit Zip Code and Post Office Directory* lists all five-digit zip codes in the United States and is available for purchase from some post offices, and some bookstores or by writing the Superintendent of Documents, U.S. Government Printing Office, Washington, DC 20402.

Save as much as a full day in delivery by mailing in the morning instead of late in the afternoon. If this is not possible, mail as early as possible to avoid congestion at the end of the business day.

Metered Mail

Metered mail is mail with an imprinted meter stamp in place of a postage stamp. Postage meters are convenient for many offices because postmark, date, and cancellation are imprinted by the meter directly on envelope. This takes much less time than applying stamps. Time is also saved when the mail reaches the post office because metered mail does not have to be canceled and postmarked. If you sort outgoing metered mail with the stamp facing the same way, even more time is saved at the post office. In addition, using metered mail protects against loss, waste, and stamp borrowing.

Postage meter equipment consists of two parts — an office mailing machine and a detachable postage meter. The U.S. Postal Service licenses the meter. The mailing machine is purchased, but the meter is leased from an authorized manufacturer. This manufacturer is responsible for the proper operation, maintenance, and replacement of the machine if necessary.

ABBREVIATIONS FOR STATES, TERRITORIES, AND CANADIAN PROVINCES

Alabama	AL	Kentucky	KY	Oklahoma	OK
Alaska	AK	Louisiana	LA	Oregon	OR
Arizona	AZ	Maine	ME	Pennsylvania	PA
Arkansas	AR	Maryland	MD	Puerto Rico	PR
California	CA	Massachusetts	MA	Rhode Island	RI
Canal Zone	CZ	Michigan	MI	South Carolina	SC
Colorado	CO	Minnesota	MN	South Dakota	SD
Connecticut	CT	Mississippi	MS	Tennessee	TN
Delaware	DE	Missouri	MO	Texas	TX
District of Columbia	DC	Montana	MT	Utah	UT
Florida	FL	Nebraska	NE	Vermont	VT
Georgia	GA	Nevada	NV	Virginia	VA
Guam	GU	New Hampshire	NH	Virgin Islands	VI
Hawaii	HI	New Jersey	NJ	Washington	WA
Idaho	ID	New Mexico	NM	West Virginia	WV
Illinois	IL	New York	NY	Wisconsin	WI
Indiana	IN	North Carolina	NC	Wyoming	WY
Iowa	IA	North Dakota	ND		
Kansas	KS	Ohio	OH		
Alberta	AB	Newfoundland	NF	Prince Edward Island	PE
British Columbia	BC	Northwest Territories	NT	Quebec	PQ
Labrador	LB	Nova Scotia	NS	Saskatchewan	SK
Manitoba	MB	Ontario	ON	Yukon Territory	YT
New Brunswick	NB				

Personnel at the nearest post office set the meter to the amount of postage purchased. (The U.S. Postal Service offers on-site setting for an additional fee over cost of postage. Contact the local post office to determine in what areas this service is available.)

For large packages or envelopes that will not fit into the meter, an adhesive strip is available for imprinting. The strip is then placed on the package.

Mail Classifications

First-class mail is sealed (with the exception of postcards and postal cards) and cannot be opened for postal inspection. First-class mail includes

- Handwritten and typewritten messages
- Bills and statements
- Postcards and postal cards (postal cards are the ones printed by the U.S. Postal Service)
- Cancelled and uncancelled checks
- Business reply mail

NOTE: Stamp large envelopes or packages "first class" to avoid confusion with third-class mail.

Second-class mail includes

- Magazines and newspapers issued at least four times a year with a permit to mail at second-class rates
- Individual, complete copies of a publication, clearly marked second-class mail, from mailers other than publishers

Third-class mail is often called advertising mail. It has a weight limit of 16 ounces and usually is not sealed so it can be opened for postal inspection. It includes

- Circulars, catalogs, and other printed material
- Merchandise and photographs

Fourth-class mail, or parcel post, is for sending packages or parcels that weigh more than 16 ounces. Rates are calculated according to the weight of the package and distance it is being mailed. An envelope may be taped to the outside of a fourth-class package so long as first-class postage is paid. Fourth-class mail includes

- Special catalog mailings
- Special fourth-class mailings
- Library mailings

Priority mail is given full airmail handling. All first-class mail that exceeds 13 ounces is rated as priority mail. Maximum weight is 70 pounds.

Information concerning international mail is contained in *Publication 41, International Mail,* which can be requested from the Superintendent of Documents, U.S. Government Printing Office, Washington, DC 20402.

Overseas military mail to Armed Forces Post Offices and Fleet Post Offices is not considered international mail.

Special Services

Certified Mail. Certified mail provides proof that mail was delivered. A signature from the addressee is required on a receipt form, which is retained for 2 years by the addressee's post office. There is a fee for this service. For an additional fee, a return receipt will be provided to the sender. This return receipt should be kept in the sender's files as proof that the addressee actually received the mail.

Express Mail. Express mail is available through the U.S. Postal Service or through independent carriers, such as Federal Express. Because it is expensive, express mail should be used only for urgent mail. Overnight delivery is guaranteed. Second-day delivery is available from some of the services and is less expensive than overnight delivery. The U.S. Postal Service has an express mail international service. This service is available to 52 foreign countries. If an addressee has moved, the Postal Service will forward the express mail via express mail free of charge. The U.S. Postal Service also has a custom-designed service for unique situations or hard-to-reach locations.

The U.S. Postal Service and most other express mail services will accept packages in the customer's container or will provide a container at no extra cost.

Insuring Mail. The U.S. Postal Service express mail is insured against loss, damage, or rifling at no additional cost. Third- and fourth-class mail can be insured against loss or damage for up to $200. Items of greater value should be sent by registered mail (see below). There are two types of insured mail—unnumbered and numbered. There is a minimal fee for unnumbered insured mail that is sent parcel post. With numbered insured mail, a receipt is given to the mailer at the point of origin by the post office. The postal service obtains a signature upon delivery. A return receipt as proof of delivery can be obtained by the mailer for insured mail over $15 in value. There is an additional fee for numbered insured mail.

Registered Mail. Domestic first-class and priority mail can be registered to protect valuable items, and this is the safest way to mail valuables. The fee for this service is based on the stated value of the mail, with an indemnity limit of $10,000. Because a receipt is given to the customer at time of mailing, registered mail cannot be posted through a regular collection box. The post office keeps records of mailing through a number assigned to the mail. A proof-of-delivery receipt can be obtained for an additional fee. Registered mail is transported under lock and is kept separate from other mail.

Special Delivery. Special delivery does not speed mail transportation from the origin post office to the designation post office. It does ensure fast delivery to the addressee once it has reached the designation post office. An extra fee in addition to regular postage is charged for special delivery. This classification is available for all classes of mail.

June 7, 1990

L.G.G., M.D.
565 Main Street
Anytown, USA 12345

Dear Dr. G.

Subject: S.T.L.

I saw and examined S.T.L. on June 6, 1990, in my office.

As you know, she has been complaining of right upper quadrant pain with some nausea. The pain has increased in severity over the past several months.

On examination, the patient was tender in the right upper quadrant; an ultrasound performed on June 5, 1990, showed the presence of stones in her gallbladder.

I have explained the treatment for cholelithiasis, and she agrees to a cholecystectomy. This has been booked for June 12, 1990.

Thank you for referring this patient. I will keep you informed of her progress.

Sincerely yours

H.G., M.D.
Professor of Surgery
University Medical Center

amg

FIGURE 2-9
Block letter style with open punctuation. All lines begin flush with left margin. Punctuation at end of salutation and complimentary close is omitted.

Special Handling. Special handling items are handled separately from the rest of the mail. The special handling designation is used for third- and fourth-class mail, and an extra fee is charged. Items that are breakable or perishable should be considered for special handling.

Letter-Writing Formats

Parts of a Business Letter

A business letter includes the following. The italicized parts are essential.

Date line
- Typed three to six lines below the letterhead
- Written as month, day, year; no Roman numerals

Reference line
- Typed one to four lines below date line
- File, control, order, invoice, or policy number

Special mail notation
- Typed in all caps two to four lines below last entry and at least two lines above inside address
- Regular mail, special delivery, certified, etc.

On-arrival notation
- Typed in all caps two to four lines below last entry and at least two lines above inside address
- Specifies confidential or personal

Inside address
- Typed three to eight lines below date line
- Contains no more than five lines
- Should not overrun center of page

                                                                               June 7, 1990

L.G.G., M.D.
565 Main Street
Anytown, USA 12345

Dear Dr. G.:

                            Subject: S.T.L.

I saw and examined S.T.L. on June 6, 1990, in my office.

As you know, she has been complaining of right upper quadrant pain with some nausea. The pain has increased in severity over the past several months.

On examination, the patient was tender in the right upper quadrant; an ultrasound performed on June 5, 1990, showed the presence of stones in her gallbladder.

I have explained to her the treatment for cholelithiasis, and she agrees to a cholecystectomy. This has been booked for June 12, 1990.

Thank you for referring this patient. I will keep you informed of her progress.

                                                        Sincerely yours,

                                                        H.G., M.D.
                                                        Professor of Surgery
                                                        University Medical Center

amg

FIGURE 2-10

Modified semi-block letter style with mixed punctuation. Inside address, salutation, identification initials, enclosure notation, and carbon copy notations are flush with left margin. Indent first line of each paragraph. Center or place on page in best relation to letterhead. Mixed punctuation calls for colon at end of salutation and commonly after complimentary close.

- Lengthy organization names or business titles are carried over to a second line and indented two spaces

Attention line

- Typed two lines below inside address
- Should not be underlined or typed in all caps
- Names specific person in organization to receive letter when letter is addressed to an organization

Salutation

- Typed two to four lines below inside address or two lines below attention line
- Omitted in simplified style

Subject line

- Typed three lines below inside address in a simplified letter or two lines below salutation in other styles
- Should be short and to the point
- Must be included in a simplified letter
- Typed in all caps and not underlined, or underlined with just main words capitalized
- Word subject may be included

Message

- Begins two lines below salutation or subject line

Complimentary close

- Typed two lines below last line of message
- Omitted in simplified letter style

Signature block

- Typed at least five lines below last line of a simplified letter or four lines below complimentary close
- Mr., Mrs., Miss, and Ms. are the only titles to appear before name and should be in parentheses

Identification initials

- Typed two lines below end of signature block

Enclosure notation

- Typed one to two lines below last entry
- Indicate number of enclosures, if more than one, in parentheses after word enclosure

Carbon copy notation

- Typed two lines below last entry
- Blind carbon copies are no longer recommended

Postscript

- Typed two to four lines below last entry
- Omit redundant P.S. and P.S.S.

Figures 2–9 to 2–11 show various acceptable formats of business letter writing.

Letters Written by Office Personnel

When writing letters for a physician's signature, office personnel should follow the writing style of the physician as close as possible.

SPECIAL HINT

An internal code is useful to indicate which letters were written by office personnel for the physician's signature and which ones were actually written by the physician. One code is to omit the typist's initials on all letters written by office personnel and to include them in all letters written by the physician.

Envelope Addresses

An example of a properly addressed envelope is shown in Figure 2–12. The procedure for correctly addressing an envelope is as follows:

1. Always use a return address.
2. Machine print or typewrite the address in all capitals.
3. Omit all punctuation.
4. Type ATTENTION line, if used, above name of firm.
5. Delivery address line includes:
   a. street address, P.O. box number, rural route number, or highway contract route number, plus room, apartment, or suite number
   b. indicate whether street is: west (W), east (E), south (S), or north (N)
6. Use the following abbreviations:

ST	street
AVE	avenue
DR	drive
LN	lane
PL	place
RD	road
CIR	circle
RM	room
STE	suite
APT	apartment

June 7, 1990

L.G.G., M.D.
565 Main Street
Anytown, USA 12345

Subject: S.T.L.

I saw and examined S.T.L. on June 6, 1990, in my office.

As you know, she has been complaining of right upper quadrant pain with some nausea. The pain has increased in severity over the past several months.

On examination, the patient was tender in the right upper quadrant; an ultrasound performed on June 5, 1990, showed the presence of stones in her gallbladder.

I have explained to her the treatment for cholelithiasis, and she agrees to a cholecystectomy. This has been booked for June 12, 1990.

Thank you for referring this patient. I will keep you informed of her progress.

H.G., M.D.
Professor of Surgery
University Medical Center

amg

FIGURE 2-11
Simplified letter. Begin all lines flush with left margin. Omit salutation and complimentary close.

---

7. The last line is reserved solely for the city, state, and zip code.

SPECIAL HINT

Address for Success brochure can be obtained for free by writing the Manager, Merchandise and Promotions, U.S. Postal Service, 900 East Fayette Street, Room 510B, Baltimore, MD 21233-9611.

Attending Physician Statements

Insurance Payment

Insurance companies can request additional information not included on the insurance claim form. This request may include such things as

- Copies of operative reports
- Date of onset of illness
- Information on previous treatments

```
SURGICAL ASSOCIATES
234 S MAIN ST
ANYTOWN USA 12345-0567




                            C T SMITH MD
                            UNIVERSITY MEDICAL CENTER
                            1345 MAIN ST STE 7890
                            ANYTOWN USA 56789-8901
```

FIGURE 2-12
Example of properly addressed envelope.

Disability

Disability claim forms request diagnosis, any hospitalization, surgical procedures, and dates of estimated disability. When a return-to-work date is indicated, state whether or not this means full or part time and if there are any work limitations, such as no heavy lifting. If disability is long term, insurance companies will require an updated form periodically, usually on a monthly basis.

Life Insurance

Life insurance companies request medical records from treating physicians before they issue policies to applicants. Indicate in the chart what parts of records were sent to the insurance company and the date they were sent.

Life insurance companies often subcontract the requesting of information to other companies, such as Equifax. Verify that the consent form signed by the patient authorizes release of information directly to Equifax; the form often authorizes release of information specifically to the insurance company and not Equifax.

Second Opinion

Insurance companies are now requiring second opinions for many surgical procedures. Usually the second opinion is performed by a surgeon not associated with the operating surgeon. In some rural areas, this may not be possible.

A second-opinion statement asks for the name of operating surgeon, the name of the second-opinion surgeon, diagnosis, and surgical procedure, and whether the second surgeon agrees with the procedure to be performed. Sometimes the date of proposed surgery is requested also.

Medical Reports

Letter of Referral

A letter of referral is sent when a physician refers a patient for evaluation and treatment. In this letter, the reasons for referral are detailed, as well as previous treatment and findings. A referral letter may be drafted by office personnel and approved by the physician. An alternative is to send copies of the patient's records. If the records are extensive, a summary letter can save the consultant's time.

Consultant's Letter

A physician who is acting as a consultant should send a letter to the referring physician immediately after a patient has been evaluated. The letter should include the consultant's findings and recommendations for further treatment. Office personnel need to make sure this letter is sent as soon as possible after a patient is examined in a consultant's office.

Report to Patient

A written report can be sent to patients regarding the results of testing. This letter can be written by office personnel for approval by the physician. It should include the results of testing and any recommendations the physician has for further testing or treatment.

Manuscript Preparation

Research

Research can be original clinical research done by the physician or research performed in a library. Office personnel may be called on to research literature in a medical library. Research is greatly facilitated if one is aware of the following resources.

Index Medicus. The major index for medical literature is the *Index Medicus*. This book contains an index to current medical articles in journals from all major countries in the world. The index lists publications by both author and subject.

Journal Indexes. Each journal has an index issue, usually every 6 months or at the end of a year, in which it lists articles published in that journal by author and subject.

Computer Searches. Hospital and medical school libraries can do computer searches for literature on a particular subject. A computer search saves time because it provides a list of all the articles on a topic and the journals in which they were published. After review of the computer list, pertinent articles can be researched.

Interlibrary Loan. If the journal desired is not one that is carried by the library, the library can request a copy from another library through a system of interlibrary loans.

The Abstract

The *abstract* gives, in briefest possible form, the nature of the paper, the most important points, and the conclusions. It contains the name of the author; the title of the article; and the journal title, year, volume, and page number. There are journals that publish only abstracts. Usually these abstracts relate to one particular field. Read abstracts to determine whether or not the entire article should be obtained for review.

The Summary

Abstracts and summaries are similar, but a *summary* is usually referred to when the contents of an article are summarized as a whole. An abstract gives brief summaries of only each section of an article that leads to a conclusion.

Drafts

Manuscript drafts should be double spaced with wide margins on both sides to allow space for changes. Triple spacing can also be used in drafts to allow generous space for corrections and additions.

> **SPECIAL HINT**
>
> Typing each draft on a different color of paper (first on blue, second on pink, etc.) is an easy way to identify different versions.

Headings

Provide headings throughout a manuscript to mark the beginning of new subjects or ideas. The format of headings (flush with left margin, indented, underlined, or all caps) depends on the requirements of the journal or book publisher to whom the manuscript is being submitted.

Quotations

Previously published material included in a manuscript must be either enclosed in quotations or indented and printed in smaller-sized type. If quoted material is brief, quotations marks are acceptable. If it is a long quotation, the other method is preferred.

Omissions in quoted material are indicated by ellipsis points (three periods with one space between each) followed by punctuation normally required (for example, ...). The writer's insertions within quoted material are added in brackets.

Footnotes

Footnotes appear at the bottom of a page on which the citation of a reference occurs or on a separate page at end of the manuscript. Consult the requirements of the journal or book publisher for the preferred method.

Many word-processing programs have the capability of preparing footnotes.

Illustrations and Tables

Illustrations and tables should not be mounted in the manuscript. All illustrations and tables need to be kept separate, and on each piece indicate the page in the manuscript where it should appear. On that page, a corresponding notation needs to be made in the margin where the illustration or table should be printed. Legends or captions for illustrations are typed on a separate sheet of paper with notations specifying the illustration with which each legend belongs.

Bibliography

The format for bibliographies depends on the individual journal or publisher. In general, references to books should include the following:

- Name of author or editor
- Title of book
- Name of publisher
- Location of publisher (city and sometimes state)
- Year of publication

References to articles should include

- Name of author
- Title of article
- Name of journal in which it appears
- Page numbers on which it begins and ends
- Date of issue

Consult the requirements of the journal or book publisher for the specific format.

Index

Technical books require an index. Some books have separate subject and author indexes. The more complete the index, the more valuable the book is as a reference. Many word-processing programs have the capability of preparing indexes. If a physician is going to be publishing many books, it would be beneficial to purchase a program that has this capability.

Proofs of Books or Articles

Proofs are sent to the author for corrections. Proofs should be read for typographical errors and checked with original manuscript. Any corrections are made in margins. Two people should check the proof. One can read original manuscript aloud and the other can check the proof. If three people are available, one can read and two can check for corrections.

Special Requirements for Specific Journals

Each journal has requirements for submission of manuscripts, illustrations, and tables as well as the format for footnotes and the bibliography. These requirements are usually printed at the front of the journal near the table of contents. Deadline dates are also included.

Reprints

Reprints of articles published in journals can be obtained. Order at the time the corrected proof is returned to the publisher. Reprints can be mailed as third-class printed matter within the United States.

Remember to count reprints upon receiving them to make sure the number received is same as the number billed for.

Bibliography

Buckner F: The Uniform Health-Care Information Act: A physician's guide to record and health care information management. *Journal of Medical Practice Management* 5:207–212, 1990.

Chamberlain M, Cramer-Hong A, Miller M, Opel R: *Confidentiality of Medical Records.* Eau Claire, WI: Lorman Business Center, 1988.

Cooper MG, Cooper DE: *The Medical Assistant.* New York: McGraw-Hill, 1988.

Doris L, Miller BM: *Complete Secretary's Handbook,* 4th ed (revised by M DeVries). Englewood Cliffs, NJ: Prentice Hall, 1977.

Eckersley-Johnson AL (Ed): *Webster's Secretarial Handbook.* Springfield, MA: Merriam-Webster, 1976.

Kahn G, Yerian T, Steward J Jr: *Progressive Filing and Records Management.* New York: McGraw-Hill, 1962.

Practice management. *Medical Economics* 9(3):33, 1990.

Quinn WH: Statutes of limitation on malpractice claims. *Vermont State Medical Society Reporter,* 5–7, June 1990.

Chapter 3

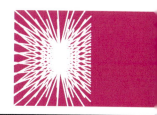

FACILITIES MANAGEMENT

JULIANNA S. DRUMHELLER

OPENING A PRACTICE
Suggested Time Frame for Opening a Practice
Renting Versus Owning
Site Selection
Space Planning
Construction and New Site Design
Supplies and Furniture

OBTAINING NEW OR ADDITIONAL SPACE
CLOSING A PRACTICE
LANDLORD RELATIONS
COMMUNITY RELATIONS

Facilities management is defined as the maintenance of the environment for the orderly conduction of business. It is important for all personnel to have a clear understanding of who is responsible for making decisions concerning the operation of the physical surroundings. It should be established with the employer how much authority the facilities manager will have in establishing and continually evaluating the environmental standards.

Responsibilities are determined by the type of practice that is being managed. Responsibilities differ for a small one-physician office as opposed to a multiple-physician office or a practice with satellite offices throughout the city. In a single location solo-practice facility, management is most likely a part-time activity. In a multiple-physician practice with or without satellite locations, management becomes a full-time responsibility.

The art of facilities management is to plan and direct decor, select and maintain equipment, and improve work flow for the complete harmony of the organization. The facilities manager establishes rules and regulations and coordinates the operation of the workplace with other managers. If the goals of the business are adhered to, the practice should run smoothly.

OPENING A PRACTICE

Planning a new facility is a joint effort among outside professionals, the physician, and the staff. A new or remodeled area must be functional and promote the concept of quality patient care as well as employee morale and productivity. Decisions to be made include design, construction, equipment, financing, operations, maintenance, security, and training. A good plan will include medical and scientific developments as well as future developments so that the facility designed today will be functional in the years to come. The physician and the facilities manager establish a chain of authority for each category of decisions to be made and a time frame as to when the tasks need to be accomplished.

Suggested Time Frame for Opening a Practice

One Year before Starting Practice

- Decide type of practice (group or solo)
- Decide physical location (city, county, state)

Nine Months before Starting Practice

- Choose support services (accountant, attorney, banker, insurance broker, etc.)
- Obtain appropriate licenses, such as state licenses to practice and Drug Enforcement Administration approvals

Six Months before Starting Practice

- Decide on participation for various insurance carriers
- Obtain county and city licenses

Three Months before Starting Practice

- Hire an office manager

One Month before Starting Practice

- Set up office
- Start making appointments

SPECIAL HINT

The American Medical Association (AMA) Department of Practice Development has an excellent information kit called "Starting Your Practice" available through the AMA's order department.

Renting Versus Owning

Two factors the physician needs to consider in deciding whether to own or rent are long-term and short-term liability.

Factors	Own	Rent
1. Equity	Yes	No
2. Short-term liability	No	Yes
3. Facility growth and change	No	Yes
4. Depreciation expense tax deduction	Yes	No
5. Property appreciation	Yes	No
6. Low initial investment	No	Yes

Site Selection

Factors the physician needs to consider when selecting a site include the following:

Area of specialty
    Neighborhood setting
    Proximity to hospital
Public transportation
Adequate parking
    Pay or free
    Validation of parking
Safety (patients and employees)
    Lighting for evening hours
Accessibility

Space Planning

Considerations involved in space planning are as follows:

Type of practice
    Family practice
    Specialty
Handicapped access
Play area for children
Two patient waiting areas
    Sick patients
    Well patients
Number of physicians
    Number of examination rooms needed
    Number of examination rooms per physician
Atmosphere
    Relaxed and professional
    Formal and professional
Work space arrangement
    Administrative
    Clinical
Traffic flow
    Easy arrival
    Registration
    Examinations
    Laboratory testing
    Insurance verification
    Accounting
    Departure

Construction and New Site Design

Factors to consider in the design and construction of a new site are (1) time, (2) the architect, and (3) the contractor.

1. How long will the entire project take?

    Time required to draw plans
    Time needed for architect selection
    Time needed for contractor selection

2. Who will be selected as the architect?

    Make sure the architect is licensed.
    Choose an architect who has a good reputation for commercial building design.
    Choose an architect who will have a good working relationship with the contractor.
    Ask to see other projects.
    Talk to other clients of the architect.
    How much service, working plans, and supervision of job will the architect supply?

3. Who will be selected as the contractor?

    Make sure the contractor is licensed.
    Choose a contractor who has a good reputation for commercial building.
    Choose a contractor who has a reputation for prompt, efficient completion.
    Obtain references from other clients of the contractor.
    Offer a completion bonus, penalty, or both.

SPECIAL HINT

An attorney should be consulted before a contract of this magnitude is negotiated and signed.

Supplies and Furniture

Determine how much and what type of equipment will be needed. Obviously, an ophthalmologist would use different instruments from those required by an OB/GYN physician. Consider how many examination rooms will need to be equipped and how the rooms should be furnished. Perhaps two rooms will be used for routine care and one for surgery. In some instances, the larger, more expensive pieces of equipment can be shared with another physician in the building. If the office is not convenient to a hospital, consider doing a certain amount of laboratory work in the office. Medicine is a service industry; consequently, it is important to be attentive to the needs of the patients. Elderly and handicapped patients find it is much easier to go to one location where everything can be accomplished at one time.

Most equipment should be purchased, but leasing is also an option. Larger pieces of equipment are quite expensive and quickly become outdated; leasing ensures that new equipment will be available as it comes on the market. Select a reputable supplier who will provide prompt repair or replacement when needed. Check the supplier's credibility. Check with other physicians' offices to determine the supplier's dependability in providing expendable items as well as leasing and purchasing of major equipment.

Supplies and furniture are discussed in more detail in Chapter 4 of this reference manual.

OBTAINING NEW OR ADDITIONAL SPACE

New or additional space is required if the physician decides to remodel, relocate, or open a satellite office. Questions to ask when considering any of these ventures are

1. Has the practice changed?
2. Are there too many patients for the amount of office space?
3. Are there too few patients for the amount of office space?
4. Is the environment no longer conducive to the practice?
5. Can additional services be added at the present location?
6. Is there more than one location?
7. Does the practice need to slow down?

Before deciding which direction will be best for the practice, conduct a survey like the following one to find out what the patients think.

PATIENT SURVEY

1. How long have you been a patient?
   Years _____ Months _____
2. Are other family members patients?
   Yes _____ No _____
3. Do you find this office convenient?
   To your home: Yes _____ No _____
   To your pharmacy:
   Yes _____ No _____
   To your outside laboratory:
   Yes _____ No _____
   To the hospital: Yes _____ No _____
   To your business: Yes _____ No _____
4. Do you feel safe in this neighborhood?
   Yes _____ No _____
5. Would you like to see more services provided?
   Yes _____ No _____
   If yes, which ones? _____
   _____
6. If you are handicapped, do you find access to this office convenient?
   Yes _____ No _____

Please make comments or explain any No answers in the space provided at the bottom of this page.

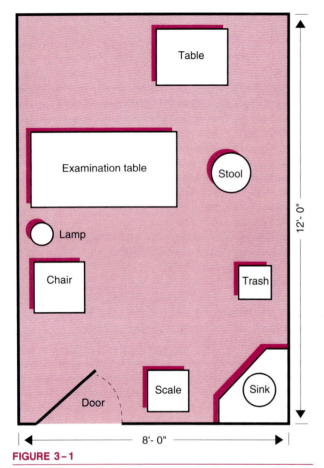

FIGURE 3-1

Examination room before redesign.

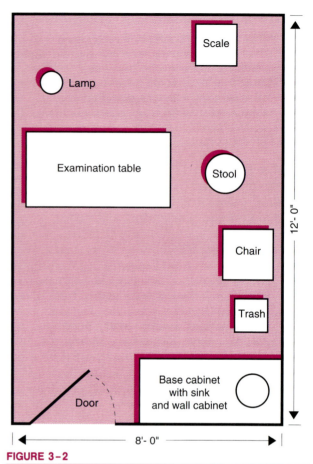

FIGURE 3-2

Examination room after redesign.

Once the decision has been made to remodel, relocate, or establish a satellite office, consider the following:

- Make plans so that the remodeling does not cut into the business activities and interfere with cash flow.
- Make sure that the ability to provide services to your patients is maintained.
- Plan to add more space than needed. This will allow for future expansion without interruption.
- Consider storage for bulk buying and saving.
- Consult the staff in the office for advice on improving work areas.

SPECIAL HINT

Select an architect and a contractor and follow all the guidelines outlined earlier in this chapter. It may be cost efficient to consult the original architect and contractor because they are already familiar with the structure.

Figures 3-1 and 3-2 are before and after drawings of an examination room that has been redesigned to offer more storage and efficiency.

CLOSING A PRACTICE

Take into consideration the ease with which closing a practice can be accomplished for the physician as well as the patient. Employees should be considered in any decision to close a practice. Once the decision to close the practice has been made, the closing date must be established. Then patients are notified of the closing date and told why the practice is closing, for example:

- Retirement
- Relocation
- Illness
- Death

Patients may be notified of the closing in the following ways:

- Send a letter to all patients.
- Publish an announcement in the local newspapers several times.

Disposal of practice can occur by sale, partner takeover, or simply, closing the doors.

When a practice is being closed, patients' medical records must be transferred to other physicians at the patients' requests. Patients must request in writing for transfer of records. It is legally acceptable to transfer originals. Keep a record of when and to whom records were transferred. Make certain the announcement states the deadline for transfer of records.

Allow for records that are not requested by the patient to be transferred elsewhere. Another physician may be willing to be custodian. If so, make certain the announcement states that fact.

Disposal of equipment may occur in any of the following ways:

- The physician may sell the equipment.
- The medical equipment supplier may help sell it.
- The equipment may be donated to a teaching institution (this may be tax deductible).

The physician then settles with suppliers. Leased equipment not purchased by another physician must be paid off. Disposable supplies may be taken back by the supplier. Large equipment may be sold, perhaps with the supplier's help. Advertise equipment for sale in medical journals.

Finally, when a practice is being closed, accounts receivable must be collected. In addition, continuation of liability insurance in the form of a one-time purchase should be considered.

LANDLORD RELATIONS

When leasing space for the medical office, consider the landlord's reputation. Other tenants can be informative as to whether the landlord performs repairs and routine maintenance in a timely and efficient manner. A *lease* is a contract by which one conveys real estate or equipment for a specified period of time for a specified sum of money (Figures 3–3 and 3–4).

THIS LEASE AGREEMENT made this ____ day of _____, 19 ____, between _____, hereinafter called Lessor, and _____ hereinafter called Lessee.

WITNESSETH:

The Lessor hereby demises, leases, and lets to the Lessee, its successors and assigns, and the Lessee does hereby rent from the Lessor, the following premises:

Office comprising approximately _____ square feet located at _____ with the appurtenances, to be used for office purposes. The term of this lease shall be _____ months beginning _____ and ending _____; provided, however, Lessor shall give Lessee notice of its intentions to renew the lease no later than _____ months prior to the expiration of this lease.

The rent shall be _____ monthly, payable in advance on the first business day of each and every month.

THE PARTIES HERETO COVENANT WITH EACH OTHER AS FOLLOWS:

1. The Lessee will pay the rent at the times and in the manner aforesaid, and at the expiration of the term will remove its goods and effects, and will peacefully yield up to Lessor said premises in as good

FIGURE 3–3

Lease agreement, example 1.

order and repair as when delivered to it, damage by fire or casualty, damage beyond its reasonable control, and ordinary wear and tear excepted.

2. Premises shall be kept in reasonable repair by the Lessor, except that repairs or service calls made necessary through the negligence of the Lessee shall be paid for by the Lessee.

3. Premises shall be used for office only and Lessee may assign or sublet in writing all or any part of the premises, sublet tenant to be approved by Lessor. Lessee to remain responsible for collection and payment of all rents.

4. Lessee agrees to use only a reasonable amount of parking spaces and to cooperate in keeping out unauthorized vehicles.

5. The Lessee shall not use the leased premises for any unlawful purpose. No use shall be made or permitted to be made of the leased premises, or any part thereof, and no acts done therein that may unreasonably disturb the quiet enjoyment of any other tenant in the building of which the leased premises are a part.

6. The Lessor shall for the rent reserved furnish at its own expense electric current for air conditioning and lighting said premises, replacement of electric light bulbs and fluorescent tubes, janitor service, hot and cold water, sufficient heat whenever necessary to make the demised premises comfortable for occupation, and shall furnish all janitor supplies and all supplies for toilets and lavatories. Lessor shall not be liable for temporary interruptions in electricity, air conditioning, water, etc. beyond Lessor's control, so long as Lessor is making diligent efforts to have repairs made so that the affected service can be returned to normal.

7. The Lessor may, during the term at reasonable times and during the usual business hours, enter to view the premises and may show said premises to others.

8. If the demised premises shall be damaged by fire or other casualty as to be substantially destroyed, then this lease shall cease and come to an end, and any unearned rent paid by the Lessee shall be apportioned and refunded to it.

9. If the Lessee shall neglect or fail to perform or observe any of the covenants contained herein in its part to be observed and performed for _____ days after notice by the Lessor, or if the Lessee shall be adjudicated bankrupt or insolvent according to law, or shall make an assignment for the benefit of creditor (except where the term hereby granted has been lawfully assigned as permitted by paragraph 3 hereof to an assignee who has assumed the covenants of this lease), then and in any of said cases, the Lessor may lawfully enter into and upon the said premises or any part thereof in the name of the whole, and repossess the same as of the former estate of the Lessor and expel the Lessee and those claiming under and through it and remove its effects (forcibly if necessary), without being deemed guilty of any manner of trespass, and without prejudice to any remedies which might otherwise be used for arrears of rent or breach of covenant, and upon entry as aforesaid this lease shall terminate, and the Lessee covenants that in case of such termination it will indemnify the Lessor against all loss of rent, costs expended and reasonable attorney's fees which the Lessor may incur by reason of such termination, during the residue of the term specified.

10. All notices to be given hereunder by either party shall be in writing and may be served in person or by certified mail, return receipt requested, addressed to the party intended to be notified at the post office address of such party last known to the party giving such notice.

11. The Lessor covenants that the Lessee, on paying the rent as it falls due and performing the covenants aforesaid, shall and may peaceably and quietly have, hold and enjoy the demised premises for the term aforesaid.

12. Any improvements (including, but not limited to carpeting, doors and doorways, lighting fixtures, ceiling, etc.) made by Lessee to the leased premises shall, when made, become the property of the Lessor.

13. All painting, recarpeting, and other architectural and cosmetic changes made by the Lessee shall be at Lessee's own expense and without reimbursement from Lessor.

14. No architectural change shall be made without the prior written approval of the Lessor.

The covenants and agreements contained in the foregoing lease are binding upon the parties hereto and their respective heirs, executors, administrators, successors, legal representative and assigns.

WITNESS the following signatures and seals:

_____ (SEAL)
Lessor

_____ (SEAL)
Lessee

FIGURE 3–3 Continued

THIS LEASE AGREEMENT, executed in duplicate this _____ day of _____, 19 ___, _____ by _____ and between _____, hereinafter referred to as the "Landlord," and _____, hereinafter referred to as the "Tenant."

WITNESSETH:

Landlord hereby lets unto the Tenant and the Tenant hereby hires from the Landlord the following described property, hereinafter referred to as the "premises":

1. TERM: The term of this lease shall be _____ for _____ commencing on the ___ day of _____, 19 ___, and ending on the _____ day of _____, 19 ___.

2. RENT: The Tenant agrees to pay to the Landlord as rent for the term of this lease $_____, payable in consecutive monthly installments of $_____ each, commencing on the ___ day of _____, 19 ___, and following on the first day of each month thereafter throughout the term.

3. DUTIES AND OBLIGATIONS OF THE TENANT:

   a. Tenant shall pay all charges for electricity, water, sewerage, and gas used during the term of this lease or any renewal thereof.

   b. Tenant shall not keep or have on the premises any article or thing of dangerous, flammable, or explosive character that might increase the danger of fire upon said premises or that might be pronounced "extra hazardous" by any reasonable insurance company.

   c. Tenant shall provide and maintain appropriate receptacles for the collection and storage of garbage and other waste.

   d. Tenant shall maintain the premises by performing the following:

   1. Keeping all outside yard areas clean and in safe condition and keeping all walks free from ice and snow, trash and rubbish.

   2. Keeping in good and safe working order and condition all electrical, plumbing, sanitary, heating, ventilating, air conditioning and other facilities and appliances, normal wear and tear excepted, it being understood that all the above are in good working order on the day of execution of this lease, and it being further understood that Tenant shall be responsible for repairs required by reason of negligence by the Tenant.

   3. Complying with all obligations primarily imposed upon Tenant by applicable provisions of building and housing codes materially affecting health and safety.

   4. At the termination of the term, whether by expiration of this rental agreement or by reason of default by the Tenant, promptly vacate the premises, removing all items of personal property and leaving the premises in good and clean order and repair, reasonable wear and tear excepted.

4. ALTERATIONS, ADDITIONS AND IMPROVEMENTS: Tenant shall make no alterations, additions or improvements to the premises except with the written consent of the Landlord, and all alterations, additions and improvements shall inure to the benefit of and be the property of the Landlord.

5. SUBLEASE OR ASSIGNMENT: It is agreed that the Tenant shall have no right to sublease the premises or assign this lease without the prior written consent of the Landlord, which consent may be arbitrarily and unreasonably withheld by the Landlord if the Landlord so chooses.

6. ACCESS: Landlord shall have the right to enter the premises in order to inspect the premises, make necessary or agreed repairs, decorations, alterations or improvements, supply necessary or agreed services or exhibit the dwelling either to prospective or actual purchasers, mortgagees, tenants, workmen or contractors. The Landlord may so enter without the consent of the Tenant in case of emergency.

7. DESTRUCTION BY FIRE: If the premises are damaged or destroyed by fire or casualty to an extent that the unit is substantially impaired the Tenant may immediately vacate the premises and notify the Landlord in writing within _____ days thereafter of his intention to terminate the rental agreement, in

FIGURE 3-4

Lease agreement, example 2.

which case this rental agreement terminates as of the date of vacating or, if the premises are not damaged to the extent that the unit is substantially impaired, and therefore no termination occurs, then the Landlord shall properly repair the damage and an abatement be made for the rent corresponding to the time during which and the extent to which said premises may have been damaged, but in any event, if the premises shall be so damaged that the Landlord shall decide not to rebuild or repay, the term of this lease shall cease at the time of the damage and the aggregate rent be paid up to the time of the damage.

8. RENEWAL: Either party to this agreement shall have the right to terminate this lease at the expiration of any term, or any extension or renewal thereof, by giving the other party _____ days' notice in writing prior to the expiration of said term, or any extension or renewal thereof, and absent said notice, this lease shall continue from term to term, having been automatically renewed on the same conditions as herein set out.

9. NONCOMPLIANCE WITH RENTAL AGREEMENT: FAILURE TO PAY RENT: If there is a breach of this agreement by the Tenant, the Landlord may deliver a written notice to the Tenant specifying the acts and/or omissions constituting the breach, and stating that the rental agreement will terminate upon a date not less than _____ days after the receipt of the notice, if the breach is not remedied in _____ days. If the breach is remedied by repairs or the payment of damages or otherwise and the Tenant adequately remedies the breach prior to the date specified in the notice, the agreement shall not terminate. If rent is unpaid when due and the Tenant fails to pay the rent within _____ days after written notice by the Landlord specifying the nonpayment and specifying the Landlord's intention to terminate the rental agreement, the Landlord may terminate this agreement and proceed to obtain possession, recover damages, and/or obtain injunctive relief as allowed, and in all cases requiring legal action, the Landlord may recover reasonable attorneys' fees as allowed.

10. INCREASE OF RENT: If during the term of this lease real property taxes or the special assessments as to the premises or as to the real property upon which the premises are located are increased by the governing body of the political subdivision within which jurisdiction the premises are located, Landlord shall have the right to increase the rent proportionally, upon _____ days' notice to the Tenant.

11. WATER DAMAGE: The parties agree that Landlord shall not be responsible for any water damage to Tenant's personal property whether the damage is caused by water originating on the interior of the premises or originating from an exterior source. It is understood that it shall be the responsibility of Tenant to obtain his own insurance to cover losses to his personal property caused by water damage.

12. ENTIRE AGREEMENT: This lease embodies the entire contract between the parties and shall not be altered, changed or modified in any respect without and excepting an instrument of equal dignity to this instrument.

13. BINDING EFFECT: The covenants and conditions and agreements herein shall apply to and bind the heirs, executors, representatives, successors and assigns of the parties hereto.

WITNESS the following signatures and seals.

_____ (SEAL)
Landlord

_____ (SEAL)
Tenant

FIGURE 3-4 *Continued*

> **SPECIAL HINT**
>
> Always read the lease completely line by line and understand all the terms and agreements.

Terminology that needs to be understood includes

Landlord or lessor or owner: One who gives a lease

Tenant or lessee or renter: A person to whom a property is leased

Make certain the lease specifies exactly whether the lessor or the lessee is responsible for the following items:

  Cleaning services
  Janitorial service
  Biomedical waste
  Normal upkeep
  Painting
  Routine maintenance
  Security choices
    Alarm system
    Security guards
    Maintenance of security system
  Repair of fixtures
  Regular vendors — repairs
  Lawn care
  Snow removal: Parking lot and sidewalks
  Water
  Phone system
  Electricity
  Sewer
  Fire insurance
  Disaster insurance
  Liability

Vendors of these services need to be updated to determine the best service and price.

COMMUNITY RELATIONS

The medical practice can become a vital force in building a good sense of community in the neighborhood. Some programs that are available to participate in are:

  Crime Stoppers
  Health fairs
  Neighborhood awareness programs

Participation in these kinds of programs can help the practice to grow.

Bibliography

American Medical Association: *The Business Side of Medical Practice*. Chicago, 1989.

Sloane RM, Sloane BL: *A Guide to Health Facilities: Personnel and Management*, 2nd ed. St. Louis: C.V. Mosby Company, 1977.

Chapter 4

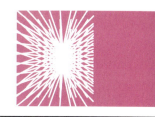

OFFICE EQUIPMENT AND SERVICES

JANE B. SEELIG

LEASE AND PURCHASE AGREEMENTS
Financial and Tax Advantages
Depreciation
Policy and Procedure Development
Policy/Procedure Manuals and Updating Procedures
Maintenance Agreements

SECURITY
Access and Activation
Sensor Placement
Options

GROUNDS AND PARKING SYSTEMS
Waste Disposal
Custodial and Housekeeping Services
Security Violation, Incident Handling, Reporting, and Follow-up

PURCHASING AND INVENTORY CONTROL
Purchasing Control
Storage and Inventory
Inventory Control

OFFICE EQUIPMENT AND MAINTENANCE
Telephone Systems and Services
Photocopy Machines and Services
Facsimile (Fax) Machines and Services
Computers

SALES REPRESENTATIVES
Sample Handling
Recourse from Suppliers

LEASE AND PURCHASE AGREEMENTS

The financial position of the practice is the major determining factor when the decision whether to purchase or lease a major equipment item is being made. Tax advantages are based on the type of equipment being purchased; the purpose of the item's use; whether the business is a proprietorship, partnership, or corporation; and the current interest deduction allowance laws. The best source of advice on whether to lease or purchase an item is your accountant. Your accountant is also in the best position to assess the value of using capital versus obtaining a financial institution loan to fund the purchase, if this is your decision. When assessing the advantages of lease versus purchase, many factors must be considered. The comparison checklist in the chart below will assist you in making the decision.

PURCHASE VERSUS LEASE FACTORS

	Purchase	Lease
Quoted price		
Finance charge		
Time period for payment		
Discount for prepayment		
Coverage		
Terms		
Total expense		

Down payment: This allows for lower lease payments or may be required to serve as "earnest money" when purchasing high-cost items such as a computer system. If the equipment order is cancelled, the earnest money payment is usually forfeited.

55

- **Time period for payment:** Some suppliers offer a "ninety (90) days same as cash" advantage when purchasing an item. When leasing, there may be options for monthly, quarterly, semiannual, or annual payments; each has its advantages and disadvantages.
- **Coverage:** Frequently suppliers offer additional options or extended maintenance coverage with full purchase plans. Lease agreements either include or exclude option coverage or disposable item coverage. Insurance coverage may be mandatory as part of the purchase or lease agreement with expandable benefits, or the choice of insurance coverage may be left to you.
- **Negotiated terms:** Fixed payments for the term of the lease or the option to reduce payments at a future date if interest rates drop may be included as a term of the lease. It is advisable to verify that early payment of the contract does not incur a penalty. Frequently a penalty clause is included for terminating the lease before the negotiated end date. If equipment upgrade is a possibility, be sure to review the contract for allowance of credit toward the upgrade.

An example of a purchase and lease situation is the postage meter. The postage meter/letter-sealing base may be purchased, whereas the metering portion must be leased with a separate maintenance agreement.

Financial and Tax Advantages

The specific tax laws that apply to your individual practice situation are best identified by your accountant. There have been many changes over recent years applicable to the tax law regulations for business purchases. An example is the regulations currently governing the decision of lease versus purchase of an automobile used for business purposes. If you own an automobile that you use only for business purposes, a deduction for depreciation and operating expenses can be taken, but no deduction can be taken for the payments to finance the purchase. In contrast, if you lease the automobile, you may deduct the monthly payments, but not the depreciation.

After you have received the quotation from your equipment sales representative and have settled on the model that fits your needs, you should assess the various prices for the features and options quoted. When exploring the financing options, take into consideration the state tax as it is applied to the total expense of the item. Taxes cannot be overlooked whenever a decision is made regarding a major purchase item. The total purchase price, including applicable taxes, could make the difference in the final decision of financing versus using available capital to purchase the item.

Depreciation

There are a variety of ways of depreciating an item. The basis for the depreciation time period or term is usually the expected period of the item's usefulness or the life of the item. Usual terms of depreciation are 5, 10, 15, or 25 years. Depreciation can be taken as an equal amount for every year of the estimated usefulness or life (flat line) or as a percentage of decreasing amounts (appreciation) per year taken over the time of usefulness or life. Depreciation is deducted from taxes as a business expense for the full term of the usefulness of the item or the determined period of depreciation. Again, your accountant is the best authority for determining the term and method of depreciation. Frequently financing is obtained for the term of depreciation to give the purchaser tax advantages for deduction of interest and depreciation expense.

A word of caution regarding depreciation: If you sell an item before the end of its term of depreciation, the depreciation deductions taken must be adjusted to conform with the actual time of ownership. Therefore, it is most important that you provide information regarding such a sale or any disposal of a major purchase item to your accountant so the proper accounting procedures can be followed and adjustments made for the next tax filing. If this is not done, a tax penalty may be levied.

Policy and Procedure Development

A policy should be put into place for periodic evaluation of the lease agreements and contracts that have been entered into by the practice. Evaluation should consider the effectiveness, cost, and current market situation, as well as the practice's financial position. This evaluation process can also be followed before signing any agreement. The following questions should be answered before entering into an agreement or when evaluating one currently in place:

- How does the total cost compare with the income expected to be generated or saved by the item?
- Does the term of payment fit into the practice's expectation of its future financial situation?
- Can the agreement be terminated or paid early without penalty? If there is a penalty, how is it determined?
- Who is involved in the decision-making process and who is to sign the agreement?
- What is the policy regarding upgrading of the item or the trade-in value within the terms of the agreement?
- Are there tax credits available for the purchase?
- Is there an advantage to purchase over lease (provided the financial position of the practice makes this an option)?

When answering these questions, research must be done. Frequently the information gathered can be used to answer multiple questions. Purchase decisions must be researched thoroughly and the following items considered before the final decision is made:

- The financial status of the practice
- The cost of the item per annum for the long term, including upgrade costs, appreciation, and depreciation
- Benefits anticipated
- The future needs of the practice anticipated with the growth that is expected

When forecasting growth, consideration must be given to the growth of the geographic area, the traffic flow, and the location of the practice. Careful care must be taken to remain current with the regulations, laws, and tax benefits for these decisions. To ensure that you are not in conflict with any regulations, it is wise to seek legal

Date	Item	Activity	By Whom

Final Decision: Purchase   Lease   Price: _____

Preparation needed: _____

Financing by: _____ Terms: _____ years _____ percentage

Service requirements: _____

Renewal dates: _____

FIGURE 4-1

Equipment purchase information.

counsel. If consideration is being given to physical expansion to accommodate expansion of services offered by the practice, city and state regulations must be reviewed. Any time expansion is undertaken that increases the capacity of the building for patients or employees, adequate parking and restroom facilities must be provided to conform with zoning regulations. Legal counsel should periodically review all leases regarding office space and equipment, especially the provisions regarding provider bankruptcy, claim procedures, and malpractice or liability for both lessee and lessor.

Policy/Procedure Manuals and Updating Procedures

As decisions are made regarding the purchase or lease of equipment, they should be summarized in a manual for future reference. The policy manual would outline the decisions made regarding the purchase or lease of each piece of equipment, with the reasoning behind each decision as well as the terms of the agreement. A copy of each agreement could be placed in this manual for easy reference.

This procedure manual outlines the decision-making process, who the decision makers were, the information upon which the decision was based, a timetable for the decision process, and the projected financial benefits of the purchase as they relate to the projected costs. The expense breakdown would include the price quoted, related taxes, financing expense, discounts provided, maintenance costs, and estimated schedule, as well as any expenses related to installation and preparation of the physical facility (Figure 4–1).

Maintenance Agreements

The purpose of the maintenance agreement is to provide adequate service and repair at the most economical price. The agreement usually becomes effective after the expiration of the warranty or, if there is no warranty, upon purchase of the item. The following table is a summary of items that should be considered when evaluating a maintenance contract.

MAINTENANCE/SERVICE CONTRACT FEATURES

Renewal time frame
Frequency limitations
Effectiveness
Contract terms
  Labor
  Travel time
  Guaranteed response time
  Exclusions
    Parts
    Labor
  Limitations/restrictions
  Temporary replacement provisions
Upgrade provisions
Depreciation rate

ITEMS REQUIRING REVIEW

Physical plant—insurance
Heating—installation warranty and service restrictions
Ventilation—service provisions
Cooling—service provisions
Plumbing—installation warranty and service restrictions
Structure—builder's records, schematics, and floor plans
Outlot—landscaping care, parking area, and sprinkler system
Electrical—building schematic, dedicated outlets, and contractor

EQUIPMENT ISSUES FOR REVIEW

Insurance coverage requirements
Subcontractor/contractor insurance limitations
Extraordinary physical plant needs (x-ray and laboratory)
Liability responsibility or specific need coverage by insurance

SECURITY

Protection of the physical contents of the medical practice is no longer an option. Pharmaceuticals as well as expensive medical and office equipment present the need for more sophisticated security than a locked door, drawer, or safe. There are many electronic systems to choose from that are designed for business and residence use. These can easily be modified for the medical practice. The sophistication of the system chosen determines not only the level of security provided, but also the cost of installation, equipment, and maintenance.

Access and Activation

The first security systems were key activated. The systems available today are activated by touch keypad with individual access codes or electronically coded identification strip cards. Each employee is provided a personal access code, which eliminates the need to physically change the locks when an employee departs. Today's systems allow for individual access as well as for zone security. Specific physical areas of the facility can be independently secured with zone enunciation. Alarm activators can be audio detectors for wood or glass breakage or can be heat or motion sensitive, using infrared rays.

Sensor Placement

The placement of the sensors is extremely important. More than a few security systems have been disrupted by an electrical storm or furniture leg. Floor sensors need to be placed in an entry or high-traffic area that is not at risk of having furniture placed directly on the sensor and damaging it. Wall sensors should not be placed directly facing a window or hot air register. Many late-night false alarms have been activated by severe storms and lightning. Placing a sensor in the door frame requires consideration of the door's fit into the frame as well as the tightness of the lock fittings.

Options

Standard options include auxiliary power by battery, smoke detection systems, and connection to the police and fire stations. The following chart serves as a checklist for system features and options; however, it is not inclusive of all options available. Technology progresses too rapidly to propose that any such listing would be complete.

SECURITY SYSTEM FEATURES

Basic cost
Option cost
Maintenance cost
Exterior alarms
Exterior sensors
Interior alarms
Interior sensors
Activation key/card/code
Insurance requirements
Wireless/wire
Alarm/silent/audio
Zone enunciator
Movement: Forced-air heat/floor sensor/doorway
Selectable/individual alarm
Maintenance
Power source
    Monitoring and test
    Auxiliary system
Downloading/uploading
Remote capabilities
Activity log
Police alarm connection
Fire alarm connection
Smoke detector
Panic system (button)
Training for system use
Power loss interference

GROUNDS AND PARKING SYSTEMS

The security of the exterior of the building, the grounds, and parking areas of the medical practice cannot be ignored. As large medical facilities and multispecialty clinics replace solo practitioners, parking for patients and employees requires formal security. The automated gate with timed parking ticket for entry has become commonplace. This requires the additional expense of a parking attendant to collect the fees or validated passes at time of exit. Some practices avoid the need for a parking lot attendant by issuing special tokens for exit. Regardless of the system chosen, parking security is expensive and a burden to the patients. Patient access to the building is a concern that cannot be ignored. Handicapped parking and building entrance access are now government mandated. Again, zoning regulations dictate the requirements for parking and the entrances to the facility. When the parking lot is being designed, parking for the facility employees and physicians should be designated.

The parking area and grounds need to be maintained. Arrangements should be made with reputable and reliable companies for the care of the lawn, shrubbery, trees, and flowers, as well as leaf removal and snow removable if applicable to your area of residency. The parking lot surface should be blacktop, and periodically (once every 3 to 5 years) it should be patched and sealed to preserve the surface. A service should be employed to promptly clear snow and ice from the parking lot surface as well as periodically sweep the parking lot surface. These expenses must be budgeted into the planned expenses for the physical upkeep of the practice. Insurance coverage must also be budgeted. It is advisable that each practice owner, whether a proprietor, partner, or corporation board member, have umbrella insurance in addition to the building or condominium insurance for protection of personal assets against loss in the case of a liability claim. If such a claim is filed or there is the possibility that a claim will be filed, the issuing insurance agent and agency must be immediately notified. Complete details of the incident should be documented, and, if appropriate law enforcement records should be obtained and forwarded to the insurance carrier. When purchasing insurance coverage, the policy limitations and claim-filing restrictions must be clearly understood. A copy of the insurance policy and a summary of filing procedures should be filed in your insurance reference manual.

Waste Disposal

Disposal of trash and medical waste has become not only a moral but an environmental issue. Many medical offices are initiating recycling systems for trash disposal. Because of the volume of paper used in meeting government regulations and the number of aluminum cans and glass and plastic receptacles used, the health care industry can make a noticeable contribution to the national recycling effort. Disposable items must be collected with a frequency that corresponds to the volume of waste produced. The waste disposal dumpster must have a secure structure surrounding it in an unobstructed area. This allows your properly licensed medical waste disposal company easy access to the dumpster. The cost of waste disposal has risen in recent years because of these needs. Caution needs to be taken to not shortcut these expenses, because such a decision could incur enormous expenses should a violation of the current regulations occur.

Custodial and Housekeeping Services

As with the employment of anyone, it is imperative that references be checked for any custodial personnel or service employed. Employment may take the form of subcontracting or direct employment. Employees' insurance coverage must be verified. Notation should be made of any exclusions or waivers of liability within the insurance policy that may place you at risk. A copy of this insurance coverage should be placed in your insurance manual. As with all employees or subcontractors, you should provide a concise description of responsibilities and procedures to your custodial and housekeeping personnel. A periodic evaluation and update should be performed on an established schedule. The frequency of service should be outlined and adjusted as appropriate. The general contract of employment should contain the following items:

- The area of coverage
- The supplies needed, who is to provide them, and usage control
- The cost compared with the value of the service
- Security provisions
- Confidentiality guidelines
- Infection control procedures
- Disposal of waste guidelines
- Medical waste disposal guidelines
- Consequences of violation of guidelines and procedures

Security Violation, Incident Handling, Reporting, and Follow-up

The employee handbook, policy manual, and procedure manual should contain information regarding the consequences of policy or procedure violations. Security violation has varying degrees of severity, as dictated by the following regulating bodies or documents:

- Contract (whether implicit or explicit)
- Insurance
- Local regulations
- State regulations
- Federal regulations

All violations should be handled internally before being brought before any outside authority. Depending on the severity of the infraction, this may involve the office manager or practice administrator, the personnel manager, the Board of Directors, or a committee comprised of any or all of the practice authorities listed. The following procedure is recommended:

1. Identify the violator(s) and specific violation.
2. Assess the liability risk resulting from the violation.
3. Notify the violator of his or her violation.
4. Provide a forum for a hearing of the violation circumstances.
5. Document the violation with witness testimony.
6. Substantiate witness testimony with written documentation.
7. Review options for violation consequences, including legal action.

Should the severity of the violation require the involvement of an external authority, the following procedure should be followed:

1. Assess the level of severity of the violation:
   - Contract/agreement,
   - Tort or wrong-doing, or
   - Criminal law (local, state, or federal).

2. Determine authority for reference:
   - Attorney or
   - Prosecutor.

3. Review internal authority documentation.

4. Assess action to be taken:
   - Reprimand,
   - Dismissal,
   - Legal action.

After any type of violation, it is appropriate to review the procedure that was followed and how the situation was handled. If necessary, any procedures in place should be updated. Action options to prevent recurrence should be assessed and put into effect.

PURCHASING AND INVENTORY CONTROL

Management of materials should be under the control of one person who has the responsibility for cost comparison, inventory control, and purchase control.

Purchasing Control

One person should be responsible for all purchasing. If a large volume of items are purchased, a purchase order system should be used. The system can have alphabetical identification for departments and sequential numerical identification for further control. The least expensive item may not be the most cost-effective; therefore standards should be established regarding the expections of the quality of the item. Quantity guidelines should also be established. A high-volume purchase at a discounted price is not cost-effective if there is not a corresponding high volume of use of the item. Storage costs must be evaluated whenever a high-volume purchase is being considered.

The importance of educated vendor selection cannot be overrated. There are a variety of source options available, such as local vendors, mail-order catalog vendors, vendors who send representatives to the office on a regular basis, and telephone solicitors.

SPECIAL HINT

Excessive caution must be exercised with telephone solicitors. There are many pirate companies that present a special sale with rising prices scheduled to become effective in the near future. Usually they offer copier or office supplies. Frequently these materials are inferior or do not meet manufacturer specifications. Use of these items may violate your maintenance contract because of damage to the equipment that may occur with use. Frequently the office supply order will generate a gift to thank you for your patronage, such as a toaster oven, coffee maker, or blender. The quantity usually needed to receive a gift is a case or gross, which greatly reduces the cost-effectiveness of the purchase. Therefore, care must be exercised when special buys or discounts are considered for purchase.

The cost of the form of payment needs to be considered. Delivery charges can be included in the item price, added to the order price, or added as a COD (cash on delivery) charge, or a discount of delivery charges may be allowed if payment is made within a specific period of time. Such terms warrant evaluation in the assessment of the total cost of the purchase. If the cash flow position of the business allows for high-volume purchase only after the first of the month, care must be taken that payment is due at this time so advantage can be taken of the payment discount offer.

In choosing a vendor, consideration must be given to the availability of the product in the case of urgent need for the item. Delivery of ordered supplies requires evaluation of scheduling, timeliness, and cost:

Scheduling. Do the deliveries arrive at a convenient time for the office personnel?

Timeliness. Is the vendor able to guarantee delivery as scheduled, as well as in the case of urgent need?

Cost. Are the freight/delivery charges in addition to the item price, or does the vendor absorb these costs? An attractive item price can be enormously inflated if the guaranteed next-day delivery cost is at your expense.

Discount. Are discounts allowed for early payment, volume purchases, or preferred customer rating?

Storage and Inventory

The availability of storage space is an ever constant issue in the medical practice, whether for patient files that are considered inactive, for medical supplies that do or do not require refrigeration, for office supplies, or for medical books and journals. Identification of space allotments for these supplies and materials is beneficial when planning purchases. Careful organization is imperative for good inventory control.

INVENTORY DIRECTORY

Item	Supplier	Purchase Date	Volume	Cost	Cost per Unit	Reorder Date

SPECIAL HINT

When selecting storage areas, consider the security of the area, climate control, sprinkler protection against fire damage, and, correspondingly, protection against water damage. Helpful tips may be provided by your local fire department, such as elevation of the supplies off the floor and plastic covering of the top surface.

Inventory Control

Precise inventory control is of prime importance. Maximization of physical space allowances and purchasing power, determination of the rate of use, and the avoidance of supply shortage are the basic reasons for inventory control. The person responsible for purchasing should maintain a purchasing directory detailing the item, supplier, date of purchase, volume purchased, and total and per-unit cost, such as the example given below. Rate of use may also be recorded on this document. This provides a definite basis for expense projections. A calendar notation can be made for reordering based on this information.

Cases of copier paper, envelopes, or stationery may have an inventory record placed on the outside of the case (Figure 4–2). An additional inventory record may be on index cards showing

SAMPLE 1

Item	Volume Purchased	Purchase Date	Available Volume	Date Used	Date Reordered

SAMPLE 2

Item	Supplier		Purchase Date
Volume Available		Date Removed from Inventory	
12			
11			
10			
9			
8			
7			
6			
5			
4			
3			
2 ***Reorder			
1			

FIGURE 4–2

Inventory control.

the item name, purchase date, volume purchased, remaining inventory, and use dates. Naturally, anyone authorized to replenish supplies, and thereby reduce inventory, must be held responsible for completing the inventory control form. This cooperation is essential to maintain an effective inventory system.

Review of the inventory should be scheduled at regular intervals. The inventory records should be used to verify the review. Proper accounting methods recommend that the individual authorized to place the orders not be the individual responsible for verification of receipt of the goods or payment of the bills. In smaller practices this is not always practical; however, some type of system should be implemented to ensure against improper use of purchasing authority. The inventory directory should be used to analyze inventory needs on a regular basis. This enables the purchaser to best assess the volume used as well as identify any changes in the pattern of use.

OFFICE EQUIPMENT AND MAINTENANCE

Telephone Systems and Services

The divestiture of the AT&T telephone system has provided the opportunity to choose the long-distance service that best fits the practice's needs. Many factors, from expectations of use to expansion capabilities, must be considered when making this decision. The local telephone carrier provides intrastate service, while the long-distance carrier provides interstate service. The physical service to the system, which includes line and outlet installation, is usually provided by a third company that must coordinate their work with your selected carriers. Failure to notify each carrier of the activities of the others causes a delay in service as well as increased expense. The following listing is offered to provide direction in selecting a telephone system.

	Available	Cost
Line capacity		
Number available		
Expansion capacity		
Fax line		
Computer provisions		
Intercom system		
Internal		
Overhead		
Hands-free response/speakerphone		
Number of sets needed		
Wall mount		
Desk set		
Features		
Redial		
Three-way/conference calling		
Privacy calling		
Silent ring		
Self-programmed speed dialing		
Battery backup		
Maintenance agreement		
Insurance requirements		
Answering service/machine		

Photocopy Machines and Services

When selecting a copier, as when selecting a telephone system, you must determine the needs the copier is expected to fill. The following table may provide direction in making this selection.

	Available	Cost
Usage estimate		
Zoom lens for reduction and enlargement		
Collating 10–20–40 bins		
Stapling		
Automatic feed		
Multiple colors		
Individual		
Simultaneous		
Computer form feed		
Book/magazine copying (dual side)		
Paper size variation		
Identification of jam location		
Noise reduction		
Two-sided copying		
First copy speed		
Copy speed		
Warm-up time		
Size/weight of machine		
Stationary top versus moving top		
Paper cassette/drawer capacity		
Image shift/editing		
Key counter		
Supplies needed		
Paper		
Toner		
Wire		
Developer		

The copier requires routine maintenance. For this reason, it is advisable to negotiate a maintenance contract. Special note should be made of the parts not covered; if a separate contract or rider is available to cover these, there may be value in obtaining such coverage. The depreciation advantage of the purchase and the capacity of the copier to provide for the practice needs as it grows should be considered. As with every maintenance contract, frequency of service, provisions for emergency needs such as replacement equipment, additional costs related to service calls, and provisions for renewal need to be evaluated.

Facsimile (Fax) Machines and Services

Purchase of a fax machine directly involves the telephone company because the transmissions are made over telephone lines. The telephone line requires fax capabilities, tone control, and singular dedication without line rollover capabilities.

```
                                    Available   Cost
Paper
    Automatic roll
    Individual sheets
    Thermal paper
    Minimum/maximum length capacity
Features
    Redial
    Automatic time/date stamp
    Daily listing with numbers dialed and time
    Speed dial
    Phone hookup
    Resolution adjustment
    Coping capacity
    Memory capacity
    Interrupted transmission capacity
    Multistation transmission
    Storage of transmission during paper interruption
    Delayed transmissions
    Confidential communication
    Capacity for interfacing with other fax machines
    Error correction
    Copy contrast control
    Individual transmission journal
```

The maintenance contract for the fax machine has the same evaluation points as those for other equipment:

- Frequency of service
- Emergency coverage with equipment loan provisions
- Estimated cost of parts that are not covered and whether a rider or separate contract is available
- Upgrading provisions
- Depreciation value (life expectancy)

Computers

Computers are discussed thoroughly in Chapter 9. Basic physical requirements include space, climate control, ventilation, electrical requirements and static control. When assessing the need for a computer, do not overlook the system's capacity for growth.

SALES REPRESENTATIVES

The medical practice is contacted by a variety of sales representatives who require communication with persons responsible for separate duties within the office. For smooth office operation, scheduling of these representatives is recommended. The mechanics of the scheduling are determined by individual preference. Some offices prefer to have the receptionist responsible or have specific time parameters set within which representatives can schedule themselves. Scheduling limitations may be established. For example, no more than one representative may be seen per day, or the frequency of appointments per individual may be limited to one visit every 6 to 8 weeks. The appointments may be scheduled before, during, or after patient hours or during lunch, since many representatives choose to provide the meal and use the time to discuss their product with the physician(s) without interruption of patient care.

Sample Handling

The physician samples provided by the pharmaceutical representatives need to be handled in the same manner as other controlled substances. The organization can be by trade name alphabetically or by clinical purpose. A log should be kept of all medications and corresponding distribution. This log serves the dual purpose of controlling inventory and revealing a pattern of use. It provides the clinical coordinator with a referral point for reordering purposes. Frequently representatives bring in samples when there is no scheduled appointment in response to a telephone call or letter.

Recourse from Suppliers

It is appropriate to seek recourse from a supplier when

- The supplier fails to live up to a contract,

- The supplier fails to provide the service,
- The product is unreliable,
- The supplier repeatedly fails to keep scheduled appointments,
- The supplier fails to make deliveries on a timely basis, or
- The supplier fails to keep current on market regulations.

Because of the competitive nature of sales, close attention needs to be paid to the ethics of the sales representative as well as the firm represented. False representation of product capabilities may be avoided by demanding a complete demonstration before purchasing the equipment. A listing of references should be provided and customer satisfaction confirmed. Any business that does not adhere to proper corporate ethics should be reported to the appropriate authorities and the Better Business Bureau. Although the Bureau does not take legal action, a written record is maintained.

Bibliography

Alert II Pictorial Brochure. Ademco, A Division of Pittway Corp., 1984.

Legend-100 Specifications Brochure. Fire Burglary Instruments, Inc., An FBX Company, 100 Engineers Rd., Hauppague, NY 11788.

Minolta EP 4300 Zoom Copier, EP 4301 Zoom Copier, EP 4230 Copier, EP 3120 Zoom Copier, EP 2100 Copier, EP 8600 Copier, 5400 Series Pictorial Specification Brochures. Minolta Corporation, Business Equipment Division, 101 Williams Drive, Ramsey, NJ 07446, 1988.

Panafax UF-170, UF-160, UF-260 Pictorial Specification Brochures. Panasonic Communications & Systems Company, Division of Matsushita Electric Corporation of America, Two Panasonic Way, Secaucus, NJ 07094.

Star XL4800EZ, Star XL4600 Residential Pictorial Specification Brochure. Fire Burglary Instruments, Inc., An FBX Company, 100 Engineers Rd., Hauppague, NY 11788.

Chapter 5

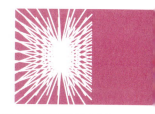

QUALITY ASSURANCE

LOIS E. WOLFGANG

QUALITY ASSURANCE
Purpose of Quality Assurance
Quality Assurance Process

QUALITY OF CARE
Qualifications of Allied Health Personnel
Continuing Education
Job Performance

MEDICAL RECORDS
RISK MANAGEMENT
Incident Report and Follow-up

QUALITY CONTROL
Safety Management
Laboratory and Radiology
Infection Control

QUALITY ASSURANCE

Quality patient care is the goal of the medical practice, whether it be in the physician's office, a clinic, or a hospital. In order to improve and provide quality patient care, a system of monitoring the health care environment, the health care practitioners, and the results of the care provided must be developed, used, and reviewed on a regular basis.

All medical offices should have a plan for the monitoring and evaluation of the quality of care delivered by their practice. Quality assurance and risk management programs are as important for small medical offices as they are for large clinics and hospitals. Hospitals have a long history of recognized standards of care for quality assurance and accreditation. The mandating of the Professional Standards Review Organization (PSRO) to review necessity, quality, and appropriateness of federally funded hospital care initiated formal quality assurance programs. Ambulatory care facilities are relatively new to this process. The first ambulatory care manual was published by the Joint Commission on Accreditation of Health Care Organizations in 1975. The edition of the *Ambulatory Health Care Standards Manual* referred to in this chapter is the 1990 edition.

Accreditation by the Joint Commission of Health Care Organizations for ambulatory care is voluntary but serves as a positive tool in evaluating, improving, and maintaining quality patient care. Accreditation forces the practice into self-assessment methods for continuing quality patient care.

With the exception of physicians in solo practice, any health care organization may apply for accreditation. The accreditation program is intended for:

- Ambulatory care clinics
- Ambulatory surgery centers
- Group practices
- Community health centers
- Cardiac catheterization centers
- Primary care centers
- Urgent/emergency care centers
- College or university health programs
- Armed services programs
- National American Health Service Centers[1]

The Joint Commission determines whether the standards can be applied appropriately to a given applicant. If the organization does not meet the requirements for accreditation, some type of quality assurance/risk management program can be developed to provide and assure quality patient care.

With the increased use of ambulatory health care, there is an increase in the acuity level of the patients and even a greater need for quality assurance and risk management programs.

Purpose of Quality Assurance

The purpose of a quality assurance program is to ensure that practices and organizations deliver health care services that demonstrate a high level of quality care and that the services are provided in a manner consistent with the principles of professional practice and reflect concern for the consumer.

It is important to understand the following terms before beginning the process of developing a quality assurance program.

Quality: A degree of excellence or superiority in kind. The Joint Commission defines quality as "the degree of adherence to generally recognized contemporary standards of good practice and anticipated outcomes for a particular service, procedure, diagnosis or clinical problem."[2]

Quality assurance: Primarily a professional function designed to identify and resolve problems in patient care and to identify and take advantage of opportunities for improvement in care. A quality assurance program includes ongoing monitoring, evaluation, and improvement in care.[2]

Quality patient care: According to the Joint Commission, "The degree to which patient care services increase the probability of desired patient outcomes and reduce the probability of undesired outcomes, given a current state of knowledge."[1]

Risk management: Primarily, efforts to prevent physical and emotional injury to the patients, staff, and visitors; also to protect the financial assets of the organization by preventing those events that are most likely to lead to liability, reducing liabilities when untoward events do occur, and assuring adequate financial protection against potential liability through appropriate insurance coverage. According to the Joint Commission, "Poor quality creates a risk and is likely to lead to a liability."[2]

Utilization review: Ensuring appropriate allocation of the organization's resources by striving to provide high-quality patient care in the most effective and efficient manner. Cost and effectiveness, staffing, and distribution of goods and services are mechanisms used to achieve quality.[2]

Quality control: An aggregate of activities designed to ensure adequate quality.

The viewpoints of quality care may vary slightly, depending on whether the health care consumer, the practitioner, or the purchaser of health care is prioritizing the important elements of care. Quality may mean different things to each of these groups; for example:

Consumer: Responsiveness to perceived care needs; level of communication, concern, and courtesy; degree of symptom relief; and level of functional improvement.

Practitioner: Degree to which care meets the current technical state of the art and freedom to act in the full interest of the patient.

Purchaser: Efficient use of funds available for health care, appropriate use of health care resources, and the maximum contribution of health care possible toward reducing lost productivity.[2]

Quality Assurance Process

The monitoring and evaluation process is designed to help health care organizations focus on high-priority, quality-of-care issues and thus effectively use their quality assurance resources. This process involves:

- Identification of the most important aspects of care provided by the practice,
- Development of indicators for the systematic, ongoing monitoring of aspects of care,
- Evaluation of care to identify problems or opportunities for improvement in the quality and appropriateness of care, and
- Development of corrective action to improve the care or solve problems and evaluation of the effectiveness of those actions.[2]

The collection and aggregation of data about a series of events or activities allow trends or patterns of care to be identified. Patterns or single events help to efficiently identify situations in which case review is most likely to identify opportunities to improve care or correct deficiencies in care. The monitoring and evaluation process cannot identify every case of substandard care, but it does help the practice to identify situations on which its attention could be most effectively focused.[2]

The monitoring and evaluation process involves the following 10 steps:

1. Assign responsibility for monitoring and evaluation activities.
2. Delineate the scope of care provided by the practice.

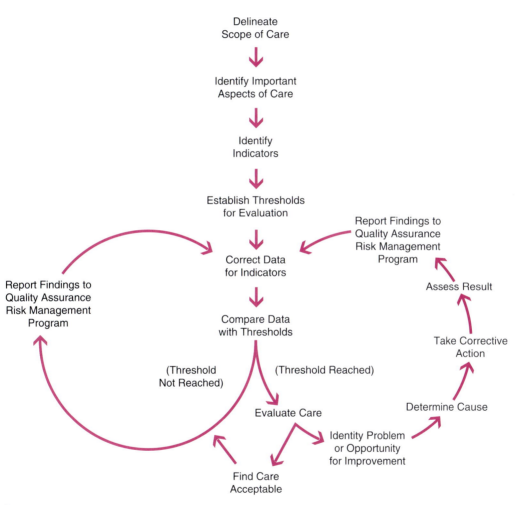

FIGURE 5-1

The monitoring and evaluation process as it functions from Step 2 to Step 10. Appropriate staff members delineate scope of care, identify important aspects of care, identify indicators, and establish thresholds for evaluation to facilitate monitoring and evaluation of care provided in a particular department. Data pertaining to the indicators are collected, and the cumulative data are compared with the thresholds for evaluation. If the threshold is not reached, no further evaluation as part of monitoring and evaluation is performed, and the findings are included in the information reported to the organization-wide quality assurance program. When the threshold is reached, the important aspect of care is evaluated to determine whether a problem or opportunity for improvement is present. If a problem or opportunity for improvement is identified, the cause is determined and corrective action is taken. After a sufficient period of time, the effectiveness of the actions is assessed, and findings are reported to the organization-wide quality assurance program. Monitoring and evaluation are continued to identify any future deficiencies in care. (Copyright 1988 by the Joint Commission on Accreditation of Health Care Organizations, Chicago. Redrawn by permission.)

3. Identify the most important aspects of care provided by the practice.
4. Identify indicators for monitoring the important aspects of care.
5. Establish thresholds at which the indicators trigger evaluation of care.
6. Monitor the important aspects of care by collecting and organizing data for each indicator.
7. Evaluate care when thresholds are reached to identify problems or opportunities to improve the care.
8. Take actions to improve care or correct identified problems.
9. Assess the effectiveness of the actions and document the improvement in care.
10. Communicate the results of the monitoring and evaluation process to relevant individuals or services and to the practice-wide quality assurance program[2] (Figures 5–1 and 5–2).

An effective quality assurance program is implemented throughout an organization and is designed to objectively and systematically monitor and evaluate the quality and appropriateness of patient care, pursue opportunities to improve patient care and clinical performance, and resolve identified problems in care and in performance.[3]

Monitoring and evaluation activities are ongoing, to ensure that improvements in care and performance are sustained and integrated. In addition to being ongoing, monitoring and evaluation activities are:

- Planned, systematic, and comprehensive;
- Use indicators and related thresholds for evaluation that are agreed on by the staff and accepted by the organization; and
- Accomplished by the routine collection of data related to the indicators and periodic comparisons of the level of performance with thresholds for evaluation.[3]

Aspect of care	Accidents/injuries
Indicator	The number of accidents/injuries attributed to environmental factors shall not exceed 1% of the total number of patient visits per month.
Threshold	100%
Data	Source and method of collection: All accident report forms will be monitored on a monthly basis for cause, result, and trends.

FIGURE 5–2

An example of how to establish the guidelines for monitoring and measuring specific aspects of quality of patient care.

QUALITY OF CARE

Qualifications of Allied Health Personnel

The qualifications, licensure, and certification of all office staff should be specified in the office policy and procedure manual. Personal qualifications, licensure, and certification credentials should be maintained in an individual personnel file. Both the policy and personnel file validate the scope of practice for the individual practitioner. The scope of practice determines the quality of patient care provided by the ambulatory care setting. The chart on the facing page indicates educational and licensure requirements for various health care personnel.

Continuing Education

Continuing education is a major part of professional development in the medical office because research provides medical professionals with new knowledge on a daily basis. Each professional's participation in continuing education should be documented and recognized in annual job performance evaluation.

Continuing education activities should relate to the type and nature of medical care provided by the practice as well as the specific individual responsibilities within the practice. In large practices the continuing education may be offered on site; in addition, programs are provided by health care providers in the local community, at state and national conventions of professional organizations, and in professional journals.

Several states require continuing education for renewal of licenses, and some professional organizations require continuing education for recertification. The length of time varies with each state and professional organization. Responsibility for maintaining licensure and certification lies with the practitioner. Requirements are available to medical practices, and each practice should

Title	Education	Certificate/Licensure
MD	Medical school—residency Residency—specialty	License
PA	Bachelor's degree	PA-C certification and National Registration State-level registration
RN	Diploma 3 years-hospital based Associate degree Bachelor's degree	License by examination
LPN	9 months–1 year post high school	License by examination
MA	9 months–2 years (associate degree) post high school	Certification encouraged but not required
Radiology technician	Associate degree Bachelor's degree	License by examination (ARRT*) License by examination (ARRT)
Medical technologist (MT)	Bachelor of science degree	Registration by examination (ASCP†)
Medical laboratory technician (MLT)	1–2 years post high school	Registration by examination

* ARRT, American Registry of Radiologic Technologists.
† ASCP, American Society of Clinical Pathologists.

maintain a file of requirements for the types of practitioners employed.

Continuing education activities of practitioners improves the quality of care by keeping the practice and practitioners up to date on disease processes and new treatments available.

Job Performance

Evaluation of practitioners assists in promotion of quality patient care. The quality of patient care is affected by the performance of the practitioner, not just his or her credentials. Job performance evaluation should include knowledge base, communication skills, technical skills, and documentation in the medical record.

The provision of high-quality health care services can be demonstrated by having:

- Available and accessible health services;
- A description of the intake system for patients during and after normal hours of operation;
- Provisions for and information about emergency and after-hours care;
- A mechanism for informing patients of the names, specialties, and titles of the professionals providing and/or responsible for their care;
- Appropriate diagnostic procedures;
- Treatment consistent with clinical impression or working diagnosis;
- Availability and appropriate use of consultative services;
- Patient education;
- Timely and adequate transfer of appropriate patient care documents when patients are transferred to or from other health care providers;
- Reasonable follow-up regarding patient compliance with a plan of care;
- Timely identification and notification of patients who require additional follow-up, including laboratory and radiology studies;
- Available resources for medical emergencies that may arise in connection with the services provided to patients;
- Concern for cost of care by:
  - Making sure health care services are relevant to the needs of patients;
  - Not duplicating diagnostic procedures;
  - Ensuring that treatment frequency is appropriate;
  - Using the least expensive resources when available; and
  - Using ancillary services.[1]

Patients are to be treated in a manner that recognizes their basic human rights—with respect, consideration, and dignity.

The following information is vital for quality patient care and patient compliance with treatment and should be readily available to staff and patients:

- Policy on patient rights and responsibilities;
- The services available at the organization;
- Provisions for after-hours and emergency coverage;
- Conduct and responsibilities of patient, including the consequences of refusing treatment or therapy;
- Policy on treatment of an unemancipated minor not accompanied by an adult;
- Patients' right to refuse to participate in experimental research;

- Fees for service;
- Policies concerning payment of fees;
- Resources for grievance to the organization's staff and governing body for recommending changes in policies and services; and
- Mechanism for resolving complaints by patients and families, including a response or correction action.[1]

Information should be provided to all patients concerning their diagnoses and treatment as well as the opportunity to participate in discussions involving their health care. Confidentiality of records and release of information also contribute to the quality of care. Patient confidence in the organization increases the quality and decreases the risks of the organization.

MEDICAL RECORDS

A medical record system permitting prompt retrieval of information must be maintained. Medical records must be legible, documented accurately in a timely manner, and readily accessible to health care practitioners. The ambulatory care facility must do the following:

- Maintain a system for the collection, processing, maintenance, storage, retrieval, and distribution of medical records.
- Provide prompt availability of all clinical information relevant to patients.
- Treat all patient information in a strictly confidential manner and protect from loss, tampering, alteration, destruction, and unauthorized or inadvertent disclosure of information.
- Designate an individual to be in charge of medical records whose responsibilities include:
  - Maintaining of confidentiality, security, and physical safety of records;
  - Maintaining the identification of each patient's record;
  - Maintaining a predetermined, organized medical record format;
  - Supervising the collection, processing, maintenance, storage, timely retrieval, and distribution of medical records.
- Develop written policies concerning medical records, including:
  - Confidentiality;
  - Provision against loss, tampering, alteration, or destruction;
  - Retention of active records;
  - Retirement of inactive records;
  - Legible, appropriate, accurate, and timely entry of data into the medical record;
  - Release of information; and
  - Consents for treatment.
- Provide a summary list of significant past medical diagnoses, procedures, or problems in each record to facilitate ongoing effective medical care, including:
  - Surgical procedures,
  - Medical conditions,
  - Allergies, and
  - Current medications.
- Document the following information during each visit:
  - Date;
  - Department;
  - Practitioner's name and profession (for example, MD, RN, PA, or MA);
  - Chief complaint;
  - Objective findings;
  - Diagnosis/medical impression;
  - Diagnostic studies ordered;
  - Therapies administered;
  - Disposition, recommendations, and instructions to patient; and
  - Signature of practitioner.
- Secure clinical summaries of patient treatment in hospitals, ambulatory surgical facilities, nursing homes, consultant's offices, etc. for promotion of continuity of care.[1]

INCIDENT REPORT FORM

Patient: _____   Name: _____

Visitor: _____   Address: _____

Staff: _____   _____

Telephone: _____

Age _____ Sex _____ Location of Incident _____

Describe the Incident: _____

_____

_____

_____

Signature of Person Writing Report:

_____

Follow-up: _____

_____

_____

Signature of Person Writing Report:

_____

Result:			
	Injury:	Yes _____	No _____
	Treated by Physician:	Yes _____	No _____
	Taken to Hospital:	Yes _____	No _____
	Follow-up MedCare:	Yes _____	No _____
	Insurance Covered:	Yes _____	No _____
	Worker's Compensation:	Yes _____	No _____

DO NOT PLACE IN PATIENT'S RECORD OR REPRODUCE BY XEROX

FIGURE 5-3

Monitoring of accidents/incidents in the medical office is a valuable tool used to measure risk management and safety issues in the office setting. As specific policy, procedures and format will ensure data collection and corrective actions are taken to improve quality of patient care.

RISK MANAGEMENT

As defined in the beginning of the chapter, risk management is the prevention of physical and emotional injury to patients, visitors, and staff. To prevent physical and/or emotional injury, the practice must identify potential new risks and monitor all incidents to help reduce current risks.

Frequent risk management issues include the following:

Administration

- Appointment delays
- Lack of follow-up appointment system and recall
- Lack of telephone time spent with patient
- Lack of telephone time spent with family
- Lack of sensitivity to patient concerns (for example, waiting time)
- Lack of continuity of care providers
- Unsafe facilities
- Failure to obtain consultations
- Large volumes of patients treated, resulting in lack of time with patient and family.

Clinical

- Improper injection sites
- Minor surgical errors
- Specimen collection/labeling errors
- Drug abuse detection in patients
- Improper prediagnostic test instructions
- Use of improper infection control techniques

Monitoring of the risk management issues in the office is an important tool to improving quality patient care. The areas with marked incidences should be evaluated and corrective action taken to eliminate or decrease these risks. One method of monitoring is the use of an incident report form.

Incident Report and Follow-up

An incident report form is used to document any occurrence that is not consistent with routine office practice or patient care. It is a method of reducing risk factors and improving patient care, and is not meant to be a negative report kept on employees (Figure 5–3). Incident reports are completed on visitors, patients, and/or staff when occurrences are known by any staff members of the practice. Incidents also include accidents and environmental conditions that could result in illness or injury.

Developing an appropriate reporting form is important in establishing a procedure for managing patient, visitor, and/or staff occurrences as well as collecting and documenting information on occurrences to be used in quality assurance risk management as a part of ongoing efforts to improve patient care and safety in the office. All incident report forms are to be maintained in a separate file from other records. They are not a part of the patient or employee records.

QUALITY CONTROL

Quality control involves three major areas of the ambulatory care setting: safety management, laboratory and radiology services, and infection control.

Safety Management

The ambulatory safety care setting should provide a safe environment for patients, visitors, and personnel. The safety plan should include:

- Reporting of accidents, injuries, and safety hazards
- Provision of safety-related information to all employees
- Designation of one person to be responsible for management of the program
- Policies and procedures addressing the distribution of, storage of, and access to abusable supplies, such as drugs, needles, and prescription pads
- Emergency plans for times of disaster
- Fire safety systems and plans as well as an emergency plan
- A plan for safe management of hazardous materials
- An organization-wide smoking policy
- A plan for ensuring that patient care equipment performs properly and safely and that individuals are trained to operate the patient equipment

- Systems for electrical distribution (heating, air conditioning, medical gases, etc.) that are designed, stabled, operated, and maintained to provide safe and adequate service
- Safety devices and operational procedures for the safety of patients and personnel, including restrooms, bathing areas, storage areas, floor coverings, examination rooms, etc.
- Security measures for patients, personnel, and the public that are consistent with the conditions and risks inherent in the location of the facility[1]

Laboratory and Radiology

Medical laboratory and radiology services are to be designed to meet the needs of patients in accordance with professional practices and legal requirements. The medical laboratory and radiology plan should include:

- Medical laboratory and radiology service that is conducted in a timely manner and appropriate to the needs of patients
- Performance and documentation of quality control, including calibration of equipment and validation of test results through control specimens
- Timely insertion of documentation of laboratory and radiology results in patients' records
- Competent personnel available to complete the tests
- Policies and procedures for all laboratory tests performed and for the safety and quality of radiology
- Space, equipment, and supplies sufficient for performing the volume of work with optimal accuracy, precision, efficiency, and safety.[1]

Infection Control

Infection control includes measures to prevent, identify, and control infections acquired in the ambulatory care setting or brought into the ambulatory care setting from the community. All areas and aspects of the practice setting are affected by infection control.

Infection control includes the establishment of oral and written procedures relating to the control of infectious disease hazards which may affect employees, visitors, and patients.

The basic elements of an infection control program are:

- Definitions of ambulatory setting infections, for surveillance purposes; to provide for early, uniform identification and reporting of infections; and to determine pertinent infection rates
- A practical system for reporting, evaluating, and maintaining records of infections among patients and personnel (includes ongoing data collections, review, and follow-up)
- Ongoing review and evaluation of all aseptic, isolation, and sanitation techniques employed in the practice
- Written policies on isolation of specific patients as they make an office visit (quality of care should not be interrupted)
- Orientation of all new employees regarding the importance of infection control and personal hygiene, as well as their responsibility in the control of infection, and instruction of all employees on the Centers for Disease Control Universal Precautions, protective equipment, and specific work plan practices
- Written policies and procedures regarding collection of specimens, performance of laboratory tests, and disposal of infectious material.[2]

Injury and illness records should be carefully inspected and analyzed and corrective action implemented. All levels of personnel (from housekeeper to physician) should follow procedures for infection control in providing quality patient care (including the completion of incident report forms as a tool for monitoring and correcting the incidence of infection).

For example, gloves should be worn by:

- All health care workers who have cuts, abrasions, chapped hands, dermatitis, etc;[1]
- All health care workers involved in the procedure of instrumental examination of the otopharynx, gastrointestinal tract, and genitourinary tract;
- All health care workers involved in examination of abraded or nonintact skin and active bleeding;
- All health care workers involved in cleaning of body fluids and decontaminating procedures;
- All health care workers involved in any invasive procedure.[4]

Assessment of the infection control plan in the ambulatory care setting should include review of infections by type and incidence and the follow-up of each case.

References

1. *Ambulatory Health Care Standards Manual*. Chicago: Joint Commission on Accreditation of Health Care Organizations, 1990.
2. *Guide to Quality Assurance*. Chicago: Joint Commission on Accreditation of Health Care Organizations, 1988.
3. *Sample Indicators for Evaluating Quality Ambulatory Care*. Chicago: Joint Commission on Accreditation of Health Care Organizations, 1987.
4. *Centers for Disease Control, Guidelines for Prevention and Transmission of HIV and Hepatitis B Virus to Health Care Workers*. US Department of Health and Human Services, 1989.

Bibliography

Accreditation Manual for Hospitals. Chicago: Joint Commission on Accreditation of Health Care Organizations, 1990.

Accreditation Manual for Hospitals. Chicago: Joint Commission on Accreditation of Health Care Organizations, 1991.

Ambulatory Health Care Standards Manual. Chicago: Joint Commission on Accreditation of Health Care Organizations, 1990.

Guide to Quality Assurance. Chicago: Joint Commission on Accreditation of Health Care Organizations, 1988.

Primer on Indicators: Development and Application. Chicago: Joint Commission on Accreditation of Health Care Organizations, 1990.

Quality Review Bulletin. Chicago: Joint Commission on Accreditation of Health Care Organizations.

Simple Indicators for Evaluating Quality Ambulatory Care. Chicago: Joint Commission on Accreditation of Health Care Organizations, 1987.

Chapter 6

BOOKKEEPING, CREDIT, AND COLLECTIONS

VICKI S. SANDERS

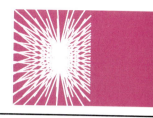

BOOKKEEPING SYSTEMS
Starting a System
Bookkeeping Methods
Double-Entry Accounting
Bookkeeping Systems
Maintaining an Accounts Receivable Bookkeeping System
Posting Special Accounting Entries
Completing an Accounts Receivable Trial Balance
Maintaining an Accounts Payable Bookkeeping System
Completing a Disbursements Journal Trial Balance
Completing a Year-to-Date Cash Disbursements Summary
Maintaining Petty Cash Records

BANKING
Opening a Checking Account
Selecting Checks
Writing Checks
Accepting Checks for Payment
Endorsing Checks
Making Bank Deposits
Reconciling a Bank Statement

CREDIT AND COLLECTIONS
Establishing a Credit and Collection System
Billing Patients
Collecting Past Due Accounts
Collection Ratio
Preparing an Accounts Receivable Aging Record
Preparing a Monthly Accounts Receivable Analysis

BOOKKEEPING

Starting a System

A physician's office must maintain a financial record system that keeps track of the income and expenditures of the practice. The income consists of the fees paid by patients for services rendered by the physician. The expenditures are the costs incurred from operating the practice. A typical bookkeeping system consists of at least four basic elements:

- A daily record that shows charges and payments
- An account for each patient (or family unit) showing individual charges, payments, and balance owed
- A record of disbursements, including payroll
- A petty cash record for small expenditures

The system must also be capable of providing information to the federal government for income tax purposes as well as information from which the financial status of the practice can be determined. Other factors to be considered are

- What will be the initial cost of the system, and what will be the ongoing cost of maintaining the system?
- Does the system have an effective audit trail?
- Does the system facilitate the handling of insurance claims?

- Will the system permit conversion to a computerized program?
- Does the system provide proof of posting and year-to-date accounts receivable totals?
- How time consuming is the system to use and maintain?

A variety of bookkeeping systems are available from which to choose. Select a system that fits the needs of the practice and has the capability of expanding. A professional management consultant or accountant can offer guidance in selecting an appropriate system for the practice.

A new medical practice may begin with a manual system and then later convert to a computerized bookkeeping program; however, if cost-effective, it may be desirable to computerize the office from the beginning. Refer to Chapter 9 for the use of computers in business applications.

Bookkeeping Methods

Two methods of bookkeeping in the medical practice include accounts receivable and accounts payable bookkeeping. Accounts receivable bookkeeping involves the recording of charges for services rendered, payments received, and the collection of what is owed. The term *accounts receivable* refers to the amounts owed by patients.

Accounts Receivable

The financial records of accounts receivable bookkeeping generate information on the daily charges and payments received, an individual record for each patient or family unit, and data for reports that reflect the financial status of the practice.

The recordkeeping forms in a typical accounts receivable bookkeeping system consist of the following:

Daily journal: Also called a *general journal* or *day sheet*, this is a record of the total fees charged and payments received per day.

Charge slip (numbered sequentially): Also called a *transaction slip*, this is a form of routing ticket on which procedures and fees are recorded as the service is performed. Numbering each charge slip sequentially provides an audit trail in the event a charge slip is lost or not posted on the daily journal.

Ledger card: Also called a *patient account* or *accounts receivable ledger*, this consists of an individual record by patient name (or family unit) that shows the current balance owed. The accounts receivable ledger is also used for billing and collection purposes.

Patient receipt (in duplicate): A receipt written for a patient who pays cash, a copy of which is retained as an office record. To minimize paperwork, some bookkeeping systems combine the patient receipt with the charge slip in one form.

Additional materials and equipment needed to maintain the system include a file tray for the ledger cards and a binder for the daily journal sheets. The bookkeeping records may be stored in various ways, depending on the facilities available and the particular needs of the practice.

Accounts Payable

Accounts payable are amounts owed by the medical practice to individuals or suppliers. Accounts payable bookkeeping involves accounting for expenses incurred from operating the medical practice, similar to the expenses of operating any business. For example, because the medical practice requires one or more employees, the accounts payable system must incorporate payroll records. Payroll disbursements require additional recordkeeping functions in order to document the earnings and payroll deductions of each employee, as well as provide a summary of income and deductions for all employees.

To satisfy the basic requirements of maintaining an accurate accounts payable system, the recordkeeping forms must consist of

Disbursement journal (check register): Records the expenses paid out, including payroll.

Payroll records: Reflects earnings and deductions for each employee and provides a summary of the total earnings and deductions of all employees.

Petty cash record: Provides a system of keeping a small cash fund for paying out minor expenses.

Additional materials needed to maintain the system include a binder or file folder for payroll records and a locked cash box for petty cash or envelope for storing in the office safe.

Double-Entry Accounting

Even though the typical medical office bookkeeping system is capable of documenting the daily transactions of the practice, additional summaries that document the financial status of the practice must be prepared. These summaries are elements of the formal accounting process and therefore are customarily prepared by an accountant rather than the medical assistant. However, the medical assistant may be asked to submit financial data on which the accountant's financial statements will be based. It is therefore beneficial for the medical assistant to understand his or her role in the accounting process.

The operation of the physician's practice, from a financial viewpoint, is classified by the terms *assets, liabilities,* and *owner's equity.* Assets are anything of monetary value, liabilities are what is owed by the practice, and owner's equity is the value of the practice after liabilities have been deducted from the assets. This relationship can be expressed by the standard accounting equation:

$$\text{ASSETS} = \text{LIABILITIES} + \text{OWNER'S EQUITY}$$

Using the accounting equation, the medical assistant can prepare reports summarizing the operations of the practice. One such report is called a *balance sheet*; this indicates the status of the practice at a particular time. Another necessary report is the *income statement,* which summaries those activities involving revenues and expenses for a particular time period, usually a month.

Although medical assistants are not expected to handle the entire accounting process, they are the primary link in the accounting cycle and should have a clear understanding of their role in the accounting process. See Chapter 7 for additional guidance in carrying out accounting processes.

Bookkeeping Systems

Two of the most commonly used bookkeeping systems in medical offices are single-entry and pegboard bookkeeping. Which system a practice chooses depends largely on the size, special accounting needs, and personal preferences of the practice.

Single-Entry System

Single-entry bookkeeping, sometimes called the *daily log,* is a simple system of recording the transactions of a business. The basic recordkeeping forms in a single-entry bookkeeping system are as follows:

Accounts Receivable Records	Accounts Payable Records
Daily journal	Disbursements journal
Patient ledger cards	Payroll records
Receipts	Petty cash journal
	Petty cash vouchers

Physicians who have a low-volume patient load are more likely to use single-entry bookkeeping than a large medical clinic. The system is inexpensive to purchase and works well in a small practice. However, the system requires that each entry be posted separately on each recordkeeping form. This is time consuming and increases the possibility of errors. Single-entry bookkeeping does not provide a daily proof of posting or clear audit trail, which further increases the possibility of errors being made (Figure 6–1).

Pegboard System

Pegboard bookkeeping, also called the *one-write system,* includes all the forms listed in the box below. Some systems combine the transaction slip and receipt in one form (Figure 6–2). Blank receipts may also be purchased and used to post payments when no other transaction occurs.

Pegboard bookkeeping also requires the use of an aluminum or Masonite pegboard constructed with pegs used for positioning and holding the recordkeeping forms. A binder for the day sheets and a file tray for the ledgers are among the additional equipment needed to maintain the pegboard system.

When posting charges and payments with pegboard, a day sheet and bank of transaction slips are mounted over the pegs of the pegboard. The

Accounts Receivable Records	Accounts Payable Records
Day sheet (daily journal)	Disbursements/payroll journal with one-write check-writing capacity
Patient ledger cards (accounts receivable ledger)	Petty cash journal
Transaction slips*	Petty cash vouchers
Receipts	

* May be combined with receipt in a single form

DATE: _____ DAILY JOURNAL

NAME	DESCRIPTION/SERVICE CODE		AMOUNT CHARGED			AMOUNT PAID	
William Green	OV		35	00		35	00
D. B. Brown	OV, Inj.		50	00		35	00
Betty Kendrick	Dressing Change		15	00		0	
Wallace Dunn	OV, serology		55	00		15	00
James Jones	OV, CBC, UA		57	00		57	00
Donald Day	FBS		12	00		12	00
Joe Swanson	Comprehensive		85	00		15	00
Catherine Riley	Brief, CBC, Inj		42	00		0	
Michael Steves	Intermediate OV		35	00		15	00
Rusty Owens	Intermediate OV		35	00		0	
M. R. Watkins	Limited OV		20	00		20	00
Barbara Hopkins	Intermediate OV, X-ray		70	00		25	00
Mary Nell Hill	Minor surgery		125	00		0	
Roger Green	Brief OV		15	00		10	00
Stephanie Lett	Comprehensive, lab		117	00		85	00
Charlotte Mason	Payment		—			30	00
J. T. Watkins	Payment		—			40	00
Sheila Nichols	Hosp admission x 2 visits		155	00		0	
DeWayne Chumley	ER Visit		75	00		0	

FIGURE 6-1
Daily journal.

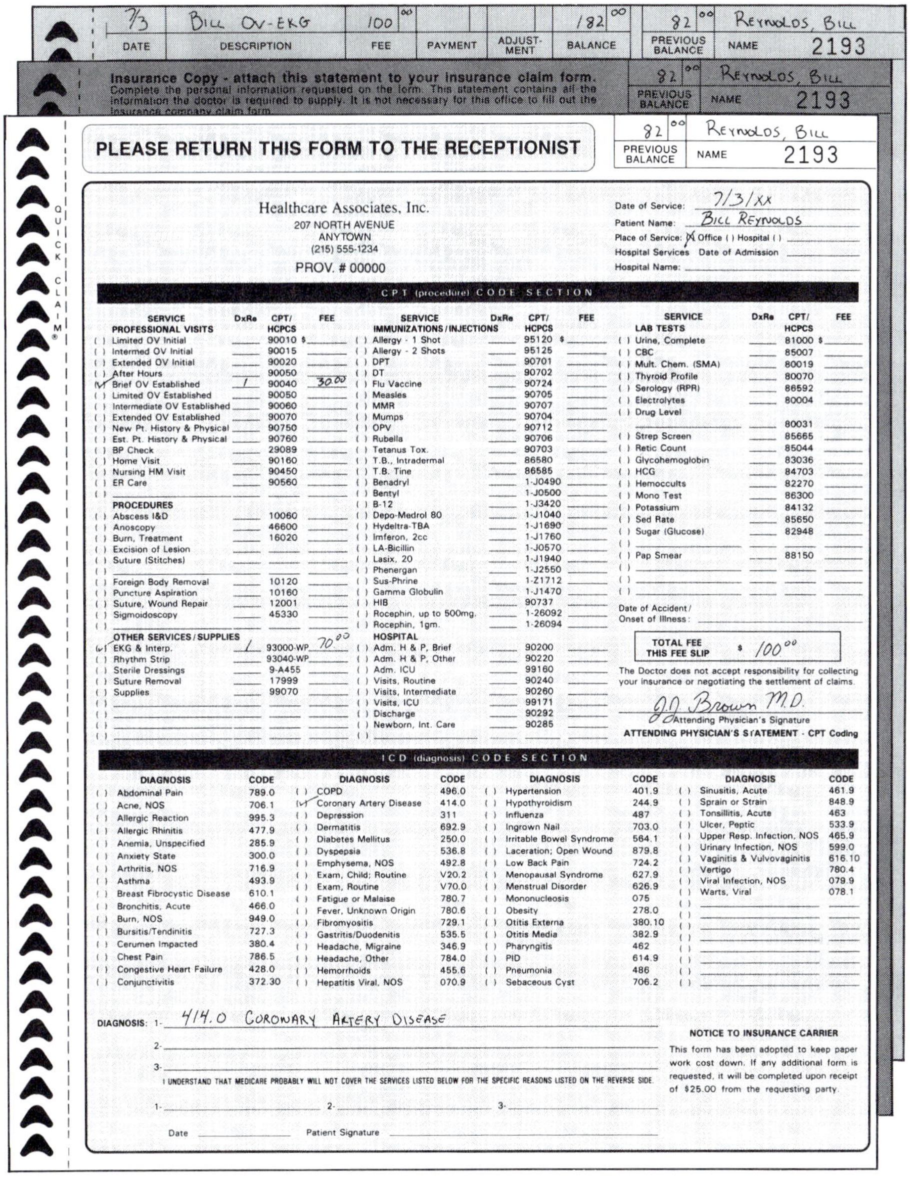

FIGURE 6-2

Pegboard transaction slip and receipt combined. (Reproduced with permission from Safeguard Business Systems, Inc.)

patient ledger is placed between the day sheet and charge slip. As the charges and payments are recorded, the information is simultaneously transferred to the charge slip, ledger and day sheet (Figure 6-3).

Recording expenses to the disbursements journal with the pegboard system likewise simultaneously records all necessary information in one step. A bank of checks and a disbursement sheet are placed over the pegs of the pegboard, and as the check is being written for disbursement, the entry to the disbursements journal is transferred simultaneously. When a paycheck is written, a payroll summary record is inserted between the check and disbursement journal. As the paycheck is written, the payroll gross, deductions, and net pay are recorded on the check and disbursement journal simultaneously (Figure 6-4).

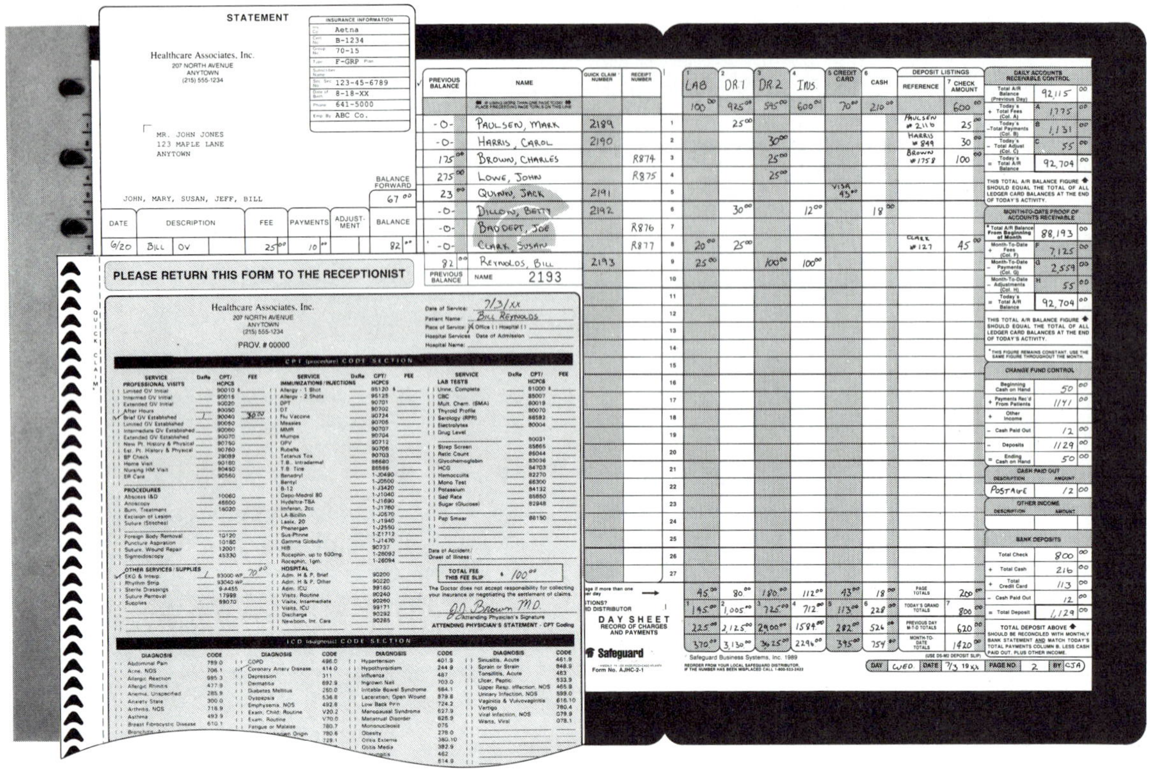

FIGURE 6–3

Pegboard accounts receivable system. (Reproduced with permission from Safeguard Business Systems, Inc.)

The pegboard bookkeeping system is designed especially to reduce the burden of paperwork and increase efficiency. The pegboard is appropriate for a high-volume medical practice. However, the initial startup cost is more expensive than that of the single-entry system, and learning how to use the system may seem complex to someone who has little experience in bookkeeping (although it can be learned in a relatively short period of time).

Maintaining an Accounts Receivable Bookkeeping System

Initiating a Patient Ledger Card

A patient ledger card is initiated at the time of a patient's first visit to the office and is accomplished by extracting data from the patient's registration form and typing or handwriting the information onto the ledger card (Figure 6–5). Below is a list of the basic information that should be included on every ledger card.

- Name of responsible party;
- Complete mailing address and zip code;
- Telephone number;
- Name, address, and phone number of health insurance company (both spouses' insurance companies, if applicable), insured's policy number, and summary of coverage, such as copay required per visit, yearly deductible, etc.

Other billing information may be necessary, depending on the practice's particular needs. It may be necessary to include the names of the family members whose charges will appear on the responsible party's account, or to identify ledgers with special notations, such as those to whom the physician gives professional discounts.

SPECIAL HINTS

Maintain all patient ledger cards in protective metal trays that are designed for easy storage and retrieval.

Maintain all ledger cards in alphabetical order by the name of the responsible party. Type

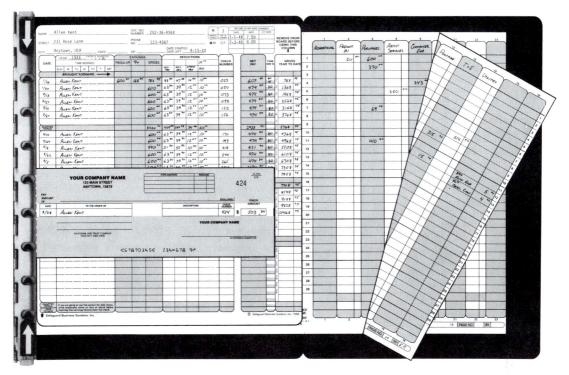

FIGURE 6-4

Pegboard accounts payable system. (Reproduced with permission from Safeguard Business Systems, Inc.)

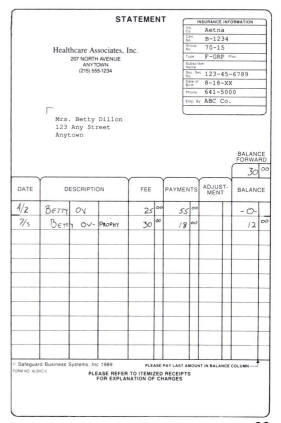

FIGURE 6-5

Accounts receivable ledger. (Reproduced with permission from Safeguard Business Systems, Inc.)

the responsible party's name with first or last name first, according to office policy. Typing the name in all capital letters will make it stand our for ease in filing and retrieval.
- When several family members are being seen in the office, one ledger card may be kept in the name of the responsible party and the names of the other family members placed visibly on the front or back of the ledger card.
- When an account is being established for the children of divorced parents, place the ledger card in the name of the person identified on the divorce decree as the responsible party. Ask for the responsible party's address, home, and business phone number if different from the children's home address. If both parents are jointly responsible, it is best to place the ledger card in the name of the parent who most often accompanies the children to the physician's office.
- Some accounts are best maintained by company name. An example of this is when a company sends their employees to the physician's office for work-related injuries under Worker's Compensation. The charges are entered on the company ledger card, including the name of the employee treated; then a monthly bill of all services rendered to referred employees can be readily submitted. Other examples of company accounts include employee physicals, life and health insurance physicals, and referrals for disability determination.
- Before leaving the office every day, secure patient ledger cards to prevent theft, water damage, or fire. The best safety for ledger cards is to place them in a locked fireproof safe. If this is not possible, place the ledger cards into a locked file cabinet, or at least tightly close the file trays to lessen the chance of total destruction in the event of a fire. Built-in, fireproof drawers situated near the cashier's window provide easy access and safety and omit the need to move the ledger cards from one place to another.

Recording Charges and Payments to the Daily Journal

Each patient visit usually results in a fee charged (a *debit* in bookkeeping terms) for the services rendered by the physician and must be accounted for. The fees collected are recorded as payments (a *credit* in bookkeeping terms) and represents the income of the practice. Fees charged *(debited)* but not collected *(credited)* represent the balance owed or accounts receivable. The accounts receivable balance usually represents a debit balance. If an overpayment appears on a patient's account, the balance becomes a credit and must be distinguished from debit balances by encircling or placing brackets around the amount in the balance column. The formula for recording charges and payments may be represented as follows:

$$\begin{array}{c} \text{Fees charged} - \text{Fees collected} = \text{Accounts receivable} \\ \text{or} \\ \text{Debits} - \text{Credit} = \text{Balance owed} \\ \$35 - \$10 = \$25 \text{ (a debit balance)} \\ \$35 - \$50 = [\$15] \text{ (a credit balance)} \end{array}$$

A daily journal sheet is used for each day's transactions. A ledger card is used to keep track of the balances owed by each patient or family unit.

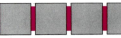

PROCEDURE

POSTING CHARGES AND PAYMENTS USING SINGLE-ENTRY BOOKKEEPING

PURPOSE

To provide a record of charges and payments for services rendered by the physician.

EQUIPMENT AND MATERIALS:

Daily journal sheet
Patient ledger cards

Chapter 6: BOOKKEEPING, CREDIT, AND COLLECTIONS 85

Receipts
Pen or pencil

PROCEDURAL STEPS

1. Post entry to daily journal (see Figure 6–1).

   - Enter the patient's name and service code or abbreviation.
   - Enter the total fee in the charge column.
   - Accept payment from patient and post it in the payments column.

2. Write a patient receipt for amount paid, if any.

   - Give receipt to patient.

   - Keep one file copy, if applicable.

3. Post entry to patient's ledger card (Figure 6–5).

   - Enter date of visit, service code, or abbreviation.
   - Enter the total fee in the charge column.
   - Enter payment received, if any.
   - Add previous balance, if any and less today's payment, to charges and enter balance in the current balance column.

4. Repeat steps 1–3 for each patient seen.
5. At end of day, total all columns on day sheet. The payments column total should equal the total currency and checks in the cash drawer.

PROCEDURE

POSTING CHARGES AND PAYMENTS USING PEGBOARD BOOKKEEPING

PURPOSE

To provide a record of charges and payments for services provided by the physician.

EQUIPMENT AND MATERIALS

Daily journal sheet (Figure 6–6)
Patient ledger cards
Combination transaction slips
Pen or pencil

PROCEDURAL STEPS

Preparation

1. Place a new day sheet on the pegboard.
2. Enter today's date.
3. Bring forward control balances from the previous day.
4. Insert bank of transaction slips over pegs, with the first charge slip aligned with the first line of entry.

Performance

5. Pull ledger cards for patients being seen.
6. Assign receipt number and preenter on pegboard.

   - Insert patient ledger card between the day sheet and transaction slip, aligning it with the first line of entry.
   - Preenter patient's name, date, and receipt number.
   - Preenter any balance owed in the previous balance column.
   - Remove transaction slip from the pegboard and attach to the front of the patient's medical record.
   - Remove patient ledger card and set aside until end of visit.
   - Repeat step 6 until each patient being seen has been preentered on the day sheet.

7. Post charges and payments.

   - At the end of patient's visit, the transaction slip is returned and fees entered on the transaction slip from the fee schedule.
   - Reinsert transaction slip and patient ledger card on pegboard.
   - On the receipt portion of transaction slip, enter procedure code or abbreviation and fee for each service rendered.
   - Total fees and enter in the charge column.
   - Accept payment from patient and enter in

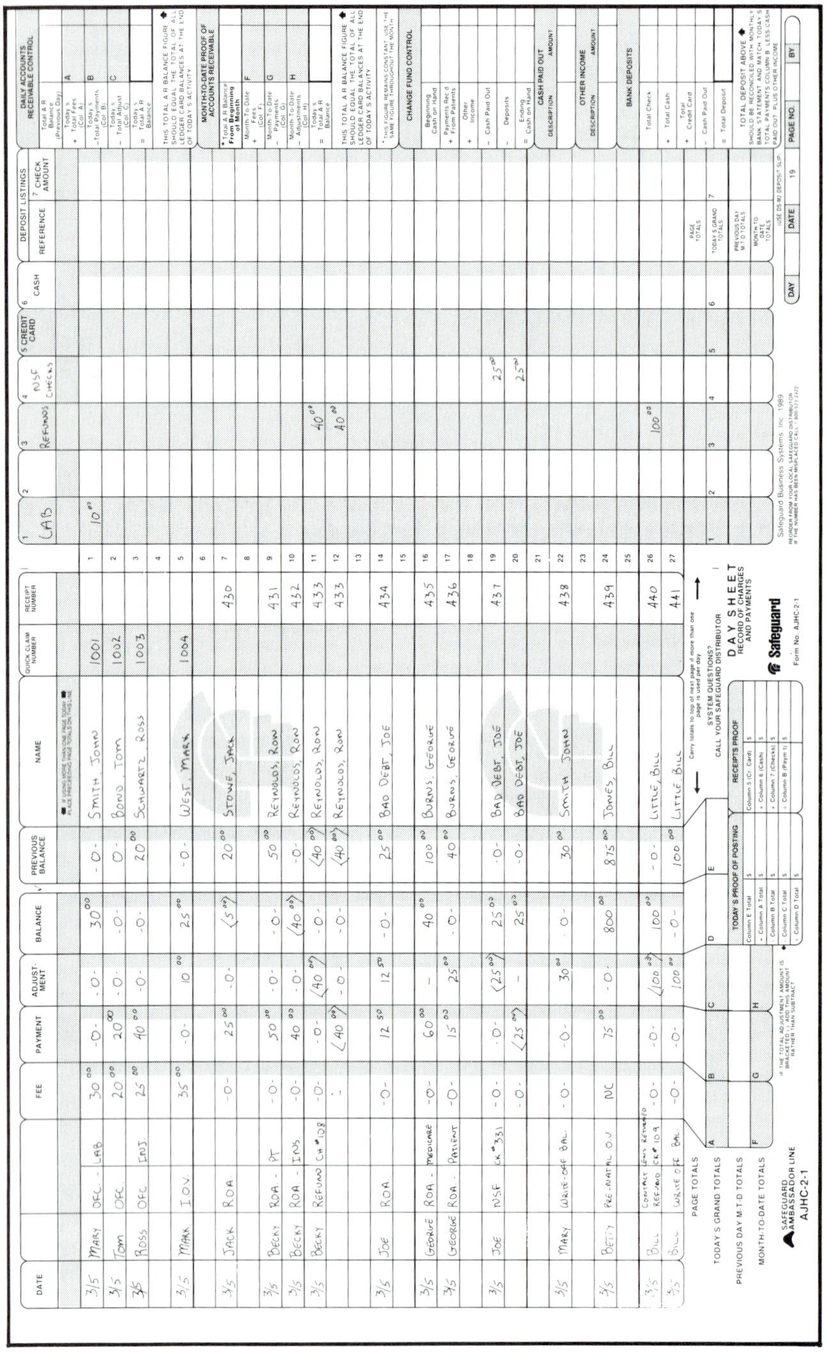

FIGURE 6-6

Pegboard day sheet. (Reproduced with permission from Safeguard Business Systems, Inc.)

payment column and in the deposit column under check or cash.
- Bring forward new balance in the balance column.
- Remove charge slip and ledger card from pegboard, giving one copy of the receipt to patient, retaining one for file copy. NOTE: If insurance is filed for charges, an additional copy of the charge slip is attached to the claim form and routed to the insurance clerk.
- Repeat step 7 for each patient seen.

8. Refile all patient ledger cards.
9. File transaction slip copies numerically by receipt number.
10. Complete day sheet summaries.

- At end of day, total all columns on day sheet using a pencil.
- Complete proof of posting by day sheet directions or the following formula:

Previous balance column total
+ Charge column total
− Payments and adjustments
= Current balance column.

NOTE: If proof-of-posting balance is not same as the balance column total, an error in posting has occurred. Recheck each entry posted for error.

- Complete accounts receivable control by day sheet directions or the following formula:

Previous accounts receivable balance
+ Today's total charges
− Today's total payments and adjustments
= Accounts receivable year to date.

- Complete cash control by day sheet directions or the following formula:

Cash on hand + Cash received
= Total deposit − Total amount deposited
= Current cash on hand.

11. File day sheet in binder.

Posting Special Accounting Entries

Occasionally, unusual circumstances occur that require special accounting entries. Examples of some of these entries are described below. The accountant for the medical practice can also provide assistance in determining how to handle these and other special entries, whether the single-entry or pegboard bookkeeping system is used.

Adjustments

Adjustments usually include delinquent accounts, insurance nonallowed amounts, or professional discounts. When an adjustment is posted, the entry must be entered on both the daily journal and patient ledger.

Delinquent Accounts. Patient accounts that are delinquent require special handling. The office manager or accountant may eventually turn over unpaid accounts to a collection agency who in turn charges a percentage fee, usually up to 50% of the amount recovered. In Figure 6–7, the fee of $128 was collected from the patient by the collection agency who retained 50% as fee for recovery of the delinquent account. To record collection agency fees, post an entry to the patient ledger and day sheet as follows:

1. Enter date and a description.
2. Enter the amount paid to the practice.
3. Enter amount retained by the collection agency in the adjustment column.
4. Bring forward current balance.

Some practices elect to write off delinquent accounts as uncollectable when turning the account over to the collection agency and reinstating any amounts recovered by the collection agency. Only the percentage amount paid to the practice is reinstated and not the percentage retained by the agency. See the patient ledger in Figure 6–8 for a sample entry.

At some point, a patient's account may be deemed uncollectable and is written off to bad debt. To post an entry to the patient ledger and day sheet to write off a delinquent account, see Figure 6–9 and follow these steps:

1. Enter date and a description.
2. Enter amount to be written off in the adjustment column.

SUSAN JOHNSON
2331 First Avenue NW
Anytown, USA 99999

DATE	REFERENCE	DESCRIPTION	CHARGE	CREDITS PAYMENTS	ADJ.	CURRENT BALANCE
		BALANCE FORWARD →				
1/10/9-		90015, 71020, 85025	158 00	30 00	—	128 00
7/13/9-		Collection Recovery	—	64 00	64 00	0

FIGURE 6-7
Entry posted to show recovery of a delinquent account.

SUSAN JOHNSON
2331 First Avenue NW
Anytown, USA 99999

DATE	REFERENCE	DESCRIPTION	CHARGE	CREDITS PAYMENTS	ADJ.	CURRENT BALANCE
		BALANCE FORWARD →				
1/10/9-		90015, 71020, 85025	158 00	30 00	—	128 00
6/25/9-		Write off	—	—	128 00	0
7/13/9-		Collection Recovery		64 00	[64 00]	0

FIGURE 6-8
Entry posted to show recovery of a write-off.

		TAMMY GRAYSON 277 Oxford Road Anytown, USA 99999				

DATE	REFERENCE	DESCRIPTION	CHARGE	CREDITS PAYMENTS	ADJ.	CURRENT BALANCE
		BALANCE FORWARD →				
1/14/9-		90017, 82800	47 00	—	—	47 00
8/13/9-		Write off	—	—	47 00	0

FIGURE 6-9

Entry posted to write off an uncollected balance.

		BOBBY WILSON 761 Hilside Cirle Anytown, USA 99999				

DATE	REFERENCE	DESCRIPTION	CHARGE	CREDITS PAYMENTS	ADJ.	CURRENT BALANCE
		BALANCE FORWARD →				
7/24/9-		90015	35 00	—	—	35 00
8/11/9-		Medicare Pymt	—	26 40	2 00	6 60

FIGURE 6-10

Entry posted to show insurance payment with nonallowed adjustment.

3. Bring forward new balance in the balance column.

Insurance Nonallowed Amounts. Some physicians are under contract with various insurance companies to accept the allowable fee as payment for services. The patient cannot be billed for the difference between the allowable fee and the actual charge and, therefore the difference must be adjusted off the patient's account. Figure 6–10 is a Medicare insurance payment for a $35 office fee, $2 of which has been determined by the insurance company to be above the allowable charge. This amount cannot be collected from the patient and is adjusted off the patient's account. Follow the steps below to post an entry to the patient ledger and day sheet for insurance payments with nonallowed amounts:

1. Enter date and description.
2. Enter amount paid by insurance in the payment.
3. Enter nonallowed amount in the adjustment column.
4. Bring forward new balance.

Professional Discounts. Some physicians are accustomed to giving professional discounts to medical assistants, nurses, dentists, members of the clergy, etc. Figure 6–11 shows an entry for a patient who received a 25% discount on a comprehensive office visit. Physicians may or may not apply the discount to other procedures, such as laboratory tests or x-rays. Follow the steps below to post an entry to the patient ledger and day sheet for professional discounts:

1. Enter date and a description.
2. Enter total fee in the charge column.
3. Figure percentage to be discounted and enter amount in the adjustment column.
4. Enter payment from patient, if any, in the payment column.
5. Bring forward new balance in the balance column.

Reversing Entries

Reversing an entry is an action taken to cancel or reverse a previous charge or payment posted. When an amount is posted to reverse a charge or payment, the amount is circled or enclosed with brackets. When the columns are totaled at the end of the day, the amount in brackets is subtracted rather than added. Several kinds of situations require reversing entries. As an alternative, the ac-

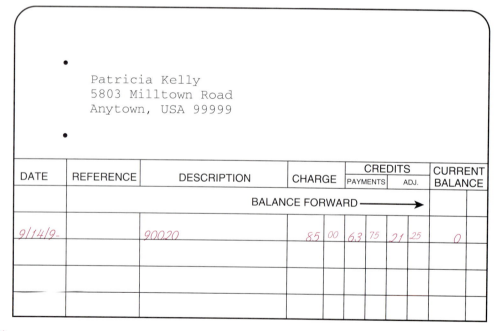

FIGURE 6–11

Entry posted to show professional discount adjustment.

countant may suggest using the adjustments column rather than reversing the entry.

Returned Checks. A check received from a patient in payment of office fees may be returned by the bank marked "Not Sufficient Funds" (NSF). The check is reinstated to the patient ledger and daily journal by posting a reversing entry. The check should also be deducted from the deposits column in the checkbook. Refer to Figure 6–12 and follow the steps below to post a returned check.

1. Deduct the amount of the returned check on the checkbook stub.
2. Post an entry to the patient ledger and day sheet.

- Enter date and a description.
- Enter amount of returned check in the payment column in brackets.
- Bring forward the new balance.

Patient Refunds. A refund to the patient may be warranted when there has been an overpayment resulting in a credit balance (credit balances are represented by placing brackets around the amount in the balance column). An example of this is when a patient pays an office fee and then later the insurance pays for the same service; this results in a duplication because both payments are credited to the same charge. Refer to Figure 6–13 and follow the steps below for posting a payment that results in duplicate payment.

1. Post an entry to the patient ledger and day sheet.
2. Enter date and a description.
3. Enter payment received in the payment column.
4. Bring forward new balance.

The overpayment may result in a credit balance on the patient's account. If this is the case, the credit balance may remain on the patient's account and applied to future charges, or if the patient requests a refund, post a reversing entry to the patient ledger and day sheet as follows:

1. Enter date and brief explanation.
2. Enter the credit balance with brackets in the previous balance column.
3. Enter the amount of the refund in the payment column with brackets.
4. Bring forward the current balance.

RUSSELL WILLIAMS
P.O. Box 2717
Anytown, USA 99999

DATE	REFERENCE	DESCRIPTION	CHARGE	CREDITS PAYMENTS	ADJ.	CURRENT BALANCE
		BALANCE FORWARD →				
6/10/9-		90010	20 00	—		20 00
7/03/9-		12011	45 00	30 00		35 00
7/11/9-		Returned Check	—	[30 00]		65 00

FIGURE 6–12
Entry posted to reinstate balance due to a returned check.

DATE	REFERENCE	DESCRIPTION	CHARGE	CREDITS PAYMENTS	ADJ.	CURRENT BALANCE
		BALANCE FORWARD →				
6/13/9-		Minor Surgery	85 00	85 00	—	0
7/11/9-		Insurance pymt	—	85 00	—	[85 00]
7/11/9-		Patient Refund	—	[85 00]	—	0

ROBERT ABRAMS
9336 Lonesome Bend Rd.
Anytown, USA 99999

FIGURE 6–13
Entry posted to show a patient refund.

Completing an Accounts Receivable Trial Balance

A trial balance, performed at the close of each month, discloses any errors between the daily journal and the patient ledgers. For example, if an entry has been posted to the day sheet but not to the patient ledger, the totals from the patient ledgers will not balance with the day sheet totals. The trial balance does not prove accuracy of total accounting but detects posting or mathematical errors.

PROCEDURE

COMPLETING AN ACCOUNTS RECEIVABLE TRIAL BALANCE

PURPOSE

To ensure accuracy in recordkeeping and detect errors in posting.

MATERIALS AND EQUIPMENT

Adding machine with tape
Ledger cards of all patients

PROCEDURAL STEPS

1. Pull all patient ledger cards that show a balance owed.
2. Enter the balance from each ledger on the adding machine and total the figures.
3. Compare the ledger account total with the accounts receivable month-end balance. The two totals should be the same.

If a single-entry bookkeeping system is used and no accounts receivable control is kept, use the following computation to obtain a current accounts receivable control total:

Accounts receivable at first of month: $_____
+ total charges of current month: $_____
− total payments and adjustments: $_____
= accounts receivable at end of month: $_____

Maintaining an Accounts Payable Bookkeeping System

Accounts payable bookkeeping involves the recording of expenses for the practice. Purchases for supplies, equipment, etc. are paid by check or petty cash at the time of purchase, or a statement or invoice is mailed from which payment is made. Copies of all statements and invoices paid should be kept in a folder by expense category. Unpaid invoices are kept in a folder marked "accounts payable." Expenses may be paid as the statement or invoice is received or may be saved and paid only once or twice per month.

The expenses of a medical practice are recorded in a disbursements journal with columns for the date, payee's name, check number, check amount, and numerous columns into which the different kinds of expenses are categorized (see Figure 6–14). Expense accounts may include but are not limited to

- Salaries
- Rent
- Clinical supplies
- Laboratory fees
- Books/journals
- Travel
- Professional dues
- Instruments/equipment
- Office supplies
- Utilities
- Laundry/cleaning
- Taxes and licenses
- Insurance
- Miscellaneous

SPECIAL HINT

An expense account labeled "sundry accounts" may be added and used to record expenses that are not tax deductible for business expenses but may be applicable to the physician's personal income tax deductions.

A disbursements journal is customarily maintained on a monthly basis, with totals calculated at the end of each month and a new disbursements journal sheet begun at the beginning of the next month. Posting may be done at the end of each day, week, or month; however, pegboard systems are designed so that as the check is written the disbursements journal is posted simultaneously in one step. Following are the procedures for posting to a disbursements journal for both single-entry and pegboard systems.

PROCEDURE

RECORDING EXPENSES TO A SINGLE-ENTRY DISBURSEMENTS JOURNAL

PURPOSE

To maintain a monthly record of business expenses.

MATERIALS AND EQUIPMENT

Disbursements journal sheet
Checkbook
Pen or pencil

PROCEDURAL STEPS

1. Prepare the disbursements journal form.

   - At the beginning of the month, enter the month and year on the disbursements journal.
   - Label each expense column with the expense accounts established by the practice.

2. Post each check written to the disbursements journal chronologically by check number.

   - Enter date of check.
   - Enter to whom check was written.
   - Enter amount of check.
   - Enter check number.
   - Post check amount in the appropriate expense account(s).

3. Repeat step 2 for every check written during the month. NOTE: Use the petty cash journal and check written to replenish fund to post the total expenses paid out during the month, then spread the amount among the appropriate expense categories (for example, postage and office supplies).

4. Total all columns of the disbursements journal.

PROCEDURE

RECORDING EXPENSES TO A PEGBOARD DISBURSEMENTS JOURNAL

PURPOSE

To maintain a monthly record of business expenses.

MATERIALS AND EQUIPMENT

Disbursements journal sheet (Figure 6–14)
Payroll record form for each employee
Bank of checks
Pegboard
Pen or pencil

PROCEDURAL STEPS

1. Prepare the pegboard.

   - Place a bank of checks and a disbursements journal over the pegs of the pegboard with the first check lined up with the first line of entry on the disbursements journal sheet.
   - Enter the appropriate month, year, and page number.
   - Label each expense column with the expense account categories established by the practice.
   - If applicable, bring forward last month's column totals and post in the appropriate line at the bottom of the journal.

2. Write checks for disbursement.

   - Starting with the first check, enter the date, payee name, and amount of check.
   - Enter check number and amount for which the check is written.
   - Enter check amount in the appropriate expense account. If necessary, distribute the amount among the appropriate expense categories.
   - Remove the check from the pegboard.
   - Write the amount of the check in words on the appropriate line.
   - Have the check signed by the physician or an individual with the power of attorney.
   - Staple a duplicate of the check, if any, to a copy of the invoice and file under the name of the expense account to which the check is posted.

3. Write payroll checks.

   - Insert an employee payroll summary record between the bank of checks and the disbursements journal sheet, lining it up with the next available line of entry.
   - Enter total hours worked, date, employee name, gross pay, deductions, and net pay which is the amount the check is to be written. The gross pay and deductions are usually entered on the stub or duplicate copy of the check and not on the original.
   - Enter check amount in the appropriate expense account(s).
   - Remove the check from the pegboard.
   - Write the amount of the check in words on the appropriate line.
   - Have the check signed by the physician or individual with power of attorney.
   - Insert check in sealed envelope for mailing or interoffice distribution. The duplicate copy of the check is given to the employee to serve as a pay stub.

4. At the end of the month, total all columns of the disbursements journal.

Completing a Disbursements Journal Trial Balance

Complete a trial balance of the disbursements journal after the last check of the month has been entered and all columns of the journal have been totaled. The trial balance ensures that each check posted has been correctly distributed among one or more of the expense account categories. To perform a trial balance, do the following:

> Add together the totals from each expense account category. Do not include the payroll deduction column totals. The total should equal the total of the "check amount" column.

DISBURSEMENTS JOURNAL (Check Register)

MONTH ENDING Sept. 19___   PAGE 1 OF 1

DAY	PAYEE	CHECK NO	AMOUNT	SALARIES	RENT	CLINICAL SUPPLIES	OFFICE SUPPLIES	LAB FEES	EQUIP-MENT	POWER	WATER	PHONE	GAS	PROF. DUES	JOURNALS	TRAVEL EXPENSE	TAXES	SUNDRY CHECKS DESCRIPTION	AMOUNT
9/1	State Realty Co.	282	900 00		900 00														
9/6	Wilcox Medical Supply	283	279 40			279 40													
9/8	O'Hara Office Supply	284	51 73				51 73												
9/9	JAMA	285	35 00												35 00				
9/15	Cathy Brown	286	531 50	531 50															
9/15	Dorothy Webb	287	650 40	650 40															
9/15	Dawn Foster	288	741 22	741 22															
9/18	Post Office	289	29 00				29 00												
9/18	Board Medical Co.	290	87 60						87 60										
9/18	Wilcox Medical Supply	291	47 30			47 30													
9/22	Professional Laboratory	292	165 00					165 00											
9/28	Power Company	293	118 20							118 20									
9/28	Telephone Company	294	89 70									89 70							
9/28	Water & Sewer Board	295	51 04								51 04								
9/28	Gas Corporation	296	77 19										77 19						
9/30	AMGA	297	85 00											85 00					
9/30	Internal Revenue	298	1,940 50														1,940 50		
9/30	Cathy Brown	299	550 43	550 43															
9/30	Dorothy Webb	300	675 81	675 81															
9/30	Dawn Foster	301	741 22	741 22															
9/30	Office Warehouse	302	133 75				133 75												
	MONTH END TOTALS		7980 99	3890 58	900 00	326 70	214 48	165 00	87 60	118 20	51 04	89 70	77 19	85 00	35 00	-0-	1940 50		
	TOTALS BROUGHT FWD																		
	YEAR TO DATE TOTALS																		

FIGURE 6–14

Accounts payable disbursements journal.

PETTY CASH JOURNAL

PERIOD BEGINNING _March 1_ 19 ____ ENDING _March 31_ 19 ____

DATE	VOUCHER NO.	PAID TO	FOR	EXPENSE CATEGORY	AMOUNT	BALANCE
3/01		BALANCE BRO'T FWD				14.86
3/01		cash replenished			35.14	50.00
3/14	1	post office	stamps	office supplies	5.80	44.20
3/19	2	Watts Hardware	batteries	maintenance	4.71	39.49
3/25	3	office warehouse	labels	office supplies	12.80	26.69
		ENDING BALANCE				26.69

RECEIPT VOUCHER

DATE _3/19_ NO. _2_

PURCHASED FROM: _Watts Hardware_

ITEM(S) PURCHASED:

batteries

AMOUNT PAID.................$ _4.71_

Cristy Welch
Purchaser signature

FIGURE 6-15

Petty cash journal and receipt voucher.

Completing a Year-to-Date Cash Disbursements Summary

When the disbursements journal is maintained on a monthly basis, it is helpful to know the total expenses for the year, especially if the office operates under a budget. The accountant also needs year-to-date totals when preparing the deductions on income tax forms.

Some disbursements journals provide space at the bottom of the journal sheet. If a space is not provided, a blank journal sheet may be used by transferring the month end totals to the blank journal sheet and total. To keep a year-to-date summary of expenses month by month, follow these steps:

1. Total the columns of the disbursement journal for the current month.
2. Bring forward the column totals from the previous month and enter in the space provided.
3. Add current month's total to previous month's total and enter in year-to-date columns.

At the end of every month, repeat the steps above. Begin a new year-to-date total at the beginning of the new accounting year.

Maintaining Petty Cash Records

The purpose of a petty cash fund is to have cash readily accessible for making small purchases that do not warrant writing a check. Examples of these types of expenses are postage-due fees or fees for cleaning or office supplies. The amount of cash maintained in the fund varies, usually from $25 to $50, but should be large enough to cover small expenses that occur during 1 month. Figure 6–15 shows the petty cash forms included in a typical system. These forms are

Petty cash record form: Lists separately every disbursement paid from the fund each month. The format varies but should show at least the date of purchase, description of purchase, payee's name, and amount paid.

Petty cash voucher: Substituted from the sales receipt and is a short form completed in the absence of a sales receipt.

The currency for the petty cash fund should be kept separate from the main cash drawer, in either a cash box or an envelope stored in the office safe.

To set up the petty cash fund, write a check for cash for the amount deemed appropriate for the office. Post the check to the disbursements journal in the miscellaneous expense account column. Future checks written to replenish the fund are posted on the disbursements journal and spread among the appropriate expense categories. Figure 6–14 shows a sample entry of petty cash distributions on check number 1438 for $23.50.

Each time petty cash is used to make a purchase, a sales receipt should be obtained and kept with the petty cash records. If a sales receipt is not available, have the purchaser fill out a petty cash voucher as a substitute for the sales receipt (Figure 6–15).

The petty cash journal should be periodically balanced to the total receipts and vouchers, usually once per month or when the fund becomes depleted. The following procedure provides general guidelines for establishing and maintaining accurate records for petty cash.

PROCEDURE

ESTABLISHING AND MAINTAINING A PETTY CASH FUND

PURPOSE

To provide a record for business expenses paid for in cash.

MATERIALS AND EQUIPMENT

Petty cash journal form
Petty cash vouchers and receipts of expenditures (Figure 6–15)
Current month's disbursement journal
Checkbook
Pen or pencil

PROCEDURAL STEPS

1. Establish petty cash fund.

   • Write a check for the determined amount.

- Post the check to the petty cash journal as the beginning balance.
- Post the check also to the current month's disbursements journal in the miscellaneous expense account column.

2. Record expenses in the petty cash journal.

- Post a separate entry to the petty cash journal for each sales receipt and petty cash voucher received, entering payee's name, expense category, and amount paid.
- Bring forward the new balance after each entry.

3. Balance petty cash fund.

- At end of the month or when fund becomes depleted, total the expense column in the petty cash journal.
- Write a check for the amount of expense paid out to replenish the fund.
- Post total expense amount to the current month's disbursements journal in the appropriate expense account columns.
- Add the total expense amount shown in the petty cash journal to the total currency left in the fund. The total should equal the beginning fund balance.

BANKING

Opening a Checking Account

Most full-service banks offer a wide range of services. When the practice opens a checking account, first investigate the various services available. There are several options from which to choose:

Regular account: An individual checking account that may require a monthly service charge. Some banks waive the charge if the checking account balance remains above a certain amount.

Joint account: More than one person's name appears on the account and each person is authorized to make deposits or withdrawals.

Special account: Services vary but may involve charging an amount for each check rather than a set monthly service charge. Special accounts of this type are feasible only when a few checks are written each month.

Business account: The owner or authorized representatives of the business may make deposits or withdrawals.

Other types of checking accounts include interest-bearing accounts, overdraft protection accounts, and senior citizens' checking accounts.

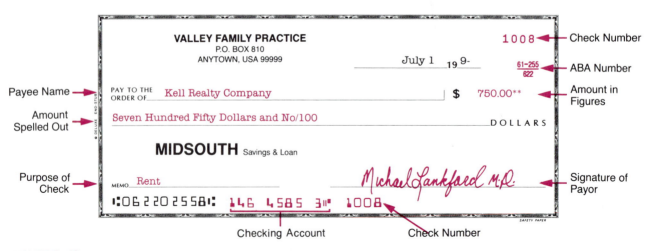

FIGURE 6-16
Personal check with parts identified.

Chapter 6: BOOKKEEPING, CREDIT, AND COLLECTIONS 99

FIGURE 6-17

Commercial checks.

In addition to checking, banks offer many other services, including night depositories, banking by mail, safe deposit boxes, traveler's checks, cashier's and certified checks, international currencies, international banking, notary service, and 24-hour minibanks. Trust services are also available that involve investment services; custody services; escrow service; estate planning; and trustee, guardian, and executor services.

Selecting Checks

The check-writing system chosen for the office varies with personal preference but is usually compatible with the type of bookkeeping system used. Examples of check writing systems include

- Regular checks (see Figure 6–16)
- Commercial checks, printed with three or four checks per page and stored in a spiral or three-ring binder (Figure 6–17)
- Pegboard one-write system, with checks in banked sets of 10–15 per set (see Figure 6–4)

All of the checks in these systems are usually prenumbered in sequence; preprinted with the practice account number; and personalized with the practice name, address, phone number, tax identification number, etc.

Writing Checks

Special care should be taken when writing checks. If not written properly, the check may not be honored by the bank. Refer to the procedure below for writing checks. Figure 6–16 identifies the parts of a completed check.

PROCEDURE
WRITING CHECKS

PURPOSE

To create a negotiable instrument to pay for business expenses.

MATERIALS AND EQUIPMENT

Checkbook
Pen or typewriter

PROCEDURAL STEPS

1. Complete check stub.

   - Enter date the check is being written, amount of check, to whom check is written, and purpose of check.
   - Bring forward the new balance by subtracting previous check balance from amount of check being written.

2. Complete the check.

   - Date the check as it appears on check stub.
   - Write out the full name of the payee, using abbreviations only when commonly accepted.
   - Enter the amount of the check, in numerals, close to the dollar sign. Place an asterisk or straight line across any remaining space to prevent tampering.
   - Spell out the dollar amount of the check in words. Separate the cents by the word *and* then write the cents in fraction. Write the fraction as "No/100" if there are no cents or write the word *only* in place of the fraction.

3. Obtain the signature of the physician or a person who has the power of attorney.

SPECIAL HINTS

Postdated checks should not be written unless permission is given by the payee.
Keep the checkbook balance up to date so that the current balance is available at all times.
If checks are typewritten, avoid using correctable carbon ribbon that a skillful forger can alter.
The amount written out in words is the amount the bank usually pays, so make sure it agrees with the amount written in figures.

Store the checkbook in a secure place that can be accessed only by authorized persons.

Make no corrections on the check. If you make an error, write *VOID* on the stub and check. File the voided check with the canceled checks for verification should banking records be audited.

Accepting Checks for Payment

Accepting checks for payment of services rendered in the physician's office is common practice. It is convenient for patients and provides another record of proof of payment. In an office whose clientele does not change frequently, accepting checks for payment is quite safe if information such as phone numbers, address, employer, etc. is kept current; however, a few precautions should be observed when accepting checks:

- Make sure the check is dated correctly, shows the correct amount, and is signed properly.
- Preprinted personal checks are safer to accept than blank or counter checks. If a blank check is accepted, make sure the check has account numbers printed at the bottom and the bank's name and American Banker's Association number, expressed in a fraction (for example, $\frac{61-91}{620}$), appears on the check. It is a good idea to call the bank to verify that the patient has a checking account.
- Do not accept out-of-town checks unless you are acquainted with the patient or person presenting the check.
- A check that has "Paid in Full" written on the face of it should not be accepted unless the check does pay the total balance due. If the medical office accepts such a check, it cannot legally collect for any balance remaining.

The office may also establish a policy to not accept some or all of the following third-party checks:

- Checks with two endorsements;
- Payroll checks;
- Money orders, unless made out to the practice;
- Government income tax refunds;
- Insurance checks made out to the patient.

Such checks often require that change be paid back to the patient. Cash reserve can become depleted quickly, and if the check is returned for any reason, you lose not only the amount owed but also the amount of change paid back to the patient.

Endorsing Checks

Before checks can be cashed or deposited, the check must have an appropriate endorsement on the reverse side (Figure 6-18). The three ways in which checks may be endorsed are

Blank endorsement: Requires only the name of the payee's signature.
Full endorsement: Transfers payment from original payee to someone else, and endorsement specifies to whom the check is payable.
Restricted endorsement: Limits the use of the check to a specific purpose such as "For Deposit Only." Restricted endorsement is appropriate to use if checks are mailed or deposit of the check is delayed. The check is then protected from fraudulent use.

SPECIAL HINTS

Endorse a check with a blank endorsement only at the time of presentation at the bank. If lost or stolen, the check with such an endorsement can still be presented for payment.

Use restrictive endorsement on all checks received from patients. Stamp the endorsement on back of the check when it is received. This protects the check from fraudulent use if it is lost or stolen before deposit is made.

If the practice accepts insurance checks made out to the patient, make sure patient correctly signs with a full endorsement.

Some insurance companies accept only handwritten rather than stamped endorsements, which will be indicated on the back of the check if required.

Making Bank Deposits

The office manager or designated medical assistant is generally responsible for making deposits and maintaining an accurate deposit record. The deposits should be made frequently, usually on a daily basis. The total amount of payments received and posted on the daily journal is the amount deposited.

Patients often ask to write a postdated check, which requires the office to delay deposit until the future date written on the check. If permis-

102 Chapter 6: BOOKKEEPING, CREDIT, AND COLLECTIONS

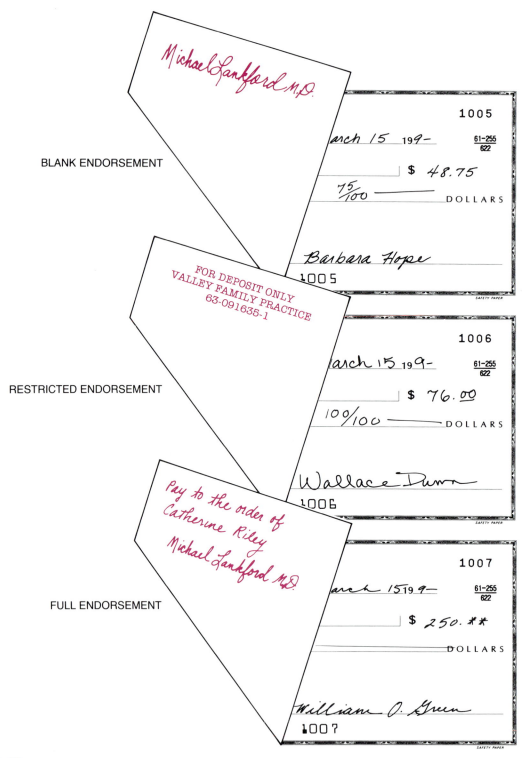

FIGURE 6-18
Types of check endorsements.

sion to write a postdated check is given, the payment should not be entered on the daily journal until the date of the check. This allows the total payments to balance with the daily journal total and prevents the postdated check from being accidentally deposited.

You may use the deposit slips that come with the checkbook or check-writing system or purchase commercial deposit slips that are larger if the office receives a large quantity of checks. One-write systems include deposit slips that are placed on the pegboard, and the check is posted to the deposit slip at the time payment is received.

Establish a systematic method of preparing deposits. The number of errors and the time it takes to complete preparation of a deposit will decrease.

Deposits are generally made in person by transporting the deposit to the bank and presenting it to the teller; however, it may be necessary to make deposits to the night depository if the bank is closed. If so, place the office phone number and contact person's name on the outside of the envelope in case the bank has a question regarding the deposit. Most banks mail a transaction slip that verifies receipt of the night deposit.

To prepare a deposit, refer to Figure 6–19 and use the following procedure as a guideline.

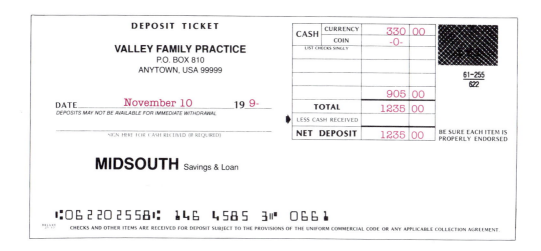

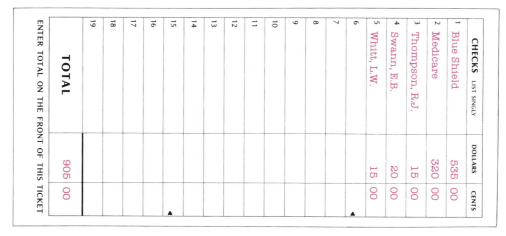

FIGURE 6–19

Bank deposit ticket, front and back.

PROCEDURE

PREPARING A BANK DEPOSIT

PURPOSE

To deposit funds into a business checking account.

MATERIALS AND EQUIPMENT

Deposit slip (Figure 6-19)
Daily receipts
 Checks
 Currency
Pen or typewriter
Adding machine
Endorsement stamp

PROCEDURAL STEPS

1. Verify total cash with the daily journal and separate checks from currency. Arrange the currency with larger bills on top and all bills facing the same direction.
2. Record the total currency and coins onto the deposit slip.
3. Make sure each check is dated correctly and signed.
4. Write or stamp endorsement on the back of each check.
5. Handwrite or type each check separately, entering the patient's name or account number and the amount of the check.
6. Total the check column on the deposit slip, making sure the total agrees with the total amount in checks.
7. Enter total amount of checks.
8. Add total currency and total checks and enter on deposit slip in total deposit column. Make sure total deposit agrees with the total in actual cash and checks. NOTE: Photocopy a file copy of deposit slip back and front or make a carbon copy when completing the deposit slip.
9. Place deposit slip, currency, and checks in an envelope or bank bag for transport to the bank. (Using a bank bag makes one an obvious target. Camouflage the bank bag by putting it in a tote bag, purse, or briefcase during transport.)
10. Enter the deposit amount in the checkbook.

Reconciling a Bank Statement

Each month the bank mails a bank statement that shows the current balance of the checking account as well as a list of the daily transactions, including checks written, deposits, and any other credits such as service charges (Figure 6-20). The purpose of the bank statement is to verify that the balance shown by the bank agrees with the amount shown in the practice checkbook. The balances do not ordinarily agree due to delay in the bank statement reaching the office before other transactions occur. Therefore, a bank reconciliation should be performed to reach an agreement between the bank statement and checkbook.

STATEMENT

Midsouth
Savings and Loan

ACCOUNT NUMBER

4610449

STATEMENT PERIOD

10/31 - 11/29

RESULTING IN A BALANCE OF

BALANCE LAST STATEMENT	WE HAVE ADDED		WE HAVE SUBTRACTED		
	NO.	DEPOSITS/CR	NO.	CHECK/DEBITS	
$3176.42	6	$9460.25	18	$5012.20	$7624.47

SER.CHG.	ITEMS ENCLOSED	MINIMUM BAL.	AVERAGE BAL.	YTD INTEREST
	18	$2309.00	$3896.00	

TYPE OF ACCOUNT..........BUSINESS ACCOUNT

DATE	AMOUNT	DESCRIPTION
11/03	3200.50	DEPOSIT
11/08	1119.00	DEPOSIT
11/12	235.00	DEPOSIT
11/15	2367.75	DEPOSIT
11/18	843.00	DEPOSIT
11/21	1695.00	DEPOSIT

CHECKS

DATE	NO.	AMOUNT	DATE	NO.	AMOUNT
11/01	680	26.97	11/20	689	675.00
11/01	681	800.00	11/21	690	360.20
11/02	682	40.00	11/23	691	55.31
11/03	683	136.11	11/25	692	24.70
11/08	684	17.76	11/26	693	435.33
11/09	685	20.40	11/26	694	614.20
11/14	686	246.89	11/26	695	823.13
11/14	687	541.57	11/27	696	75.00
11/16	688	30.00	11/27	697	89.63

Notice: See reverse side for important information

FIGURE 6-20

Typical bank statement.

PROCEDURE

RECONCILING A BANK STATEMENT

PURPOSE

To verify the accuracy of the bank statement and that the checkbook balance and the bank statement agree.

MATERIALS AND EQUIPMENT

Bank statement/reconciliation form (Figure 6–21)
Checkbook
Calculator or adding machine
Pen or pencil

PROCEDURAL STEPS

1. Enter the amount shown on statement for "Ending Balance."
2. Enter any deposits that have not been credited on the statement.

   - To determine the amounts not credited on the bank statement, compare the statement with the checkbook, placing a checkmark on the checkbook stub beside each deposit credited.
   - Any deposits not checked off have not been credited on the bank statement.

3. Total the amounts in steps 1 and 2 and enter the balance.
4. List separately any checks, payments, transfers, or other withdrawals from your account that are not on the bank statement.

   - To determine the checks, payments, transfers, etc. not credited on the bank statement, compare the statement with the checkbook stub and place a checkmark on the checkbook stub by each amount credited. Verify that the check amount agrees with the amount on the checkbook stub.
   - Any amounts not checked off have not been credited on the bank statement.

5. Enter total amount not credited on bank statement.
6. Subtract line 5 from line 3 and enter balance. This amount is the adjusted bank statement balance.
7. Check the adjusted bank statement balance with the amount shown in the checkbook. The amounts should be the same. If they do not agree, follow the steps below to reconcile the checkbook to the adjusted bank statement balance.

   - Enter the ending checkbook balance.
   - Add any deposits, interest payments, etc. shown on the bank statement but not on checkbook.
   - Subtract service charges, automatic teller charges, etc. not shown on checkbook.
   - The resulting balance is the adjusted checkbook balance and should agree with the adjusted bank statement balance.

8. If the balances still do not agree, check your addition and subtraction on the statement worksheet and checkbook. Recheck all checks and deposits and verify that the amount on the statement is the same on the checkbook.

COMMON ERRORS THAT PREVENT RECONCILIATION OF A BANK STATEMENT

- Deposits made but omitted from the checkbook
- Checks omitted from checkbook
- Incorrect recording of checks or deposits on checkbook (if the amount of the error is divisible by 9, a transposition of figures may be the problem)
- Addition and subtraction errors on the statement worksheet or checkbook

BANK STATEMENT RECONCILIATION
MONTH OF _July_ 19 _____

BANK STATEMENT

Current balance on statement........ $ _17,858.82_

Total deposits not on statement...... + _1,645.50_

SUBTOTAL................................ _19,504.32_

Total checks not on statement........ − _824.15_

BALANCE................................ [_18,680.17_]

CHECK BOOK REGISTER

Current balance in register............ $ _18,687.17_

Total deposits not in register.......... + _-0-_

SUBTOTAL................................ _18,687.17_

Total checks not in register............ − _-0-_

Service charges or other debits...... − _7.00_

BALANCE................................ [_18,680.17_]

[OUTSTANDING CHECKS]	
[CK NO]	AMOUNT
[366]	14.56
[367]	52.01
[368]	175.00
[369]	44.54
[370]	81.00
[371]	16.98
[372]	17.43
[373]	339.22
[374]	54.81
[375]	28.60
[ ]	.
[ ]	.
[ ]	.
[ ]	.
[ ]	.
[ ]	.
[ ]	.
[ ]	.
[ ]	.
[TOTAL	824.15]

FIGURE 6–21
Bank statement with reconciliation.

FEE COLLECTION POLICY

OFFICE VISITS

We ask that you pay for routine office fees, laboratory tests, x-rays, etc. at the time service is rendered. If you have insurance coverage for such services with whom the physician has a participating agreement, you must pay the copayment and deductibles at the time service is rendered. If the insurance claim is rejected, you are responsible for paying the entire fee. If someone other than you is responsible for paying office fees but will not be present with you, advance arrangements must be made.

SURGERY

In the event that you require surgery whether in the office or in the hospital, we will file a claim with your insurance company. You are responsible for any amount not covered under the insurance policy.

HOSPITALIZATION

The physician will charge a separate fee from the hospital fee for services rendered while you are in the hospital. We will file a claim with your insurance company. You are responsible for any amount not covered under the insurance policy.

CREDIT ARRANGEMENTS

If you require extensive treatment resulting in a large fee, not otherwise covered by your insurance policy, we will cooperate with you by agreeing to a credit arrangement.

You will be required to complete a credit application, and if the agreement results in payments being made in more than four installments, you will be required to sign a Truth In Lending Statement as required by federal law. We request that you ask to see the office manager as soon as you realize the need for credit arrangements.

ELECTIVE PROCEDURES

If you have a procedure performed that is considered elective and not covered by your insurance policy, you are asked to pay for the procedure in advance. Credit arrangements are not available for elective procedures.

INSURANCE POLICY

The physician has a participating agreement with Blue Cross Blue Shield and Medicare only. We do not routinely accept Medicaid, Champus, or other commercial insurance (Aetna, Prudential, etc.). However, in the event of surgery or hospitalization, we will file a claim with your insurance company.

You are responsible for paying copayments and deductibles for office fees at the time of service, and for any services rejected by the insurance company.

FIGURE 6-22
Typical fee collection policy.

CREDIT AND COLLECTIONS

Establishing a Credit and Collection System

Issues involved in establishing a credit and collection system include (a) educating the office staff and distributing tasks, (b) discussing fees with patients, (c) establishing fee collection policies (fee for service, credit card billing, and third-party reimbursement), (d) establishing credit terms and conditions, (e) setting up billing methods and a timetable for follow-up, (f) considering the use of outside agencies for collection follow-up, and (g) monitoring the effectiveness of billing and collection procedures.

Educating the Office Staff

The best way to prevent poor collections is to make sure the staff is well informed. Designate one staff member to coordinate the credit and collection system, implement policy, and educate the rest of the staff. Regular staff meetings improve interoffice relations, promote teamwork, and reduce errors. Staff meetings can be used to

- Review credit and collection policies,
- Define staff responsibilities and assign tasks,
- Discuss problems and consider alternative solutions,
- Offer suggestions on how to communicate professionally with patients when discussing fees,
- Set collection goals,
- Motivate and recognize staff accomplishments.

Setting Fees

The criteria used by physicians to set fees may include some or all of the following:

- Fees charged by other physicians in the geographic area.
- Location of the practice.
- Size of the practice or clinic, number of services offered, cost of operating the practice such as salaries, utilities, rent, equipment & supplies, etc.
- Experience and education of physician.

The fee schedule should be typed and updated periodically as fees change. The fee schedule must be made available to patients if requested. When fees change, a notice should be posted in the waiting room and at the cashier's window.

Discussing Fees with Patients

In addition to educating the staff, taking the time to inform patients of the fee policy results in fewer misunderstandings, reduces the possibility of embarrassment, and improves rapport between all parties concerned. If patients feel they received discourteous treatment, they may initiate litigation or seek treatment elsewhere.

The appropriate time to inform patients of office policy is in advance of their first office visit. This can be done several ways, including

- On the telephone when appointment is first made
- In an information brochure (Figure 6–22)
- On the patient registration form
- In a welcome letter mailed in advance of first visit
- In person with designated staff member before the patient is called back to see physician

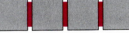

PROCEDURE

DISCUSSING FEES WITH PATIENTS

PURPOSE

To reduce misunderstandings about the costs of medical care and to increase the effectiveness of collections.

MATERIALS AND EQUIPMENT

Private area where discussion can be confidential
Patient's ledger card
Fee schedule
Insurance form
Pen

PROCEDURAL STEPS

1. Speak slowly, clearly, and distinctly. Display professionalism at all times, but try to make the patient feel comfortable.

2. Refer to the fee schedule and make a copy available to the patient if requested.
3. Inform the patient of the fee collection policy:

   - Fee for service,
   - Credit card billing,
   - Third-party reimbursement.

4. Allow the patient to respond and ask questions.
5. If insurance assignment is accepted, have appropriate claim form completed and signed by patient. Make assignment notation on the patient's ledger card.
6. If other third-party reimbursement is accepted as payment, ask for proper authorization form, etc. Make appropriate notation on the patient's ledger card.
7. End the conversation if no potential problems are detected.

If a patient indicates that he or she is unable to pay, the physician will have to decide whether to treat the patient and discount the fee or refer the patient to an appropriate resource agency that provides indigent patient care. However, it may be possible to counsel the patient and set up credit arrangements (see MAKING CREDIT ARRANGEMENTS procedure).

Collecting Fees

Fee for Service. Fee for service is the process of requesting payment at the time services are rendered. This system of collection ensures constant cash flow, reduces time and cost of billing, and eliminates the time-consuming process of seeking third-party reimbursement.

Credit Card Billing. Another method of paying for fees is through credit card billing such as Visa, MasterCard, or American Express. This method allows patients to charge their bill on a credit card so that payment in full is made to the physician, and the patient makes payments to the credit card company.

The practice can accept credit cards for payment of office fees by applying at the bank where the practice normally does business. The bank may charge a handling fee to the practice for credit card billing.

Third-Party Reimbursement. Third-party reimbursement involves billing someone other than the patient for payment of services rendered. The most common third-party reimbursers are insurance companies and Worker's Compensation.

Insurance reimbursement requires handling through a billing process separate from the regular billing cycle. Instructions for insurance billing are given in Chapter 8.

Worker's Compensation programs are mandatory according to state law and provide medical benefits for workers involved in accidents or unintended conditions resulting from employment. The patient usually presents a letter from the employer that authorizes payment of services. Coverage is limited to the patient's Worker's Compensation case, and any unrelated services provided will not be paid.

SPECIAL HINT

The patient is responsible for paying for the unrelated services and should be informed of this in advance.

The charges for authorized services are entered on a ledger card in the company's name. Unrelated charges are posted on the patient's ledger card. All billing is sent to the company, not the patient. Each company may have specific requirements in submitting Worker's Compensation claims, but this can usually be integrated into the routine billing process.

Credit Arrangements. The terms and conditions for extending credit must be fair and applicable to the majority of the patient population served. The Federal Equal Credit Opportunity Act prohibits discrimination in extending credit on the basis of race, color, religion, national origin, sex, marital status, or age. The same credit terms that are extended to one patient must also be extended to all other patients. Refusal to extend credit can be based only on the patient's ability or inability to pay. Patients have the right to ask for an explanation in writing if credit is refused.

When there is a specific agreement between the patient and practice for payments to be made in more than four installments, Regulation Z of the Truth in Lending Act mandates that the practice provide written documentation in the form of a disclosure statement. Figure 6–23 meets the requirements of such an agreement.

Whether the practice charges interest or not, the form must be completed and signed by the patient. If no specific agreement is made and the practice bills the patient on open account, no disclosure form is necessary, even if more than four installments are made.

Complete personal and financial information should be on file to facilitate collection follow-up. The patient registration form (Chapter 2) may be adequate; however, some practices prefer to have the patient complete a credit application.

Because changes in addresses, phone numbers, employment, etc. occur periodically, frequent update is necessary. Updating may be achieved by:

- Developing an update form that can be kept at the receptionist's window where patients sign in;
- Providing space on the sign-in sheet for changes in address, phone number, insurance benefits, etc.; or
- Making it a habit to ask patients when they sign in if there has been a change in their address, phone number, insurance benefits, etc.

(Practice Name and Address Here)

FEDERAL TRUTH IN LENDING STATEMENT

PATIENT NAME: Deborah Moore

ADDRESS: 2360 Rayburn Street

Anytown, USA 99999

NAME OF RESPONSIBLE PARTY: Same as patient

* * * * * * *

1. Total Fee For Services	$ 800.00
2. Less Down Payment	200.00
3. Unpaid Balance	600.00
4. Amount Financed	600.00
5. FINANCE CHARGE	NONE
6. ANNUAL PERCENTAGE RATE	NONE
7. Total Number of Payments	6
8. Total Payment Due	600.00

The total payment (#8 above) is payable to Dr. Joan Saye, at the above practice address, to be paid in 6 monthly installments of $100.00 each. The first installment is due on May 1, 199-, and all subsequent payments on the same date each month until paid in full.

April 16, 199-
Date

Signature of Patient or Responsible Party

FIGURE 6-23

Truth in lending statement.

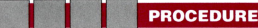

PROCEDURE
MAKING CREDIT ARRANGEMENTS

PURPOSE

To secure payment yet accommodate the patient's financial situation if possible.

MATERIALS AND EQUIPMENT

Private area where conversation can be confidential
Patient's ledger card
Truth in Lending form
Typewriter
Calendar

PROCEDURAL STEPS

Discussion should be between responsible party and designated staff member.

1. Allow the patient to discuss his or her financial situation and ask questions.
2. Inform the patient of credit terms and conditions.
3. Allow the patient to suggest a payment amount.
4. If acceptable within scope of credit policy, accept patient request. If not, suggest alternative and reach agreement.
5. Make necessary notations on the patient's ledger.
6. Have the patient complete a credit application, if necessary.
7. If payment arrangement is for more than four installments, prepare Truth in Lending Statement and ask the patient to sign it.
8. Make a carbon or photocopy of the Truth in Lending statement for the patient and keep original in a confidential file.

Billing Patients

Billing involves the process of mailing patients statements reflecting the balance owed. Statements are usually mailed to patients once a month, near the same date each month, and at a time that most other household bills are being mailed. Figure 6–24 is a sample statement prepared on a statement form. Other types of statements are

- A photocopy of the patient's ledger cards reflecting all transactions
- Handwritten or typed statements generated from the patient's ledger card showing only the current month's transactions
- Handwritten or typed statements reflecting only the balance due
- Statements prepared from the patient's ledger card by an outside billing service
- Computer-generated statements (see Chapter 9)

Billing Methods

Monthly billing: All patients' statements are mailed out at one time.

Cycle billing: Patient accounts are divided into two to four alphabetical sections, and statements are mailed at two to four specified time periods during the month. For example, the accounts may be divided into A–L and M–Z, with A–L statements being mailed on the 15th of the month and M–Z statements on the 25th of the month.

STATEMENT

Date July 25, 199-

Betsy S. Putnum
1212 Stark Street
Anytown, USA 99999

TERMS:

PLEASE DETACH AND RETURN WITH YOUR REMITTANCE

$ ....
AMOUNT ENCLOSED

DATE	DESCRIPTION	CHARGES	CREDITS	✓	BALANCE
	BALANCE FORWARD ▷				35.00
07/1/9-	Office Visit, X-ray	70 00	-0-		105 00
	-PLEASE REMIT-				
7/24/9-	CURRENT BALANCE				$105 00

⇧
PAY LAST
AMOUNT
IN THIS
COLUMN

Thank You

FIGURE 6–24

Patient statement. (Redrawn with permission from Colwell Systems, Inc.)

PROCEDURE

BILLING PATIENTS MANUALLY

PURPOSE

To secure payment when fees were not paid at the time of visit.

MATERIALS AND EQUIPMENT

Patient ledger cards
Blank statement forms
Collection timetable
Typewriter

PROCEDURAL STEPS

Current Accounts

1. Review patient ledger to determine current status. If past due, transfer ledger to the file for past due accounts.
2. Prepare patient statement (see Figure 6–24).

   - Insert blank statement form into typewriter.
   - Type name and address of responsible party.
   - Type patient's name if different from responsible party.
   - Enter balance at beginning of month.
   - Enter all transactions for the current month (date, description, fee, payment, and balance).
   - Add appropriate citation ("Please Remit," "Insurance Pending," etc.)

3. Fold statement and insert into a window envelope along with a return envelope.
4. Repeat steps 1–3 for all current accounts.

Past Due Accounts

1. Review patient ledger card and determine action to be taken (check timetable for collection follow-up).
2. Make notation on patient ledger card or use colored tab.
3. Prepare statement as in step 2 in Current Accounts.
4. Prepare collection letter, if appropriate.
5. Fold statement and collection letter and insert into a window envelope along with a return envelope.
6. Repeat steps 1–5 for all past due accounts.

Collecting Past Due Accounts

Figure 6–25 shows a typical timetable used to facilitate collection follow-up. The timetable allows the aging of patient accounts to determine the number of days an account is past due. As long as payments are being made regularly on open account or per agreement, the account remains current and aging is delayed. On accounts that are past due, a series of collection letters mailed with the statement often prompts the patient into action. The request for payment becomes stronger with each letter mailed. Figure 6–26 shows a series of typical collection letters.

SPECIAL HINT

Always make a notation on the ledger indicating action taken, such as "Letter #1 mailed April 25." Different-colored tabs or sticky labels, representing the type of action taken at each billing cycle, may be used to mark the accounts. Using a color-coded system saves time over writing a notation on each ledger and serves as a reminder of what action will be needed at the next billing cycle.

Tips for Tracing Skips

When a billing statement is returned undeliverable, the practice should immediately begin a trace to locate the patient's correct address. Some problems in skip tracing can be resolved by having the billing envelopes preprinted with the statement "Address Correction Requested." For a fee, the post office will forward bills to a new address and notify the practice of the change. The following are suggestions for tracing skips:

Review the address for typing errors, correct zip code, etc.

TIMETABLE FOR COLLECTION FOLLOW UP

Time of Service

First request: Ask for payment and/or confirm fee collection agreement (fee for service, statement billing, credit card billing, third-party reimbursement, or credit arrangements). Collect copayments and deductibles on insurance claims.

Less Than 30 Days

Second request: Mail statement marked "Please Remit."

30 to 60 Days

Third request: Mail billing statement and collection letter 1. Make notation (or place colored tab) on patient ledger card. Within 15 days of collection letter, telephone patient to inquire and obtain commitment for date when payment will be made. Make notation on patient ledger card.

60 to 90 Days

Mail collection letter 2: Make notation (or use colored tab) on patient ledger card.

90 to 120 Days

Mail collection letter 3: Final notice. Give patient 15 days to respond, then turn account over to collector. Make notation (or use colored tab) on patient ledger card.

FIGURE 6-25

Typical timetable for collection follow-up.

- Compare the address with data shown on the patient's registration form.
- Send the patient the statement in a plain envelope by certified mail with return receipt, which requires the patient's signature. The patient will be curious enough to sign for the envelope. The receipt is returned to the office, verifying the correct address.
- Call the patient's employer to inquire if the patient is currently employed; however, do not disclose reason for call.
- Call the person listed to contact in case of emergency, being careful not to disclose any personal or financial information.
- Call referring physician's office, if applicable, to request most recent address and phone number on file.
- If the patient has been recently hospitalized, check with the admissions office for current address and phone number.
- Checking the city directory, locate neighbors to find out if the patient has moved.
- If the patient is a member of a community or professional organization, call and leave a message for the patient, being careful not to disclose the reason for call. The member who answers the phone may unconsciously volunteer information that will be helpful.
- Call the patient's health insurance company. Supply the patient's policy number and ask if the patient is still covered under the policy. Ask if the patient has submitted a change of address.
- If the practice is a member of the local credit bureau, call and request most recent address and phone number on file for the patient.
- Check also with schools, banks, utility companies, and moving companies.

Telephone Collection

Guidelines

1. Verify current information for accuracy before making the call.
2. Review previous payment habits of patient and success of previous collection steps, such

COLLECTION LETTER #1

[Current date]

[Patient name]
[Street address]
[City, state, zip]

Dear

We did not receive your payment last month, and thought that perhaps you just overlooked it.

Unfortunately, the account is now past due, but immediate payment will bring it back up to current status.

Please telephone me now if you intend to delay payment more than ten days so that further action to collect will not be undertaken.

Sincerely,

Nedra Woodress
Business Manager

FIGURE 6-26A-D

Various sample collection letters.

COLLECTION LETTER #2

[Current date]

[Patient name]
[Street Address]
[City, state, zip]

Dear

Since you did not respond to the previous correspondence, I assume that an unusual situation is preventing you from making payment.

You may be relieved to know that our office extends credit terms to patients with unusual circumstances. We also accept Visa, Mastercard, and American Express.

In order for your credit to be protected, you must contact us to make credit arrangements or mail payment immediately to delay further action against your account.

Sincerely,

Nedra Woodress
Business Manager

FIGURE 6-26 *Continued*

COLLECTION LETTER #3

[Current date]

[Patient name]
[Street address]
[City, state, zip]

Dear

We regret that you have not responded to previous requests for payment. We provided service in good faith with the understanding that you would pay on a timely basis.

Because you have not fulfilled your obligation, we must now submit your name to the credit bureau and turn your account over to a professional collection agency.

We will protect your account for _____ more days before taking action, should you wish to clear your balance.

Sincerely,

Nedra Woodress
Business Manager

FIGURE 6-26 *Continued*

---

as letters, personal interviews, or telephone calls.
3. Determine a strategy for obtaining a promise to pay.
4. Speak only with the individual responsible for the bill.
5. Identify yourself.
6. Give the reason for the call.
7. Be courteous but firm; speak naturally but confidently.
8. Be sympathetic, but remain poised and in control.
9. Ask for payment in full then wait for a response.
10. Obtain a commitment, summarize the payment plan, and then end the call.
11. Make a note of the payment plan with the date and your initials on the back of the patient's ledger card.

Situations to Avoid

- Using words or phrases that incite defensive behavior, argument, or anger from the patient.
- Calling so frequently that the patient claims harassment.
- Calling the patient after 9:00 P.M. and before 8:00 A.M.
- Discussing the nature of the call with anyone other than the person responsible for the bill, including employers, relatives, neighbors, and co-workers.
- Calling the patient's place of employment repeatedly or at all if you know it is prohibited.

Collection Agencies

If the physician agrees that delinquent accounts will be turned over to a collection agency, a few considerations should be observed. Only an

COLLECTION LETTER #4

[Current date]

[Patient name]
[Street address]
[City, state, zip]

Dear

Because you have failed to pay for services rendered to you, I must withdraw from extending further medical care to you.

Regretfully, your refusal to pay has resulted in your name being given to the credit bureau and to our collection agency.

For a period of _____ days, I will provide emergency care and treatment during which time you should select another physician. With your written authorization, I will forward a copy of your medical record to your new physician.

Sincerely,

_____, M.D.

FIGURE 6-26 *Continued*

agency that is licensed and bonded should be selected. The agency's reputation should be investigated, to make sure it adheres to collection laws, and references of clientele who have used the agency in the past 2 years should be requested. The agency should be required to submit weekly or monthly reports itemizing the collection status of each patient account. Terms and conditions should be put in writing, and a record of the agency's success rate in collecting what is owed should be kept.

Once the patient's account is turned over to a collector, the practice is not to mail any further statements or make any payment arrangements with the patient. If payments are mistakenly mailed to the practice, the collection agency must be notified.

At this point, the physician may want to dismiss the patient from his or her care, and a certified letter with return receipt should be mailed (see Figure 6-26D). In addition, the accountant may suggest that the account be written off to bad debt (see Special Accounting Entries).

Small Claims Court

If the practice does not use a collection agency, the physician may choose to file a claim in small claims court. However, there is a minimum amount per claim that can be presented in court for judgment. The amount varies according to state regulations. Once a judgment has been issued, it is final, and the physician still must collect the amount owed from the patient, which is often difficult.

Starting a Claim in Small Claims Court

1. The practice must file a Statement of Claim (Figure 6-27), which can be obtained from the small claims court clerk.

120 Chapter 6: BOOKKEEPING, CREDIT, AND COLLECTIONS

| State of Alabama
Unified Judicial System
Adm. Office of Courts
Form SM-1 Rev 8/77 | STATEMENT OF CLAIM
(Complaint)
General | Case Number
SM ___ _____
ID   YR   Number |

IN THE SMALL CLAIMS COURT OF _____ COUNTY

Plaintiff   Against   Defendant
Address   Address

Attorney   Attorney
Address   Address

Date of
  Filing _____   Additional
                                                Defendants

NOTICE TO EACH DEFENDANT—READ CAREFULLY

You are being sued in the Small Claims Court by the Plaintiff(s) shown above, THE JUDGE HAS NOT YET MADE ANY DECISION IN THIS CASE, AND YOU HAVE THE RIGHT TO A TRIAL TO TELL YOUR SIDE.

HOWEVER, IF YOU FAIL TO TAKE ANY ACTION TO PROTECT YOUR RIGHTS WITHIN 14 DAYS AFTER THESE PAPERS WERE DELIVERED TO YOU, A COURT JUDGMENT CAN BE TAKEN AGAINST YOU FOR THE MONEY OR PROPERTY DEMANDED IN THE FOLLOWING COMPLAINT. THIS COULD LEAD TO GARNISHMENT OF YOUR PAYCHECK AND/OR SALE OF YOUR HOME OR OTHER BELONGINGS, UNLESS PROTECTED BY LAW, TO SATISFY THAT JUDGMENT.

TO PREVENT THIS, YOU OR YOUR LAWYER MUST FILL OUT THE ENCLOSED ANSWER FORM, AND DELIVER OR MAIL A COPY TO THE COURT, AT THE ADDRESS SHOWN ABOVE, SO IT WILL ARRIVE AT THE COURT WITHIN 14 DAYS AFTER THESE PAPERS WERE DELIVERED TO YOU. INSTRUCTIONS FOR THIS ARE ON THE BACK OF THE ANSWER FORM ITSELF. (If you did not receive an Answer form, call the Court IMMEDIATELY to obtain another form.) YOU WILL THEN BE NOTIFIED OF THE DATE AND TIME OF YOUR TRIAL. If you have questions or need assistance with your Answer, see a lawyer or call or come by the Court.

COMPLAINT

1. Plaintiff claims the defendant owes _____ the sum of $_____ because:

2. Plaintiff also claims from the defendant court costs in the sum of $_____ (see note below), plus $_____ for interest and $_____ for lawyers fees (**only** if plaintiff is represented by a licensed, practicing attorney.)

   NOTE: The total amount of court costs may be more than this amount when the case is finally settled. The clerk will inform you of any additional costs at the close of the case.

_____   [   ]   _____
Clerk (Signature)   (Deputy Clerk   Plaintiff or Attorney (Signature)
                               Initials)

ADDRESS:
                                               PHONE NO. _____
PHONE NO. _____
                        COURT RECORD (White)   SEE INSTRUCTIONS ON THE BACK

FIGURE 6-27

Statement of claim. (Reprinted with permission from Supreme Court, State of Alabama.)

COLLECTION RATIO		
Total payments year to date		$ 74,893
Divided by charges year to date	$ 81,280	
Less adjustments (insurance nonallowed, discounts, etc.)	$ 1,126	$ 80,154
Equals collection ratio		93%

FIGURE 6-28
Collection ratio computation.

ACCOUNTS RECEIVABLE AGING RECORD

Date: Prepared By: Page ____ of ____

No.	Account Name	1–30	30–60	60–90	90–120	120+	Balance Owed

FIGURE 6-29
Accounts receivable aging record.

2. Type the information requested on the form. Make sure the claim is accurate and complete.
3. Submit the completed form to the small claims court clerk.
4. A court date will be set, and the clerk will send the patient a summons to appear in court, usually delivered by the county sheriff.
5. On the day of court, be present with patient's account and other documentation (disclosure statement signed by patient, etc.).
6. The trial will be a simple, informal hearing before the judge, who will review the claim and issue judgment.
7. If the judge requires the patient to pay amount owed, ask the patient to pay immediately.
8. If patient refuses to pay, the practice may obtain a court order to garnish the patient's wages.

Collection Ratio

Compute the collection rate each month to determine the success of overall collection efforts. Most accountants agree that the average collection ratio should be better than 90%. Figure 6–28 shows the computation of a collection ratio.

Preparing an Accounts Receivable Aging Record

The accounts receivable aging record is a report derived from the patient ledgers. The record reflects the status of individual patient accounts, with the amount owed designated in the appropriate column for the number of days past due (Figure 6–29). Preparing the report is time consuming, but it is beneficial in evaluating the results of collection efforts and making decisions for action to be taken.

Preparing a Monthly Accounts Receivable Analysis

Preparing a monthly accounts receivable analysis provides the physician with a status of the

MONTHLY ACCOUNT ANALYSIS	
Period Ending: June 199-	
LESS THAN 60 DAYS	$ 21,260
60 TO 90 DAYS	13,866
90 TO 120 DAYS	7,344
OVER 120 DAYS (COLLECTIONS)	$ 11,592
TOTAL OUTSTANDING	$ 54,062

FIGURE 6–30

Monthly accounts analysis.

amounts owed and reflects the effectiveness of the credit and collection procedures. Figure 6–30 shows a sample account analysis with the amounts owed broken down by the number of days past due. If the total of amounts owed is greater than 2 months' average charges, the credit and collection procedures should be reevaluated.

Bibliography

American Medical Association: *The Business Side of Medical Office*. Chicago: American Medical Association, 1989.

Fordney M, Follis J: *Administrative Medical Assisting*, 2nd ed. Media, PA: Harwal, 1988.

Frew M, Frew D: *Comprehensive Medical Assisting: Administrative and Clinical Procedures*, 2nd ed. Philadelphia: F.A. Davis, 1988.

Kinn M, Derge E: *The Medical Assistant: Administrative and Clinical*, 6th ed. Philadelphia: W. B. Saunders, 1988.

Medical Management Institute: *Collections, Coding and Insurance Management*. Alpharetta, GA: Medical Management Institute, 1987.

Safeguard Business Systems: *How to Improve Medical Office Financial Controls*. Fort Washington, PA: Safeguard Business Systems,

Chapter 7

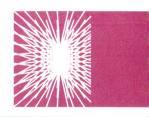

ACCOUNTING AND TAXES

DEBORAH A. STANDEFER

ACCOUNTING
Accounting Methods
Chart of Accounts
Revenue
Expenditures
Balance Sheet
Income Statement
Analysis of Profit and Loss

Cost Analysis of Services and Cost Procedures
Budget

TAXES
Property Tax
State Tax
Federal Taxes

Accounts payable: These are short-term liabilities, arising from the purchase of merchandise or services.
Accounts receivable: Services or goods have been received by the customer, but payment in full has not been made. This is the unpaid balance.
Assets: Things of value owned, including cash, accounts receivable, land, buildings, equipment, etc.
Budget: The annual estimate of revenue and expenditures.
Capital: Represents the amount by which the assets exceed the liabilities.
Cost accounting: The process of accumulating the costs and identifying with the services rendered.
Cost analysis: The practice of matching receipts and expenses of like kind.
Expense: Costs incurred by the business in the process of earning revenue.
Income (revenue): Earned by providing a service for patients. The revenue earned is measured by the assets received in exchange, usually in the form of cash or an account receivable.
Income statement: Shows the revenues and the costs and expenses associated with those revenues. The net effect of this statement is the net income or loss of a company for the operations of a specific period of time.
Liabilities: Debts, that is, the amounts owed to others.

ACCOUNTING

Keeping accurate records in the medical practice is critical to its success, and a degree in accounting is not required to do it! A medical assistant can gather information and prepare reports, which saves a considerable amount of money in accounting fees and is a valuable asset to any practice.

Accounting Methods

An *accounting method* is a systematic recording and evaluating of business activities. This information provides a basis to plan, coordinate, and control the growth and direction of a medical practice.

There are basically two methods of accounting: *accrual* (reporting of all revenues in the period earned, all expenses in the period consumed, all assets in the period purchased, and all liabilities in the period incurred; this method is generally used by a business that sells goods) and cash basis accounting. In this chapter, our primary focus is on cash basis accounting.

Cash basis accounting recognizes revenue when it is received and expenses when they are paid out. This method is most often used in service-related businesses, for example, a medical practice. The primary order of business is providing a service in return for payment. For example,

- A patient receives service on February 25. The charge is posted to accounts receivable.
- The patient makes payment on March 10. The payment is posted as taxable income.

After selecting a method of accounting, it becomes necessary to decide on practice goals. As is true with any business, the medical practice needs to know where it wants to go in order to get there. Set goals similar to those illustrated in Figure 7–1. Goal setting is an important first step in establishing an effective accounting system. Draw on the expertise of the staff, accountant, attorney, financial advisor, and others entrusted with practice information. After goals are identified, they should be written down.

After you have set the goals of the practice, select the reports that will help track those goals. Then determine what data are needed to produce each report. The computer is especially useful because of its ability to generate a great variety of reports and statistics at the touch of a button (see Chapter 9).

Chart of Accounts

The *chart of accounts* is a listing of all accounts used in the practice. It should be as detailed and flexible as necessary to itemize the points of interest you want to track in your practice and revised annually to add new accounts or to delete categories no longer needed.

Each different type of income or expense that makes up the day-to-day operation of the practice is assigned a category (asset, liability, capital, income, or expense) and account title with a number. The account number corresponds to the category, for example,

assets — 1000
liabilities — 2000
capital — 3000
income — 4000
expense — 6000

The list of these accounts by category is the *chart of accounts* (Figure 7–2).

Referring to the chart of accounts in Figure 7–2, notice the numbers assigned for "Accounts Receivable" (#1210) and "Accounts Payable" (#2200). In the cash basis of accounting, no figures are actually posted to these general ledger accounts during the day-to-day business. However, these categories should remain on the chart of accounts to indicate to a bank or investor that there are additional monies that affect the financial position of the practice.

Revenue

Revenue can be recorded on a computer or manually. Within the framework of either method of entry, payments are received and recorded as revenue. It is important to record revenue so there is a permanent record for income taxes, planning, and monitoring the business.

Recording Transactions

All transactions for the day are recorded on a *day sheet* (Figure 7–3). The day sheet contains the names of the patients seen each day, the amount charged for medical services rendered, any money collected, and any adjustment made on an account (for example, refund, Medicare or Medicaid write-off, etc.). Tailor the day sheet to include columns to break down laboratory or x-

Goal	What I Need to Reach It
Income tax preparation	Income statement
	Balance sheet (with all items reconciled)
	List of any assets purchased or sold
	New loan, rent, or lease agreements
Time off with my family	Adequate income
	Schedule office hours 4 days
	Leave office by 5:00 P.M.
Retire at age 55	Adequate income
	Pension plan
Healthy practice	Happy patients
	Physician currency in field
	Stocked and comfortable facility
	Well-trained, well-compensated staff

FIGURE 7–1

Tailor your own practical goals.

N.O. Payne, M.D., Solo Practice
Chart of Accounts

Account #	Account Title	Category
1012	Savings in ABC Bank	Checking/Savings
1020	Checking Account XYZ Bank	Checking/Savings
1210	Accounts Receivable	Accounts Receivable
1710	Machinery and Equipment	Fixed Assets
1810	Accumulated Depreciation—Machinery and Equipment	Other Assets
2200	Accounts Payable	Accounts Payable
2320	Payroll Tax (Federal, Medicare, and Social Security) Payable	Other Current Liabilities
2330	Payroll Tax (State Employment Security) Payable	Other Current Liabilities
2340	Payroll Tax (Federal Unemployment—FUTA) Payable	Other Current Liabilities
3999	Retained Earnings (for Corporation) or Owner's (or Partner's) Equity (for Owner/Partner)	Capital
4100	Professional Services—Fees	Income
4101	Laboratory Income	Income
4110	Refund	Income
4200	Recovery of Bad Debts	Income
4201	Other Income	Income
6050	Conference and Training	Expense
6060	Depreciation	Expense
6080	Drugs and Medical Supplies	Expense
6090	Dues and Subscriptions	Expense
6100	Employees' Benefits and Expenses	Expense
6110	Equipment Leased	Expense
6130	Bank Charges and NSF checks	Expense
6140	Insurance	Expense
6160	Janitorial	Expense
6165	Laboratory Expense	Expense
6170	Legal and Accounting	Expense
6200	Office Supplies	Expense
6210	Outside Laboratory	Expense
6250	Rent	Expense
6260	Repairs and Maintenance	Expense
6270	Salaries	Expense
6320	Taxes—Payroll	Expense
6350	Taxes and License	Expense
6370	Utilities and Telephone	Expense
6380	Miscellaneous	Expense

FIGURE 7-2
Chart of accounts.

Chapter 7: ACCOUNTING AND TAXES

Day sheet for 03/12/92

Account/Name	Starting Bal	Charges	Payments	Adjustments	Final Bal	Cash	Checks	Credit Card
1337 Able Body	0.00	36.00	36.00	0.00	0.00	0.00	36.00	0.00
1322 Martha Crock	0.00	208.00	0.00	0.00	208.00	0.00	0.00	0.00
1198 Tom Jones	828.00	0.00	622.40	0.00	165.60	0.00	662.40	0.00
1186 Elvis Presley	1800.00	0.00	1440.00	0.00	360.00	0.00	1440.00	0.00
0956 Mario Andreti	1170.00	0.00	1170.00	0.00	0.00	0.00	1170.00	0.00
0440 Vicki Best	391.20	0.00	271.20	0.00	120.00	0.00	271.20	0.00
1122 John Better	1061.00	0.00	1008.00	0.00	53.00	0.00	1008.00	0.00
0105 Mary Ledger	83.60	0.00	50.00	0.00	33.60	0.00	50.00	0.00
1155 Jean Label	6.60	0.00	6.60	0.00	0.00	0.00	6.60	0.00
1304 Shawn Piper	36.00	828.00	0.00	0.00	864.00	0.00	0.00	0.00
1338 Doris Treestem	0.00	53.00	0.00	0.00	53.00	0.00	0.00	0.00
1174 Lois Lane	36.00	489.00	0.00	0.00	525.00	0.00	0.00	0.00
1317 Clark Kent	0.00	684.00	0.00	0.00	684.00	0.00	0.00	0.00
1320 Martha Maple	36.00	1170.00	0.00	0.00	1206.00	0.00	0.00	0.00
1339 Ray Cheddar	0.00	36.00	36.00	0.00	0.00	0.00	36.00	0.00
1192 Timothy Bear	187.20	0.00	187.20	0.00	0.00	0.00	187.20	0.00
1339 Ted Baer	0.00	0.00	165.60	0.00	(165.60)	0.00	165.60	0.00
1341 April Showers	0.00	36.00	36.00	0.00	0.00	36.00	0.00	0.00
1343 June Bugg	0.00	36.00	0.00	0.00	36.00	0.00	0.00	0.00
TOTALS	5635.60	3576.00	5069.00	0.00	4142.60	36.00	5033.00	0.00

FIGURE 7-3

Day sheet.

ray income or, in a group practice, to separate income by physician. Separate numbers may be used to code each physician's income or to code income and expense by facility and/or department.

Computerized systems (like the one illustrated in Figure 7-3) include a column for the patient's account receivable number. This number offers another method to retrieve the account.

Revenue Sources

Payments come from either a patient or a third-party payer. Some examples of third parties are

Medicare; Medicaid; Worker's Compensation; and companies contracted to provide service, such as a health maintenance organization or a preferred provider organization. In cash basis accounting, *revenue* is the amount of money actually received, regardless of the amount charged.

In cash basis accounting the amount charged is not taxed when billed, but the amount charged is tracked. This amount is called *accounts receivable*. It is systematically tracked through a record, sometimes referred to as *accounts receivable control*.

Accounts Receivable Control. At the day's end, an accounts receivable control is generated, using the transactions from the day sheet (Figure 7–4). This record begins with the balance carried forward from the close of the prior day *(beginning accounts receivable balance)*. It contains a cumulative total of the day's charges, payments, and adjustments. The calculation of all of these figures results in the *New Accounts Receivable Balance*.

Accounts receivable are tracked throughout the life of the practice by carrying this procedure forward from one day to the next. The dollar amount in the month-to-date total payments column at month's end should balance with the amount of money deposited into the bank under #4100 "Professional Services—Fees" for the same time period (see Figure 7–2). This "mini-audit" ensures against embezzlement and is a cross-check that deposits throughout the month were entered correctly.

SPECIAL HINTS

- In order for the month-to-date total payments column and the amount of money deposited under number 4100 to balance, it is critical the amount of money in the change drawer be constant and cash deposits made daily.
- Both the day sheet and the accounts receivable control should be completed each day there is activity on any account.

Aged Accounts Receivable. The record for balancing individual patient accounts with the amount carried on the day sheet is an *aged accounts receivable,* or *aging*. The sample shown in Figure 7–5 is for generating a manual report. On a computer, the report can be generated by following program instructions.

Aging is a method of

- Balancing the total outstanding accounts that are uncollected (the total of all aged accounts) with the accounts receivable balance being carried on the day sheet (in Figure 7–5, that number is $74,610.64),
- Providing a visual monitor to what patients' accounts are outstanding,
- Listing account activity (the date the last payment was made and when insurance was filed),
- Providing a collection tool to see what accounts are overdue and need to be followed up.

ACCOUNTS RECEIVABLE CONTROL
Dr. N.O. Payne

DATE   1-17-92

	DAILY	MONTH TO DATE	YEAR TO DATE
Beginning Accounts Receivable Balance	77535.64		
Total Charges	125.00	5969.00	84631.00
Total Payments	3050.00	9939.93	70939.44
Adjustments	.00	1484.09	5827.94
New Accounts Receivable Balance	74610.64		

FIGURE 7–4
Accounts receivable control.

ACCOUNTS RECEIVABLE AGING RECORD

ENTER CREDITS IN PARENTHESES ( ) AND SUBTRACT WHEN TOTALING COLUMNS AND PAGE.

NAME _____ AS OF DATE _____ PREPARED BY _____ PAGE ___ OF ___ PAGES

NO.	ACCOUNT NAME	INSURANCE INFORMATION		DATE OF LAST PAYMENT	CURRENT 1 TO 30 DAYS	31 to 60 DAYS	61 to 90 DAYS	91 to 120 DAYS	121 DAYS & OVER	TOTAL
		DATE CLAIM FILED	AMT. OF CLAIM							
	AMOUNTS BROUGHT FORWARD									
1	Andreti, Mario	3/14/90	1 170 00		1 170 00					1 170 00
2	Baer, Ted			3/12/90				265 60		265 60
3	Bear, Timothy			3/9/90	200 00	42 00				242 00
4	Best, Vicki			2/24/90			391 20			391 20
5	Better, John	2/26/90	1 008 00	3/12/90		1 008 00	53 00			1 061 00
6	Body, Able			1/16/90				36 00		36 00
7	Bugg, June			3/22/90	36 00		36 00	10 00		82 00
8	Cheddar, Ray	3/16/90	2 495 00	3/12/90	2 400 00		20 00		75 00	2 495 00
9	Crock, Martha				208 00					208 00
10	Jones, Tom	2/2/90	828 00	3/12/90			165 60			165 60
11	Kent, Clark	1/19/90	684 00				684 00			684 00
12	Label, Jean			2/9/90					6 60	6 60
13	Lane, Lois	3/18/90	489 00	3/12/90	489 00		36 00			525 00
14	Ledger, Mary			3/10/90				50 00	33 60	83 60
15	Maple, Martha	3/10/90	1 170 00	3/12/90	1 170 00	36 00				1 206 00
16	Piper, Shawn	2/26/90	828 00	3/20/90	828 00	36 00				864 00
17	Presley, Elvis	2/18/90	1 800 00	3/12/90		360 00				360 00
18	Showers, April			3/12/90	53 00					53 00
19	Treestem, Doris			1/22/90					182 40	182 40
20	Balance from prior pages				28 940 07	19 450 88	10 857 21	3 718 44	1 563 04	64 529 64
21	Accounts Receivable Balance				35 494 07	20 932 88	12 243 01	4 080 04	1 860 64	74 610 64
22										
23										
24										
	AMOUNTS CARRIED FORWARD				47.57%	28.06%	16.41%	5.47%	2.49%	

FIGURE 7-5

Accounts receivable aging record. (Courtesy of Practice Productivity, Inc., Atlanta, GA.)

Complete and balance the aging report with the day sheet monthly. To balance, check that the grand total achieved at the end of recording all ledger cards (if a manual system is used) or patient accounts (if a computerized system is used) on the aging report is the same as the final accounts receivable amount on the accounts receivable control for that same day. If there is a discrepancy, it *must* be found and corrected. If the aging report does not balance, here is what you can do to find the discrepancy:

1. Go back to the last point balanced (you will know what that is because of the note you made to yourself on the day sheet when it did balance) and re-add the day sheets to rule out an addition error. If there is no problem there,
2. Run a calculator tape of the ledger cards again to double check that no card was missed while recording them that would be picked up when adding.
3. Make sure all ledger cards are in the file. Separate ledger cards into "cards with balances" and "zero balance cards," and check through the -0- balance cards to make sure a card with a balance was not misfiled.
4. Check the day sheets for anything that was written in and not carboned through from a ledger card. If such an entry is found, double check it against the ledger card to make sure they are the same.
5. Start at the last point balanced and item by item check off each transaction against the ledger cards.
6. As a last resort, put it down and come back another day, starting from scratch. The elves will come in the night and straighten it all out, but only after you have toiled and stewed for a day or two.

Aging before sending out statements ensures all accounts are present and accounted for.

SPECIAL HINT

A computer can inadvertently drop accounts from the aging and the accounts will not balance.

Take the information gained from the aging report one step further, and apply percentages to each column. This offers an excellent method of monitoring accounts and

- Detects timely insurance billing
- Targets slow-paying insurance groups

Using the sample in Figure 7-5, calculate the percentage of each column to the total by dividing the column total into the overall total. (Example: $35,494.07/$74,610.64 = 47.57\%$.) Repeat this for each column. The total of all percentages should equal 100%. Compare percentage totals from month to month. Establish a normal or average percentage total for the practice. Any deviation from that normal should be investigated and explained.

Monies for Outside Medical/Financial Services. Whatever the source of revenue, the chart of accounts should reflect an income account that defines the source. All monies received from that source should be posted into the respective account.

Outside Medical Services. There are additional revenue-generating sources within a practice. Such revenue might be outside medical services. For example, in a radiology practice, a physician may interpret x-rays for another facility. Revenue may be generated from that service. A pathologist may contract with other clinics to interpret their specimens.

DEBIT
$1,000.00 #1020 Checking Account

CREDIT
$ 500.00 #4102 Radiology income
$ 500.00 #4101 Laboratory income

Outside financial services may be another source of revenue. For example, the practice may own a computer with a large capacity and employ a staff with the expertise to provide a billing service to another clinic.

DEBIT
$500.00 #1020 Checking Account

CREDIT
$500.00 #4105 Billing Service Income

Credit and Collections. Revenue may come from collection, that is, recovery of a bad debt (see Chapter 6). When a balance is turned over to a collection agency, that balance is then written off as a bad debt. The account balance is reduced to zero. The recommended way to post this pay-

ATTENDANCE RECORD

NAME _Betty Jones_ EMPLOYEE NUMBER _123-45-6789_

DEPARTMENT _Administrative_

VACATION BALANCE CARRIED FORWARD FROM LAST YEAR # DAYS _0_

SICK LEAVE BALANCE CARRIED FORWARD FROM LAST YEAR # DAYS _0_

NOTES _____

CODES FOR ATTENDANCE

1. PERSONAL ACCIDENT OFF DUTY
2. PERSONAL ILLNESS
3. FAMILY ILLNESS
4. LEAVE OF ABSENCE
5. LAYOFF
6. ACCIDENT ON DUTY
7. VACATION
8. LATE
9. EXCUSED
10. UNEXCUSED
11. ____
12. ____
13. ____
14. ____
15. ____

YEAR	1	2	3	4	5	6	7	8	9	10	11	12	13	14	15	16	17	18	19	20	21	22	23	24	25	26	27	28	29	30	31
JAN.	4	8	8	—	—	9	7	8	8	8	—	—	9	8	8																
FEB.																															
MAR.																															
APRIL																															
MAY																															
JUNE																															
JULY																															
AUG.																															
SEPT.																															
OCT.																															
NOV.																															
DEC.																															

TOTAL

	1	2	3	4	5	6	7	8	9	10	11	12	13	14	15	TOTAL

FIGURE 7–6

Attendance record. (Courtesy of Practice Productivity, Inc., Atlanta, GA.)

ment is to *not* run it through accounts receivable, but rather deposit it into an income account to reflect the collection of a bad debt, for example, #4200 "Recovery of Bad Debts."

DEBIT
$200.00 #1020 Checking Account

CREDIT
$200.00 #4200 Recovery of Bad Debt

Expenditures

In generating revenue, expenses are incurred. At the very least, operating a medical practice requires

- a facility
- staff
- insurance coverage
- equipment
- supplies

Referring back to the chart of accounts (see Figure 7–2), accounts #6000 to #6999 represent expenses. These items cover the day-to-day items necessary to operate a business.

Expenses for Physical Plant

Property management is discussed in detail in Chapter 3; however, it is mentioned here because the expense of rent or ownership is substantial. Practice goals play a major role in this category. Information gathered from accounting records (historical and current) provides the tools to decide the financial feasibility of building, renting, remodeling, or expanding with a satellite office.

Wages and Salaries

Money spent on wages/salaries and benefits constitutes a major portion of a practice's expenses.

Figuring the Payroll. The number of hours worked by each employee is recorded. Some practices prefer using a timeclock where employees are monitored by having the employees "punch the clock." These are more common in larger facilities. In a smaller practice, each employee can keep track of hours on an "attendance record" similar to the one illustrated in Figure 7–6. From the attendance record, figure the number of hours for which each employee is entitled to be paid.

According to federal wage and hour regulations, employees must receive overtime pay for hours worked in excess of 40 per week at a rate not less than one and a half times the regular rate of pay. State wage and hour laws may be more stringent with overtime definitions, such as mandating overtime for more than 8 hours in any one day. Be familiar with individual state requirements. Some state labor laws require employers to pay wages to all employees *in full* at least twice a calendar month. (See also Chapter 10, Wages and Salaries.)

SPECIAL HINT

If you have a computer program for payroll, follow the program instructions for payroll.

In a manual payroll system, each employee has an earnings card (Figure 7–7) from which calculations are made and payroll deductions figured. The earnings card is used to record

- Pay rate
- Federal withholding allowance, from the W-4 (Figure 7–8) completed each year, for federal tax withheld
- Social security tax
- Medicare tax
- State income tax
- State unemployment tax
- Local income tax

Referring to Betty Jones's attendance record (see Figure 7–6), calculate earnings for the first pay period in January. The personnel policy states Betty is eligible for 8 hours of Holiday pay for working New Years Day, and she has 5 paid sick days each year, payable at 8 hours per day.

Betty would be eligible for straight-time pay of $10.00 per hour for 87 hours (24 hours for the first week, 39 hours for the second week, and 24 hours for the third week), and overtime pay of $15.00 per hour for 2 hours (the second and third Mondays, on which she worked 9 hours).

Under federal regulations, Betty is not eligible to receive overtime for 9 hours of work on January 6th because this was compensated for on the following day of 7 hours of work. *However,* this particular state has an overtime law to compensate overtime pay for any hours over 8 hours per day. The gross wages for the pay period ending

NAME Betty Jones
CLOCK NUMBER
DEPT.

M	2
MARITAL STATUS	NO. OF EXEMPT.

☐ M. ☒ F.

STREET 123 Main Street
SOC. SEC. NUMBER 123-45-6789

CITY Anytown, AK
PHONE NO.
DATE STARTED
DATE LEFT

RECORD OF PAY RATE CHANGES	
DATE	RATE
	$10./hr

YEAR ______ ENCIRCLE QUARTERS 1 2 3 4

TIME WORKED	DATE PAY PERIOD ENDING	TIME WORKED: SUN	M	TU	W	TH	F	SAT	GROSS PAYROLL	F.W.T.	SOC. SEC.	D. INS.	S.W.T.	ESC	MEDICARE	CHECK NO.	← DEDUCTION AMOUNTS / NET PAY	
										DEDUCTIONS								
		BROUGHT FORWARD →																
	1/15/92	87 straight time 2 o.t.							900.00	85.00	55.80	-	-	4.50	13.05	7902	741.65	1
																		2
																		3
																		4
																		5
																		6
																		7
																		8
																		9
																		10
																		11
																		12
																		13
																		14
																		15
																		16
	QTR.																	
	TO DATE																	
																		1
																		2
																		3
																		4
																		5
																		6
																		7
																		8
																		9
																		10
																		11
																		12
																		13
																		14
																		15
																		16
	QTR.	If you are going to use this section for daily hours, write employees name on face of check before inserting this earnings record under the check.																
	TO DATE																	

FIGURE 7-7

Earnings card. (Reprinted with the permission of Safeguard Business Systems, Inc., Fort Washington, PA.)

1990 Form W-4

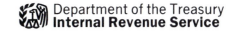
Department of the Treasury
Internal Revenue Service

Purpose. Complete Form W-4 so that your employer can withhold the correct amount of Federal income tax from your pay.

Exemption From Withholding. Read line 6 of the certificate below to see if you can claim exempt status. *If exempt, complete line 6; but do not complete lines 4 and 5.* No Federal income tax will be withheld from your pay. This exemption expires February 15, 1991.

Basic Instructions. Employees who are not exempt should complete the Personal Allowances Worksheet. Additional worksheets are provided on page 2 for employees to adjust their withholding allowances based on itemized deductions, adjustments to income, or two-earner/two-job situations. Complete all worksheets that apply to your situation. The worksheets will help you figure the number of withholding allowances you are entitled to claim. However, you may claim fewer allowances than this.

Head of Household. Generally, you may claim head of household filing status on your tax return only if you are unmarried and pay more than 50% of the costs of keeping up a home for yourself and your dependent(s) or other qualifying individuals.

Nonwage Income. If you have a large amount of nonwage income, such as interest or dividends, you should consider making estimated tax payments using Form 1040-ES. Otherwise, you may find that you owe additional tax at the end of the year.

Two-Earner/Two-Jobs. If you have a working spouse or more than one job, figure the total number of allowances you are entitled to claim on all jobs using worksheets from only one Form W-4. This total should be divided among all jobs. Your withholding will usually be most accurate when all allowances are claimed on the W-4 filed for the highest paying job and zero allowances are claimed for the others.

Advance Earned Income Credit. If you are eligible for this credit, you can receive it added to your paycheck throughout the year. For details, obtain Form W-5 from your employer.

Check Your Withholding. After your W-4 takes effect, you can use **Publication 919**, Is My Withholding Correct for 1990?, to see how the dollar amount you are having withheld compares to your estimated total annual tax. Call 1-800-424-3676 (in Hawaii and Alaska, check your local telephone directory) to order this publication. Check your local telephone directory for the IRS assistance number if you need further help.

Personal Allowances Worksheet

A Enter "1" for **yourself** if no one else can claim you as a dependent . . . . A _____

B Enter "1" if:
1. You are single and have only one job; or
2. You are married, have only one job, and your spouse does not work; or
3. Your wages from a second job or your spouse's wages (or the total of both) are $2,500 or less.
. . . . . . B _____

C Enter "1" for your **spouse**. But, you may choose to enter "0" if you are married and have either a working spouse or more than one job (this may help you avoid having too little tax withheld) . . . . C _____

D Enter number of **dependents** (other than your spouse or yourself) whom you will claim on your tax return . . . . D _____

E Enter "1" if you will file as a **head of household** on your tax return (see conditions under "Head of Household," above) . . E _____

F Enter "1" if you have at least $1,500 of **child or dependent care expenses** for which you plan to claim a credit . . . . F _____

G Add lines A through F and enter total here . . . . ▶ G _____

For accuracy, do all worksheets that apply.
- If you plan to **itemize or claim adjustments to income** and want to reduce your withholding, turn to the Deductions and Adjustments Worksheet on page 2.
- If you are **single** and have **more than one job** and your combined earnings from all jobs exceed $25,000 OR if you are **married** and have a **working spouse or more than one job**, and the combined earnings from all jobs exceed $44,000, then turn to the Two-Earner/Two-Job Worksheet on page 2 if you want to avoid having too little tax withheld.
- If **neither** of the above situations applies to you, **stop here** and enter the number from line G on line 4 of Form W-4 below.

- Cut here and give the certificate to your employer. Keep the top portion for your records. -

Form **W-4**
Department of the Treasury
Internal Revenue Service

Employee's Withholding Allowance Certificate
▶ For Privacy Act and Paperwork Reduction Act Notice, see reverse.

OMB No. 1545-0010
19**90**

1 Type or print your first name and middle initial | Last name | **2** Your social security number

Home address (number and street or rural route)

City or town, state, and ZIP code

3 Marital status:
☐ Single ☐ Married
☐ Married, but withhold at higher Single rate.
Note: *If married, but legally separated, or spouse is a nonresident alien, check the Single box.*

4 Total number of allowances you are claiming (from line G above or from the Worksheets on back if they apply) . . **4** _____

5 Additional amount, if any, you want deducted from each pay . . . . **5** $ _____

6 I claim exemption from withholding and I certify that I meet **ALL** of the following conditions for exemption:
- Last year I had a right to a refund of **ALL** Federal income tax withheld because I had **NO** tax liability; **AND**
- This year I expect a refund of **ALL** Federal income tax withheld because I expect to have **NO** tax liability; **AND**
- This year if my income exceeds $500 and includes nonwage income, another person cannot claim me as a dependent.

If you meet all of the above conditions, enter the year effective and "EXEMPT" here . . . ▶ **6** 19 _____

7 Are you a full-time student? *(Note: Full-time students are not automatically exempt.)* . . . . **7** ☐ Yes ☐ No

Under penalties of perjury, I certify that I am entitled to the number of withholding allowances claimed on this certificate or entitled to claim exempt status.

Employee's signature ▶ _____ Date ▶ _____, 19____

8 Employer's name and address (**Employer:** Complete 8 and 10 **only if sending to IRS**) | **9** Office code (optional) | **10** Employer identification number

FIGURE 7-8

W-4 form.

Form W-4 (1990) Page **2**

Deductions and Adjustments Worksheet

Note: *Use this worksheet only if you plan to itemize deductions or claim adjustments to income on your 1990 tax return.*

1. Enter an estimate of your 1990 itemized deductions. These include: qualifying home mortgage interest, 10% of personal interest, charitable contributions, state and local taxes (but not sales taxes), medical expenses in excess of 7.5% of your income, and miscellaneous deductions (most miscellaneous deductions are now deductible only in excess of 2% of your income) . . . . **1** $ _____

2. Enter:
   - $5,450 if married filing jointly or qualifying widow(er)
   - $4,750 if head of household
   - $3,250 if single
   - $2,725 if married filing separately
   . . . . **2** $ _____

3. **Subtract** line 2 from line 1. If line 2 is greater than line 1, enter zero . . . . **3** $ _____
4. Enter an estimate of your 1990 adjustments to income. These include alimony paid and deductible IRA contributions . . **4** $ _____
5. **Add** lines 3 and 4 and enter the total . . . . **5** $ _____
6. Enter an estimate of your 1990 nonwage income (such as dividends or interest income) . . . . **6** $ _____
7. **Subtract** line 6 from line 5. Enter the result, but not less than zero . . . . **7** $ _____
8. **Divide** the amount on line 7 by $2,000 and enter the result here. Drop any fraction . . . . **8** _____
9. Enter the number from Personal Allowances Worksheet, line G, on page 1 . . . . **9** _____
10. **Add** lines 8 and 9 and enter the total here. If you plan to use the Two-Earner/Two-Job Worksheet, also enter the total on line 1, below. Otherwise, **stop here** and enter this total on Form W-4, line 4 on page 1 . . . . **10** _____

Two-Earner/Two-Job Worksheet

Note: *Use this worksheet only if the instructions at line G on page 1 direct you here.*

1. Enter the number from line G on page 1 (or from line 10 above if you used the Deductions and Adjustments Worksheet) . **1** _____
2. Find the number in **Table 1** below that applies to the **LOWEST** paying job and enter it here . . . . . . **2** _____
3. If line 1 is **GREATER THAN OR EQUAL TO** line 2, subtract line 2 from line 1. Enter the result here (if zero, enter "0") and on Form W-4, line 4, on page 1. **DO NOT** use the rest of this worksheet . . . . . . **3** _____

Note: *If line 1 is **LESS THAN** line 2, enter "0" on Form W-4, line 4, on page 1. Complete lines 4–9 to calculate the additional dollar withholding necessary to avoid a year-end tax bill.*

4. Enter the number from line 2 of this worksheet . . . . **4** _____
5. Enter the number from line 1 of this worksheet . . . . **5** _____
6. **Subtract** line 5 from line 4 . . . . **6** _____
7. Find the amount in **Table 2** below that applies to the **HIGHEST** paying job and enter it here . . . . . . **7** $ _____
8. **Multiply** line 7 by line 6 and enter the result here. This is the additional annual withholding amount needed **8** $ _____
9. Divide line 8 by the number of pay periods each year. (For example, divide by 26 if you are paid every other week.) Enter the result here and on Form W-4, line 5, page 1. This is the additional amount to be withheld from each paycheck . . **9** $ _____

Table 1: Two-Earner/Two-Job Worksheet

Married Filing Jointly		All Others	
If wages from **LOWEST** paying job are—	Enter on line 2 above	If wages from **LOWEST** paying job are—	Enter on line 2 above
0 - $4,000	0	0 - $4,000	0
4,001 - 8,000	1	4,001 - 8,000	1
8,001 - 19,000	2	8,001 - 14,000	2
19,001 - 23,000	3	14,001 - 16,000	3
23,001 - 25,000	4	16,001 - 21,000	4
25,001 - 27,000	5	21,001 and over	5
27,001 - 29,000	6		
29,001 - 35,000	7		
35,001 - 41,000	8		
41,001 - 46,000	9		
46,001 and over	10		

Table 2: Two-Earner/Two-Job Worksheet

Married Filing Jointly		All Others	
If wages from **HIGHEST** paying job are—	Enter on line 7 above	If wages from **HIGHEST** paying job are—	Enter on line 7 above
0 - $44,000	$310	0 - $25,000	$310
44,001 - 90,000	570	25,001 - 52,000	570
90,001 and over	680	52,001 and over	680

Privacy Act and Paperwork Reduction Act Notice.—We ask for this information to carry out the Internal Revenue laws of the United States. We may give the information to the Department of Justice for civil or criminal litigation and to cities, states, and the District of Columbia for use in administering their tax laws. You are required to give this information to your employer.

The time needed to complete this form will vary depending on individual circumstances. The estimated average time is: **Recordkeeping** 46 min., **Learning about the law or the form** 10 min., **Preparing the form** 70 min. If you have comments concerning the accuracy of these time estimates or suggestions for making this form more simple, we would be happy to hear from you. You can write to the **Internal Revenue Service,** Washington, DC 20224, Attn: IRS Reports Clearance Officer, T:FP; or the **Office of Management and Budget,** Paperwork Reduction Project (1545-0010), Washington, DC 20503.
✮U.S. Government Printing Office: 1989-245-063

FIGURE 7-8 Continued

January 15th would then be $900.00 ($870.00 straight time and $30.00 overtime).

If Betty worked in a state where there were no laws regulating overtime, the compensation would be according to federal regulations, or 88 straight-time hours (24 hours for the first week, 40 hours for the second week, and 24 hours for the third week) at $10.00 per hour and 1 overtime hour (the third Monday, on which she worked 9 hours) at $15.00 per hour.

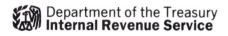

Department of the Treasury
Internal Revenue Service

Circular E
Employer's Tax Guide

1990 Social Security Tax Rate and Wage Base

The social security tax rate is 7.65% each for employers and employees on the first $50,400 of wages paid in 1990.

1990 Federal Unemployment (FUTA) Tax Rate

The Federal Unemployment (FUTA) tax rate is 6.2% for 1990.

New Form 940-EZ for 1989

Beginning in 1989, you may be able to use new Form 940-EZ instead of Form 940, Employer's Annual Federal Unemployment (FUTA) Tax Return. You can generally use new Form 940-EZ if: (1) you paid unemployment taxes ("contributions") to only one state; (2) you paid these taxes timely; and (3) all wages that were taxable for FUTA tax were also taxable for your state's unemployment tax.

New Reporting Requirement for Employee Business Expenses

Beginning in 1989, new rules apply to the amounts you pay your employees for business expenses. See "What to Include on the 1989 Form W-2" on page 11 for more details. A per diem chart is on page 51 to be used in calculating the amount to report on Form W-2.

Dependent Care Assistance

For 1989 and future years, employers must report dependent care benefits paid (or incurred) under section 129 of the Code on Form W-2. See "Dependent Care Benefits" on page 12 for more details.

1990 Form W-2

At the time this publication went to print, IRS was considering several changes to the 1990 Form W-2, Wage and Tax Statement. The form and separate instructions will be available at the beginning of 1990.

1990 Form W-4

The 1990 Form W-4, Employee's Withholding Allowance Certificate, is available. You may order copies by calling 1-800-424-3676.

Pending Legislation

At the time this publication went to print, Congress was considering legislation that would: (1) retroactively extend the exclusion from income for employer-provided educational assistance until December 31, 1991; (2) repeal section 89 nondiscrimination rules; (3) revise the information reporting penalties; (4) require income tax withholding on the wages of certain agricultural workers; and (5) revise the payroll tax deposit requirements on deposits of $3,000 or more. If such legislation is enacted, IRS will issue further guidance.

Internal Revenue Service
P.O. Box C-32121
Richmond, VA 23261-2121

Official Business
Penalty for Private Use, $300
Do Not Forward

Table of Contents

Section no.	Page no.
1. Purpose	2
2. Are You an Employer?	2
Federal, State, Local Government Employers	3
3. Employer Identification Number	3
4. Who Are Employees?	3
5. Employee's Social Security Number	3
6. Taxable Wages	4
7. Taxable Tips	5
8. Supplemental Wage Payments	6
9. Payroll Period	6
10. Withholding From Employees	6
11. Figuring Withholding	7
12. Income Tax Withholding From Pensions and Annuities	7
13. Depositing Taxes	8
14. Filing the Quarterly Return of Withheld Income Tax and Social Security Taxes	9
15. Filing the Federal Unemployment (FUTA) Tax Return	11
16. Reporting Withheld Income Tax	11
17. Reporting to Employees	11
18. Advance Payment of the Earned Income Credit	12
19. Social Security and Income Tax Withholding, and FUTA Tax Payments, on Sick Pay	13
▶ Chart for Special Rules of Various Types of Services and Payments	15–20
▶ Methods of Income Tax Withholding	20–21
▶ Recordkeeping	21
▶ Income Tax Withholding—Percentage Method Tables	22–23
▶ Income Tax Withholding—Wage Bracket Tables	24–43
▶ Social Security Employee Tax Tables	44–45
▶ Advance EIC—Percentage Method Tables	46–47
▶ Advance EIC—Wage Bracket Tables	48–50
▶ Reporting Employee Business Expenses	51
▶ Business Expense Per Diem Rates	51
▶ Guide to 1989 Information Returns	52–53
▶ Federal Tax Deposit (FTD) Checklist	54–55
▶ Index	Back cover

Bulk Rate
Postage and Fees Paid
Internal Revenue Service
Permit No. G-48

FIGURE 7–9

First page of Circular E of the Employer's Tax Guide from the Internal Revenue Service.

Sample Payroll

1. Make an entry for $900.00 under gross wages.
2. Look up the federal withholding in Circular E, *Employer's Tax Guide* (Figure 7-9), a yearly revised circular provided by the Internal Revenue Service. Because Betty is paid twice monthly, the married, semimonthly table (Figure 7-10) is used. There are separate withholding tables for single and married employees. Consider all taxable wages as outlined in Circular E. Betty's federal withholding for this pay period is $85.00. Make this entry to her earnings card under the column "FWT" for federal withheld tax.
3. Next, figure the first part of social security (or FICA—Federal Insurance Commission Administration) withholding. Again, Circular E is the reference for the percentage withheld. In 1992, the social security tax rate was 6.2% for the employers and for the employee on the first $55,500 of wages paid in 1992. The second part of the social security tax is for Medicare and beginning in 1991, employers could no longer combine and report the two parts as a single amount. In 1992, the Medicare tax rate was 1.45% for both employer and employee on the first $130,200 of wages paid in 1992. This means that whatever amount is calculated as withholding for the employee, the employer must match (see section on payroll taxes in this chapter). If any employees make in excess of $55,500 and $130,200, respectively, this year, any wages over those amounts are exempt from this tax and you stop withholding additional monies. Quarterly tax reports are discussed in more detail elsewhere in this chapter. Monitor the accumulated salaries as they approach these limits.
4. To figure Betty's social security tax without using the table provided in Circular E, multiply $900.00 (gross wages) $\times$ 6.2% = $55.80. Enter this figure in the column on her earnings card under "social security withheld."

    To figure Medicare tax without using the table provided in Circular E, multiply $900.00 (gross wages) $\times$ 1.45% = $13.05. Enter this figure on her earnings card under "Medicare Withheld."
5. Some states have an income tax. Follow state guidelines for this amount withheld. In Betty's state, the only other payroll tax is from the state for unemployment, and it is called the employment security contribution (ESC) tax. This is .5% of wages to a maximum wage of $22,600.00 for the year. Multiply Betty's wages of $900.00 by .5% and you have an ESC withholding of $4.50. Label a column on the earnings card and make this entry.
6. Subtract all withholding from gross salary to arrive at the net salary ($900.00 − $85.00 − $55.80 − $13.05 − $4.50 = $741.65).
7. Write a check following the guidelines in Chapter 6.

Benefits

Good benefit packages offered by a medical practice can add incentives for present staff and attract new employees to a practice. Benefits offered should be written in the personnel policy (see Chapter 10) so that all employees understand them. Be consistent with benefits and do not offer select employees what others do not receive.

SPECIAL HINT

There may be exceptions to the number or amount of benefits offered, but *caution* should be used and any decision to exempt certain employees should be cleared with the practice attorney.

Benefits may include all or any combination of the following:

- Paid vacation
- Sick days and/or personal days
- Health and/or life insurance
- Free health care in the practice
- In-house babysitting
- Pension and profit-sharing plans
- Bonuses (Christmas, birthday, or practice production)
- Uniforms
- Parking fees
- Vehicle
- A dollar allowance for child care
- A dollar allowance for education
- Professional dues

Be as imaginative as practice policy and finances allow.

Communicate in dollars what benefits the employees actually receive. Use a form similar to that shown in Figure 7-11. This serves two purposes:

- Employees are aware of the actual dollars, over wages, they receive.
- It is an accounting tool.

MARRIED Persons—SEMIMONTHLY Payroll Period
(For Wages Paid After December 1991)

And the wages are—		And the number of withholding allowances claimed is—										
At least	But less than	0	1	2	3	4	5	6	7	8	9	10
		The amount of income tax to be withheld shall be—										
$0	$155	$0	$0	$0	$0	$0	$0	$0	$0	$0	$0	$0
155	160	1	0	0	0	0	0	0	0	0	0	0
160	165	1	0	0	0	0	0	0	0	0	0	0
165	170	2	0	0	0	0	0	0	0	0	0	0
170	175	3	0	0	0	0	0	0	0	0	0	0
175	180	4	0	0	0	0	0	0	0	0	0	0
180	185	4	0	0	0	0	0	0	0	0	0	0
185	190	5	0	0	0	0	0	0	0	0	0	0
190	195	6	0	0	0	0	0	0	0	0	0	0
195	200	7	0	0	0	0	0	0	0	0	0	0
200	205	7	0	0	0	0	0	0	0	0	0	0
205	210	8	0	0	0	0	0	0	0	0	0	0
210	215	9	0	0	0	0	0	0	0	0	0	0
215	220	10	0	0	0	0	0	0	0	0	0	0
220	225	10	0	0	0	0	0	0	0	0	0	0
225	230	11	0	0	0	0	0	0	0	0	0	0
230	235	12	0	0	0	0	0	0	0	0	0	0
235	240	13	0	0	0	0	0	0	0	0	0	0
240	245	13	0	0	0	0	0	0	0	0	0	0
245	250	14	0	0	0	0	0	0	0	0	0	0
250	260	15	1	0	0	0	0	0	0	0	0	0
260	270	17	2	0	0	0	0	0	0	0	0	0
270	280	18	4	0	0	0	0	0	0	0	0	0
280	290	20	5	0	0	0	0	0	0	0	0	0
290	300	21	7	0	0	0	0	0	0	0	0	0
300	310	23	8	0	0	0	0	0	0	0	0	0
310	320	24	10	0	0	0	0	0	0	0	0	0
320	330	26	11	0	0	0	0	0	0	0	0	0
330	340	27	13	0	0	0	0	0	0	0	0	0
340	350	29	14	0	0	0	0	0	0	0	0	0
350	360	30	16	1	0	0	0	0	0	0	0	0
360	370	32	17	3	0	0	0	0	0	0	0	0
370	380	33	19	4	0	0	0	0	0	0	0	0
380	390	35	20	6	0	0	0	0	0	0	0	0
390	400	36	22	7	0	0	0	0	0	0	0	0
400	410	38	23	9	0	0	0	0	0	0	0	0
410	420	39	25	10	0	0	0	0	0	0	0	0
420	430	41	26	12	0	0	0	0	0	0	0	0
430	440	42	28	13	0	0	0	0	0	0	0	0
440	450	44	29	15	1	0	0	0	0	0	0	0
450	460	45	31	16	2	0	0	0	0	0	0	0
460	470	47	32	18	4	0	0	0	0	0	0	0
470	480	48	34	19	5	0	0	0	0	0	0	0
480	490	50	35	21	7	0	0	0	0	0	0	0
490	500	51	37	22	8	0	0	0	0	0	0	0
500	520	53	39	25	10	0	0	0	0	0	0	0
520	540	56	42	28	13	0	0	0	0	0	0	0
540	560	59	45	31	16	2	0	0	0	0	0	0
560	580	62	48	34	19	5	0	0	0	0	0	0
580	600	65	51	37	22	8	0	0	0	0	0	0
600	620	68	54	40	25	11	0	0	0	0	0	0
620	640	71	57	43	28	14	0	0	0	0	0	0
640	660	74	60	46	31	17	3	0	0	0	0	0
660	680	77	63	49	34	20	6	0	0	0	0	0
680	700	80	66	52	37	23	9	0	0	0	0	0
700	720	83	69	55	40	26	12	0	0	0	0	0
720	740	86	72	58	43	29	15	0	0	0	0	0
740	760	89	75	61	46	32	18	3	0	0	0	0
760	780	92	78	64	49	35	21	6	0	0	0	0
780	800	95	81	67	52	38	24	9	0	0	0	0
800	820	98	84	70	55	41	27	12	0	0	0	0
820	840	101	87	73	58	44	30	15	1	0	0	0
840	860	104	90	76	61	47	33	18	4	0	0	0
860	880	107	93	79	64	50	36	21	7	0	0	0
880	900	110	96	82	67	53	39	24	10	0	0	0
900	920	113	99	85	70	56	42	27	13	0	0	0
920	940	116	102	88	73	59	45	30	16	1	0	0
940	960	119	105	91	76	62	48	33	19	4	0	0
960	980	122	108	94	79	65	51	36	22	7	0	0

Page 38

FIGURE 7-10

Semimonthly payroll chart from Circular E.

Benefit	Company Pays	You Pay
Medical		
Life insurance		
Holiday pay		
Vacations		
Sick leave		
Personal leave		
Worker's Compensation		
Retirement		
Education		
Incentive bonus		
Child care allowance		
Other:		
Total Benefits		

Gross wage for 19__ $_____
Total benefits paid by employer $_____

Your employer is currently providing _____% over your current wage for your benefits.

Date: _____

FIGURE 7-11

Summary of employee benefits.

Communicating benefits in dollars will help in making decisions on future benefits, that is, whether it is appropriate to add more or delete some. The practice may be in an industrial area where employees are covered by spouses' company plans. To offer health insurance as a benefit would not necessarily appeal to this staff. As an alternative, a decision could be made to place the money that would have been put into a health insurance plan into a benefit that would be more appealing to these employees, possibly child care or vehicle allowance.

Some practices may include employee benefits as a payroll expense and not assign a separate expense account in their chart of accounts (see Chapter 10 for more details about benefits). However, beginning in 1989, new rules apply to the amounts employees are paid for business expenses. Refer to "What to Include on the 1989 Form W-2" in Circular E for more details.

CAUTION: There is a legal requirement to report as wages and pay the federal and social security tax on the dollar value of some benefits. The practice accountant should review this annually for tax changes. See federal publication 525, *Taxable and Nontaxable Income,* for items that require payroll tax withholding, such as vacation pay, child care payments, etc., that are calculated within the pay structure and need *not* have a separate expense category.

Items such as parking fees, job-related education, professional dues, etc. can legally be considered practice expenses and not "taxable wages" to the employee. These can be grouped under an expense account title such as "Employees' Benefits and Expenses," #6100, or be considered as separate expense items; for example, education may be put into account #6050 "Conference and Training" (see Chart of Accounts, in Figure 7-2).

Insurance Premiums

Another major expense to a practice is the cost of insurance premiums.

Types of Insurance

Professional Liability, or Malpractice Insurance. This provides coverage in the event litigation is brought against the practice or physician. Suits can be brought about by a negligent act that adversely affects the patient. Examples include

- Unanticipated foreign bodies left within the patient
- Wrong medication or wrong dosage with adverse sequelae
- Operation on wrong side or at wrong level
- Any major unanticipated fetal damage
- Any unanticipated death
- Any unanticipated major surgical complication
- Failure to diagnose

Depending on the type of practice and the location, premiums range from thousands to hundreds of thousands of dollars annually.

Business Owners' Insurance Package. This policy provides coverage in the event someone slips and falls and is injured on the practice's property, or to cover the loss of equipment.

Bond. A bond offers coverage for employees handling money in a practice. If money is missing, a claim can be filed under the bond policy.

Worker's Compensation. This insurance covers employees in the case of on-the-job injury.

Group Health and/or Life. This type of insurance is a benefit to employees. Policies may be purchased to cover employees and family members for health care and hospitalization in the event of illness or death.

Life/Disability. Many group practices and corporations carry life/disability insurance on the practitioners, listing the other partners or the corporation as the beneficiary. This is done to lessen the financial burden after the death or disablement of a partner.

Commercial Auto. If company-owned vehicles are used by the practice, a commercial auto insurance policy will provide comprehension and collision coverage.

Knowing practice goals helps in making insurance decisions. Because premiums are not free, practitioners have to weigh peace of mind and the legal requirements of providing these policies against their cost.

The decision to carry insurance is not always elective. Some hospitals require professional liability insurance before granting privileges, some state laws require Worker's Compensation insurance of all employers, and corporate by-laws may require life insurance of all officers.

With any insurance policy, it is important to review it annually. Most will be renewed automatically by the insurance agent. Review practice needs and make sure policies cover those needs. A trusted, competent agent can be a valuable asset in helping conduct the review. Be aware and watchful of the commission the agent gets on the separate policies. Motives for recommending re-

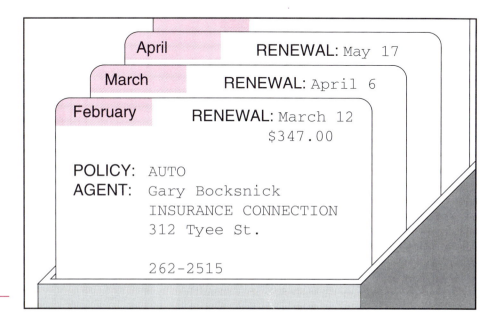

FIGURE 7-12

Insurance tickler file.

140 *Chapter 7: ACCOUNTING AND TAXES*

newals should be based on your needs and not agent commissions.

> **SPECIAL HINT**
>
> Watch that policy coverage does not lapse. A "tickler file," similar to the one illustrated in Figure 7–12, can take the form of 3 × 5 cards. The heading for each card is the type of insurance up for renewal. The name, address, and phone number of the agent, and last year's premium make up the contents of the card. File them in a box by month. If the policy expires in March, file the card in February. This will provide an alert to call and set up the review and potential renewal of the policy.

Supplies

Supplies are ordered and arrive at various times during the month. It is not efficient use of time to write checks as each invoice is received. Instead, accumulate the bills into an accounts payable folder. An A–Z expanding "every day file/sorter" is recommended. When an invoice or bill is received in the mail, check it over to verify it is a valid bill.

Verifying a valid bill. When supplies are ordered, a purchase order is generated (Figure 7–13). A three-part form provides an original to the ordering company, a second copy to attach to the purchase order book for reference, and a third copy to give to the bookkeeper as notification to expect an invoice. When merchandise is received

FIGURE 7–13

Sample of a purchase order (Courtesy of Rediform, Dallas, TX.)

and checked off on the packing slip, it too goes to the bookkeeper to be matched with the purchase order. When the time comes to write checks, these three items (purchase order, packing slip, and invoice) are matched and there is no question that the bill is valid and should be paid.

Getting the Most out of Practice Funds

The accounting system chosen should incorporate a method for paying operating expenses to take advantage of using practice funds to their fullest. One way to do this is to have two accounts—a savings account (interest-bearing checking account or money market fund, with limited check-writing privileges) and a checking account in which a minimum balance is kept from which to pay bills. Deposit daily revenue into the savings account and let it draw interest. When checks are written, twice monthly, from the checking account, figure out the total of the amount needed to cover those checks. Make a withdrawal of that amount from the interest-bearing account and deposit that amount to cover the checks.

Writing Checks

1. When the time arrives to generate checks, take out the payables file and payroll information.
2. Review the invoices. Each valid invoice is assigned an account number from the chart of accounts according to the expense category it falls in. For example, an electric bill would be assigned #6370 "Utilities," and an invoice for copy paper would be assigned #6200 "Office Supplies."
3. Payroll calculations are made using the method described under Wages and Salaries.
4. Payroll tax deposits should be made as outlined under Payroll Tax.

N.O. Payne, M.D.
Balance Sheet
April 1, 1992

Assets
1012	Savings in ABC Bank	10,257.92
1020	Checking Account XYZ Bank	1,087.00
1210	Accounts Receivable	54,496.47
1710	Machinery and Equipment	98,932.33
1810	Accumulated Depreciation—Machinery and Equipment	47,955.19
	Total Assets	$212,728.91

Liabilities
2200	Accounts Payable	-0-
2320	Payroll Tax (Federal, Medicare, and Social Security) Payable	1,352.78
2330	Payroll Tax (State Employment Security) Payable	237.06
2340	Payroll Tax (Federal Unemployment—FUTA) Payable	10.79
	Total Liabilities	$1,600.63

Capital
3999	Retained Earnings/Owner's Equity	$211,128.28
	Total Liabilities and Capital	$212,728.91

FIGURE 7-14
Balance sheet.

Balance Sheet

In well-managed practices accounting activities are reviewed on a monthly basis, as soon as possible after the end of business for that month.

Assets, liabilities, and capital comprise the financial position of a company. The balance sheet tells the financial position of the business on a given date (a historical view) (Figure 7–14).

Assets represent economic resources that are owned by the business. *Liabilities* represent the economic obligations. *Capital* (or *owner's equity*) is the interest of the owners in the business. There are two types of capital: (1) that contributed by the owner and/or stockholder and (2) that earned and accumulated through profitable operations (*retained earnings*).

N.O. Payne, M.D.
Income Statement
April 1, 1992

Income
4100	Professional Services–Fees	32,929.24	
4101	Laboratory Income	5,287.41	
4110	Refund	(493.80)	
4200	Allowance for Bad Debts Collected	400.00	
4201	Other Income	1,000.00	
	Total Income		$39,122.85

Expenses
6050	Conference and Training	85.00	
6060	Depreciation	-0-	
6080	Drugs and Medical Supplies	346.04	
6090	Dues and Subscriptions	185.00	
6100	Employees Benefits and Expenses	176.00	
6110	Equipment Leased	746.20	
6130	Bank Charges and NSF checks	7.20	
6140	Insurance	1,525.00	
6160	Janitorial	304.41	
6165	Laboratory Expense	294.00	
6170	Legal and Accounting	105.00	
6200	Office Supplies	507.75	
6210	Outside Laboratory	71.40	
6250	Rent	1,800.00	
6260	Repairs and Maintenance	-0-	
6270	Salaries	12,958.73	
6320	Taxes–Payroll	1,535.27	
6350	Taxes and License	25.00	
6370	Utilities and Telephone	369.70	
6380	Miscellaneous	-0-	
	Total Expenses		$21,041.70
	Net Income		$18,081.15

FIGURE 7–15
Income statement.

Income Statement

The income statement adds income and subtracts expenses to arrive at net income/loss for a given period—month, quarter, or year (a current view). Although it is important to know the amount of net income, it is equally important to know where it comes from and what it costs to generate (Figure 7-15).

Revenue

The practice earns revenue by providing medical services for patients. *Revenue* is measured in the form of accounts receivable collected. In a medical practice, revenues represent gross increases in assets, either by a larger balance in the practice's bank account or a balance in an accounts receivable account.

Expense

Costs incurred in the process of earning revenue are *expenses*. Expenses represent gross decreases in assets (for example, the checking account balance would be less as a result of paying bills) or gross increases in liabilities (for example, payroll taxes are withheld from employees and held in these accounts until the end of the quarter, when they are paid to the government).

Net Profit/Loss

Net Profit = Income > Expense
Net Loss = Expenses > Income

Select a time each month to generate this report, after the bank statement has been balanced. Compare each income and expense item. Watch

N.O. Payne, M.D.
Profit and Loss Analysis

For the Month of _____

Current Period

	Last Year	This Year	Budget	% Last Year	% Budget
Total Income					
Total Expense					
Net Income/Loss					

Year to Date

	Last Year	This Year	Budget	% Last Year	% Budget
Total Income					
Total Expense					
Net Income/Loss					

FIGURE 7-16

Profit and loss analysis.

for a large increase or decrease in any one item. There should be an explanation for each. For example, it would be expected for the insurance expense account to be larger in January than in other months, because the annual professional liability premium is paid then. If a sudden increase or decrease is reflected for the same account, look at all of the items posted to that account. If an explanation is found, there is no problem. If there is no justification for the variation, a problem is indicated. Through the budgeting process, expenses are anticipated for the following year.

Analysis of Profit and Loss

Another format for reviewing profit and loss is demonstrated in Figure 7–16. This form offers a condensed version of the income statement. This may be a more visual way to compare figures and percentages with the same time last year and amount budgeted. Some computerized accounting systems produce an income statement to include these columns.

This completed report provides a planning tool for securing a loan or monitoring progress over a period of time. It also can be used as a marketing tool to attract another practitioner to the practice.

Cost Analysis of Services and Procedures

Cost accounting is the practice of matching receipts and expenses of like kind. This process can be used to monitor each department or each facility. If there are one or more satellite clinics, it is important to know what each facility generates in expenses and income (see Chapter 3 for additional information). It is important to know whether an in-house laboratory or x-ray service is making or losing money. By analyzing this information, as illustrated in Figure 7–17, a sound business decision can be made as to whether it would be more profitable to send the laboratory work to an outside laboratory or continue to do it in-house.

When using cost analysis, it is important that all costs be considered, including the percentage of rent each department occupies. When allocating facility expenses, consider an appropriate percentage of management salary and benefit expense, malpractice premiums, legal and accounting fees, and any other expense indirectly involved in the cooperative management of multiple departments or facilities. Other additional intangible considerations might be convenience to your patients and what competitors offer.

Cost analysis can be a useful tool when setting practice goals. If one goal is to convert an in-house laboratory to one that collects specimens and prepares them for transport, this information would provide some insight as to the financial impact of that decision on the practice. Ask the accountant to point out areas where cost accounting can help analyze other areas in the practice.

Budget

Goals can be set, but an operating budget provides a tool for making those goals happen. A *budget* is the operational planning and control system. The most effective and accurate budget is prepared with input and participation from all department heads in the practice. Communicate practice goals to all staff members and let them know there is a budget process in place to accomplish those goals. Figure 7–18 illustrates a "proposed monthly budget."

Consider projected needs:

- New equipment
- Additional practitioner
- Additional support staff

SPECIAL HINT

Check the budget periodically to see how close it comes to projected figures. Be willing to modify and revise the budget as new information becomes available. The operating statement of profit and loss monitors this. Constantly ask questions and be watchful of new and added information.

Reading and Analyzing Financial Statements

In a seminar done by B. Wright Associates of Midvale, Utah, four uses of a budget were identified:[*]

Detailed Operational Plan. The operating budget provides the plan by which management will attain the company goals. It is not just a forecast. It is planning for a result and controlling to maximize the chances of achieving that result.

Cash Requirements Forecasting. Operational budgets provide the final step in forecasting the

---

[*] From *Reading and Analyzing Financial Statements.* Copyright 1986, B. Wright & Associates, Midvale, UT 84047.

N.O. Payne, M.D.
Cost Analysis

LABORATORY IN-HOUSE

Account #			
4101	MONTHLY LAB INCOME		$5,000.00
	EXPENSES:		
6165	Supplies	$ 300.00	
1710	Equipment	800.00	
6270	Salary	1,800.00	
6100	Benefits	450.00	
6250	Rent (% of space used)	480.00	
6260	Maintenance	50.00	
	Total expenses		$3,880.00
	Net profit		$1,120.00

LABORATORY–OUTSIDE

Account #			
4101	MONTHLY LAB INCOME		$5,000.00
	EXPENSES:		
6270	Salary	$1,000.00	
6100	Benefit	250.00	
6250	Rent	200.00	
6210	Laboratory fee	1,500.00	
	Total expenses		$2,950.00
	Net profit		$2,050.00

FIGURE 7-17
Cost analysis.

timing and amount of cash required. The operational budget, along with the accounts payable system, accounts receivable system, and capital budget, provides the tools necessary to keep close control on cash requirements.

Operating Targets Determination. Operational budgets provide the detail required to assess the viability of corporate targets and give the areas of personal requirements, capacity requirements, revenue targets, and profit goals. Preparation of the operating budget helps the manager make more realistic appraisals of overall goals and objectives.

Managerial Performance Tool. The budget is management's best assessment of conditions that will develop during the operating year and provides a tool for the measurement of the effectiveness of the manager in determining how developing conditions will affect operations.

It is important to compare the projected budget with actual results. Any significant variance should be investigated and corrected for the following year. Goals and target objectives may have to be adjusted according to the results of the assessment.

<u>N.O. Payne, M.D.</u>
Proposed Monthly Budget
April 1, 1992

<u>Income</u>

4100	Professional Services–Fees	30,000.00
4101	Laboratory Income	5,000.00
4201	Other Income	1,500.00
	Total Income	$36,500.00

<u>Expenses</u>

6050	Conference and Training	100.00
6080	Drugs and Medical Supplies	450.00
6090	Dues and Subscriptions	250.00
6100	Employees' Benefits and Expenses	600.00
6110	Equipment Leased	750.00
6130	Bank Charges and NSF checks	25.00
6140	Insurance	2,200.00
6160	Janitorial	350.00
6165	Laboratory Expense	300.00
6170	Legal and Accounting	150.00
6200	Office Supplies	500.00
6210	Outside Laboratory	150.00
6250	Rent	1,800.00
6260	Repairs and Maintenance	300.00
6270	Salaries	15,000.00
6320	Taxes–Payroll	2,000.00
6350	Taxes and License	30.00
6370	Utilities and Telephone	450.00
6380	Miscellaneous	1,095.00
	Total Expenses	$26,500.00
	Net Income	$10,000.00

FIGURE 7–18

Proposed monthly budget.

TAXES

Property Tax

Property tax rates are determined by locality. Check with the practice's accountant and/or local government offices for details and dates and filing information.

State Tax

State tax rates are determined by each individual state. Some states have income taxes; others do not. Check with the practice's accountant and/or local government offices for details on the proper reporting and withholding of any state taxes that might affect the practice. For an example of a state-imposed employment tax on payroll, see Quarterly Tax Reports.

Federal Taxes

Federal Income Tax

The amount of federal income tax paid by the practice depends on whether it operates as a corporation, partnership, or proprietorship. There are numerous rules and regulations governing each type of business. These rules and regulations are subject to changes annually. An accountant or other trained professional can prepare the practice's federal income tax return. By keeping timely, accurate records as discussed in this chapter, you can minimize the amount of time necessary to prepare the return.

Payroll Tax

Wages subject to federal employment taxes include all pay given to an employee for services performed. This includes salaries, vacation allowances, bonuses, and commissions. You must be familiar with the federal Circular E and state laws for withholding on fringe benefits. The practice's accountant can clarify any questions. The total of all of these is considered *gross wages* and is the figure needed to calculate withholding.

Payroll tax deposits are calculated after each pay period. The amount of taxes determines the frequency of deposits. Taxes are due when the wages are paid, not when the payroll period ends.

SAMPLE: The decision to pay a third-quarter bonus is made, but not until after the quarter-end financial report is reviewed on October 15. The end of the pay period in this case is September 30, and the check will not be written until October 15. Those payroll taxes are then due from the October 15 date, the day the money was issued to the employee.

The rules for timely payment of payroll taxes for federal and social security withheld as taken from Circular E are as follows:

- **Rule 1—Less than $500 at the end of the quarter.** If at the end of the calendar quarter the total undeposited taxes for the quarter are less than $500, taxes do not have to be deposited. Pay the taxes to the IRS with Form 941 or deposit them by the end of the next month.
- **Rule 2—Less than $500 at the end of any month.** If at the end of any month the total undeposited taxes are less than $500, a deposit is not required but can be carried over to the following month within the quarter.
- **Rule 3—$500 or more but less than $3000 at the end of any month.** If at the end of any month the total undeposited taxes are $500 or more but less than $3000 the taxes must be deposited within 15 days after the end of the month. There are exceptions to this. Become familiar with them.
- **Rule 4—$3000 or more but less than $100,000 at the end of any 8-month period.** Each month is divided into eight deposit periods that end on the 3rd, 7th, 11th, 15th, 19th, 22nd, 25th, and last day of the month. If at the end of any 8-month period the total undeposited taxes are between $3000 and $100,000, deposit the taxes within 3 banking days after the end of that 8-month period. There are exceptions here also, so become familiar with your situation as stated in Circular E.

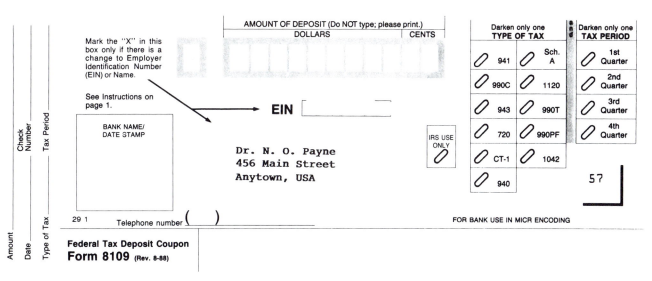

FIGURE 7–19
Federal tax deposits at your bank.

Additional guidelines for undeposited taxes in excess of $100,000 are outlined in a separate section of Circular E.

Deposits. Deposits are made using form 8109 (Federal Tax Deposit Coupon), shown in Figure 7–19. Coupon books are mailed to all employers who have a tax ID number. Call the IRS for number assignment. Mark the box to indicate the type of deposit. Federal tax withheld, Medicare taxes, and social security are marked 941. This corresponds to the form number (941) used to report information quarterly. Deliver each deposit coupon and payment to a financial institution qualified as a depositary for federal taxes. Make checks payable to the bank and include the practice tax ID number on the check. Write the pay period involved on the check stub.

Depositing on Time. The timeliness of deposits is determined by the date they are received by an authorized depositary. A deposit received after the date due is considered timely if shown it was mailed by the second day before the due date. (There are exceptions to this rule.)

Penalties. A 2–15% penalty is charged when taxes are not deposited by the date due or when federal tax deposits are mailed or delivered to IRS offices rather than the authorized depositaries. The penalty amount is determined by the amount of underpayment and/or the number of days the deposit is late. Penalties are defined in detail in Circular E.

Because of penalties involved in missing a deposit, consider writing the check for payroll taxes at the time payroll checks are written. Obtain a bank receipt stamped with the date of each deposit.

The procedure for making payroll tax deposits is detailed in Wages and Salaries. Use the earnings card (pay period ending January 15th), as illustrated in Figure 7–7.

To figure the amount of tax, add:

Federal tax withheld for *all* employees	$ 85.00
FICA withholding (withheld)	$ 55.80
FICA matched funds (employer expense)	$ 55.80
Medicare witholding (withheld)	$ 13.05
Medicare matched funds (employer expense)	$ 13.05
Total	$222.70

CREDIT
$222.70 #1020 — Checking Account

DEBIT
$153.85 #2030 — Payroll Tax Withheld
$ 68.85 #6320 — Payroll Tax Expense

Quarterly Tax Reports. At the close of every quarter, payroll tax reports are to be filed.

1st Quarter: January 1–March 31
2nd Quarter: April 1–June 30
3rd Quarter: July 1–September 30
4th Quarter: October 1–December 31

Complete these reports and mail by April 30th, July 31st, October 31st, and January 31st, respectively, after the close of the quarter. As an extra precaution, if time permits, consider having them in the mail by the 15th. If an error is discovered when doing the reports and additional payments are due and are paid by the 15th, there is often no penalty, unless the amount falls under Rule 4 ($3000 or more). Use the following guidelines:

1. Total the individual earnings cards (see Figure 7–7).
2. Write up a worksheet (Figure 7–20) to include the following:

   - Employee's name
   - Employee's social security number
   - Taxable FICA wages*
   - Taxable Medicare wages*
   - Taxable ESD wages*
   - Taxable federal unemployment tax wages*
   - Gross wages
   - Federal tax withheld
   - FICA tax withheld
   - Medicare tax withheld
   - ESD withheld
   - Net payroll

3. With the information in step 2 on this worksheet, sketch out the bottom half of the work-

---

* Maximum taxable wages are set annually (and often change in January—check with the accountant for any changes). Only withhold up to that point for each employee. The maximum is the only amount on which taxes are charged.

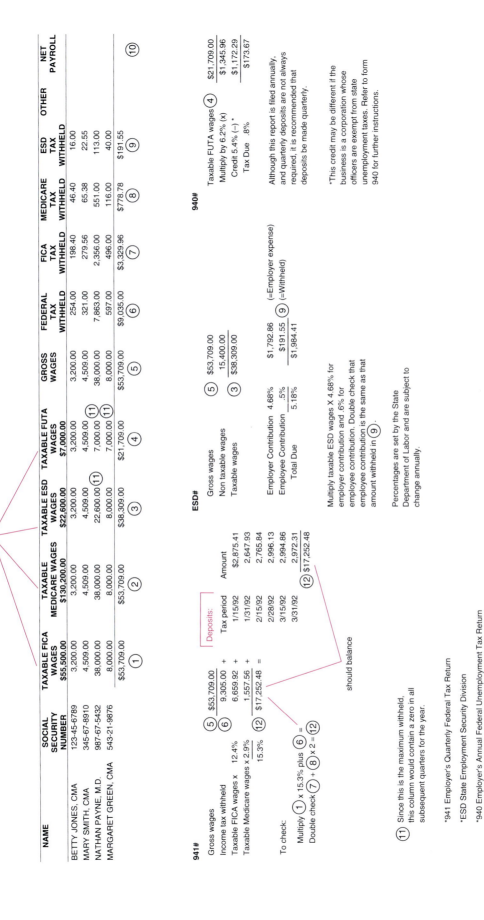

FIGURE 7-20

Quarterly payroll worksheet.

150 *Chapter 7: ACCOUNTING AND TAXES*

1 Control number	22222	For Paperwork Reduction Act Notice, see separate instructions OMB No. 1545-0008	For Official Use Only ▶				
2 Employer's name, address, and ZIP code			6 Statutory employee □ Deceased □ Pension plan □ Legal rep. □ 942 emp. □ Subtotal □ Deferred compensation □ Void □					
			7 Allocated tips		8 Advance EIC payment		
			9 Federal income tax withheld		10 Wages, tips, other compensation		
3 Employer's identification number		4 Employer's state I.D. number	11 Social security tax withheld		12 Social security wages		
5 Employee's social security number			13 Social security tips		14 Nonqualified plans		
19a Employee's name (first, middle, last)			15 Dependent care benefits		16 Fringe benefits incl. in Box 10		
			17 See Instr. for Forms W-2/W-2P		18 Other		
19b Employee's address and ZIP code							
20		21		22		23	
24 State income tax	25 State wages, tips, etc.	26 Name of state	27 Local income tax	28 Local wages, tips, etc.	29 Name of locality		

Copy A For Social Security Administration   Dept. of the Treasury—Internal Revenue Service

Form **W-2 Wage and Tax Statement 1990**

FIGURE 7-21

W-2 form: Wage and tax statement.

1 Control number 33333 OMB No. 1545-0008	For Official Use Only ▶		3 Employer's state I.D. number	5 Total number of statements
☐ Kind of Payer	2 941/941E ☐ CT-1 ☐	Military ☐ 942 ☐ 943 ☐ Medicare gov't. emp. ☐	4	
6 Establishment number	7 Allocated tips		8 Advance EIC payments	
9 Federal income tax withheld	10 Wages, tips, and other compensation		11 Social security tax withheld	
12 Social security wages	13 Social security tips		14 Nonqualified plans	
15 Dependent care benefits	16 Adjusted total social security wages and tips		17 Deferred compensation	
18 Employer's identification number			19 Other EIN used this year	
20 Employer's name			21 Gross annuity, pension, etc. (Form W-2P)	
			23 Taxable amount (Form W-2P)	
			24 Income tax withheld by third-party payer	
22 Employer's address and ZIP code (If available, place label over boxes 18 and 20.)				

DO NOT STAPLE

Under penalties of perjury, I declare that I have examined this return and accompanying documents, and to the best of my knowledge and belief, they are true, correct, and complete.

Signature ▶ _____ Title ▶ _____ Date ▶ _____

Telephone number (optional) _____

Form **W-3 Transmittal of Income and Tax Statements 1990** Department of the Treasury Internal Revenue Service

Please return this entire page with the accompanying Forms W-2 or W-2P to the Social Security Administration address for your state as listed below. **Household employers filing Forms W-2 for household employees should send the forms to the Albuquerque Data Operations Center.**
Note: Extra postage may be necessary if the report you send contains more than a few pages or if the envelope is larger than letter size. Do NOT order forms from the addresses listed below. You may order forms by calling 1-800-424-3676.

If your legal residence, principal place of business, office or agency is located in ▼	Use this address ▼
Alaska, Arizona, California, Colorado, Hawaii, Idaho, Iowa, Minnesota, Missouri, Montana, Nebraska, Nevada, North Dakota, Oregon, South Dakota, Utah, Washington, Wisconsin, Wyoming	Social Security Administration Salinas Data Operations Center Salinas, CA 93911
Alabama, Arkansas, Florida, Georgia, Illinois, Kansas, Louisiana, Mississippi, New Mexico, Oklahoma, South Carolina, Tennessee, Texas	Social Security Administration Albuquerque Data Operations Center Albuquerque, NM 87180
Connecticut, Delaware, District of Columbia, Indiana, Kentucky, Maine, Maryland, Massachusetts, Michigan, New Hampshire, New Jersey, New York, North Carolina, Ohio, Pennsylvania, Rhode Island, Vermont, Virginia, West Virginia	Social Security Administration Wilkes-Barre Data Operations Center Wilkes-Barre, PA 18769
If you have no legal residence or principal place of business in any state	Social Security Administration Wilkes-Barre Data Operations Center Wilkes-Barre, PA 18769

Paperwork Reduction Act Notice.—We ask for this information to carry out the Internal Revenue laws of the United States. We need it to ensure that taxpayers are complying with these laws and to allow us to figure and collect the right amount of tax. You are required to give us this information.

The time needed to complete and file this form will vary depending on individual circumstances.

The estimated average time is 26 minutes. If you have comments concerning the accuracy of this time estimate or suggestions for making this form more simple, we would be happy to hear from you. You can write to the **Internal Revenue Service,** Washington, DC 20224, Attention: IRS Reports Clearance Officer T:FP; or the **Office of Management and Budget,** Paperwork Reduction Project (1545-0008), Washington, DC 20503.

FIGURE 7-22

W-3 form: Summary of W-2s.

sheet with the figures needed to fill the blanks on each tax report. These include

- *941*—Employer's quarterly federal tax return. This form is used to report gross wages, federal tax withheld and deposited, FICA (social security) and Medicare withheld and deposited, and the dates deposits are made. *Penalties are stiff for not filing within the proper time frames.* See Circular E for details.
- *ESD*—This refers to the form used to report to the Alaska Department of Labor the amount allocated to go into the Employment Security Division (state unemployment is partially financed by this means). The employer's contribution is determined by the State Department of Labor for each individual employee based on a prior wage paid by that employer. The state department of labor will notify the employer at the beginning of each year of the new rates. There is a maximum wage rate (also subject to change annually).
- **Federal Unemployment Tax (FUTA)**—This is an employer expense only. No amount is withheld from the employee's check for this tax. The rule for deposits from Circular E is to deposit FUTA tax if it is more than $100.00 annually. This is a cumulative total, so if the first-quarter liability is $80.00, no deposit is required; however, that added to the second-quarter liability requires a deposit because it exceeds $100.00. This tends to be very confusing, and it is recommended to make deposits quarterly—to the same federal depositary bank—using the coupons (Form 8109 as illustrated in Figure 7–19; mark the 940 oval) supplied by the IRS. Although deposits are made quarterly, the federal tax report (Form 940) is filed at the end of the year, for the year ending December 31. This report is due to the IRS by January 31. *Please note*: There is a different formula used to figure the amount of FUTA tax due from a corporation whose officers are exempt from paying state unemployment taxes. Detailed instructions can be found on Form 940.

Year-End Payroll Reports. Form W-2, as illustrated in Figure 7–21, is a statement to each employee of the yearly total of wages and taxes withheld. This should be supplied to the employee by January 31 of the following year. The employer keeps a copy, and the remaining W-2s are forwarded to the Social Security Administration after being summarized on form W-3 (Figure 7–22) by February 28.

If payments of $600 or more are made to persons not treated as employees for services performed for the business (for example, janitorial

FIGURE 7–23

Form 1099: Miscellaneous report "nonemployee compensations."

Chapter 7: ACCOUNTING AND TAXES 153

| Form **W-9**
(Rev. December 1987)
Department of the Treasury
Internal Revenue Service | **Request for Taxpayer
Identification Number and Certification** | Give this form
to the requester. Do
NOT send to IRS. |

Name (If joint names, list first and circle the name of the person or entity whose number you enter in Part I below. **See instructions if your name has changed.**)

Please print or type

Address

City, state, and ZIP code

List account number(s)
here (optional) ▶

Part I Taxpayer Identification Number		**Part II** For Payees Exempt From Backup Withholding (See Instructions)
Enter your taxpayer identification number in the appropriate box. For individuals and sole proprietors, this is your social security number. For other entities, it is your employer identification number. If you do not have a number, see *How To Obtain a TIN*, below. **Note:** *If the account is in more than one name, see the chart on page 2 for guidelines on whose number to enter.*	Social security number OR Employer identification number	Requester's name and address (optional)

Certification.—Under penalties of perjury, I certify that:

(1) The number shown on this form is my correct taxpayer identification number (or I am waiting for a number to be issued to me), **and**

(2) I am not subject to backup withholding either because I have not been notified by the Internal Revenue Service (IRS) that I am subject to backup withholding as a result of a failure to report all interest or dividends, or the IRS has notified me that I am no longer subject to backup withholding (does not apply to real estate transactions, mortgage interest paid, the acquisition or abandonment of secured property, contributions to an individual retirement arrangement (IRA), and payments other than interest and dividends).

Certification Instructions.—You must cross out item (2) above if you have been notified by IRS that you are currently subject to backup withholding because of underreporting interest or dividends on your tax return. (Also see *Signing the Certification* under *Specific Instructions*, later.)

Please Sign Here   Signature ▶   Date ▶

Instructions

(Section references are to the Internal Revenue Code.)

Purpose of Form.—A person who is required to file an information return with IRS must obtain your correct taxpayer identification number (TIN) to report income paid to you, real estate transactions, mortgage interest paid, the acquisition or abandonment of secured property, or contributions you made to an individual retirement arrangement (IRA). Use Form W-9 to furnish your correct TIN to the requester (the person asking you to furnish your TIN), and, when applicable, (1) to certify that the TIN you are furnishing is correct, (2) to certify that you are not subject to backup withholding, and (3) to claim exemption from backup withholding if you are an exempt payee. Furnishing your correct TIN and making the appropriate certifications will prevent certain payments from being subject to the 20% backup withholding.

Note: *If a requester gives you a form other than a W-9 to request your TIN, you must use the requester's form.*

How To Obtain a TIN.—If you do not have a TIN, you should apply for one immediately. To apply for the number, obtain **Form SS-5**, Application for a Social Security Number Card (for individuals), or **Form SS-4**, Application for Employer Identification Number (for businesses and all other entities), at your local office of the Social Security Administration or the Internal Revenue Service. Complete and file the appropriate form according to its instructions.

To complete Form W-9 if you do not have a TIN, write "Applied For" in the space for the TIN in Part I, sign and date the form, and give it to the requester. For payments that could be subject to backup withholding, you will then have 60 days to obtain a TIN and furnish it to the requester.

During the 60-day period, the payments you receive will not be subject to the 20% backup withholding, unless you make a withdrawal. However, if the requester does not receive your TIN from you within 60 days, backup withholding, if applicable, will begin and continue until you furnish your TIN to the requester.

Note: *Writing "Applied For" on the form means that you have already applied for a TIN* **OR** *that you intend to apply for one in the near future.*

As soon as you receive your TIN, complete another Form W-9, include your new TIN, sign and date the form, and give it to the requester.

What Is Backup Withholding?—Persons making certain payments to you are required to withhold and pay to IRS 20% of such payments under certain conditions. This is called "backup withholding." Payments that could be subject to backup withholding include interest, dividends, broker and barter exchange transactions, rents, royalties, nonemployee compensation, and certain payments from fishing boat operators, but do not include real estate transactions.

If you give the requester your correct TIN, make the appropriate certifications, and report all your taxable interest and dividends on your tax return, your payments will not be subject to backup withholding. Payments you receive will be subject to backup withholding if:

(1) You do not furnish your TIN to the requester, or

(2) IRS notifies the requester that you furnished an incorrect TIN, or

(3) You are notified by IRS that you are subject to backup withholding because you failed to report all your interest and dividends on your tax return (for interest and dividend accounts only), or

(4) You fail to certify to the requester that you are not subject to backup withholding under (3) above (for interest and dividend accounts opened after 1983 only), or

(5) You fail to certify your TIN. This applies only to interest, dividend, broker, or barter exchange accounts opened after 1983, or broker accounts considered inactive in 1983.

For other payments, you are subject to backup withholding only if (1) or (2) above applies.

Certain payees and payments are exempt from backup withholding and information reporting. See *Payees and Payments Exempt From Backup Withholding*, below, and *Exempt Payees and Payments* under *Specific Instructions*, on page 2, if you are an exempt payee.

Payees and Payments Exempt From Backup Withholding.—The following lists payees that are exempt from backup withholding and information reporting. For interest and dividends, all listed payees are exempt except item (9). For broker transactions, payees listed in (1) through (13), and a person registered under the Investment Advisers Act of 1940 who regularly acts as a broker are exempt. Payments subject to reporting under sections 6041 and 6041A are generally exempt from backup withholding only if made to payees described in items (1) through (7), except that a corporation that provides medical and health care services or bills and collects payments for such services is not exempt from backup withholding or information reporting. Only payees described in items (2) through (6) are exempt from backup withholding for barter exchange transactions, patronage dividends, and payments by certain fishing boat operators.

(1) A corporation.

(2) An organization exempt from tax under section 501(a), or an individual retirement plan (IRA), or a custodial account under 403(b)(7).

(3) The United States or any agency or instrumentality thereof.

Form **W-9** (Rev. 12-87)

FIGURE 7–24

W-9 form, which is used for address and taxpayer ID# of 1099 prospects.

DO NOT STAPLE	6969 ☐ CORRECTED	
Form **1096** Department of the Treasury Internal Revenue Service	**Annual Summary and Transmittal of U.S. Information Returns**	OMB No. 1545-0108 **1990**

ATTACH IRS LABEL HERE

⌈ Type or machine print FILER'S name (or attach label)

Street address

City, state, and ZIP code ⌋

If you are not using a preprinted label, enter in Box 1 or 2 below the identification number you used as the filer on the information returns being transmitted. Do not fill in both Boxes 1 and 2.

Name of person to contact if IRS needs more information

Telephone number ( )

For Official Use Only

1 Employer identification number	2 Social security number	3 Total number of documents	4 Federal income tax withheld $	5 Total amount reported with this Form 1096 $

Check only one box below to indicate the type of form being transmitted. If this is your FINAL return, check here . . . . ☐

☐ W-2G 32	☐ 1098 81	☐ 1099-A 80	☐ 1099-B 79	☐ 1099-DIV 91	☐ 1099-G 86	☐ 1099-INT 92	☐ 1099-MISC 95	☐ 1099-OID 96	☐ 1099-PATR 97	☐ 1099-R 98	☐ 1099-S 75	☐ 5498 28

Under penalties of perjury, I declare that I have examined this return and accompanying documents, and, to the best of my knowledge and belief, they are true, correct, and complete.

Signature ▶ .... Title ▶ .... Date ▶ ....

Please return this entire page to the Internal Revenue Service. Photocopies are NOT acceptable.

Instructions

Purpose of Form.—Use this form to transmit paper Forms 1099, 1098, 5498, and W-2G to the Internal Revenue Service. DO NOT USE FORM 1096 TO TRANSMIT MAGNETIC MEDIA. See **Form 4804,** Transmittal of Information Returns Reported on Magnetic Media.

Use of Preprinted Label.—If you received a preprinted label from IRS with Package 1099, place the label in the name and address area of this form inside the brackets. Make any necessary changes to your name and address on the label. However, do not use the label if the taxpayer identification number (TIN) shown is incorrect. **Do not prepare your own label. Use only the IRS-prepared label that came with your Package 1099.**

If you are not using a preprinted label, enter the filer's name, address, and TIN in the spaces provided on the form.

Filer.—The name, address, and TIN of the filer on this **form must be the same as those you enter in the upper left area of Form 1099, 1098, 5498, or W-2G.** A filer includes a payer, a recipient of mortgage interest payments, a broker, a barter exchange, a person reporting real estate transactions, a trustee or issuer of an individual retirement arrangement (including an IRA or SEP), and a lender who acquires an interest in secured property or who has reason to know that the property has been abandoned.

Transmitting to IRS.—Group the forms by form number and transmit each group with a **separate** Form 1096. For example, if you must file both Forms 1098 and Forms 1099-A, complete one Form 1096 to transmit your Forms 1098 and another Form 1096 to transmit your Forms 1099-A.

Box 1 or 2.—Complete only if you are not using a preprinted IRS label. Individuals not in a trade or business must enter their social security number in Box 2; sole proprietors and all others must enter their employer identification number in Box 1. However, sole proprietors who are not required to have an employer identification number must enter their social security number in Box 2.

Box 3.—Enter the number of forms you are transmitting with this Form 1096. Do not include blank or voided forms in your total. Enter the number of correctly completed forms, not the number of pages, being transmitted. For example, if you send one page of three-to-a-page Forms 5498 with a Form 1096 and you have correctly completed two Forms 5498 on that page, enter 2 in Box 3 of Form 1096.

Box 4.—Enter the total Federal income tax withheld shown on the forms being transmitted with this Form 1096.

Box 5.—No entry is required if you are filing Form 1099-A or 1099-G. For all other forms, enter the total of the amounts from the specific boxes of the forms listed below:

Form W-2G	Box 1
Form 1098	Box 1
Form 1099-B	Boxes 2 and 3
Form 1099-DIV	Boxes 1a, 5, and 6
Form 1099-INT	Boxes 1 and 3
Form 1099-MISC	Boxes 1, 2, 3, 5, 6, 7, 8, and 10
Form 1099-OID	Boxes 1 and 2
Form 1099-PATR	Boxes 1, 2, 3, and 5
Form 1099-R	Box 1
Form 1099-S	Box 2
Form 5498	Boxes 1 and 2

For Paperwork Reduction Act Notice, see the separate Instructions for Forms 1099, 1098, 5498, and W-2G. Form **1096** (1990)

FIGURE 7-25

Form 1096: Summary of 1099s.

service or a mover), file a form 1099-Misc (Figure 7–23). This form is similar to a W-2 and requires the recipient's name, address, and social security or tax ID number and amount paid. Form W-9 (Figure 7–24) is filled out by the taxpayer and provides the information needed to complete the 1099. The total of 1099s are summarized on a form 1096 (Figure 7–25) and submitted to the IRS. If the service is performed by a business that is incorporated, no 1099 is required.

Bibliography

Beck (Ed): *Physician's Advisory Newsletter.* Plymouth Meeting, PA: MCA Publications, 1989.

Bocksnick, Gary, Insurance Connection. 312 Tyee Street, Soldotna, Alaska 99669 (907)262-2515.

Fess P, Niswonger C: *Accounting Principles,* 13th ed. Cincinnati, Ohio: South-Western Publishing, 1981.

Lincoln National Life Insurance Company, Fort Wayne, Indiana 46801.

Lindsey B: *The Administrative Medical Assistant.* Englewood Cliffs, NJ: Prentice-Hall, 1980.

MICA – Medical Indemnity Corporation of Alaska, Aleut Plaza Office Bldg., Old Seward Hwy., Suite 203, Anchorage, AK 99503 (907)563-3414.

Practice Productivity, Inc., 5076 Winters Chapel Road, Suite 700, Atlanta, Georgia 30360-1832. 1-800-241-6228.

Reading and Analyzing Financial Statements (II-F86/036). Midvale, UT: B. Wright & Associates, 1986.

Rediform 16801 Addison Rd., Dallas, TX 75248.

Schmiedicke R, Naagy C: *Principles of Cost Accounting,* 7th ed. Cincinnati, Ohio: South-Western Publishing, 1983.

Stein, George CPA, P.O. Box 3466, Soldotna, Alaska 99669 (907)262-1455.

Talahaski Fordney M, Johnson Follis J: *Administrative Medical Assisting.* New York: John Wiley & Sons, 1982.

Tuter, Janice CPA, *Obendorf, Tuter & Lambe,* 189 So. Binkley Suite 201, Soldotna, Alaska 99669 (907)262-9123.

Chapter 8

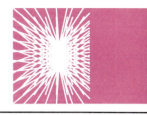

INSURANCE AND CODING

NANCY VINES CAMPBELL
MARY KLINGE

COVERAGE AND POLICIES
Types of Health Insurance Coverage
Types of Health Insurance Policies
CLAIMS PROCESSING
Information from the Medical Record/Patient
Assignments
Claim Forms
Claim Filing Deadline
Insurance Log
PAYMENTS AND REJECTIONS
Methods of Payments
Resource-Based Relative Value Scale
Explanation of Benefit
Rejections
Refiles
HEALTH MAINTENANCE ORGANIZATIONS

Types of HMOs
ICD-9-CM CODING
History
Impact of the *ICD-9-CM* on Physicians' Offices
Prerequisites for Accurate Coding
The *ICD-9-CM* Coding Books
Remembering the Basics: Some Guidelines
The Employee's Role in Coding
Physician Education
Validation of the Diagnosis in the Medical Record
Guidelines for Coding Specific Conditions
Additional Coding Information
Diagnosis-Related Groups
The Future of the ICD

COVERAGE AND POLICIES

Types of Health Insurance Coverage

Health insurance plays a vital role in the physician's office. Among the many problems the medical assistant may encounter is that most of the patients have no idea what type of insurance coverage they have. There are at least four types of health insurance coverage:

- Basic medical
- Major medical
- Hospitalization
- Surgical

Health insurance is considered by many to be a game. It is important that all pieces and players work together to provide the physician and the hospital with the best reimbursement possible. An understanding of the definitions of the four types of health insurance will help you play the game more efficiently.

Basic Medical

The basic medical portion of the patient's insurance varies according to the options chosen by the patient or the patient's employer. Depending on individual coverage, basic medical may include an office visit, diagnostic x-ray, and laboratory work. Other plans may cover only diagnostic x-ray and/or laboratory work. Many insurance companies have a deductible ranging from $100 to as much as $750, $1000, or $2000. In some instances this deductible must be met before the basic medical portion of the insurance paying. The basic medical portion of the insurance is exactly what it says — *basic*.

Today with the many preferred provider organizations (PPOs), if a patient sees a physician other than one participating in the PPO the policy reverts back to basic and major medical coverage. (PPOs are discussed later in this chapter.)

Major Medical

The major medical portion of the patient's policy comes into play in several ways. If a patient is involved in an accident and seeks medical care, this care is considered under the major medical portion. There can be a dollar amount maximum per accident (this could be somewhere around $300) and the stipulation that the patient seek medical care within a specified time period after the accident. As stated previously, this information varies according to the patient's individual policy. Remember, the patient is the best source of information concerning insurance coverage. Although many patients do not know much about their coverage, make a copy of the insurance card (front and back) for future use.

The major medical portion of insurance may also cover drug expenses. Once again, depending on the individual patient's coverage, the drug expense will be applied toward the major medical and reimbursed at a percentage set by the insurance company (normally 80%).

Hospitalization

The hospitalization portion of the patient's insurance policy covers charges that are incurred during a hospital stay. With the many changes in short-stay admissions, a hospital stay is defined as inpatient services rendered beyond a 24-hour stay. The hospitalization portion can be subject to a deductible for each hospital stay. This deductible varies depending once again on the amount listed by the insurance company (a ballpark figure is $200–$500).

Preadmission Certification. Preadmission Certification (PAC) is required for all admissions except maternity and emergency admissions. The patient is responsible for making sure a written PAC is completed before admission into the hospital.

Many insurance companies will not pay the physician's charges or any hospital charges if the subscriber and the physician do not complete the PAC form before admission.

Emergency Admission. The hospital should be advised that the admission is an emergency to assure that proper documentation is placed in the chart. The claim will need to reflect the admission as emergent (Figure 8–1).

Surgical

The surgical portion of the patient's insurance is used when the physician renders surgical care to the patient. This can range from services rendered on an outpatient basis in the physician's office, services rendered in a one-day surgery ambulatory care center, or services rendered during an inpatient hospital stay.

Types of Health Insurance Policies

Blue Cross/Blue Shield

Blue Cross/Blue Shield is a nationwide insurance company. There are more than 75 local Blue Cross/Blue Shield organizations, each operating under state law as a nonprofit organization. Your local Blue Cross/Blue Shield organization works closely with the physician and hospital to provide assistance in interpreting policies and procedures. This task is handled by the provider and professional relations staff at Blue Cross/Blue Shield. Besides interpreting policies and procedures, they conduct workshops and seminars, always providing both the physician and medical assistant with up-to-date information. It is important to maintain a good working relationship with this group, especially your own representative.

> **SPECIAL HINT**
>
> Insurance is changing rapidly, and a good medical assistant must be well informed of all changes taking place.

Blue Cross/Blue Shield coverage comprises two parts. Physicians and professional services are paid for their services under the Blue Shield portion of the contract, while hospitals are paid under the Blue Cross portion. Patients may be covered under both Blue Cross and Blue Shield or either Blue Cross or Blue Shield.

If a patient has only Blue Shield coverage, another company may be providing coverage for the hospital services, and vice versa. Medicare, Medicaid, or CHAMPUS may be administered by the local Blue Cross/Blue Shield group of your state. Blue Cross/Blue Shield would be the fiscal intermediary for these programs, with Blue Cross han-

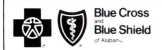

PREADMISSION CERTIFICATION

P.O. Box 2504
Birmingham, Alabama 35201-2504

Dear Doctor:

Preadmission Certification is designed to promote the utilization of outpatient service in place of the inpatient hospital setting, when appropriate. Prior to the admission, Blue Cross and Blue Shield of Alabama must review the medical necessity of the inpatient setting. Please complete Section II of this page to facilitate this process. Failure to obtain preadmission certification may result in denial of benefits. Please telephone Blue Cross and Blue Shield of Alabama at the telephone number listed below for emergency admissions within 24-48 hours of the admission date.

I. PATIENT INFORMATION

Patient Name	Subscriber Name *(If not Patient)*	Contract Number	Group-Division Number
Street Address	City State ZIP	Home Telephone Number	Work Telephone Number
Date of Birth	Signature of Subscriber or Dependent of Legal Age		

II. ADMISSION INFORMATION

Primary Admitting Diagnosis	ICD-9 Code	Secondary Admitting Diagnosis	ICD-9 Code
Proposed Admission Date	Proposed Surgery Date	Name Of Admitting Hospital Or Facility	Recommended Length Of Stay
Brief Summary Of Previous Outpatient Treatment		Proposed Surgical Procedure(s)	CPT Code(s)
☐ Continued On Attached Sheet		☐ Continued On Attached Sheet	
Medical Factors Indicating Need For Hospitalization		Outline Of Proposed In Hospital Treatment Plan	
☐ Continued On Attached Sheet		☐ Continued On Attached Sheet	

III. PHYSICIAN INFORMATION

I certify that this inpatient admission is medically necessary for the diagnosis given. I also certify that this patient could not use any of the alternatives to inpatient coverge available to him/her. I understand that this inpatient admission is subject to medical review.

Attending Physician's Name	Ala. Provider # (If Applicable)	Office Telephone	Mailing Address, City, State, ZIP
Contact Person	Doctor's Signature		Date

Please return this form to:
BLUE CROSS AND BLUE SHIELD OF ALABAMA
ATTENTION: Preadmission Certification
P.O. Box 2504
Birmingham, Alabama 35201-2504

In Birmingham (205) 988-2245
Outside Birmingham Call:
1 800 248-2342
Telefax 205 985-5820

PRO-70-1 (Rev. 1-92)

FIGURE 8-1

Preadmission Certification form. (Courtesy of Blue Cross and Blue Shield of Alabama.)

dling Medicare Part A and Blue Shield handling Medicare Part B.

Always ask to see the Blue Cross/Blue Shield card, because there are many types of identification cards. Each state, as well as some foreign countries, has its Blue Cross/Blue Shield organizations identified by its own card.

Federal Employee Program

The Federal Employee Program (FEP) is a plan administered by Blue Cross and Blue Shield to provide health care insurance to federal government employees.

FEP cards can be identified by the words "Government-Wide Service Benefit Plan" followed by the subscriber's name and identification number (Figure 8–2). The identification number always begins with an *R* followed by eight digits. The enrollment code is either 101, 102, 104, or 105. The effective date of current coverage is in the card's right lower corner.

Enrollment codes 101, 102, 104, and 105 are coverage codes defined as follows:

101	self-only high option
102	family high option
104	self-only low option
105	family low option

Besides telling you the type of coverage the patient has, the enrollment code also lets you know the amount of copayment due.

Central Certification

Another variation in coverage and cards is central certification.

The central certification card is identified by the words "central certification" located in the top right corner of the card (Figure 8–3). The particular coverage is administered by a control plan and provides coverage for companies whose employees are located all over the country in many cities and states. Having the control plan administer the recordkeeping of all employees who may travel extensively or relocate frequently benefits the subscriber and physician greatly. The medical assistant files the patient's claim directly with the local Blue Cross/Blue Shield organization.

When filing a central certification plan, it is important to remember to include the following:

- Subscriber's name (as listed on card)
- Identification code and number
- Group number

Including these three items on claim forms ensures payment from the local carrier.

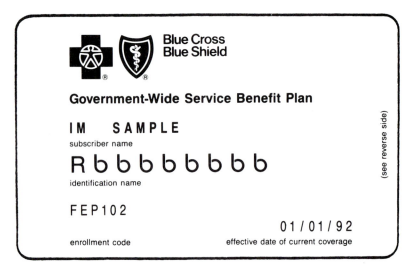

FIGURE 8–2

Blue Cross Federal Employee Program card. (Courtesy of Blue Cross and Blue Shield of Alabama.)

Chapter 8: INSURANCE AND CODING **161**

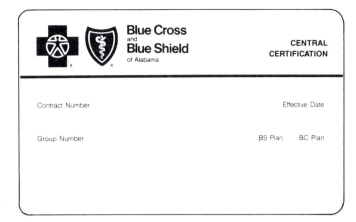

FIGURE 8-3

Blue Cross central certification card. (Courtesy of Blue Cross and Blue Shield of Alabama.)

Blue Shield Permanent Reciprocity Program

A double-ended red arrow on a patient's identification card indicates coverage under the Blue Shield Permanent Reciprocity Program. The arrow is located in the upper left corner of the card. Inside the arrow is an *N* followed by three digits (Figure 8-4). Coverage under the Permanent Reciprocity Program involves a method in which out-of-area claims may be paid by the local Blue Shield plan where the services are rendered. When preparing a claim, be sure and include the subscriber's name and the information contained in the double-ended red arrow (*N* plus three digits). These claims are filed with the local Blue Shield plan.

Medicare, United Mine Workers of America, and Travelers Medicare

These policies are all forms of health insurance for the elderly or disabled. Eligibility for Medicare coverage actually begins at age 65 or when a person becomes disabled. The patient must contact Social Security to enroll in Medicare for coverage to begin. Medicare is administered by the federal government, and each state has a intermediary carrier that administers the rules and regulations set down by the federal government. For many states, the local Blue Cross/Blue Shield insurance company is the carrier.

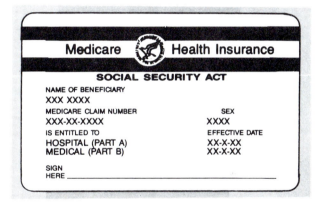

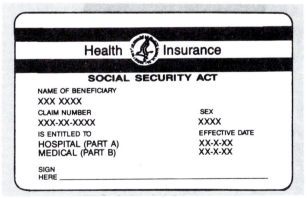

FIGURE 8-5

Medicare cards. (Courtesy of Blue Cross and Blue Shield of Alabama.)

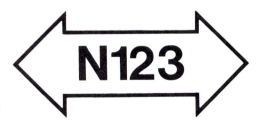

FIGURE 8-4

Blue Shield permanent reciprocity program symbol. (From Fordney, M.: *Insurance Handbook for the Medical Office*, 2nd ed. Philadelphia: W.B. Saunders, 1981.)

Most Commonly Used Medicare Suffix Codes

A	Wage earner
B	Wife, not dependent on having child in her care
B3	Second claimant
B1	Husband
B4	Second claimant
B2	Wife, dependent on having child in her care
B5	Second claimant
B6	Divorced wife
B9	Second claimant
C1	Child (youngest child is C1, next youngest is C2, etc.)
D	Widow, at least age 60
D2	Second claimant
D1	Widower, at least 62
D3	Second claimant
D4	Widow, remarried after age 60 (benefit 50% of PIA)
D5	Widow, remarried after age 62 (benefit 50% of PIA)
D6	Surviving divorced wife
D7	Second claimant
E	Mother (widow with child in her care)
E2	Second claimant
E1	Surviving divorced mother
E3	Second claimant
F1	Father
F7	Second alleged father
F2	Mother
F8	Second alleged mother
F3	Stepfather
F4	Stepmother
F5	Adopting father
F6	Adopting mother
G	Lump sum claimant (first claimant is G1, second claimant is G2, etc.)
H	Precedes claim symbol when payment is made from Disability Trust Fund
J	Special Age 72 beneficiary ($40.00 benefit)
K	Spouse of J ($20.00 benefit)
J1 or K1	entitled to HIB, less than 3 Q/C's
J2 or K2	entitled to HIB, 3 or more Q/C's
J3 or K3	not entitled to HIB, less than 3 Q/C's
J4 or K4	not entitled to HIB, 3 or more Q/C's

FIGURE 8-6

Medicare suffix codes.

T	HIB entitlement; no RSDI entitlement, not qualified RR beneficiary, may or may not be entitled to SMIB
M	SMIB entitlement ONLY; not eligible for any type of OASI monthly benefit or HIB (Deemed Insured) and is not a "qualified RR beneficiary"
M1	SMIB entitlement ONLY; appears to be eligible for HIB through entitlement to monthly benefits or under deemed insured provision but elects to file for SMIB only
W	Disabled widow
W2	Second claimant
W1	Disabled widower
W3	Second claimant
W6	Disabled surviving divorced wife
W7	Second claimant

When a female spouse of a wage earner, drawing social security benefits because of her husband's contribution, becomes a widow, her Medicare suffix may change from a B to a D. If you know of a recently widowed beneficiary with a B suffix, ask if a new Medicare card has been issued so that your records can be updated.

FIGURE 8-6 Continued

Medicare. The Medicare card is white with red and blue stripes (Figure 8-5). There have been revisions made to the Medicare card. As of September 1990, the new cards use the terms *hospital* (Part A) and *medical* (Part B). The changes were made because beneficiaries and the medical community had shown a preference for these terms when referring to medicare coverage. Additional revisions to the Medicare card occurred in Spring 1991. Medicare appears as part of the header and the health insurance claim number (contract number) is identified as the Medicare claim number.

The card is labeled "Health Insurance" or "Medicare Health Insurance." According to the Health Care Financing Administration (HCFA), the cards issued before the implementation of the revisions are still valid. Medicare's health insurance number can be identified by the patient or the patient's spouse's social security number followed by a suffix (Figure 8-6).

United Mine Workers of America. United Mine Workers of America (UMWA) is administered by Blue Cross of California, located in Van Nuys. The address is

> UMWA Health Retirement Funds
> P.O. Box 9924
> Van Nuys, CA 91409

This type of medicare is available to retired mine workers and their spouses. The card looks different from other Medicare cards (Figure 8-7).

It generally takes longer to receive payment or denial from UMWA than from other carriers.

Travelers Medicare. Travelers Medicare is filed in Augusta, Georgia. The address for this insurance is

> Travelers Insurance Company
> Railroad Medicare Claim Department
> Interstate West Office Park
> P.O. Box 10066
> Augusta, GA 30903

Once again the Medicare card looks almost the same, but the numbers are different. The words "Railroad Retirees" appears on the Travelers Medicare card. The patient who is covered by Travelers Medicare can be identified by the prefixes shown in Figure 8-8.

Explanation of Medicare Benefits. Medicare is very basic in its coverage, although the rules and regulations administered by the federal government keep changing. The basic parts of Medicare coverage are Part A and Part B.

Medicare Part A. Part A is hospital insurance,

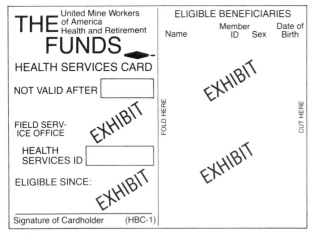

FIGURE 8-7

United Mine Workers of America card.

which covers inpatient hospital services, outpatient diagnostic services, some posthospital care, and care received in an extended-care facility. If the patient is covered under this portion of Medicare when hospitalized, Medicare pays the hospital charges.

Medicare Part B. Part B is for medical services and must be purchased by the patient. It covers most physician services, end-stage renal disease, and home health services. This pays for physician charges, durable medical equipment, home health care, and stay in an extended-care facility (Figure 8-9).

Home health care covers skilled care that is medically necessary and certified by the doctor. Medicare only partially covers skilled nursing care, and this care must be administered at a nursing home certified by Medicare as a skilled nursing facility.

All Medicare patients must sign the Extended Patient Signatures Authorization form. The patient signs once, and the signature is good for a lifetime. By having patients sign this form, the physician agrees to file all Medicare claims, assigned or nonassigned.

> **SPECIAL HINT**
>
> The signed form is kept on file in the physician's office.

Medicare Deductible. Part A is subject to a deductible for each hospital admission. This can vary from year to year and is set by the federal government. In 1992, the deductible was $652. Part B is subject to a deductible of $100 of approved charges. The deductible runs from calendar year to calendar year. In dealing with many elderly patients, it becomes difficult to explain Medicare benefits. It is important that they understand that the $100 is of approved charges rather than incurred charges. Figure 8-10 shows an example of Medicare's calculation of a submitted charge.

Medicare Supplement. Patients may carry a supplemental insurance to Medicare. Medicare supplemental insurance policies are sometimes referred to as "Medigap" policies because they are intended to fill the gap in health care protection that Medicare does not cover. This can vary according to the type of coverage the patient chooses. Some supplemental insurances pay the patient's deductible or a portion thereof. This pertains to the inpatient deductible for hospital admissions as well as the deductible for medical services.

Medicaid

Medicaid is insurance regulated by the state government, and each recipient must meet certain income requirements. Medicaid recipients are issued a Medicaid card each month depending on their eligibility.

> **SPECIAL HINT**
>
> Always verify effective dates of coverage.

The eligibility of the Medicaid patient is reevaluated each month. The Medicaid card lists the eligible recipients, their names, dates of birth, and Medicaid number. The Medicaid number consists

MA	CA	WH	WCH
WA	A	WCA	WCD
PA	PD	PH	JA
H	MH	WD	

NOTE: Six or nine digits should follow the prefixes listed above.
For example MA-000000

FIGURE 8-8

Travelers Medicare prefixes.

Medicare Part B

Extended Patient Signature Authorization

TO BE COMPLETED BY PROVIDERS OF SERVICE—Please PRINT or TYPE

Provider's Name *(If you are a DME supplier, please complete certification at bottom of page)*	Provider's I.D. Code
Provider's Address *(Street, City, State, ZIP Code)*	

Beneficiary's Name	Medicare HI Number	Applicable MEDIGAP Group Number

TO BE COMPLETED BY BENEFICIARY OR AGENT—Directions For Payment Of Benefits And Release Of Medical Information

STATEMENT FOR PAYMENT OF MEDICARE BENEFITS

I request that payment of authorized Medicare benefits be made either to me or on my behalf to

Dr. _____ or to _____ (the Suppler) for any services or items furnished to me by the physician or supplier. I authorize any holder of medical information about me to release to Health Care Financing Administration and its agents any information needed to determine these benefits or the benefits payable for related services.

STATEMENT FOR PAYMENT OF MEDIGAP BENEFITS

I request that payment of authorized MEDIGAP benefits be made either to me or on my behalf to

_____ for any services furnished to me by the physician/supplier. I authorize any holder of medical information about me to release to (name of MEDIGAP Insurer)

_____ any information needed to determine these benefits or the benefits payable for related services.

_____ _____
Signature of Beneficiary or person signing for Beneficiary   Date Signed

Address of Person Signing For Beneficiary *(Street, City, State, ZIP Code)*	Relationship Of Agent To Beneficiary

Reason Beneficiary Is Unable To Sign

IMPORTANT INFORMATION FOR PHYSICIANS

In submitting claims under this procedure, PHYSICIANS undertake:
1. To complete and submit promptly the appropriate Medicare billing form for all services covered by the request for payment—**even those in which the physician has not accepted assignment.**
2. To incorporate, by stamp or otherwise, information to the following effect on any bills they send to Medicare patients: "DO NOT USE THIS BILL FOR CLAIMING MEDICARE BENEFITS. A CLAIM HAS BEEN OR WILL BE SUBMITTED TO MEDICARE ON YOUR BEHALF." This requirement is necessary to prevent patients from submitting duplicate claims.
3. To cancel the authorization on request by the patient.
4. To make the patient signature files available for carrier inspection upon request.

IMPORTANT INFORMATION FOR SUPPLIERS

1. Only use this extended patient signature authorization for **assigned** claims.
2. Renew the patient signature agreement if a new item is rented or purchased.
3. Place alongside the beneficiary's signature the following statement: "RESPONSIBLITY FOR OVERPAYMENT ON ASSIGNED CLAIMS ACCEPTED."

DURABLE MEDICAL EQUIPMENT SUPPLIERS AGREEMENT

NOTE: THE FOLLOWING STATEMENT MUST BE SIGNED BY THE DME SUPPLIER PRIOR TO AUTHORIZATION OF PAYMENT FOR RENTAL OF DURABLE MEDICAL EQUIPMENT IN ASSIGNMENT CASES.

This supplier assumes unconditional responsibility for refunding of all overpayments for assigned claims for rental of durable medical equipment that may result from the failure of the Carrier to receive prompt notice of the return of, or the end of need for the rental of equipment, or the death or institutionalization of the Beneficiary.

_____ _____
Signature of Durable Medical Equipment Supplier   Date Signed

MCB-56 (Rev. 4-89)   Form Approved OMB 0938-0222

FIGURE 8-9

Medicare Part B extended patient signature authorization. (Courtesy of Blue Cross and Blue Shield of Alabama.)

Level 2	99212	$45.00
Medicare nonallowed		10.00
Medicare approved		35.00
Medicare payment at 80% of approved charge (if deductible met)		$28.00

FIGURE 8-10

Example of Medicare's calculation of a submitted charge.

of 13 digits. Normally, the Medicaid number is three zeros followed by the patient's social security number, followed by a check digit (Figure 8-11).

Limitations. The Medicaid patient is limited as to the number of inpatient and outpatient services received. Medicaid limits hospital inpatient days to 12 per calendar year. Medicaid also limits outpatient visits to 12 per calendar year, and services must be medically indicated.

Civilian Health and Medical Program of the Uniformed Services

The Civilian Health and Medical Program of the Uniformed Services (CHAMPUS) provides families of Uniformed Services personnel and retirees supplemental medical services in military, Public Health Service facilities, and the private sector. CHAMPUS is a comprehensive health benefits program funded by Congress. Eligible personnel may seek care from a Navy or Army hospital near home. Patients are also able to have care rendered to them outside the military facilities. Patients may choose a private physician. Patients are responsible for some inpatient and outpatient cost sharing. Each eligible CHAMPUS patient 10 years of age or older is required to have a Uniformed Services Identification and Privilege card.

Commercial (Independent, Private) Policies

Each physician's office decides which insurance should be filed for patients. This can vary according to the patient clientele of the individual physician. For example, a physician may set up practice in a small town where the local and largest employer for that area participates in Aetna (this could be Provident, Mailhandlers, etc.) for its employees. It may be wise for that physician to file Aetna for the patients.

Commercial or private insurances require the same information as required by Blue Cross, Medicare, and Medicaid. Most can be submitted on the standard insurance form (HCFA-1500). Many insurance companies now require use of diagnosis codes in the *International Classification of Diseases, 9th Revision, Clinical Modifications (ICD-9-CM)* and procedure codes in the *Current Procedural Terminology (CPT-4)* (these are discussed later in this chapter).

When completing commercial insurance form for the patient, make sure the patient has completed his or her portion and has signed the release of information and/or the assignment, if needed. This standard form can be ordered through the American Medical Association (Figure 8-12), whose address is

> 515 North State Street
> Chicago, IL 60610.

Health Maintenance Organization

Under a health maintenance organization (HMO) plan, participating physicians render certain medical services to a group of enrolled people who make fixed periodic payments to the plan. HMOs are popular with many employers and employees because they provide preventive care and offer lower premiums and predictable medical expenses.

For further reading on HMOs, see Richards in the Suggested Readings.

Preferred Provider Organizations

A preferred provider organization (PPO) varies from the standard HMO. Patients can choose from a panel of physicians who have agreed (through contract) to provide services. Patients can go to these physicians and experience less out-of-pocket expense. Many PPOs offer a plan whereby the patient pays a small copayment for each visit. Unlike many other insurance carriers, PPOs waive any preexisting condition clauses and cover many services pertaining to preventive medicine. Most PPOs require the patient to use only the hospitals that have signed PPO contracts. This could cause inconvenience for some patients. If the patient chooses to seek care from a physician outside the PPO, the patient becomes responsible for the bill.

Independent Practice Associations

The independent practice association (IPA) is similar to an HMO. This health care plan is made

Chapter 8: INSURANCE AND CODING **167**

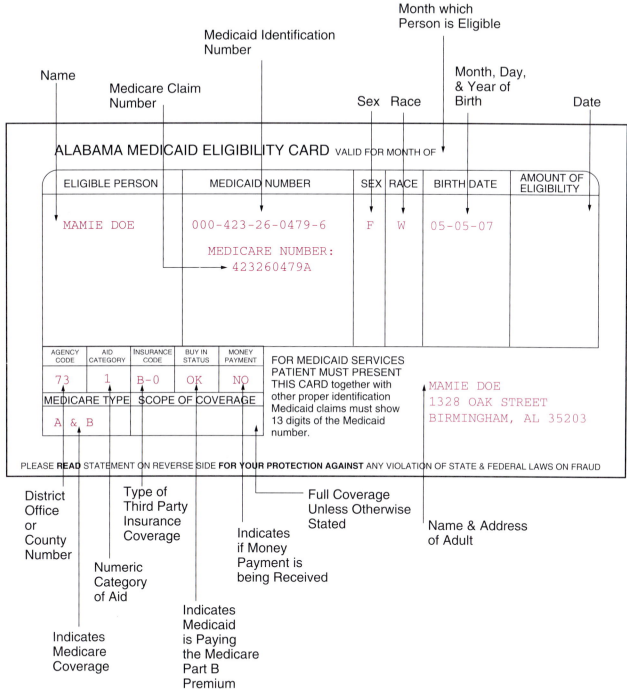

FIGURE 8-11
Medicaid card. (Courtesy of Alabama Medicaid Agency.)

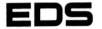

FIGURE 8-12

Standard HCFA-1500 insurance claim form. (Courtesy of Alabama Medicaid Agency.)

REFERS TO GOVERNMENT PROGRAMS ONLY

MEDICARE AND CHAMPUS PAYMENTS: A patient's signature requests that payment be made and authorizes release of medical information necessary to pay the claim. If item 9 is completed, the patient's signature authorizes releasing of the information to the insurer or agency shown. In Medicare assigned or CHAMPUS participation cases, the physician agrees to accept the charge determination of the Medicare carrier or CHAMPUS fiscal intermediary as the full charge, and the patient is responsible only for the deductible, coinsurance, and noncovered services. Coinsurance and the deductible are based upon the charge determination of the Medicare carrier or CHAMPUS fiscal intermediary if this is less than the charge submitted. CHAMPUS is not a health insurance program and renders payment for health benefits provided through membership and affiliation with the Uniformed Services. Information on the patient's sponsor should be provided in those items captioned "Insured"; i.e., items 3, 6, 7, 8, 9 and 11.

BLACK LUNG AND FECA CLAIMS: The provider agrees to accept the amount paid by the Government as payment in full. See Black Lung FECA instructions regarding required procedure and diagnosis coding systems.

SIGNATURE OF PHYSICIAN OR SUPPLIER (MEDICARE, CHAMPUS, FECA AND BLACK LUNG)

I certify that the services shown on this form were medically indicated and necessary for the health of the patient and were personally rendered by me or were rendered incident to my professional service by my employee under immediate personal supervision, except as otherwise expressly permitted by Medicare or CHAMPUS regulations.

For services to be considered a 'incident' to a physician's professional service, 1) they must be rendered under the physician's immediate personal supervision by his/her employee, 2) they must be an integral, although incidental part of a covered physician's service, 3) they must be of kinds commonly furnished in physician's offices, and 4) the services of nonphysicians must be included on the physician's bills.

For CHAMPUS claims, I further certify that neither I nor any employee who rendered the services are employees or members of the Uniformed Services (refer to 5 USC 5536). For Black Lung claims, I further certify that the services performed were for a Black Lung related disorder.

No Part B Medicare benefits may be paid unless this form is received as required by existing law and regulations (20 CFR 422 510).

NOTICE: Any one who misrepresents or falsifies essential information to receive payment from Federal funds requested by this form may upon conviction be subject to fine and imprisonment under applicable Federal laws.

BECAUSE THIS FORM IS USED BY VARIOUS GOVERNMENT AND PRIVATE HEALTH PROGRAMS, SEE SEPARATE INSTRUCTIONS ISSUED BY APPLICABLE PROGRAM.

NOTICE TO PATIENT ABOUT THE COLLECTION AND USE OF MEDICARE, CHAMPUS, FECA, AND BLACK LUNG INFORMATION

We are authorized by HCFA, CHAMPUS and OWCP to ask you for information needed in the administration of the Medicare, CHAMPUS, FECA, and BLACK LUNG programs. Authority to collect information is in section 205(a), 1872 and 1875 of the Social Security Act as amended and 44 USC 3101, 41 CFR 101 et seq and 10 USC 1079 and 1086; 5 USC 8101 et seq; and 30 USC 901 et seq.

The information we obtain to complete claims under these programs is used to identify you and to determine your eligibility. It is also used to decide if the services and supplies you received are covered by these programs and to insure that proper payment is made.

The information may also be given to other providers of services, carriers, intermediaries, medical review boards and other organizations or Federal agencies as necessary to administer these programs. For example, it may be necessary to disclose information about the benefits you have used to a hospital or doctor.

With the one exception discussed below, there are no penalties under these programs for refusing to supply information. However, failure to furnish information regarding the medical services rendered or the amount charged would prevent payment of claims under these programs. Failure to furnish any other information, such as name or claim number, would delay payment of the claim.

It is mandatory that you tell us if you are being treated for a work related injury so we can determine whether workers' compensation will pay for treatment. Section 1877(a)(3) of the Social Security Act provides criminal penalties for withholding this information.

MEDICAID PAYMENTS (PROVIDER CERTIFICATION)

I hereby agree to keep such records as are necessary to disclose fully the extent of services provided to individuals under the State's Title XIX plan and to furnish information regarding any payments claimed for providing such services as the State Agency or Dept. of Health and Human Services may request. I further agree to accept, as payment in full, the amount paid by the Medicaid program for those claims submitted for payment under that program, with the exception of authorized deductibles and coinsurance.

SIGNATURE OF PHYSICIAN (OR SUPPLIER): I certify that the services listed above were medically indicated and necessary to the health of this patient and were personally rendered by me or my employee under my personal direction.

NOTICE: This is to certify that the foregoing information is true, accurate, and complete.

I understand that payment and satisfaction of this claim will be from Federal and State funds, and that any false claims, statements, or documents, or concealment of a material fact, may be prosecuted under applicable Federal or State laws.

PLACE OF SERVICE CODES:
1 — Hospital as Inpatient
2 — Hospital as Outpatient
3 — Physician's Office
4 — Patient's Home
5 — Day Care Facility—Psychiatric
6 — Night Care Facility—Psychiatric
7 — Nursing Home/Domiciliary Facility
8 — Extended Care Facility/Skilled Nursing Facility
9 — Ambulance
0 — Other Locations
A — Independent Laboratory
B — Other Medical, Surgical Facility
C — Dental Office
D — Residential Substance Abuse Treatment Facility
E — Outpatient Substance Abuse Treatment Facility
F — Psychiatric Day Care—Inpatient

TYPE OF SERVICE CODES:
0 — Surgical Assistance
1 — Nurse Midwife, Dialysis Center, PreNatal Clinic, State Lab
2 — Surgery
3 — Maternity
4 — Anesthesia
5 — X-Ray/Diagnostic
6 — Medical
6 — Consultation
6 — Emergency Medical Care
6 — Concurrent Care
6 — Psychiatric Care
6 — Physical Therapy/Medicine
6 — Chemotherapy (Antineoplastics)
7 — Dental Care
8 — Clinical Laboratory or Pathology
8 — Radioimmunoassay (R.I.A.)
E — X-Ray Therapeutic
F — Ambulance Service
G — Physical Accessories (purchase)
H — Physical Accessories (rental)
M — Vision Care
N — Injectable Drugs
P — Radiology and Pathology (Professional Component)
R — Family Planning Clinic
V — Hearing Care

FIGURE 8-12 *Continued*

up of a group of physicians and other health care providers who form a corporation to offer health care coverage for their patients. After collecting premiums from the subscribers, the physicians are paid on a fee-for-service, per-patient basis. Funds for operating the IPA are obtained by holding out a certain percentage of the premium fund. At the end of the year, physicians share in the excess or pay if there is a deficit.

CLAIMS PROCESSING

Information from the Medical Record/Patient

The best source of information concerning a patient's insurance is the patient. Depending on the size of the physician's office, there may or may not be direct contact with the patient. The patient's medical record can be an excellent place to obtain insurance information. The patient set-up sheet (this may be called several different names, but refers to the information sheet the patient completes on the first visit to the physician) can list the pertinent insurance information for each patient. This can be updated and referred to as often as needed.

Assignments

Assignment: The patient, by agreement, authorizes the insurance company to pay benefits directly to the physician for services rendered.

Regarding Medicare, the physician must choose to be either participating or nonparticipating. This may be decided at one of two times:

1. Within 90 days of
   a. Being newly licensed to practice.
   b. First opening an office in a particular carrier area
   c. Becoming a physician for whom a hospital previously billed services but who is now billing his or her own services.
2. Before December 31 of a current year (the physician files with the local fiscal intermediary his or her agreement to participate or not participate for the following calendar year).

The local carrier that administers Medicare issues the physician a provider number to be used regarding all claims and correspondence.

Participating

If the physician chooses to participate, he or she agrees to not bill the Medicare patient for the difference between the actual charge for a particular service and the amount allowed by Medicare. The physician will be in violation with Medicare if he or she does so. Participating physicians can increase their fee schedule at any time. The physician who accepts assignment for Medicare patients must also file claims for services rendered on behalf of the patient.

Recent legislation passed by the Congress (the Omnibus Budget Reconciliation Act of 1989) included a new Medicare claims filing requirement. Effective September 1, 1990, all physicians must file with the Medicare carrier all claims for services provided to Medicare beneficiaries.

- The claims-filing requirement applies to all physicians who provide covered services to Medicare beneficiaries.
- Physicians are not required to take assignment of Medicare benefits unless they are enrolled in the Medicare Participating Physician Program or the Medicare beneficiary is also a recipient of state medical assistance (Medicaid).
- Physicians may not charge the beneficiary for preparing and filing a Medicare claim.
- Physicians who do not submit Medicare claims for Medicare beneficiaries may be subject to a civil monetary penalty of up to $2000 for each violation.
- Most claims submitted by a participating physician are processed within a ceiling of 17 days, or else interest is paid.

Nonparticipating

If the physician chooses not to participate, there are many more rules and regulations that must be complied with.

- The physician is able to bill the patient for the entire charge amount.
- The fee schedule for nonparticipating physicians is based on 95% of the fee schedule amount.
- Nonparticipating physicians are subject to limits on their actual charge. These limits are referred to as limiting charges.

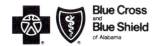

FIGURE 8-13

Blank Medicaid and Blue Cross claim forms. (Courtesy of Blue Cross and Blue Shield of Alabama.)

Illustration continued on following page

Chapter 8: INSURANCE AND CODING

BLUE SHIELD CLAIMS

SIGNATURE OF PHYSICIAN: Your signature in this box is certification that the services listed on this form were medically indicated and necessary to the health of this patient and were personally rendered by yourself or were rendered by another person under your personal direction.

PAYMENT TO PHYSICIAN: For direct payment to you, your signature and the date signed are required in block 31, and a checkmark in the box captioned "YES" is required in block 27 otherwise, payment will be made to the subscriber.

PLACE OF SERVICE CODES

1 - Inpatient Hospital
2 - Outpatient Hospital
3 - Doctor's Office
4 - Patient's Home
5 - Day Care Facility (PSY)
6 - Night Care Facility (PSY)
7 - Nursing Home
8 - Skilled Nursing Facility
9 - Ambulance

O - Other Location
A - Independent Laboratory
B - Other Medical, Surgical Facility
C - Dental Office
D - Residential Substance Abuse
    Treatment Facility
E - Outpatient Substance Abuse
    Treatment Facility
F - Psychiatric Day Care - Inpatient

TYPE OF SERVICE CODES

0 - Surgical Assistant
2 - Surgery
3 - Maternity
4 - Anesthesia
5 - X-ray/Diagnostic (Total Fee)
6 - Medical Care
7 - Dental Care
8 - Clinical Laboratory or Pathology
   (Total Fee)
9 - Consultation
A - Emergency Medical Care
B - Concurrent Care
C - Psychiatric Care
D - Physical Therapy/Medicine
E - X-ray Therapeutic
F - Ambulance Service
G - Physical Accessories (purchase)
H - Physical Accessories (rental)
I - Dental Surgery
J - Home Care Program Services

L - Visiting Nurse Services
M - Vision Care
N - Emergency Accident Care
P - Radiology and Pathology
   (Professional Component)
Q - Chemotherapy (Antineoplastics)
R - Donor Surgery & Related Services
T - Radioimmunoassay (R.I.A.) or
   Competitive Protein Binding Analysis
U - Supplemental Accident
V - Hearing Care
W - Second Opinion Consultation/Surgery
X - Alcohol/Rehabilitation
Z - Portable X-ray—Technical

FIGURE 8-13 Continued

- In 1992, the limiting charges could not exceed 120% of the nonparticipant fee schedule amount.
- Beginning in 1993 and thereafter, the limiting charges cannot exceed 115% of the nonparticipant fee schedule.
- Nonparticipating physicians' Medicare claims will be processed within a ceiling of 24 days compared with 17 days' process time for participating physicians.

Claim Forms

There are several different types of claim forms. Some carriers may require using their form, and others allow use of a standard insurance form. The standard form is commonly referred to as HFCA-1500. Medicare, Medicaid, and CHAMPUS use the HCFA-1500 form. CHAMPUS, however, has its own form that may be used to complete insurance information. Its name and number are CHAMPUS/CHAMPVA claim form 500 (Rev. 4-87). See Figure 8–13 for copies of insurance claims.

Processing claim forms is a very simple task. There are two ways a claim form can be processed:

- Electronic
- Manual (also referred to as hardcopy)

There are three methods used to submit claims electronically:

- Computer to computer
- Magnetic tape
- On line terminals

More information regarding the computer applications can be found in Chapter 9.

PROCEDURE

PROCEDURE: COMPLETING THE MANUAL CLAIM FORM (HCFA-1500)

For an example of a completed form, see Figure 8–14.

EQUIPMENT AND MATERIALS

The patient's insurance information and copy of card
The patient's medical record
The patient's charge ticket (encounter form) for the date of service to be filed (This charge ticket should contain all charges incurred through the physician's office, including x-ray and laboratory work if performed. In some physicians' offices, the charge tickets have been coded with the proper *ICD-9-CM* code, and this code can be taken from the charge ticket directly to the insurance form.)
Typewriter
Claim form
CPT-4
ICD-9-CM

PROCEDURAL STEPS

1. In block 1 ("Patient's name"), enter the patient's last name, first name, and middle initial as they appear in the medical record.
2. In block 2 ("Patient's date of birth"), enter the patient's month, day, and year of birth expressed in numbers (e.g., 06/20/53 for June 20, 1953).
3. In block 3 ("Insured's name"), enter the insured's last name, first name, and middle initial as they appear on the insurance card.
4. In block 4 ("Patient's address"), enter the patient's complete street address. All claims *must* include zip codes.
5. In block 5 ("Patient's sex"), indicate the patient's sex by placing an *X* in the appropriate box.
6. In block 6 ("Insured's ID number"), enter the patient's number listed on the insurance card. For Medicaid enter the patient's 13-digit Medicaid recipient number as it appears on the white monthly eligibility card.
7. Block 7 ("Patient's relationship to the insured") is completed as appropriate.
8. In block 8 ("Insured's group number"), enter group number, if applicable, as it appears on the insurance card.
9. In block 9 ("Other health insurance coverage"), if the patient has other health insurance coverage, enter all pertinent information.
10. In block 10 ("Was condition related to: (A)

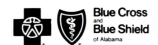

FIGURE 8–14

Completed Blue Cross claim form. (Courtesy of Blue Cross and Blue Shield of Alabama.)

BLUE SHIELD CLAIMS

SIGNATURE OF PHYSICIAN: Your signature in this box is certification that the services listed on this form were medically indicated and necessary to the health of this patient and were personally rendered by yourself or were rendered by another person under your personal direction.

PAYMENT TO PHYSICIAN: For direct payment to you, your signature and the date signed are required in block 25, and a checkmark in the box captioned "YES" is required in block 26 otherwise, payment will be made to the subscriber.

PLACE OF SERVICE CODES

1 - Inpatient Hospital
2 - Outpatient Hospital
3 - Doctor's Office
4 - Patient's Home
5 - Day Care Facility (PSY)
6 - Night Care Facility (PSY)
7 - Nursing Home
8 - Skilled Nursing Facility
9 - Ambulance

0 - Other Location
A - Independent Laboratory
B - Other Medical, Surgical Facility
C - Dental Office
D - Residential Substance Abuse
     Treatment Facility
E - Outpatient Substance Abuse
     Treatment Facility
F - Psychiatric Day Care - Inpatient

FIGURE 8–14 Continued

patient's employment or (B) an accident, auto or other?"), place an *X* in the appropriate boxes. For Medicaid, if "yes" to any of these questions is checked, complete and attach an XIX-TPD-1-76 form (Figure 8–15). If the accident was home related, indicate "home accident" or if the visit is not related to an accident, use "treatment due to disease" in block 11.

11. In block 11 ("Insured's address"), give the complete address.
11a. In block 11a (CHAMPUS sponsors), indicate the insured's status and enter the branch of service.
12. In block 12 ("Patient's or authorized person's signature"), the patient's signature and the date are required after he or she has read the statement on the back of the claim form. If billing on computer, you may write "signature on file." Medicare patients are required to sign the Medicare Part B Extended Patient Signature Authorization (see Figure 8–9). NOTE: Radiologists, pathologists, and anesthesiologists may use the statement "signature not required."
13. In block 13 ("Authorization of payment"), the patient's signature is required if payment is to be sent to the provider. This does not apply to Medicaid patients.
14. Block 14 ("Date of illness, injury, or pregnancy") is completed only if the information pertains to the patient's condition.
15. Block 15 ("Date first consulted you for this condition") is completed only if the information pertains to the patient's condition.
16. In block 16 ("Has the patient ever had same or similar symptoms?"), place an *X* in the appropriate box if the information pertains to the patient's condition. NOTE: For "emergency," place an *X* only if the condition is an emergency.
17. Block 17 ("Date patient able to return to work") is completed as appropriate.
18. Block 18 ("Dates of total disability/dates of partial disability") is completed only if the patient is eligible for disability benefits. For Medicaid patients, leave blank.
19. In block 19 ("Name of referring physician or other source"), enter the complete name and provider number of the referring physician or agency if the service rendered is a referral or consultation. Enter "none" if there is no referring physician or agency.
20. In block 20 ("For services related to hospitalization, give hospitalization dates"), for inpatient hospitalization, indicate the patient's admission and discharge dates.
21. In block 21 ("Name and address of facility where services rendered"), if the services were provided other than in the patient's home or the provider's facility, enter the name, address, and zip code of that facility.
22. In block 22 ("Was laboratory work performed outside your office?"), place an *X* in

Chapter 8: INSURANCE AND CODING

ALABAMA MEDICAL ASSISTANCE PLAN—TITLE XIX
FORM XIX-TPD-1-76
MEDICAID AUTHORIZATION ASSIGNMENT

I. Patient's Name: _____ Medicaid #: _____

II. Provider: _____

III. **TO BE COMPLETED IF INSURANCE INVOLVED:**

   A. Name of Insurance Company: _____

   B. Address of Insurance Company: _____

   C. Policy #: _____ Policyholder: _____

   D. Name & Address of Employer if Group Insurance: _____
   _____

IV. **TO BE COMPLETED IF SERVICES RENDERED AS A RESULT OF AN ACCIDENT:**

   A. Date of Accident: _____ Location: _____
   (LIST CITY & COUNTY FOR AUTO ACCIDENT,
   _____
   SITE (HOME, SCHOOL, ETC.) & ADDRESS FOR OTHER TYPE)

   B. Describe Accident: _____

   C. If auto accident, give name & address of driver(s): _____
   _____

   D. Was auto insurance carried? Yes _____ No _____ (If yes, complete Item III)

   E. If school accident, was school insurance carried? Yes _____ No _____ (If yes, complete Item III)

   F. Has an attorney been retained? Yes _____ No _____ Name of attorney: _____

V. **COMPLETE THE FOLLOWING IF ANY MEMBER OF YOUR HOUSEHOLD IS EMPLOYED:**

   Employee: _____ Relationship: _____

   Employer: _____ Address: _____

VI. **TO BE COMPLETED IF THERE IS OTHER INSURANCE AND/OR IF AN ACCIDENT WAS INVOLVED:**

AUTHORIZATION AND ASSIGNMENT

I authorize any holder of medical or other information about me to release information needed for this or a related Medicaid claim to the Alabama Medical Services Administration, and I authorize the further release of any such information to any other parties who may be liable for any of my medical expenses. I hereby assign to the Alabama Medical Services Administration all claims against third parties, including tortfeasors and insurance companies, who may be liable for any of my medical expenses to the extent that such expenses are paid by Medicaid; I also assign all rights in any settlement made by me and arising out of any claim of which this is a part to the extent of medical expenses paid by Medicaid, whether or not a portion of such settlment is designated as being for medical expenses. Any such funds received by me shall be paid to the Alabama Medical Services Administration. I permit a copy of this Authorization and Assignment to be used in place of the original.

_____   _____
SIGNATURE OF PATIENT (OR PARENT IF PATIENT IS UNDER 19)   WITNESS SIGNATURE BY MARK MUST BE WITNESSED

_____   _____
SIGNATURE OF POLICYHOLDER   WITNESS SIGNATURE BY MARK MUST BE WITNESSED

_____
Date

MCD-16
380-206

EDS-3
Alabama Diversified Health Services / Alabama Hospital Association

FIGURE 8–15

Medicaid XIX-TPD-1-76 authorization form. (Courtesy of Alabama Medicaid Agency.)

the appropriate box. If "no" is checked, do nothing further. If "yes" is checked, be sure that the name, address, and zip code of the facility that performed the service is entered in block 21. For Medicaid, the physician is permitted to bill for routine venipuncture for collection of specimens tested outside the office.

23. In block 23A ("Diagnosis or nature of illness or injury"), enter the code and a narrative description that is complete, concise, and specific for injury or illness (the *ICD-9-CM* and *CPT-4* are discussed later in this chapter). For Medicaid, only two diagnosis codes are allowed per claim form. Radiologists and pathologists are not required to enter a written diagnosis or *ICD-9-CM* code. These providers should print "Diagnosis not required — radiologist or pathologist" in block 23A.

24. In block 23B ("EPSDT and family planning"), for Medicaid place an *X* in the appropriate box. For "Prior authorization," if the service performed was specifically prior authorized, indicate the six-digit number supplied by the state Medicaid agency.

25. In block 24A ("Date of service"), for each service performed, enter the date of service. Express all dates in numbers (e.g., 03/25/90). In the event that identical services and charges are performed on the same day, enter the same date of service in both the "from" and "to" columns, and enter the number of services or units performed in block 24F. When identical services and charges are performed on consecutive days of service, enter the first date of service in the "from" column and the last date of service in the "to" column, and enter the number of services or units performed in block 24F.

26. In block 24B ("Place of service"), for each service, enter the appropriate "place of service" code. These codes can be found on the back of the claim form.

27. In block 24C ("Fully describe procedures, medical services or supplies furnished for each date given"), enter the appropriate five-digit *CPT-4* procedure code. Enter a narrative description that is complete, concise, and specific for each billed service. Also recognized are HCPCS (Health Care Financing Administration Common Procedure Coding System) codes for injectable drugs administered by the physician. For anesthesiologists, the *ASA Relative Value Guide* must be used when billing anesthesia procedures.

28. In block 24D ("Diagnosis treated code"), for each service stated in block 24C, enter the line item reference of the diagnosis that it relates to (i.e., 1 or 2) from block 23A. If a procedure is related to more than one diagnosis, the primary diagnosis to which the procedure is related should be the one referred to in this section. For Medicaid, if the services rendered relate to more than two diagnoses, a separate claim must be completed.

29. In block 24E ("Charges"), indicate the usual and customary charges to the public for each line of service listed.

30. In block 24F ("Number of units of service"), enter the number of units of service or visits in the appropriate column for each service rendered. A unit of one is assumed unless otherwise indicated.

31. In block 24G ("Type of service"), for each service, enter the appropriate "type of service" code listed on the back of the claim form. When filing Medicaid only, use the type of service codes on the back of the HCFA-1500 (Rev. 1-84) form.

32. Block 24H should be left blank.

33. In block 25 ("Signature of physician or supplier"), after reading the provider certification on the back of the claim form, the physician should sign the claim.

34. In block 26 ("Accept assignment"), the provider checks "yes" or "no" to indicate his or her decision to accept assignment of benefits when a claim is filed. For Medicaid, the provider agrees to accept the Medicaid reimbursement as payment in full for those services covered under the Medicaid program.

35. In block 27 ("Total charge"), enter the sum of the charges shown in block 24E. The total should reflect on the charges for each page.

36. In block 28 ("Amount paid"), enter the amount paid by other insurance, if applicable. Do not list the copayment amount collected.

37. In block 29 ("Balance due"), subtract block 28 from block 27 and enter the balance in this block.

38. In block 30 ("Physician's social security number"), enter the social security number of the physician or supplier.

39. In block 31 ("Physician's or supplier's name, address, zip code, telephone number, and provider number"), enter the physician's or supplier's name, street, city, state, zip code, and telephone number. Also enter the physi-

CHAMPUS/CHAMPVA CLAIM FORM

For services or supplies provided by civilian sources of medical care
Read cover instructions and the back of this form **before completing and signing!**

OMB No. 0704-0084

Patient/Sponsor Information (Items 1 through 18 to be completed by the beneficiary/patient or sponsor.)

1. PATIENT'S NAME (Last, First, Middle Initial)
2. PATIENT'S DATE OF BIRTH — MONTH | DAY | YEAR
7. SPONSOR'S NAME (Last, First, Middle initial)
3. PATIENT'S ADDRESS (Street, City, State, ZIP Code)
PHONE NO. (include area code)
4. PATIENT'S SEX ☐ MALE ☐ FEMALE
8. SPONSOR'S SOCIAL SECURITY NO. OR VA FILE NO.
9. VA STATION NO.
5. MILITARY/VA IDENTIFICATION CARD
CARD NO.
ISSUE DATE MONTH DAY YEAR | EFFECTIVE DATE MONTH DAY YEAR | EXPIRATION DATE MONTH DAY YEAR
6. PATIENT'S RELATIONSHIP TO SPONSOR
☐ SELF ☐ SPOUSE
☐ NATURAL or ADOPTED CHILD ☐ STEPCHILD
OTHER (Specify):
10. SPONSOR'S DUTY STATION OR ADDRESS FOR RETIREES.
PHONE NO. (Include area code)
14. DO YOU HAVE OTHER HEALTH INSURANCE? ☐ YES ☐ NO
IF YES, ENTER NAME OF OTHER PLAN OR PROGRAM:
ADDRESS
CITY STATE ZIP
15. IS CONDITION WORK RELATED? ☐ YES ☐ NO
MILITARY SERVICE RELATED? ☐ YES ☐ NO
AUTOMOBILE ACCIDENT RELATED? ☐ YES ☐ NO
11. SPONSOR'S BRANCH OF SERVICE
☐ USA ☐ USAF ☐ USMC ☐ USN
☐ USCG ☐ USPHS ☐ NOAA ☐ VA
12. SPONSOR'S GRADE/RANK
13. SPONSOR'S STATUS
☐ ACTIVE DUTY ☐ RETIRED ☐ DECEASED
16. INPATIENT/OUTPATIENT CARE
☐ OUTPATIENT ☐ INPATIENT-EMERGENCY ☐ PROGRAM FOR THE HANDICAPPED ☐ INPATIENT HOSPITAL-OUTSIDE CATCHMENT AREA
☐ INPATIENT-SKILLED NURSING FACILITY
☐ INPATIENT HOSPITAL WITHIN CATCHMENT AREA (ATTACH DD FORM 1251) ☐ INPATIENT-OTHER
14a. TYPE OF COVERAGE:
☐ EMPLOYMENT (GROUP) ☐ MEDICAID ☐ STUDENT PLAN
☐ PRIVATE (NON-GROUP) ☐ MEDICARE ☐ OTHER:
14b. OTHER IDENTIFICATION NUMBER
14c. EFFECTIVE DATE MONTH DAY YEAR
17. DESCRIBE CONDITION FOR WHICH YOU RECEIVED TREATMENT. IF AN INJURY, NOTE HOW IT HAPPENED.
14d. OTHER PROGRAM THROUGH EMPLOYMENT?
EMPLOYER NAME:
18. SIGNATURE OF PATIENT OR AUTHORIZED PERSON, CERTIFIES CLAIM INFORMATION AND AUTHORIZES RELEASE OF MEDICAL OR OTHER INSURANCE INFORMATION. READ INSTRUCTIONS AND BACK OF THIS FORM BEFORE SIGNING.
SIGNED: DATE: RELATIONSHIP TO PATIENT:

Physician/Other Provider (Items 19 through 33 are to be completed by the physician or other provider.)

19. NAME, ADDRESS & PHONE NO. OF REFERRING PHYSICIAN
☐ PRIVATE PRACTICE or ☐ UNIFORMED SERVICES
20. NAME & ADDRESS OF FACILITY WHERE SERVICES RENDERED (other than home or office)
21. PROVIDER OF SERVICES
☐ ATTENDING PHYSICIAN
☐ OTHER:
22. HOSPITALIZATION INFORMATION
ADMITTED MO DAY YEAR | DISCHARGED MO DAY YEAR
23. LAB WORK OUTSIDE YOUR OFFICE? ☐ YES ☐ NO CHARGES:
24. DIAGNOSIS, SYMPTOM OR NATURE OF ILLNESS OR INJURY, RELATE DIAGNOSIS TO PROCEDURE IN COLUMN "D" BY REFERENCE TO NUMBERS 1,2,3 or DX CODE
1.
2.
3.

25A. DATES OF SERVICE MO/DAY/YEAR	B* PLACE OF SERVICE	C PROCEDURE CODE IDENTIFY:	D. DESCRIBE PROCEDURES/SUPPLIES FOR EACH DATE, SUBMIT REPORT EXPLAINING UNUSUAL SERVICES OR CIRCUMSTANCES.	E DIAGNOSIS CODE	F CHARGES	LEAVE BLANK

26. PATIENT'S ACCOUNT NO.
27. PROVIDER'S SOCIAL SECURITY NO.
28. PROVIDER'S EMPLOYER I.D. NO.
29. PHYSICIAN'S OR OTHER PROVIDER'S NAME, ADDRESS, ZIP CODE & PHONE NO. (INCLUDING AREA CODE)
PROVIDER NO.
G. TOTAL CHARGES $
30. AMOUNT PAID BY BENEFICIARY $
31. AMOUNT PAID BY OTHER INSURANCE $
32. **AGREEMENT TO PARTICIPATE** (READ BACK OF THIS FORM)
☐ YES ☐ NO
33. SIGNATURE OF PHYSICIAN OR OTHER PROVIDER (READ BACK OF THIS FORM BEFORE SIGNING)
SIGNED: DATE:

*PLACE OF SERVICE CODES
1— (IH)—INPATIENT HOSPITAL
2— (OH)—OUTPATIENT HOSPITAL
3— (O)—DOCTOR'S OFFICE
4— (H)—PATIENT'S HOME
5— (DCF)—DAY CARE FACILITY (PSY)
6— (NCF)—NIGHT CARE FACILITY (PSY)
7— (NH)—NURSING HOME
8— (SNF)—SKILLED NURSING FACILITY
9— (AMB)—AMBULANCE
0— (OL)—OTHER LOCATIONS
A— (IL)—INDEPENDENT LABORATORY
B— (OF)—OTHER MEDICAL/SURGICAL FACILITY
C— (RTC)—RESIDENTIAL TREATMENT CENTER
D— (STF)—SPECIALIZED TREATMENT FACILITY

CHAMPUS FORM 500 REV. Apr 87—Previous editions may be used.

FIGURE 8-16

Blank CHAMPUS form.

cian's or supplier's provider number. The provider name, number, and signature must match.
40. In block 32 ("Patient's account number"), enter the patient's account or medical record number. Entries appearing in this block will be referenced on the "Explanation of payment."
41. In block 33 ("Physician's employer ID number"), enter the physician's or supplier's employer ID federal tax number.

NOTE: The CHAMPUS form (Figure 8–16) varies in that lines 1–18 are to be completed by the patient with information obtained from the CHAMPUS card. The standard HCFA-1500 claim form is also accepted by CHAMPUS.

Claim Filing Deadline

Most insurances have claim filing deadlines. For Medicare and CHAMPUS, all claims must be submitted no later than December 31 of the calendar year after the year in which the medical service was provided. For example, a claim for medical service received during the calendar year 1992 must be filed no later than December 31, 1993. Medicaid has a claim filing deadline of 1 year from the date of service. Blue Cross/Blue Shield time limits for filing claims vary according to the individual group. For most groups, claims must be filed within 24 months from the date of service.

Insurance Log

The insurance log is a very important document that can be used by the medical assistant to recoup otherwise-overlooked monies owed to the physician by the insurance companies. This log maintains a list of claims that are outstanding with each insurance carrier (Figure 8–17). There are several variations of insurance logs. It is best to find one that works best for you. Be creative and design your own insurance log if you do not find the exact information you need.

SPECIAL HINT

The important thing to remember is that the log has to work for you in order to be effective.

By looking at the insurance log, the medical assistant can quickly see the status of each claim — whether it is outstanding and needs follow-up with the insurance company, or can be crossed off as paid. When crossing off a claim that has been paid, do so carefully, making sure all important data can still be read.

SPECIAL HINT

The medical assistant may want to log the claims according to insurance carrier. This may simplify follow-up on delinquent claims by reviewing each carrier's list and sending one letter stating the delinquent claims for that particular physician. Each month's unpaid claims can be set aside, suspending them in a file, and reviewed on a monthly to bimonthly basis.

PAYMENTS AND REJECTIONS

Methods of Payments

- Usual, customary, and reasonable (UCR)
- Resource-based relative value scale (RBRVS)
- Fee schedule
- Diagnosis-related groups (DRGS)

The medical assistant must be familiar with these four methods of payments. Blue Cross/Blue Shield may use a variety of reimbursement methods. The most common type of payment used is UCR. In many states, the local Blue Cross/Blue Shield carriers have developed PPOs. PPOs (referred to in Alabama as Preferred Care) are very popular and rank second to UCR, with payments being made according to a fee schedule.

Usual, Customary, and Reasonable

An understanding of UCR payment is helped by a knowledge of the terminology involved:

INSURANCE LOG

INSURANCE CO.	DATE FILED	PATIENT'S NAME	ADDRESS	$ OF CLAIM	DATE PAID	AMT PAID	REFILE	FOLLOW-UP DATE

FIGURE 8-17
Insurance log.

Usual fee: The fee normally charged by the physician for a specific service rendered to the patient.

Customary fee: The fee charged by the physician in the same or similar specialty that is in the range for the same services within the same geographical location.

Reasonable fee: The fee is considered reasonable even if it does not meet customary and usual criteria. This would include unusual circumstances requiring additional skill or time regarding a specific service.

UCR payment can be determined by taking the normal fee charged by the physician, taking the fee charged by other physicians in the same locale and specialty and comparing the two fees, considering unusual circumstances, if any. The insurance carrier will not reimburse a charge that is lower than the community's UCR at the higher UCR rate, however.

SAMPLE: A physician sees an established patient for a routine office visit and charges $25.00. The physician gets reimbursed at the $25.00 rate, even though the customary fee for that particular level of service is higher ($35.00). The insurance carrier reimburses the physician the actual charge submitted or the UCR charge or the customary charge, whichever is the lowest.

- Under Blue Cross/Blue Shield plans, a physician can either be participating or nonparticipating. When a physician is participating, payment is made directly to the physician. The physician accepts this amount (which will be a usual, reasonable, or customary fee) as payment in full.
- Nonparticipating physicians' payment can vary according to the subscriber's policy/plan. Some Blue Cross/Blue Shield plans have the patient paying a percentage of the charge as copayment. This percentage can range from 5% to 25%.

Resource-Based Relative Value Scale

As part of the legislation passed by Congress (Omnibus Budget Reconciliation Act [OBRA] of 1989) in an effort to create more equity and consistency in payments to physicians, a new Medicare physician payment system was developed.

The new Medicare fee schedule, which began January 1, 1992, replaces the customary, prevailing, and reasonable charge payment system. This fee schedule is based on the relative value of resources that physicians spend to provide services for Medicare patients.

The fee schedule amount for a service is calculated based on the following three factors:

- Relative value units (RVU)
- Geographical practice cost indices (GPCI)
- National conversion factor (CF)

There will be no payment differentials for a service based on the physician's specialty. The new Medicare fee schedule assigns higher relative values to visits and includes a new set of codes known as evaluation and management (E and M) codes. The E and M codes replace the former visit code system and also provide physicians with a more accurate description of the relative amount of effort they use to perform these services.

The Health Care Financing Administration (HCFA) states that there will be a 5-year transition period for implementing the Medicare fee schedule. After 1992, the transition is as follows:

- 1993 — 25% of the fee schedule amount is added to 75% of the 1992 payment rate.
- 1994 — 33% of the fee schedule amount is added to 67% of the 1993 payment rate.
- 1995 — 50% of the fee schedule amount is added to 50% of the 1994 payment rate.
- 1996 — full fee schedule paid for all physician services.

Fee Schedule

The fee schedule is a list of accepted charges for specific services rendered by the physician. For more information concerning fee schedules, see Chapter 6.

Diagnosis-Related Group

In 1985 DRGs began as a means to control hospital costs. There are now 492 DRGs. These inpatient services are paid under Medicare Part A. These are categorized according to diagnosis. These classifications group the patients whose medically related diagnosis and treatment and length of stay are about the same. Regardless of the length of stay, the hospital is reimbursed one set amount relating to the particular DRG(s) for the patient. (See Appendix, Diagnosis-Related Groups Listing.)

Explanation of Benefit

The explanation of benefit (EOB) can also be referred to as explanation of payment (EOP). Both the EOB and EOP refer to the statement

PROVIDER REMITTANCE EXAMPLE

```
                    ALABAMA MEDICARE PART B PROVIDER REMITTANCE                11/01/90
                                                                              PAGE:    1
                    PROVIDER NAME:    DR JOHN DOE
                    PROVIDER NUMBER:  012345

DR JOHN DOE
123 MAIN STREET
ANYTOWN, AL 35000
                                                                                   ACCT.
BROWN, ANN D      (123121234D)     CLAIM #902886101010000
PROVIDER NAME SVC DATE(S)   PROCEDURE P T NUM SUBMITTED  NON-ALWD  DEDUCT  CO-INS  PAY BENE  PAY PROV  AC  AB
DR J DOE      0831 08310    7311026   3 4  1    12.84      12.84    0.00    0.00     0.00      0.00    39
                            7313026   3 4  1    12.84      12.84    0.00    0.00     0.00      0.00    39
CLAIM REMARKS                 CLAIM TOTALS      25.68      25.68                                0.00
                                                                            NET PAY:           0.00

                                                                                   ACCT.
JONES, TOM B      (123456789A)     CLAIM #902865101020000
PROVIDER NAME SVC DATE(S)   PROCEDURE P T NUM SUBMITTED  NON-ALWD  DEDUCT  CO-INS  PAY BENE  PAY PROV  AC  AB
DR J DOE      1205 12059    7016026   5 4  1    12.58       2.52    0.00    2.01     0.00      7.88    82
CLAIM REMARKS 6               CLAIM TOTALS      12.58       2.52                                7.88
ADJUSTMENTS - P: 0.00                 G:  0.17    O:  0.00                  NET PAY:           7.88

                                                                                   ACCT. AB12345-0001
SMITH, JANE A     (987654321A)     CLAIM #902851101030001
PROVIDER NAME SVC DATE(S)   PROCEDURE P T NUM SUBMITTED  NON-ALWD  DEDUCT  CO-INS  PAY BENE  PAY PROV  AC  AB
DR J DOE      0921 09210    7101026   3 4  1    13.24       2.65    0.00    2.12     0.00      8.47    82
                                                CLAIM TOTALS 13.24  2.65                       8.47
CLAIM REMARKS
ADJUSTMENTS - P: 4.00                 G:  0.00    O:  0.00                  NET PAY            4.47

                                    INTEREST SUBMITTED  NON-ALWD          CO-I  PAY BENE   PAY PROV
TOTAL CLAIMS    3                        0.00    51.50    30.85            4.     0.00      12.35
CHECK NUMBER:       001234567890
```

FIGURE 8-18

Example of Medicare remittance. (Courtesy of Blue Cross and Blue Shield of Alabama.)

mailed from the insurance carrier to either the provider or the subscriber that explains the action taken on each claim. This EOB shows a breakdown and explanation of payment or denial for each line item submitted. A check for the amount listed on the remittance will accompany the explanation of benefits. Many insurance companies list the rejection code descriptions on the last page of each remittance. The EOB varies according to insurance carrier. Most physician's remittances have similar information. On an average remittance (Figure 8–18), the following information appears:

Patient name
Claim number
Contract number
Date of service
Place of service
Procedure code
Total charge
Noncovered charges
Patient deductible
Copay
Nonallowed
Other coverage
Payment

Blue Cross/Blue Shield along with Medicare send remittances for each provider (physician). Medicaid pays under a group number if you are submitting claims for more than one physician. Medicaid remittances are divided into six separate sections.

- Medicaid-only paid claims
- Medicaid-only claims pending
- Medicaid-only claims denied
- Medicare-related paid claims
- Medicare-related denied claims
- Claims pending adjudication

The rejection codes used in the remittance are listed in the remittance. The last page of the remittance is a summary of the physician's payments. This includes payment totals for the present payroll and the year-to-date payment total. Figures 8–19 and 8–20 are examples of Blue Cross/Blue Shield and CHAMPUS remittances.

Contractual Nonalloweds

Nonallowed amounts occur when the physician participates in the Medicare participating physician program. Nonallowed amounts also occur when the physician participates in managed-care programs where, by signed contract, the physician agrees to write off the difference between the charge submitted and the allowed charge.

Rejections

The rejections for each claim or for a particular line item are listed on the EOB or EOP. The reasons for rejects vary widely. Often a denied claim results from something as simple as the misspelling of the patient's name or an invalid contract number. Referring to a copy of the insurance card can make refiling a claim with this particular type of rejection easy. With repeated experience with the EOB, the medical assistant will be able to quickly glance at an EOB to determine if any refiles are necessary.

A list of rejection codes may be obtained from the insurance carrier. A typical rejection code may be 903, defined on the last page of the remittance as "903—Contract Discontinued."

Refiles

A *refile* can be defined as any claim being resubmitted to the insurance company. The refile can be a claim for which there has been no response or a corrected claim. Refiles can be sent back to the insurance company with corrected information. It is best to write "REFILE" at the top of the resubmitted claim. Submit only the charge or charges you want considered, remembering to change the total amount of the claim. It can be really frustrating to resubmit a claim only to have it rejected by the insurance company as either a duplicate or as previously processed.

> **SPECIAL HINT**
>
> Develop a form letter stating that this is a reconsideration of a previously denied charge. This form letter can be attached to the resubmitted claim.

Time Limit on Refiling Claims

Medicaid and Medicare have a time limit for refiling a denied charge. A denied Medicaid or Medicare charge can only be reconsidered within six months after denial.

Follow-Up Delinquent Unpaid Claims

The insurance log (see Insurance Log section) will help in following up on delinquent unpaid insurance claims. Depending on the particular in-

CHAMPUS/CHAMPVA Explanation Of Benefits

CHAMPUS/CHAMPVA EXPLANATION OF BENEFITS
Blue Cross and Blue Shield of South Carolina

"Appeals must be filed within ninety (90) days of the receipt of this notice."

Internal Control Number		Date of Notice
Sponsor's Name		SSN or VA
Patient Beneficiary		Benefit Period Beginning Date
Name		
Date of Birth	S&R	Services From	Services To

THIS IS NOT A BILL. THIS IS A STATEMENT OF THE ACTION TAKEN ON YOUR CHAMPUS/CHAMPVA CLAIM. KEEP THIS NOTICE FOR YOUR RECORDS.

Services Were Provided By	Dates of Service From Mo. Day Yr.	Dates of Service To Mo. Day Yr.	Number of Services	Description of Services	Amount Billed	Amount Not Covered	Amount Allowed	Paid by Beneficiary	Reason Code
				FACSIMILE					
TOTAL				▶					

REMARKS/REASON CODE

TOTAL AMOUNT COVERED

CHECK NUMBER

DEDUCTIBLE INFORMATION

"Claims payments are subject to the provision that the beneficiary cost-share is collected by the provider. The provider's failure to collect the cost-share can be considered a false claim and/or may result in reduction of payment."

(32164)4/85

FIGURE 8-19

Example of CHAMPUS remittance. (Courtesy of Blue Cross and Blue Shield of South Carolina.)

CLAIM NUMBER	PATIENT NAME	CONTRACT NUMBER	CASE NUMBER	DATES OF SERVICE FROM	DATES OF SERVICE THRU	PL SR	PROC CODE	DISP CODE	TOTAL CHARGE	NONCOVERED CHARGES	PATIENT PAYABLE DEDUCT	PATIENT PAYABLE COPAY	NON-ALLOWED	OTHER COVERAGE	PAYMENT
						PREFERRED CARE CLAIMS									
555-1111111	BROWN J	000112222		01/01/89	01/01/89	3	690060	P10	40.00	0.00	0.00	15.00	5.00	0.00	20.00
				01/01/89	01/01/89	3	GL0111		30.00	0.00	0.00	5.60	2.00	0.00	22.40
							CLAIM TOTALS		70.00	0.00	0.00	20.60	7.00	0.00	42.40
555-1111112	RICHARDS L	000122222		01/01/89	01/01/89	3	885025	PMD	10.00	0.00	0.00	3.00	3.20	0.00	3.80
555-1111113	JONES A	000132222		01/01/89	01/01/89	3	217777	P25	200.00	0.00	0.00	0.00	−50.00	0.00	250.00
						PREFERRED CARE MEDICARE SUPPLEMENT CLAIMS									
667-0010001	MCCORD B	011011111		01/01/89	01/01/89	2	245678	P10	300.00	0.00	0.00	0.00	100.00	0.00N	96.00
667-0010002	SMITH H	021011111		01/01/89	01/01/89	2	245678	P10	300.00	170.00	0.00	0.00	0.00	104.00A	26.00
667-0010003	RUSSELL F	031011111		01/01/89	01/01/89	3	690020	PMD	50.00	20.00	0.00	6.00	0.00	24.00A	0.00

FIGURE 8–20

Example of Blue Cross/Blue Shield remittance.

surance carrier, the amount of time it takes for insurance reimbursement greatly varies. The following are periods of time from the date a claim is submitted to the date payment is made:

Blue Cross and Blue Shield	3–4 weeks
Medicare	2–3 weeks
Medicaid	4–6 weeks
Private insurance companies	6–8 weeks
CHAMPUS	60–90 days

There is one form of recourse the medical assistant can take if it is thought that the insurance carrier is paying too slowly.

SPECIAL HINT

A letter may be written to the insurance carrier requesting the status of the outstanding claim. A copy of this letter can be sent to the insurance commissioner in your state.

HEALTH MAINTENANCE ORGANIZATIONS

HMOs are considered an alternative to traditional insurance plans. Traditional insurance plans combine how care is paid for with how that care is delivered. Under an HMO plan, participating physicians provide comprehensive medical services to a group of enrollees who make fixed periodic payments to the plan. HMOs are popular with many employers and employees because they provide preventive care.

Claims are not submitted either by the patient/insured or the physician. HMOs usually require their enrollees to receive care only from physicians who belong to the HMO. If referral to a specialist is needed, the HMO doctors decide which specialist is to be seen and under what circumstances.

Types of HMOs

Closed HMOs

Prepaid Group Practice Model. A prepaid group practice model is one of the closed types of HMO and is designed to allow the physician to practice medicine without being concerned about the business end of his or her practice. Physicians who have formed an independent group contract with a health plan, and members enrolled by the plans are provided medical treatment. The physician works for a salary that is paid by the independent group. Services are provided at one or more locations by a group of physicians. These select physicians, who are employees of the HMO, are under contract with the HMO to render care.

Staff Model. The staff model is similar to the prepaid group practice model in that the physicians are salaried. The health plan hires the physicians who work exclusively for the HMO.

Advantages of HMOs

- There is no need to pay money out of pocket.
- There is no need to file claims.
- Medical expenses are predictable, because the care is paid for in advance by a fixed fee.
- Routine physical examinations are often covered.
- A wide range of services are covered for a fixed fee.

Disadvantages of HMOs

- Patient may be required to change from personal physician to one who works for the HMO.
- Travel may be required to a central clinic, which may be inconvenient.
- Approval may be needed from the HMO physician before a specialist can be seen.
- Patient may be required to see only specialists who are HMO members.

Open HMOs

Independent Practice Association. The IPA offers a wide range of services for a preestablished price. These services usually require no deductible or little or no co-insurance. Patients enrolled in this type of HMO can receive care from either the HMO physician or from physicians who have signed agreements to see patients enrolled in the plan. In addition to the IPA patients, the IPA physicians continue seeing their regular patients on a fee-for-service basis. The physicians are not employed by the HMO and are not paid salaries by the HMO.

Network HMO. The network HMO insurance plan provides health care services for a fixed price, usually paid for in advance. The physician who participates in this particular HMO may be referred to as the "gatekeeper." Primary care physicians, such as family practitioners, internists, pediatricians, and general practitioners provide services exclusively. Patients enrolled in this plan must see their primary care physician before consulting any specialist. The patient may not get to see the specialist of his or her choice. In any of the HMO plans, a patient who wishes to see a physician who is not participating in the network may do so—but may be responsible for the entire cost of the services received.

ICD-9-CM CODING

History

The most widely used statistical classification system for the study of disease is the *International Classification of Diseases* (*ICD*) developed by the World Health Organization. The World Health Organization defines a classification of diseases as a system of categories to which morbid conditions are assigned according to some criteria.

The *ICD* has its early beginnings in 1893 when Dr. Jacques Bertillon developed the *Bertillon Classification of Causes of Death*. The American Public Health Association recommended in 1898 that this classification system be adopted by registrars in Canada, Mexico, and the United States and that it be revised every 10 years. In 1938, the fifth revision became known as the *International Classification of Diseases*. After the sixth revision, hospitals began experimenting with this system for classifying diseases. In 1956, a pilot study was undertaken by the American Hospital Association and the American Medical Record Association using a modified version of the *ICD*. This study concluded that the use of the *ICD* for hospital coding and indexing was feasible with modification. Modifications have evolved through the years since 1956.

In 1978, the World Health Organization published the 9th revision of the *ICD* (*ICD-9*). In that same year, the *International Classification of Diseases, 9th Revision, Clinical Modification* (*ICD-9-CM*) was issued in the United States.

Originally, codes were assigned to permit retrieval of medical records by diagnosis and operation for the purpose of medical research and education. Today government programs such as Medicaid and Medicare as well as other third-party payers require these codes to be placed on claim forms not only by hospitals but also by providers of ambulatory care services, including physicians' offices.

Impact of the *ICD-9-CM* on Physicians' Offices

The Catastrophic Coverage Act of 1988 has had a great impact on physicians' offices because of the changes that took effect on April 1, 1989. One of the most notable changes is that *ICD-9-CM* coding is required on all Medicare claims whether the physician is participating or not.

The Catastrophic Coverage Act mandates submission of an appropriate diagnosis code (or codes) for each item or service furnished by a physician under Part B of Medicare on every bill or request for payment submitted.

If a participating physician repeatedly fails to provide the requested codes, payment can ultimately be denied. For the nonparticipating physician, fines can be levied up to $2000 for each incidence of noncompliance, and repeat violations may ultimately result in exclusion from Medicare.

As a result of this act, specific coding guidelines have been developed for physicians' offices, which had not been previously in effect.

SPECIAL HINT

It is extremely important that both the employers and employees responsible for coding activities are aware of what is needed in order to make the billing process smooth and keep the cash flow constant.

VOLUME I

Acknowledgements x
Preface xi
Introduction xiii
Conventions xxi
Guidance In Use xxiv

DISEASES TABULAR LIST—PART I

Chapter

(1)	Infectious and Parasitic Diseases	1
(2)	Neoplasms	97
(3)	Endocrine, Nutritional, and Metabolic Diseases and Immunity Disorders	201
(4)	Diseases of the Blood and Blood-Forming Organs	237
(5)	Mental Disorders	255
(6)	Diseases of the Nervous System and Sense Organs	311
(7)	Diseases of the Circulatory System	407
(8)	Diseases of the Respiratory System	457
(9)	Diseases of the Digestive System	483
(10)	Diseases of the Genitourinary System	535

OPERATIONS TABULAR LIST

Chapter

(1)	Operations on the Nervous System	583
(2)	Operations on the Endocrine System	595
(3)	Operations on the Eye	601
(4)	Operations on the Ear	620
(5)	Operations on the Nose, Mouth, and Pharynx	626
(6)	Operations on the Respiratory System	640
(7)	Operations on the Cardiovascular System	650
(8)	Operations on the Hemic and Lymphatic System	678
(9)	Operations on the Digestive System	681
(10)	Operations on the Urinary System	721
(11)	Operations on the Male Genital Organs	736
(12)	Operations on the Female Genital Organs	744
(13)	Obstetrical Procedures	757
(14)	Operations on the Musculoskeletal System	763
(15)	Operations on the Integumentary System	793
(16)	Miscellaneous Diagnostic and Therapeutic Procedures	803

DISEASES TABULAR LIST—PART 2

Chapter

(11)	Complications of Pregnancy, Childbirth, and the Puerperium	871
(12)	Diseases of the Skin and Subcutaneous Tissue	913
(13)	Diseases of the Musculoskeletal System and Connective Tissue	939
(14)	Congenital Anomalies	979
(15)	Certain Conditions Originating in the Perinatal Period	1025
(16)	Symptoms, Signs, and Ill-Defined Conditions	1047
(17)	Injury and Poisoning	1073

SUPPLEMENTARY CLASSIFICATION

V Codes Classification of Factors Influencing Health Status and Contact With Health Service 1235
E Codes Classification of External Causes of Injury and Poisoning 1273

FIGURE 8-21
Table of contents in the tabular list. (Reprinted with permission from Puckett CD: *The Educational Annotation of ICD-9-CM*. Reno, NV: Channel, 1989.)

APPENDICES

A	Morphology of Neoplasms	1373
B	Glossary of Mental Disorders	1393
C	Classification of Drugs by American Hospital Formulary Service List Number and Their *ICD-9-CM* Equivalents	1395
D	Classification of Industrial Accidents According to Agency	1403

REFERENCE LIST

Reference List 1409

FIGURE 8–21 *Continued*

We can be certain that coding—*ICD-9-CM* for diagnoses and *Current Procedural Terminology* (*CPT*) for procedures—is here to stay. The 10th revision of *ICD* is now underway. It is anticipated that the earliest the *ICD-10* will be ready for use is October 1, 1994.

Prerequisites for Accurate Coding

In order to code accurately, it is essential that the person coding have an understanding of medical terminology. An understanding of the terminology as well as the coding rules should be mandatory before a person is given the responsibility for coding.

SPECIAL HINT

In order to remain up to date, it is essential to attend coding workshops. Those employees with primary responsibility for coding should make it their goal to attend, at a minimum, one *CPT* and one *ICD-9* coding class each year. One can never know too much about coding.

In addition to attending workshops specifically related to coding, it is essential that someone in the office be assigned the responsibility for reading and disseminating information contained in the newsletters/bulletins that are sent from Medicare as well as other insurance carriers. The coder will find valuable information in these communications that will assist him or her in billing accurately the first time. If an insurance carrier sends out new guidelines for billing, this mailing is considered notification of change. Failure to read and follow these guidelines could result in lost payments to the physicians.

The *ICD-9-CM* Coding Books

The coding books for coding diseases and injuries are arranged in two volumes.

Volume 1—Tabular List

Volume 1 (Figure 8–21) is organized into 17 chapters dealing with conditions that affect a body system, such as Chapter 7, "Diseases of the Circulatory System," or conditions classified according to etiology, such as Chapter 1, "Infectious and Parasitic Diseases."

Each chapter has the following subdivisions:

- Sections—groups of three-digit categories
- Categories—three-digit code numbers
- Subcategories—four-digit code numbers

SPECIAL HINT

The fourth digits have been added to the category codes to provide more information or specificity about the etiology (cause), site, or manifestation (indication). These are called "subcategory codes."

- Fifth-digit subclassifications—five-digit code numbers. Even greater specificity has been added to some categories by use of the fifth digit. Fifth-digit codes may appear in several places: (a) the beginning of the chapter, (b) the beginning of the section, (c) the beginning of the three-digit category, or (d) the fourth-digit category.

In addition to 17 chapters, there are two supplementary classifications in volume 1:

- "Factors influencing health status and contact with health service"—V codes
- "External cause of injury and poisoning"—E codes

Volume 1 contains the following appendices:

- "Morphology of Neoplasms"—M codes
- "Glossary of Mental Disorders"

TABLE OF CONTENTS

VOLUME II

INTRODUCTION vii

SECTION 1
Alphabetic Index to Diseases and Injuries 1

SECTION 2
Table of Drugs and Chemicals 769

SECTION 3
Index to External Causes of Injuries and Poisonings (E Code) 877

SECTION 4
Index to Procedures 925

FIGURE 8-22
Table of contents in the alphabetical index. (Reprinted with permission from Puckett CD: *The Educational Annotation of ICD-9-CM.* Reno, NV: Channel, 1989.)

- "Classification of Drugs by the American Hospital Formulary"
- Classification of Industrial Accidents According to Agency"

Volume 2—Alphabetical Index

Volume 2 is organized into three main sections (Figure 8-22):

"**Index to Diseases and Injuries.**" This index is organized alphabetically by main term (terms in bold letters). Main terms generally indicate the disease condition or injury; however, there are exceptions, and one such example is the obstetrical conditions. These can be found under such terms as "delivery," "labor," "pregnancy," and "puerperal." Terms indented under the main term are called subterms.

"**Table of Drugs and Chemicals.**" See Figure 8-23.

"**Index to External Causes of Injuries and Poisonings.**" This is the index used for assigning E codes.

Volume 3

The coder should be aware that *ICD-9-CM* code books contain a third volume, which is used by hospital coders to code procedures. Because physician offices use *CPT* coding for coding their procedures, this volume is not used for coding in the medical office.

Types of Coding Books

Today, there are many types of *ICD-9-CM* code books on the market, such as:

- The traditional bound books without coding enhancements

Chapter 8: INSURANCE AND CODING   191

| Substance | Poisoning | External Cause (E-Code) |||||
		Accident	Therapeutic Use	Suicide Attempt	Assault	Undetermined
Adalin (acetyl)	967.3	E852.2	E937.3	E950.2	E962.0	E980.2
Adenosine (phosphate)	977.8	E858.8	E947.8	E950.4	E962.0	E980.4
Adhesives	989.8	E866.6	—	E950.9	E962.1	E980.9
ADH	962.5	E858.0	E932.5	E950.4	E962.0	E980.4
Adicillin	960.0	E856	E930.0	E950.4	E962.0	E980.4
Adiphenine	975.1	E855.6	E945.1	E950.4	E962.0	E980.4
Adjunct, pharmaceutical	977.4	E858.8	E947.4	E950.4	E962.0	E980.4

FIGURE 8-23

Table of drugs and chemicals. (Reprinted from *St. Anthony's ICD-9-CM Code Book for Physician Payment,* © 1990, with permission of St. Anthony Publishing, Inc., Alexandria, VA.)

- Loose-leaf code books with various coding enhancements

Most books published now contain some type of coding enhancement to assist the coder.

SPECIAL HINT

The physician's office coder needs to be aware that many of the enhancements are for the hospital coder to assist him or her in arriving at the correct DRG.

There are coding books with enhancements specifically with the coder in the physician's office in mind. These books provide the coder with some of the following guides (Figure 8-24):

- Highlighted codes that should never be used
- Highlighted codes that may cause delayed, reduced, or disallowed claims
- Highlighted codes that require additional information

In addition, there are books on the market that explain the meaning of various conditions cov-

GLOSSARY

(COLOR CODING)
(LIGHT RED)   Restricted codes. Three digit codes that require fourth or fifth digit.

✓ 5th   Codes that require a fifth digit.

(YELLOW)   Caution—unspecified code. These codes should be used only if a more specific code is NOT available. Contact the physician to determine if a more specific diagnosis is available.

(ORANGE)   Nonspecific codes. These codes are acceptable to third-party payers but a more explicit narrative should be documented on the claim.

(BLUE)   Signs, symptoms, and ill-defined condition codes. These codes can be used to justify certain CPT levels of service and/or procedures when a more specific diagnosis has not been established.

(PURPLE)   External causes of injury and poisoning codes. These codes should not be used alone, but in conjunction with the sign, symptom, or condition code that was the result of the adverse effect.

FIGURE 8-24

Glossary. (Reprinted from *St. Anthony's ICD-9-CM Code Book for Physician Payment,* © 1990, with permission of St. Anthony Publishing, Inc., Alexandria, VA.)

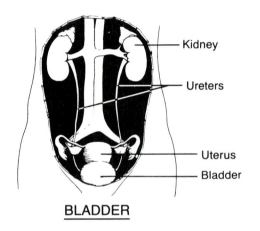
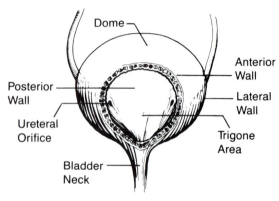

ANATOMY OF THE BLADDER — The *urinary bladder* is a hollow, collapsible musculomembranous organ, and is located within the pelvic cavity, behind the symphysis pubis. In the male, it lies against the rectum, and in the female it lies against the vagina and uterus. When filled it may contain 500 ml. of urine and pushes upward indenting the abdominal cavity. The *trigone* area is the floor of the bladder formed by three points, the two *ureteral orifices* and the *urethral orifice*. The *dome* is the expandable superior surface of the bladder. The *bladder neck* is that area surrounding the urethral orifice. The *ureteric orifice* is that area surrounding the ureteral openings. The *urachus* in the adult forms the middle umbilical ligament of the bladder.

PHYSIOLOGY OF THE BLADDER — The *urinary bladder* functions as a reservoir for the urine produced by the *kidneys* until the individual expells the urine (micturition). Micturition occurs when the bladder becomes distended with urine and stretch receptor nerves signal the micturition center in the sacral spinal cord. Parasympathetic nerve impulses start rhythmically contracting the bladder and the individual senses an urgency to urinate. Following the midbrain decision to urinate, the external urethral sphincter is relaxed, and urination begins as the bladder muscle contracts.

> *Excludes:* *carcinoma in situ (233.7)* — NOTE: Carcinoma in situ of the bladder is a neoplastic entity wherein the tumor cells have not progressed beyond the transitional epithelium of the bladder, and lack the property of invasion to the basement membrane.

188.0 TRIGONE OF URINARY BLADDER — The area of the bladder floor formed by the ureteral orifices and the urethral orifice.

188.1 DOME OF URINARY BLADDER — The expandable superior surface of the bladder.

188.2 LATERAL WALL OF URINARY BLADDER — The side walls of the bladder.

188.3 ANTERIOR WALL OF URINARY BLADDER — The front wall of the bladder.

188.4 POSTERIOR WALL OF URINARY BLADDER — The back wall of the bladder.

ANAPLASIA — A loss of differentiation of cells and of their orientation to one another and to their axial framework and blood vessels.
CONTIGUOUS — In contact or conjunction with adjacent sites.

FIGURE 8–25
Example of enhanced coding book with explanation of terminology. (Reprinted with permission from Puckett CD: *The Educational Annotation of ICD-9-CM*. Reno, NV: Channel, 1989.)

ered by the codes (Figure 8–25). Encoders, computerized programs to assist the coder in arriving at the correct code, are also available. The coder must remember that enhanced books contain the same codes as the unenhanced versions. These books are designed as helps to the coder.

Since the *ICD-9-CM* was published, there have been numerous advancements in the medical field. It is important that the coder keep the books up to date. Each year since 1986, an *Official Authorized Addendum to ICD-9-CM* has been published with coding changes. These addenda are effective October 1 of each year.

Many publishers of coding books offer a subscription service to help coders keep their books up to date. It is important that the subscription service not be allowed to lapse. Coders using the loose-leaf notebooks receive the revised pages to replace the outdated pages. Coders using the hardbound books must *write in* the changes. At any rate, it is important to obtain a current addendum before October 1 of each year.

If one does not have a subscription service with one's books, addenda can be ordered through the American Hospital Association in Chicago for a nominal charge as well as through various companies specializing in the sale of coding books. In addition, one can check with the Medicare carrier to see if these changes are available.

When deciding on which coding books an office should have, the coder must weigh not only the cost of the code books but also the benefits of such things as

- Availability of subscription service for updates
- Ease of updating books
- Enhancements offered
- Value of having each term explained.

PROCEDURE

CODING

PURPOSE

To maximize reimbursement

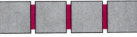
MEDICAL ASSISTING ALERT

Taking time to code correctly saves time spent recoding and shortens the turnaround time for reimbursement.

EQUIPMENT AND MATERIALS

ICD-9-CM code books
Medical dictionary
Pencil
Medical record
Form containing diagnosis

PROCEDURAL STEPS

1. Analyze the medical terminology.
   RATIONALE: It is important to make certain the coder understands what the physician is saying.
2. Locate the main term in the Alphabetic Index. For example, if you are coding acute bronchitis, look up "bronchitis."
3. Refer to any notes under the main term. These notes are in ruled off boxes in the Alphabetic Index.
   RATIONALE: These boxes provide important information to assist the coder in proper code assignment.
4. Refer to any modifiers (terms in parentheses) immediately following the main term.
5. Refer to any subterms indented under the main term. In the example of the diagnosis of acute bronchitis, the word *acute* is the subterm.
   RATIONALE: Subterms make the code specific.
6. Follow any cross-reference instructions that might be given, such as "see" or "see also."
   RATIONALE: These instructions help guide the coder to look under the correct term.
7. Verify the code assignment by checking the Tabular List (volume 1).
   RATIONALE: It is always important to use Volume 1 to assure proper code assignment.
8. Read and be guided by any instructional phrases in the Tabular List. Examples of instructional phrases are "code if desired," "code also," as well as inclusion and exclusion notes.
   RATIONALE: Instructional phrases guide the coder in determining whether proper code assignment has been made and if additional codes should be used.
9. Assign the code.

Remembering the Basics: Some Guidelines

Regardless in what specialty the coder is employed, certain basic guidelines must be followed to assure coding accuracy.

Nonessential Modifiers. The words in parentheses are called "nonessential modifiers." Their presence or absence in a diagnosis has no effect on the selection of the code number (Figure 8–26).

Gastroenteritis (acute) (catarrhal) (chronic)
  (congestive) (hemorrhagic)
  (noninfectious) (*see also* Enteritis)   558.9
    aertrycke infection   003.0
    allergic   558.9
    chronic   558.9
      ulcerative   556
    dietetic   558.9
    due to
      food poisoning (*see also* Poisoning,
        food)   005.9
      radiation   558.1
    epidemic   009.0
    functional   558.9
    infectious (*see also* Enteritis, due to, by
      organism)   009.0
      presumed   009.1
    salmonella   003.0
    septic (*see also* Enteritis, due to, by
      organism)   009.0
    toxic   558.2
    tuberculous (*see also* Tuberculosis)   014.8
    ulcerative   556
    viral NEC   008.8
      specified type   008.6
    zymotic   009.0

FIGURE 8-26

Use of the parenthesis. (Reprinted from *St. Anthony's ICD-9-CM Code Book for Physician Payment,* © 1990, with permission of St. Anthony Publishing, Inc., Alexandria, VA.)

E Codes. E codes stand for "external cause of injury." These can never be used as a principal diagnosis. They merely tell what the cause of the accident was, such as a "fall down stairs." These codes are generally used with a trauma code (codes 800–999), for example, "fracture of the head of right radius due to a fall from a ladder 813.05, E881.0." However, there are exceptions, the most notable being adverse drug reactions. One such example would be "drowsiness due to side effects of Chlor-Trimeton." The coder would code drowsiness (code 708.0), and in order to show that it was due to Chlor-Trimeton the E code from the "Therapeutic Use" column in the Table of Drugs and Chemicals would be used (code E933.0).

V Codes. The acceptability of V codes varies from insurance company to insurance company. Some situations can be coded only with V codes, such as chemotherapy. Often situations covered under the V codes are not reimbursable by insurance companies, such as a prophylactic injection or routine physical examination.

Coders employed by either a radiology billing service or a laboratory billing service must remember to use the appropriate V code (V72.5 for radiology and V72.6 for laboratory) as the reason for the encounter and then code the diagnosis/symptom to the level of specificity known for the encounter.

When an internist performs a preoperative evaluation before a patient undergoes a cholecystectomy for cholelithiasis, this evaluation can be coded using code V71.7 (observation for suspected cardiovascular disease). The reason for the surgery would be a secondary diagnosis and in this case would be coded 574.xx.

Uncertain Diagnosis. When a diagnosis is listed as "suspected," "probable," "questionable," "possible," or "rule out," *do not* code it as if the disease or injury or pregnancy is established. Instead, code the condition to the highest degree of certainty that may be found in symptoms, signs, abnormal test results, or other reason for the visit. (*This applies to coding in ambulatory settings only.*)

When the physician does not identify a definitive symptom/diagnosis at the conclusion of a patient care visit or identifies a "suspected," "questionable," "problem" condition, the coder should code the *chief complaint* as the reason for the visit.

Condition Appearing under More Than One Term in Alphabetical Index. Many conditions can be found under more than one term in the Alphabetical Index; for example, Wolff-Parkinson White syndrome can be found under "Wolff" and also under the word "syndrome." However, the coder should arrive at the same code regardless of which term is used.

"See" and "See Also" Instructions. The instruction "See" in the Alphabetical Index is a mandatory instruction to the coder to look elsewhere for the code (Figure 8-27). The instruction "see also" in the Alphabetical Index directs the coder to look under another main term if all

Bronchitis (diffuse) (hypostatic) (infectious)
  (inflammatory) (simple)—*continued*
    Castellani's   104.8
    catarrhal   490
      acute—*see* Bronchitis, acute
      chronic   491.0
    chemical (acute) (subacute)   506.0
      chronic   506.4
      due to fumes or vapors (acute)
        (subacute)   506.0
        chronic   506.4
    chronic   491.9
      with
        airway obstruction   491.2
        obstruction   491.2
        tracheitis (chronic)   491.8

FIGURE 8-27

Use of the *see* instruction. (Reprinted from *St. Anthony's ICD-9-CM Code Book for Physician Payment,* © 1990, with permission of St. Anthony Publishing, Inc., Alexandria, VA.)

Gastritis—continued
  glandular 535.4
    chronic 535.1
  hypertrophic (mucosa) 535.2
    chronic giant 211.1
  irritant 535.4
  nervous 306.4
  phlegmonous 535.0
  psychogenic 306.4
  sclerotic 535.4
  spastic 536.8
  subacute 535.0
  superficial 535.4
  suppurative 535.0
  toxic 535.4
  tuberculous (see also Tuberculosis) 017.9
Gastrocarcinoma (M8010/3) 151.9
Gastrocolic—see condition
Gastrocolitis—see Enteritis
Gastrodisciasis 121.8
Gastroduodenitis (see also Gastritis) 535.5
  catarrhal 535.0
  infectional 535.0
  virus, viral 008.8
    specified type 008.6
Gastrodynia 536.8

FIGURE 8–28

Example of the *see also* instruction. (Reprinted from *St. Anthony's ICD-9-CM Code Book for Physician Payment*, © 1990, with permission of St. Anthony Publishing, Inc., Alexandria, VA.)

the information cannot be located under the first main entry (Figure 8–28).

NEC. NEC (Not Elsewhere Classifiable) signifies that the category number is to be used only when no other category is provided for this condition in the Tabular List, for example, "infection, respiratory upper (acute) NEC (465)," or when there is insufficient information to enable the coder to classify the condition to a more specific category. This is *not* a "catch-all" code, however.

NOS. NOS (Not Otherwise Specified) is equivalent to "Unspecified" and "Unqualified." When no modifying adjective or other specification is stated in the diagnosis, the code of NOS may be used, for example, "465.9, unspecified site, includes upper respiratory infection (acute) NOS."

Use of Three-Digit Disease Codes. The three-digit disease category codes are used only if there are no decimal digits listed in that category.

Use of Four-Digit Subcategory Codes. The four-digit subcategory codes are used only if no fifth-digit subdivisions are provided.

When a Fifth Digit Is Required But There Is No Fourth Digit. When a category does not have a fourth digit but requires a fifth digit, use a zero for the fourth digit and add the appropriate fifth digit, for example, polyhydramnios 657.0x.

Two Diagnoses or a Diagnosis with a Complication. Two diagnoses or a diagnosis with an associated complication may often be coded adequately with only one code, for example, "Acute appendicitis with peritonitis, 540.0." This is identified in the subterms under "appendicitis."

Using Two or More Codes. Use two or more codes if necessary to completely classify a diagnosis or procedure. The "Code Also" instruction in the Tabular List provides the best guide in determining whether two codes are necessary.

Instruction in the Tabular List to "Use an Additional Code if Desired." This should be interpreted as mandatory.

Expression of Symptoms. When a confirmed diagnosis is present, it is not necessary to code expressions of the symptoms that accompany the diagnosis. For example, for acute gastroenteritis with nausea and vomiting, the nausea and vomiting are not coded.

After Coding a Diagnosis. After the diagnosis is coded, evaluate the codes to make sure that the code numbers convey the patient's condition accurately.

The Employee's Role in Coding

Coding virtually controls the purse strings of the business, because the *CPT* and *ICD-9-CM* codes that are submitted to the third-party payers determine the payment the physician receives. In order to help ensure prompt and accurate payment from third-party payers, *submit claims as soon as possible after service is rendered and diagnosis determined.*

Review superbills to ensure that the *ICD-9* and *CPT* codes are accurate. For example, if diabetes mellitus is the diagnosis, make certain that it is submitted on the superbills as a five-digit code and not a three- or four-digit code.

Third-Party Payers' Rules for Coding

Follow the coding rules outlined by the third-party payers. These are as follows:

Sequencing. The main reason the patient saw the physician on a given day should be sequenced first. This could be a diagnosis, condition, problem, complaint, or other reason.

Principal Diagnosis. For ambulatory care, this is the diagnosis documented in the patient's medical record to be chiefly responsible for the outpatient services performed during the visit. The code should be consistent with the physician's understanding of the patient's problem at the conclusion of the visit.

Uncertain Diagnoses. The coder should *not* code outpatient diagnoses documented as "suspected," "probable," "questionable," "possible," or "rule out" as if they were established.

Specificity. The coder *should* code the condition to the highest degree of certainty. These codes could be symptoms, abnormal test results, or other reasons for the visit.

Number of Codes to Submit. The HCFA-1500 claim form will allow for submission of a total of *four ICD-9* codes. It is important to submit the principal diagnosis first, as described above. The additional codes should be for conditions that co-exist at the time of the visit or subsequently develop and that have an effect on the treatment that is received. Conditions previously treated and no longer existing are not coded.

Use of Valid Codes. It is important to use the maximum number of digits that have been assigned to a condition.

SAMPLE: Normal delivery is always a three-digit code, code 650. However, the code for duodenal ulcer is always a five-digit code. If a code does not contain the correct number of digits specified, the third-party payer will return the claim form for correction. This causes a delay in payment to the physician.

Physician Education

The following are some tips to help ensure proper coding, which in turn will lead to proper reimbursement.

1. The term "rule out" cannot be coded—use symptoms to their highest degree of specificity (including possible, probable, or suspected). (NOTE: This guideline for ambulatory coding differs significantly from inpatient hospital coding. In an inpatient setting, "rule out" is coded as if it were present.) The term "ruled out" also cannot be coded. This indicates that the suspected condition is not present.
2. If an alternative condition is diagnosed, this should be coded. Otherwise, code the appropriate symptom or use the appropriate V71 code—"Observation without need for further medical care."
3. If there is a confirmed diagnosis, encourage the physician to be specific. For example, with the diagnosis of duodenal ulcer, is it acute or chronic and is there hemorrhage or perforation involved?
4. If the diagnosis is acute and/or chronic, this should be specified. Both conditions are coded if there are entries for both conditions. The acute is sequenced first.
5. Diagnoses should be sequenced listing the main reason for which the patient is coming to see the physician on this occasion, then giving any other diagnosis (up to three) for which the patient is being treated.
6. If your physician is the consultant on a hospitalized patient, submit the primary diagnosis as the main reason for which the consultation is done. This may not be the principal reason the patient was admitted to the hospital, however.
7. It is most important to make certain that all procedures performed in the office have a related diagnosis. For example, if a patient comes in for an upper respiratory tract infection and for some reason a urinalysis is done, make certain that at least symptoms are listed to justify the urinalysis, or this procedure will not be reimbursed.
8. Do not submit codes for diagnoses that have no impact on the current treatment, such as status posthysterectomy 1 year ago, when no treatment is involved.
9. With the diagnosis of diabetes, if the diabetes is uncontrolled the physician should state it as such. Use the appropriate fifth digit to designate whether the patient is insulin dependent.
10. When the physician is the primary attending physician on an inpatient, it is important that the principal diagnosis submitted for physician charges and principal diagnosis submitted by the hospital be the same.
11. Do not automatically send reports with the claim form unless specifically requested, because the claim form and reports are often separated when they reach the insurance carrier. Hence, reports do not always end up with the claim form and will likely have to be resubmitted.
12. It is true that in spite of all of the changes, the *CPT* code (procedure code) still forms the basis of the physician's payment. However, the diagnosis code must now relate to the *CPT* codes submitted. Therefore, it is im-

perative that the diagnoses submitted be as accurate as possible.

Validation of the Diagnosis in the Medical Record

Not to be forgotten is the importance of medical record documentation. It is essential to ensure correct payment should questions be raised by a third-party payer or an audit be performed by the Inspector General's Office. Adequate documentation in office medical records is no less important than it is in hospital records.

The diagnosis must be validated in the office record just as it is in the case of a hospital patient. It must not look like it came floating out of the air.

In addition, the level of service must also be documented. Failure to adequately document the level of service could result in downcoding (lowering level of service) by Medicare and can result in the charge of "fraud" and a $2000 fine per infraction. The following is an example of what needs to be documented in the office medical record when an *intermediate* level of service is being billed.

Five of the following seven items must be documented:

- Complaints and/or symptoms
- Duration and/or course of illness
- Details of illness
- Limited examination (two or more areas)
- Laboratory and/or x-ray values and findings
- Diagnosis and/or problem
- Treatment, injection, or advice

SPECIAL HINT

Remember, when records are reviewed by third-party payers, "If it is not documented, it was not done." Office personnel should keep the physician informed of what documentation is necessary to ensure the physician receives the maximum reimbursement that is due.

Guidelines for Coding Specific Conditions

After coders have become familiar with the basic coding guidelines, which affect all areas of coding regardless of specialty, they must then familiarize themselves with guidelines for coding specific diseases and/or injuries. Although it is impossible to cover all of the coding guidelines for each of the systems, the following are key areas the coder should know.

Alcohol and Drug Abuse

Alcohol and drug dependence/abuse codes always require fifth digits. Use of the fifth digits is as follows:

Fifth Digit	Description
0	Unspecified—Course unknown or first signs of illness with course uncertain
1	Continuous—More or less regular maladaptive use for over 6 months
2	Episodic—A fairly circumscribed period of maladaptive use, with one or more similar periods in the past
3	In remission—Previous maladaptive use, but not using substance at present

Alcohol Dependence. There is, in addition to the characteristics described under "Alcohol Abuse," physiological dependence or pathological pattern of use and either the development of tolerance or withdrawal that results from its use (category 303).

Alcohol Abuse. This is a continuous or episodic use of alcohol for at least one month with reported instances of acute intoxication and the social implications of its use (code 305.x– with the appropriate fifth digit). Category 305 is used to classify the conditions resulting from nondependent abuse of drugs.

Burns

Except for burns of the eye and of internal organs, burns are classified according to the degree of burn, as follows:

Condition	Degree	Fourth Digit
Erythema	First	1
Blisters, epidermal loss	Second	2
Full-thickness skin loss	Third	3
Deep necrosis of underlying tissue	Deep third	4
Deep necrosis of underlying tissues with loss of body part	Deep third	5

Code 948 indicates extent of body surface involved. Use the fifth digit to indicate percentage of third-degree burns. If the burn is not third degree, use zero for the fifth digit. The fourth digit indicates total percentage of body surface involved in the burns.

If there are multiple degrees of burns present at the same site, code only the most severe degree of burn of that site. If multiple degrees of burns are present at several sites, code the most severe degree of burn at each site.

Complications

1. Locate the main term for the complication in the Alphabetic Index, for example, thrombophlebitis.
2. Check the subterms for an indication that the condition is the result of medical or surgical complications such as "postoperative."

   SAMPLE: "Thrombophlebitis — postoperative, 997.2."

3. If there is not a specific code identified, consult the main term "Complication"; for example, for postoperative wound infection, look under "Complication," "surgical procedures," "wound infection" (998.5).
4. Use a second code to identify a specific complication if such a code is available.

   SAMPLE: "Postoperative atelectasis of the lung 997.3 [for postoperative respiratory complications] and 518.0 [for atelectasis]."

If a condition stated in the diagnosis as a "postoperative complication" is specifically excluded from the 996–998 codes, code 998.8 ("Other specified complications of procedures, not elsewhere classified") may be used as an additional code if the title of the category or subcategory in Chapters 1–16 does not specifically identify it as a "postoperative" condition or "due to surgery."

Circulatory System

Hypertension

Benign Hypertension. This type of hypertension remains fairly stable over the years, but if untreated can be an important risk factor in coronary heart disease and cerebrovascular disease. Effective antihypertensive drug therapy is the treatment of choice.

Most hypertension is benign, but make certain that the physician specifies this. If it is not specified, the correct code is 401.9.

Malignant Hypertension. This type of hypertension occurs in about 5% of the patients with a diagnosis of hypertension. This form is frequently abrupt in onset, runs a course measured in months, and often ends with renal failure or cerebral hemorrhage.

Hypertension as the Cause of Other Disease. Hypertension is frequently the cause of various forms of heart and vascular disease; however, ICD-9-CM does not presume a cause-and-effect relationship. To determine if there is a cause-and-effect relationship, the coder must pay close attention to the wording of the diagnosis. The words *due to* and the adjective *hypertensive* indicate a causal relationship. When this is the case, the statement can be coded as one code.

SAMPLE: "Hypertensive heart disease with congestive failure, 402.91."

The words *with* and *and* indicate there is no causal relationship, and each statement is coded separately.

SAMPLE: "Benign hypertension and congestive heart failure, 401.1 [benign hypertension] and 428.0 [congestive heart failure]."

Myocardial Infarction. As of October 1, 1989, when using the 410 series of codes, the coder must assign a fifth digit to indicate episode of care. When coding acute myocardial infarction, do not use 410.9x if the site of the infarct can be determined (Figure 8–29).

SAMPLE: "Acute myocardial infarction, anterolateral wall, 410.00."

Code 412 indicates an old infarction that is no longer presenting symptoms. Code 414.8 is a chronic infarction — one that is generally older than 8 weeks and presenting symptoms.

Diabetes Mellitus

Diabetes Mellitus, Type I. This type of diabetes (previously called juvenile diabetes) is insulin dependent. The patient requires insulin therapy to live. Diabetes mellitus Type I without complications would be coded 250.01.

Diabetes Mellitus, Type II. This type of diabetes (previously called adult onset) is not insulin dependent. Diabetes mellitus Type II without complications would be coded 250.00.

Diabetes Mellitus with a Systemic Manifestation. Diabetes mellitus of either Type I or Type II with systemic manifestation requires an additional code to further identify the manifestation.

410 ACUTE MYOCARDIAL INFARCTION — A severe, sudden onset of myocardial necrosis due to formation of a thrombus in the coronary arterial system obstructing arterial blood flow to that section of cardiac muscle.

The following fifth-digit subclassification is for use with category 410:

0 EPISODE OF CARE UNSPECIFIED
Use when the source document does not contain sufficient information for the assignment of fifth digit 1 or 2.

C.V. COMP
DRG #121

1 INITIAL EPISODE OF CARE
Use to designate the acute phase of care regardless of the location of treatment. Includes cases that are transferred for care and treatment within the acute phase of care. Any subsequent episode of care for another (repeat) myocardial infarction is also assigned the fifth digit 1.

2 SUBSEQUENT EPISODE OF CARE
Use to designate observation, treatment or evaluation of myocardial infarction within 8 weeks of onset, but following the acute phase, or in the healing state where the episode of care may be for related or unrelated condition(s).

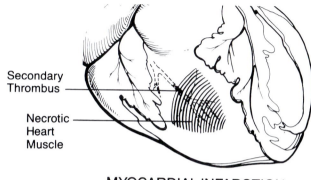

Includes: Cardiac infarction — See Acute Myocardial Infarction above.
Coronary (artery):
Embolism — An obstructing blood clot in the coronary arteries.
Occlusion — An obstruction of a coronary artery by thrombosis or as a result of a spasm.
Rupture — Forcible tearing of a coronary artery.
Thrombosis — The formation, or presence of an aggregation of blood factors, primarily platelets and fibrin forming a blood clot.
Infarction of heart, myocardium, or ventricle — Necrosis of cardiac muscle.
Rupture of heart, myocardium, or ventricle — Forcible disruption of cardiac muscle.
Any condition classifiable to 414.1–414.9 specified as acute or with a stated duration of 8 weeks or less

FIGURE 8–29
Example of the section on acute myocardial infarction with explanation of terms. (Reprinted with permission from Puckett CD: *The Educational Annotation of ICD-9-CM.* Reno, NV: Channel, 1989.)

Both codes are required to completely classify the condition, with the diabetes code being sequenced first.

SAMPLE: "Diabetes mellitus (250.7×) with gangrene (785.4)."

Uncertainty Regarding Insulin Dependency. Diabetes always requires a fifth digit to specify whether or not the patient is insulin dependent. If the type of diabetes cannot be determined, the coder should use a zero for the fifth digit.

Drug Poisonings versus Adverse Reactions

Poisoning by drugs is defined as either the wrong drug or the wrong dosage being given or taken. NOTE: A poisoning can be accidental, such as a medication taken in error. It can also be purposeful, such as a suicide or homicide attempt.

Poisoning by drugs differs from an "adverse reaction." An adverse reaction occurs when the right drug and dosage are given, and, in spite of this, an untoward reaction occurs, such as an allergic reaction or anaphylactic response.

The Table of Drugs and Chemicals is used for poisoning. However, the column titled "Therapeutic Use" is used when describing an external cause (E code) of an adverse reaction to a properly administered drug. When coding an adverse reaction to a correct substance properly administered, code the nature of the adverse reaction or manifestation.

SAMPLE: "Vertigo due to Librium, 780.4."

An E code ("Therapeutic Use" column) would be used to describe the substance ("Librium, E939.4").

The codes for toxic effects of substances that are chiefly nonmedicinal, such as poisoning due to soap (989.6), are also included in the Table of Drugs and Chemicals.

Fractures and Dislocations

When coding skull fractures, an attempt should be made to specify the level of consciousness.

SAMPLE: Closed fracture of base of skull without intracranial injury and with no loss of consciousness, 801.01."

The coder should read the beginning of Chapter 17 to clarify fracture terminology, that is, closed fractures versus open fractures.

Closed fracture: Bone does not penetrate the skin.

Open fracture: Bone penetrates the skin (compound fracture).

Both Closed and Open Fracture. When a fracture includes both closed and open descriptors (for example, compound, comminuted fracture of distal radius), code it as an open fracture (813.52).

Pathological Fractures. Pathological fractures are coded as 733.1. The site cannot be specified.

Fracture and Dislocation. Fracture–dislocations are coded as fractures.

Infectious Disease

In order to accommodate the coding of human immunodeficiency virus (HIV) infections, new categories were assigned in October, 1986. These are as follows:

Code	Description
Category 042	Acquired immune deficiency syndrome (AIDS)
Category 043	AIDS-like syndrome
Category 044	HIV infections

Late-Effect Coding

A late effect may be defined as a current condition, usually long term, that resulted from a previous acute illness or injury.

Adenocarcinoma (M8140/3)—see also Neoplasm, by site, malignant

> Note—The list of adjectival modifiers below is not exhaustive. A description of adenocarcinoma that does not appear in this list should be coded in the same manner as carcinoma with that description. Thus, "mixed acidophil-basophil adenocarcinoma," should be coded in the same manner as "mixed acidophil-basophil carcinoma," which appears in the list under "Carcinoma."
>
> Except where otherwise indicated, the morphological varieties of adenocarcinoma in the list below should be coded by site as for "Neoplasm, malignant."

with
   apocrine metaplasia (M8573/3)
   cartilaginous (and osseous) metaplasia (M8571/3)
   osseous (and cartilaginous) metaplasia (M8571/3)

FIGURE 8–30

Example of how to begin coding a neoplasm. (Reprinted from *St. Anthony's ICD-9-CM Code Book for Physician Payment,* © 1990, with permission of St. Anthony Publishing, Inc., Alexandria, VA.)

SAMPLE: "Paralysis (344.9) resulting from a previous cerebrovascular accident (CVA) (438)."

A late effect is composed of two parts—residual and cause. The *residual* is coded as the current condition, and the *cause* is coded as an additional diagnosis. A late-effect E code is used to describe the cause of the late effect. For example, if the late effect were the result of a motor vehicle accident, the appropriate E code would be E929.0.

Neoplasms

When coding neoplasms (abnormal growths, such as tumors), first look in the Alphabetical Index for the name of the neoplasm. Do not automatically go to the Table of Neoplasms (Figures 8–30 and 8–31). The guidance in the Alphabetical Index may be overridden if a descriptor is present that contradicts the usual tumor behavior.

Classification of Neoplasms

Malignant. Malignant neoplasms are neoplasms that can invade and destroy adjacent structures and spread to distant sites to cause death.

Primary. The site where a neoplasm originated.

Secondary. Site to which the primary site has spread (metastatic site).

	Malignant			Benign	Uncertain Behavior	Unspecified
	Primary	Secondary	Ca in situ			
Neoplasm, neoplastic	199.1	199.1	234.9	229.9	238.9	239.9

Notes—1. *The list below gives the code numbers for neoplasms by anatomical site. For each site there are six possible code numbers according to whether the neoplasm in question is malignant, benign, in situ, of uncertain behavior, or of unspecified nature. The description of the neoplasm will often indicate which of the six columns is appropriate: e.g., malignant melanoma of skin, benign fibroadenoma of breast, carcinoma in situ of cervix uteri.*

Where such descriptors are not present, the remainder of the Index should be consulted where guidance is given to the appropriate column for each morphological (histological) variety listed: e.g., Mesonephroma—see Neoplasm, malignant; Embryoma—see also Neoplasm, uncertain behavior; Disease, Bowen's—see Neoplasm, skin, in situ. However, the guidance in the Index can be overridden if one of the descriptors mentioned above is present: e.g., malignant adenoma of colon is coded to 153.9 and not to 211.3 as the adjective "malignant" overrides the Index entry "Adenoma—see also Neoplasm, benign."

2. Sites marked with the sign * (e.g., face NEC*) should be classified to malignant neoplasm of skin of these sites if the variety of neoplasm is a squamous cell carcinoma or an epidermoid carcinoma and to benign neoplasm of skin of these sites if the variety of neoplasm is a papilloma (any type).

abdomen, abdominal	195.2	198.89	234.8	229.8	238.8	239.8
cavity	195.2	198.89	234.8	229.8	238.8	239.8
organ	195.2	198.89	234.8	229.8	238.8	239.8
viscera	195.2	198.89	234.8	229.8	238.8	239.8
wall	173.5	198.2	232.5	216.5	238.2	239.2

FIGURE 8–31
Table of neoplasms. (Reprinted from *St. Anthony's ICD-9-CM Code Book for Physician Payment,* © 1990, with permission of St. Anthony Publishing, Inc., Alexandria, VA.)

In Situ. Cells undergoing malignant changes but still confined to the point of origin, without invasion of surrounding normal tissue.

Benign. In a benign neoplasm, growth does not invade adjacent structures or spread to distant sites but may displace or exert pressure on adjacent structures.

Uncertain Behavior. The pathologist is not able to determine whether the tumor is benign or malignant because some features of each are present.

Unspecified Nature. Neither the behavior nor the histological type of tumor is specified in the diagnosis.

Treatment of the Primary Site. When treatment is directed only at the primary site of the malignancy, the primary site can be designated as the principal diagnosis.

SAMPLE: "Carcinoma of the lung (162.9) with metastasis to the brain (198.3) (patient admitted for thoracentesis)."

Treatment of Secondary Site. When treatment is directed toward the secondary site only, this site is designated as the principal diagnosis, even though the primary malignancy might still be present. In this case, the secondary site would be sequenced first and the primary site would be coded as an additional diagnosis.

SAMPLE: "Metastatic carcinoma to the lung (197.0) from breast (174.9), patient admitted for lung biopsy."

Chemotherapy or Radiotherapy. If the visit

is primarily for chemotherapy (V58.1) or radiotherapy (V58.0), the reason for the visit is sequenced first and the primary site, if still present, would be sequenced next, with any secondary sites following.

SAMPLE: "Chemotherapy (V58.1) for carcinoma of the prostate (185)."

Possible Malignancy. The diagnosis of possible malignancy is coded to the highest degree of certainty in ambulatory care.

Cysts. Cysts are not neoplastic. Look under the term *cyst* for proper coding.

Asterisks in Table of Neoplasms. When there is an asterisk next to an anatomical site in the Table of Neoplasms, the site is coded as a squamous cell or epidermoid carcinoma of the skin.

SAMPLE: "Squamous cell carcinoma of the calf (173.7)."

Do not use the code by the asterisk but rather look under neoplasm, skin, and then go to the particular site.

Papilloma. If the neoplasm is a papilloma, it is coded as a benign neoplasm of the skin.

SAMPLE: "Papilloma of the abdominal wall (216.5)."

Primary Site. If the primary site is still present or was removed during the current episode of care, code the primary site and then any secondary sites that might be present.

SAMPLE: "Carcinoma of the lung (162) with metastasis to the liver (197.7), patient seen for a lung biopsy."

V Codes. If the primary site was previously removed and there is no evidence of recurrence of the primary site, use a V code to indicate personal history of malignant neoplasm (V10.11).

SAMPLE: "History of malignancy of lung (V10.11)."

If secondary sites are present, code them. In this case, the secondary site codes would be listed before the V code.

SAMPLE: "Metastatic carcinoma to the liver (197.7) with previous history of carcinoma of the lung (V10.11)."

If a patient is coming in for a check-up with no evidence of recurrence, then the V code would be used as the principal diagnosis.

SAMPLE: "Routine check-up (V70.0) with history of carcinoma of the colon (V10.05)."

A V code is also used if the primary reason the patient is coming to the physician is chemotherapy (V58.1) or radiation therapy (V58.0).

Location of Primary or Secondary Site Unknown. If the primary or the secondary site is known to be present but the location is unknown, use the code 199.1.

Recurrent Malignancy. Recurrent malignancy in the same site as a previous malignant neoplasm is generally coded as a new primary lesion.

SAMPLE: "Recurrent carcinoma of the colon (153.9)."

Pregnancy, Childbirth, and Puerperium

Abortions. There are certain maternal and fetal complications associated with abortions, and these can be found in categories 640–676. A fifth-digit subclassification must be used with all codes 640–676, except code 650.

The fourth digit of .7 is used with the abortion code when a specified maternal complication is present and not covered by other fourth digits in categories 634–638.

The abortion is the primary diagnosis, with the complication being secondary. When coding the maternal complication, use the fifth digit of .0 with the obstetric condition.

SAMPLE: "Incomplete spontaneous abortion (634.71) due to placenta previa (641.00)."

When dealing with a fetal complication as the reason for the abortion, code the abortion first using the fourth digit of .9, which indicates that there is no maternal complication present. The appropriate fifth digit for the fetal complication portion of the code is .0.

SAMPLE: "Abortion (635.92) due to chromosome abnormality in the fetus (655.10)."

Normal Delivery. Code 650, "Delivery in a completely normal case," can be used only when no other code is used. It includes only normal spontaneous delivery, cephalic (vertex) presentation, of one live fetus, full-term gestation. The delivery may be accompanied by an episiotomy but no other manipulation or application of forceps to assist delivery. It excludes multiple births and stillbirths.

Code 669.5, "Forceps or ventouse delivery"

without mention of indication, is used for normal delivery, cephalic presentation, routine application of low or outlet forceps or vacuum extraction, or one liveborn fetus without mention of complication of labor or delivery.

Multiple Pregnancy. Every multiple pregnancy is considered a high risk, even if the delivery is completely normal. Code 650 cannot be used.

Other Conditions. If an obstetrical condition is not found under "Delivery" ("Complicated by"), then the coder should look under "Pregnancy" ("Complicated by").

The presence of such conditions as anemia, diabetes mellitus, drug dependence, rubella, or thyroid dysfunction is considered a complication of pregnancy because it requires investigation not needed in a normal pregnancy. These are coded to categories 647 and 648.

The Respiratory System

Chronic Obstructive Pulmonary Disease (COPD) NOS. This is coded as 496.

COPD with Other Condition. If there is COPD mentioned with emphysema, chronic bronchitis, allergic alveolitis, asthma, or bronchiectasis, code the component condition rather than 496, for example, COPD with emphysema (492.8).

When a patient has an acute exacerbation of the COPD, the coder should code the acute condition that caused the exacerbation first and the COPD second.

SAMPLE: "Acute pneumonitis (486) with COPD (496)."

Additional Coding Information

The coding guidelines discussed above are by no means all inclusive, but are only meant to give the coder some guidance in the coding process. There are numerous coding references on the market, and coders should make certain that they have at least one coding reference book in the medical office to assist with problem areas and help ensure accurate coding. In addition, the coder in the medical office should consider consulting the Medical Records Department of the local hospital to assist with difficult coding situations.

Coding for reimbursement is here to stay, and the coder in the medical office should make it a goal to be the very best coder that he or she can be. Early on, the office personnel should strictly follow the established coding guidelines; then if an audit should occur, the coding procedures will be defensible.

SPECIAL HINT

One last reminder: No matter how accurate the coding, if the medical necessity for the services provided is not documented in the patient's record and the diagnosis validated in the record, it is likely that correct reimbursement will not be received, because it will be assumed that if it was not documented, the service was not provided.

Diagnosis-Related Groups

As a result of the Tax Equity and Fiscal Responsibility Act of 1982, the prospective payment system became a reality. With the dawning of the 1984 fiscal year, the health care industry saw wide-sweeping changes in the method of third-party reimbursement. These changes primarily affected acute care hospitals and were an attempt by the government to control the rising costs of health care.

As a result, hospitals are now paid a predetermined rate per discharge, rather than being reimbursed on the basis of reasonable costs.

As mentioned earlier in this chapter, the cornerstone of the prospective payment system is the DRG. This system was developed as a result of a Yale University study. This study broke 23 major diagnostic categories, based on organ systems such as the nervous system, respiratory system, cardiovascular system, etc., into 467 distinct medically meaningful groups. As of October 1992 there are now 492, DRGs. In other words, every diagnosis fits into one of the 492 DRGs. Each DRG is assigned a weight and a dollar rate, and those two figures multiplied together equal the payment the hospital receives. In some cases this payment may be greater than the actual charges; in other cases, the payment received may be less than the actual charges.

This has led to a decreased length of stay in hospitals across the country. The reimbursement rate is designed to cover the acute phase of an illness or injury and not the total recuperation period. In addition, Medicare as well as other third-party payers no longer pay for admission to the hospital when treatment and/or procedures can safely be done on an outpatient basis.

Hospitals are expected to provide high-quality

care. To assure that patients are not discharged prematurely and that the care is of high quality, Peer Review Organizations closely monitor hospitals through periodic review of medical records. In addition, failure to have justified admission and incorrect DRG assignment can also result in hospitals being reprimanded and even sanctioned. Meaningful documentation validating each diagnosis is a must if a hospital expects to receive maximum reimbursement. Proper coding is essential to the correct assignment of a DRG.

The Future of the ICD

Several changes are being planned for *ICD-10*, including a name change. It will be called the *International Statistical Classification of Diseases and Related Health Problems*.

There will also be changes in the structure of the codes. An alphanumeric coding scheme will be used, with one letter and two numbers at the three-character level.

This change more than doubles the size of the coding frame and enables the vast majority of chapters to be assigned a unique letter or group of letters, each capable of providing 100 three-character categories.

It is proposed that ICD-10 will have 21 chapters. The supplementary classifications "External Causes of Injury and Poisoning" (E codes) and "Factors Influencing Health Status and Contact with Health Services" (V codes) will be included as part of the core classification.

> **SPECIAL HINT**
>
> It should be a priority for employers and employees to attend continuing education seminars on coding procedures.

Bibliography

INSURANCE

Blue Cross and Blue Shield of Alabama: *Blue Shield and Medicare Physician's Manual*. Birmingham: Blue Cross and Blue Shield, 1990.
EDS Federal Corporation: *The Alabama Administrative Medicaid Code Book*. Montgomery: EDS Federal Corporation, 1989.
Richards C: *Managing Managed Care*. Chicago, American Association of Medical Assistants, 1991.

ICD-9-CM CODING AND DIAGNOSIS-RELATED GROUPS

Books

American Hospital Association: *Coding Clinic*. Chicago, IL: 1984–1989.
American Hospital Association: *ICD-9-CM Coding Handbook with Answers*. Chicago, IL: American Hospital Association, 1989.
American Medical Association: *A Guide for Physicians—Diagnosis Related Groups and the Prospective Payment System*. Chicago, IL: American Medical Association, 1984.
American Medical Association: *Medical Carrier Review*. Chicago, IL: American Medical Association, 1988.
American Medical Record Association. *Medical Record Management*, Berwyn, IL: Physicians' Record Company, 1985.
Code Book for Physician Payment, Volumes 1 and 2. Alexandria, VA: St. Anthony Publishing, 1989.
Finnegan R: *A Basic ICD-9-CM Coding Workshop*, Units 1 and 2. Chicago, IL: American Medical Record Association, 1989.
Finnegan R: *Coding for Prospective Payment*. Chicago, IL: American Medical Record Association, 1984.
Finnegan R: *ICD-9-CM Basic Coding Handbook*. Chicago, IL: American Medical Record Association, 1989.
International Classification of Diseases, 9th Revision, Clinical Modification. vols. 1 and 2. Ann Arbor, MI: Commission on Professional and Hospital Activities, 1980.
Jones MK: *Training Manual for Physician Coding*. Alexandria, VA: St. Anthony Publishing, 1990.
Joseph ED, Tuckler JH, Fox LA: *Documenting Ambulatory Care*. Chicago, IL: Care Communications, 1986.
Puckett C: *The Educational Annotation of ICD-9-CM*. Reno, NV: Channel Publishing, 1989.
Tucker J: *Learning to Code with ICD-9-CM*. Chicago, IL: Care Communications, 1986.

Periodicals

Finnegan R: Coding notes. *Journal of American Medical Record Association* 59(8):22–25, 1988.
Finnegan R: Coding notes. *Journal of American Medical Record Association* 59(10):26–27, 1988.
Finnegan R: Coding notes. *Journal of American Medical Record Association* 60(2):22–23, 1989.
Finnegan R: Coding notes. *Journal of American Medical Record Association* 60(8):18–19, 1989.
Finnegan R: Coding notes. *Journal of American Medical Record Association* 60(10):19–20, 1989.
Finnegan R: Coding notes. *Journal of American Medical Record Association* 60(12):18–21, 1989.
Finnegan R: Coding notes. *Journal of American Medical Record Association* 61(4):24–25, 1990.
Finnegan R: Coding notes. *Journal of American Medical Record Association* 61(8):30, 1990.
Klinge M: A basic review of ICD-9 coding for the medical office. *The Professional Medical Assistant* 25–29, July/August, 1987.
Klinge M: Assist the physician with coding know-how. *The Professional Medical Assistant* 8–12, July/August, 1989.
O'Gara S: Coding notes—data sets and coding guidelines: Sequencing vs. classification rules. *Journal of American Medical Record Association* 61(2):20–21, 1990.
Renfro J: New ICD-9-CM coding requirements—a challenge for medical assistants. *The Professional Medical Assistant* 16–18, July/August, 1989.

Chapter 9

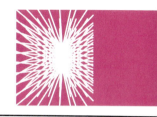

COMPUTERIZATION AND PRACTICE MANAGEMENT FOR THE HEALTH CARE PROVIDER

NANETTE HOFFMAN

BENEFITS OF COMPUTERIZING A MEDICAL PRACTICE
Efficient Patient Billing
Efficient Third-Party Reimbursement
Efficient Patient Recall and Scheduling
Evaluation of the Practice
Better Patient Care
More Efficient Office Staff
Flexibility of the Software to Grow with the Practice and Handle Changes in the Health Care Industry

HARDWARE CONSIDERATIONS
SOFTWARE CONSIDERATIONS
Flow of the Program
Keeping Additional Records
Preparing Practice Management Reports
Security
Summary of Software
CHOOSING THE VENDOR
TRAINING AND SUPPORT
UPGRADES

The decision for a medical practice to automate is an important decision that deserves careful analysis. Often the decision about automation is avoided out of fear, uncertainty, and doubt. This is unfortunate, because outside forces including the government, insurance companies, and consumers are demanding that physicians become more efficient. These demands are being enforced by controlling the prices physicians can charge. Therefore, it is incumbent on physicians to manage their practices more efficiently. This is where the computer helps.

Computerizing your office is a decision that deserves thoughtful planning and careful implementation. The benefits of computerizing will be noticed in a variety of ways, such as increased time for patient care, decreased accounts payable, increased staff efficiency with less paper chasing, and an improvement in management of the practice.

BENEFITS OF COMPUTERIZING A MEDICAL PRACTICE

Efficient Patient Billing

- Statements are sent in a scheduled, timely manner.
- Statements are clear and descriptive, reducing the amount of time the staff spends explaining the statements to patients.
- Better aging tools increase cash flow and decrease bad debt write-offs.
- Reports are easily generated for evaluating ac-

counts receivable and identifying potential credit problems.
- Month-end workload is reduced because the computer prints the patient statements and month-end practice management reports.

Efficient Third-Party Reimbursement

- The computer requires valid procedure and diagnosis codes, which result in faster reimbursement and fewer rejected claims.
- Insurance claims are generated automatically. There is less time between the patient's visit and the filing of the claim.
- Computers allow electronic claim submission and scan forms for faster reimbursement and better cash flow.
- On-line history of patient accounts allows for easy refiling of rejected claims.

Efficient Patient Recall and Scheduling

- Patient recall letters can be generated automatically.
- Computers allow flexibility of patient recall based on parameters set by the individual practice.
- Searching for patient appointments is made easy and less time consuming by creating accessible records.

Evaluation of the Practice

- Reports are available to show revenues generated by procedure or diagnosis as well as by referrals, location (if a multilocation practice), and provider (if more than one provider).

Better Patient Care

- Access to patient records is faster.
- Less administrative time permits more time for patient care.
- Computers permit access to hospital records, medical database services, and cross-referencing of the patient database.

More Efficient Office Staff

- The computer is ready for work every day and does not need a vacation.
- Computers help to ease the paper chase.
- Computers demand a high level of discipline that results in fewer mistakes.

Flexibility of Software to Grow with the Practice and Handle Changes in the Health Care Industry

- Computers provide an efficient way to handle growth of the medical practice.
- Flexibility in design of software allows for individual needs of varying medical specialties.
- Flexibility in design also provides for changes, which are a continuous part of the health care industry.

HARDWARE CONSIDERATIONS

It is important to evaluate the practice's present and future needs so that the appropriate hardware is obtained. Although it does not pay to go overboard, upgrading equipment is expensive and time consuming, so it is prudent to buy more powerful equipment than appears necessary. Be careful to avoid both the salesman who will "lowball" in hopes of getting the sale and the salesman who tries to oversell you. The specific equipment needed for the practice must be defined.

Number of Computer Workstations Needed. In determining the number of workstations needed, consider the number of physicians, the size of the office staff, and the number of patients seen in a typical day.

Size of the Hard Disk Drive. What kinds of information will be stored in the computer? If your plan is to use the computer for practice management, accounting, word processing, and other programs, consider a larger capacity hard disk. If the office will use the computer only for practice management, a smaller hard disk may suffice. The price of hard disks has fallen dramatically in the last few years. Therefore, always buy a larger drive than seems necessary.

Type of Printer Needed. Will you be printing the patient statements and insurance claims? Are you required to print letters to referring practitioners and attorneys? By analyzing the uses of your printer, you will be able to choose the appropriate printer, whether it be dot matrix, inkjet, or laser printer.

SPECIAL HINT

Be aware that a laser printer's greatest expense is not the purchase price but the cost of each individual copy.

Will You Need a Modem, Fax, or Any Other Hardware? Modems allow your computer to dial into another computer over the telephone line to share information. If your office will be using electronic medical databases or if your vendor provides on-line support, a modem is a necessary piece of equipment. A computer fax allows your computer to dial into a fax at another site.

SPECIAL HINT

The fax is a time-saving piece of equipment if your office is in an area where pharmacies have fax machines to receive prescriptions from physicians.

SOFTWARE CONSIDERATIONS

When looking at software packages, be sure to note the following points:

- Good software is easy to use, logical, and concise.
- It is flexible and able to handle your office's special situations.

Flow of the Program

The computer program should follow a pattern similar to the normal flow of work in your practice. In the simplest of cases this means that

1. A new patient will come into the office for a visit.
2. He or she will fill out a new patient information sheet to be kept in the chart.
3. A copy of the patient's insurance card will be made.
4. The chart will be prepared.
5. The patient will be seen by the physician and will have procedures done.
6. The patient will pay for the visit and will leave.

There is a definite flow in this scenario that a good practice management package will also follow. The following steps will illustrate how a particular software program (in this case, HDS* Medical Assistance Professional) will efficiently handle this situation.

Step 1. A new patient is entered. In Figure 9–1 the patient list is shown. Notice that the list is in alphabetical order and does not require the user to remember an account number for a patient. However, patients' most important identifying information appears on the list. Notice that the age, social security number, and chart number are displayed on the list.

To add a new patient to the list the operator presses the "insert" key. A question appears (Figure 9–2) asking if the patient will be responsible for paying the bill. After a yes response, a patient record (Figure 9–3) appears for the operator to fill in. This record requires some very important information, such as the full name, social security number, birth date, and sex of the patient as well as the patient's mailing address and phone numbers. A chart number may also be added to the patient's record. This record is saved, and a new question appears (Figures 9–4 and 9–5) asking if the patient has insurance coverage. If the operator answers yes, another question appears (Figure 9–6) asking if the patient is the policy holder. After these questions are answered, the patient's insurance information (Figures 9–7 and 9–8) is entered into the database, and the new patient's information is complete.

Step 2. The next step is to enter today's charges for a new patient. The patient is chosen from the patient list, and the patient information menu appears (Figure 9–9). Procedures are chosen from the menu and a blank record appears (Figures 9–10 and 9–11). From this point a diagnosis record also appears (Figures 9–12 and 9–13) so that the diagnosis information and the procedure information can be added at the same time. Note that only valid *International Classification of Diseases, 9th Revision, Clinical Modifications (ICD-9-CM)* and *Current Procedural Terminology (CPT-4)* codes should be kept in the system (Figure 9–14). This greatly reduces the chance of insurance claim rejections.

After all of the necessary information is entered into the diagnosis and procedure records, they will be saved and the Charge and Payment Entry screens will appear (Figures 9–15 and 9–16). These screens show the information that was entered for the new patient's visit today for verification of charges and any changes that may need to be made at this point. The payment for today's visit is also entered. This information is saved.

---
* Health Data Services, Inc., Charlottesville, VA.

Text continued on page 216

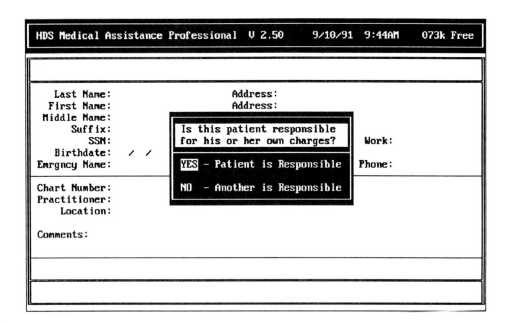

FIGURE 9-1
Sample listing of names in a patient database. (Courtesy of Health Data Services, Inc., Charlottesville, VA, 1992.)

FIGURE 9-2
Computer prompt screen for determining patient financial responsibility. (Courtesy of Health Data Services, Inc., Charlottesville, VA, 1992.)

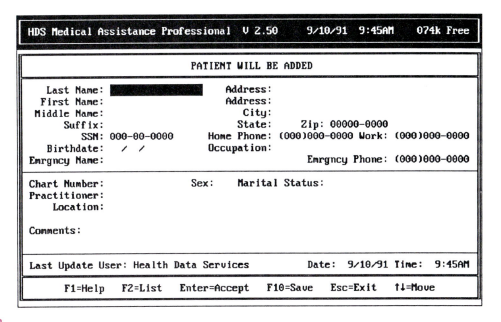

FIGURE 9-3
Patient information screen display. (Courtesy of Health Data Services, Inc., Charlottesville, VA, 1992.)

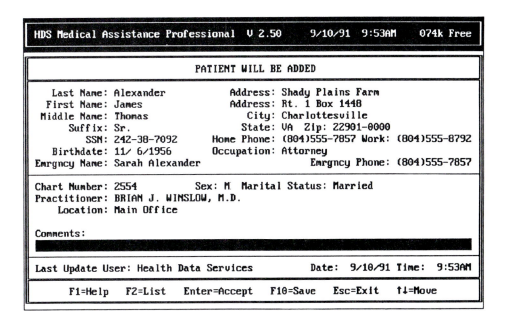

FIGURE 9-4
Completed patient information screen. (Courtesy of Health Data Services, Inc., Charlottesville, VA, 1992.)

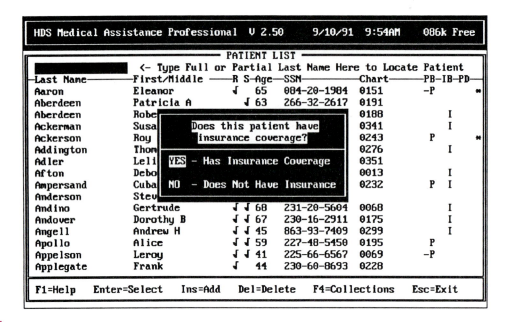

FIGURE 9-5
Computer prompt screen for determining patient insurance coverage. (Courtesy of Health Data Services, Inc., Charlottesville, VA, 1992.)

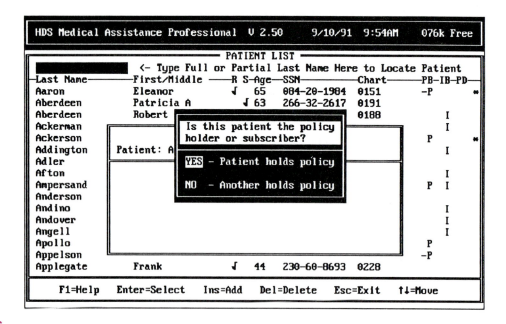

FIGURE 9-6
Computer prompt screen for determining policy ownership. (Courtesy of Health Data Services, Inc., Charlottesville, VA, 1992.)

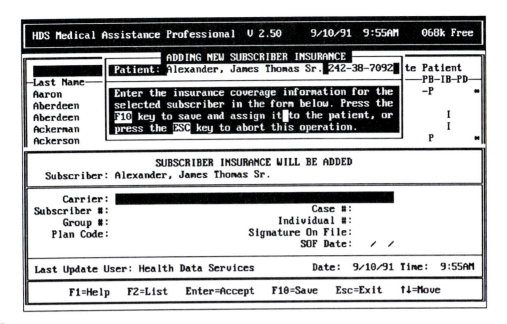

FIGURE 9-7

Patient insurance screen display. (Courtesy of Health Data Services, Inc., Charlottesville, VA, 1992.)

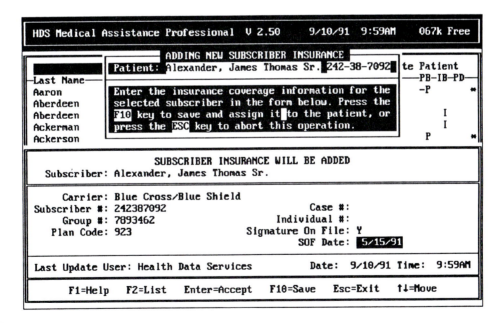

FIGURE 9-8

Completed patient insurance screen. (Courtesy of Health Data Services, Inc., Charlottesville, VA, 1992.)

212 *Chapter 9: COMPUTERIZATION AND PRACTICE MANAGEMENT FOR THE HEALTH CARE PROVIDER*

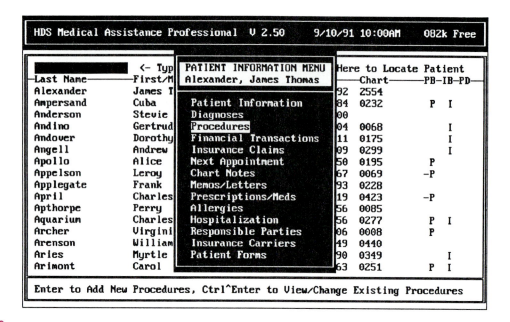

FIGURE 9-9

Patient information menu display. (Courtesy of Health Data Services, Inc., Charlottesville, VA, 1992.)

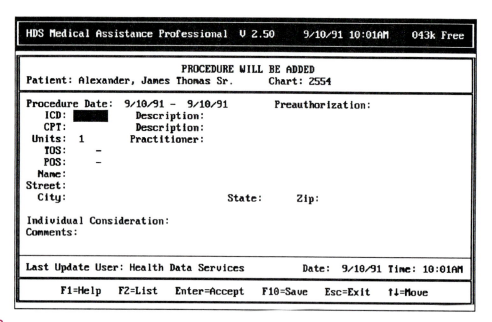

FIGURE 9-10

Screen display for procedure records. (Courtesy of Health Data Services, Inc., Charlottesville, VA, 1992.)

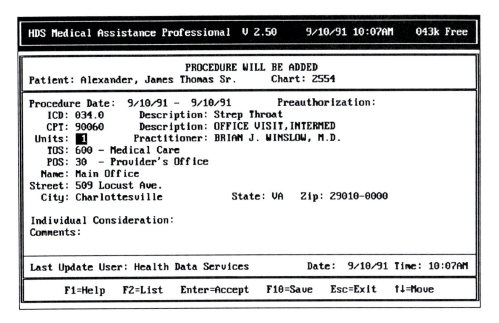

FIGURE 9-11

Completed procedure record screen. (Courtesy of Health Data Services, Inc., Charlottesville, VA, 1992.)

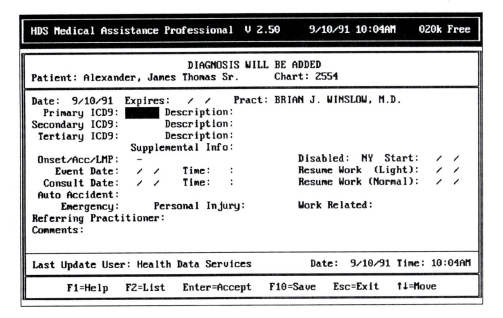

FIGURE 9-12

Screen display for diagnosis records. (Courtesy of Health Data Services, Inc., Charlottesville, VA, 1992.)

214 *Chapter 9: COMPUTERIZATION AND PRACTICE MANAGEMENT FOR THE HEALTH CARE PROVIDER*

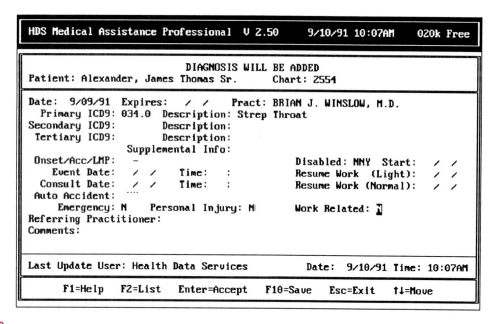

FIGURE 9–13

Completed diagnosis record screen. (Courtesy of Health Data Services, Inc., Charlottesville, VA, 1992.)

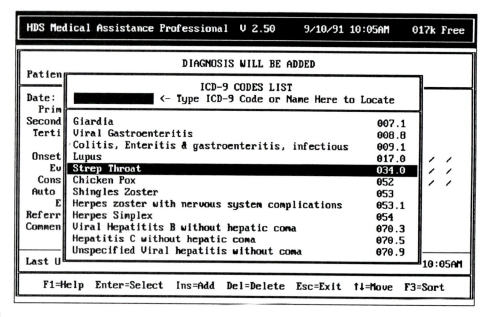

FIGURE 9–14

ICD-9 menu display. (Courtesy of Health Data Services, Inc., Charlottesville, VA, 1992.)

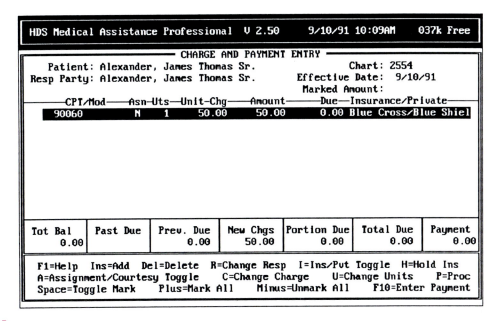

FIGURE 9–15
Charge and payment entry screen. (Courtesy of Health Data Services, Inc., Charlottesville, VA, 1992.)

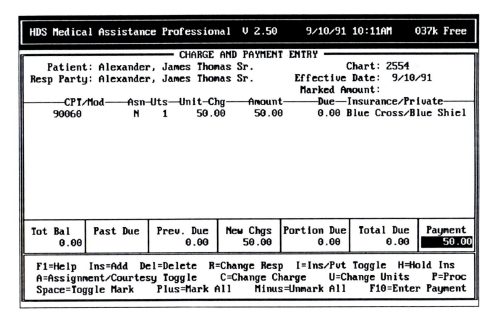

FIGURE 9–16
Sample payment entry. (Courtesy of Health Data Services, Inc., Charlottesville, VA, 1992.)

The HDS Medical Assistance Professional software package is capable of handling very simple (as this example is) as well as very complex situations. This program easily and efficiently handles such scenarios as a patient who is a minor whose father pays the bills while the patient is covered by the mother's insurance. This same program has the ability to accept assignment on laboratory charges for Medicare patients when the provider does not participate with Medicare, and many more special cases.

Step 3. After statements have been sent to the patients, payments begin to come to the office. Posting these checks is done quickly and easily. The responsible party (the person responsible for paying the bill) appears on the responsible party list (Figure 9–17). This responsible party is chosen, and the responsible party menu appears (Figure 9–18). Financial transactions are chosen, and a list of the financial transactions, including charges, insurance claims, previous payments, previous statements, and any other transactions the responsible party had in the past, appears (Figure 9–19). The statement transaction should be chosen at this time. After the statement is selected from the list, a transaction menu appears (Figure 9–20). There are a number of transactions on the menu from which to choose. Private payment is chosen in this case, and a payment transaction record appears (Figure 9–21) and the amount of the payment is entered (Figure 9–22). This record is saved, and the posting is complete.

Step 4. After insurance claims have been filed, the checks and remittances or explanations of benefits come to the office. These are posted in our sample system according to the patient who incurred the charges. Once again, the patient is chosen from the patient list. The insurance claims menu option (Figure 9–23) is selected, and a list of all outstanding claims appears (Figure 9–24). The correct claim is selected from the list. An insurance claim processing screen appears (Figures 9–25 and 9–26). The screen shows the first procedure that appeared on the claim. This procedure is posted. The amount considered by the insurance company or the Medicare allowable amount should be entered. The insurance payment is entered next, followed by the deductible, if any, and the copayment amount if any, which will be automatically transferred to the responsible party's private account. The computer then calculates the amount to be adjusted off or charged off. This record is saved, and the next procedure that appeared on the claim appears on the screen to be posted. If that charge has not been paid with this check, it can be posted at a later time.

Text continued on page 221

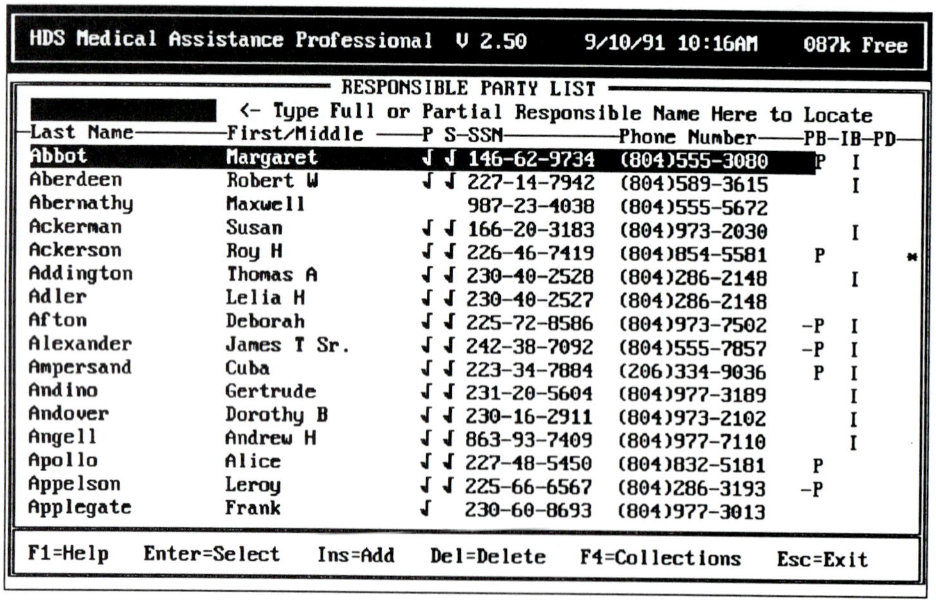

FIGURE 9–17

Responsible party display screen. (Courtesy of Health Data Services, Inc., Charlottesville, VA, 1992.)

Chapter 9: COMPUTERIZATION AND PRACTICE MANAGEMENT FOR THE HEALTH CARE PROVIDER   **217**

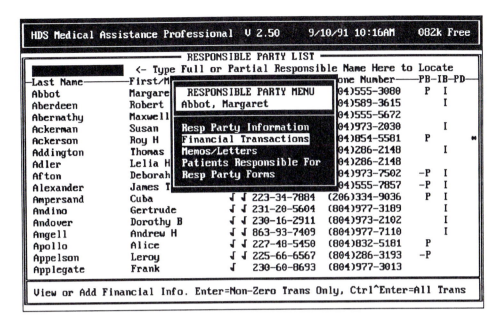

FIGURE 9-18
Responsible party menu display. (Courtesy of Health Data Services, Inc., Charlottesville, VA, 1992.)

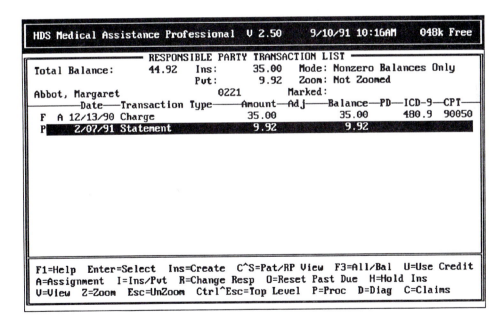

FIGURE 9-19
Screen listing for responsible party transactions. (Courtesy of Health Data Services, Inc., Charlottesville, VA, 1992.)

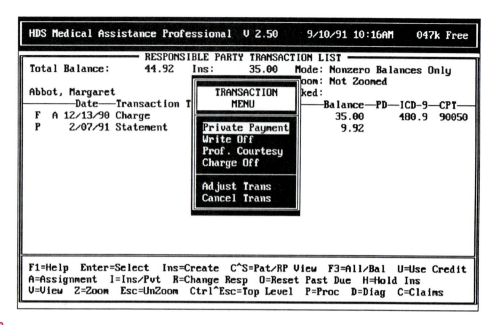

FIGURE 9-20

Transaction menu display. (Courtesy of Health Data Services, Inc., Charlottesville, VA, 1992.)

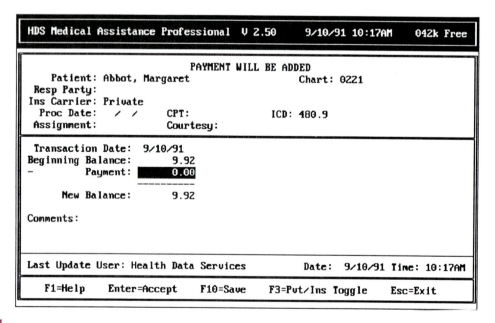

FIGURE 9-21

Payment record. (Courtesy of Health Data Services, Inc., Charlottesville, VA, 1992.)

Chapter 9: COMPUTERIZATION AND PRACTICE MANAGEMENT FOR THE HEALTH CARE PROVIDER

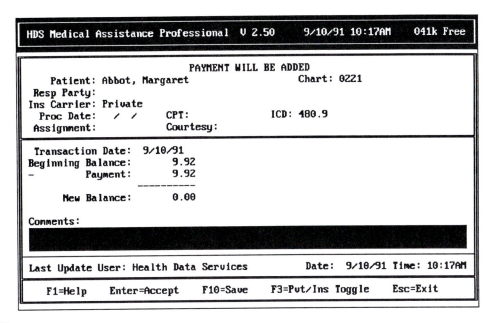

FIGURE 9-22
Payment entry. (Courtesy of Health Data Services, Inc., Charlottesville, VA, 1992.)

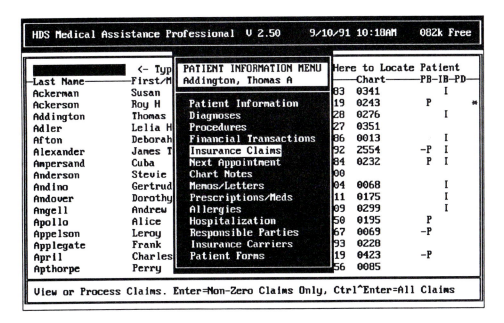

FIGURE 9-23
Patient information menu for insurance claims. (Courtesy of Health Data Services, Inc., Charlottesville, VA, 1992.)

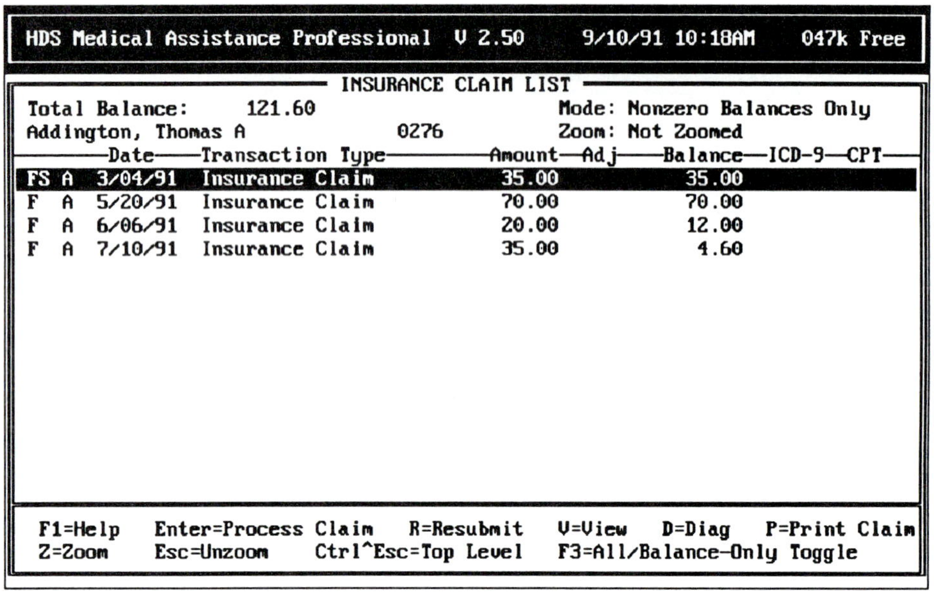

FIGURE 9-24

Screen listing for outstanding insurance claims. (Courtesy of Health Data Services, Inc., Charlottesville, VA, 1992.)

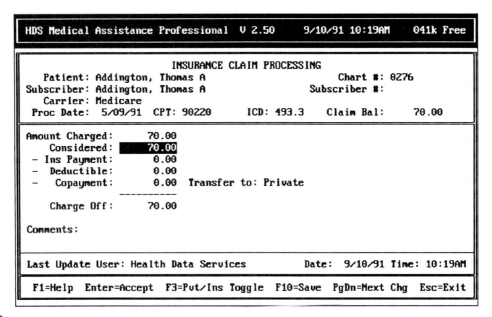

FIGURE 9-25

Insurance claim entry display. (Courtesy of Health Data Services, Inc., Charlottesville, VA, 1992.)

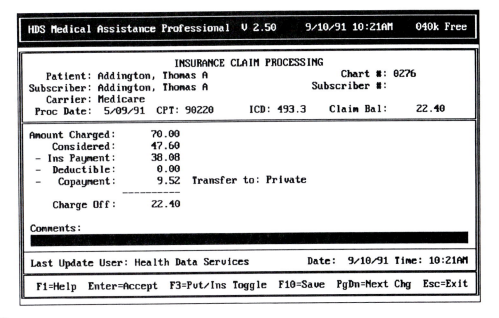

FIGURE 9-26

Completed insurance claim processing screen. (Courtesy of Health Data Services, Inc., Charlottesville, VA, 1992.)

Keeping Additional Records

The sample software, HDS Medical Assistance Professional, also has the ability to keep patient chart notes in the patient's record. This system is organized so that when a new chart note is entered into the computer it can be printed onto the previously used chart note paper at the exact line on the sheet. This reduces wasted paper.

The patient's next appointment can be entered into the patient's record, which creates a recall report allowing all of the patients in any given time period to be sent a reminder of an upcoming appointment. This feature can reduce missed appointments and remind patients that it is time for their check-ups.

The patient's allergies, prescriptions and medications, and hospitalization records are also kept in his or her record. Keeping this information in the computer greatly reduces the time spent looking in the chart for information when an insurance processor is on the telephone. It can also be a safeguard if something were to happen to the chart itself.

Memos and letters can also be written from within a patient's record with the memos/letters word processing feature. These can then be printed onto the physician's stationery and mailed off, with a copy saved in the computer.

Preparing Practice Management Reports

A good practice management program will provide reports concerning a variety of topics, such as

- Financial reports
- Analysis reports
- Patient reports
- Summary reports
- Insurance reports

Within the realm of financial reports, there should be such reports as

- Activity or day sheets
- Accounts receivable
- Past due accounts
- Outstanding insurance claims
- Revenue generated reports
- Income reports

There should also be analysis reports such as diagnosis and procedure reports to show information such as the number of procedures done in a given period of time and the amount of revenue generated. The package should also have the ability to print the *CPT-4* codes list with fees and the *ICD-9-CM* list. The ability to print patient, responsible party, insurance subscriber, and insurance carrier lists should exist.

Security

The security and integrity of the data kept in the computer should be guarded. The use of passwords to gain entry to the program is a must, as is a routine of daily backups of all data files, program files, and any other files that would be difficult to replace.

Summary of Software

It is important to consider the ease of use or "friendliness" of the software. The software illustrated in this chapter uses drop-down menus and is list driven. This style is user friendly and requires no memorization of commands or codes to perform tasks. All special keys used in this package are listed for the user on the lower portion of the screen. These keys change on each screen according to the availability of their use. This program also guides the user through the system with clear questions in a yes-or-no format. This ensures that no necessary information falls through the cracks.

CHOOSING THE VENDOR

When choosing the vendor, be sure to consider the following characteristics.

Knowledge. Be sure the vendor has a good working knowledge of the health care industry as well as of practice management. The vendor should stay abreast of coming changes in the industry. A qualified vendor knows about changes and is planning the approach to any changes that will affect the software so that the changes are addressed in a timely manner.

Experience. A good vendor has been in the field of health care and computers for a reasonable amount of time. Ask candidates the following questions:

What kind of track record does the vendor hold?

What references does the vendor have, and may they be contacted to ensure that the qualifications are valid?

How many systems does the vendor have in place? For how long?

Are updates done in a timely manner?

Support Staff Qualifications and Experience. Staff should be educated in the health care and computer industries and knowledgeable about changes taking place that will affect those fields.

Flexibility. The vendor should be able to fulfill any special needs your practice or specialty may have. The vendor should listen to your suggestions for improvements. Many innovative ideas have come from medical practices that have made improvements in practice management software.

TRAINING AND SUPPORT

Training and support are very important considerations. It is essential that the kind of support, the amount of support, and the fees for support are agreed on before any contracts are signed. Support can vary from little or none to total. It varies from free, to very expensive monthly payments, to pay per call. Free support is sometimes the most effective kind. Pay per call can be very expensive. There may be a choice between total support for hardware and software and partial support for only certain aspects of your system.

Thorough training is essential to an efficient transition from a manual system to computerization. The vendor should provide guidance in organizing patient account records and charts to ensure the smoothest possible installation. Trainers should be accessible to answer all questions.

UPGRADES

Regarding upgrades, ask these questions:

Will the computer hardware and software be upgraded automatically, or will upgrades be optional and/or expensive?

Will the upgrades be part of the initial cost, or will there be a fee attached to each upgrade?

There are several alternative choices for computerizing your office. You can buy all the equipment and software for a set fee, which could be costly. Purchasing expensive hardware that can become obsolete in a short period of time may be less cost-effective than leasing equipment. Another alternative is to subscribe to a service that provides hardware, software, upgrades, training, support, and auxiliary services (such as patient and/or insurance billing).

Chapter 10

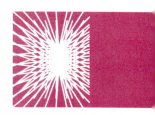

EMPLOYMENT PRACTICES

JOAN B. CONRAD

RECRUITMENT AND HIRING
The Planning Process
Job Descriptions
Sources of Job Candidates
Interviewing Process
Selection of Candidates

WAGES AND SALARIES
Determining and Evaluating Pay Scales
Federal Wage and Hour Regulations

BENEFIT PACKAGES
Required Programs
Retirement Programs
Health Insurance Programs
Life Insurance Programs
Disability Insurance Programs
Sick Leave and Personal Leave Programs
Other Benefits
Legal Requirements

RECRUITMENT AND HIRING

Recruitment and hiring practices require attention to established personnel procedures and legal requirements. Many options exist for the practice manager and the physician employer. By defining authority limits and responsibilities, developing a practice philosophy with regard to employment matters, and consulting with employees and other ancillary support persons, the manager and physician can simplify the decision-making process and achieve more effective results.

The Planning Process

Many situations could occur in an office practice that create a vacancy. Perhaps a vacancy occurs because a problem employee has been terminated; perhaps an employee has left to have a child; perhaps a physician has died, retired, or quit; or perhaps a new physician has been introduced into the practice. Such situations offer either the opportunity for confusion and chaos or the opportunity to reassess and review the office personnel structure. In all situations, the key is to plan and to organize materials. In either a large, multiphysician office or a small, single-physician office, the position's title, workweek, job duties, requirements, and pay scale may be predetermined. The management process will be one of selecting a qualified and potentially compatible employee. Even with this simple scenario, development of a "position vacancy checklist" is a good organizational tool (Figure 10–1).

As a manager's authority may vary from office to office, so may his or her opportunity or ability to provide input. However, in these times of increasing governmental involvement and restriction of fees, resulting in loss of practice income, all managers may use any vacancy as an opportunity to reevaluate the status quo to see if opportunities exist to economize and increase the office's efficiency.

Points to Consider

1. Can the position be modified to allow for part-time personnel with reduced benefits and

_____ Announce position available
_____ Set deadline for filling vacancy
_____ Make temporary coverage arrangements
       Job descriptions
       _____ Create
       _____ Review
_____ Select resource to obtain candidates
_____ Implement resources
_____ Conduct screening process
_____ Schedule interviews
       Organize interview materials
       _____ Employment application
       _____ Interview checklist
       _____ Review guidelines
_____ Conduct interviews
_____ Make job offer
       Assemble new hire package
       _____ Employee handbook
       _____ Policies manual
       _____ Procedure manual
       _____ Required employee forms
       Orientation
       _____ Select staff member to orient
       _____ Specify amount of time devoted to orientation
       Training
       _____ Select staff to train
       _____ Specify length of training

FIGURE 10-1

Position vacancy checklist.

cost compared with full-time personnel with more substantial benefits and costs?
2. Would designating this a job-shared position open up opportunities to tap a larger labor force — for example, former office personnel who left to have children and may not want or need full-time employment?
3. What is the current status of the labor force in the community? Study the classified ads on Sundays to determine whether similar positions are being offered and if they repeat from one week to the next. Multiple openings may mean a lack of qualified applicants for your position. You may need to modify the pay scale, benefits, hours, etc. as an attraction. Survey other practices by calling their managers and asking if they would share any current experiences with you about availability and quality of applicants.
4. Are existing personnel flexible, qualified, and/or willing to perform different or additional duties?
5. Is this the time to switch from a physician-specific to a duty-specific work assignment?
6. Can the existing office personnel be retained but the salaries/wages, benefits, or hours modified to accommodate the situation?

Once you have evaluated your needs and established the position and the parameters for employment, the next step is to develop a job description.

Job Descriptions

The Michigan Department of Civil Rights has written, "One of the most effective ways to ensure sound selection procedures and to avoid unlawful discrimination is for employers to carefully develop written, job-related position descriptions which outline the required skills and abilities for each position. Obviously, the purpose of a sound selection process is to obtain good employees who can meet specific work requirements and successfully perform the particular job duties."[1]

A job description is a summary of the basic tasks performed on the job and relevant parameters for performing the job. A sample form to develop a job description is offered in Figure 10-2. The format may vary according to the style of the description writer. Job descriptions are excellent tools to determine if there is overlapping and/or duplication of responsibilities and what the job priorities are. The process of writing job descriptions can also create understanding between the employees and the employer. In practices that have no job descriptions, employees may be asked to complete a preprinted form that details their activity. An office manager could conduct a personal interview with each employee. In practices with established job descriptions, reviewing them with each employee can serve to update the description and remind the employee of his or her responsibilities.

Job descriptions are translated into job specifications that include the following:

- Experience — length of time and previous activities performed
- Education — amount of schooling and specific knowledge required
- Responsibility — degree of accountability and the decision making necessary

Position (Describe by title, e.g., "medical assistant—generalist")
Licensure requirements (Specify, e.g., no licensure required)
Education requirements (Specify, e.g., associates' degree from an accredited medical assisting program)
Specific work experience (Specify, e.g., entry-level position, no experience necessary)
Required work skills (Specify, e.g., ability to type XXX/words per minute using IBM Correcting Selectric II; alpha digit filing experience; knowledge of medical terminology; computer data entry experience (specify type); surgical assisting experience (specify specialty); physical ability necessary to lift XXX pounds)
Duties of position (List)
Personal requirements (List your needs; e.g., legible handwriting, pleasant telephone voice, team player, bilingual abilities)
Workweek (Define, e.g., "Mondays through Fridays")
Hours (Specify, e.g., "9:00 A.M. to 6:00 P.M. One-hour lunch period off or on premises, staggered")
Salary/wage range (Specify, e.g., "This is classified as a nonexempt position by federal regulations. The starting salary range will be $6.00–$8.50 per hour.")
Authority limits (Specify, e.g., "Will report directly to the office manager, may not purchase or commit to purchase without countersignature or office manager and/or physician employer.")
Benefits (Define. May refer to a separate list. Some practices offer limited benefits for part-time or half-time personnel, so separate listing may be indicated.)

FIGURE 10-2

Job descriptions.

- Physical effort—physical activity requirements and requirements for bona fide discrimination
- Authority—who employee reports to and what boundaries of authority are
- Supervision—number of persons supervised
- Other parameters—specification of workweek as full- or part-time, hours, and salary range.

Once needs and opportunities for restructuring have been determined, consideration of where candidates can be located must be made.

Sources of Job Candidates

Classified Ads

Classified advertising is a commonly used source for obtaining job applicants. Writing a classified ad is not a time to be stingy with dollars, because a sparsely worded advertisement signifies many negative things to the applicant about the management and the employer. A well-designed, thoughtful advertisement can catch the eye of the reader and present a professional image of your practice.

Points to Consider

A border or frame of white is an effective attention getter. Contact the newspaper for alternatives of ad design, assistance with copy, and cost experience.

The Sunday personnel wanted section is commonly the most comprehensive. If cost is a factor, consider spending your dollars on one large Sunday ad rather than a smaller one that runs throughout the week.

Survey and compare current classified ads to see what catches your eye. Ask co-workers their opinions.

Add a statement in your advertisement that says "All replies are confidential" and honor that statement.

Include a deadline for application submissions.

Blind Ads. In blind ads, responses are directed to a box number. Practice identity is not revealed. This is a common custom, especially when other employees do not know of the vacancy.

Direct Responses. Consider offering not only your practice name, but the address and person to whom the resume is to be sent. Potential employees appreciate this because there are, in every community, employers with whom an experienced applicant may have already worked or with whom the applicant may not wish to be associated. This also signifies that current personnel are aware of the vacancy and offers candidates the opportunity for networking with your current employees.

Phone Responses. Consider segregating blocks of your time and entertain direct phone responses between specific hours on specific days. This is a relevant practice if the position requires phone work with a triage system. Regardless of the position, telephone screening will bring response. Have a simple form ready for each phone applicant so that you can ask the same questions and say the same thing to all applicants and note their answers. Possible questions include "What attracted you to the advertisement?", "Do you really prefer part-time [or full-time] work?", and

SUBJECT	LAWFUL PRE-EMPLOYMENT INQUIRIES	UNLAWFUL PRE-EMPLOYMENT INQUIRIES
NAME:	Applicant's full name. Have you ever worked for this company under a different name? Is any additional information relative to a different name necessary to check work record? If yes, explain.	Original name of an applicant whose name has been changed by court order or otherwise. Applicant's maiden name.
ADDRESS OR DURATION OF RESIDENCE:	How long a resident of this state or city?	
BIRTHPLACE:		Birthplace of applicant. Birthplace of applicant's parents, spouse or other close relatives. Requirement that applicant submit birth certificate, naturalization or baptismal record.
AGE:	*Are you 18 years old or older?	How old are you? What is your date of birth?
RELIGION OR CREED:		Inquiry into an applicant's religious denomination, religious affiliations, church, parish, pastor, or religious holidays observed. An applicant may not be told "This is a Catholic (Protestant or Jewish) organization."
RACE OR COLOR:		Complexion or color of skin.
PHOTOGRAPH:		Requirement that an applicant for employment affix a photograph to an employment application form. Request an applicant, at his or her option, to submit a photograph. Requirement for photograph after interview but before hiring.
HEIGHT:		Inquiry regarding applicant's height.
WEIGHT:		Inquiry regarding applicant's weight.
MARITAL STATUS:		Requirement that an applicant provide any information regarding marital status or children. Are you single or married? Do you have any children? Is your spouse employed? What is your spouse's name?
SEX:		Mr., Miss or Mrs. or an inquiry regarding sex. Inquiry as to the ability to reproduce or advocacy of any form of birth control.
HEALTH:	Do you have any impairments, physical, mental, or medical which would interfere with your ability to do the job for which you have applied? Inquiry into contagious or communicable diseases which may endanger others. If there are any positions for which you should not be considered or job duties you cannot perform because of a physical or mental handicap, please explain.	Inquiries regarding an individual's physical or mental condition which are not directly related to the requirements of a specific job and which are used as a factor in making employment decisions in a way which is contrary to the provisions or purposes of the Michigan Handicappers' Civil Rights Act. Requirement that women be given pelvic examinations.

FIGURE 10-3

Sample preemployment inquiry guide. (Courtesy of Michigan Department of Civil Rights, Detroit, MI.)

CITIZENSHIP:	Are you a citizen of the United States?	Of what country are you a citizen?
	If not a citizen of the United States, does applicant intend to become a citizen of the United States?	Whether an applicant is naturalized or a native-born citizen; the date when the applicant acquired citizenship.
	If you are not a United States citizen, have you the legal right to remain permanently in the United States? Do you intend to remain permanently in the United States?	Requirement that an applicant produce naturalization papers or first papers.
		Whether applicant's parents or spouse are naturalized or native born citizens of the United States; the date when such parent or spouse acquired citizenship.
NATIONAL ORIGIN:	Inquiry into languages applicant speaks and writes fluently.	Inquiry into applicant's (a) lineage; (b) ancestry; (c) national origin; (d) descent; (e) parentage, or nationality.
		Nationality of applicant's parents or spouse.
		What is your mother tongue?
		Inquiry into how applicant acquired ability to read, write or speak a foreign language.
EDUCATION:	Inquiry into the academic, vocational, or professional education of an applicant and the public and private schools attended.	
EXPERIENCE:	Inquiry into work experience.	
	Inquiry into countries applicant has visited.	
ARRESTS:	Have you ever been convicted of a crime? If so, when, where, and nature of offense?	Inquiry regarding arrests.
	Are there any felony charges pending against you?	
RELATIVES:	Names of applicant's relatives, other than a spouse, already employed by this company.	Address of any relative of applicant, other than address (within the United States) of applicant's father and mother, husband or wife and minor dependent children.
NOTICE IN CASE OF EMERGENCY:	Name and address of person to be notified in case of accident or emergency.	Name and address of nearest relative to be notified in case of accident or emergency.
MILITARY EXPERIENCE:	Inquiry into an applicant's military experience in the Armed Forces of the United States or in a State Militia.	Inquiry into an applicant's general military experience.
	Inquiry into applicant's service in particular branch of United States Army, Navy, etc.	
ORGANIZATIONS:	Inquiry into the organizations of which an applicant is a member excluding organizations the name or character of which indicates the race, color, religion, national origin, or ancestry of its members.	List all clubs, societies, and lodges to which you belong.
REFERENCES:	Who suggested that you apply for a position here?	

*This question may be asked only for the purpose of determining whether applicants are of legal age for employment.

FIGURE 10-3 Continued

"What do you want me to know about yourself?" This method is so popular with applicants that you may wish to consider the impact of multiple, continual calls on your practice. Assigning another person to answer the phone and take down names and telephone numbers of potential candidates may be advisable in order to keep your lines open to patients!

With any telephone screening, a word of caution: Do not pursue any disclosures an applicant may make about his or her marital status, age, or any of the protected characteristics (see Legal Requirements). Just note that the information was volunteered. For example, the question "Do you require coverage in a group health plan?" allows for a yes or no answer, which certainly is appropriate, but most applicants will discuss their personal situation with you and volunteer answers to questions you legally may not ask (Figure 10-3). At the beginning of each conversation, after identifying yourself, tell each applicant that you are screening by phone because a good phone voice is essential to the position. Tell them that you are unable to call all applicants back, but at the end of the day (state time) you will call back candidates you wish to interview. Get the correct spelling of the applicant's name and the phone number at which he or she can be reached at the determined time.

Resume. Regardless of the type of ad you use, request a typewritten resume and a handwritten, not typed, cover letter that provides a response to the advertisement. For example, "Send (or bring) a typed resume and a handwritten cover letter that details why you wish to be considered for this position."

Cover Letters. Requesting a handwritten cover letter not only affords an opportunity to check legibility and written communication skills, but also permits elementary handwriting analysis. Just as the stylus of an electrocardiograph machine transmits electrical impulses of the heart, so does the pen transmit the writer's emotional and physical well-being. The interpretive skills of the examiner determine the validity of the analysis with both the electrocardiographic tracing and the handwriting sample. Short of extensive reading and practice, trust your instincts! For example, does it not make sense that sloppy writing may be the sign of a sloppy thinker? Does it not follow that close attention to legibility and punctuation is the sign of a careful person or a perfectionist? An original handwriting style often signifies an innovative personality who is independent and may chaff against a structured, regulated position.

Alternate Sources

Employee Referrals. Ask current employees if they know of anyone who might be interested in the position. Consider implementing a finder's fee or monetary award for the referral of a successful candidate.

Employment Agencies. Call a variety of private agencies to determine their procedures and policies. Determine if this will be an employer-paid, fee-shared, or applicant-paid position. Consider scheduling an on-site visit to make a personal assessment of the agency's style to determine if they will be able to attract the kind of applicant you require. You may even ask for references.

College Posting Systems. Colleges in your community may have a job posting system available at little or no cost to you or the applicant. Contact your local college to determine their resources.

Trade School Externship Programs. Many medical assisting programs require a number of hours of externship before granting a diploma or certificate. Participating in the externship programs may give you an opportunity to break in a potential team member before making the commitment to hire.

Resource Centers. Larger communities may have a woman's resource center that offers training to the displaced homemaker or those not previously employable for a variety of reasons. This may prove to be an excellent resource if your office supplies comprehensive on-the-job training.

Unsolicited Resumes by Mail or Walk-ins. In many communities it is customary to receive unsolicited resumes by mail or have assertive job hunters walk into a practice with a resume when no vacancy exists. Do not throw those resumes away! Keep them on file for a period of time — for example, 3 months — especially if the position is one that is difficult to find a replacement for, such as a transcriptionist or nurse practitioner.

Interviewing Process

This process is designed to assess qualities that cannot be objectively measured to determine whether a candidate is suitable for a position. Effective interviewing requires one to follow general principles. Before applying those principles, predetermine the limits of authority as with all management issues. Large office or small, there must be agreement on who will conduct initial and subsequent interviews, who will be involved in the hire process, and who will extend the job offer. A manager with little or no interviewing experience may wish to develop an interview form.

Recommended Interviewing Practices

After a group of potential candidates has been collected, interviews will need to be scheduled.

- Allow ample time for these interviews in a private location free from interruptions.
- Allow for introductory small talk, helping to put the candidate at ease.
- Have the applicant complete a job application. Be prepared to have a plan of action if the

candidate refuses to sign an authorization for a reference and employment history investigation.
- Control the interview. Do not allow either the candidate or yourself to be distracted from the process at hand.
- Provide a job description to the applicant. Collect it at the end of the interview.
- Discuss the position available, ask your questions, and answer any questions the applicant may have.
- Close the interview after double-checking you have all the information on which to make a decision.
- Thank the candidate for his or her interest.
- Evaluate the candidate before conducting the next interview. A sample evaluation form is shown in Figure 10–4.
- Pay attention to courtesies such as paying for parking, if applicable.

Job Applications

An employment application, whether created in house or purchased, should be reviewed against the preemployment inquiry guide (see Figure 10–3). An employment application should include a release of liability based on the former employer's disclosure of information. It is advisable to include a request for permission to contact a former employer. The application should

---

Name of applicant _____ Date _____

IMPORTANT CHARACTERISTICS	IMPRESSIONS, FACTS, INFERENCES
Personal Qualities Appeared healthy? Grooming appropriate? Enthusiastic? At ease? Nervous? Problem areas?	
Intelligence Meets basic skills requirements? Meets experience requirements? Any areas that require training? Has an effort been made to maintain current competency?	
Motivation What are employment goals? What are personal goals? Can we satisfy candidate's employment goals?	
Attitude How does candidate react to authority? How does candidate feel about assuming responsibility? Does candidate seem negative or positive?	
Communication Skills Is correct grammar used? What is quality of self-expression? Does candidate listen or interrupt? Is handwriting legible? Were instructions in cover letter followed? Were spelling and punctuation correct in cover letter?	
General impression	

FIGURE 10–4
Sample interview evaluation form.

also contain a statement that certifies the information supplied is true and that any misinformation, if discovered, will result in immediate dismissal. Rulings in the Toussaint case, a Michigan Supreme Court decision on wrongful discharge, make it advisable that the employment application is a good place to inform candidates that employment is on an "at will" basis. It is also advisable to request your practice's legal counsel to confirm that the job application does not infringe on any of the protected characteristics (discussed in Legal Requirements).

SPECIAL HINT

Make no notations, symbols, etc. on the job application. These are legal pieces of paper and are to be retained for 1 year. Notes and symbols, even time of appointments, have been determined to be evidence of discrimination in some discrimination hearings. The best advice is to keep those clean and do any notations on your evaluation forms, which you may destroy after selecting and hiring a candidate.

Resumes

It is becoming more and more common to find applicants using commercially prepared resumes. If your candidate is using such a resume, you may want to ask the candidate to restate items in his or her own words. This practice will help you to determine if an item has been inflated by the commercial preparer for presentational purposes.

Letters of Reference

If the candidate has a letter of reference to offer, or a copy of an evaluation form from a previous employer, beware. Leaving a previous employer with some of his or her stationery and creating a glowing letter of reference about one's employment is a simple and, unfortunately, frequent practice.

SPECIAL HINT

Always double-check with the person who signed the letter, if such a letter is presented. Read the letter to the former employer to determine if the statements have been altered. A letter may have been provided but changed substantially.

Inappropriate Dress

If the candidate's appearance is inappropriate by community standards for interviews (for example, the person is dressed in blue jeans, T-shirt, and red hightops tennis shoes when most would present in a skirt, suit, or uniform), you may note that on any evaluation form you are using. You may even communicate your surprise to the applicant and note their response. At this time, there are no laws protecting applicants from their own follies with regard to dress. However, *ask for an explanation*.

In American society, the way a candidate dresses for a job interview can be a significant statement of his or her attitude toward the position. On the other hand, do not automatically rule out an applicant who is dressed eccentrically. Do not miss a potentially excellent employee who showed up for the interview wearing Army fatigues and combat boots because he or she had just come from Reserve duty and you were too embarrassed to find an explanation for the attire!

Legal Requirements

Although one might yearn for a time past when the employment waters were less difficult to navigate, the reality is that managers and physicians, incorporated or not, big town or small, assume a potential target for costly liability in the employment process. The risks can be minimized by understanding legal requirements. To quote from the Michigan Department of Civil Rights:

> A person's race, sex, marital status, handicap, cetera are not indicators of an individual's potential to be a good worker. Keeping in mind the specific job requirements and the pertinent skills required to perform the particular job, employers may elicit adequate information on their employment applications which will aid in making good selection. Employers can deprive themselves of valuable employees by stereotyping rather than judging applicants on an individual basis. In screening . . . assumptions should not be made based on an applicant's identity or status. For example, it should not be assumed that because a woman has small children she will not be able to work odd hours. The issue is whether she can, in fact, work odd hours and not whether she has children.[1]

Protected Characteristics. Beware of unlawful discrimination. Both state and federal laws prohibit any consideration of race, color, national origin, sex, religion, or age in the hiring process. Considerations of height, weight, marital status, and handicaps that are unrelated to the individual's ability to perform the job are also prohibited in some states. Handicap protection is discussed in Chapter 11. There should be *no expression of preference* for candidates according to such protected characteristics. Because of their tendency to depict protected characteristics, photographs of a prospective employee may not be used.

Preemployment Tests. Preemployment test performance designed to measure skill, aptitude, or psychological characteristics must be validated according to Equal Employment Opportunity Commission (EEOC) guidelines. These regulations ensure that test performance correlates with job success. EEOC regulations may be obtained by writing:

> EEOC
> 1400 L Street NW
> Suite 200
> Washington, DC 20005

Or you may write, call, or visit a local EEOC office. A plea to a local member of congress can also help you to obtain these documents. For instance, a typing test for a clinical position that does not require a typewriter is inappropriate but is highly appropriate for a transcriptionist.

SPECIAL HINT

If you are in doubt as to whether or not a test you require is valid, call your legal counsel to determine whether you must submit it to the EEOC for validation.

Reference Checks

Many employers are reluctant to release any information because of the potential for expensive litigation. However, absenteeism, length and dates of employment, and duties performed are items that must be validated. Although there are serious weaknesses in reference checks, their usefulness cannot be ignored.

SPECIAL HINT

Letters are generally poor vehicles to transmit information, because most people are reluctant to put anything that could be construed as incriminating in writing. However, telephone calls can be revealing. What is left unsaid and the inflection used in a voice can be clues as to problem areas.

If a position calls for handling money, it is imperative that your insurance carrier providing bonding insurance be consulted. The insurance carrier's resources for obtaining reference checks on credit, character, and legal violations can be extensive. The insurance carrier will operate within the parameters of legislation in those areas.

Points to Consider

If a job applicant specifies who may not be called for a reference at a former place of employment, be wary. If you are instructed to call not the office manager but a physician in the practice, you may be dealing with a candidate who was terminated for insubordination. Ask the candidate specifically why he or she does not want the office administrator called. It is unlikely that the physician could validate the questions you need to ask.

If a job applicant refuses to sign a release from liability or authorization, terminate the interview and tell the candidate he or she cannot be considered for the position.

Beware of intercepted calls. If, when calling a candidate's former place of employment, you are asked by a receptionist to state the reason for the call and are told, "I can help you," be certain with whom you are talking. Situations have occurred where a friendly former co-worker gives an unsolicited opinion or even alters existing facts. If you believe that has happened to you, call the physician directly by placing the call from your physician employer. Although the former physician employer might not be able to validate facts, he or she can validate the authority of the person with whom you spoke.

Courtesies

- Tell the job candidates up front whether or not you will be calling them back.
- If reasonable, write candidates you are not considering and thank them for their interest.
- If applicable, pay for candidates' parking.

Selection of Candidates

After you have interviewed and evaluated candidates, consulted with any other persons involved in the hiring process, checked references, and made a decision as to whom the position will be offered, an administrator may either schedule another meeting, at which time the job offer will be presented, or may offer the position by telephone. Some larger organizations use offer letters. Before an offer is tendered, the starting salary must be calculated and the starting date determined. If an agency has been used, coordination with the agency must occur. Keep a copy of the advertisement and the job applications on hand for 1 year. It is advisable to have back-up candidates on hand. A candidate may have several job offers and is trying to determine which will fulfill his or her needs best. There are often occasions when the applicant will let you know in several days. You have the right and often the responsibility to deliver an ultimatum in terms of time. If an offer is made and the employee tells you that he or she would prefer to work for your practice but another practice has offered her more, your practice philosophy will determine whether you make a counter offer or withdraw the offer. There are candidates who will use this technique as a ploy to raise their starting salary or get more vacation time.

WAGES AND SALARIES

A structured, well-thought-out wages and salaries policy can provide both employers and employees with tools for motivation and satisfaction. By understanding federal wage and hour regulations, the employer can minimize the risk of legal action and financial liability and the costs associated with unemployment compensation.

Determining and Evaluating Pay Scales

An effective wage and salary program is designed to attract, retain, and motivate employees. Programs that do not set these goals may be ineffective and costly to the practice. An administrator must take into account supply and demand, the labor market, legislation, organizational productivity, and the practice's philosophy.

A variety of methods are available to determine what a job is worth. One tries to be competitive with wages and salaries, but there are intrinsic factors to consider as well. These may include a reputation the office has for friendliness, for closing on time each day, for no weekend or evening hours, or for the physician's respect for employees' intelligence and contributions to patients' well-being. There are many documented cases of an employee's changing from a highly paid job to one offering less money because the hours were better or the physicians involved treated their office personnel as thinking professionals.

Suggested Methods

- The percentage point yardstick plan is one way to determine starting salary. In this plan, illustrated in Figure 10–5, various percentage points for credentials necessary to perform the job satisfactorily are rated.
- Another method is to assess the current market value by calling or visiting the local community hospital personnel department and discussing their salary ranges for similar job descriptions.
- Many publications offer salary surveys that are geographically and specialty specific.
- Networking resources available through professional organizational affiliations—such as office managers—can provide relevant data.
- Speaking with the program director of local nursing programs and/or medical assisting programs is a good way to find what they are recommending to their new graduates.

Points to Consider

Some practices prefer to develop a formal salary range for each position. These specify the minimum and maximum amounts that will be paid for a position. Salary ranges are, in theory, reviewed at selected intervals. In larger organizations it is common for these salary ranges to be posted. When this attitude is taken, everyone in an office can be aware of what everyone else is making.

Other practices believe salaries/wages are personal and private matters, and office personnel are cautioned not to discuss what they are making with each other. Incidentally, this can only be a recommendation and cannot be cause for dismissal. It is the office management's responsibility to discuss the reasons for this approach; for

STARTING SALARY DETERMINATION—PERCENTAGE CALCULATIONS SAMPLE*

3%	for each year of relevant experience
5%	certification from American Association of Medical Assistants, Inc. (CMA) or American Medical Techologists (RMA)
5%	continuing education validation from American Association of Medical Assistants, Inc. or American Medical Technologists
20%	baccalaureate degree

All percentage points are totaled. Calculate the range of starting salary, e.g., $6.00–$8.50 per hour. The difference between these two figures—$2.50—is used by which the number of percentage points earned are multiplied.

Three years of relevant experience plus national certification would earn the candidate 24% points, calculated as .24 × $2.50 = 60¢. From the low end of the scale, $6.00 per hour, 60¢ would be added, making the starting salary for that position $6.60 per hour.

* *Salary* is used synonymously with *wages* for demonstrational purposes. Avoid crediting minimum education requirements.

FIGURE 10–5

Starting salary determination—percentage calculations sample.

example a worker who earns XX dollars more than his or her co-worker might find that he or she is expected to do more work.

SPECIAL HINT

There is no right or wrong philosophy. However, if a practice has many personnel tied to an old salary range and newer employees are brought in at an updated figure with no revisions for the older employees, a practice manager can expect serious morale problems. In developing a philosophy, fairness should be a major consideration.

Federal Wage and Hour Regulations

Federal Fair Labor Standards Act of 1939 as Amended

One specific law all practice managers should be familiar with is the Fair Labor Standards Act. This delineates the standards of minimum wage, overtime pay requirements, equal pay requirements, record-keeping requirements, and child labor. This act applies to practices that have gross receipts of more than $25,000 per year or more than two employees. In an amendment to this law that became effective May 1, 1974, the scope of the standards was broadened to include medical practices. In 1977, the 4th Court of Appeals upheld that medical practices were *not* exempt from overtime pay, minimum wage, etc.

Overtime Compensation. Overtime compensation is a rate of not less than one and one half times the regular rate of pay for hours worked over 40 hours in a workweek unless a specific exemption is met. Because the amount of money an employee should receive under the minimum wage and overtime provisions cannot be determined without knowing the number of hours, records must be kept.

Time Record Keeping. Time clocks are often used in order to avoid errors and are highly recommended for practices that have different sites or employ many part-time personnel.

Management rules should be posted near the time cards, for example, "Sign in and out in ink," and "Employees are prohibited from checking other employees out."

Hours worked include *all the time* the employee is required to be on premise or on duty, even time spent waiting. Work permitted is counted as work time. The law says that management has the responsibility to enforce these regulations, so an announcement that the overtime was not authorized in advance will not impair the employee's right to overtime compensation.

Other forms of record keeping are permitted. For example, one employer hands out Hallmark date books to each employee at the start of the year. Employees note the number of hours worked each day in the boxes, sign the book attesting to the accuracy of the data, and at each pay cycle hand it in.

Without the employees' signature on the time card, the process is invalid.

Exemptions from Overtime

> **SPECIAL HINT**
>
> Neither title nor designation that the position is salaried makes an employee exempt.

There are specific exemptions from overtime, but they are dependent on specific, clearly defined criteria as set forth in Wage and Hour Publication 1363, *Executive, Administrative, Professional and Outside Sales Exemptions Under the Fair Labor Standards Act*. These criteria are

- An employee's duties and responsibilities
- The salary paid, except in the case of doctors, lawyers, teachers, and outside sales people. For example, registered nurses are exempt because they meet clearly defined criteria of having completed a formalized educational process of a certain duration, whereas a licensed practical nurse or a medical assistant with an associate degree doing "RN work"—even the same work that an office RN is doing—is not exempt.

Executive Exemption. For an employee to be exempt as a bona fide executive, all the following tests must be met:

1. The employee's primary duty must be management of the enterprise or a customarily recognized department or subdivision.
2. The employee must customarily and regularly direct the work of at least two or more other employees therein.
3. The employee must have the authority to hire and fire or recommend hiring and firing, or the employee's recommendations on these and other actions affecting employees must be given particular weight.
4. The employee must customarily and regularly exercise discretionary powers.
5. The employee must devote no more than 20% of his or her hours worked (less than 40% if employed by a retail or service establishment) to activities not directly and closely related to the managerial duties.
6. The employee must be paid on a salary basis at a rate of at least $155.00 per week.

Administrative Exemption. For an employee to be employed in a bona fide administrative capacity, all the following tests must be met:

1. The employee's duty must be either

    - responsible office or nonmanual work directly related to the management policies or general business operations of the employer or the employer's customers; or
    - responsible work that is directly related to academic instruction or training carried on in the administration of a school system or educational establishment.

2. The employee must customarily and regularly exercise discretion and independent judgment, as distinguished from using skills and following procedures, and must have the authority to make important decisions.
3. The employee must

    - regularly assist a proprietor or a bona fide executive or administrative employee;
    - perform work under only general supervision along specialized or technical lines requiring special training, experience, or knowledge;
    - execute under only general supervision special assignments.

4. The employee must not spend more than 20% of the time worked in the workweek (less than 40% if employed by a retail or service establishment) on nonexempt work, that is, work not directly and closely related to the administrative duties.
5. The employee must be paid on a salary or fee basis at a rate of not less than $155.00 a week.

The following are examples of duties that are managerial when performed by an employee managing a department or supervising other employees:

- Interviewing
- Selecting and training employees
- Setting and adjusting pay rates and work hours
- Directing work
- Evaluating the employees' efficiency and productivity
- Planning and distributing work
- Determining work techniques.

Nonexempt duties might include

- Performing the same kind of work as the employees supervised

- Performing any work as the employees supervised
- Performing any work, even if it is not like that performed by subordinates, that is not part of supervisory functions
- Preparing payrolls
- Performing routine clerical duties such as bookkeeping, billing, filing, operating business machines, or transcribing

NOTE: *Job titles are not yardsticks of exemption from overtime compensation.* Also, *salaried, nonexempt workers are, by law, still eligible for overtime.*

General Provisions

No Waiving of Overtime Pay. The requirement that overtime must be paid after 40 hours a week may not be waived by agreement between the employer and the employees. Similarly, an agreement that only 8 hours a day or 40 hours a week will be counted as working time will clearly fail. An announcement by the employer that no overtime work will be permitted or that overtime work will not be paid for unless authorized in advance will not be allowed.

Salary for Workweek Exceeding 40 Hours. A fixed salary for a regular workweek longer than 40 hours does not discharge the statutory obligation. For example, an employee might be hired to work a 44-hour workweek for a weekly salary of $200.00. In this instance, the regular rate is obtained by dividing the $200.00 or straight-time salary by 44 hours, which results in a regular rate of pay $4.55 per hour. The employee is then due additional overtime computed by multiplying the 4 overtime hours by half the regular rate of pay ($2.275, for overtime pay of $9.10).

Pay for Foregoing Holidays and Vacations. In some instances employees are entitled to holiday or vacation pay but forego the holiday or vacation and work on that day or period. If they receive their customary rate (or higher) for their work on the holiday or vacation day, the additional sum given as holiday or vacation pay is excluded from the regular rates of pay.

Salary for Periods Other Than a Workweek. Where the salary covers a period longer than a workweek, such as a month, it must be reduced to its workweek equivalent. A monthly salary can be converted to its equivalent weekly wage by multiplying by 12 (the number of months) and dividing it by 52 (the number of weeks). A semimonthly salary is converted to its equivalent weekly wage by multiplying by 24 and dividing by 52.

Time of Payment (of Overtime). There is no requirement that overtime compensation be paid weekly. The general rule is that overtime pay earned in a particular workweek must be paid on the regular pay day for the period in which the workweek ends. If the correct amount of overtime pay cannot be determined until some time after the regular pay period, the employer must pay the overtime compensation as soon after the regular pay period as practicable. Payment may not be delayed for a period longer than is reasonably necessary for the employer to compute and arrange for payment, and in no event may payment be delayed beyond the next pay day after such computation can be made.

Time Off in Lieu of Pay. The overtime pay requirement may not be waived. However, it is common for an employee to have an employee work 44 hours one week to include Saturday morning and then 35 hours the next week, which is more than one and one half the hourly amount. The employee's salary would be the same for both weeks. The employee would have to agree to that as terms of employment. It would be better if the employer had the person working Saturday morning take compensatory time off the week of the Saturday, not the next week, so that no more than 40 hours occur.

Docking Pay. An employer paying an hourly or salaried nonexempt employee may penalize that employee for excessive lateness. The manager should warn the offender that he or she is going to be docked 1 or 2 hour's pay for every hour late. Wage and hour law says an employer may double-dock in accordance with these three rules:

1. The deduction cannot bring an employee's pay below the minimum hourly wage.
2. The deductions must be made at the regular hourly rate of the employee, not his or her overtime rate.
3. The maximum permitted weekly deduction is based on a regular workweek.

Obviously, an employee who is earning the minimum wage cannot be double-docked.

Rest and Meal Periods. Although rest periods of short duration, running from 5 to about 20 minutes, are common, there is no law in the United States that says employers must give either rest or meal periods. Both of these breaks promote employee efficiency and are valid considerations of potential employees when evaluating a job offer. However, rest periods must be counted as working time. If it is a requirement of employment that a lunch break be taken on premise to be available for an emergency or work, that time must be considered as working time. The key is that the employee is not completely relieved from duty and cannot use the time effectively for his or her own purposes unless the employee is definitely told in advance that he or she may leave the job and not have to commence work until a definitely specified hour has arrived. A transcriptionist who reads a book while waiting for dictation is considered to be working because he or she is engaged to wait.

Holiday and Vacation Pay. There are no holidays that an employer is required to give as time off with or without pay. It is unlikely, however, that Thanksgiving or Christmas would be considered as a regular working day in the physician office because of the difficulty that would present in finding employees to work for such an employer! With more and more ambulatory care centers available to people, the necessity for staffing these centers on those holidays grows. Generally a type of premium pay is used to attract employees but there is no legal requirement for this custom.

As with holidays, there is no law mandating vacation pay. The entitlement is one of the employer's making, not a legal requirement.

If an office manager comes into a practice where the physician employer is not knowledgeable of existing laws, it is the responsibility of the manager to acquaint him or her with the law, because the monetary penalties that exist are severe and will be enforced.

Penalties. U.S. Department of Labor Publication 1282, *Handy Reference Guide to the Fair Labor Standards Act* states, "the Fair Labor Standards Act provided for the following methods of recovering unpaid minimum and/or overtime wages:

1. The Division may supervise payment of back wages;
2. The Secretary of Labor may bring suit for back wages and the equal amount as liquidated damages;
3. The employee may file a private suit for back pay and an equal amount as liquidated damages, plus attorneys fees and court costs; and
4. The Secretary may obtain an injunction to restrain any person from violating the law, including the unlawful withholding of proper overtime compensation . . . and a two year statute of limitations applies to the recovery of back pay except in the case of willful violation, in which a three year statute applies."

An employee can file a complaint with a federal and/or state agency and that agency can legally audit the employer's required records. The name of the employee is protected. In a small office it might be easy to determine who filed the complaint, but any employer who attempts to retaliate faces heavy fines and penalties. The employee is protected from retaliation under Section 604A of the Civil Rights Act of 1964 as amended.

Record-Keeping Requirements

Every employer shall maintain and preserve payroll or other records containing the following information and data with respect to each and every employee who is subject to minimum wage or wage and overtime provisions:

1. Name in full and, on the same record, the employee's identifying symbol or number if such is used in place of name on any time, work, or payroll records. This shall be the same name as that used for Social Security record purposes.
2. Home address, including zip code.
3. Date of birth, if under 19.
4. Sex and occupation in which employed.
5. Time of day and day of week on which the employee's workweek begins.
6. Regular hourly rate of pay for any week when overtime compensation is due.
7. Hours worked each workday and total hours worked each workweek.
8. Total daily or weekly straight-time earnings or wages exclusive of overtime compensation.
9. Total overtime compensation for the workweek.
10. Total additions to or deductions from wages paid each pay period.
11. Total wages paid each pay period.
12. Date of payment and the pay period covered by payment.

All items except those referring to overtime compensation also apply to bona fide executives and administrative and professional employees.

Records to be preserved 3 years include

- Payroll records—from the last date of entry, all those payroll or other records containing the employee information and data listed above
- Certificates, agreements, plans, notices, etc.—these generally apply to individual contracts or collective bargaining agreements that include any memoranda
- Oral agreements—these must be written in terms of a summary.

Records to be preserved 2 years include

- Basic records
- Wage rate tables
- Work-time schedules
- All records used by the employer in determining wage deductions—e.g., savings bonds payroll deduction flow sheet, employee request for $2.00 additional to be withheld for state income tax.

BENEFIT PACKAGES

Supplementary benefits can account for a large percentage of payroll costs. Physician employers and office managers can study other firms' benefits, their own organizational needs and budget, and federal/state legislation to determine which benefits they should consider. Supplemental benefits can be tailored to meet a practice's needs, to compete in the marketplace, and to provide for security for office personnel.

Required Programs

Contribution toward Social Security, Worker's Compensation, and unemployment compensation can be significant costs to an employer, but many employees may not recognize these programs as benefits. Consider itemizing and relating these costs to employees.

Retirement Programs

Many physician groups have incorporated for tax advantages for federally qualified retirement plans. Pension plans must meet very specific requirements determined by federal legislation. Obtaining consultation from an attorney who specializes in pension plan requirements is advisable.

Health Insurance Programs

Health care costs are increasing rapidly. This is due to inflation, the economics of the health care industry, an aging population, and the introduction of new and expensive treatments for many illnesses as well as the spiraling costs of malpractice insurance. It has been estimated that in the past 5 years employer health insurance costs for premiums have increased 80–90%. Because health care costs are increasing so rapidly, employers are looking for alternative strategies to contain these costs.

Methods of Cost Containment

Auditing and Minimizing Costs. Employee auditing of hospital bills to discover errors of services billed and not received does not return huge savings in a health care cost containment strategy, but it is an excellent way to get employees involved in the issue, especially when those employees are employed by a health care provider. Offering a financial incentive would complement this strategy; for example, the company might pay the employee up to 20% of the amount recovered. Large physician groups can contract with a Professional Review Organization and Utilization Review panel to audit and question the need for hospitalization, the length of stay in a hospital, and the type of care provided. Managed care plans require physicians and hospitals and even patients to take procedural steps for full benefits to be paid. These steps are intended to result in better care and cost savings. These programs include

- Preadmission certification for hospitalization benefits
- Concurrent review of extended hospitalizations
- Discharge planning for hospitalized patients
- Catastrophic care assistance, incentive or mandatory second surgical opinions, and incentive or mandatory ambulatory surgery

Alternative Provider Arrangements. Health maintenance organizations (HMOs) offer a flat fee for all care provided. The employees must receive their medical care from certain physicians who have contracted with the HMO. HMOs encourage preventive medicine. In addition to whatever state requirements HMOs must meet to operate, about two-thirds of them must comply with the federal Health Maintenance Organization Act. An HMO qualifies under the HMO Act if it is established with federal grants or loans. The HMO Act requires employers to make a dual choice available to employees if there are at least 25 employees who live in the HMO's service area. The absence of federal qualification is not any indication that an HMO is deficient, and federal qualification is not any guarantee that an HMO is adequate either fiscally or medically.

There are two types of HMOs: group and individual practices. In the group type, a group of physicians from multiple specialties formally organize and practice as a single entity at a single location. In the individual practice type, physicians organize into the HMO on paper and continue to practice out of their private offices. Generally, HMO members form only a part of their total practice. Although HMO participants rate HMOs as effective in controlling costs, many participants perceive that their HMO physician is less willing to refer a patient to a specialist than is a physician under traditional medical plans. The drawback of HMOs is the limit on choice.

In a Preferred Provider Organization (PPO), employees receive discounted fees or higher levels of reimbursement if they obtain care from certain physicians or hospitals. Employees are free to obtain care from other physicians or hospitals, but the fee is not discounted. PPOs are unregulated and, therefore, more flexible than HMOs.

Alternative Funding Methods. Conventional group insurance contracts can be modified by an agreement for the employer to assume an increased share of the risk in exchange for lower premiums. Cost sharing—employees paying for a greater portion of personal health care expenses through either an increased annual deductible amount or an increased employee copayment—is a way to decrease the cost of health care for the employer.

Besides shifting costs from the employer to the employee, many believe that cost sharing decreases the overall cost of health care because employees are deterred from using some services they would otherwise have used. In addition, in theory, employees become more careful consumers, choosing lower cost services. However, there are adverse reactions that could come from increased cost sharing in the form of high deductibles and larger copayments. Employees may put off obtaining needed medical care because of costs, and the result could adversely affect their employment by increased absenteeism.

Where employees pay a fixed contribution to their health insurance premium costs, the employee's use of health care services is not affected because the payments are independent of their usage.

Changing or Designing Benefits. If the majority of your employees would not use psychiatric coverage, why offer an insurance policy that includes it? If the employees are past childbearing age, why offer maternity benefits? If you have a small office and all the office personnel have had their tubes tied, why offer sterilization benefits? In smaller, more intimate offices custom-designing insurance coverage is a workable option that can net savings.

Wellness Programs. Working in the health care industry is no guarantee that our life-styles reflect healthy choices. There is a growing trend toward developing wellness programs with the aim of achieving and maintaining employees' good health and subsequent job productivity. Wellness programs are long-term investments. Such programs can be formally or informally structured. They can range from fitness centers in the workplace and assistance with alcohol and substance abuse, to simple encouragement to sign up for a marathon walk as an office team or participating in a nonsmoking clinic.

Congress has exacerbated cost control problems for employers by enacting the Consolidated Omnibus Budget Reconciliation Act of 1985 (COBRA) and Medicare cost-shifting laws. COBRA affects employers who have more than 20 employees and mandates, among other things, continued access to group plans for retired employees. If your practice has more than 20 employees, consultation with legal counsel regarding requirements of COBRA and other legislation should be ongoing.

The Medicare cost-shifting laws require that working persons 65 years and older be covered by the employer plan, with Medicare secondary.

Life Insurance Programs

Term life insurance is most commonly offered. The manager and/or employer would review insurance carriers' rate structures and reputations and develop a life insurance program that specifies what age a person has to be to participate, the months of service required for participation, and the amounts of insurance available.

> SAMPLE: After 6 months of continued full-time employment defined as 40 hours per week, the following term life insurance is offered to employees who qualify under the insurance carrier's guidelines:
>
> | Salary/Wages per Year | Benefit |
> |---|---|
> | $10,000–15,000 | $15,000 term life |
> | $15,000–25,000 | $25,000 " " |
> | $25,000–40,000 | $50,000 " " |
> | $40,000 plus | $75,000 " " |

Disability Insurance Programs

The insurance industry will tell you that it is more likely for an employee to become disabled while under your employment than die while employed. Many employers have considered disability insurance to be more important than life insurance for their employees' security. For many practices, however, the costs of disability insurance are prohibitive. An important fact that could make it affordable under a premium cost shift is to make employees aware that if they pay the premium the benefits are not taxed, whereas if the employer pays the premium, the benefits are taxed.

Sick Leave and Personal Leave Programs

Many offices offer sick leave and personal leave; many others do not formally offer these programs. The general attitude is to use time offered, especially if there is no incentive for not using it. If an office can accommodate such unscheduled absences, implementation of such a plan can be considered. However, many groups cannot make such accommodations without hardship, and the physician employers prefer to use their own judgment in matters relating to sick and personal leave.

In many states, an employee is ineligible for unemployment benefits if he or she requests and is given a leave of absence. A bona fide leave of absence should permit reinstatement to the employee's job or a similar position at the same rate of pay on expiration of the leave. No guarantee or reinstatement should be made for extended leaves of absence; rather, reinstatement should be conditioned on the availability of the job for which the employee is qualified. There is no law that defines "extended period of absence." Some offices may consider 6 weeks extended, whereas others may consider 6 months extended. Once an employer maintains a leave-of-absence policy, definite leave-of-absence rules must be established and recorded on a printed form so that employees may read them at the time they sign the application for a leave of absence. The leave-of-absence rules (including sick leave/personal leave) should set forth the following information:

- The length of leave permitted
- Whether the employee should call in periodically and, if so, how often and to whom
- Medical reports required, if any
- Steps that can be taken to extend or terminate the leave

The employee should be given a copy of the leave of absence form. If the employee fails to report as requested or does not return to work when the leave expires, an effort should be made to learn the reason before he or she is separated from employment. Failure to follow these rules can land an employer and manager in the deep waters of wrongful discharge, discrimination, and a host of other charges that may not be valid but can cause a lot of paperwork, grief, and money.

Pregnancy is often a reason for voluntary separation and a request for a leave of absence.

> **SPECIAL HINT**
>
> *A pregnant employee must be allowed to continue working as long as she is able to work.*

An employer does not have to make allowances for repeated absenteeism caused by oversleeping, nausea and vomiting, or "not feeling well." These are considered as pregnancy-related disabilities and considered as a "quit without good cause" attributable to the employer or as unavailability for work. However, the nondisabled pregnant employee must be allowed to decide, in conjuction with her doctor's opinion, when her leave or separation will commence. If an employer does not have a sick leave or leave-of-absence policy and an employee requests 6 weeks off after the baby is born, there is no law mandating that the employer hold her job for her. However, if an employee wishes to work until delivery, use 2 weeks' earned vacation time and then return, an employer must accommodate her request unless a policy to the contrary is in writing and applicable to nonpregnant employees as well.

Other Benefits

Paid vacations, holiday pay, tuition aid plans, educational awards, uniform allowances, professional liability insurance, professional organization dues, costs of licensure, certification, recertification, paid parking and structured bonuses tied in with unused sick days are among the benefits employers have offered their employees. In some communities, there are employers who offer child care assistance plans, group legal service plans, and savings bond plans (at the employee's expense).

Legal Requirements

Although Section 89 of the Tax Reform Act of 1986 was repealed in 1989, every administrator and employer should be aware that federal tax laws are not only complicated, but also ever changing. Figure 10–6 is an illustration of the complexity involved in a repeal. There is a growing trend toward considering benefits as taxable when there is a difference between the value of the benefits the employer receives versus those the employees receive. Bills requiring mandated benefits such as maternity and paternity leave are also commonly introduced by legislators.

In order to meet Internal Revenue Service requirements, write out your plans. Specific requirements are for health and accident plans, group term life insurance plans, tuition reduction plans, cafeteria plans, dependent care assistance, and group legal service plans.

Health and accident plans include dental, vision, hearing, prescription drug plans, medical reimbursement arrangements, accidental death or dismemberment plans, business travel accident plans, wellness programs, and drug and alcohol treatment or counseling programs. The general practice is to buy an insurance plan and have a written plan description in addition to the benefits booklet provided by the insurance company. The plan should include who is eligible after how long and any other requirements. The amount of benefits should be included as well as any compliance with COBRA.

Cafeteria plans are choices between cash/salary contributions and health or other nontaxable benefits. Companies may provide a pool of funds that employees can use to "purchase" a benefits package tailored to fill their specific needs. The company would say, "Here is a credit of XXX dollars to spend on total benefits offered by this company. You will decide what benefits are best for you and your family." The company could allow employees to use the credit for child care assistance, employee contributions to the pension plan, life insurance, vision, long-term-care coverage, health insurance, etc. Credits not "spent" are not distributed to the employee in the form of income. Again, consult with a management expert or legal counsel before implementing this approach, because there are specific regulations involved.

The office manager of a small practice or the business administrator of a very large practice has many rules and regulations to follow in developing even "simple" items like fringe benefits.

> **SPECIAL HINT**
>
> Continual reading of management journals, continuing education in the form of seminars, and networking with other management professionals are necessary to stay current to protect yourself and your employer.

Internal Revenue Code Section 603D, which was amended in conjunction with now-repealed Section 89, requires the filing of annual reports for

- group term life insurance (Code Section 79)
- medical expense reimbursement plans, both insured and self-insured (Code Sections 105 and 106);
- dependent care assistance programs (Code Section 129).

As of March 26, 1990, Notice 90-24, IRB 1990-13 countermanded the 1989 Form 5500 Instructions. However, employers who provide

- legal service plans (Code Section 120),
- cafeteria plans (Code Section 125),
- qualified educational assistance programs (Code Section 127)

are still required to file Form 5500.

FIGURE 10–6

Internal Revenue Code Section 603D.

Reference

1. Michigan Department of Civil Rights: *Pre-Employment Inquiry Guide*. Detroit: Michigan Department of Civil Rights, 1985.

Bibliography*

WH Publication 31563: *Executive, Administrative, Professional and Outside Sales Exemptions Under the Fair Labor Standards Act*. Reissued December 1983.

WH Publication 1281: *Regulations, Part 541: Defining the terms "Executive," "Administrative," "Professional" and "Outside Salesman."* Revised June 1983.

WH Publication 1325: *Overtime Compensation Under the Fair Labor Standards Act*. Revised April 1985.

WH Publication 1262: *Regulations, Part 778: Interpretive Bulletin on Overtime Compensation*. Revised February 1981, printed July 1983.

WH Publication 1261: *Records to be Kept by Employers Under the Fair Labor Standards Act of 1938 as Amended*. Reprinted September 1984.

WH Publication 1282: *Handy Reference Guide to the Fair Labor Standards Act*. Revised June 1987.

---

* All of these publications may be purchased from the Superintendent of Documents, U.S. Government Printing Office, Washington, DC 20402. They are often available free of charge at your local Department of Labor or through your congressperson.

Chapter 11

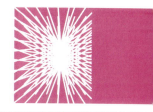

PERSONNEL AND OFFICE POLICIES

JOAN B. CONRAD

POLICY MANUAL
The Outline
Contents of the Manual
Writing the Manual
Updating the Manual

EMPLOYMENT AND LABOR LAWS
Worker's Compensation
Issues in the Workplace

SELECTION OF ANCILLARY SERVICES
Criteria for Selection of Attorneys, Accountants, and Consultants

SEPARATION FROM EMPLOYMENT
Warnings
Suspensions
Discharges
Exit Interviews

POLICY MANUAL

The practice of stating employment policies in writing, often in the form of an employment manual or employee handbook, has become commonplace in medical practices of all sizes. Personnel policy manuals are written codes of etiquette, intended to make people comfortable in their day-to-day interactions with one another. If people know what is expected from them behaviorly, they can concentrate on other matters of importance.

The manual writer is often an employee, usually the manager, working in conjunction with his or her employer. Together they determine the policies to be set in force. Regardless of the expertise of the writer and/or the employer, it is advised that policy manuals be reviewed by an employment specialist, either an attorney who specializes in employment issues or a practice consultant with a proven track record. Putting a policy down in writing should have the effect of clarifying issues; however, it can create confusion if it lends itself to more than one interpretation.

Different interpretations have the potential to create hostile feelings and lower employees' morale. Care must be taken not only with the content, but with the tone or style of writing. A manual can be explicitly detailed, right down to "Gum chewing is not allowed on premises," or general in its summary. Before writing begins, a general outline should be drafted. The contents will depend on a variety of issues: the experiences of the writer/employer, the location and size of the practice, and the requirements of the physician owner. If you have developed a network of practice managers, perhaps some of them would consider lending you their manual.

The Outline

To begin the outline, you might select the basic points that need clarification: what the practice expects from its employees and what the employees can expect from the practice. If a medical practice has determined that it is an at-will employer during a 3 month probationary period, but a just-cause employer after permanent employment is offered and accepted, the manual would contain this statement, with clarifying definitions as to the terms "just cause" and "at will."

Just-cause items might be categorized as "Summary dismissal will occur when [list the behaviors]". A manager should be advised that a just-cause employee has the right to a jury trial in many states. Check with your practice attorney or your state Department of Labor.

When writing a policy manual, just-cause employers should consider how something that sounds reasonable does not always end up that way. For example, you might state, "Summary dismissal will occur when the employee steals from the practice, another employee, or a patient." If the employee were caught red-handed (even signing a statement of guilt), had his or her employment terminated, and the office did not prosecute, the employee could still bring suit for wrongful discharge. The jury could find the employee not guilty because, in their eyes, no criminal act was committed and/or proven. They might believe the employee's claim that he or she was intimidated into signing the confession. There have been cases of an employee saying he or she had taken money but gave most of it to the employer, who then did not have to pay income tax on it, when, in fact, nothing of the sort happened.

If the jury is composed of successful business/management individuals, it is doubtful the employee would be believed, but this type of juror is not always available. Picture the psychological machinations of the jurors when a tearful employee sobs, "Doctor X needed a new Porsche and told me that if I took the money I could keep 20% of it. I'm sorry I did it, but I was afraid I'd lose my job if I didn't." Morally outrageous? Sure, but effective in placing doubts about the employee's guilt. Again, discussion with a legal advisor as to what constitutes immediate dismissal is advised. The statement in question might better read, "Summary dismissal will occur when the employee is proven guilty in a court of law of stealing from the practice, another employee, or from a patient. The employer retains the right to place the employee in question in the status of having been laid off from work without pay while the issue is being resolved. The employee has the right to file for unemployment benefits."

If the practice has purchased an employee dishonesty bond, the manager must be certain to notify the insurance company and coordinate the actions to be taken. The insurance policy will probably mandate action regarding prosecution and recovery. The insurance policy language may be a good source for the wording of this clause in the manual.

At this point, you might be thinking that one way to avoid being liable would be to not put anything in writing! It would be a valid point for consideration; however, the attorney who deals on behalf of the aggrieved employee could subpoena all past employment records of terminated employees and go over every single reason the employer had for firing past employees. Any inconsistencies could result in the manager's, and/or employer's looking unprofessional, arbitrary, or even malicious. Whatever the result, even a good result, the process of litigation will take valuable time away from the practice of medicine. Litigation also has the potential of tying up office personnel so that they are unable to provide care to patients and support to the physician. Moreover, a trend is developing in American society that puts not only the employer but also the manager at risk of personal liability in employment litigation. There is no insurance available to protect the practice or the manager from liability with regard to employment practices.

With the potential for litigation and personal liability, many employers are making their offices at-will offices. Although stating that employees can lose their employment at the employer's will understandably might lower your personnel's morale, it could also save the practice from the difficulties associated with litigation.

Contents of the Manual

Figure 11–1 illustrates the many types of items to be considered in a policy manual. The list is not inclusive. One might also have to consider whether there will be different rules for different types of employees, for example, part-time, full-time, and half-time employees. There is a strong probability that fringe benefits would be significantly different. Perhaps the consideration will be made based on the employee's exemption status. For example, a registered nurse performing nursing functions is considered to be exempt from federal wage and hour laws regarding overtime. If it is the office policy that all office personnel have an unpaid hour for lunch, but a patient's emergency medical treatment prevents the RN from having an hour off — perhaps because of vacationing peers — there might be some policy considering compensating him or her for the lost time. If a receptionist were to be placed in the same situation of a lost lunch hour, he or she

1. Welcome
2. Statement of orientation procedures
3. Brief description of the structure of the organization (Also, a description of your policy as to being an "at will" employer or a "just cause" employer)
4. A history of the organization and/or a credentializing or personalization of the practice's medical staff
5. Summary dismissal criteria
6. Administrative policies regarding paydays, advances of salary for emergencies, vacations
7. Time cards/time clock rules/overtime policies
8. Lunch periods/breaks/lunchroom policies
9. Jury duty policy
10. Smoking policy
11. Personal appearance/dress codes
12. Chronic lateness/absenteeism policy
13. Parking policies
14. Emergency, bereavement, sick leave policies
15. Policy on moonlighting, second jobs
16. Policy on personal phone calls
17. Solicitations policy
18. Performance reviews policy
19. Resignations policy
20. Benefits (indirect compensation)

    Vacations
    Holidays
    Health insurance
        Hospitalization
        Dental plans
        Vision plans
        Prescription drug coverage
    Life insurance
    Disability insurance
    Pension programs/profit-sharing programs
    Uniform allowances
    Education reimbursement plans
    Professional licensure, professional dues payment
    Malpractice insurance
    Meeting/seminar reimbursement plans

FIGURE 11–1
Contents of a typical employee manual.

would have the opportunity for being compensated at the rate of one and one half times his or her normal hourly rate in the form of overtime, whereas the RN would not. Perhaps the employer has even considered a system of quarterly assessment of actual time worked over 40 hours per week for exempt personnel and has translated this into a plan whereby extra vacation time would be earned or actual cash in the form of a quarterly bonus would be paid.

Defining parameters of behavior, codes of conduct, and employee rewards and benefits can also be valuable in terms of marketing your practice to prospective employees. In addition, a practice that "has its act together" in the form of carefully thought-out and written policies can provide strong leadership that facilitates good patient care. If a practice attracts the best, it provides better service.

Writing the Manual

Now that you have discussed items with your employer and formed an outline, it is time to put the actual policies into words. Keep your sentences short and to the point. Avoid complicated sentence structures. Be careful that by using concise statements, the manual does not become adversarial in its tone. Figure 11–2 illustrates this caution.

Both approaches say the same thing—that smoking is hazardous to your health and no smoking is permitted in the office. However, the non-adversarial approach acknowledges human nature and says that smokers may have a need to smoke during a break and the management acknowledges this need. The key is consideration.

One suggestion proven to be effective is to take the draft of a policy statement and have co-workers, friends, or family review its effect. Even if they disagree with the policy, they should not let this affect their ability to say how it makes them feel. These feelings are good indicators of how a cross section of your employees might read the statement. Sometimes these discussions provide good insight into the policy statement itself. Is it too rigid? Does it violate a law? Is it clear? Does it bring to mind another, nonaddressed issue?

Updating the Manual

After the manual is written, date it. As employment laws change, as the practice's experiences change, and as the employer's and the employees' needs change, the effective manager revises and updates the manual to reflect these changes. When making your timetable of things to do, consider reviewing the employee handbook at least annually. Any change should be dated as to when it became effective. Many management consultants recommend that employees review and sign

Smoking Policy

Adversarial approach:

As health care professionals, you should be aware that smoking is not healthy. Smoking causes odors on your body that are offensive to nonsmokers, both employees and patients. There will be no smoking on premises. Violators will be disciplined.

Nonadversarial approach:

As health care professionals, you are aware that our physicians caution their patients on the medical risks associated with smoking. They extend the same caution to you, their employee. They have requested that there be no smoking on premises. However, one may, with permission from one's supervisor, take an off-premise break of 10 minutes twice daily for this purpose. Please be considerate of your co-workers and patients. Be aware that smoking odors do linger on clothing, hands, and breath. Please take appropriate personal hygienic measures to prevent complaints.

FIGURE 11-2
Example of how to avoid using adversarial tone when writing the employee manual.

---

the updates, indicating their understanding and their acceptance of the new policies. New employees can sign that they have read the manual and understand the policies during the orientation phase of their employment. If employees do not have their own copies, an office copy should be completely accessible to them. An employee should be able to consult this copy without having to ask the manager for it.

EMPLOYMENT AND LABOR LAWS

It is only by broadening your awareness, continuing your education, and communicating that you can stay on top in the continuously changing world of health care. The trends in health care financing and employment/labor regulations require not only vigilance but ongoing assessment of your ability to effectively function in your position. Still, a doctoral degree in management is no guarantee of being able to deal effectively with the office personnel who are providing patient care. The job of the manager is not only to provide effective personnel and processing systems and financial management, but also to focus on the basic issue of providing quality medical care in the health care delivery system. Simply put, there is a patient out there who needs the wisdom, skills, and nurturing your physician and his or her support staff can provide. Your job as manager is to accommodate the process, enabling everyone to do his or her job effectively. The caveat in medicine is "do no harm." That is an appropriate perspective for the manager to take as well. Only by enlarging your sphere of awareness can you accomplish this goal.

Worker's Compensation

Worker's Compensation is an employment benefit mandated by state legislation. States referred to as "labor intensive" often have stronger legislation than agricultural-based states. Worker's Compensation insurance provides compensation for disability or death as a result of a work-related accidental injury or disease, *regardless of fault*. Benefits are paid by employers (either directly or through their insurance company) and should not be confused with unemployment insurance or group insurance for illness/accident/hospital/health insurance. Payments to the injured party are made by the insurance carrier, not the state's Worker's Compensation bureau. Because state laws vary, only a general summary can be given here.

SPECIAL HINT

It is advisable that you contact your state's Department of Labor, Bureau of Workers' Disability, for a copy of the legislation specific to your state.

With Worker's Compensation, employees are entitled to reasonable medical care to cure or relieve the effects of work-related injuries and diseases. They are also entitled to weekly compensation benefits that may be claimed as long as the disability and wage loss continue. Entitlements may also include entities such as transportation costs to and from the physician's office or hospital. The specific amount of weekly compensation depends on the date and type of injury. For example, if a worker returns to work at a different job that pays less than the one at which he or she was working at the time of the injury, and the reason is that he or she is still unable to work at the previous job, the employee is entitled to partial compensation benefits. Prompt payment of benefits is required by law. If there is any dispute about a worker's claim, the Bureau of Workers' Disability will resolve it. Most states have a clause for employees who work for more than one employer. In such cases, the injured employee gets credit for all wages reported to the Internal Revenue Service for benefit computation purposes. The liable employer must pay the total benefit.

Vocational rehabilitation is a goal of many states' legislation. The goal of vocational rehabilitation is to assist a worker to return to appropriate employment as soon as reasonably possible. Direct job placement is often provided. Vocational rehabilitation may be provided by one's employer or insurance carrier, by the state's rehabilitation agency, or by a private rehabilitation facility. If the injured employee and the employer or carrier cannot agree on a rehabilitation program, the injured party has a right to a hearing with the Bureau of Workers' Disability. If either the employee or the employer disagrees with the decision of the bureau, either may exercise their right of appeal.

Many states require injured workers to notify their employer or insurance carrier of any additional wages earned during a benefit period. They must submit to reasonable periodic medical examinations and cooperate with reasonable rehabilitation efforts directed toward helping them to return to appropriate competitive employment. No person may receive full Worker's Compensation benefits and unemployment insurance benefits for the same period of time from the same employer.

Accident prevention is the key to a low loss record and reduced insurance costs. New employees should be given proper instruction and training so they will know and understand the requirements of the job to be performed. As new methods are introduced or a product change is made, it is necessary to retrain employees to the new procedure. Diligence and care should be exercised to ensure that all functions of a new procedure are fully understood. Retraining is also needed to keep able employees from becoming sloppy in their approach to safety. A complete record of employee performance should be maintained. This should include basic employment records, attendance records, and attainment and promotional achievements. Attendance records should show the exact reasons for absence from duty, such as vacations, illnesses, funeral attendance, accidents, etc. This record can be of tremendous importance in the event it is necessary to challenge an employee at a later date. Recognizing an employee's outside activities and lifestyle may also provide valuable information about alleged injuries and disabilities at a later date.

Every employee should be provided a reasonably clean and safe place to work. This is furnished primarily by the employer, but it is also the responsibility of the employees to maintain a clean and safe environment. Good housekeeping is the first rule of safety. All places of employment should be kept clean to the extent that the nature of the work allows and clear of obstacles that could cause hazard. The safety and proper maintenance of buildings, grounds, equipment, and fire safety materials are also important. A person trained in first aid and first aid equipment and supplies should be available at all times. One might assume that a medical facility would be in compliance with this last recommendation, but, surprisingly, there is negligence in some medical offices.

Termination of Compensation Payments

Because there are very few defenses in terms of compensability left to the employer, the early termination of Worker's Compensation benefits is one of the best ways to reduce the total expense of Worker's Compensation claims. Compensation is terminated as the result of several events; the most common of these is the end of the disability and the employee's return to work at his or her regular job and/or a different job. Returning to work at light duty is a form of vocational rehabilitation. If the employee refuses reasonable vocational rehabilitation, payments may be terminated. Weekly compensation also ends in the event of the death of the employee from a cause unrelated to the compensable disability. If the death is due to the original injury/disease, benefits must be paid to the employee's dependents up to a specified period of time. Benefits may also cease when the case is resolved by settlement through an agreement approved by an administrative law judge. This agreement is to redeem liability. The amount of the settlement is usually based on a compromise of any benefits due to that date, any future weekly benefits, and/or an allowance for future medical expenses. After this redemption of liability is final, there is no more exposure of the employer or the insurance carrier to liability of subsequent loss. Such redemption of liability usually requires the employee to submit his or her unqualified resignation to the employer.

If a former employee's claim for Worker's Compensation benefits overlaps with a claim for wrongful discharge or discrimination, it is common for the claims to be handled separately, with insurance counsel representing the employer in the compensation proceedings and the company's regular labor attorney defending it against the other charges. A coordinated effort is essential to the company's success. Be certain your attorneys are talking to one another. Approve nothing until you are satisfied it includes the broadest release possible.

Issues in the Workplace

Today's society has created a work environment that is complex, challenging, and changing. What is a commonplace employment practice in the office of today may be illegal tomorrow. Managers must stay aware of legislation that relates to their practice. Whether a medical practice is located in a rural community or a cosmopolitan city, whether it is a one-physician practice or a megagroup, the issues of acquired immune deficiency (AIDS) testing, drug use, mandatory drug screening, alcohol and substance abuse, and smoking have the potential to try your management skills.

Drug Testing/Substance Abuse/Alcohol Abuse

A neighboring state may have definitive standards that relate to all of these issues, whereas your state may have weak standards or no standards. Generally, however, it is believed that employers are allowed to test an employee who they have reasonable grounds to believe is impaired from performing his or her job. Some states allow widespread or random testing of an employer's work force. Most states have protected the employee against the possibility of false-positive tests by requiring that an independent laboratory test a sample twice before determining that it is positive. Other legislators have passed bills that say an employee may, at his or her own expense, pay for a third laboratory test. Some pending state legislation wants to require an employer to give advance notice to employees of the intention to test. For all employees, it is important that policies and practices not violate their right to privacy. Remember, managers serve both employees and the employer. Employers must also be concerned about possible claims of defamation. Michigan's Department of Civil Rights asserts that individuals suffering from drug addiction or alcoholism may be handicapped for purposes of the Michigan Handicapper's Civil Rights Act. However, Michigan courts did concede that if an employee is unable to perform work because he or she is impaired by the use of alcohol or drugs, the employee is not protected by the antidiscrimination statutes of Michigan.

Legislation protecting the worker often seems uncoordinated on some issues. The problem with drug testing is that there is no legal definition of drug intoxication. For example, if a test's sensitivity is set incorrectly, the test may detect passive marijuana smoke inhaled by a person! There must be good testing procedures to ensure that the proper sample is tested. Mere presence of the drug in the blood or urine only proves that the employee used the drug within some number of hours before the test, not necessarily while on premise. Most employers have policies prohibiting the use of alcohol or drugs on company time or premises. In addition, these policies often forbid employees from working under the influence of drugs and/or alcohol.

Some employers are attempting to deal with substance abuse by directing employees to community service organizations or Employee Assistance Programs (EAPs). EAPs are either in-house programs or outside contractors. There may be some employers and managers who choose to avoid confrontation with a substance abuser; however, there can be legal consequences to avoiding the issue. In *Otis Engineering Corp v. Clark,* 668 SW2d 307 (Tex 1983), an employer sent an employee home because he looked intoxicated. One the way home, the employee had an auto accident and killed two women with his car. The court held that the husbands of the two dead women could bring suit against the employer and recover if it were found that a reasonably prudent employer under similar circumstances would have taken other steps to prevent the employee from the possibility of causing harm to others. You may have a carefully thought-out and written policy checked by legal counsel with regard to these issues, but have you given thought to what steps you, as manager, might take if your employer or one of the physicians in your group is substance impaired? Does your practice have a written policy for the physicians in your group? In one corporation, an impaired physician was let off the hook by the state's Medical Board because the Board was "sensitive to the issue of the physician's right to earn a living" and the issue of litigation.

Smoking in the Workplace

Former Surgeon General Koop has stated that cigarette smoking is clearly the largest single preventable cause of illness and premature death in the United States. Correct or not, there is increasing pressure from anti-smoking groups to restrict smoking in public places and in private workplaces. Again, state laws vary. Smokers claim the right to be free from regulation of their tobacco use, while nonsmokers claim the right to be free from secondary smoke. There has long been a ban on smoking in certain places where there is risk of fire. Now, many states are implementing regulations that restrict smoking in public places, including private places of employment.

Many employers have voluntarily adopted a variant of a nonsmoking policy because of health concerns and the complaints of nonsmokers. A middle-of-the-road approach may help to satisfy both factions by providing a designated area for those who smoke. A number of companies refuse to hire applicants who smoke, even off the job. They argue that this makes it easier to enforce on-the-job smoking bans and reduces costs in insurance, Worker's Compensation and sick pay. In a tight labor market, however, an employer may not want to adopt this stringent a policy because of the difficulty this poses in finding capable office personnel. There are some risks in not hiring smokers. Some states may determine that smokers are handicapped, and a refusal to hire them may be a violation of the law. Although there is little doubt about the health risks associated with smoking, there is doubt about the right of an employer to violate a person's right to choose his or her own risk, life-style, or habits as long as they are legal.

Issues Related to Acquired Immune Deficiency Syndrome

Human immunodeficiency virus (HIV) positivity in our patient population and within the medical support team has become an issue that affects all of us. The Americans With Disabilities Act of 1990 (ADA), federal legislation, offers employment protection for individuals with AIDS or AIDS-related disease. At this time, there is controversy over mandating HIV testing for health care workers and the subsequent release of results to patients who feel they need to know. Health care practitioners, especially those with greater exposure risks, insist on a right to privacy. This issue is a profound one that involves the potential of liability and litigation, and any policy on this subject should be carefully worded.

Equal Opportunity Developments

Many employers have developed policies on equal opportunity (nondiscrimination) practices and affirmative action programs. Federal, state, and local laws may mandate the development of such a written policy. A nondiscrimination policy is intended to prevent discriminatory practices on the basis of race, sex, creed, color, religion, national origin, age, marital status, sexual preference, source of income, physical or mental handicaps when the individual is otherwise qualified, status of disabled veterans, and any other non-job-related factor. Affirmative action policies are intended to commit the employer to *affirmatively act* in those special areas relating to social distinction or protected classes where past discrimination has denied equality of opportunity.

Protection of Handicapped Individuals. Congress adopted new handicapped protection statutes in 1990 with the passing of the ADA, perhaps the most significant civil rights legislation in decades. The ADA requires barrier-free public accommodations and commercial facilities as well. As of January 13, 1992, alterations to existing buildings must be designed to permit handicapper use to the most feasible extent possible. Newly constructed facilities must be readily accessible to handicapped individuals unless the owner can show that it would be structurally impractical.

ADA only applies to businesses employing 15

or more persons; however, some states have already enacted stronger legislation that applies to all employers in the state. Michigan amended their Michigan Handicappers' Civil Rights Act (MHCRA) in 1990 to include all employers. The principal emphasis of both the ADA and the MHCRA is the duty to accommodate. The law obligates employers to accommodate conditions that substantially limit one or more of an individual's major life activities, but that, when accommodated, do not prevent the individual from performing the essential functions of the job he or she desires. The required accommodations may include removing barriers to wheelchairs, providing special adaptive devices on equipment, modifying machinery, furnishing readers or interpreters, restructuring jobs, and altering work schedules.

Accommodation is necessary only to the extent that it does not impose an undue hardship on the employer. ADA defines undue hardship as "significant difficulty or expenses" and requires the employer to prove undue hardship. MHCRA uses a specific formula to cap the employer's costs.

Significantly, the ADA prohibits preemployment physical examinations until after an offer of employment has been made and unless all entering employees are examined. Medical information obtained about applicants must be recorded on separate forms and kept in confidential medical files accessible only to those who need to know of job restrictions. Of interest, although handicapped applicants may be denied employment if they pose a direct threat to the health or safety of others, there is not an exception for persons whose handicaps may endanger themselves.

The federal statutes exclude from protection persons discharged, disciplined, or denied employment for current use of illegal drugs. However, former drug users and those undergoing rehabilitation may not be denied employment opportunities on account of their past practices. This latter requirement may cause difficulties to the large medical practice that keeps drugs on premise. Job qualification standards, employment tests, and selection criteria that tend to screen out handicapped persons may not be used unless they are job related and consistent with business necessity. Handicapped applicants who believe that they have been discriminated against can file a complaint with the state Department of Civil Rights and/or the Equal Employment Opportunity Commission. Claims of failure to accommodate may be raised only if the handicapped individual has first notified the employer in writing of the need for accommodation. Such notice must be given within 182 days of the date the handicapped individual knew or should have known that accommodation was needed. Employers are required by ADA to post notices advising employees and applicants of their rights and obligations.

Sexual Harassment

Title VI of the Civil Rights Act provides for protection of employees from gender-based discrimination. The most frequent type of sexual harassment claim is that sexual requests were made as an express or implied condition to economic benefit (such as a raise or promotion). This kind of claim is called *quid pro quo*. The other kind of sexual harassment claim is for conduct that creates an intimidating, hostile, or offensive work environment. The plaintiff, male or female, must prove he or she was subjected to unwelcomed sexual advances, requests for sexual favors, or other verbal or physical conduct of a sexual nature. These may be unsolicited verbal comments, patting, pinching, or unnecessary touching as well as the obvious, physical assault. The question is whether the alleged advances were unwelcomed.

In *quid pro quo* cases, the alleged advances must be made by one of the employee's superiors. In hostile-environment cases, the prohibited conduct may also be committed by co-workers, customers, or the public if the employer is responsible for the environment. In any case, the conduct must have the effect of unreasonably interfering with an individual's work performance. All offices should have an internal reporting mechanism. If not, it will be assumed that the employer had knowledge but failed to act.

Under the legal principle of *respondeat superior,* the employer is strictly liable for a supervisor's conduct toward employees. In hostile-environment cases, the issue is whether the employer knew or should have known of the hostile environment. Sexual harassment claims are frequently difficult to prevent from the manager's point of view, because they can be based on one incident by one person. With the addition of the word "implied," a single joke in poor taste could be construed as sexually harassing. Courts have held that an employee's psychological well-being is a privilege. If sexual conduct is sufficiently severe or persistent to harm an employee's psychological well-being, substantially affecting his or her working environment, it may be actionable. Theoretically at least, employers should not be liable for the extreme reactions of an unusually sensitive employee to conduct which would not offend the average person. An interesting twist is that any employee who did not submit to requests for sexual favors, and therefore did not receive any employment benefit that an employee who did submit received, may have an actionable case of discrimination!

When an allegation of sexual harassment is made against a nonemployee such as a drug representative, a supplier, or a party providing ancillary services, management must be notified at once so that appropriate action can be taken. In such cases, it is advised that the company's attorney be contacted by the office manager for instructions in how to deal with the situation.

Pregnancy Leave

This issue affects those females of childbearing age only. Legislation has been passed in many states, which can be summarized as follows: An employee who is pregnant should be treated like any employee who is not. It is not up to the employer to determine the employee's ability to report to work. That decision is the right of the employee to be made in conjunction with her physician. If nonpregnant employees can have their pay docked for excessive tardiness, then pregnant employees can also have their pay docked for excessive tardiness. If a pregnant employee abuses a sick-day policy that specifies termination after a certain number of sick days and applies to all employees, she is at risk for losing her job, just like anyone else.

Employers offering health and hospitalization insurance to their employees should consider the stage of the pregnancy and what the cessation of insurance benefits may do the mother-to-be. A pregnant woman in her eighth month probably would have difficulty finding other work and subsequent insurance coverage. Even if the reason for termination of employment were valid, a pregnant employee so deprived of insurance/hospitalization coverage may well claim discrimination in hopes of receiving a cash settlement to cover her costs. Offices with less than 20 employees are not obligated under the Consolidated Omnibus Budget Reconciliation Act of 1985 to provide continuation of insurance benefits (that the employee would pay for) under the group policy rates. If an office offers disability insurance to their employees, in some states it is illegal not to carry pregnancy protection riders on all females of childbearing age.

Does an employer have to hold a job for a pregnant woman to return to, regardless of her length of absence? If the practice of the employer is that no other employee has a job held for him or her, probably not. However, the U.S. Supreme Court upheld a California statute that requires employers to provide 4 months of unpaid pregnancy leave and reinstatement to the same job (*California Federal Savings and Loan Association v. Guerra,* 55 USLW 4077, 1987). Check with your attorney as to what your state's statutes are regarding pregnancy leave.

Immigration Reform

In 1987, Alan C. Nelson, Commissioner of the U.S. Immigration and Naturalization Services (INS) prefaced the U.S. Government Printing Office's *Handbook for Employers on Instructions for Completing Federal Form I-9* with these statements:

When the Congress passed and the President signed into law the Immigration Reform and Control Act of 1986, the result was the first major revision of America's immigration laws in decades. The new law seeks to preserve jobs for those who are legally entitled to them: American citizens and aliens who are authorized to work in our country . . . Put briefly, the law says that you should hire only American citizens and aliens who are authorized to work in the United States. You will need to verify employment eligibility of *anyone* hired after November 6, 1986, and complete and retain a one-page form (I-9).

Figure 11–3 reproduces this form in its entirety.

The *Handbook* also states:

The new immigration law also prohibits discrimination. Under this law, if you have four or more employees, you may not discriminate against any individual (other than an unauthorized alien) in hiring, discharging, or recruiting or referring for a fee because of that individual's national origin, or, in the case of a citizen or intending citizen, because of his or her citizenship status.

There are serious and severe penalties for employers found noncompliant, ranging from fines to imprisonment. Figure 11–4 reproduces the acceptable documents for verifying employment eligibility. Form I-9, which is reproduced in the *Handbook,* may be photocopied and used by employers. However, if you want a limited number

254 *Chapter 11: PERSONNEL AND OFFICE POLICIES*

U.S. Department of Justice
Immigration and Naturalization Service

OMB No. 1115-0136
Employment Eligibility Verification

Please read instructions carefully before completing this form. The instructions must be available during completion of this form. ANTI-DISCRIMINATION NOTICE. It is illegal to discriminate against work eligible individuals. Employers **CANNOT** specify which document(s) they will accept from an employee. The refusal to hire an individual because of a future expiration date may also constitute illegal discrimination.

Section 1. Employee Information and Verification. To be completed and signed by employee at the time employment begins

Print Name: Last	First	Middle Initial	Maiden Name

Address (Street Name and Number)	Apt. #	Date of Birth (month/day/year)

City	State	Zip Code	Social Security #

I am aware that federal law provides for imprisonment and/or fines for false statements or use of false documents in connection with the completion of this form.

I attest, under penalty of perjury, that I am (check one of the following):
☐ A citizen or national of the United States
☐ A Lawful Permanent Resident (Alien # A _____)
☐ An alien authorized to work until ___/___/___
   (Alien # or Admission #)

Employee's Signature	Date (month/day/year)

Preparer and/or Translator Certification. *(To be completed and signed if Section 1 is prepared by a person other than the employee.)* I attest, under penalty of perjury, that I have assisted in the completion of this form and that to the best of my knowledge the information is true and correct.

Preparer's/Translator's Signature	Print Name

Address (Street Name and Number, City, State, Zip Code)	Date (month/day/year)

Section 2. Employer Review and Verification. To be completed and signed by employer. Examine one document from List A **OR** examine one document from List B **and** one from List C as listed on the reverse of this form and record the title, number and expiration date, if any, of the document(s)

	List A	OR	List B	AND	List C
Document title:	_____		_____		_____
Issuing authority:	_____		_____		_____
Document #:	_____		_____		_____
Expiration Date (if any):	___/___/___		___/___/___		___/___/___
Document #:	_____				
Expiration Date (if any):	___/___/___				

CERTIFICATION - I attest, under penalty of perjury, that I have examined the document(s) presented by the above-named employee, that the above-listed document(s) appear to be genuine and to relate to the employee named, that the employee began employment on (month/day/year) ___/___/___ and that to the best of my knowledge the employee is eligible to work in the United States. (State employment agencies may omit the date the employee began employment).

Signature of Employer or Authorized Representative	Print Name	Title

Business or Organization Name	Address (Street Name and Number, City, State, Zip Code)	Date (month/day/year)

Section 3. Updating and Reverification. To be completed and signed by employer

A. New Name (if applicable)	B. Date of rehire (month/day/year) (if applicable)

C. If employee's previous grant of work authorization has expired, provide the information below for the document that establishes current employment eligibility.

Document Title: _____ Document #: _____ Expiration Date (if any): ___/___/___

I attest, under penalty of perjury, that to the best of my knowledge, this employee is eligible to work in the United States, and if the employee presented document(s), the document(s) I have examined appear to be genuine and to relate to the individual.

Signature of Employer or Authorized Representative	Date (month/day/year)

Form I-9 (Rev. 11-21-91) N

FIGURE 11-3

Employment Eligibility Verification form.

LISTS OF ACCEPTABLE DOCUMENTS

LIST A
Documents that Establish Both Identity and Employment Eligibility

1. U.S. Passport (unexpired or expired)

2. Certificate of U.S. Citizenship *(INS Form N-560 or N-561)*

3. Certificate of Naturalization *(INS Form N-550 or N-570)*

4. Unexpired foreign passport, with *I-551 stamp or* attached *INS Form I-94* indicating unexpired employment authorization

5. Alien Registration Receipt Card with photograph *(INS Form I-151 or I-551)*

6. Unexpired Temporary Resident Card *(INS Form I-688)*

7. Unexpired Employment Authorization Card *(INS Form I-688A)*

8. Unexpired Reentry Permit *(INS Form I-327)*

9. Unexpired Refugee Travel Document *(INS Form I-571)*

10. Unexpired Employment Authorization Document issued by the INS which contains a photograph *(INS Form I-688B)*

OR

LIST B
Documents that Establish Identity

1. Driver's license or ID card issued by a state or outlying possession of the United States provided it contains a photograph or information such as name, date of birth, sex, height, eye color, and address

2. ID card issued by federal, state, or local government agencies or entities provided it contains a photograph or information such as name, date of birth, sex, height, eye color, and address

3. School ID card with a photograph

4. Voter's registration card

5. U.S. Military card or draft record

6. Military dependent's ID card

7. U.S. Coast Guard Merchant Mariner Card

8. Native American tribal document

9. Driver's license issued by a Canadian government authority

For persons under age 18 who are unable to present a document listed above:

10. School record or report card

11. Clinic, doctor, or hospital record

12. Day-care or nursery school record

AND

LIST C
Documents that Establish Employment Eligibility

1. U.S. social security card issued by the Social Security Administration *(other than a card stating it is not valid for employment)*

2. Certification of Birth Abroad issued by the Department of State *(Form FS-545 or Form DS-1350)*

3. Original or certified copy of a birth certificate issued by a state, county, municipal authority or outlying possession of the United States bearing an official seal

4. Native American tribal document

5. U.S. Citizen ID Card *(INS Form I-197)*

6. ID Card for use of Resident Citizen in the United States *(INS Form I-179)*

7. Unexpired employment authorization document issued by the INS *(other than those listed under List A)*

Illustrations of many of these documents appear in Part 8 of the Handbook for Employers (M-274)

Form I-9 (Rev. 11-21-91) N

FIGURE 11-3 *Continued*

LIST A
Documents That Establish Identity and Employment Eligibility

- United States Passport
- Certificate of United States Citizenship. (INS Form N-560 or N-561)
- Certificate of Naturalization. (INS Form N-550 or N-570)
- Unexpired foreign passport which:
  — Contains an unexpired stamp which reads "Processed for I-551. Temporary Evidence of Lawful Admission for permanent residence. Valid until ____. Employment authorized;" or
  — Has attached thereto a Form I-94 bearing the same name as the passport and contains an employment authorization stamp, so long as the period of endorsement has not yet expired and the proposed employment is not in conflict with any restrictions or limitations identified on the Form I-94
- Alien Registration Receipt Card (INS Form I-151) or Resident Alien Card (INS Form I-551), provided that it contains a photograph of the bearer.
- Temporary Resident Card. (INS Form I-688)
- Employment Authorization Card. (INS Form I-688A)

LIST B
Documents That Establish Identity

For individuals 16 years of age or older:

- State-issued driver's license or state-issued identification card containing a photograph. If the driver's license or identification card does not contain a photograph, identifying information should be included, such as name, date of birth, sex, height, color of eyes, and address.
- School identification card with a photograph
- Voter's registration card
- United States military card or draft record
- Identification card issued by federal, state or local government agencies
- Military dependent's identification card
- Native American tribal documents
- United States Coast Guard Merchant Mariner Card
- Driver's license issued by a Canadian government authority

For individuals under age 16 who are unable to produce one of the documents listed above:

- School record or report card
- Clinic doctor or hospital record
- Daycare or nursery school record

LIST C
Documents That Establish Employment Eligibility

- Social Security number card, other than one which has printed on its face "not valid for employment purposes."
  Note: This must be a card issued by the Social Security Administration; a facsimile (such as a metal or plastic reproduction that people can buy) is not acceptable.
- An original or certified copy of a birth certificate issued by a state, county, or municipal authority bearing an official seal
- Unexpired INS employment authorization
- Unexpired re-entry permit. (INS Form I-327)
- Unexpired Refugee Travel Document. (INS Form I-571)
- Certification of Birth issued by the Department of State. (Form FS-545)
- Certification of Birth Abroad issued by the Department of State. (Form DS-1350)
- United States Citizen Identification Card. (INS Form I-197)
- Native American tribal document
- Identification Card for use of Resident Citizen in the United States. (INS Form I-179)

FIGURE 11-4

Acceptable documents for verifying employment eligibility.

of fresh copies, you may obtain them by writing the INS. In bulk, they may be ordered from:

> U.S. Department of Justice
> Immigration and Naturalization Service
> 425 I Street NW
> Washington, DC 20536

Retention of Employees' Records

Federal, state, and local laws mandate employers to keep various records for employees for certain lengths of time. Basically, the records that must be retained by medical practices are as follows:

- Job applications
- INS form I-9
- Preemployment testing and results
- Reference letters
- W-4s
- Performance review
- Salary history
- Time and attendance records
- Any material that pertains to either promotion or demotion
- All reprimands, warnings, and incident reports
- Signatures attesting to having received and accepted policies
- If appropriate, letters of resignation.

A normal practice is to maintain an employee file in which these materials are kept and to maintain that file's accessibility for 3 years after an employee is discharged or voluntarily leaves the practice.

In some communities, a manager may be asked to verify employment of employees who left their practice 5 years earlier, so it may be helpful to maintain these files longer. Other than the legal requirement of 3 years for most documents, keeping old employee files longer depends on the size of the practice, the number of employees coming and going, the age of the practice and the space available for storage. Many smaller practices have their physician owners store the material off premise in their own houses after the period of 3 years. Other practices systematically destroy the material. Copies of an employee's W-2 income transmittal forms should be saved for 7 years; however, these are generally kept in a separate section than the employee's file. The Occupational Safety and Health Act (OSHA) requires employers to keep accurate and timely records of work-related injuries and accidents in accordance with its rules. An employer may also be required to maintain records of employee exposure to potentially toxic substances or harmful physical agents. An employer need not record injuries or illnesses that do not result in lost time or are of a first-aid nature.

SPECIAL HINT

Because state laws vary, often depending on the number of employees an employer has, it is incumbent on the employer or the manager to find out what these laws are.

Summary

The days when an employer is allowed to control the welfare of his or her employees have ended. Legislation on all levels of government has guaranteed much protection to the worker. With the *Toussaint v. Blue Cross and Blue Shield of Michigan,* 408 Mich 1980, decision, the Michigan Supreme Court ruled that employers may be bound by employment contracts they never intended to make, if employees believe that the employer policies, publications, or verbal statements are commitments.

In today's society, an employer's right to terminate an unproductive and/or uncooperative employee has been severely compromised. From an employee's view, this is very good; from a manager's point of view, it has the potential to create ulcers!

For example, bills are pending in legislatures that would mandate not just pregnancy leave, but parental/family leave. In one such case, the bill would require employers to provide 60 working days of paid leave and an additional 120 days of unpaid leave for 2 years. Benefits would continue during these leaves of absence. The leave could be taken for newborn, newly adopted, or seriously ill dependents (which might include ill parents supported by the employee or those who are over 65 years of age). The bill additionally complicates a manager's life by adding that an employee could take this leave by working a fewer number of work days per week than scheduled or a fewer number of hours per work day. When the employee returns from his or her leave, the employee must be given their original or equivalent position!

Can you imagine trying to arrange for staff support for your physician employer under those kinds of conditions? Furthermore, if you manage a large multiphysician practice where physicians are not employers, can you foresee the disastrous financial results in continuing their salaries when they are not producing income? This legislation could be disastrous for an office with few personnel. With increasing limitations on reimbursement for health care services, the potential for no job to come back to takes on a reality. To be prepared and effective, then, the office manager must know not only the legal responsibilities of his or her position, but also what other legislation is pending.

SELECTION OF ANCILLARY SERVICES

It is apparent that the effective office manager needs an off-premise support and counsel team either contracted for or obtained by networking. Networking is simply the development of a contact system of friends and peers for support and interchange of ideas. The criteria for selection of your networking contacts usually include the individuals' effectiveness in their position, their intelligence and sensitivity, their listening and communication skills, and their willingness to share. Professional organizations such as the American Association of Medical Assistants provide an excellent networking source on a national level. Other professional organizations may include the Medical Group Management Association, the American Group Practice Association, and the Group Health Association of America.

It also has become apparent that what you don't know *will* hurt you. Therefore, it is imperative that you and your staff continue education and training, either by in-service or by formal classes, seminar attendance, and reading. There are many flyers sent to medical offices which peddle marginal programs in hopes of exploiting these needs for a profit. If you belong to a professional organization, you have the opportunity of calling or writing that organization to get some assistance in determining the educational validity of the programs offered by these flyers. Many managers scan the material in the flyer and, because it seems relevant, register for the program. Attendance either confirms the validity of their choice or leaves them wondering why the time and money were spent. Word of mouth from your peers is also a good source for determining a seminar's merit. In some larger cities that have large multispecialty medical office buildings, managers have been known to informally group for a weekly hour-long breakfast to discuss items of relevance. All it takes is for one person to write a proposal or invitation stating purpose, time, date, and place, on an 8½ × 11 inch sheet of paper, make copies, and distribute the invitation to offices in the building. If only one person shows up, fine. The next week there might be three others who attend, and so on. The philosophy is similar to the calm pond disturbed by a rock thrown into it.

Criteria for Selection of Attorneys, Accountants, and Consultants

The selection process of your networking group is far easier than the selection of attorneys, accountants, and consultants the practice must use. In this evaluation process, you must take into account whether you have the authority to offer input into this process at all. Many managers come into a practice and find these ancillary personnel already established. If they are effective, fine; but what if you find that they are ineffective? You need to consider how to evaluate this finding and present it to your employer. Often, physicians have developed a working relationship with these support persons and have developed a degree of trust based on experience. Disturbing that relationship because you, as manager, find it difficult to work with that party is not sufficient cause to insist that the relationship be terminated. Incompetency or lack of result is sufficient. The effective manager does not create a void. You must offer options for replacement, with specific criteria developed and presented.

Attorneys

It makes no sense in today's times to have an attorney who is a tax specialist giving advice on issues dealing with employment. How much more effective it is to have a firm that has not only corporate lawyers but also pension plan specialists, tax specialists, and labor specialists. Your contact lawyer, the "company" lawyer, could refer you to the appropriate specialist within the firm. On a practical level, the manager who has been promoted from within because he or she has shown herself to be capable and responsible may read this chapter and wonder how she will cope with all of this. Develop criteria? Where to begin? It really is easier than it sounds. Try, "Doctor, I've been reading this manual on medical assisting, and I think we have some problems. Can we schedule some time to talk about some of my concerns?"

When the meeting occurs, simply state your position, which may be that you do not think the practice's tax attorney is as helpful to the practice as he or she could be. Listen to your employer and hear what he or she has to say. Offer to do research. If an attorney provides good corporate service but is weak on other issues, the State Bar Association or local Bar Association can give you names of competent specialists in the field of law you require.

Accountants

Accountants come in all varieties. The one you want is the one who provides the services you need at a price you can afford. There are specialists in accounting as well. The methods used to find an attorney work with finding an accountant, too. Here, however, one needs to interview candidates to determine their educational background, experience, and additional professional credentials. When certified by an accrediting body, accountants must continue their education to renew their credentials just like certified medical assistants must. Accountants may be willing to share with you who their other clients are, providing references. Check up on these references. The following are questions that may be asked of the reference:

- Does the accountant do work on or off premises?
- Does he or she provide you with service promptly?
- Is the material provided relevant and easily understood?
- Have you had problems with his or her tax forms?
- Is the accountant easily accessible?

You have already determined what services the candidate is able to provide. All you have to do is to verify with others that they were provided in a timely, accurate, and professional manner.

Consultants

After 20 years in the field, this writer is aware that consultants come in all shapes and sizes and wear a variety of disguises. This is both an indictment and a recognition that there are lots of so-called experts out there.

SPECIAL HINT

Word of mouth is a method for finding who is right for your practice. Interviewing the consultant is a must. Your physician's state medical association or specialty affiliation association is an excellent resource to access.

There are multiple national consulting companies available. If you hear of one that has provided excellent service to an office in your area, contact it by phone. On the phone, inquire as to its availability and charge structure.

- Will you be paying for mileage, room, and board in addition to an hourly fee?
- Is it a bulk fee?
- Do they provide a written plan of recommendation?
- What is involved?
- Do they come on premise and interview all office personnel and do time/work flow studies and review the practice's financial status?
- Do they also talk with the practice's attorney and accountant, perhaps reviewing the corporation's records?

This last practice has the potential of incurring additional costs to you not included on the consultant's bill, in the form of attorney fees.

- When a consultant is chosen and performs the service for which you have contracted him or her, is your physician employer going to be amenable to change?
- If you work with a group of physicians who have rigid ideas, is it even financially advisable to have a consultant work with you if the physicians would veto all suggestions for change?
- Is the consultant empowered by the employer? If so, does he or she have specific knowledge of employment/labor laws? There have been many cases where a consultant has evaluated a practice and recommended firing the wife who works for her husband, the physician, or terminating the manager's employment!

All over the United States, there are medical office managers who have decided to free-lance on their own, providing contracted services as consultants. Some of these are very knowledgeable; many are not. The rule of Rs is a tool to use when evaluating consultants.

> **Rule of Rs**
>
> References
> Results
> wRitten recommendations

If a consultant will not put his or her recommendations in writing and sign it, do not use the consultant. If you act on a recommendation made in writing from a consultant, there is the possibility that in any subsequent litigation shared liability might get your employer and you off the hook for unknowingly violating the law. It could be presumed in court that someone purporting to be an expert would have knowledge of employment law, for example, and their written recommendation to you (which subsequently violated the law) was taken on good faith by you. If you lose the lawsuit, you might at least have the opportunity to recover costs by countersuing the consultant for malpractice.

SEPARATION FROM EMPLOYMENT

Cases of employees who decide they can no longer work at their current employment, employees whose behavior is threatening their employment, and employees whose employment must be terminated arise for every employer. Employment practices have been developed to help the manager in this regard.

Warnings

The effective use of warnings can change a marginal employee into a desirable one. If not, the warnings can be used as evidence to prove the employee's disqualification for benefits if separation from employment is planned because of misconduct. Warnings should be in writing, and the employee should sign and date the form in order to document the fact that he or she received the warning. If unsigned, the employee can always charge that the warnings were concocted after the fact. Unless the employee commits a serious offense requiring immediate discharge, he or she should be warned at least once, preferably twice, and informed in writing that the next act will result in discharge. (DO NOT, however, establish a policy of progressive discipline unless you are prepared to be bound by it in all cases.) Make certain that employee evaluations and wage increases accurately reflect any problems with the employee and are consistent with any disciplinary warnings given to the employee.

Suspensions

Suspension is another disciplinary measure that can possibly salvage a marginal employee. If not, suspension can also be a means of disqualifying an employee for benefits if he or she is suspended for misconduct. An employee should be notified of the suspension in writing, and the written notice should include the reason for suspension, the inclusive dates, and the date the employee is to return to work. This can prevent many problems if the employee files a claim and gives distorted facts to any board, commission, or attorney.

Discharges

Thorough Investigation of the Facts. Complete facts should be assembled before an employee is discharged. Never act on hearsay. The decision should involve as many managerial levels as possible, and the person authorizing the discharge should make certain to have complete knowledge of the situation. The employee's personnel file should be reviewed to determine whether there is sufficient documentation to support the discharge. If immediate action is necessary before the facts can be thoroughly investigated, place the employee on suspension before making the discharge decision.

Definition of Misconduct. Although there are statutory acts of misconduct listed by many states as warranting disqualification for unemployment benefits, a discharge based on work-connected misconduct will be defined as conduct that is deliberate with willful disregard of the employer's interests. Some acts that may constitute misconduct are the following:

- Insubordination
- Deliberate and unwarranted refusal to obey instructions
- Excessive unexcused tardiness
- Excessive unexcused absenteeism
- Gross neglect of duty
- Actions on the job specifically prohibited, such as fighting, theft, making defamatory remarks about co-workers, sexual harassment, drug use, or alcohol use
- violation of a well-established and important company policy

SPECIAL HINT

Remember, the burden of proof rests on the employer.

Written Warnings. An employee should have received prior written warnings for violations of company policy in order to be disqualified from receiving unemployment benefits on that basis. In a wrongful-discharge case, the jury might believe the employer if written warnings had been issued and signed by the employee.

When to Act. Act immediately following the last incident, instead of allowing an employee to work after it occurs.

Informing the Employee. Always inform the employee in writing of the reason for discharge. Try to have the terminated employee sign that he or she acknowledges this is the reason for discharge.

Exit Interviews

Conducting an exit interview is a good way to learn the cause of an employee's separation when a resignation is voluntary. If the employee has given a written resignation that is general in content, the exit interview might elicit information that points out a company deficiency or a personnel problem of which the manager was unaware. When an employee resigns or is terminated, the exact reason for the separation should be recorded and maintained in the personnel file. Maintaining specific information not only is necessary to combat unjustified unemployment claims, but also provides defense against possible discrimination or wrongful-discharge claims. Avoid general statements.

Accurately and completely record all the facts and in the form of a memo or other document, and have anyone with first-hand knowledge of the facts review, sign, and date the document. Even if the terminated employee refuses to sign the document, a permanent record for future use is available. By the time an employee might start litigation, facts could be forgotten or supervisors and witnesses no longer available, so this document is very valuable. If at all possible, the signature of the employee should be obtained on the separation report/memo in order to gain his or her acknowledgment of the reason for separation.

Chapter 12

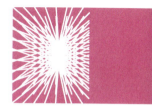

ETHICS

MARCIA LEWIS

INTRODUCTION
What Are Ethics?
Why Ethics?
Ethical Conflicts
Moral Principles

ETHICS AND PROFESSIONALISM FOR MEDICAL PERSONNEL
Code of Ethics
Ethics Related to the Analysis of the Profession

THE ETHICS OF CONFIDENTIALITY

THE ETHICS OF CONSENT

BIOETHICAL ISSUES IN AMBULATORY CARE
Patients' Right to Health Care
Patients' Right to Live or to Die
Patients' Right to Procreate or to Abort

PRACTICAL IMPLICATIONS OF ETHICS AND BIOETHICS FOR MEDICAL PERSONNEL IN AMBULATORY CARE
The "Ethics Check" Questions
What to Do When You Don't Know What to Do
Ethical Dos and Don'ts

INTRODUCTION

Say "medical ethics" to a group of medical office employees, and their reactions will be varied. Some will say, "Medical office personnel don't need to know about that. They don't deal with medical ethics. That's for hospital employees to worry about." Some will say, "Office patients have such minor problems with ethics in the medical office that employees don't concern themselves." Still others may say, "Yes, employees in the medical office have ethical dilemmas, but they sure don't know how to handle them!"

Most would agree that the majority of literature on medical ethics, news coverage included, concerns the major ethical dilemmas that occur in the hospital and acute care settings. However, ethical problems do occur in ambulatory care settings. And ethical issues in the medical office do affect patients, employees, and the community.

Indeed, ethical issues occur in the medical office with greater frequency than many would believe. A descriptive study was done by Julia E. Connelly, M.D., and Steven DalleMura, M.Div.,[1] to determine the prevalence and range of ethical problems encountered in the office practice of medicine. They concluded that in almost a third of the patients seen in the office, one to six ethical problems were present. The authors identified three major ethical issues: (1) psychological factors that influence the patient's preference, (2) socioeconomic factors, and (3) problems relating to the quality of life. Furthermore, they concluded that although ethical problems occurred at any age, they occurred more frequently in those patients over 60 years of age.

What Are Ethics?

Ethics are standards of conduct and moral judgments. Ethics are values. Ethics concern what is good, what is right, what is virtue, and what is vice. Children learn right from wrong by action, misaction, and example. Children may be told "It is wrong to lie," "Share," "Do not steal," and "Children should never. . . ." Parents, teachers, and other authority figures model good behavior and poor behavior. Individuals learn by seeing and by doing. Religion may influence ethical beliefs. Education may determine what one believes to be good and right. Life experiences are varied yet shape individuals' ethical foundations. Thus, personal ethics are developed at a very young age, although they may change as one grows and lives.

When one enters the work world, whatever the job, one develops a sense of business ethics. One learns the value of money, about inter- and intraorganizational business ethics, about the work ethic and society, and about interpersonal relationships. One learns a sense of right and wrong about work and business.

When an individual becomes a medical office employee, he or she enters another ethical arena — medical ethics. Employees bring to the medical office the ethical foundation they developed as children and as young adults. Again, their ethics may change, but their basic foundation remains intact.

Medical ethics is defined as "a system of principles governing medical conduct. It deals with the relationship of a physician to the patient, the patient's family, fellow physicians, and society at large."[2] If individuals are medical personnel, then, their medical ethics deal with the relationship of them as medical professionals with the patient, the patient's family, fellow professionals, and society. It is an awesome charge to be involved with the ethics of caring for patients — one to be taken seriously and one to be taken with the same awareness and understanding of, for example, disease processes or any clinical skills office personnel undertake.

Why Ethics?

Professionals need to be equipped with strong values and decision-making skills to successfully deal with the ethical challenges they and their patients encounter. Medical dilemmas do exist; knowledge and understanding of ethics allow professionals to act responsibly. Medical employees are able to recognize and anticipate ethical dilemmas. Many medical employees have felt uncomfortable in a situation and not known why they feel that way. Perhaps it is because they are in the midst of an ethical dilemma.

Consider, for example, the case of an elderly patient. Would this situation make you feel uncomfortable? An 85-year-old woman comes in for her annual check-up, and it is noted that the facial tumor anterior to her right ear is enlarged and somewhat grotesque appearing. She is afraid of the surgical risk and refuses to consider its removal. This is an ethical dilemma.

Ethical awareness and knowledge allow medical personnel to become more tolerant of others' ethical stances, whether they be their fellow employees, their employer(s), or their patients. Occasionally, medical personnel feel frustrated because they do not agree with the actions of fellow employees or their employers. Patients' behavior may be the cause of consternation, too. Medical personnel may be willing to change their behavior or to accept another's behavior once they become more aware and cognizant of another's views.

What if a 16-year-old unmarried pregnant woman refuses prenatal care because she denies her pregnancy? Would most office employees agree with this patient's stance? What are the health risks to this patient? Who decides what is good and right for this patient?

Knowledge of ethics may help reduce conflicts between employees, and between employees and employers with differing values. Once medical personnel understand another's reasoning, they may be better equipped to resolve arguments. Learning about ethics does not necessarily make professionals more moral, but it can help increase understanding and tolerance, and can help place ethical issues in perspective.

Ethical Conflicts

Ethical dilemmas exist in the medical office. The conflict may be minor, merely causing discomfort and frustration, or it may be major, giving cause to consider leaving the medical profession. The conflict may be between the medical employee's personal code of ethics and the professional code he or she has assumed. For example, the employee may believe that abortion is wrong for any reason, yet knows that abortions are performed. The conflict may be between the medical employee and the employer. For instance, the physician may refuse to accept welfare patients, whereas the medical employee believes this is wrong according to his or her personal code of ethics. Finally, the conflict may be between the medical employee and the patient. For example, if the patient smokes, abuses drugs, and is obese, the medical employee may find this totally unacceptable behavior.

When ethical problems exist, patient care and

treatment may be affected. Patients may refuse treatment because of previous poor medical care; physicians may not relate information to the patient if a poor physician–patient relationship exists. Only when ethical issues are recognized can better medical decisions be made. Physicians, medical personnel, and patients must realize the import of ethical dilemmas.

How are ethical dilemmas such as these resolved? Are there any standards or principles that provide a foundation on which to build? Are there guidelines that can be used when medical personnel are faced with moral dilemmas?

Ethical theories offer a basis for reasoning and analysis but are too complex for inclusion in this chapter. A bibliography of such theories is listed at the end of the chapter. In ordinary life, medical personnel rarely have the time or the opportunity to engage in an elaborate process of reasoning and analysis of ethical issues. Therefore, a more practical approach is needed. That approach is to employ moral principles that are derived from and justified by ethical theories.

Moral Principles

In this section, five moral principles, taken from a well-known ethicist, Ronald Munson, are presented. Munson's book, *Intervention and Reflection: Basic Issues in Medical Ethics*,[3] details both the ethical theories that are not included here and the moral principles that follow.

FIVE MORAL PRINCIPLES

1. Above all, do no harm. We ought to act in ways that do not cause needless harm or injury to others.
2. We should act in ways that promote the welfare of other people. That is, we should help other people when we are able to do so.
3. We should act in such a way as to bring about the greatest benefit and the least harm.
4. Similar cases ought to be treated in similar ways. This principle expresses the notion that justice involves fairness of treatment.
5. Rational individuals should be permitted to be self-determining. . . . We act autonomously when our actions are the result of our own choices and decisions. Thus, autonomy and self-determination are equivalent.

The five moral principles provide a foundation on which to base individual moral decisions. When reading through these principles, try them on. How do they fit? Do they seem right? Are they acceptable? Are they wrong? Note any reactions.

Let's examine each of these principles.

Above all, do no harm. . . . We ought to act in ways that do not cause needless harm or injury to others.[3]

Medical personnel need to be aware of their actions so that they do not unintentionally cause harm to patients. There is a standard of care to which *all* medical employees must adhere. Of course, mistakes will occur, but patients can expect medical employees to be diligent, cautious, and thoughtful in their work. Medical personnel must possess the skill and knowledge necessary or they may be charged with ethical or legal maleficence (the act of committing harm).

The American Association of Medical Assistants (AAMA), the nationally recognized professional organization for medical assistants, may indeed set the standard of care for medical assistants. This standard, based on a certification examination, a continuing education program, and its accreditation of medical assisting education programs, is the yardstick for medical assistants. By using this national standard, medical assistants should cause no harm or injury to patients.

We should act in ways that promote the welfare of other people. That is, we should help other people when we are able to do so.[3]

Part of the physician's Hippocratic oath states, "As to diseases, make a habit of two things—to help or at least do no harm." The first—"to help"—is part of this moral principle. Some medical personnel may agree that the first moral principle of "do no harm" is correct, but may wonder if "to help" is a clear duty. Does this go beyond the standard of care? Is it implicit in the standard of care? Are health care professionals called "helping professionals" with reason? Proponents of this moral principle certainly believe that helping patients is an essential moral principle. Society expects medical employees to make reasonable sacrifices for their patients.

Society certainly adheres to this principle of helping or beneficence by providing immunization programs, dental fluoride programs, and water treatment plants, to name a few examples. Medicare and Medicaid programs are further examples of beneficence by society. There are limits, however. How helpful shall office personnel be?

> *We should act in such a way as to bring about the greatest benefit and the least harm.*[3]

Sometimes called the principle of utility, this principle means that "Actions are right in proportion as they tend to promote happiness, wrong as they tend to produce the reverse of happiness.... The 'utility' or the 'usefulness' of an action is determined by the extent to which it produces happiness."[3]

An action by itself may be right or wrong. What is important is the consequence of the act. For example, performing a diagnostic test is not correct or right in all cases. The risk may be too great for some patients. The consequence of performing the diagnostic test is the determining factor rather than the act (the diagnostic test) itself.

What should be done in the following case? A 56-year-old woman requests further diagnostic testing because she believes she may have cancer. The physician sees no medical need. According to the utility principle, this patient's happiness is dependent on her receiving the additional testing. The cost, the risks, or the medical necessity of further diagnostic testing may not enter into this patient's thought processes. What should be done?

A 36-year-old woman with severe angina refuses a medically needed stress test because a friend experienced a cardiac arrest a few months ago during such a test. What should happen in this case? Who decides? What is the greatest benefit? What is the least harm?

> *Similar cases ought to be treated in similar ways. This principle expresses the notion that justice involves fairness of treatment.*[3]

Patients can expect—even demand—to be treated justly by medical employees. This principle of justice, however, leaves unanswered questions. What about *equality*? Is everyone treated the same in all respects? What about *need*? If services are to be doled out according to individual need, do those who have a greater need receive a greater share? What about people's *contribution* to society? When not everyone can receive an equal portion or has an exact need, do physicians and office personnel consider what contribution that person can make to society? What about individual *effort*? Does someone living a healthy life-style deserve more than someone who abuses his or her body? What is fair? What is just?

Consider, for example, a 45-year-old man who has hypertension. His condition requires frequent office visits and medications, neither of which he can afford. Should the office employee make appointments for this patient? Should the physician be obligated to see this patient?

> *Rational individuals should be permitted to be self-determining.... We act autonomously when our actions are the result of our own choices and decisions. Thus, autonomy and self-determination are equivalent.*[3]

In other words, patients are qualified to decide what is best for them. Patients are their own moral agents, able to assume responsibility for their own actions.

Medical personnel need to act without threat of coercion to their patients. Medical personnel need to offer any and all available options to patients without duress. Medical employees need to clarify information provided to patients by physician employers. Medical personnel are agents of their physician employer and, as such, need to act according to their employer's wishes.

What about a 76-year-old man who requests medical verification that he is competent to drive his car? He has Alzheimer's disease with severe intellectual impairment. Is this patient rational? Who determines his competency if the courts refuse? Whose choice is it, the physician's or the patient's?

Consider a 25-year-old mentally retarded man who refuses medical treatment for gonorrhea. He insists he does not need the care or any follow-up. Who is responsible for this patient? Who should make the choices? What are the implications of the decision?

There seem to be more questions than answers. Physicians and office personnel find themselves in these ethical dilemmas daily. Moral principles are necessary to help them consider their options and their patients' choices.

The five moral principles offer some guidelines for rational actions. The principles provide food for thought, a basis for analysis.

Readers may already have adopted some of these principles without being aware of it. Some may choose to ignore all principles in lieu of their own morals. No principle by itself can solve all ethical dilemmas. Some, however, are stronger for individuals to adopt. Medical personnel need to think through these principles. They need to clarify their personal and medical ethics.

ETHICS AND PROFESSIONALISM FOR MEDICAL PERSONNEL

A profession must have a code of ethics to profess its general, cultural, and moral trends, that is, its own personal conviction. If medicine had no ethical code, this profession would be vulnerable to whatever religious, popular, or legal trends were fashionable. It would succumb to whatever the most powerful forces are. Ethics provide a tradition to medicine, one that can withstand the whims of society.

A code of ethics is essential to inform the public what the practice of medicine means. Health care practitioners are not merely technicians; rather, patterns of practice exist. A code of ethics provides the central point of orientation for professional life in medicine and for medical personnel.

The reasons for the continuation of a code of ethics for medical employees do not imply that such a code means there are no conflicts or that the practice of medicine remains unchanged. Rather, the contrary exists. A code of ethics demands conflicting views and encourages tension and debate. There is no one answer for medicine and its practices. However, medicine is unique, which requires the code to be unique too.

Medicine is notable because health care professionals are dealing with sick persons who are dependent and vulnerable. Patients generally are in an exploitable state. Think about the patient in the white gown, lying down on the examination table, undergoing a physical examination. Who is in control? Who is dependent?

Further, medical knowledge is obtained through the privilege of a medical education. Physicians' knowledge is not proprietary. Society says it is acceptable to invade a person's privacy, to experiment with human subjects. Therefore, physicians' knowledge is not individually owned; rather, it is to be used for the good of the sick. Care of the ill is certainly unique.

Medical personnel working with physicians need to remember how patients feel when in the medical office. They also need to be aware of how to use their skill and knowledge to benefit patients rather than for any self-interest. Patients need to make their own decisions based on medical information offered by physicians and medical personnel. Medical personnel need standards by which to care for the ill.

Code of Ethics

Medical assistants have a code of ethics adopted by their professional organization, the AAMA. It is as follows:

AMERICAN ASSOCIATION OF MEDICAL ASSISTANTS CODE OF ETHICS

The Code of Ethics of the AAMA shall set forth principles of ethical and moral conduct as they relate to the medical profession and the particular practice of medical assisting.

Members of the AAMA dedicated to the conscientious pursuit of their profession, and thus desiring to merit the high regard of the entire medical profession and the respect of the general public which they serve, do pledge themselves to strive always to:

A. render service with full respect for the dignity of humanity;
B. respect confidential information obtained through employment unless legally authorized or required by responsible performance of duty to divulge such information;
C. uphold the honor and high principles of the profession and accept its disciplines;
D. seek to continually improve the knowledge and skills of medical assistants for the benefit of patients and professional colleagues;
E. participate in additional service activities aimed toward improving the health and well-being of the community.

CREED

I believe in the principles and purposes of the profession of medical assisting.
I endeavor to be more effective.
I aspire to render greater service.
I protect the confidence entrusted to me.
I am dedicated to the care and well-being of all patients.
I am loyal to my physician employer.
I am true to the ethics of my profession.
I am strengthened by compassion, courage, and faith.

The code of ethics is general in nature yet sets specific parameters for the medical assistant. Medical assistants should respect patients. Medical assistants should maintain patient confidentiality. Medical assistants must act professionally. Medical assistants should continue their education in an effort to benefit patients. Lastly, medical assistants are obligated to become active in their community in an effort to improve its health and well-being.

Another code of ethics applies to Registered Medical Assistants and is provided by the American Medical Technologists. Their code is similar to AAMA's in that it is general in nature and encourages medical assistants to adhere to the highest of standards, principles, and traditions.

To consistently adhere to these codes of ethics, medical assistants would be superhumans. All professionals must strive for such perfection. Ethical standards are values. They are the *shoulds,* the *oughts,* of the practice of medicine and of medical assisting.

"Developing Ethics Related to the Analysis of the Profession"

An ethical code provides standards by which to measure a profession such as medical assisting. But how does one analyze whether a professional has the competencies needed to practice? The AAMA devised a tool, called *"Developing A Curriculum"* (DACUM), which defines eight general areas of competency.[4] These competencies are

- Display professionalism
- Communicate
- Perform administrative duties
- Perform clinical duties
- Apply legal concepts to practice
- Manage the office
- Provide instruction
- Manage practice finances

Entry-level skills and advanced skills of medical assisting are identified within each competency. How does this relate to ethics?

The DACUM provides an occupational analysis with ethics as a common thread through all eight competencies. For instance, "Display professionalism" includes "perform within ethical boundaries." The code of ethics tells medical assistants how to behave. Included in the "Communicate" competency is the skill "treat all patients with empathy and impartiality." How do medical assistants do that? Obviously, they need to be unbiased. They need to know their personal codes of ethics and have thought through their codes of medical ethics. Are they acting within their physicians' codes of ethics?

Within the competency "Perform administrative duties" is "prepare and maintain medical records." Once all the legal ramifications are followed, the ethical issues of medical records pervade. For example, medical assistants read data in medical records. Can they discuss such information at lunch with other medical assistants? Is this a legal and ethical issue?

The competency "Perform clinical duties" contains the skill "prepare patients for procedures." What if the procedure is one medical assistants find offensive? Do medical assistants exhibit behavior to the patient that might indicate their dislike for the procedure? What should medical assistants do?

All other competencies have ethical implications. "Apply legal concepts to practice": Can a law be unethical? Yes, for some medical assistants it may be legal but unethical. For instance, abortion is legal but a medical assistant may firmly believe that abortion is wrong. "Manage the office" spells out the skill "operate and maintain facilities and equipment safely." What if the medical assistant forgets to clean a particular piece of equipment and, when asked to use it, decides it is "OK this time" and does not tell anyone it is not clean? "Provide instruction" to patients with special needs is a skill in the DACUM. What if the medical assistant does not like handicapped patients? Will the assistant's attitude be conveyed to such a patient? Is this treatment ethical? Lastly, the competency "Manage practice finances" includes "implement current procedural terminology and ICD-9 coding." What if the medical assistant codes incorrectly and receives money for procedures the physician did not perform? Does it make a difference if the assistant did not know initially, but discovers it later?

Medical ethics permeate most of the competencies that medical assistants are asked to possess. If medical assistants are to be ethical in deed and act, they need to be skilled and willing to use those skills in a manner that is not in conflict with their professional code of ethics.

THE ETHICS OF CONFIDENTIALITY

Confidentiality is a legal and ethical issue in medicine. The term *confidential* means imparted in secret; therefore, the information the patient shares with the physician is to be kept confidential. No one is to know the information, and no one is to share the information unless the patient gives permission. The right to privacy is the patient's right, not the physician's. This means the patient determines when the information can or cannot be shared.

> **SPECIAL HINT**
>
> Some state laws do not recognize the patient–physician relationship, so medical personnel need to be knowledgeable about their state laws concerning confidentiality.

The ethics of confidentiality begin with trust. The patient trusts the physician and office employees to keep the information confidential. The patient may feel shame or vulnerability if any information is subsequently shared inappropriately by physicians or office employees. Medical personnel can do much to increase the confidentiality of information obtained from patient records, telephone calls, and in-office visits. Meticulous care must be taken to ensure privacy of patients. Of course, third parties may have access to patient information. However, medical personnel need to know when it is necessary to obtain the patient's authorization to release information. It is prudent, too, to inform patients when information is released.

For example, is it necessary to obtain permission to release the following information? Is this an ethical question? A 24-year-old wife asks the family physician what her husband was treated for last week. She had received her husband's medical bill and was curious as to why he was seeing the physician.

Most patients, especially those who have worked in the medical field, worry about the rather mundane breaches of confidentiality that occur in hallways, elevators, cafeterias, neighborhoods, and social gatherings. Medical personnel need to be aware of who they are sharing medical information with and when they are sharing the information.

> **SPECIAL HINT**
>
> Remember to maintain confidentiality at all times.

THE ETHICS OF CONSENT

Giving informed consent is a legal and ethical issue. The ethics are detailed here. In ambulatory care, medical personnel may assist physicians in numerous treatments and procedures during a day. In most cases, the patient risks are negligible, so the ethical conflicts are few. Also, patients may informally receive treatment information over a period of several visits to the physician's office, rather than at one single visit.

Does this mean patients in ambulatory care do not need to be expressly informed? Quite the contrary. Patients do have to make choices about their care. Patients need to be autonomous. What is needed for ambulatory patients and informed consent is a "transparency model" as described in the *Hastings Center Report*.[5] This report is one in which "disclosure is adequate when the physician's basic thinking has been rendered transparent to the patient."[6] The physician tells the patient about the treatment, allowing the patient to participate by asking questions and entering into the reasoning process with the physician so that the patient can see how the physician arrived at the recommended treatment. The transparency model is one where physicians disclose information as required by the law but in a more conversational mode. Ethically, informed consent is "an ongoing process of conversation designed to maximize patient participation after adequately revealing the key facts."[5]

BIOETHICAL ISSUES IN AMBULATORY CARE

Medical office employees face bioethical issues. The prefix *bio* indicates a relationship to life, emphasizing the values or ethics of life issues. "Bioethics refers to the moral issues and problems that have arisen as a result of modern medicine and research."[6] Bioethics involve both ethical and medical issues.

News reports keep individuals abreast of the latest and hottest bioethical issues. Think, for example, about surrogacy. Baby M is now old news. Remember Karen Ann Quinlan? Euthanasia and the right to remove or withhold treatment to allow death with dignity are old news. But what about assisting in suicide? What are the issues now?

Medical personnel working in ambulatory care face patient rights and responsibility issues every day. The American Hospital Association (AHA) developed a Statement on a Patient's Bill of Rights that addresses patient rights when patients are hospitalized.[6] Patient rights include the right to

- Confidentiality
- Informed consent
- Information concerning their care
- Continuity of care
- Respectful care

The Bill of Rights does not, however, directly address patient responsibility. Does that mean patients do not have responsibility? Is a patient's responsibility understood? Whatever the reason for AHA's omission of patient responsibility, it is important to remember when caring for patients that patients have rights *and* responsibilities. They should be in control of their lives. Also, medical employees are agents of their physician employers, which means medical personnel act on their employers' behalf. Perhaps this places medical personnel in a precarious position, but, viewed positively, medical personnel are agents of patients and agents of their physician employers' acting on behalf of both.

Patients' Right to Health Care

Is health care a right or a privilege? Many would argue that basic health care is a right. But who defines "basic health care"? In 1983 the President's Commission for the Study of Ethical Problems in Medicine and Biomedical and Behavioral Research published a report entitled *Securing Access to Health Care.*[7] The report concluded that health care is not a right; rather, health care is a societal ethical obligation balanced without excessive individual obligation. Who determines what is fair and what is just health care?

Oregon has defined a model of rationing of health care that may prove to be a first.[8] The Oregon Legislative Assembly passed a bill to guarantee access to a basic level of health care for all Oregonians. The bill provides economic incentives to providers for employing those services and procedures that are effective and appropriate in preference to those that are marginal or unproven. Oregon says that every citizen is guaranteed access to the health care system.

Is Oregon's model one that the rest of the nation should emulate? Is Canada's model better? Canada has a universal health care coverage policy that is publicly administered with a single-payer program. The Canadian government negotiates the price of all major medical services with the various doctor groups. Is either of these two health programs better than what commonly exists in the United States, where health care costs are soaring? Couple the high cost of medical care with the rapid increase in medical technology and ask, "Should all patients have access to health care?" Should one refer to the moral principles defined earlier and pass legislation that only those who can contribute to society receive health care? Shall only the rich receive adequate health care? Who decides?

Medical office personnel need to be aware that they, too, make microallocation decisions regarding patients' access to health care. For instance, when employees have two or more patients vying for one appointment slot, how do they decide who gets the appointment when two patients are similar in medical need? On what basis is that decision made? Also, what about the hypertensive patient described earlier who needs to see the physician and needs prescribed medication but can afford neither? Should that patient receive medical attention even though he cannot afford it? Is health care a right or a privilege?

The type of medical insurance coverage may determine whether patients receive medical care. Some physicians may refuse to see patients who do not have full medical insurance benefits; others may want cash up front. Who makes decisions about whether physicians in a particular medical office are participating or nonparticipating physicians for some types of insurance? Who talks to the patients on the telephone and informs them that they can or cannot see the physician? Do office personnel bill the insurance company or does the patient? Is health care a right or a privilege?

Patients' Right to Live or to Die

Early in June 1990, Dr. Jack Kevorkian assisted Janet Adkins, 54 years old, in her effort to kill herself.[9] Mrs. Adkins, diagnosed with Alzheimer's disease, wanted to die with dignity. Dr. Kevorkian inserted an intravenous (IV) device into Mrs. Adkins's arm. When Mrs. Adkins wanted to die, she pressed a button that stopped the IV salt water and replaced it with a barbiturate used in executions. After a minute, the IV solution switched to potassium chloride which caused cardiac arrest and death. Dr. Kevorkian designed the device. He was charged with murder but under public pressure, the charges were dropped. He subsequently assisted another person to die using his device. Is this legal? Is it ethical?

There are patients who wish to live even though they are very ill. These patients may require artificial means to keep them alive such as kidney dialysis or life support systems. Who decides what is artificial and what is not? Are food and water considered artificial? Is medication to relieve pain considered artificial?

Medical personnel generally do not enter into the decision-making process of allowing patients to live or permitting patients to die. Their physician employers, however, may. What medical personnel need to be concerned about is discussing with patients their thoughts about death and life, their right to live and their right to die.

Most states have living wills, sometimes referred to as natural death acts, which are legal documents defining patients' right to die preferences.

SPECIAL HINT

Medical personnel must be knowledgeable about their state laws concerning living wills.

Some states require a lawyer to draw up such a contract; others allow patients to prepare their own fashioned after the state law. If in doubt about your state laws, ask your legal counsel.

Patients may have a durable power of attorney, which means that they have designated another person as their attorney when they can no longer speak or act on their own behalf. The person who acts on the patient's behalf knows what the patient desires and will communicate with the patient's physician.

SPECIAL HINT

Each state has its own definition of durable power of attorney, and it would behoove medical personnel to be knowledgeable of their state laws.

Patients' Right to Procreate or to Abort

With the advent of high technology in medicine, the choice to procreate poses many options formerly unknown. Now women may choose a surrogate to offer them a birth option. Women may select artificial insemination by husband or by donor. Procreation may occur as a result of in vitro fertilization (IVF). Frozen sperm may be used. The options are numerous. Technology will continue to pose alternatives in and questions about procreation.

Who should decide what method(s) to use? Will surrogacy or IVF pose any problems to the babies born? What about the effects of such options on society? Are there ethical and legal ramifications? Who will pay? Who can afford such technology? Who deserves such technology?

SPECIAL HINT

Medical personnel need to be knowledgeable about the methods of procreation and their uses and the state laws concerning procreation. Once medical personnel know about birth options, they must clarify their values and ethical stance.

Abortion is an ethical dilemma for some and a political issue for many. When does life begin? Does life begin at conception, at the time of birth, or somewhere in between? Lewis and Warden describe three ethical issues concerning abortion: (1) "Are there any reasons to justify abortions?" (2) "Are current laws regarding abortions consistent, fair, and just?" (3) "Are abortions an appropriate method of birth control?"[6] Obviously, these three questions create more questions than answers.

> **SPECIAL HINT**
>
> Medical personnel need to be aware of federal and state laws concerning abortion and medical personnel rights as caregivers as well.

Medical personnel need to clarify for themselves where they stand on abortion issues. Will they assist in an abortion? Will they care for patients who want an abortion? As with most ethical dilemmas, there are no uniform right answers—only answers that medical personnel clarify for themselves.

PRACTICAL IMPLICATIONS OF ETHICS AND BIOETHICS FOR MEDICAL PERSONNEL IN AMBULATORY CARE

The "Ethics Check" Questions

Situations that pose ethical questions occur with enough frequency in the medical office that practical approaches are necessary. The "Ethics Check" questions, posed by Blanchard and Peale,[10] offer a practical approach to solving ethical dilemmas. When you are faced with an ethical dilemma, ask the following three questions:

1. Is it legal?
2. Is it balanced?
3. How will it make me feel about myself?[10]

If the answer to any one of the three questions is no, the situation is unethical, according to Blanchard and Peale. The first question asks if the situation violates any federal or state law or any office policy. If, for instance, state law deems the act illegal, the situation is unethical. If a physician employer or office policy views the situation as wrong, it is considered unethical.

The second question addresses the fairness of the situation. Does it cause someone to win and someone to lose? If so, it is unethical. The situation as should promote a win–win relationship.

The third question focuses on an individual's morality or personal code of ethics. Ask yourself, "If the situation is published in the local newspaper, will I feel good?" On a more personal level, ask yourself, "If my family knows about the situation, will I feel good?" If the answer is yes, the situation is ethical. If the answer is no, then it is unethical.

To summarize Blanchard and Peale's "Ethics Check": If the answer to any one of the three questions is no or maybe, the situation is unethical. Use these three questions when in doubt about the ethicality of a situation. The questions may help to clarify your ethical position.

What to Do When You Don't Know What to Do

Medical personnel need to be knowledgeable about ethical and bioethical issues in the ambulatory care setting. Personal values clarification and verification of ethical beliefs help medical personnel recognize ethical dilemmas when they occur in themselves, patients, and co-workers. Ethical dilemmas need to be recognized, discussed, and faced so that effective patient care can continue.

If medical personnel find themselves in an uncomfortable ethical situation and do not know what to do, several options exist. They may select to do nothing, but just "be there" for the patient. A caring attitude may be all that is necessary. Or, they may choose to confront the patient or physician and patient with the ethical issue. Acknowledgment and discussion of the ethical dilemma may be essential for its resolution. Or medical personnel may decide to discuss the ethical issue with fellow employees or employer. Discussion with others sometimes alleviates anxiety and fear. It is wise, too, to realize that ethical issues may not be resolved. Ethical issues may cause frustration and confusion, regardless of what is tried.

Sometimes talking is not enough. Sometimes outside help is needed. Referrals to outside agencies may be necessary. Medical personnel may need to discuss with their employers an appropriate referral.

Actions speak louder than words. Medical employees' ethics may "show" even though they may wish to hide them from patients. Medical employees may have been taught that neutrality is the best policy.

> **SPECIAL HINT**
>
> No matter what stance is taken, remember, nonverbal behavior speaks and, many times, speaks louder than verbal language.

Ethical Dos and Don'ts

Office personnel are encouraged to wear their own ethics, not someone else's. Medical personnel function as professionals much better if they know their beliefs and work with them rather than against them.

Too many times medical office personnel get "should" upon. Employers, fellow employees, and patients may tell personnel how they should act, what they should do, and what they should say. When someone tries to tell employees what to do ethically, they begin to feel uncomfortable. It is then time to clarify one's individual stance and act on it, but not at the expense of others, especially patients.

- When patients ask for advice, office personnel need to be careful. Listen. Let patients make their own decisions and permit them to assume responsibility for their own behavior. Offer options and information, not opinions.
- It is best to be caring and nonjudgmental. What works for oneself may not work for patients. Each patient has his or her own circumstances. One needs to allow patients to decide their best action.
- Office personnel need to allow patients independence, not dependency. People feel confidence when they make their own decisions. They feel self-worth. People can become self-sufficient. Allow for success and for failure.
- It is best not to moralize for, or to, patients. Patients are people with rights and responsibilities. Patients have their own personal code of ethics. They know what is right for them.
- Lastly, medical personnel need to take care of themselves. Being healthy and loving oneself allow one to care for others.

Medical personnel work in an arena of ethical dilemmas. Sometimes answers to ethical dilemmas are obvious and fairly easy to define. Other times, answers may be nonexistent. It helps to clarify one's values, to be nonjudgmental with patients, and to be caring.

References

1. Connelly JE, DalleMura S: Ethical problems in the medical office. *Journal of the American Medical Association* 260:812–815, 1988.
2. Thomas CL (Ed): *Taber's Cyclopedic Medical Dictionary*, 16th ed. Philadelphia, F.A. Davis, 1989, p. 626.
3. Munson R: *Intervention and Reflection: Basic Issues in Medical Ethics*. Belmont, CA: Wadsworth, 1988.
4. Seibert ML, Amos PA: DACUM revisited: The 1990 update on the profession of medical assisting. *The Professional Medical Assistant* 23(3):17–20, May/June, 1990.
5. Brody H: Transparency: Informed consent in primary care. *Hastings Center Report* 19(5):5–9, 1989.
6. Lewis M, Warden CD: *Laws and Ethics in the Medical Office, Including Bioethical Issues*. Philadelphia: F.A. Davis, 1988, p. 215.
7. Sass HM: Justice, beneficence, or common sense?: The President's Commission's Report on Access to Health Care. *The Journal of Medicine and Philosophy* 8:383, 1983.
8. Hasnain R, Garland M: *Health Care in Common: Report of the Oregon Health Decisions Community Meetings Process*. April, 1990.
9. Atman LK: Janet Adkins' death intensifies the debate. *The Sun* [Bremerton, WA], June 14, 1990.
10. Blanchard K, Peale NV: *The Power of Ethical Management*. New York: William Morrow, 1988.

Bibliography

Altruism, self-interest, and medical ethics (editorial). *Journal of the American Medical Association* 258:1939–1940.
American Association of Medical Assistants: *Law for the Medical Office*. Chicago: American Association of Medical Assistants, 1984.
Beauchamp TL, Childress JF: *Principles of Biomedical Ethics*, 2nd ed. New York: Oxford University Press, 1983.
Blocker JN: Ethics: Fundamental to professionalism. *The Professional Medical Assistant* 23(3):25–27, May/June 1990.
Childress JF: The place of autonomy in bioethics. *Hastings Center Report* 20(1):12–17, 1990.
Christie RJ, Hoffmaster CB: *Ethical Issues in Family Medicine*. New York: Oxford University Press, 1986.
Christie RJ, Hoffmaster CB, Bass MJ, McCracken E: How family physicians approach ethical problems. *Journal of Family Practice* 16:1133–1138, 1983.
Churchill LR: Reviving a distinctive medical ethic. *Hastings Center Report* 19(3):28–34, 1989.
Dayringer R, Paiva REA, Davidson GM: Ethical decision making by family physicians. *Journal of Family Practice* 17:267–272, 1983.
Dolenc Emery D, Schneiderman LJ: Cost-effectiveness analysis in health care. *Hastings Center Report* 19(4):8–13, 1989.
Evans RW: Health care technology and the inevitability of resource allocation and rationing decisions, part I. *Journal of the American Medical Association* 249:2047–2053, 1983.
Evans RW: Health care technology and the inevitability of resource allocation and rationing decisions, part II. *Journal of the American Medical Association* 249:2208–2219, 1983.
Flight MR: Setting a standard of care for medical assistants, part I. *The Professional Medical Assistant*, January/February, 1985, pp. 10–19.
Flight MR: Setting a standard of care for medical assistants, part II. *The Professional Medical Assistant*, March/April, 1985, pp. 12–19.
Glendon MA: Abortion: Searching for common ground. Is there life after Roe v. Wade? *Hastings Center Report* 19(4):22–29, August 1989.
Kitzhaber J: Rationing health care: The Oregon model. *The Center Report* [The Center for Public Policy and Contemporary Issues, Vol. 2, No. 1, University of Denver] 2(1):1–6, 1990.
Lewis-Chermak MA: *Applications of Case Law in Selected Bioethical Issues Related to the Medical Office Setting*. Doctoral dissertation in education, Seattle University, Seattle, WA, 1987.

President's Commission for the Study of Ethical Problems in Medicine and Biomedical and Behavioral Research: *Deciding to Forego Life-Sustaining Treatment: A Report on the Ethical, Medical, and Legal Issues in Treatment Decisions.* Washington, DC: U.S. Government Printing Office, 1983.

President's Commission for the Study of Ethical Problems in Medicine and Biomedical and Behavioral Research: *Making Health Care Decisions: A Report on the Ethical and Legal Implications of Informed Consent in the Patient-Practitioner Relationship* (3 vols). Washington, DC: U.S. Government Printing Office, 1982.

President's Commission for the Study of Ethical Problems in Medicine and Biomedical and Behavioral Research: *Securing Access to Health Care: The Ethical Implications of Differences in Availability of Health Services* (3 vols). Washington, DC: U.S. Government Printing Office, 1983.

Chapter 13

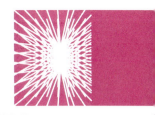

MEDICAL LAW

LISA McCOLLUM

REGULATION OF MEDICAL OFFICES
Sources of Information Regarding Federal and State Laws
Branches of Law

CREDENTIALING OF HEALTH CARE PERSONNEL
Licensure
Certification
Registration

MEDICAL ASSISTING PRACTICE
Laboratory Testing
Venipuncture and Injections
Radiography

MEDICAL PROFESSIONAL LIABILITY
Contracts
Standard of Care
Statute of Limitations
Insurance

PATIENT CARE
Emergency Aid
Appointments
Consent
Minors

MEDICAL RECORDS
Ownership and Access
Retention
Confidentiality
Disposal

PUBLIC HEALTH REPORTING REQUIREMENTS

COMPREHENSIVE DRUG ABUSE PREVENTION AND CONTROL ACT OF 1970
Registration
Record-Keeping
Inventory
Prescriptions

DRUG SCREENING

UNIFORM ANATOMICAL GIFT ACT OF 1968

DEATH AND DYING
Living Wills
Durable Power of Attorney for Health Care
Withdrawal of Life Support

MONITORING LEGISLATION

This chapter is intended to be a reference source for medicolegal information that is frequently needed by medical assistants. It does not contain the depth of information included in a medical law course or text and should not take the place of either. If more information is needed on a topic, resources are listed at the end of this chapter. A glossary of legal terms is also included.

REGULATION OF MEDICAL OFFICES

Medical offices are regulated by federal, state, and local laws. Federal laws are the same for every state. State laws, called *statutes* or *statutory laws,* may be different in each state.

> **SPECIAL HINT**
>
> It is vital that physicians and medical office personnel know what the law is in their state. In situations where a state law is deemed to be equivalent to the requirements of a federal law, the state law is enforced.

The Supremacy Clause of the U.S. Constitution holds that federal law is supreme to state law in cases of conflict. This chapter offers information that is generally applicable to all medical offices. However, know the laws that regulate medical and business practices in your state to ensure compliance.

Sources of Information Regarding Federal and State Laws

Public Library

Federal, state, and local laws and regulations are in the reference section of the library. State laws usually are contained in two sets of books. One set is the actual text of the law itself, usually

Public Law

Criminal Law	Constitutional Law	Administrative Law	International Law
Arson	Civil rights	Consumer protection	Arms control
Bribery	Federal and State powers	Environmental protection	Extradition
Burglary	Relations between states	Interstate commerce	Hijacking and piracy
Extortion	Separation of executive, judicial and legislative powers	Public safety	Human rights
Forgery		Social welfare	Territorial waters
Kidnapping		Taxation	Uses of outer space
Larceny		Workers' wages and hours	Uses of ocean
Manslaughter			War crimes
Murder			
Perjury			
Rape			
Robbery			

Private Law

Contract and Commercial Law	Tort Law	Property Law
Credit purchases	Invasion of privacy	Landlord-tenant relations
Employment contracts	Personal injury	Mortgages
Guarantees	Professional malpractice	Transfer of ownership
Insurance policies	Slander and libel	Unclaimed property
Patents	Traffic accidents	
Promissory notes	Trespass	
Sales contracts	Unfair competition	
Subscriptions		

Inheritance Law	Family Law	Corporation Law
Estates	Adoption	Corporation finance
Probate	Annulment	Documents of incorporation
Trusts	Divorce	Mergers and acquisitions
Wills	Marriage	

Excerpted from: World Book Encyclopedia, 1983 edition, volume 12, 120e and 120f.

FIGURE 13-1

Branches of the law. (Excerpted from *World Book Encyclopedia*, vol. 12. Chicago: World Book, 1983, p. 120e, 120f; in American Association of Medical Assistants: *Law for the Medical Office,* Chicago, 1984, p. 6.)

called the "registered code." The other set is the rules and regulations that are written to help administer the law, usually called the "administrative code." Both sets of information should be consulted.

State Medical Association

Many state medical associations publish a booklet that identifies and interprets state laws that affect physicians' practices in that state. They may also have a legislative department that can provide information on state and federal laws and legal forms specific to that state.

The Physician's Professional Liability Insurance Carrier

The physician's liability insurance company has information on the laws in that state. Many companies have risk management departments that can provide you with information, recommendations, and legal forms.

State Medical Assistant Society

The legislation committee of the State Medical Assistant Society may have information available or may direct you to a source that can answer your questions.

State Attorney General's Office

The State Attorney General's office can answer questions regarding existing state law and how it is interpreted in that state. This office can be found in your state office listings in the telephone book.

Branches of Law

Laws in the United States can be divided into two broad categories: public and private law. Public law defines and enforces the rights and responsibilities of the government to its people and the rights and responsibilities of the people to the government. Private law, or civil law, governs the activities between and among private cit-

---

EMPLOYMENT LAWS
    Health and safety:
        Occupational Safety and Health Act of 1970 (OSHA)
    Wages and hours:
        Fair Labor Standards Act
    Collective bargaining and union activities:
        National Labor Relations Act (Wagner Act)
        Labor Management Relations Act (Taft-Hartley Act)
    Discrimination in employment:
        Title VII, The Civil Rights Act of 1964
        Equal Pay Act of 1963
        Age Discrimination in Employment Act
    Retirement:
        Employment Retirement Income Security Act (ERISA)
ANTITRUST LAWS
    Sherman Act
    Federal Trade Commission Act
    Clayton Act
    Robinson-Patman Act
CONSUMER PROTECTION LAWS
    Federal Trade Commission Act (1914)
    Consumer Credit Protection Act (Truth in Lending Act, 1969)
    Fair Credit Reporting Act (1974)
    Equal Credit Opportunity Act (1977)
    Fair Debt Collection Practices Act (1977)
    Bankruptcy Act, Revised (1978)

FIGURE 13-2
Federal laws that regulate medical office business.

Medical practice acts
   Physician
   Nursing
   Other allied health professionals
Confidentiality
Informed consent
Statute of limitations on tort actions
Abortion
Sterilization
Natural death acts/living wills
Removal of life support
Public health reporting requirements
   Births
   Deaths
   Communicable diseases
   Sexually transmitted diseases
   Human immunodeficiency virus and acquired immune deficiency syndrome
   Injuries
      Gunshot and knife wounds
      Assault
      Rape
   Abuse and neglect
      Children
      Elderly
   Industrial poisoning
   Controlled substance abuse
Worker's Compensation
Wage statutes

FIGURE 13-3
Subsections found in most state laws that regulate medical practices.

izens. Each of these categories can be subdivided further (Figure 13-1).

Medical offices are affected by almost every branch of law. Some of the most important federal laws that regulate business and employment are listed in Figure 13-2. Other chapters in this book can provide you with information on how these laws apply to a medical practice. Laws that regulate the practice of medicine are primarily state laws. These laws can be very different in each state.

SPECIAL HINT

Medical office personnel should be familiar with the state laws pertinent to the subjects listed in Figure 13-3. (See Appendix D.)

CREDENTIALING OF HEALTH CARE PERSONNEL

Regulation of an occupation involves some form of credentialing. Credentialing in health care is the recognition of professional or technical competence by the state or federal government, private or professional organizations, and certifying organizations. Regulation may

- Control entry into the field
- Limit the performance of certain procedures to a specific occupation
- Establish a minimum standard of training, knowledge, and skill
- Ensure the competence of health care personnel

Licensure

The primary responsibility for regulating the health care professions remains with the states, by virtue of their right to legislate to protect the health, welfare, and safety of their citizens. Licensing is the mechanism that states have used for this purpose, and each state has the right to establish its own licensing standards.

Occupational licensure laws have traditionally regulated the quality of services provided by independent practitioners or occupations that have little or no supervision. Licensure laws have been spreading to many of the dependent allied health occupations, in which workers work under the supervision of a licensed health care practitioner.

Licensure is the most restrictive form of regulation. It prohibits anyone from engaging in activities covered by the prescribed scope of practice in a license without permission from a government agency.

State Medical Practice Acts

A medical practice act is a state statute governing the practice of medicine. Physicians are licensed under the medical practice act of their state. Practicing medicine is generally defined as diagnosing, treating, and/or prescribing treatment for a physical or mental condition. A person cannot perform any of the activities outlined in a state's medical practice act unless he or she is licensed to do so in another practice act in that state, such as the nursing practice act or the physician's assistant practice act.

Certification

Certification, a voluntary credential, is the process by which a nongovernmental agency or association grants recognition to persons meeting predetermined qualifications specified by that agency or organization. This is the credentialing mechanism used by most professional associations.

Certified Medical Assistant

The Certified Medical Assistant Examination is offered by the Certifying Board of the American Association of Medical Assistants (AAMA). For an application or more information, contact:

> AAMA Certification Department
> 20 North Wacker Drive, Suite 1575
> Chicago, IL 60606
> 1-800-228-2262

Registration

Registration is the least restrictive form of regulation. It is the process by which qualified individuals are listed on an official roster maintained by a governmental or nongovernmental agency or board. This listing is to identify the practitioner and may not require any qualification examinations.

Registered Medical Assistant

The Registered Medical Assistant Examination is offered by American Medical Technologists. For an application or more information contact:

> Registered Medical Assistants
> 710 Higgins Road
> Park Ridge, IL 60068-5765
> (708) 823-5169

MEDICAL ASSISTING PRACTICE

Medical assistants are not licensed as an occupation in any state. Many states grant physicians the right to delegate certain clinical tasks to qualified allied health care personnel by a clause in the medical, nursing, or physician assistant practice act. The language in the statute would exempt medical assistants from licensure requirements and allow them to perform certain clinical tasks under the delegation and supervision of a licensed health care practitioner.

According to Donald Balasa, staff legal counsel for the AAMA, there are currently 19 states that have no statutory language authorizing the doctor's right to delegate clinical procedures to unlicensed health care personnel (Balasa D: *State Health Legislation Report* 18(1):5, 1990). If no legal challenge to medical assisting practice is raised in these states, the current delegation practice can continue.

Laboratory Testing

In 1987 Congress passed the Omnibus Budget Reconciliation Act, which required physician's office laboratories (POLs) to meet health and safety standards that would be issued by the Department of Health and Human Services. In 1988 the Clinical Laboratory Improvement Amendments (CLIAs) were passed. The regulations to implement the requirements of these two laws address the areas of quality control, quality assurance, record-keeping, and the qualifications of personnel who perform testing procedures in a POL.

The CLIA 1988 Final Rule was published in the *Federal Register* on February 28, 1992. It went into effect on September 1, 1992. The CLIA 1988 regulations apply to anyone who performs laboratory testing for the diagnosis, disease prevention, or treatment of humans.

A copy of the CLIA 1988 Final Rule is found in Appendix D–3 or may be obtained from:

> Superintendent of Documents
> U.S. Government Printing Office
> Washington, DC 20402-9325
> (202) 783-3238

Request the *Federal Register* dated February 28, 1992, stock number 069-001-00042-4. A fee of $3.50 for each copy is required.

States may seek exemption from the federal standards if they have regulations that are equivalent to the CLIA 1988 regulations. Some states have passed their own laws to regulate laboratory work performed in a physician's office. These laws may have more stringent standards that laboratories in that state must meet.

Venipuncture and Injections

Some states require unlicensed health care personnel to have a permit or be registered with the state if they perform venipunctures, injections, or allergy testing, or in some other way pierce human tissue. There could be minimum training standards, testing, and payment of a fee associated with this permit, or registration. In some states it may be illegal for a medical assistant or other allied health care personnel to perform these tasks.

Radiography

Some states require unlicensed health care personnel to obtain a limited permit to expose patients to ionizing radiation. The minimum training standards, testing, and fees vary. According to Donald Balasa, staff legal counsel for the AAMA, the following states have statutes or regulations that affect allied health care personnel who take x-rays:

California
Illinois*
Iowa
Kentucky
Maine
Massachusetts
New Jersey
Oregon
Pennsylvania
Vermont

---

* Medical assistants may not take x-rays in Illinois.

MEDICAL PROFESSIONAL LIABILITY

Contracts

A contract is an agreement between two or more competent people to do or not do something lawful in exchange for payment of some kind. There are three parts to every contract: the offer, the acceptance, and the consideration.

In a medical office the patient offers him- or herself for medical treatment, the physician accepts the patient, and the patient agrees to pay a fee to the doctor for those services. No contract exists until the patient arrives for treatment, and the physician accepts the patient by providing medical care or treatment.

Types of Contracts

Express contracts may be written or verbal and describe specifically what each party to the contract will do. Implied contracts are not indicated by words but by the actions of the parties involved. The majority of physician–patient contracts are implied contracts.

The Statute of Frauds is a law that dictates which contracts must be written in order to be enforceable. Because physician–patient contracts are implied, they are not required to be written to be enforceable. If someone other than the patient agreed to pay the bill for the physician's services, that agreement would need to be in writing to be enforceable.

Termination of Contracts

A breach of contract occurs when one of the parties fails to meet his or her contractual obligations. A physician is obligated to treat a patient until

- The patient's condition no longer needs treatment

or
- The patient discharges the physician

or
- The physician withdraws from the patient's care

Discharge by a Patient. If a patient discharges a physician from his or her care, the physician should send a letter to the patient to confirm and document the termination of the physician–patient contract. An example of such a letter is shown in Figure 13–4. The letter should be mailed by certified mail with a return receipt requested. A copy should be retained in the patient's chart.

FIGURE 13-4

Letter confirming discharge by patient. (Reprinted with permission from *MedicoLegal Forms with Legal Analysis*. Chicago, American Medical Association, 1991.)

Date: _____

Dear _____:

This will confirm our telephone conversation today during which you discharged me from attending you as your physician in your present illness. In my opinion, your condition requires continued medical treatment by a physician. If you have not already obtained the services of another physician, I suggest that you do so without delay. You may be assured that, upon your authorization, I will furnish that physician with information regarding the diagnosis and treatment that you have received from me.

Very truly yours,

_____, M.D.

Withdrawal by a Physician. A physician who withdraws from a patient's care without proper notification can be sued for abandonment if the patient suffers an injury from lack of access to medical care. If a physician chooses to withdraw from a patient's care, he or she must send a letter to the patient to document the termination of the contract. Examples of letters regarding a physician's withdrawing from care are given in Figures 13-5 and 13-6. In situations where the withdrawal from a patient's care is due to noncompliance by the patient, the letter must be sent certified with a return receipt and a copy filed in the chart.

Standard of Care

Malpractice is generally defined as the negligence or carelessness of a professional. Medical liability claims are made for one of three reasons:

Malfeasance: Doing something that is wrong or unlawful.
Misfeasance: Improper performance of a lawful act.

FIGURE 13-5

Letter of withdrawal from attendance. (Reprinted with permission from *MedicoLegal Forms with Legal Analysis*. Chicago, American Medical Association, 1991.)

Date: _____

Dear _____:

I find it necessary to inform you that I am withdrawing from further professional attendance upon you because you have persisted in refusing to follow my medical advice and treatment. Since your condition requires medical attention, I suggest that you place yourself under the care of another physician without delay. If you desire, I shall be available to attend you for a reasonable time after you receive this letter, but in no event for more than ____ days.

This should give you ample time to select a physician of your choice from the many competent practitioners in this city. With your authorization, I will make available to this physician your case history and information regarding the diagnosis and treatment you have received from me.

Very truly yours,

_____, M.D.

```
Date: _____

Dear _____:

Because of _____ (my retirement, reasons of health, etc.)
I am discontinuing the practice of medicine on _____,
19____. I will not be able to attend you professionally after that date.

I suggest that you arrange to place yourself under the care of another
physician. If you are not acquainted with another physician, I suggest
that you contact the _____ (local) Medical Society.

I shall make my records of your case available to the physician you
designate. Since the records of your case are confidential, I shall re-
quire your written authorization to do so. For this reason, I am in-
cluding at the end of this letter an authorization form. Please complete
the form and return it to me.

I am sorry that I cannot continue as your physician. I extend to you
my best wishes for your future health and happiness.

                                          Yours very truly,

                                          _____, M.D.
```

FIGURE 13-6

Letter to discontinue practice. (Reprinted with permission from *MedicoLegal Forms with Legal Analysis*. Chicago, American Medical Association, 1991.)

Nonfeasance: Failure to do something that should have been done.

There are four elements to be proved in a malpractice case. Sometimes these have been called the "Four *D*s" of negligence; see Figure 13-7.

Statute of Limitations

The statute of limitations is the time limit within which people can initiate a lawsuit. These statutes vary greatly from state to state both in how they are determined and the length of time allowed. The statute of limitations in each state determines the length of time a physician must retain medical records on patients. Some common methods used to set time limits are

- Occurrence of negligence—The statutory period would begin when the negligence occurred.
- Last treatment rule—The statutory period

THE FOUR *D*S OF NEGLIGENCE

DUTY
A duty to provide care existed. There is a physician–patient relationship.

DERELICT
The physician was derelict in that duty and failed to adhere to the standard of care.

DAMAGES
The patient must have suffered damages or injuries.

DIRECT CAUSE
The harm suffered by the patient was directly caused by the physician's breach of duty to that patient.

FIGURE 13-7
The four *D*s of negligence.

TABLE 13-1

STATUTES OF LIMITATIONS, TORT ACTIONS*

State	Limitation Period	Minors	Comments
Alabama	2 years after occurrence or 6 months after discovery, with maximum of 4 years after occurrence.	Under 4 until 8th birthday; otherwise adult law.	
Alaska	2 years after discovery.	Adult law applies.	
Arizona	3 years after occurrence.	Until 7th birthday or death; otherwise adult law.	Discovery of foreign objects and intentional concealment extend statutory period.
Arkansas	2 years after occurrence.	1 year after 18th birthday.	Foreign objects or suspicion thereof extends period 1 year from date of discovery.
California	3 years after occurrence or 1 year after discovery, whichever is first.	Under 6 within 3 years or before 8th birthday, whichever is longer; otherwise within 3 years of occurrence. Period extended if parent, guardian, or physician's insurer commits fraud in not acting on behalf of minor.	Fraud, intentional concealment, and foreign objects extend statutory period.
Colorado	2 years from discovery; maximum of 3 years after treatment.	2 years after 6th birthday; otherwise adult law.	Intentional concealment or foreign objects extend beginning date to time of discovery.
Connecticut	2 years from discovery, with maximum of 3 years after occurrence.	Same as adult law.	
Delaware	2 years from occurrence; 1 more year allowed if injury could not have been discovered with reasonable diligence.	Under age 6, three years from occurrence or age 6; otherwise, adult law.	
Florida	2 years from discovery, with maximum of 4 years from occurrence.	Same as adult law.	
Georgia	2 years from occurrence.	Period begins on 18th birthday.	1 year from discovery of foreign object.
Hawaii	2 years from discovery; maximum of 6 years from occurrence.	Period begins on 18th birthday.	Intentional concealment extends period.
Idaho	2 years from occurrence.	6 years from occurrence.	Foreign bodies and intentional concealment extend period. Ionizing radiation injuries must be filed within 3 years of discovery, with maximum of 30 years from occurrence.
Illinois	2 years from discovery; maximum of 4 years from occurrence.	2 years after 18th birthday.	Fraudulent concealment extends period 5 years after discovery.
Indiana	2 years from occurrence.	Under 6 until 8th birthday.	

Table continued on following page

TABLE 13-1
STATUTES OF LIMITATIONS, TORT ACTIONS* Continued

State	Limitation Period	Minors	Comments
Iowa	2 years from discovery; maximum of 6 years after occurrence.	1 year after 18th birthday.	Foreign objects and intentional concealment extend period.
Kansas	2 years from occurrence; maximum of 4 years if it could not have been discovered during first 2 years.	1 year after 18, provided not more than 8 years after occurrence.	2 years after discovery of ionizing radiation injury, with maximum of 4 years after occurrence.
Kentucky	1 year after discovery, with maximum of 5 years after occurrence.	1 year after 18th birthday or 5 years from occurrence.	
Louisiana	1 year after occurrence; 3 years if it could not have been discovered during first year.	Adult law applies.	
Maine	2 years after occurrence.	2 years after 18th birthday.	Intentional concealment and foreign objects extend period to 2 years after discovery.
Maryland	3 years after discovery; 5 years after occurrence, whichever is first.	Period begins on 16th birthday.	
Massachusetts	3 years after occurrence.	Under 6, until 9th birthday; otherwise adult law.	
Michigan	2 years from end of treatment or 6 months from discovery, whichever is later.	1 year after 18th birthday.	2 years after discovery of intentional concealment.
Minnesota	2 years after end of treatment.	2 years after 18th birthday.	Intentional concealment and foreign objects extend period.
Mississippi	2 years after discovery.	2 years after 21.	
Missouri	2 years after occurrence.	Under 10 until 12th birthday.	2 years after discovery of foreign body, with maximum of 10 years after occurrence.
Montana	3 years after occurrence or discovery, whichever is later, with maximum of 5 years after occurrence.		Fraudulent concealment suspends limitation period.
Nebraska	2 years after occurrence or 1 year after discovery with maximum of 6 years after occurrence.		
Nevada	4 years after occurrence or 2 years after discovery, whichever occurs first.	Adult law applies unless injury is brain damage or birth defect, either of which extends period until 10th birthday. Sterility extends period for 2 years after discovery.	Fraudulent concealment suspends period.
New Hampshire	2 years after occurrence.	Period begins after 8th birthday.	Fraudulent concealment and foreign objects extend period 2 years after discovery.

TABLE 13-1

STATUTES OF LIMITATIONS, TORT ACTIONS* *Continued*

State	Limitation Period	Minors	Comments
New Jersey	2 years after discovery.	Until age 23.	
New Mexico	3 years after occurrence.	3 years after 6th birthday.	
New York	2½ years after occurrence or date of last treatment when treatment was continuous.	10 years after discovery.	Foreign objects extend period to 1 year after discovery; fraudulent concealment also extends period.
North Carolina	3 years after occurrence or 1 year after discovery, with maximum of 4 years after occurrence.	1 year after 18th birthday.	Foreign objects extend period 1 year after discovery, with maximum of 10 years after occurrence.
North Dakota	2 years after discovery, with maximum of 6 years after occurrence.	1 year after 18th birthday.	
Ohio	1 year after discovery, with maximum of 4 years after occurrence.	Under 10, until 14th birthday; otherwise adult law applies.	
Oklahoma	2 years after discovery, with maximum of 3 years after occurrence.	Period begins with 18th birthday.	Foreign objects and fraudulent concealment extend period to 2 years after discovery.
Oregon	2 years after discovery, with maximum of 5 years after occurrence.	1 year after 18th birthday or 5 years after discovery.	
Pennsylvania	2 years from discovery.	Same as adult law.	
Rhode Island	2 years after occurrence; if not discovered, within 1 year of discovery.	1 year after 16th birthday.	
South Carolina	3 years after occurrence or discovery, with maximum of 6 years after occurrence.	1 year after 18th birthday.	2 years after discovery of foreign body.
South Dakota	2 years after occurrence.	3 years after occurrence unless under 6; otherwise adult law.	
Tennessee	1 year after occurrence or 1 year after discovery with maximum of 3 years after occurrence.	Until 21.	Fraudulent concealment and foreign objects extend period to 1 year after discovery.
Texas	2 years after occurrence.	Under 12, until 14th birthday.	
Utah	2 years after discovery with maximum of 4 years after occurrence.		1 year after discovery of fraudulent concealment or foreign object.
Vermont	7 years after occurrence.	7 years after 18th birthday.	Foreign objects suspend period.
Virginia	2 years after treatment.	2 years after 18th birthday.	

Table continued on following page

TABLE 13–1
STATUTES OF LIMITATIONS, TORT ACTIONS* Continued

State	Limitation Period	Minors	Comments
Washington	3 years after occurrence or 1 year after discovery, with maximum of 8 years after occurrence.	Period begins on 18th birthday.	Fraudulent concealment suspends statute.
West Virginia	2 years after discovery.	Same as adult law.	
Wisconsin	3 years after occurrence.	3 years after occurrence or until 10.	Foreign objects and fraudulent concealment suspend period.
Wyoming	2 years after occurrence or discovery.	Until 8th birthday or 2 years after injury, whichever is longer.	Plaintiff must establish that injury could not have been discovered within 2 years of occurrence.
District of Columbia	3 years after discovery.	3 years after 21st birthday.	

* From Chapman S: How long should you keep your patients' medical records? *Legal Aspects of Medical Practice,* New York, August 1979; Appeared in American Association of Medical Assistants: *Law for the Medical Office,* Chicago, 1984, pp. 257–263.

would begin when the course of treatment ended.
- Discovery rule—The statutory period would begin when the patient discovers, or should have discovered the negligence.
- Combination policy—A more complex system that sets various time limits depending on the type of injury.

A chart of state statutes of limitations for tort actions is provided in Table 13–1.

SPECIAL HINT

Although these statutes rarely change, it is advisable to verify this information for your state.

Insurance

Professional liability insurance is designed to pay for the cost of defending a malpractice case and to pay any awards to the plaintiff if the case is lost. Physicians must have proof of liability coverage to practice in most hospitals.

Physicians must bear the responsibility for any negligence of their employees if the negligence occurs during the course of their employment. As an agent of the physician, medical office personnel are usually covered under their physician employer's professional liability insurance.

This does not prevent a medical assistant from purchasing a liability policy. According to Myrtle Flight, J.D., CMA:

Problems arise when an assistant is named co-defendant in a lawsuit and the physician's insurance will not represent the assistant, or the positions of the assistant and the physician conflict. The cost of hiring an attorney is high, especially in a lengthy malpractice action, and it is important that any legal defendant have legal representation. The value of malpractice insurance for the medical assistant is that of having an attorney appointed and financed by the insurance company (Flight M: *Law, Liability, and Ethics.* Albany, NY, Delmar, 1988, pp 81–82).

PATIENT CARE

Emergency Aid

Good Samaritan laws protect volunteers from being sued if they respond to an emergency situation such as an automobile accident. Emergencies in a medical office are not usually covered by Good Samaritan laws. It is prudent to treat someone who presents in your office as an emergency as though they were a patient until transportation to an emergency room can be arranged.

Appointments

The appointment book can be considered a legal document if it is written in ink. Many offices use pencil due to the number of appointments rescheduled. Cancellations and failed appointments must be documented in the patient's chart to prove noncompliance or contributory negligence on the part of the patient.

Consent

A patient must voluntarily consent to be touched, examined, or treated by medical personnel. Consent can be implied by a person's actions and behavior, or it can be expressed verbally or in written form. Before a procedure is performed on a patient, it is important to have the patient's informed consent.

```
                                                        A.M.
                Date: _____ Time _____ P.M.


    1. I authorize the performance upon _____
                                         (myself or name of patient)
    of the following operation _____
                                   (state name of operation)
    to be performed by or under the direction of Dr. _____.

    2. The following have been explained to me by Dr. _____:

       A. The nature of the operation _____
                                          (describe the operation)
       _____

       _____

       B. The purpose of the operation _____
                                          (describe the purpose)
       _____

       C. The possible alternative methods of treatment _____
       _____
                         (describe the alternative methods)
       D. The possible consequences of the operation _____

       _____
                        (describe the possible consequences)
       E. The risks involved _____

       _____
                           (describe the risks involved)
       F. The possibility of complications _____

       _____
                        (describe the possible complications)
    3. I have been advised of the serious nature of the operation and
    have been advised that if I desire a further and more detailed explana-
    tion of any of the foregoing or further information about the possible
    risks or complications of the above-listed operation it will be given to
    me.
    4. I do not request a further and more detailed listing and explana-
    tion of any of the items listed in paragraph 2.

    Witness _____   Signed _____
                                       (Patient or person authorized to
                                             consent for patient)
```

FIGURE 13-8

Surgical informed consent. (Reprinted with permission from *MedicoLegal Forms with Legal Analysis*. Chicago, American Medical Association, 1991.)

Physicians are legally responsible for obtaining informed consent from patients before performing a procedure. Obtaining informed consent may not be delegated to medical office personnel. Informed-consent laws vary from state to state. The basic information a patient must be given to make a knowledgeable decision is as follows:

- The nature of their illness or injury
- The proposed treatment
- The expected results of the treatment
- The risks and possible side effects of the treatment
- Possible alternatives to the treatment
- The result if no treatment was done

Informed consent is a process of communication between the physician and the patient and not just the signing of a consent form. An example of an informed-consent form is given in Figure 13–8. Each state has its own requirements for the forms used in obtaining informed consent. An example of a consent for a sterilization procedure is provided in Figure 13–9. Figure 13–10 is an example of a consent for human immunodeficiency virus (HIV) testing.

Minors

A *minor* is defined as a person who has not yet reached the age of majority, usually 18 to 21 years of age. In most states, a minor may not give consent for medical care except in special circumstances. There can be difficult issues related to confidentiality and financial responsibility.

Date: _____ Time _____ A.M. / P.M.

We the undersigned husband and wife, each being more than twenty-one years of age and of sound mind, request

Dr. _____, and assistants of his choice, to perform upon

_____, the following operation:
(name of patient)

_____*
(state nature and extent of operation)

It has been explained to us that this operation is intended to result in sterility although this result has not been guaranteed. We understand that a sterile person is NOT capable of becoming a parent.

We voluntarily request the operation and understand that if it proves successful the results will be permanent and it will thereafter be physically impossible for the patient to inseminate, or to conceive or bear children.

Signed _____
(Husband)

Signed _____†
(Wife)

Witness _____

* This form is intended to be used where the primary purpose rather than the incidental result is sterilization.
† The question of the necessity of the consent of the patient's spouse to a voluntary sterilization has never been litigated. It would appear that such consent is not necessary, although it may be desirable. The statutes in Georgia, North Carolina, and Virginia, which specifically authorize voluntary sterilization, require the written consent of the patient's spouse.

FIGURE 13–9

Sterilization informed consent. (Reprinted with permission from *MedicoLegal Forms with Legal Analysis*. Chicago, American Medical Association, 1991.)

I voluntarily give my consent to be tested for exposure to the Human Immunodeficiency Virus (HIV). HIV is the term used for the virus that is thought to cause AIDS. I understand that my blood will be drawn for the purpose of determining whether I have been exposed to this virus.

I understand that the exact meaning of an HIV antibody test result may not be clear in my case. A positive result does not mean that I will come down with AIDS. A negative result does not ensure that I do not have early HIV infection or that I cannot transmit the infection.

I understand that all reasonable efforts to provide confidentiality and/or anonymity to the extent provided by law will be made. However, I understand that the results of this test will be recorded in my medical record. As medical record information, these test results will be regarded as confidential, and the Hospital will not disclose these test results to unauthorized third parties without my express written authorization. I understand, however, that confidentiality cannot be absolutely guaranteed, and that the results will be available to physicians and other health care professionals responsible for my care and treatment.

I understand that Illinois law requires that if this test result in combination with other data leads my physician to make a presumptive diagnosis of AIDS, then my case must be reported to the public health authorities and may be investigated by them.

I have been informed that if this test is positive a physician will provide counselling for follow up care and for precautions against transmitting this infection.

I understand that if I refuse this test my exposure to the HIV will remain unknown. My ability to infect others with this virus will also remain unknown.

I warrant that I freely give my informed consent and that I have not been forced, coerced, or subjected to any constraint or inducement. I understand that I may withdraw this consent anytime prior to having my blood drawn.

    _____ I hereby give consent for the performance of the HIV antibody test.

    _____ I refuse consent for the performance of the HIV antibody test. I understand that this refusal may limit the clinical data available to my physician. However, this refusal will not affect my access to further care.

_____ _____
Signature   Date

_____
Witness

Editor's Note: *This form is reproduced with permission of Northwestern Memorial Hospital, Office of General Counsel, 750 N Lake Shore Drive, Chicago, IL 60611.*

FIGURE 13-10

Human immunodeficiency virus (HIV) testing informed consent. (Courtesy of Northwestern Memorial Hospital, Chicago, IL.)

> **SPECIAL HINT**
>
> You must consult your state's laws regarding the treatment of minors for:
>
> - Contraception
> - Termination of pregnancy
> - Sexually transmitted diseases
> - Substance abuse

Treatment Authorization

The minor's legal guardian must give consent for most medical treatment. If the minor is brought to the physician's office by someone other than the legal guardian, the physician should obtain a written treatment authorization before providing treatment. In an emergency situation, consent is assumed and the parent or legal guardian should be contacted as soon as possible to obtain consent.

Emancipated and Mature Minors

Emancipated minors are self-supporting and away from the custody and control of parents or legal guardians. They could be married or in the armed forces. An emancipated minor may consent to medical care.

Mature minors are deemed to be sufficiently aware of the nature and consequences of their medical care. Capacity to consent is determined on a case-by-case basis by the court.

Divorce Agreements

Responsibility for treatment authorization and financial responsibility for minors can be difficult to determine in cases of divorce and remarriage. Without a copy of the divorce agreement, it is difficult to verify these issues. If you are billing a noncustodial parent for a minor's medical care, it would be prudent to have that agreement in writing.

MEDICAL RECORDS

Ownership and Access

In a physician's office the medical record belongs to the physician. Patients should be allowed access to the information in their record unless prohibited by law or unless the physician feels the information would harm the patient. Many state medical associations recommend that physicians provide patients with a summary of the medical record or a copy of the chart when requested. Patients may be expected to pay the reproduction costs. It is not recommended that you refuse access to or transfer of records because a patient has an unpaid account.

Retention

The ideal would be to retain medical records indefinitely. However, because that is not practical, records should be kept until the statute of limitations has run out for your treatment of that patient. For most records, this would be the period of time from the last contact with the patient until the statutory time limit has elapsed. As a

---

To Dr. _____:

I authorize you to furnish a copy of the medical records of
_____, covering the period
(state name of patient or "myself")
from _____, 19____ to _____, 19____ or to
allow those records to be inspected or copied by _____.
I release you from all legal responsibility or liability that may arise from this authorization.

Witness _____   Signed _____
                            Date _____

FIGURE 13–11

General authorization to release records. (Reprinted with permission from *MedicoLegal Forms with Legal Analysis.* Chicago, American Medical Association, 1991.)

Confidentiality

The patient's right to privacy is related to the right to confidentiality of the medical record. No information should be released from the medical record without written authorization from the patient. An example of a general release is given in Figure 13-11. Some states have confidentiality laws that require a specific release for information relating to

- Mental illness or psychiatric treatment
- HIV testing
- Acquired immune deficiency syndrome diagnosis and treatment
- Other sexually transmitted diseases
- Drug and/or alcohol abuse

If the state confidentiality laws require a specific authorization to release this type of information, a statement that includes all these possibilities should be incorporated into your general release.

There are instances when the public's need to know certain information supersedes the patient's right to privacy. Legally required disclosures could be

- required by a court order, a subpoena
- required by statute to protect the public health or welfare

> **SPECIAL HINT**
>
> Unless ordered by a subpoena or state law, no information should be transmitted to a physician, attorney, insurance company, or federal or state agency without the express, written authorization of the patient.

Disposal

When medical records are destroyed, they should be shredded or burned to preserve their confidentiality.

PUBLIC HEALTH REPORTING REQUIREMENTS

Physicians and medical facilities are generally required to report on births, deaths, communicable diseases, and injuries resulting from violence. The local or state health department can provide you with lists of diseases that are reportable or notifiable. They can also provide you with descriptions of the procedures and with the forms needed to comply with the reporting requirements. Refer to the list in Figure 13-3.

COMPREHENSIVE DRUG ABUSE PREVENTION AND CONTROL ACT OF 1970

The Drug Enforcement Agency (DEA), a division of the Justice Department, is responsible for enforcing the Comprehensive Drug Abuse Prevention and Control Act of 1970, more commonly known as the Controlled Substances Act. This act lists substances that are controlled because of their potential for abuse and physical or psychological dependence. The substances are listed in five schedules. Schedule V drugs have the least potential for abuse, and schedule I substances have no recognized medical use but have a high potential for abuse. An excellent source of information for physicians' offices is a publication that can be obtained from your regional DEA office: *The Physician's Manual: An Informational Outline of the Controlled Substances Act of 1970.*

Registration

Every physician who administers, prescribes, or dispenses controlled substances must be registered with the DEA. Application is made on form DEA-224 and mailed to:

> DEA Registration Unit
> P.O. Box 28083, Central Station
> Washington, DC 20005

DEA Offices

Atlanta, GA Division
75 Spring Street, S.W.
Room 740
Atlanta, GA
404 / 331-4401

Boston, MA Division
JFK Federal Building
Room G-64
Boston, MA 02203
617 / 565-2800

Chicago, IL Division
500 Dirksen Federal Building
219 South Dearborn Street
Chicago, IL 60604
312 / 353-7875

Dallas, TX Division
1880 Regal Row
Dallas, TX 75235
214 / 767-7151

Denver, CO Division
P.O. Box 1860
Denver, CO 80201
303 / 844-3951

Detroit, MI Division
357 Federal Building
231 W. Lafayette
Detroit, MI 48226
313 / 226-7290

Houston, TX Division
333 West Loop North
Houston, TX 77024
713 / 681-1771

Los Angeles, CA Division
Suite 800
350 South Figueroa Street
Los Angeles, CA 90071
213 / 894-2650

Miami, FL Division
8400 N.W. 53rd Street
Miami, FL 33166
305 / 591-4870

Newark, NJ Division
Federal Office Building
Suite 806
970 Broad Street
Newark, NJ 07102
201 / 645-6060

New Orleans, LA Division
1661 Canal Street, Suite 2200
New Orleans, LA 70112
504 / 598-3894

New York, NY Division
555 West 57th Street
New York, NY 10019
212 / 399-5151

Philadelphia, PA Division
600 Arch Street, Room 10224
Philadelphia, PA 19106
215 / 597-9530

Phoenix, AZ Division
One N. First Street
Suite 201
Phoenix, AZ 85004
602 / 261-4866

San Diego, CA Division
402 W. 35th Street
National City, CA 92050
619 / 585-9600

San Francisco, CA Division
Room 12215
450 Golden Gate Avenue
San Francisco, CA 94102
415 / 556-6771

Seattle, WA Division
220 West Mercer
Seattle, WA 98119
206 / 442-5443

St. Louis, MO Division
Suite 500
7911 Forsyth Blvd.
St. Louis, MO 63105
314 / 425-3241

Washington, D.C. Division
400 6th Street S.W.
Washington, D.C 20024
202 / 724-7834

FIGURE 13-12
Regional offices of the Drug Enforcement Agency (DEA).

Chapter 13: MEDICAL LAW 293

SCHEDULE	ORAL RX	WRITTEN RX	REFILLS
I	No recognized medical use		
II	NO	YES	NO
III	YES	YES	5 times or 6 months
IV	YES	YES	5 times or 6 months
V	YES	YES	YES

FIGURE 13-13
Controlled substances prescription requirements.

Registration must be renewed every 3 years. A registration form is mailed to physicians approximately 60 days before their certificate expires.

The registration certificate must be maintained at the location for which it was granted. If the physician changes locations, modification of the registration must be requested from the nearest DEA office. If a physician has more than one office location, then each office must be registered. A list of the regional DEA offices is provided in Figure 13-12.

Record-Keeping

A physician who prescribes schedules II, III, IV, and V controlled substances is not required to keep records of those transactions. However, a physician who dispenses controlled substances is required to keep a record of each transaction. All controlled substance records must be maintained for inspection by the DEA for 2 years.

Inventory

A physician who dispenses or regularly administers controlled substances must take an inventory every 2 years of all the drugs in stock. This record is maintained at the location appearing on the certificate for 2 years.

Prescriptions

Only licensed practitioners who are registered with the DEA may issue prescriptions for controlled substances. A written prescription must

- Be dated and signed on the date of issue
- Include the patient's complete name and address
- Include the physician's name, address, and DEA registration number
- Be written in ink or indelible pencil or be typewritten
- Be signed manually by the physician

Written prescriptions may be prepared for the physician's signature by medical office personnel. However, the physician remains responsible for the content of the prescription. Requirements for prescriptions are illustrated in Figure 13-13.

DRUG SCREENING

Pre-employment drug screening and random drug screening at work are controversial subjects. Many employers are requiring drug screening as part of their hiring practices. Drug screening programs at places of employment are being legally challenged by some unions and civil rights groups.

In 1988 the U.S. Department of Transportation issued rules requiring drug testing of employees in regulated safety- and security-related jobs in the transportation industry. A health care facility faces tremendous liability potential unless clear policies and procedures are observed regarding specimen collection and testing. The chain of custody of a specimen has to be documented from collection to results.

If your office is asked to collect a specimen from a patient for drug screening, you should have the patient's written consent to perform the testing, be sure the laboratory you are using is qualified to run the tests required, and carefully document the collection and chain of custody for the specimen.

UNIFORM ANATOMICAL GIFT ACT OF 1968

All 50 states have some version of the Uniform Anatomical Gift Act of 1968. Generally any person at least 18 years of age and of sound mind may consent to give all or a part of his or her body for research or transplantation. The gift may be written as part of a will or be specified by signing, in the presence of two witnesses, a card that is carried in one's wallet. An example of the Uniform Donor Card is provided in Figure 13–14.

DEATH AND DYING

The majority of states have some form of a Natural Death Act that provides guidelines and regulations for dealing with the issues faced by terminally ill patients. There are two documents that help people provide for the direction of their care if they become unable to communicate their wishes.

Living Wills

This is a document in which a person essentially states that if he or she became terminally ill he or she would want no heroic or extraordinary measures taken to prolong his or her life. An example of a living will is provided in Figure 13–15. The form is different for each state.

Uniform Donor Card

of _____
   (name of donor)

In the hope that I may help others, I hereby make this anatomical gift, if medically acceptable, to take effect upon my death. The words and marks below indicate my desires.

I give: (a) ☐ any needed organs or parts
       (b) ☐ only the following organs or parts

_____
   Specify the organ(s) or part(s)

for the purposes of transplantation, therapy, medical research, or education:

       (c) ☐ my body for anatomical study if needed.

Limitations or special wishes, if any _____

Signed by the donor and the following two witnesses in the presence of each other:

_____ _____
(Signature of donor)   (Date of Birth of Donor)

_____ _____
(City and State)   (Date Signed)

_____ _____
(Witness)   (Witness)

FIGURE 13–14

Uniform Donor Card. (Reprinted with permission from *MedicoLegal Forms with Legal Analysis*. Chicago, American Medical Association, 1991.)

Living Will Declaration

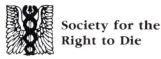

Society for the Right to Die
250 West 57th Street/New York, NY 10107

INSTRUCTIONS
Consult this column for guidance.

To My Family, Doctors, and All Those Concerned with My Care

I, _____, being of sound mind, make this statement as a directive to be followed if I become unable to participate in decisions regarding my medical care.

This declaration sets forth your directions regarding medical treatment.

If I should be in an incurable or irreversible mental or physical condition with no reasonable expectation of recovery, I direct my attending physician to withhold or withdraw treatment that merely prolongs my dying. I further direct that treatment be limited to measures to keep me comfortable and to relieve pain.

You have the right to refuse treatment you do not want, and you may request the care you do want.

These directions express my legal right to refuse treatment. Therefore I expect my family, doctors, and everyone concerned with my care to regard themselves as legally and morally bound to act in accord with my wishes, and in so doing to be free of any legal liability for having followed my directions.

You may list specific treatment you do not want. For example:
Cardiac resuscitation
Mechanical respiration
Artificial feeding/fluids by tube
Otherwise, your general statement, top right, will stand for your wishes.

I especially do not want: _____

You may want to add instructions or care you do want—for example, pain medication; or that you prefer to die at home if possible.

Other instructions/comments: _____

Proxy Designation Clause: Should I become unable to communicate my instructions as stated above. I designate the following person to act in my behalf:

Name _____
Address _____

If you want, you can name someone to see that your wishes are carried out, but you do not have to do this.

If the person I have named above is unable to act on my behalf, I authorize the following person to do so:

Name _____
Address _____

This Living Will Declaration expresses my personal treatment preferences. The fact that I may have also executed a document in the form recommended by state law should not be construed to limit or contradict this Living Will Declaration, which is an expression of my common-law and constitutional rights.

Signed: _____ Date: _____
Witness: _____ Witness: _____
Address: _____ Address: _____

Sign and date here in the presence of two adult witnesses, who should also sign.

Keep the signed original with your personal papers at home. Give signed copies to doctors, family, and proxy. Review your Declaration from time to time: initial and date it to show it still expresses your intent.

FIGURE 13-15

Living will. (Reprinted by permission of the Society for the Right to Die, 250 West 57th Street, New York, NY, 10107.)

MARYLAND

DURABLE POWER OF ATTORNEY FOR MEDICAL TREATMENT

> **INFORMATION ABOUT THIS DOCUMENT**
> This is an important legal document. Before signing this document, it is vital for you to know and understand these facts:
> This document gives the person you name as your agent the power to make health care decisions for you if you can't make decisions for yourself. Even after you have signed this document, you have the right to make health care decisions for yourself so long as you are able to do so. Your agent will be able to make decisions for you only after two physicians have certified that you are incapable of making them yourself. You have the right to revoke (take away) the authority of your agent by notifying your agent or your health care provider orally or in writing of this desire.

I, _____
(your name)

hereby appoint: _____
(agent's name)

_____
(agent's address and telephone)

as my agent to make health care decisions for me if and when I am unable to make my own health care decisions. This gives my agent the power to consent to giving, withholding or stopping any health care, treatment (including life-sustaining treatment), service, or diagnostic procedure. I specifically authorize my agent to make decisions for me about artificially supplied nutrition and hydration (tube feeding). My agent also has the authority to talk with health care personnel, get information, and sign forms necessary to carry out those decisions.

If the person named as my agent is not available or is unable to act as my agent, then I appoint the following person(s) to serve in the order listed below:

1. _____
(agent's name)

_____
(address and telephone)

2. _____
(agent's name)

_____
(address and telephone)

By this document I intend to create a power of attorney for health care which shall take effect upon my incapacity to make my own health care decisions and shall continue during that incapacity.

I have discussed my wishes with my agent, and he or she shall make all health care decisions on my behalf, including decisions to withhold or withdraw all forms of life-sustaining treatment, including artificially administered hydration and nutrition.

My particular wishes are:

_____
_____
_____
_____
_____

BY SIGNING HERE I INDICATE THAT I UNDERSTAND THE PURPOSE OF THIS DOCUMENT

I sign my name to this form on _____.
(date)

at: _____
(address)

_____
(You sign here)

WITNESSES

I declare that the person who signed or acknowledged this document is personally known to me, that he/she signed or acknowledged this durable power of attorney in my presence, and that he/she appears to be of sound mind and under no duress, fraud, or undue influence. I am not the person appointed as agent by this document, nor am I the patient's health care provider, or an employee of the patient's health care provider.

I further declare that I am not related to the patient by blood, marriage, or adoption, and, to the best of my knowledge, I am not entitled to any part of his/her estate under a will now existing or by operation of law.

FIRST WITNESS

Signature: _____

Home Address: _____

Print Name: _____

Date: _____

SECOND WITNESS

Signature: _____

Home Address: _____

Print Name: _____

Date: _____

FIGURE 13–16
Durable power of attorney. (Reprinted by permission of the Society for the Right to Die, 250 West 57th Street, New York, NY, 10107.)

Generally, anyone 18 years or older and legally competent can make a living will. It must be

- Dated and in writing
- Signed by the patient
- Signed by at least two witnesses

The witnesses may not be a relative, anyone who is financially involved with the patient, or anyone involved in the treatment of the patient. Therefore, physicians and their office personnel may not be a witness to a living will for a patient. A copy of the living will should be filed in the patient's chart and the chart labeled in some way to quickly identify that this person has signed a living will.

Durable Power of Attorney for Health Care

Durable power of attorney allows a broader scope of power than a living will. In this document a person appoints someone to act for him or her in the event the person becomes unable to act for him- or herself. This can cover financial as well as health care decisions. Each state has very specific requirements regarding a durable power of attorney. An example of a durable power of attorney form is provided in Figure 13–16.

An organization that provides information on and forms specific to the requirements of each state's laws regarding death and dying is:

> Society for the Right to Die
> 250 West 57th Street
> New York, NY 10107
> (212) 246-6973

Withdrawal of Life Support

Decisions to withdraw life support or to issue a nonresuscitation order are being challenged in court cases. Each state has regulations and guidelines you should know.

MONITORING LEGISLATION

The health care industry exists in a very dynamic legislative environment. New laws are always being proposed and old laws changed. Health professionals need to stay informed of what is happening at the state and federal levels.

Glossary

Abandonment: To terminate the physician–patient relationship without reasonable notice so the patient does not have an opportunity to arrange other health care.

Battery: The unlawful touching of a person without his or her permission.

Breach: Violation of the terms or conditions of a contract or obligation.

Claims-made insurance: A type of professional liability insurance that covers only claims made and reported within the time the insurance policy was in effect.

Common law: Law that has evolved from tradition and common custom and that has been affirmed by court judgments.

Conservator: A person appointed by the court to manage the affairs of an incompetent person.

Contributory negligence: In medical malpractice, this is any unreasonable action or inaction by the patient that contributed to the injury he or she suffered.

Damages: Compensation, usually monetary, awarded by the court to someone who has suffered a loss or injury.

Defendant: The person or party accused of wrongdoing in a court case.

Deposition: A statement by a witness written down by the attorneys for use in a trial without the witness's appearing personally.

Fraud: Willful deception with the intent of unlawful benefit or profit.

Negligence: Failure to provide the care that a reasonably prudent person would use under similar circumstances.

Occurrence insurance: A type of liability insurance policy that covers any claim that occurs while the policy is in force, no matter when it occurred or was reported.

Plaintiff: The person or party who accuses another party of wrongdoing in a court case.

Respondeat superior ("Let the master answer"): The legal principle that employers are responsible for the actions of their employees.

Statutory laws: Laws that are enacted by a governmental body.

Subpoena: A court order requiring a person to appear at a legal proceeding to give testimony.

Subpoena Duces Tecum: A subpoena that requires a party to appear in court and bring whatever documents and records are named in the subpoena.

Summons: A legal document that commands a person to appear and answer the claims in a complaint within a specified time.

Tail coverage: In liability insurance, tail coverage is a policy that protects the physician against all claims arising from professional services performed while a claims-made insurance policy was in effect, regardless of when the future claims are filed.

Tort: A wrongful act to a person or his or her property for which the law allows monetary damages to be awarded.

Bibliography

American Association of Medical Assistants: *Law for the Medical Office.* Chicago: American Association of Medical Assistants, 1984.

American Medical Association: *Medicolegal Forms with Legal Analysis.* Chicago: American Medical Association, 1991.

Balasa D: Medical assisting: An important ally of medicine in the current legislative environment. *State Health Legislation Report* 18(1): 1–8, 1990.

Balasa D: Overview of laws affecting medical assisting practice. *Professional Medical Assistant* March/April: 20, 1990.

Black H: *Black's Law Dictionary,* 5th ed. St. Paul, MN: West, 1979.

Flight M: *Law, Liability, and Ethics.* Albany, NY: Delmar, 1988.

Lewis M, Warden C: *Law and Ethics in the Medical Office: Including Bioethical Issues,* 2nd ed. Philadelphia: F.A. Davis, 1988.

U.S. Department of Justice, Drug Enforcement Agency: *Physician's Manual: An Informational Outline of the Controlled Substances Act of 1970.* Washington, DC: U.S. Government Printing Office, 1990.

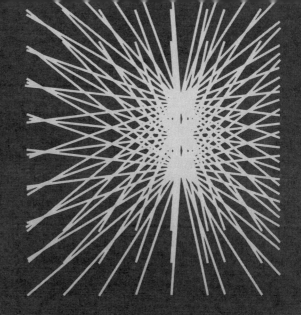

Section Two

CLINICAL PRACTICES

Chapter 14

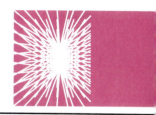

GENERAL PATIENT CARE

CAROL S. CHAMPAGNE
KAREN LANE

MEDICAL ASEPSIS
CDC Universal Blood and Body Fluid Precautions
Sanitization
Sterilization and Disinfection
PATIENT INTERVIEWING
Skills for Successful Patient Interviewing
The New Patient Interview
VITAL SIGNS
Height
Weight
Pulse
Respiration
Temperature
Blood Pressure
MEDICAL EXAMINATIONS
Preparing for a Complete Physical Examination
Preparing for a Proctological Examination
The Eye and Ear Examinations
The Neurological Examination
Employment, School, and Insurance Examinations
Patient Self-Examination

MEDICAL ASEPSIS

It is essential to employ practices in the medical office that reduce the number and hinder the transmission of pathogens. In many office settings 30–40 ill patients may be seen each day. The possibility of transmission of pathogens from one patient to another is great if care is not taken to maintain medical asepsis. The patient entering the office expects a clean environment with no evidence of the prior patient. Therefore, a clean office environment promotes good patient relations.

However, the practice of maintaining a clean office environment is much more important than just good public relations; it is vital to the health of patients and those employed in the medical office.[1] Recently the fear of acquired immune deficiency syndrome (AIDS) has caused all health care workers to become more diligent in their efforts to maintain asepsis. Health care workers are now more careful to observe all the Universal Blood and Body Fluid Precautions issued by The Centers for Disease Control (CDC). The medical assistant should be aware of these precautions and make them a part of his or her daily routine. Observing these precautions will protect the health care worker and the patient.

CDC Universal Blood and Body Fluid Precautions

1. All health care workers should routinely use appropriate barrier precautions to prevent skin and mucous membrane exposure, when contact with the blood and body fluids, mucous membranes, or nonintact skin of any patient is anticipated.

   • Gloves should be worn for touching blood and body fluids, mucous membranes, or

nonintact skin of all patients; for handling items or surfaces soiled with blood or body fluids; and for performing venipuncture and other vascular access procedures.
- Gloves should be changed after contact with each patient.
- Masks and protective eye wear or face shields should be worn during procedures that are likely to generate droplets of blood or other body fluids to prevent exposure of mucous membranes of the mouth, nose, and eyes.
- Gowns or aprons should be worn during procedures that are likely to generate splashes of blood or other body fluids.

2. Hands and other skin surfaces should be washed immediately and thoroughly if contaminated with blood or other body fluids.

- Hands should be washed immediately after gloves are removed.

3. All health care workers should take precautions to prevent injuries caused by needles, scalpels, and other sharp instruments during disposal of used needles and when handling sharp instruments after procedures.

- To prevent needle-stick injuries, needles should not be recapped, purposely bent or broken by hand, removed from disposable syringes, or otherwise manipulated by hand.
- After they are used, disposable syringes and needles, scalpel blades, and other sharp items should be placed in puncture-resistant containers for disposal; the puncture-resistant containers should be located as close as is practical to the area in which they will be used.
- Large-bore reusable needles should be placed in a puncture-resistant container for transport to the reprocessing area.

4. Saliva has not been implicated in human immunodeficiency virus (HIV) transmission. However, to minimize the need for emergency mouth-to-mouth resuscitation, mouthpieces, resuscitation bags, or other ventilation devices should be available for use in areas in which the need for resuscitation is predictable.

5. Health care workers who have exudative lesions or weeping dermatitis should refrain from all direct patient care and from handling patient care equipment until the condition resolves.

6. Health care workers who are pregnant are not known to be at greater risk of contracting HIV infection than those who are not pregnant. However, if an individual develops HIV infection during pregnancy, the infant is at risk of infection resulting from perinatal transmission. Because of this risk, pregnant health care workers should be especially familiar with and strictly adhere to precautions to minimize the risk of HIV infection.

Additional Blood and Body Fluid Precautions

Because many medical assistants work in laboratories based in physicians' offices, it is important that they be aware of all precautions developed by the CDC to supplement the universal blood and body fluid precautions listed above.

1. All specimens of blood and body fluids should be put in a well-constructed container with a secure lid, to prevent leaking during transport. Care should be taken when collecting each specimen to avoid contaminating the outside of the container and the laboratory form accompanying the specimen.
2. All persons processing blood and body fluid specimens should wear gloves. Masks and protective eye wear should be worn if mucous membrane contact with blood or body fluids is anticipated. Gloves should be changed and hands washed after completion of specimen processing.
3. For routine procedures, such as histological and pathological studies or microbiological culturing, a biological safety cabinet is not necessary. However, biological safety cabinets should be used whenever possible when generating droplets. This includes activities such as blending, sonicating, and vigorous mixing.
4. Mechanical pipetting devices should be used for manipulating all liquids in the laboratory. Mouth pipetting must not be done.
5. Use of needles and syringes should be limited to situations in which there is no alternative, and the recommendations for preventing injuries with needles outlined in the Universal Precautions should be followed.
6. Laboratory work surfaces should be decontaminated with an appropriate chemical germicide after a spill of blood or other body fluids when work activities are completed.
7. Contaminated materials used in laboratory tests should be decontaminated before reprocessing or placed in bags and disposed of in accord-

ance with institutional policies for disposal of infective waste.
8. Scientific equipment that has been contaminated with blood or other body fluids should be decontaminated and cleaned before being repaired in the laboratory or transported to the manufacturer.
9. All persons should wash their hands after completing laboratory activities and should remove protective clothing before leaving the laboratory.[2]

Sanitization

The first step in medical asepsis is sanitization. Sanitization refers to cleansing[3] and must occur before sterilization or any other form of medical asepsis takes place. After removing his or her gloves or after working with a patient, it is essential that the medical assistant practice good hand-washing technique to avoid transferring pathogens from one patient to another and for self-protection.

PROCEDURE

HAND-WASHING FOR MEDICAL ASEPSIS

PURPOSE

To wash the hands as the first line of defense in the practice of medical asepsis.

EQUIPMENT AND MATERIALS

Liquid soap in a dispenser
Hand lotion in a dispenser
At least three paper towels in a dispenser

PROCEDURAL STEPS

1. Remove all rings (except plain wedding band).
   RATIONALE: Microorganisms can colonize in the grooves of rings.
2. Turn on the faucets using a paper towel.
   RATIONALE: The sink and faucets are considered contaminated.
3. Regulate the water temperature to warm.
   RATIONALE: Warm water mixes best with the liquid soap and tends not to cause dry or chapped skin.
4. Discard the paper towel in an open waste receptacle.
5. Wet hands and apply soap to the hands.
6. Keep the hands lower than the elbows at all times.
   RATIONALE: Water and debris will flow from the wrists downward into the sink and will not contaminate the arms.
7. Lather the palms and backs of the hands with circular friction movements for 15 seconds while holding the fingertips downward.
   RATIONALE: Circular friction better removes surface microorganisms and debris.
8. Lather each finger and thumbs of both hands with circular friction movements for 15 seconds while holding the fingertips downward.
9. Rinse well, keeping the hands lower than the elbows.
10. Lather the wrists and forearms, using circular friction movements, for 15 seconds.
    RATIONALE: The wrists and forearms are washed after the hands. Washing the hands first avoids spreading microorganisms from the most contaminated to the least contaminated area during the procedure.
11. Rinse the arms and hands so that the water flows from the forearm downward into the sink.
12. Inspect the hands for cleanliness and intact skin.
    RATIONALE: Chapped or cracked skin can be a source of cross-contamination.
13. Repeat the entire procedure for the first hand-wash of the day or when the hands are contaminated with substances suspected to contain pathogens.
14. Dry hands thoroughly and gently.
    RATIONALE: Wet skin or too brisk a motion with the paper towels can cause chapping.
15. Turn off the water using a third dry paper towel.
16. Apply hand lotion.
    RATIONALE: To further reduce chapping and dry, cracked skin.

17. Cover any hangnails or broken skin with Band-Aids.
RATIONALE: Broken skin should be covered with Band-Aids and gloves worn for all procedures if the skin is not 100% intact. For larger open skin areas, patient contact should be entirely avoided until the skin is healed.

Sanitization is also a necessary step before instruments are sterilized. Care must be taken to avoid injury when working with contaminated instruments. It is imperative that gloves be worn. Care should be taken with sharp instruments because gloves will offer little protection if they are punctured. After cleansing instruments and removing gloves, hands must be washed in the manner described above.[4]

To sanitize instruments in preparation for sterilization follow these steps:

1. Wear gloves when sanitizing equipment, instruments, or materials to avoid contaminating yourself.
2. Rinse in cool water containing a blood solvent, low-sudsing detergent, or germicide solution.
3. Rinse in clear water.
4. Scrub each instrument thoroughly with brush and warm, nonionizing detergent solution.
5. Rinse all detergent off using hot water.
6. Remove excess moisture by rolling instruments in a towel.
7. Package or wrap for sterilization.

Syringes are usually disposable. However, at times special syringes made of glass may be used in the physician's office. These are sanitized and sterilized after use. Follow the procedure below when sanitizing syringes in preparation for sterilization.[5]

1. Rinse immediately by filling the syringe with cool water and flushing.
2. Disassemble the unit by removing the plunger from the barrel.
3. Place syringe in water containing a low-sudsing detergent.
4. Thoroughly brush the interior of the syringe barrel.
5. Clean the inside of the tip and the plunger.
6. Flush with tap water.
7. Flush with distilled water.
8. Wrap the barrel and syringe separately to prevent breakage.
9. Place in package or wrap.

Sterilization and Disinfection

Instruments or devices that enter sterile tissue or the vascular system of any patient, or through which blood flows, should be sterilized before they are used again.[2] Chemical sterilization involves exposure of instruments or devices to a sterilant or germicide according to the manufacturer's instructions. There are several commercial chemicals on the market. An inexpensive germi-

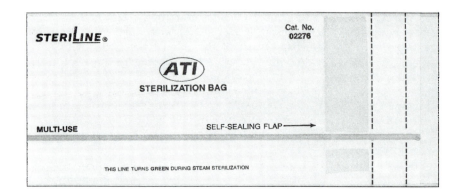

FIGURE 14–1

Instrument indicator bags have strips that change color when a minimum temperature is reached for a certain period of time. The translucency allows easy identification. (Courtesy of PyMaH Corporation, ATI Division, Somerville, NJ) cide that is readily available is a solution of sodium hypochlorite (household bleach) in a dilution of 1:100 to 1:10. This is effective if it is prepared daily. Certain commercially prepared sterilants or germicides may be incompatible with certain medical devices, so before using a chemical the medical assistant should check to be sure it is compatible with the specific device or instrument being sterilized.

Physical sterilization is usually obtained by use of an autoclave. Instruments may be wrapped to maintain the sterilization. Disposable paper bags are available for sterilization of instruments and supplies. These often have a thermoindicator that changes color when an adequate temperature has been reached for sterilization to occur (Figure 14–1).

Instruments may also be wrapped in a protective covering, such as clean muslin or special disposable paper. These materials are used because they can be permeated by steam or chemical vapor but not by airborne surface contaminants during dry handling and storage. It is very important to wrap the articles in such a way that they do not become contaminated when opened. The method for wrapping is shown below in Figure 14–2.

Generally, an autoclave is operated at approximately 15 pounds of pressure per square inch at a temperature of 250–254° F. Depending on the articles being sterilized, the time may vary as shown in Table 14–1.

When the sterilization process is completed, the autoclave must be vented if it does not vent automatically. At this time, the sterilized materials will be moist. They must be allowed to dry before they are removed from the autoclave, because microorganisms can permeate quickly through moisture, resulting in contamination. The medical assistant must be sure his or her own hands are also clean and dry to prevent moisture-caused contamination of the instruments.[2]

Sterilization indicators should be used to determine the effectiveness of the procedure. There are several forms available. The best sterilization indicator indicates whether the proper temperature was attained and the duration of that temperature. Autoclave tape will change color if it is exposed to steam. This is useful for closing and identifying a wrapped article. However, autoclave

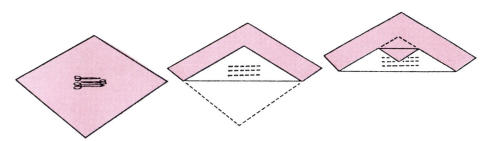

All items are placed in the center and the material folded up from the bottom, doubling back a small corner.

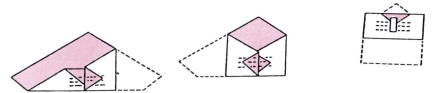

The right, then left, edges are folded over, again leaving corners doubled back. The pack is folded up from the bottom and secured with pressure-sensitive tape, then dated and labeled according to its contents. The pack should be firm enough for handling, but loose enough to permit proper circulation of steam. The materials included in each pack can be varied to suit the needs of each office, but the same wrapping pattern should be followed for all packs.

FIGURE 14–2

The method for wrapping instruments. (Reproduced from Bonewit K: *Clinical Procedures for Medical Assistants,* 3rd ed. Philadelphia: W. B. Saunders, 1990, p. 149.)

TABLE 14-1

MINIMUM STERILIZATION TIMES

Articles	Time 250 to 254°F (121 to 123°C)
Glassware, empty, inverted Instruments, metal in covered or open tray, padded or unpadded Needles, unwrapped Syringes, unassembled, unwrapped	15 minutes
Flasked solutions, 75 to 250 ml Instruments, metal combined with other materials in covered and/or padded tray Instruments wrapped in double-thickness muslin Rubber gloves, catheters, drains, tubing, etc., unwrapped or wrapped in muslin or paper	20 minutes
Dressings, wrapped in paper or muslin—small packs only Flasked solutions, 500 to 1000 ml Needles, individually packaged in glass tubes or paper Syringes, unassembled, individually packed in muslin or paper Sutures, silk, cotton, or nylon, wrapped in paper or muslin Treatment trays, wrapped in muslin or paper	30 minutes

Reprinted from Bonewit K: *Clinical Procedures for Medical Assistants*, 3rd ed. Philadelphia, W. B. Saunders, 1990, p. 148.

tape is not a sterilization indicator. It only assures that the article has been exposed to steam, not that the proper sterilization temperature and time have been attained.

Culture tests are also available and are the best way to determine the effectiveness of sterilization. Strips of paper containing heat-resistant spores are placed in the center of two different wrapped articles placed in areas of the autoclave that are the least accessible to steam penetration. After the strips have been exposed to sterilization conditions, they are removed from their wrappers and dropped into culture tubes containing a broth and are incubated for a specified period of time. If proper sterilization conditions have been met, no growth should occur.

If it is determined that instruments or devices are not being properly sterilized, the medical assistant should check the following:

- Is the autoclave properly loaded or are instruments crowded?
- Have the materials been properly prepared for sterilization?
- Is the autoclave operating properly? Is the gasket worn and not sealing?
- Is the autoclave heating properly?
- Is the load dry before removal?

PATIENT INTERVIEWING

The medical assistant is often the first person the patient sees and talks with in the medical office. This may be in the reception area. Also, once the patient is ushered to the examination room, it is often the medical assistant's responsibility to discover the reason for the visit and take the medical history. Medical assistants who perfect the art of the patient interview can put the patient at ease and at the same time obtain vital information for the physician, making his or her job less time consuming and easier.

Skills for Successful Patient Interviewing

Before a patient can be successfully interviewed, he or she must feel as comfortable as possible talking with the medical assistant. It is the medical assistant's responsibility to put the patient at ease and establish good rapport. It is important to realize that patients may be nervous and worried about their condition. Complaints that may seem minor to the medical assistant are usually causing great concern to patients, or they would not have taken the time to visit the physician.

Start by gathering all available information about the patient before you interview him or her. This eliminates unnecessary questions. Review the chart. If the patient was in the office a few days earlier, this visit may be related. You can ask the patient if he or she is feeling better and refer to the previous problem. Certain skills the medical assistant can develop increase the ability to develop a good rapport with the patient:

- Sit at eye level and use eye contact. Eye contact conveys concern.
- Sit down to take notes to convey to the patient that you are interested in listening to his or her problems. If you stand, the patient may feel rushed and cut answers short, possibly omitting

important information. If you seem preoccupied or disinterested, the patient will not confide in you.
- Convey a sense of genuine interest in the patient by your tone of voice and expression. The interview with the patient should be informal but professional.
- If the patient wanders too far off the subject, gently lead him or her back to the reason for the visit without seeming disinterested in other concerns.
- Speak to the patient using words the patient understands. Avoid using medical terminology that may be confusing.
- Ask open-ended questions to obtain more specific information. Avoid asking questions that require only a yes or no answer because this does not allow the patient to completely describe his or her condition. Some patients will not admit that they do not understand a question and will simply reply yes or no if that option is available.
- Listen closely to the patient's answers. You may find that the answers suggest other questions to ask, which can greatly aid the physician in making a diagnosis.
- Keep events in the proper time sequence as the patient discusses the problem.
- Do not insist that a patient discuss more than he or she feels comfortable discussing. The physician can finish the interview if it is incomplete.[6,7]

The New Patient Interview

When a patient comes to your office for the first time, it is necessary to obtain more information than would usually be necessary at subsequent office visits. Some physicians may choose to do this by providing a form for patients to complete before they are seen in the examination room (Figure 14-3). The medical assistant may only have to look over the form to be sure it is complete and ask patients if there are any additional facts that need to be included or explained. Other physicians may feel that the initial patient information should be obtained verbally by the medical assistant. This gives the medical assistant time to get to know the patient. It also eliminates confusion, which forms can sometimes create. The medical assistant may be asked to complete a form verbally with the patient or simply write the history in the chart. Regardless of the method, there are several topics that should be addressed in a new patient interview.

Past Medical History

- Major illnesses
- Childhood diseases
- Unusual infections
- Injuries or accidents
- Hospitalizations
- Surgeries
- Previous medical tests
- Immunizations
- Allergies
- Medications, past and present

Family History

The family history should include information that may give the physician a clue as to possible genetic illnesses or tendencies the patient may have, including the following:

- Ages and states of health of first-degree relatives
- Presence of significant diseases in relatives
- If a relative is deceased, the cause of death

Personal History

The personal history includes information regarding life-style and socioeconomic status, including the following:

- Education
- Occupational history
- Nutritional (diet) history
- Exercise habits
- Social history
- Life-style habits such as smoking, alcohol consumption, and drug use

Chief Complaint

Every patient will need to explain the reason for the visit to the physician. To obtain this information, the medical assistant should use the skills discussed in Skills for Successful Patient Interviewing. The reason for the particular visit is known as the chief complaint. The following techniques can be used to obtain the details of the chief complaint.

- Use open-ended questions to allow patients to fully describe themselves and to more accurately describe the symptoms.
- Limit the chief complaint to one or two major symptoms if possible.
- Be specific rather than vague.
- Use the patient's own words, if possible, rather

PATIENT HEALTH HISTORY

(A) IDENTIFICATION DATA Please print the following information.

Today's date ___/___/___ File no. _____

Name _____

Address _____

_____ Zip Code _____

Telephone _____ _____
            Home number   Work number

Social Security or Medicare No. _____

___ Male ___ Female ___ Race   Date of birth ___/___/___

___ Married ___ Separated ___ Divorced ___ Widowed ___ Single

Insurance provider _____

Policy number _____

Occupation _____

(B) FAMILY HISTORY:
For each member of your family, follow the grey or white line across the page and check the boxes for:
1. Their present state of health
2. Any illnesses they have had

PRINT NAMES BELOW

→ If deceased, write in age and cause of death. Include fatal accidents and suicides.

Name	Good health	Poor health	Deceased	Allergies or asthma	Anemia	Bleed easily	Diabetes	Cancer or tumor	Epilepsy	Glaucoma	Genetic disease	Alcoholism	Kidney or bladder trouble	Stomach/duodenal ulcer	Nervous breakdown	Rheumatism or arthritis	High blood pressure	Heart trouble	Gout
Father:																			
Mother:																			
Brothers/Sisters:																			
Spouse:																			
Child:																			
Child:																			
Child:																			
Child:																			
Paternal relatives (in each box, write how many affected with) →																			
Maternal relatives (in each box, write how many affected with) →																			

(C) YOUR HEALTH HISTORY (begin here with illnesses) →

PAST HISTORY

Additional Illnesses or Problems: Mark an X in the box next to any of the following that you have now or have ever had

- ☐ eye infections
- ☐ thyroid disease
- ☐ eczema
- ☐ hives or rashes
- ☐ bronchitis
- ☐ emphysema
- ☐ pneumonia
- ☐ pancreatitis
- ☐ liver disease
- ☐ diverticulosis
- ☐ hernia
- ☐ hemorrhoids
- ☐ neuralgia or neuritis
- ☐ tension/anxiety
- ☐ depression
- ☐ childhood hyperactivity
- ☐ chicken pox
- ☐ German measles
- ☐ scarlet fever
- ☐ measles
- ☐ mumps
- ☐ polio
- ☐ rheumatic fever
- ☐ malaria
- ☐ mononucleosis
- ☐ venereal disease
- ☐ yellow jaundice
- ☐ tuberculosis
- ☐ _____
- ☐ _____

Have you ever been turned down for life insurance, military service or employment because of health problems? .... ___ Yes ___ No

Major Hospitalizations: If you have ever been hospitalized for any major medical illness or operation, write in your most recent hospitalizations below. Check this box ☐ if you have had more than four such hospitalizations. (Do not include normal pregnancies)

	Year	Operation or Illness	Name of Hospital	City and State
1st Hospitalization				
2nd Hospitalization				
3rd Hospitalization				
4th Hospitalization				

Tests and Immunizations: Mark an X next to those that you have had. Enter the year when you last were given the tests or "shots."

Year
- ☐ 19___ chest x-ray
- ☐ 19___ kidney x-ray
- ☐ 19___ G.I. series
- ☐ 19___ colon x-ray
- ☐ 19___ gallbladder x-ray
- ☐ 19___ electrocardiogram
- ☐ 19___ TB test
- ☐ 19___ sigmoidoscopy

Year
- ☐ 19___ smallpox "shots"
- ☐ 19___ tetanus "shots"
- ☐ 19___ polio series
- ☐ 19___ typhoid "shots"
- ☐ 19___ flu injections
- ☐ 19___ mumps "shots"
- ☐ 19___ measles "shots"
- ☐ 19___ _____

Medicines: Mark an X in the box next to any medicines that you are now taking, or that you are sensitive or allergic to.

taking	allergic to:		taking	allergic to:
☐	☐ antibiotics		☐	☐ aspirin
☐	☐ penicillin		☐	☐ diet pills
☐	☐ sulfa		☐	☐ antacids
☐	☐ opiates/codeine		☐	☐ laxatives
☐	☐ diuretics/water pills		☐	☐ cold tablets
☐	☐ sedatives		☐	☐ _____
☐	☐ stimulants/caffeine		☐	☐ _____
☐	☐ Demerol		☐	☐ _____
☐	☐ blood pressure medicine		☐	

Your Signature: _____ CONTINUE TO NEXT PAGE

FIGURE 14-3 See legend on opposite page

than medical terminology; you may misinterpret if you try to do the latter.
- Record the duration of the patient's symptoms.
- Avoid using diagnostic terms as part of the chief complaint.

> **SPECIAL HINT**
>
> It is the medical assistant's responsibility to record the complaints, not make a diagnosis.

The physician will complete the patient's record by recording his or her own observations and diagnosis. Many physicians use a method of recording information known as SOAP. (See Chapter 2.)

Subjective information
Objective information
Assessment
Plan

The patient's chief complaint comprises the subjective portion of the record. Objective information is also recorded as the medical assistant performs vital signs. The physician then completes the objective information by examining and assessing the patient. Assessment includes the physician's diagnosis of the patient. The plan includes the physician's instructions to the patient as well as any prescriptions or medications the physician gives to the patient. It also mentions plans for future office visits as well as laboratory or radiological tests ordered for the patient.

At times, a patient may present to the physician's office in severe pain and it may be difficult to obtain a complete history from the patient. Family members may be able to answer questions. Usually when a patient presents in severe pain the primary concern is what condition is causing the pain. Nurses who work in emergency rooms have developed a plan for obtaining information necessary for the physician when a patient is in severe pain. It is known as the PQRST method of interviewing patients.

P—Provoke. What caused the pain? Did anything seem to trigger it?
Q—Quality. How does the patient describe the pain? Is it stabbing, dull, pounding, etc?
R—Region. Where is the pain located? Does it radiate to other body parts?
S—Symptoms. Are there accompanying symptoms such as nausea and vomiting, numbness, etc?
T—Time. When did the pain start? How long does it last if intermittent? Has the patient had pain like this before?

VITAL SIGNS

After the medical assistant has obtained the patient's medical history, he or she is often asked to take the vital signs—height, weight, pulse, respiration, temperature, and blood pressure. The results obtained from these simple medical tests give the physician information upon which he or she can begin to base a diagnosis. It is important that the tests be done accurately and that factors affecting the results be understood by the medical assistant.

Height

Height may not be taken on an adult at each office visit. It is, however, important to measure height on the first office visit to have a record of the height in the chart. Often this question is asked on forms the physician may be asked to complete. Having it readily available will save time for the physician.

Children need to have their height checked at regular intervals so that the physician can determine whether a proper growth rate is being maintained.

FIGURE 14-3

Example of a health history form. The health history consists of the following sections: (A) introductory data, (B) family history, (C) past history. (Reproduced from Bonewit K: *Clinical Procedures for Medical Assistants*, 3rd ed. Philadelphia: W. B. Saunders, 1990, p. 55.)

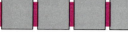

PROCEDURE

MEASURING HEIGHT

PURPOSE

To determine the patient's physical height and growth rates.

EQUIPMENT AND MATERIALS

A balance-beam scale with a measuring bar
Paper towels (optional)

PROCEDURAL STEPS

1. Place a towel on the scale.
   RATIONALE: This protects the soles of the patient's feet from cross-contamination.
2. Ask the patient to remove both shoes.
   RATIONALE: For accurate height and growth patterns, the patient should be measured in bare feet.
3. Assist the patient onto the scale and facing away from the weights.
   RATIONALE: The measuring bar better rests on the patient's head when the patient is facing away from the scale.
4. Instruct the patient to stand erect and still, looking straight ahead.
5. Lift the bar of the measuring scale above the patient's head, keeping the horizontal bar in the vertical position.
6. When high enough over the patient's head, lift the bar outward into the horizontal position.
7. Move the horizontal bar downward until it rests on the top of the patient's head.
8. Leaving the bar in position, assist the patient off the scale.
9. Read the measurement where the movable point of the horizontal bar meets the ruler. Read the ruler from the bottom up.
10. Record the height to the nearest quarter inch.
11. Return the measuring bar to zero.

SPECIAL HINT

Some scales measure height in centimeters; others measure it in inches. If your scale measures in centimeters and you wish to convert to inches, multiply the number of centimeters by 0.3937. If your scale measures in inches and you wish to convert to centimeters, multiply the number of inches by 2.54.

Weight

Most physicians request that each patient's weight be recorded at each visit. A change in weight may be significant in the physician's diagnosis. Weight changes may reflect the patient's state of health and response to medication therapy. Patients who are overweight may be evaluated for diet therapy. A sudden increase in weight may indicate that the patient is suffering from edema. Weight is also important in the prescribing of medications. Many medications are prescribed on the basis of milligram per kilogram.

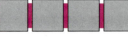

PROCEDURE

MEASURING WEIGHT

PURPOSE

To determine the patient's physical weight and growth rates.

EQUIPMENT AND MATERIALS

A balance-beam scale with a measuring bar
Paper towels (optional)

PROCEDURAL STEPS

1. Place a towel on the scale.
   RATIONALE: This protects the soles of the patient's feet from cross-contamination.
2. Place all weights to zero and check that the balance-beam pointer floats in the middle of the pointer frame.
   RATIONALE: The pointer balanced in the middle of the frame when all weights are at zero indicates that the scale is in balance.
3. Ask the patient to remove both shoes.
   RATIONALE: For accurate weight and growth patterns, the patient should be measured consistently in bare feet.
4. Assist the patient onto the scale. The scale will now be off balance and the pointer tilted to the top of the frame.
5. Instruct the patient to stand still, looking straight ahead.
6. Move the 50-lb lower weight to the groove nearest the estimated patient weight. The pointer should still be now floating somewhere between the midpoint and the top of the frame. If the pointer tilts to the bottom of the frame, the 50-lb weight has been moved too far.
7. Slide the small quarter-lb weight from left to right until the pointer floats exactly in the middle of the frame again.
8. Leaving the weights in position, assist the patient off the scale.
9. Add the numbers of the large and small weights together.
10. Record the weight to the nearest quarter lb.
11. Return the weights to zero.

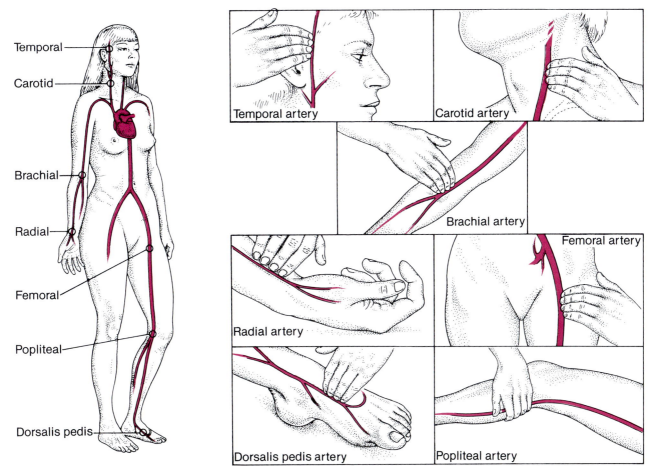

FIGURE 14–4

The pulse sites. (Reproduced from Kinn M, Derge E: *The Medical Assistant: Administrative and Clinical*, 6th ed. Philadelphia, W. B. Saunders, 1988, p. 441.)

Pulse

The pulse is the rate, rhythm, condition of arterial walls, compressibility and tension, and size and shape of the fluid wave of blood traveling through the arteries as a result of each heartbeat.[3] The heart normally beats about 70 times per minute, sending about 5 liters of blood through the adult body. The rate, rhythm, and quality of the pulse may vary, and the medical assistant must record this information on the patient's chart.

For a routine pulse the radial artery is usually the most accessible and the most commonly used (Figure 14–4). The pulse is taken using the pads of the first three fingers, never the thumb. The following chart shows normal values and how to record the pulse rate, rhythm, and quality. When abnormalities are noted, you should use the stethoscope to listen to the apical heartbeat, at the same time palpating the radial pulse. In this way you can determine if a pulse deficit is present.

THE PULSE RATE, RHYTHM, AND QUALITY

RATE

Infants	115–130 beats per minute (bpm)
Children (ages 1–7 years)	80–120 bpm
Children (ages 7 years to adult)	72–90 bpm
Adults	70–80 bpm

Factors That Affect Pulse Rate

Sex: Females tend to have a slightly faster pulse rate than male adults.
Physical activity: Exertion in the form of exercise or increased physical activity may cause increased pulse rate.
Increased body metabolism: Increased metabolism, for example, during pregnancy, will increase pulse rate.
Medications: Some medications may increase pulse rate, and others may reduce it.
Pain: Pain may increase pulse rate.
Emotions: Anger, fear, and anxiety may increase pulse rate.
Physical condition: Fever, anemia, hypoxia, shock, and congestive heart failure may increase pulse rate.
Trained athletes: These individuals may have slowed pulse rates.

RHYTHM

Normal rhythm: Intervals between beats are the same.
Premature beats: This may occur when a pacemaker fires ahead of the sinoatrial node. This initiates early systole. Because of reduced filling time, the stroke volume is decreased enough for you to feel a pause in rhythm. This may occur due to cardiac irritability, hypoxia, digitalis overdose, or potassium imbalance, or it may be a sign of a more serious arrhythmia.
Sinus arrhythmia: This is common in children and young adults and is an irregular pulse that speeds up at the peak of inspiration and slows down with expiration.
Alternating pulse: This is alternating weak and strong pulsations.
Bigeminal pulse: Two regular beats are followed by a longer pause.
Chaotic pulse: This is an extremely irregular pulse following no pattern.

QUALITY

Quality refers to the character of the pulse. It may be noted on the following 3-point scale:

3+	Bounding pulse
2+	Normal pulse
1+	Weak pulse
0	Absent pulse

Terms used to describe the quality of the pulse are as follows:

Thready: A very fine, scarcely perceptible pulse.
Vermicular: A small, rapid pulse giving to the finger a sensation of wormlike movement.
Vibrating: The sensation feels "jerky" under your finger.
Wiry: A small, tense pulse.
Abrupt: A pulse that strikes the finger rapidly; a quick or rapidly rising pulse.
Elastic: A full pulse that gives an elastic feeling to the finger.
Formicant: A pulse that is small, nearly imperceptible.
Full: A pulse that is easily felt.

PULSE DEFICIT = THE DIFFERENCE BETWEEN APICAL AND RADIAL PULSES

This information should be recorded on the chart.

Respiration

Respiration is the act of breathing, that is, inhaling and exhaling. Normal relaxed breathing is regular, effortless, and almost silent. The individual can control respiration to a certain extent.

> **SPECIAL HINT**
>
> Because patients can control respiration, the medical assistant should measure respirations without the patient's being aware of what is being done. To do this, continue to hold the wrist as if continuing to take the pulse, while measuring the respiration.

The respiratory rate for a normal, healthy adult is 16–20 respirations per minute. However, various factors affect the respiratory rate—age, physical activity, illness, drugs, and emotions. The chart below lists the terminology used to describe the various rates of respiration.

The depth of respiration indicates how much air is being inhaled or exhaled during breathing. If the depth of respiration is abnormal, it should be noted using the terminology listed in the chart.

When a patient has difficulty breathing, the medical assistant may note various sounds, such as wheezing. If these sounds are heard, they should be noted on the patient's chart using the terminology in the box below.

Temperature

Some physicians request that a patient's temperature be taken at each office visit, even if the visit is for a condition in which the temperature

---

THE SOUNDS AND RHYTHM OF RESPIRATION

Terms Used to Describe Breath Sounds

Stertorous: A snoring sound caused by secretions in the trachea and large bronchi.
Stridor: A crowing sound on inspiration. It often occurs with upper airway obstruction in laryngitis, croup in children, or lodging of a foreign body.
Wheeze: A high-pitched musical sound that occurs when the smaller bronchi and bronchioles are partially obstructed, as in emphysema or asthma.
Sigh: A deep inspiration followed by a prolonged expiration.
Rales and rhonchi: Rattling sounds that occur with secretions in the lung passageways.
Expiratory grunt: In adults this may be caused by a partial airway obstruction or a neuromuscular reflex. In an infant it may indicate imminent respiratory distress.
Absence of sound: This may result from pneumothorax, atelectasis, or local airway obstruction that prevents the ventilation of part or all of a lung field.

Terms Used to Describe Changes in Respiratory Rate and Rhythm

Eupnea: Normal respiration.
Tachypnea: Increased respiratory rate.
Bradypnea: Decreased but regular respiratory rate.
Apnea: Total absence of breathing, may be periodic.
Hyperpnea: Increased depth of respiration
Hypoventilation: Prolonged depression of respiratory center that alters both the pattern and the depth. The rate becomes irregular or slow and the depth becomes shallow.
Hyperventilation: Increase in both rate and depth of respiration.
Cheyne-Stokes: A cycle where respirations gradually increase in rate and depth and then decrease over a cycle of 30–45 seconds.
Biot's: Interrupted breathing similar to Cheyne-Stokes, except that each breath is of the same depth.
Kussmaul's: Increased rate and increased depth, panting, or labored respiration.
Apneusis: Prolonged gasping inspiration, followed by extremely short, inefficient expiration.

would not be an important factor. This is done to establish a baseline temperature in the individual. The average normal adult body temperature is 98.6° F (Table 14-2).

The average normal adult body temperature may differ according to the site used to record the temperature. Measured orally, average temperature is considered 98.6° F (37° C) and is

TABLE 14-2

TEMPERATURE CONVERSION SCALE: FAHRENHEIT TO CELSIUS*

F	C	F	C	F	C
95.0	35.0	100.2	37.9	105.4	40.8
95.2	35.1	100.4	38.0	105.6	40.9
95.4	35.2	100.6	38.1	105.8	41.0
95.6	35.3	100.8	38.2	106.0	41.1
95.8	35.4	101.0	38.3	106.2	41.2
96.0	35.5	101.2	38.4	106.4	41.3
96.2	35.6	101.4	38.5	106.6	41.4
96.4	35.7	101.6	38.6	106.8	41.5
96.6	35.9	101.8	38.7	107.0	41.6
96.8	36.0	102.0	38.8	107.2	41.8
97.0	36.1	102.2	39.0	107.4	41.9
97.2	36.2	102.4	39.2	107.6	42.0
97.4	36.3	102.6	39.3	107.8	42.1
97.6	36.4	102.8	39.4	108.0	42.2
97.8	36.5	103.0	39.5	108.2	42.3
98.0	36.6	103.2	39.6	108.4	42.4
98.2	36.8	103.4	39.7	108.6	42.5
98.4	36.9	103.6	39.8	108.8	42.6
98.6	37.0	103.8	39.9	109.0	42.7
98.8	37.1	104.0	40.0	109.2	42.9
99.0	37.2	104.2	40.1	109.4	43.0
99.2	37.3	104.4	40.2	109.6	43.1
99.4	37.4	104.6	40.3	109.8	43.2
99.6	37.5	104.8	40.4	110.0	43.3
99.8	37.6	105.0	40.5		
100.0	37.7	105.2	40.6		

* To convert degrees F to degrees C, subtract 32, then multiply by 5/9. To convert degrees C to degrees F, multiply by 9/5, then add 32.
Reprinted from Kinn M, Derge E: *The Medical Assistant: Administrative and Clinical*, 6th ed. Philadelphia: W. B. Saunders, 1988, p. 439.

TABLE 14-3

VARIANCE OF TEMPERATURE BY SITE

	Rectal ° F	Oral ° F	Rectal ° C	Oral ° C
Strenuous exercise	101-104	99.8-101.4	38.3-40	38.5
Emotion/moderate exercise	100-101.4	99.4-101.0	37.7-38.5	37.4-38.3
Active children/some adults	100-101.4	98.6-100.8	37.7-38.5	37.0-38.2
Normal range	97.2-100	96.2-99.6	36.1-37.7	36.0-37.5
Morning/cold weather	96.0-96.8	96.0-96.4	35.5-36.0	35.5-35.7

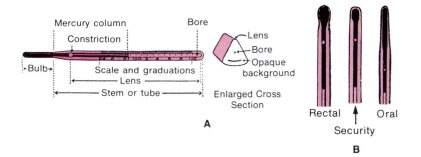

FIGURE 14-5

A, The cross-section of the clinical thermometer is triangle shaped. The lens must be held at eye level to see and read the level of mercury. **B,** Illustration of the construction of the bulbs. The rectal thermometer is stubby. The security thermometer is often used for axillary temperatures. The oral thermometer has a longer, more slender bulb. (Reproduced from Kinn M, Derge E: *The Medical Assistant: Administrative and Clinical,* 6th ed. Philadelphia, W. B. Saunders, 1988, p. 438.)

1° F (0.6° C) higher when measured rectally. Thermometers placed in the axillary region tend to register 1° F or more lower than at the oral site (Table 14-3).

Variations in body temperature can be caused by conditions other than illness.

- Strong emotions can increase body temperature.
- When body metabolism slows down, such as during sleep, body temperature is lowered.
- The temperature of the weather outdoors can affect an individual's body temperature when he or she is exposed to it.
- Physical exercise increases body temperature.
- Pregnancy raises body temperature due to increased cell metabolism.
- The age of the patient is also a factor in body temperature. Infants and young children normally have a higher body temperature and older adults have lower body temperatures.

Methods of Taking a Temperature

There are three methods for taking body temperature: oral, rectal, and axillary. These sites are used because they have an abundant blood supply, indicating the temperature of the entire body, not just the temperature of only a part of the body. Different kinds of thermometers are used for each area (Figure 14-5).

Glass thermometers are probably the most commonly used. They can be used with temperature sheaths. Electronic thermometers are becoming more popular and are also commonly used in physician's offices.

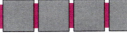

PROCEDURE

TAKING A PATIENT'S TEMPERATURE WITH AN ELECTRONIC THERMOMETER

PURPOSE

To determine a patient's body temperature.

EQUIPMENT AND MATERIALS

Electronic Fahrenheit thermometer
Swipes or tissues
Lubricant
Watch with a second hand

PROCEDURAL STEPS

1. Wash hands and follow CDC Universal Precautions (listed at the beginning of this chapter).
2. Ask the patient about hot or cold drinks or smoking within the last 15-30 minutes.
   RATIONALE: Cold drinks, hot drinks, and smoking will temporarily increase the temperature of the oral cavity.

3. Attach the proper probe to the thermometer unit.
4. Insert the probe into the face of the thermometer.
5. Remove the thermometer unit from its rechargeable base.
6. Grasp the probe by the collar and remove it from the face of the thermometer.
7. Firmly attach a disposable color-coded plastic probe cover to the probe.
   RATIONALE: This prevents cross-contamination. Covers are color coded for oral/axillary or rectal use.
8. Explain the procedure to the patient:
   a. Place the probe in the patient's mouth not under the tongue, or
   b. Place the probe in the center of the axilla, or
   c. Lubricate the end of the probe cover up to 1 inch. Spread the buttocks and place the probe approximately 1 1/2 inches into the rectum for adults and 1/2 inch for infants.
9. Hold the probe in place for 5 seconds or until the audible tone is heard.
10. Read the digital display on the screen.
11. Remove the probe from the patient.
12. Without touching the probe cover, discard the probe cover into the appropriate receptacle by pushing the ejection button.
13. Return the probe to its stored position in the thermometer unit.
14. Wash hands.
15. Record the results on the patient's chart.
16. Return the thermometer unit to its base to recharge.

Blood Pressure

Blood pressure is the force exerted on the walls of the arteries by the blood.[3] Measurements are made of the systolic and diastolic pressures. The systolic pressure is measured in the phase of the cardiac cycle known as the *systole*. It represents the highest point of blood pressure in the body. The diastolic pressure is the lower pressure measured at the point where the heart is relaxed. During contraction of the heart, the systolic pressure is measured. During relaxation of the heart diastolic pressure is measured. The first number recorded is the systolic pressure, the second number recorded, following a slash, is the diastolic pressure. The normal range for an adult's blood pressure is 110/60 – 140/90.[8]

As a person ages, blood pressure gradually increases. Blood pressure readings may vary from moment to moment. If a blood pressure reading is taken at each office visit, the physician is able to compare the readings over a period of time. Many patients also keep their own records of blood pressure readings taken at home or at other times.

Errors in Measuring Blood Pressure

To measure blood pressure, a stethoscope and a sphygmomanometer are needed. Check the stethoscope to be sure it is in good working order before use. The sphygmomanometer is an instrument that measures arterial blood pressure. It consists of a manometer containing a scale for registering pressure (this may be either a mercury or an aneroid manometer) as well as an inflatable bag surrounded by a covering known as a cuff. The cuff is available in different sizes. It is very important that the proper-size cuff be used. If the wrong-size cuff is used, it is likely that an erroneous reading will be obtained.

Errors are often made in blood pressure readings. These errors can easily be avoided if the medical assistant is careful to pay close attention to detail.

Assessing Blood Pressure by Auscultation

Blood pressure is measured by auscultatory sounds termed *Korotkoff's sounds*. These sounds are produced by the vibrations of blood against the arterial wall as the collapsed artery reopens when the cuff is deflated.

Phase I: Clear rhythmical tapping that increases in intensity. The artery first reopens.

- This first sound is noted as the systolic pressure reading.
- If the cuff is not inflated well above the systolic pressure, phase I sounds may be missed.

Phase II: Soft swishing or murmur sounds. The artery distends, creating vibrations in the vessel wall. Occasionally, sounds may completely disappear. The silence may continue for as much as 30 mm Hg.

- The loss of sound during this phase is termed

GUIDELINES TO ENSURE ACCURATE BLOOD PRESSURE READINGS

Guideline	Rationale
Use the correct-size cuff.	If the cuff is too narrow, the reading will be falsely high. If the arm circumference is less than 13 inches, a regular-size cuff should be used. If the arm is extremely small, or you are measuring the blood pressure in a pediatric patient, use a pediatric cuff. If the arm is between 13 and 16 1/2 inches, a large-size cuff should be used. If the arm is more than 16 1/2 inches, a thigh cuff should be used.
Do not deflate the cuff too slowly.	If the cuff is deflated too slowly, venous congestion can occur in the arm. This can cause an erroneous high reading. The cuff should not be deflated any slower than 2 mm Hg/heartbeat.
Be sure the cuff is wrapped tightly around the arm.	If the cuff is wrapped too loosely, a falsely elevated reading may result.
Be sure you are reading the mercury column at eye level.	If you read the column below eye level you will record a falsely low reading. If it is above eye level, you will record a falsely high level.
Be sure the mercury column is not tilted.	If the mercury column is tilted, a falsely high reading will result.
Do not overinflate the cuff.	If a cuff is overinflated, it may cause the patient pain and result in an erroneously high reading.

an *auscultatory gap*. Because an auscultatory gap can occur in hypertension and certain heart diseases, it should be noted in the recording.

- If the cuff is not inflated well above the systolic pressure or if the cuff is deflated too quickly, the sounds may be missed.

   Phase III: Crisp, sharp tapping sounds that return and continue rhythmically. The artery remains open in systole, but the sound is still obliterated in diastole.

- If the cuff is not inflated well above the systolic pressure or if the cuff is deflated too quickly, the first two phases may be missed entirely, and phase III may be misinterpreted as the systolic pressure.

   Phase IV: Soft tapping that is muffled and grows fainter. The cuff pressure falls below the blood pressure.

- Occasionally, these sounds continue to zero, especially in children, after exercise, during fever, or during pregnancy if anemia is present.
- Some physicians consider phase IV as the true diastolic reading; others consider the phase IV changes as the "fading sound" and want it recorded between the systolic and diastolic readings.
- Phase IV is usually recorded as the diastolic pressure reading for children.
- Phase IV may be recorded in adults with hypertension.

   Phase V: Disappearance of sound. It is usually recorded as the diastolic pressure reading in healthy adults.

PROCEDURE

ASSESSING BLOOD PRESSURE BY AUSCULTATION

PURPOSE

To determine a patient's blood pressure.

EQUIPMENT AND MATERIALS

Sphygmomanometer (aneroid or mercury)
Stethoscope

MEDICAL ASSISTING ALERT

Measure blood pressure before administering any medication that may affect blood pressure. At the patient's first assessment, take readings in both arms; thereafter use the arm with the higher pressure. A difference of 5–10 mm Hg is considered normal. A greater difference may indicate a condition such as arterial occlusion.

PROCEDURAL STEPS

Preparation

1. Be sure the aneroid dial points to zero or the mercury column rests at zero. Adjust in either direction.
2. Check the parts for cleanliness and leaks.
3. Choose the correct cuff size.
4. Wash hands.
5. Explain the purpose of the procedure to the patient.
6. Assist the patient into a comfortable sitting (preferred) or lying position (note position on the chart) with the arm at heart level.
   RATIONALE: Having the arm above heart level may produce a falsely low reading.
7. Remove any constricting clothing.
8. Take multiple readings on the first visit.
   RATIONALE: Blood pressure may change with position or in different extremities.

Performance

9. Palpate the brachial artery.
10. Position the cuff 1–1 1/2 inches above the antecubital space.
11. Center the arrows of the cuff over the brachial artery.
    RATIONALE: Positioning the bladder of the cuff directly over the brachial artery ensures proper compression during inflation.
12. Wrap the fully deflated cuff snugly and evenly around the upper arm.
13. Position the manometer at eye level.
14. If the patient's usual systolic pressure is unknown, palpate the patient's radial artery and inflate the cuff 30 mm Hg above the point where the radial pulse can no longer be felt.
    RATIONALE: The maximum inflation point is determined and auscultatory gap (phase II) misreadings are prevented.
15. Deflate the cuff and wait 30 seconds.
    RATIONALE: This allows the vessels to decongest and prevents false high readings.
16. Place the stethoscope earpieces in your ears, keeping the tubing free from surface noises.
17. Palpate the brachial artery and place the stethoscope bell over it.
18. Close the pressure bulb valve clockwise until it is tight.
19. Inflate the cuff to a pressure 30 mm Hg above the patient's usual blood pressure or to the maximum inflation point.
20. Open the valve and release the pressure at the rate of 2 mm Hg per second.
    RATIONALE: Too rapid or slow a release may lead to inaccurate readings.
21. Note the first Korotkoff's sound (first clear sound) as the systolic pressure.
22. Note the fourth Korotkoff's sound (fading).
23. Note the point on the manometer when the sound disappears (fifth Korotkoff's sound).
24. Deflate the cuff to zero rapidly and remove from the patient's arm.
    RATIONALE: Continuous inflation will result in numbness or tingling of the patient's arm.
25. Wait 30 seconds before repeating the procedure, if necessary.
26. Remove the cuff and store.
27. Assist the patient to a comfortable position.
28. Record the blood pressure sounds immediately by one of the following methods:

    - First/disappearance
    - First/fading sound
    - First/fading/disappearance
    - First/auscultatory gap/fading/disappearance
    - First/auscultatory gap/fading
    - First/auscultatory gap/disappearance

Assessing Blood Pressure in Children

1. Select pediatric-size cuff or choose a cuff bladder that is 40% of the circumference of the midpoint of the limb or 20% of the diameter of the limb.
2. Older children may sit; children under 5 years of age should lie flat with the arm supported at the side.
3. Wait 15 minutes if the child is upset or active.
4. Use the adult auscultatory method.

Assessing Blood Pressure by Direct Palpation

1. This method is used with patients who have a weakened brachial pulse due to severe blood loss or loss of heart contractibility.
2. Select a cuff size in the usual manner.
3. Palpate the radial artery throughout the procedure instead of using a stethoscope.
4. Record the first pulsation felt as the systolic reading.
5. Record the last thin pulse vibration as the diastolic pressure.

Assessing Blood Pressure in the Lower Extremities

1. This method is used with patients whose arms are inaccessible or who have a condition that causes a difference in blood pressure between the upper and lower extremities.
2. The site used is the popliteal artery behind the knee.
3. Position the patient in the recumbent position or standing with the knee slightly flexed.
4. Select a cuff size in the usual manner; use a wide, long cuff.
5. Position the cuff so that the bladder is over the posterior aspect of the midthigh.
6. Follow the auscultatory method.

SPECIAL HINT

Systolic pressure in the popliteal artery is usually 10–40 mm Hg higher than in the brachial artery; the diastolic pressure is usually the same as in the brachial artery.

MEDICAL EXAMINATIONS

After the medical assistant has obtained a history and performed vital signs, he or she prepares the examination room and the patient for the type of examination to be performed. Certain articles should be kept in the examination room at all times because they are used so frequently. The needs may vary according to the specialty of the physician.

Once the type of examination is determined, the medical assistant is responsible for laying out the instruments and equipment the physician will need to perform the examination. Each physician may have his or her own preferences. It is a good idea to keep a card file handy with this information listed on it.

The medical assistant may find it helpful to group items that are usually used together. For example, all items used for changing dressings or applying bandages could be placed together in a special tray. Disposable otoscope covers can often be placed in a special container that is hung on the wall. Items used for vaginal and rectal examinations can be placed together. Often a table with stirrups is used for vaginal examinations. These tables are often equipped with a warming drawer. Vaginal specula can be placed in this drawer so they will be warm when used.

The medical assistant should be familiar with the contents of the examination room, knowing exactly where everything is without having to think twice about it. This helps the physician and promotes confidence between the physician and the patient.

SPECIAL HINT

Many medical assistants have found it helpful to list on an index card the contents of each drawer or slot in a drawer and in each cabinet and attach it to the drawer or drawer divider. If this is done, then each morning before the patients come in, the examination rooms can be stocked to be sure the contents are in place. The process avoids delays for the patient, the medical assistant, and the physician.

ITEMS NEEDED IN THE EXAMINATION ROOM

Patient examination gowns	Cotton balls	Penlight flashlight	Tuning fork
Paper pillow covers	Alcohol	Waste container	Cotton swabs, large and small
Specula (vaginal and rectal)	Betadine or similar iodine-based topical medication	Drapes	Tape in varying widths
Sphygmomanometer		Examination gloves	Hydrogen peroxide
Thermometer		Gooseneck lamp	Gauze squares
Otoscope	Antibiotic ointment	Stethoscope	Specimen bottles
Ophthalmoscope	Lubricant, water soluble	Tape measure	Tissues
Tongue blades	Specimen slides	Disposable otoscope covers of varying sizes	Kidney basin (emesis basin)

POSITIONS FOR EXAMINATION

Position	Assessment
Sitting	Visualization of upper body parts; provides full expansion of lungs

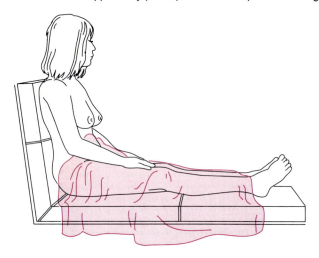

Supine	Most relaxed position; prevents contracture of abdominal muscles; provides easy access to pulse sites; facilitates breast examination

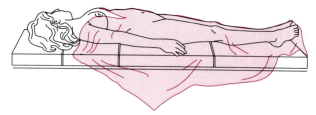

Dorsal recumbent	Provides more comfortable position for patients with painful disorders

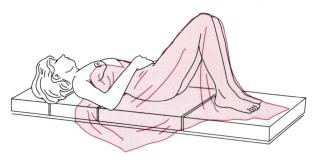

Lithotomy — Provides maximum exposure of genitalia; facilitates insertion of vaginal speculum

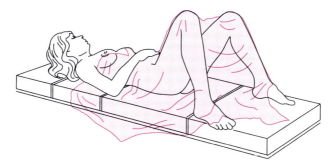

Prone — Facilitates assessment of hip joint

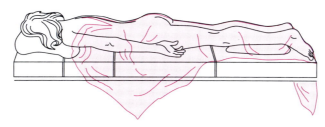

Sims — Improves exposure of the rectal area

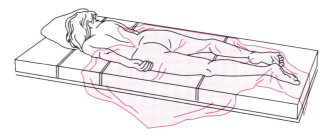

Proctological — Provides maximum exposure of rectum and facilitates insertion of proctological instruments

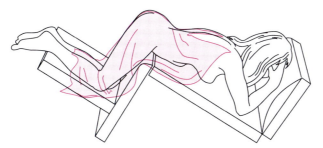

Knee–chest   Is the same as proctological in the absence of a special table for examination

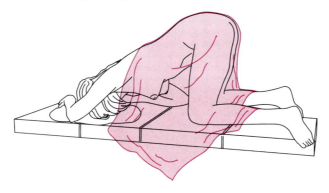

Preparing for a Complete Physical Examination

Equipment and Materials

Thermometer
Balance-beam scale
Tape measure
Otoscope
Tuning fork
Ophthalmoscope
Tonometer
Tongue blades
Percussion hammer
Speculum
Vaginal speculum (if female)
Nasal speculum
Anoscope
Lubricant
Tissues
Cotton-tipped applicator
Gooseneck lamp
Penlight flashlight
Kidney basin
Waste container
Stethoscope

Care of the Patient

1. Explain to the patient what he or she should expect.
2. Offer to answer any questions.
3. Ask the patient if he or she needs to empty the bladder before the examination (collect urine and fecal specimens at this time).
4. Explain to the patient that he or she will need to completely disrobe. Explain how to put on the examination gown, whether to place the opening in front or back as your physician prefers.
5. Ask if the patient needs any assistance with disrobing and offer your assistance.
6. If the patient does not need assistance, give him or her privacy.
7. Allow the patient time to undress and put the gown on before re-entering the examination room.
8. Provide the patient with an examination sheet and a blanket as needed.
9. Assist the patient onto and off the examination table, if necessary.
10. Do not leave confused, upset, or uncooperative patients unattended.

Preparing for a Proctological Examination

Equipment and Materials

Rectal Examination

Sheet or paper to cover the table
Tissues
Examination gloves or finger cot
Lubricant
Sponge forceps
Sponges
Rectal speculum and/or anoscope
Cotton-tipped applicators
Slide for occult blood testing

Proctosigmoidoscopy Examination

Sheet or paper to cover the table
Insufflator with bulb attachment
Metal sponge holder
Suction tip
Suction equipment
Light source
Sigmoidoscope with obturator
Examination gloves
Sponges
Lubricating jelly
Biopsy forceps
Requisitions for specimens
Containers for specimens
Rectal dressing forceps
4 × 4 inch gauze squares
Rheostat
Extension cord (if necessary)

Care of the Patient

1. Explain the examination to the patient.
2. Offer to answer any questions.
3. Ask the patient if he or she needs to empty the bladder.
4. Ask the patient to disrobe from the waist down.
5. Provide a drape for the patient.
6. Ask if the patient needs any assistance in disrobing.
7. Give the patient privacy to change.
8. Allow the patient time to disrobe before re-entering the room.
9. For the proctological examination, assist the patient to assume a knee–chest position.

   - Ask the patient to kneel with the chest resting on the examining table.
   - The buttocks are elevated with the back kept straight.
   - Be sure the patient's head, chest, and arms are supported on the table.
   - The head is turned to one side.
   - A pillow can be used for support.
   - The knees and lower legs should be separated at least a foot apart.
   - Some offices are equipped with special tables that tilt and fully support the patient in this position.

10. If only a rectal examination is to be performed, the physician may prefer that the patient be placed in the Sims position.

    - Position the patient on the left side with the left arm behind the body and the right arm forward with the elbow bent.
    - Flex both legs, with the right leg flexed sharply and the left leg flexed slightly.

11. After a patient has been in the knee–chest position, he or she may feel dizzy if allowed to stand up too quickly. It may be advisable to allow the patient to sit on the examination table for a few minutes before standing. Stay with the patient during this time.

PROCEDURE

ASSISTING WITH THE PROCTOLOGICAL EXAMINATION

PURPOSE

To provide a third person of the client's sex during the examination, to assist in the comfort of the patient, and to assist the physician in the organization of the examination.

PROCEDURAL STEPS

1. Assist the patient into position.
2. For sigmoidoscopy, record baseline vital signs and leave the blood pressure cuff on the patient's arm during the examination.
3. Drape the patient with the examination sheet.
4. Position and turn on the gooseneck or halogen lamp.
5. Hand the physician examination gloves.
6. Apply lubricant to the physician's gloves for the digital examination.
7. Instruct the patient to breathe slowly and deeply as the digital examination is performed.
8. Warm the instruments being used, if possible.
9. Provide lubricant for the instruments.
10. Hand the physician the instruments.
11. Instruct the patient to breathe slowly and deeply.
    RATIONALE: This relaxes the anal sphincters and facilitates passage of the instrument.
12. Hand the physician swabs as needed.
13. Regulate machine suction as needed.
14. Present clean containers for specimens.
15. Label the specimen with the patient's name.
16. Complete the laboratory requisition form and attach it to the specimen.
17. Record information on the patient's chart as instructed by the physician and initial the chart.
18. Clean the examination room and return instruments to the sanitization and sterilization area.

The Eye and Ear Examinations

Equipment and Materials

Eye

Snellen or other eye chart
Opaque card or eye cover
Color plate
Perimeter
Mydriatic drops
Ophthalmoscope
Tonometer
Local anesthetic for the eye
Fluorescein dye
Amsler grid
Exophthalmometer
Schirmer test kit

Ear

Otoscope
Tuning fork
Audiometer

Nose

Nasal speculum

Throat

Tongue blades
Laryngeal mirror
Head mirror
Flashlight, penlight, and/or gooseneck lamp
Culture equipment if necessary

Care of the Patient

1. Explain the examination to the patient.
2. Offer to answer any questions.
3. The patient does not usually have to disrobe for this examination. He or she may be asked to remove any jewelry, such as earrings or necklaces.

Assessment of the Eyes

The eyes are examined for visual acuity, visual field, extraocular movements, and the external eye structures. A separate ophthalmoscopic examination is also performed.

Visual Acuity. In most adults, visual acuity declines to some extent with the aging process (Table 14–4). Visual acuity can be measured in stages:

Stage I: Ask patient to read magazine or newspaper print (Figure 14–6) on the Near-Vision Acuity Chart.

TABLE 14–4

COMMON VISUAL DEFECTS CORRECTABLE WITH GLASSES

Condition	Definition
Myopia (nearsightedness)	Individual can see objects most accurately when close at hand. In myopia, the eyeball or the crystalline lens may be contoured defectively. Corrective lenses cause light to be focused directly on the retina and thus improve sight.
Hypermetropia (farsightedness)	Individual can see objects most accurately when they are at a distance. Again, the objective of the corrective lens is to allow the light to be focused on the retina.
Presbyopia	Individual can see only distant objects clearly, but the images cloud as they are drawn closer, thus resembling farsightedness. Aging appears to be a common natural cause of presbyopia as the crystalline lens which is normally elastic becomes less accommodating. Corrective lenses can improve this condition.
Astigmatism	Individual cannot focus clearly; vision is blurred. The contour of either the cornea or the crystalline lens prevents light from being projected on the retina adequately. Corrective lenses can improve the condition.
Strabismus	Individual has difficulty directing both eyes toward the same objects. Muscle coordination in the eye is affected. Eyes may cross or turn outward. Corrective lenses and specific exercises or surgery may improve the condition.

Reprinted from Frew MA, Frew DR: *Comprehensive Medical Assisting: Administrative and Clinical Procedures*, 2nd ed. Philadelphia: F. A. Davis, 1988, p. 407.

Stage II: Ask patient to read magazine or newspaper print with one eye closed or, in cases of severe impairment, to count upraised fingers.

Stage III: Ask the patient to read a Snellen eye chart (Figures 14–7 and 14–8).

Visual Field. The field of vision is the area within which stimuli will produce the sensation of sight with the eye in a straight-ahead position. Optic nerve damage or retinal disorders may block out a portion of the visual field. Any patient with visual field alterations should be referred to an ophthalmologist for a more detailed examination. Visual fields are tested by moving the finger or another object into the patient's field of vision from all four directions.

60
Nothing can take the place of "the only pair of eyes you will ever have." That is why you are exercising such good judgment in taking care of them as you are now doing.

50
For this reason, you will welcome the suggestion about lenses which are designed and made to give you "greater comfort and better appearance." In man's earliest days he had little use for glasses. He used his eyes chiefly for long distance.

40
He worked by daylight and at tasks with little detail. But now, you use your eyes for much close work—reading, writing, sewing and many other uses which the eyes of primitive man did not know. Now your eyes meet all sorts of lighting conditions, artificial and natural.

30
Many of these conditions produce "overbrightness" or glare. Sometimes it is the direct or reflected glare of sunlight; often it is direct or reflected from artificial light. And very often this glare is uncomfortable—impairs your efficiency. But special lenses, developed by America's leading optical scientists, combat this glare.

25
These lenses give you more comfortable vision and blend harmoniously with your complexion. These lenses are less conspicuous. We are glad to recommend them because they will give you greater comfort and better appearance. Thousands of satisfied wearers testify to their real benefits.

20
You are wise in taking good care of "the only pair of eyes you will ever have." You know how valuable they are, that you can never have another pair. For this reason, you will welcome the suggestion about lenses which are designed and made to give you "greater comfort and better appearance." In man's earliest days he had little use for glasses.

The above letters subtend the visual angle of 5' at the designated distance in inches.

B-858 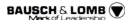 Printed in U.S.A.

FIGURE 14-6

The Near-Vision Acuity Chart of magazine and newspaper print for persons older than 40 years who have difficulty with accommodation (adjusting to changes in distance) because the eye muscles no longer respond quickly. (Reproduced from Kinn M, Derge E: *The Medical Assistant: Administrative and Clinical,* 6th ed. Philadelphia: W. B. Saunders, 1988, p. 560.)

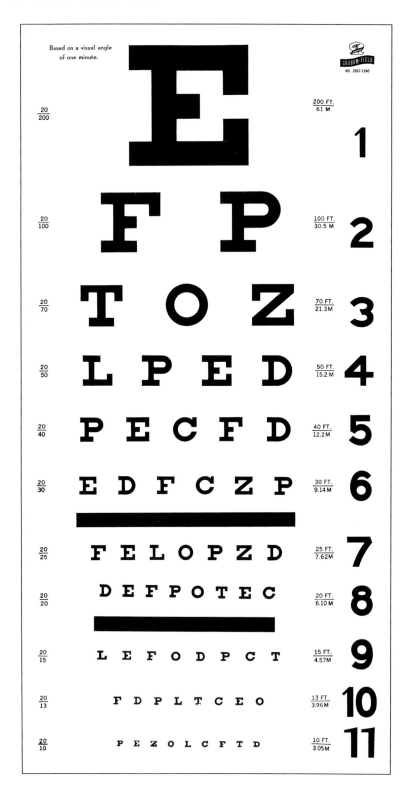

FIGURE 14-7
A Snellen eye chart consisting of letters in decreasing sizes, which is used to measure distance visual acuity. (Reproduced from Bonewit K: *Clinical Procedures for Medical Assistants*, 3rd ed. Philadelphia: W. B. Saunders, 1990, p. 83.)

Extraocular Movements. Extraocular movements are controlled by six small muscles and the innervation of cranial nerves. Altered eye movements can be an indication of eye injury or disease of the eye muscles, supporting structures, or cranial nerves. Extraocular movements are tested by observing eye movement as objects are moved through eight cardinal gazes:

- Up and down
- Right and left
- Diagonally up and down to left
- Diagonally up and down to right

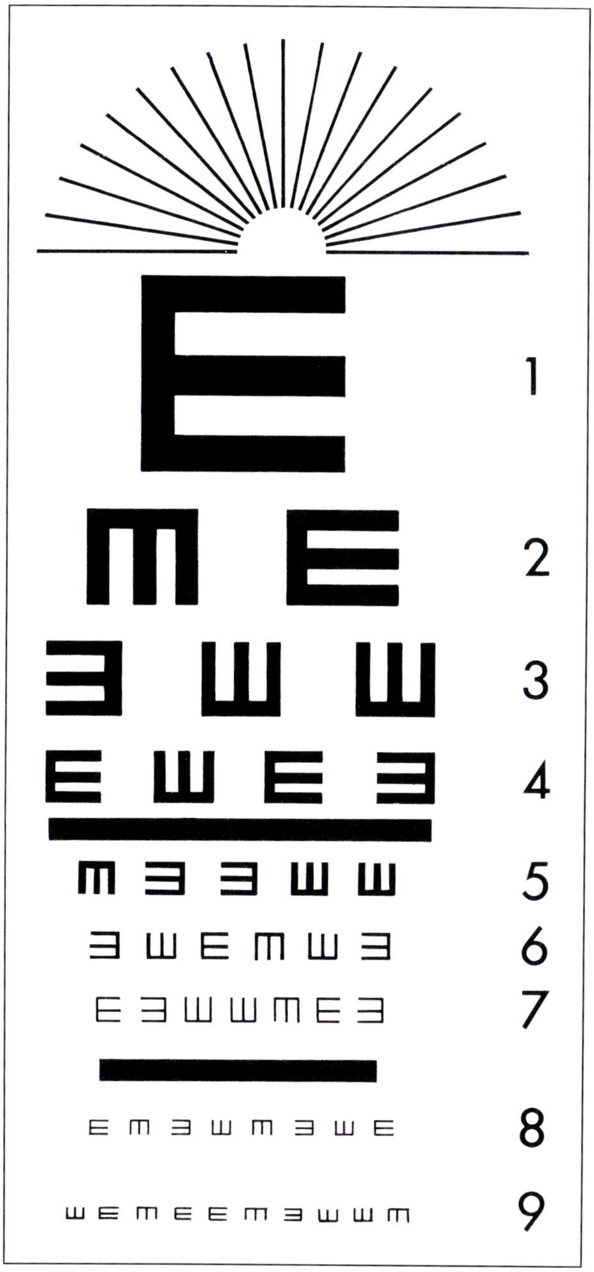

External Eye Structures. Examination of the external eye structures includes the inspection of eye alignment and position, eyebrows, eyelids, lacrimal (tear) ducts, conjunctivae, sclerae, pupils, and irises. Assessment also includes testing for the accommodation reflex by asking the patient to look at near objects, then distant objects, then near objects again.

Ophthalmoscopic Examination. The ophthalmoscopic examination is performed to inspect the internal structures of the eye, including the fundus, retina, choroid, optic nerve disc, macula, fovea centralis, and retinal vessels. Regular ophthalmoscopic examinations are very important for patients with diabetes, hypertension, and intracranial pathological conditions. Table 14-5 lists common diseases of the eye and symptoms, treatment, and the medical assistant's role associated with each.

Assessment of the Ears

The ear examination consists of the inspection of the auricle, otoscopic examination of the outer ear (ear canal) and middle ear, and hearing acuity tests. The structure of the ear is shown in Figure 14-9.

Types of Hearing Loss

Conduction loss: Sounds unable to transmit from the outer and middle ear
Sensorineural loss: Abnormalities of the inner ear, auditory nerve, or hearing center in the brain
Mixed: Conduction loss and sensorineural loss

Hearing Screening Tests

Simple Screening. Whisper random numbers to the patient, gradually increasing loudness if necessary. Normally, the patient can hear the whispers.

Weber Test for Conduction Deafness. Place the base of a vibrating tuning fork against the patient's head. Normally the patient hears the

FIGURE 14-8
A Snellen Big E eye chart consisting of the capital letter E in decreasing sizes and arranged in different directions, which is used to measure distance visual acuity. (Reproduced from Bonewit K: *Clinical Procedures for Medical Assistants,* 3rd ed. Philadelphia: W. B. Saunders, 1990, p. 84.)

TABLE 14-5
COMMON DISEASES OF THE EYE

Disease	Symptoms	Treatment	Medical Assistant's Role
Cataract (crystalline lens becomes clouded) Opacity of lens	Impaired vision: spots before the eyes. Blurred vision, halo around lights	Surgical removal (phakolysis)	General clinical medical assisting procedures. Patient education is essential before surgery
Conjunctivitis (inflammation of the conjunctiva)	Redness and swelling, pain, increased tearing (especially caused by allergy). Others are burning, itch, photophobia, and discharge	Drug therapy: ophthalmic antibiotics, antiallergic drugs such as antihistamines. Instillation of antiseptic solutions. Eye irrigation. Warm compresses. Possible allergy testing, vasoconstrictors	General medical assisting clinical procedures. Patient teaching includes instruction to prevent reinfection. Emphasis on reading and writing in good light with frequent rest periods is advised
Glaucoma (increased pressure within the eyeball with no known cause) Types: Open angle, chronic Closed angle, acute	Pain with gradual pressure and impairment of vision. Chronic pain, pressure inflammation, pupil dilation are acute symptoms	Drug therapy. Surgery. Continuous monitoring.	Patient teaching includes emphasis on avoiding the lifting of heavy objects. Emotional stress should be avoided as this tends to increase ocular pressure. Stress drug compliance
Stye (acute inflammation of the edge of the eyelid)	Stinging pain and the presence of a hordeolum (swelling) are common	Warm compresses. An incision may be made into the stye to allow drainage. Antibiotics may also be used	Teach patient warm compresses × 4 daily to promote drainage. Prevent infection by cleanliness and no rubbing. Protect eye by decreasing reading, avoiding direct sun, increasing rest by closing eyes, and avoiding strain

Reprinted from Frew MA, Frew DR: *Comprehensive Medical Assisting: Administrative and Clinical Procedures*, 2nd ed. Philadelphia, F. A. Davis, 1988, p. 408.

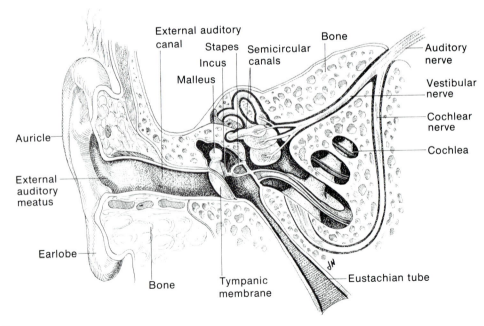

FIGURE 14-9
Structure of the ear. (From Bonewit K: *Clinical Procedures for Medical Assistants*, 3rd ed. Philadelphia: W. B. Saunders, 1990, p. 98.)

tuning fork equally in both ears at the midline of the head (negative Weber).

Rinne Test to Compare Air and Bone Conduction. Place the base of a vibrating tuning fork against the patient's mastoid bone and then close to the ear opening. Normally air conduction hearing is better than bone conduction hearing (positive Rinne).

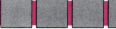

PROCEDURE
ASSESSING VISUAL FIELDS

PURPOSE

To determine normal (20/20) visual acuity for each eye.

EQUIPMENT

Snellen eye charts (regular chart, E chart, and pediatric chart)
Index card, eye patch, or eye cup

RECORDING THE VISUAL ACUITY SCORE

The visual acuity score is recorded as two numbers for each eye, for example, R:20/20, L:20/15. The numerator indicates that the patient is 20 feet from the chart. The denominator indicates the standardized number for the last line the patient is able to read accurately using one eye. Visual acuity of 20/200 is considered legal blindness.

PROCEDURAL STEPS

1. If the patient uses eye glasses, ask the patient to wear the glasses unless they are for reading purposes only.
2. Stand the patient 20 feet from the chart.
3. Ask the patient to keep both eyes open and read the smallest line of print possible.
4. Record the number of the smallest line in which the patient read more than half of the letters correctly.
5. Repeat with one eye closed.
6. Repeat with the other eye closed.
7. Record the results.
8. For patients who are illiterate, use the E chart. Ask the patient to point in the same direction as the Es.
9. Young children should use the E chart or the pediatric chart of familiar objects.

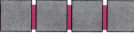

PROCEDURE
EXAMINING THE EAR CANAL

PURPOSE

To inspect the auricle(s) before, during, and after an ear lavage.

EQUIPMENT AND MATERIALS

Otoscope
Ear speculum

 MEDICAL ASSISTING ALERT

If a foreign body is present in the ear canal, be careful not to impact the foreign body any further with the use of instruments to visualize it or remove it. A reddened ear canal is an indication of inflammation. Discharge or drainage is an indication of infection.

PROCEDURAL STEPS

1. Assist the patient into the sitting position. (Infants should lie supine with the head to the side and be restrained; small children should be restrained or helped by the parent to keep the head immobile.)
2. Ask the patient about any of the following symptoms: pain, itching, discharge, ringing in the ears (tinnitus), or changes in hearing acuity.
3. Record any abnormal responses.
4. Select the largest ear speculum that comfortably fits into the ear canal.
5. Check the canal for foreign bodies before inserting the speculum.
6. Ask the patient to tilt the head toward the opposite shoulder and to keep the head still.
7. Straighten the ear canal by pulling the auricle upward and backward (for infants, pull downward and backward).
8. Insert the speculum, being careful not to scrape or injure the ear canal.
9. Look into the speculum to inspect the canal for ear wax (cerumen), foreign bodies, or discharge.
10. Inspect the ear drum (tympanic membrane) by moving the otoscope light so that it reflects the entire ear drum.
11. Note the appearance of the ear drum. It should be translucent pearly gray and free of breaks or tears.
12. Record information on the patient's chart as instructed by the physician and initial the chart.
13. Clean the examination room and return instruments to the sanitization and sterilization area.

The Neurological Examination

Equipment and Materials

Tuning fork
Ophthalmoscope
Flashlight or penlight
Tongue blades
Percussion hammer
Test tubes with hot and cold water
Bottles of sweet, bitter, salty, and sour solutions
Bottles of solutions with common familiar odors, such as cinnamon, toothpaste, etc.
Sterile safety pins
Cotton balls

Care of the Patient

1. Explain the examination to the patient.
2. Offer to answer any questions.
3. Ask the patient to disrobe, according to the physician's instructions.
4. Ask if the patient needs any assistance in disrobing.
5. Give the patient privacy for disrobing.
6. Allow time for disrobing before re-entering the room.
7. Ask the patient if he or she needs assistance in dressing.

Full assessment of the neurological system is very complex, and the physician may need assistance with note-taking and helping patients who are physically weak or limited in mobility (Table 14–6).

The full neurological examination can be lengthy. However, some aspects of the examination are integrated with parts of the routine physical examination; for example, the reflexes may be tested during assessment of the musculoskeletal system, mental and emotional status can be assessed while taking the history, and sight is assessed during the examination of the eyes.

The complete neurological assessment includes the following:

Mental and Emotional Status. Normal findings include the patient's being able to

- Respond to questions quickly
- Be aware of events around him or her
- Respond cooperatively
- Manifest good personal hygiene and appropriate dress
- Recall information immediately
- Explain common sayings and associations

SPECIAL HINT

Be careful not to question the patient about topics that are culturally or educationally discriminating. If the patient is confused or irritable, delay or skip parts of the examination and note occurrence in the patient's chart. Any sudden change in the patient's responsiveness or orientation should be immediately reported to the physician.

TABLE 14-6

THE NEUROLOGICAL EXAMINATION

Body Part and Function	Method and Equipment	Medical Assistant's Role
Mental Status Survey: Cognitive abilities	Inspection of body posture and general appearance. Interviewing with questions directed at measuring intelligence, memory, etc. Observe grooming, dress, hygiene, orientation to person, time, and place.	The medical assistant is usually not present for this portion of the examination as it might interfere with the relationship between the physician and the patient. The medical assistant, however, may provide input regarding mental status derived from time spent alone with the patient.
Face for Cranial Nerve Status: Olfactory (smell)	Patient may be asked to identify common odors with eyes closed.	The medical assistant will be present and hand the physician the items required. Patient will be sitting.
Optic (sight)	Ophthalmoscope used to examine the eye. Visual acuity test may be performed to test vision capabilities.	The visual acuity test may be the responsibility of the medical assistant.
Pupil motor reaction	Flashlight inspection. Palpation of the face. Patient clenches teeth and physician palpates muscles.	Lights out. Support unsteady patient on examining table.
Sensory	Patient closes eyes. Physician palpates the face. Safety pin may be used. Evaluate for light, touch, temperature, corneal reflex. Use sterile swab, tubes with warm and cold water.	The medical assistant may need to assemble various items that would assist the physician to test for pain or feeling sensation. Clean safety pins and cotton balls are most frequently used.
Facial motor ability	Inspection of the face as the patient is given directions such as to frown, smile, puff out cheeks, clench teeth. Observe symmetry and movement.	The medical assistant should note the degree of patient comfort. A complete examination tends to be lengthy. Rest periods are usually provided in which the physician leaves the room. The medical assistant can attend to the patient's comfort and remain for quiet conversation if time permits.
Voice	Evaluate for hoarseness/speech, tongue movements.	
Hearing	Physician may speak in various tones to test hearing capabilities. Weber and Rinne tests.	Medical assistant may be asked to perform audiometry.
Nerves of the Motor System: Coordination and muscle strength; gait	Patient will be asked to walk, do knee bends, walk on toes, raise hands above head, flex extremities, and push and pull against examiner's hands. Finger-to-nose movements. Romberg test—balance.	Medical assistant should be close to patient if balance is lost to prevent patient's falling.
Nerves of the Sensory System: Arms, trunk, legs	Inspection with pin and tuning fork, cotton balls.	The medical assistant assists the patient to assume a supine position. Patient may get very tired.
Reflexes: All points of reflexes, such as knees, elbows, ankles	Reflex hammer.	The patient is assisted to a sitting position, then again to a supine position.

Reprinted from Frew MA, Frew DR: *Comprehensive Medical Assisting: Administrative and Clinical Procedures*, 2nd ed. Philadelphia, F. A. Davis, 1988, p. 403.

Cranial Nerve Function Status. Normal findings include the patient's being able to perform the following activities:

- Smell
- See
- Taste
- Hear
- Move the jaw
- Make facial expressions
- Swallow
- Move the tongue
- Vocalize
- Move the head and shoulders

Sensory Nerve Function Status. Normal findings include the patient's being able to respond to

- Pain
- Temperature
- Light touch
- Vibration
- Up and down movements
- Two-point discrimination of touch

Motor Function Status. Normal findings include the patient's being able to

- Respond to coordinate body movements
- Maneuver movements with balance

Reflexes. Normal findings include a symmetry of reflexes on both sides of the body. Reflexes are recorded on a scale of 0–4:

0 — no response
1 — low normal or diminished response
2 — normal
3 — more active than normal
4 — hyperactive

How to examine your breasts

In the shower:

Examine your breasts during bath or shower; hands glide easier over wet skin. Fingers flat, move gently over every part of each breast. Use right hand to examine left breast, left hand for right breast. Check for any lump, hard knot or thickening.

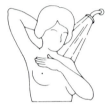

Before a mirror:

Inspect your breasts with arms at your sides. Next, raise your arms high overhead. Look for any changes in contour of each breast, a swelling, dimpling of skin or changes in the nipple.

Then, rest palms on hips and press down firmly to flex your chest muscles. Left and right breast will not exactly match — few women's breasts do.

Regular inspection shows what is normal for you and will give you confidence in your examination.

Lying down:

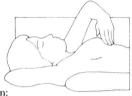

To examine your right breast, put a pillow or folded towel under your right shoulder. Place right hand behind your head — this distributes breast tissue more evenly on the chest. With left hand, fingers flat, press gently in small circular motions around an imaginary clock face. Begin at outermost top of your right breast for 12 o'clock, then move to 1 o'clock, and so on around the circle back to 12. A ridge of firm tissue in the lower curve of each breast is normal. Then move in an inch, toward the nipple, keep circling to examine *every part of your breast*, including nipple. This requires at least three more circles. Now slowly repeat procedure on your left breast with a pillow under your left shoulder and left hand behind head. Notice how your breast structure feels.

Finally, squeeze the nipple of each breast gently between thumb and index finger. Any discharge, clear or bloody, should be reported to your doctor immediately.

FIGURE 14–10

Breast self-examination. (Courtesy of the American Cancer Society, Inc., 1975.)

Employment, School, and Insurance Examinations

Employment and insurance examinations are two types of examinations performed by the physician that may entail special requirements determined by third-party requestors. There are also physical examinations for children to be admitted to school, physical examinations for adults wishing to become foster parents, and disability physical examinations. All of these physical examinations require special forms to be completed and special instructions to follow.

Medical Assistant's Role

Often the medical assistant can complete a large portion of the special form for the physician. Review the patient's record to determine information on immunizations, prior illnesses, etc. For any laboratory work that is required, the medical assistant must be careful to follow the strict requirements often stipulated on the form. At times certain companies may request that all laboratory specimens be sent to a specific address. They may also stipulate the method by which the specimen is to be collected.

SPECIAL HINT

Be sure that you understand all legal requirements and instructions before proceeding with completion of the form. If you have questions, call the individual requesting the examination report before proceeding.

Patient Self-Examination

Breast and testicular self-examinations play a major role in educating patients about cancer and screening for the presence of masses or irregularities in the breast or testicular tissues. Teach patients about the importance of monthly self-examination and ask them what methods they use and when (Figures 14-10 and 14-11). Teach patients the signs of potential abnormalities to watch for on a regular basis.

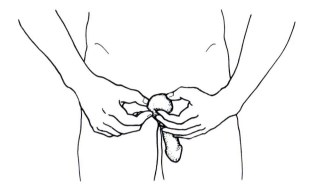
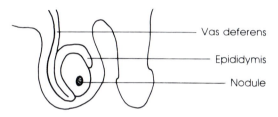

FIGURE 14-11

Testicular self-examination. (Redrawn from *For Men Only*. New York: American Cancer Society; in Kinn M, Derge E: *The Medical Assistant: Administrative and Clinical*, 6th ed. Philadelphia: W. B. Saunders, 1988, p. 538.)

References

1. Miller F, Brackman Keane C: *Encyclopedia and Dictionary of Medicine, Nursing and Allied Health,* 5th ed. Philadelphia, W. B. Saunders, 1992.
2. Bonewit K: *Clinical Procedures for Medical Assistants,* 3rd ed. Philadelphia, W. B. Saunders, 1990, pp. 9-12.
3. Thomas CL (Ed): *Taber's Cyclopedic Medical Dictionary*, 16th ed. Philadelphia, F. A. Davis, 1989, p. 1630.
4. Zakus SM: *Clinical Skills and Assisting Techniques for the Medical Assistant.* St. Louis, C. V. Mosby, 1981, p. 77.
5. Potter DO (Ed): *Practices.* Springhouse, PA: Springhouse Corporation, 1984, p. 156.
6. Sandmeyer Bootay LS: *Documenting Patient Care Responsibly.* Springhouse, PA: Intermed Communications, 1982, pp. 12-13.
7. Hall M: *Assessing Your Patients.* Horsham, PA: Intermed Communications, 1981, pp. 12-13.
8. Jarvis CM: *Assessing Vital Functions Accurately.* Horsham, PA: Intermed Communications, 1981, pp. 29-31.

Chapter 15

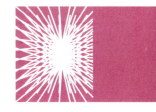

MEDICATION ADMINISTRATION

KAREN LANE

RESPONSIBILITIES IN DRUG THERAPY

READING AND UNDERSTANDING WRITTEN AND ORAL ORDERS
Abbreviations
Systems of Measurement

MEASURING AND CALCULATING DRUG DOSAGE
Measuring Medications
Drugs that Require Reconstitution

UNDERSTANDING HOW DRUGS ARE ABSORBED, DISTRIBUTED, AND EXCRETED BY THE BODY
Drug Delivery and Absorption
Factors that Influence the Effects of Drugs

ASSESSING THE PATIENT, THE DRUG, AND THE ENVIRONMENT
Patient Assessment
Drug Assessment
The Environment

CHOOSING THE CORRECT ROUTE AND SITE
Oral Medications
Mucous Membrane Medications
Topical Medications
Parenteral (By Injection) Medications

USING THE CORRECT TECHNIQUE AND EQUIPMENT FOR INJECTIONS
Advantages of Injections
Routes of Administration
Landmarks

USING SPECIAL SYRINGE TECHNIQUES
Using Syringe Dead Space and Air Bubbles
Admixing Two Drugs in a Single Syringe

ADMINISTERING PARENTERAL MEDICATIONS
Assessing the Patient Prior to Injection
Using the Z-tract Technique
Steps to Reducing Injection Pain

TUBERCULIN TESTING

RECOGNIZING POTENTIAL ADVERSE EFFECTS
Emotional Complications of Injections
Physical Complications of Injections
Managing Drug Emergencies

RESPONSIBILITIES IN DRUG THERAPY

With advancing technology in medication techniques and an increased participation of patients in their own drug administration, medical assistants have, over time, assumed an increasing responsibility in drug therapy procedures and patient care.

In the traditional medical office arrangement, the physician provides the diagnostic and medical aspects of care by prescribing or ordering drugs for administration, while the medical assistant is entrusted with the responsibility of administering the medications. Both the medical assistant and the physician, therefore, share an important role in the proper execution of medication procedures, and written office policies should outline the procedures for each type of medication administered. Written policies should include

- Patient care
- Step-by-step procedures
- Specific techniques for each type of medication administered.

The physician is legally responsible for monitoring and assessing the patient's response to drug treatment and for responding to adverse reactions or inadequate treatments associated with improperly executed orders. The physician must (a) provide written or oral orders that are accurate and clearly stated and (b) demand expertise from those entrusted with patient care.

The medical assistant must be knowledgeable about techniques of administration and the laws that specify the conditions under which medical assistants may actually administer drugs. The medical assistant must also be skilled in the physical and emotional care of the patient before, during, and after each medication administration.

The medical assistant's expertise is demonstrated by the ability to

- Read and understand written or oral orders
- Measure and calculate drug dosage accurately
- Understand how drugs are absorbed, distributed, and excreted by the body
- Assess the patient, the drug, and the environment before the administration of every medication
- Choose the correct route and site for administration
- Use the correct techniques and equipment for injections
- Determine injection sites with anatomical accuracy
- Determine when a volume of two medications can be administered in a single administration or must be divided into multiple administrations
- Recognize potential adverse effects
- Provide the physician with clinical information observed about techniques and the patient's response to treatment

Safe and effective care depends on the ability of both the physician and the medical assistant to respond to patient needs with appropriate *comfort measures, teaching* and *counseling, public education*, and positive *role modeling*.

- Comfort measures help patients cope with and adapt to the effects of drugs.
- Patient and family teaching and counseling help patients understand the importance of drug therapy and encourage them to participate in decisions about their own care.
- Public education and role modeling helps the public understand drugs and their use and abuse.

READING AND UNDERSTANDING WRITTEN AND ORAL ORDERS

Abbreviations

Drug orders and prescriptions are written with specific abbreviations that are derived from either Latin words and phrases or from systems of weights and measures (Table 15–1).

Latin phrases are most often used to denote directions for administration, for example, "every four hours" is written "q4h" *(quaque quarta hora)*.

Weights and measures are usually abbreviated in the same manner they are abbreviated in other scientific disciplines; for example, the metric weight "milligram" is abbreviated "mg" (Table 15–2).

The Drug Enforcement Agency places certain drugs and drug products under the jurisdiction of the Controlled Substances Act of 1970. These drugs and drug products are divided into five schedules. Table 15–3 lists examples.

The Food and Drug Administration assigns pregnancy categories to drugs and drug products (if known). These categories allow for assessment of the risk to the fetus when a drug or drug product is used during pregnancy or in the patient who is trying to conceive while or shortly after receiving the drug (Table 15–4).

Systems of Measurement

Drugs are weighed and measured in three systems of measurement. The systems use weight measures to determine strength and volume measures to determine amount. Each system has ap-

TABLE 15-1

COMMON PRESCRIPTION ABBREVIATIONS

Abbreviation	Latin	Translation
aa	ana	of each
a.c.	ante cibum	before meals
ad	ad	up to
ad lib.	ad libitum	as much as needed
a.m.	ante meridiem	morning
ante	ante	before
aq.	aqua	water
b.i.d.	bis in die	two times a day
c̄	cum	with
capsul.	capsula	capsule
contra	contra	against
elix.	elixir	elixir
emul.	emulsum	emulsion
et	et	and
ext.	extractum	extract
f., or ft.	Fac or fiat	make
fl.	fluidus	fluid
gm.	gramma	gram
gr.	granum	grain
gt.	gutta	drop
gtt.	guttae	drops
h	hora	hour
h.s.	hora somni	hour of sleep (bedtime)
inj.		injection (to be injected)
kg.		kilogram
M.	misce	mix
mcgm.		microgram
noct.	nocte	at night
o		other
o	omnis	every
O.D.	oculus dexter	right eye
O.S.	oculus sinister	left eye
p.c.	post cibum	after meals
p.r.n.	pro re nata	whenever necessary
pil.	pilula	pill
pulv.	pulvis	powder
q.	quaque	every
q.d.	quaque die	every day
q.h.	quaque hora	every hour
q.i.d.	quarter in die	four times a day
q.n.	quaque nocte	every night
q.n.s.	quantum non satis	quantity not sufficient
qo		every other
q.s.	quantum satis	quantity sufficient
q.2h.	quaque secunda hora	every two hours
q.4h.	quaque quarta hora	every four hours
R$_x$	recipe	take
S, or Sig	signa, signetur	write (on the label)
s̄	sine	without
sat.		saturated
sol.	solutio	solution
s.o.s.	si opus sit	if needed
sp.	spiritus	spirit
ss.	semis	one half
stat.	statim	immediately
suppos., supp.	suppository	suppository
syr.	syrupus	syrup
tab.	tabella	tablet
t.i.d.	ter in die	three times a day
tr. (tinct.)	tinctura	tincture
troc.	troche	lozenge
U.		unit
ung.	unguentum	ointment
ut dict.	ut dictum	as directed

Reprinted from Kinn M, Derge E: *The Medical Assistant: Administrative and Clinical*, 6th ed. Philadelphia: W. B. Saunders, 1988, p. 465.

TABLE 15-2
ABBREVIATIONS AND SYMBOLS FOR SELECTED WEIGHTS AND MEASURES

Apothecary System			Metric System	
♏	Min. (M.)	minim	g	gram
℈	scr	scruple	L	liter
ʒ	dr	dram	cc	cubic centimeter
fl ʒ	f dr	fluid dram	ml	milliliter
℥	oz	ounce	mg	milligram
fl ℥	fl oz	fluid ounce		
O	pt	pint		
C	gal	gallon		
	gr	grain		

Reprinted from Kinn M, Derge E: *The Medical Assistant: Administrative and Clinical,* 6th ed. Philadelphia: W. B. Saunders, 1988, p. 478.

TABLE 15-3
CLASSIFICATION OF CONTROLLED SUBSTANCES

Classification	Description	Examples
Schedule I	Drugs having a high potential for abuse and no accepted medical use. (The drug container is marked C-I.)	Heroin LSD Marihuana Mescaline
Schedule II	Drugs having a high potential for abuse but with accepted medical use. Abuse may lead to severe psychologic or physical dependence. (The drug container is marked C-II.)	Amobarbital Amphetamine Cocaine Codeine Meperidine hydrochloride (Demerol) Morphine
Schedule III	Drugs having an accepted medical use with moderate or low potential for physical dependence and high potential for psychologic dependence. (The containers are marked C-III.)	Butabarbital Codeine-containing medications Nalorphine Paregoric
Schedule IV	Drugs having accepted medical use and that may cause mild physical or psychologic dependence. (The container is marked C-IV.)	Chloral hydrate (Noctec) Chlordiazepoxide (Librium) Diazepam (Valium) Fluazepam (Dolmane) Meprobamate (Equanil) Phenobarbital
Schedule V	Drugs having accepted medical use and that have limited potential for causing physical or psychologic dependence. (The container is marked C-V.)	Drug mixtures containing small quantities of narcotics such as cough syrups containing codeine (e.g., Robitussin A-C) Diphenoxylate and atropine preparations (e.g., Lomotil)

Reprinted from Bonewit K: *Clinical Procedures for Medical Assistants,* 3rd ed. Philadelphia: W. B. Saunders, 1990, p. 231.

TABLE 15-4
CATEGORIES OF DRUGS REGARDING USE IN PREGNANCY

Category	Definition
A	Animal and human studies to date have failed to show a risk to the fetus. There appears to be no risk in any of the three trimesters of pregnancy.
B	Animal studies have shown no risk to the fetus, but clinical studies on women are inadequate or incomplete.
C	Animal studies have shown a risk to the fetus, and clinical studies on women are inadequate, incomplete, or unavailable, or no animal or human studies are available.
D	There is clinical evidence of risk to the human fetus, but drug use may be acceptable in pregnant women despite its risk.
X	There is clinical evidence that the use of a drug has a high-risk potential to the developing fetus and has resulted in birth defects. These drugs should be contraindicated in pregnancy, despite their usefulness in treatment.

TABLE 15–5
COMPARISON OF WEIGHTS AND MEASUREMENTS

Apothecary Table of Weights

APOTHECARY		APPROXIMATE METRIC EQUIVALENT		
60 grains (gr)	= 1 dram (dr ʒ)	60 to 65	milligrams (mg)	= 1 grain
8 drams	= 1 ounce (oz ʒ)	4	grams	= 1 dram
12 ounces	= 1 pound (lb)*	30 to 32	grams	= 1 ounce
		370 to 375	grams	= 1 pound
		0.37 to 0.375	kilograms	= 1 pound

Metric Table of Weights

METRIC		APPROXIMATE APOTHECARY EQUIVALENT	
1000 micrograms (mcg)	= 1 milligram (mg)	gr 1/60	= 1 mg
1000 milligrams	= 1 gram (gm)	gr 15–16	= 1 gm
1000 grams	= 1 kilogram (kg)	2.2 lb (avoir.)	= 1 kg

Apothecary Table of Volume

APOTHECARY		APPROXIMATE METRIC EQUIVALENT	
1 minim (m)		= 0.06 ml	
60 minims	= 1 fluid dram (fl dr)	4 ml	= 1 fdr (fl dr)
8 fluid drams	= 1 fluid ounce (fl oz)	30 ml	= 1 foz (fl oz)
16 fluid ounces	= 1 pint (pt or O)	500 ml or 0.5 liter	= 1 pint
2 pints	= 1 quart (qt)	1000 ml or 1 liter	= 1 quart
4 quarts	= 1 gallon (gal or C)	4000 ml or 4 liters	= 1 gallon

Metric Table of Volume

METRIC		APPROXIMATE APOTHECARY EQUIVALENT	
1000 milliliters (ml)†	= 1 liter (L)	15 minims	= 1 ml
1000 liters	= 1 kiloliter (kl)	1 quart	= 1 liter or 1000 ml

Reprinted from Falconer MW, et al: *The Drug, The Nurse, The Patient,* 6th ed. Philadelphia: W. B. Saunders, 1978, p. 57.
* Note that in the avoirdupois table there are 16 ounces in one pound. In the Troy table there are 12 ounces in one pound, as with the apothecary.
† One cubic centimeter (cc) is often used in place of one milliliter (ml). A milliliter of water occupies approximately one cubic centimeter of space.

TABLE 15–6
HOUSEHOLD MEASURES AND EQUIVALENTS*

1 minim	= 1 drop
1 teaspoon	= 5 ml or 75 drops
4 teaspoons	= 1 tablespoon (15 cc)
1 dessert spoon	= 2 drams
1 tablespoon	= 4 drams
4 tablespoons	= 1 wineglass
16 tablespoons (liquid)	= 1 cup (liquid)
12 tablespoons (dry)	= 1 cup (dry)
1 cup	= 8 fluid ounces
1 glass	= 8 fluid ounces
1 wineglass	= 2 fluid ounces
1 pint	= 1 pound
1 tablespoon	= 16 cc
1 ounce	= 1 whiskey glass

* These measure and equivalents are approximate because of the great variation in household measuring devices.
Reprinted from Kinn M, Derge E: *The Medical Assistant: Administrative and Clinical,* 6th ed. Philadelphia: W. B. Saunders, 1988, p. 479.

proximate equivalents in the other two systems. The systems are interchangeable through the use of a conversion formula. The systems of measurement are:

- Metric system (Table 15-5)
- Apothecary system (Table 15-5)
- Household measurements (Table 15-6)

MEASURING AND CALCULATING DRUG DOSAGE

Measuring Medications

"Unit Dose" Medications

Medications available in unit dose forms are premeasured in the exact amount to be administered to the patient. The volume ordered becomes the amount to administer. For example:

- Solid oral medications labeled with a specified weight (milligram or grain) are administered by the order of the number of tablets or capsules to be given.
- Parenteral solutions in a single-dose vial or syringe are administered by the order to use the vial or syringe unit.

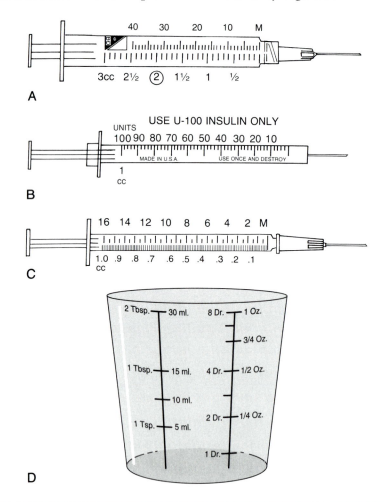

FIGURE 15-1

Various types of measures used to administer medications. **A**, Regular 3.0 cc (ml) syringe. **B**, Insulin (U-100) syringe. **C**, Tuberculin syringe. **D**, One-ounce medicine cup. (**A-C** reproduced from Bonewit K: *Clinical Procedures for Medical Assistants*, 3rd ed. Philadelphia, W.B. Saunders, 1990, p. 238.)

$$\text{Have}^* \left(\frac{\text{want}^{**}}{\text{have}^{***}} \right) = \text{Unit wanted}^{****}$$

* Unit of measurement from the written order.
** Conversion table equivalent for system of measurement on the equipment.
*** Conversion table equivalent for system of measurement in the written order.
**** Equivalent measurement in the system of measurement on the equipment.

Example:
Order: give 2 tsp
Equipment: oral syringe marked off in milliliters
Conversion (Table 15–6): 1 teaspoon = 5 ml

$$2 \text{ tsp} \left(\frac{5 \text{ ml}}{1 \text{ tsp}} \right) = 10 \text{ ml}$$

FIGURE 15–2

Universal conversion formula for converting from one unit or system of measurement to an equivalent unit or system. (Adopted from materials provided by Indiana Technical College, Human Services and Health Division, Indianapolis, IN, 1991.)

Drugs That Are Not Premeasured

Drugs that are not premeasured may require one or more of the following dosage procedures:

Measuring. A medication may be measured to an appropriate mark on a container (medicine cup, syringe, etc.) Measuring is performed without the need of further conversion or calculation. For example, oral solutions available in one strength only are administered by the order of a teaspoonful, a milliliter, or some other specified, measurable volume (Figure 15–1).

Converting. With a conversion formula, an order from one system of measurement is converted to an equivalent amount in another system of measurement before measurement is possible (Figure 15–2).

Calculating. The correct dosage is calculated by determining the volume necessary to deliver an ordered strength of a drug. Dosage problems may need to be worked to solve for:

- The unknown volume necessary to deliver an ordered strength (Figure 15–3). Drug strength/volume ratios may be microgram/milliliter, milligram/milliliter, gram/milliliter, grain/milliliter, milliequivalent, or unit/milliliter.
- A strength that can be determined only by the patient's body weight (Figure 15–4), or by using the body surface area of the patient (Figure 15–5) and the nomogram formula (Figure 15–6).
- A percentage strength stock solution. Drug strength to volume may be stated as 1%, 1 g/1000 ml, or 1:1000 (Table 15–7).

$$\frac{\text{Desired strength}}{\text{On-hand strength}} = \frac{X \left(\begin{array}{c} \text{Unknown unit} \\ \text{measure to give} \end{array} \right)}{\begin{array}{c} \text{Unit measure} \\ \text{of available strength} \\ \text{(quantity)} \end{array}}$$

$$\frac{D}{H} = \frac{X}{Q}$$
$$D \times Q = H \times X$$
$$\frac{D \times Q}{H} = X$$

FIGURE 15–3

Determining the amount of medication to give using the ratio and proportion formula.

Drugs That Require Reconstitution

Drugs in dry form must be reconstituted before use (Figure 15–7).

Oral Drugs. Oral drugs may be reconstituted with tap water.

Drugs for Stock Solutions. These should be reconstituted according to the manufacturer's directions. Usually, sterile water or distilled water is used.

Drugs for Parenteral Administration. These are reconstituted using multidose vials of sterile isotonic saline or sterile water. These multidose vials contain a small amount of bacteriostatic pre-

TABLE 15–7

MATHEMATICAL EQUIVALENTS

Percentage	Decimal	Fraction	Ratio
25%	.25	1/4	1:4
50%	.5	1/2	1:2
60%	.6	3/5 (6/10)	3:5
.5%	.005	1/200	1:200
.1%	.001	1/1000	1:1000
85%	.85	17/20	17:20
1%	.01	1/100	1:100

Reprinted from Kinn M, Derge E: *The Medical Assistant: Administrative and Clinical*, 6th ed. Philadelphia, W.B. Saunders, 1988, p. 476.

$$\frac{\text{mg}\binom{\text{Strength}}{\text{of drug}} \times \text{kg}^* \binom{\text{Body}}{\text{weight}}}{\text{Number of doses per day}} = \frac{\text{Amt. to give}}{\text{each dose}}$$

* 1 kg = weight in pounds / 2.2.

FIGURE 15-4

Determining the amount of medication to give using the mg/kg/day formula.

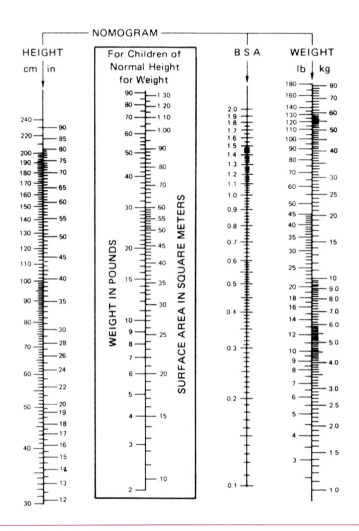

FIGURE 15-5

Using the West nomogram to determine body surface area (BSA). First, plot the height on the left vertical column. Second, plot the weight on the right vertical column. Third, draw a line to connect the plotted height and weight with a straightedge ruler. Finally, determine the BSA in square meters at the point the line crosses the surface area scale. (Modified from data of E. Boyd by C. D. West; in Behrman RE (ed.): *Nelson Textbook of Pediatrics,* 14th ed. Philadelphia: W.B. Saunders, 1992, p. 1827.)

$$\frac{\text{BSA in m}^2 \times \text{adult dose}}{1.7} = \text{Infant's or child's dose}$$

FIGURE 15-6

The formula for determining the amount of drug to give per square meter (m²) of body surface area (BSA). The "BSA in m²" is determined by first using the West nomogram (see Figure 15-5).

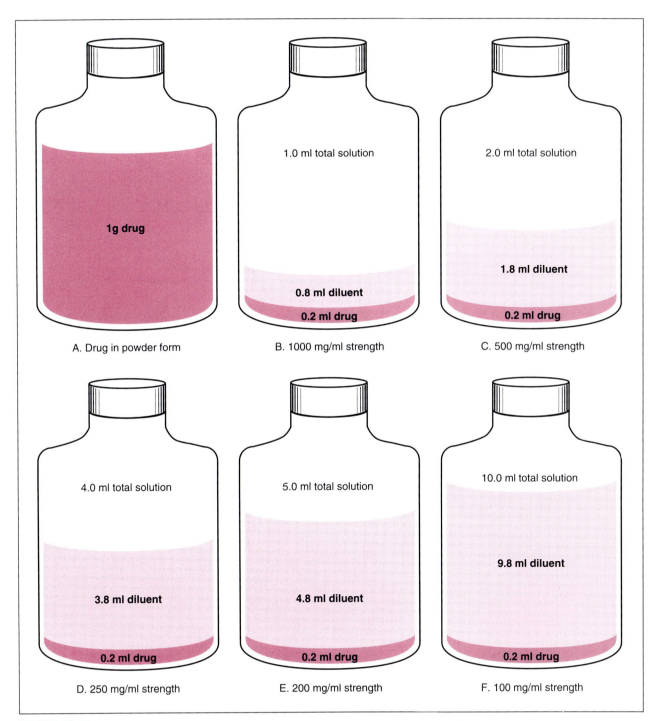

FIGURE 15–7
Reconstituting 1 g of drug that displaces (occupies) 0.2 ml of the total volume measurement after varying amounts of diluent are added.

344 *Chapter 15: MEDICATION ADMINISTRATION*

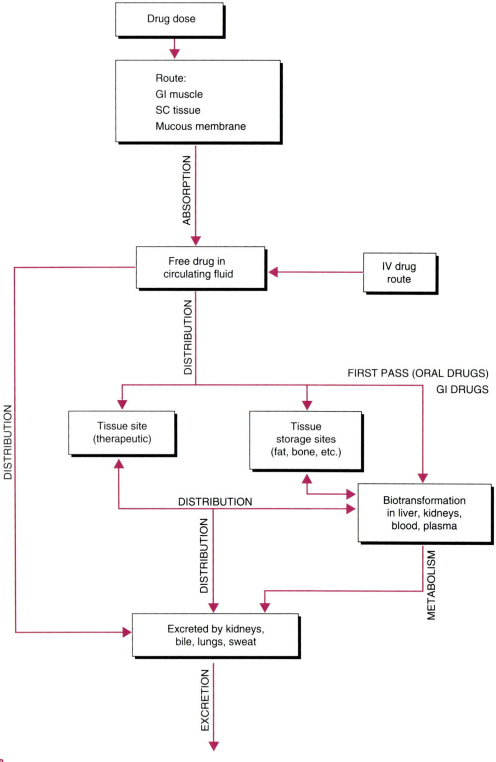

FIGURE 15-8

The processes by which the body absorbs, distributes, metabolizes, and excretes drugs.

servative. Directions for dissolving parenteral drugs can be found on the vial, on the box containing the vial, and on the package insert accompanying the vial.

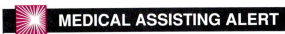

MEDICAL ASSISTING ALERT

Use *single-dose* diluents that do not contain preservatives when reconstituting pediatric medications.

SPECIAL HINT

Multidose vials of sterile isotonic saline or sterile water for injection contain bacteriostatic preservatives. Bacteriostatic preservatives have been linked to seizures in infants when used to reconstitute intramuscular drugs.

Manufacturer's directions for reconstituting drugs vary, and occasionally are inconsistent. In spite of the occasional inconsistencies, pharmacists recommend following the manufacturer's directions exactly as written.

UNDERSTANDING HOW DRUGS ARE ABSORBED, DISTRIBUTED, AND EXCRETED BY THE BODY

Drug Delivery and Absorption

For a drug to have a therapeutic effect, it must reach the intended site of action. In addition, successful therapy also depends on the drug's having no effect or only a minimum effect on other tissues or body systems. This ideal often does not occur. This is why all drugs have the capability of producing side effects or adverse reactions.

The processes by which drugs behave therapeutically or adversely depend on four factors (Figure 15–8):

- Absorption
- Distribution
- Metabolism
- Excretion

Factors That Influence the Effects of Drugs

Drug absorption, distribution, metabolism, and excretion effects are influenced by the following individual patient factors:

- Weight and height
- Age and the development and condition of body systems and organs
- Gender differences in fat tissue, hormone balance, pregnancy, and menopause
- Diurnal rhythms, acid–base balance, and electrolyte balance
- Pathology involving the kidneys, liver, or cardiovascular system, and low or high blood pressure
- Genetically caused sensitivities, resistance to drugs, and idiosyncratic reactions
- Immunological and allergic responses
- Psychological attitudes including health beliefs, placebo effects, and lack of compliance
- Environmental changes in temperature, seasons, household hygiene, and cigarette smoke
- Tolerance occurring from long-term therapy
- Cumulation (toxicity) resulting from overdose or drug accumulation in the body

ASSESSING THE PATIENT, THE DRUG, AND THE ENVIRONMENT

Patient Assessment

Drug therapy assessment begins with the patient. It is the responsibility of the entire health care team to review the patient's past history and physical condition before administering a medication.

Past History

Interview the patient for

- Chronic conditions that may contraindicate the use of a drug or require a reduced or increased dosage

- The use of other drugs (such as over-the-counter drugs, tobacco, caffeine, alcohol, and street drugs) that may intensify or interfere with the effects of a drug
- Allergies to drugs, foods, or animals (animal proteins may be contained in certain immunization products)
- Level of education for understanding prescription directions
- Level of understanding disease and therapy and pattern of health care for gaining the patient's cooperation in therapy
- Social and family support systems to help feeble, disabled, or confused patients
- Financial support to afford the cost of treatment

Physical Assessment

Weight and Height. Because most drugs are based on total body weight, the patient's body size serves as a baseline for determining dosage. Tables of desirable weights and formulas for calculating body mass can be used when the patient's height and weight are known (see Figures 15–5 and Figure 15–6).

Age. In addition to size considerations, young children and the elderly have different rates of drug absorption, distribution, metabolism, and excretion. Many usual dosages must be reduced to avoid toxicity or prolonged or exaggerated drug action.

Other Parameters. These include any special physical parameters that may relate to effective drug therapy. For example, drugs may not be adequately absorbed into systemic circulation from subcutaneous sites in patients with shock or poor tissue perfusion due to chronic circulatory conditions.

Pregnancy. During pregnancy, all drugs should be discontinued unless otherwise determined necessary for the health of the mother or to protect the fetus (see Table 15–4).

Nutrition Status. Certain foods can alter the effects of some medications, and many drugs are absorbed better on an empty stomach. Other drugs may cause gastrointestinal distress if the patient has not eaten or does not eat enough separate meals in a day.

Drug Assessment

After considering the patient's emotional and physical condition at the time of the administration, the second step in safeguarding the patient is to assess the drug order and its appropriateness to the patient. This includes ensuring that the equipment and the environment itself are in safe condition. To complete this assessment,

1. Read the package insert before preparing a medication.
2. Check the medication's expiration date.
3. Check the medication for contamination or deterioration. The solution should appear clear (or cloudy, if it is a suspension) without any debris or clumps. The package insert will give a description of what the medication should look like.
4. Ask yourself the "Seven Rights" of drug assessment. Each of the Seven Rights must be answered with a yes before medication is administered. Ask, "Do I have the . . ."

- Right patient
- Right drug
- Right dose
- Right route
- Right time
- Right technique
- Right documentation

5. The Seven Rights are confirmed during four checkpoints:

- As the medication is taken from the shelf
- As the medication is being prepared
- As the medication is being returned to the shelf
- At the time of administration

The Environment

This is the last assessment.

1. Drugs should be prepared in a quiet area without distraction by others or interruptions for other activities.
2. Medications should be given only in the presence of the physician or personnel licensed to perform all types of emergency procedures in case an emergency procedure is necessary to reverse the effects of a medication.
3. Emergency medications and treatment equipment should be available for allergic reactions and anaphylactic shock.
4. The temperature of the environment should be at a comfortable level if the patient must undress for a treatment.
5. Medications and medication equipment should be stored away from patient traffic, so that

patients cannot medicate or otherwise harm themselves.
6. Patients should be placed in safe positions and assisted to and from the treatment room.
7. Patients should be observed for 10–30 minutes after drug administration, depending on the type of drug administered.

CHOOSING THE CORRECT ROUTE AND SITE

How a drug is first absorbed is first determined by the route chosen for delivery. A route is determined by the following factors:

- Drug form
- Permeability of the site to the drug
- Absorption capability of the site
- Condition of the patient

Medications are classified by their route of administration (Table 15–8). There are four basic routes: oral, mucous membrane, topical, and injection (parenteral).

Oral Medications

The oral route is used for solid and liquid forms that are swallowed and absorbed through the process of digestion. The oral route is primarily intended for its eventual systemic effects, as well as an occasional local effect.

Whenever possible, medications should be administered orally. Check to see if an oral route is possible. Oral drugs are slow in producing their effects, but may last longer than those given by injection and are generally safer.

Unless contraindicated, provide plenty of water to the patient after taking an oral medication.

Mucous Membrane Medications

The mucous membrane route is used for solid and liquid forms that are absorbed through the mucous membranes of the nose, rectum, vagina, urethra, or oral cavity, or by inhalation into the mucous membranes of the lower respiratory tract. The mucous membrane route is primarily intended for its eventual systemic effects, although

TABLE 15–8
MEDICATION ROUTES

Route	Sites	Forms	Advantages	Disadvantages
Oral	Mouth	Liquids, tablets, capsules	Simple, safe, and the least expensive; most drugs are rapidly and completely absorbed when the stomach empties into the duodenum	Difficulty swallowing; gastrointestinal irritation; risk of aspiration; digestive secretions keep drug from being absorbed or inactivate drug
Topical	Skin, eyes, and ears	Lotions, ointments, liniments, compresses, creams, patches, drops, irrigations	Localizes effect	Lack of permeability of the skin and eye
Mucous membrane	Mouth, throat, nasal cavity, eye, inhalation, rectum, vagina, and urethra	Suppositories, solutions, droplets, vapors, sprays, sublingual and buccal tablets, drops, douche, foams, creams	Rapidly bypasses the oral route for a systemic effect or local effect	Patient misuse; membrane irritation; unwanted systemic effects from local application
Parenteral	Deltoid, ventrogluteal, and vastus lateralis muscles; forearm; subcutaneous tissues of abdomen, back, thigh, and upper arm	Sterile aqueous solutions and repository forms	Rapid and complete absorption at a steady controlled rate	Accidental overdosage; possible infections; injury; pain; fear; expense

each site may also be used for a specific local effect.

The following are points to remember when administering a mucous membrane medication:

1. Never apply solutions warmer than 100° F to the mucous membranes.
2. Clear the nasal passages before instilling or spraying nasal medications.
3. Avoid touching the patient's nose with droppers. This will contaminate the bottle and may make the patient sneeze.
4. Administer nose drops directly into the nose with the patient's head tilted back; then have the patient lean forward, head down, to prevent the medication from being swallowed.
5. Administer sprays with the patient's head upright.
6. Teach patients that nose drops should not be used more than 3 days.
7. Teach patients to use inhalation devices exactly as ordered by the physician.
8. Use gloves for inserting suppositories.
9. Have patient evacuate the bowel, if possible, before administering systemic drugs rectally.

Topical Medications

The topical route is used for liquid drug forms that are placed on the skin, in the eye, or into the ear canal for treatment of surface conditions. The topical route is used primarily for its local effect, although some drug forms, such as dermal patches, are used for a systemic effect.

The following are points to remember when administering topical medications:

1. Apply dermal medications in a thin layer by patting.
2. If rubbing is necessary, use a firm stroke. Too light a touch may cause itching.
3. Remove patient's clothing if the medication stains clothing.
4. Remove medications from jars with a tongue blade.
5. Wear gloves to prevent personal skin absorption from medications.
6. Apply medications with sterile technique if the skin is broken. Wear gloves.
7. Apply medications in a circular motion, moving from the inside to the outside.
8. Use cotton-tipped applicators for watery solutions.
9. Warm ear drops so as not to "shock" the patient when the medication is instilled into the ear canal. Cold ear drops may actually cause the patient pain.

Parenteral (By Injection) Medications

The parenteral route is used with drug forms that are either sterile solutions or suspensions or powders requiring reconstitution. The drugs are deposited in the underlying tissues for absorption. The parenteral route is primarily intended for its systemic effects, although certain sites may also be used for a specific local effect.

The following are some categories of injection routes.

- Intradermal
- Subcutaneous
- Intramuscular
- Intravenous

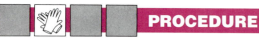

PROCEDURE

INSERTING A RECTAL SUPPOSITORY

PURPOSE

To administer a rectal medication for systemic absorption or to assist in the evacuation of the bowel.

EQUIPMENT AND MATERIALS

Warm water
Suppository
Gloves
Tissues

PROCEDURAL STEPS

Preparation

1. Confirm the date and accuracy of the order. Seek answers for any questions about technique you may have.

RATIONALE: This ensures the right time, technique, and documentation.
2. Compare the name of the patient, the name of the drug, the dose, and the route of administration against the order.
RATIONALE: This ensures the remaining five of the Seven Rights. This is the first of the four checks.
3. Check the patient's medical history for drug allergies or conditions that may contraindicate the injection.
RATIONALE: This ensures that the medication is compatible with the patient's history, condition, and other concurrent drug therapies.
4. Reread the accompanying package inscrt.
RATIONALE: You will be aware of the properties of the medication and the directions for administration.
5. Wash hands and assemble equipment.
6. Check the expiration date, the name, and the strength of the drug.
7. Inspect the medication for color and appearance. Discard any questionable solutions.
8. Compare the medication once more to the order.
RATIONALE: This is the second of the four checks.

Performance

9. Compare the medication once more to the order.
RATIONALE: This is the third of the four checks.
10. Ask the patient to state his or her name.
RATIONALE: If you simply call out a name, children, the elderly, or confused patients may respond to someone else's name.
11. Check the patient's chart to ensure the patient is the right patient.
RATIONALE: This is the fourth of the four checks.
12. Provide privacy.
13. Explain the procedure to the patient and what the medication is intended to do.
RATIONALE: Explanations help to reduce patient anxiety.
14. When administering antibiotics or analgesics, ask the patient about any allergies to these drugs.
RATIONALE: The patient may have forgotten to give this information during the history interview or may have experienced an allergy since the time the history was recorded.
15. Place the patient in a prone or the Sims position.
16. Moisten the suppository under running water.
17. Insert rounded end into the anal opening.
18. Using your gloved finger, insert the suppository 1–2 inches for children and adults or 3/4–1 inch for infants.
19. For infants and children, hold the buttocks together for the time recommended for best effect.

Follow-Up

20. Dispose of equipment properly.
21. Remove gloves and wash hands.
22. Observe the patient for any adverse effects from the medication or the injection.
23. Document the medication administration, ensuring that the record includes the date, time (if applicable), drug, dose, route, and how the patient tolerated the procedure. Complete the entry with your initials or name.

PROCEDURE
ADMINISTERING AN EYE MEDICATION

PURPOSE

To apply antiseptic solutions, antibiotic ointments, or solutions used to prepare the eye for examination.

EQUIPMENT AND MATERIALS

Ophthalmic solution or ointment in sterile container
Medication package insert

Sterile gauze
Medication order
Patient medical history

PROCEDURAL STEPS

Preparation

1. Confirm the date and accuracy of the order. Seek answers for any questions about technique.
   RATIONALE: This ensures the right time, technique, and documentation.
2. Compare the name of the patient, the name of the drug, the dose, and the route of administration against the order.
   RATIONALE: This ensures the remaining five of the Seven Rights. This is the first of the four checks.
3. Check the patient's medical history for drug allergies or conditions that may contraindicate the injection.
   RATIONALE: This ensures that the medication is compatible with the patient's history, condition, and other concurrent drug therapies.
4. Reread the accompanying package insert.
   RATIONALE: You will be aware of the properties of the medication and the directions for administration.
5. Wash hands and assemble equipment.
6. Check the expiration date, the name, and the strength of the drug.
7. Inspect the medication for color and appearance. Discard any questionable solutions.
8. Compare the medication once more to the order.
   RATIONALE: This is the second of the four checks.

Performance

9. Compare the medication once more to the order.
   RATIONALE: This is the third of the four checks.
10. Ask the patient to state his or her name.
    RATIONALE: If you simply call out a name, children, the elderly, or confused patients may respond to someone else's name.
11. Check the patient's chart to ensure the patient is the right patient.
    RATIONALE: This is the fourth of the four checks.
12. Provide privacy.
13. Explain the procedure to the patient and what the medication is intended to do.
    RATIONALE: Explanations help to reduce patient anxiety.
14. When administering antibiotics or analgesics, ask the patient about any allergies to these drugs.
    RATIONALE: The patient may have forgotten to give this information during the history interview or may have experienced an allergy since the time the history was recorded.
15. Place the patient in a sitting or supine position.
    RATIONALE: Correct positioning is important for controlling the flow of liquid medications.
16. Instruct the patient to look up as you pull the lower conjunctival sac downward with gauze-covered fingertips.
    RATIONALE: Rolling the eyeball upward reduces the chance of injuring the cornea with the dropper. The sac is pulled downward to catch the drops.

For Eye Drops

17. Instill the prescribed number of drops directly onto the center of the lower conjunctival sac. Do not touch the dropper to the eye.
18. Release the lower lid immediately and instruct the patient to rotate the eyeball. Blot excess medication.
    RATIONALE: Rotating the eyeball ensures distribution of the medication.
19. Proceed to follow-up.

For Eye Ointment

17. Squeeze a ribbon of medication along the lower lid, from the inner corner to the outer corner. Do not touch the ointment tube to the eye.
18. Release the lower lid immediately and instruct the patient to rotate the eyeball. Blot excess medication.
    RATIONALE: Rotating the eyeball ensures distribution of the medication.
19. Inspect the site to ensure the medication is distributed in the eye.

Follow-Up

20. Assist the patient into a comfortable position.
21. Inform the patient about any side effects.

22. Give the patient an opportunity to ask any questions about the medication received.
23. Close the cap on the medication without touching any parts of the opening.
RATIONALE: Ophthalmic medications are considered sterile.
24. Dispose of equipment properly.
25. Wash hands.
26. Observe the patient for any adverse effects from the medication or the injection.
27. Document the medication administration, ensuring that the record includes the date, time (if applicable), drug, dose, route, site, and how the patient tolerated the procedure. Complete the entry with your initials or name.

PROCEDURE

ADMINISTERING AN EAR MEDICATION

PURPOSE

To apply drops directly into the ear canal to soften earwax prior to irrigation or to treat bacterial infections or skin irritations.

EQUIPMENT AND MATERIALS

Otic solution, warmed slightly
Medication package insert
Sterile gauze
Medication order
Patient medical history

PROCEDURAL STEPS

Preparation

1. Confirm the date and accuracy of the order. Seek answers for any questions about technique.
RATIONALE: This ensures the right time, technique, and documentation.
2. Compare the name of the patient, the name of the drug, the dose, and the route of administration against the order.
RATIONALE: This ensures the remaining five of the Seven Rights. This is the first of the four checks.
3. Check the patient's medical history for drug allergies or conditions that may contraindicate the injection.
RATIONALE: This ensures that the medication is compatible with the patient's history, condition, and other concurrent drug therapies.
4. Reread the accompanying package insert.
RATIONALE: You will be aware of the properties of the medication and the directions for administration.
5. Wash hands and assemble equipment.
6. Check the expiration date, the name, and the strength of the drug.
7. Inspect the medication for color and appearance. Discard any questionable solutions.
8. Compare the medication once more to the order.
RATIONALE: This is the second of the four checks.

Performance

9. Compare the medication once more to the order.
RATIONALE: This is the third of the four checks.
10. Ask the patient to state his or her name.
RATIONALE: If you simply call out a name, children, the elderly, or confused patients may respond to someone else's name.
11. Check the patient's chart to ensure the patient is the right patient.
RATIONALE: This is the fourth of the four checks.
12. Provide privacy.
13. Explain the procedure to the patient and what the medication is intended to do.
RATIONALE: Explanations help to reduce patient anxiety.
14. When administering antibiotics or analgesics, ask the patient about any allergies to these drugs.

RATIONALE: The patient may have forgotten to give this information during the history interview or may have experienced an allergy since the time the history was recorded.

15. Place the patient in a sitting or side-lying position.
RATIONALE: Correct positioning is important for controlling the flow of liquid medications.
16. Tilt the patient's head toward the ear not being treated.
RATIONALE: This facilitates the flow of the medication towards the eardrum.
17. Pull the ear auricle up and back (adults and older children) or down and back (infants) and instill the warmed medication.
RATIONALE: Pulling the ear straightens the canal. Warming reduces the "shock" of the liquid in the canal.
18. Inspect the site to ensure the medication is distributed in the ear.
19. If specifically ordered, apply petroleum jelly to a cotton ball and insert in the treated ear.
RATIONALE: Petroleum jelly prevents the cotton ball from absorbing the medication.
20. Assist the patient into a comfortable position and instruct the patient to remain still for 10 minutes.
RATIONALE: The medication will be retained in the ear for absorption.
21. Inform the patient about any side effects.
22. Give the patient an opportunity to ask any questions about the medication received.

Follow-Up

23. Close the cap on the medication without touching any parts of the opening.
RATIONALE: Multiuse otic medications are considered sterile.
24. Dispose of equipment properly.
25. Wash hands.
26. Observe the patient for any adverse effects from the medication or the injection.
27. Document the medication administration, ensuring that the record includes the date, time (if applicable), drug, dose, route, site, and how the patient tolerated the procedure. Complete the entry with your initials or name.

USING CORRECT TECHNIQUES AND EQUIPMENT FOR INJECTIONS

Advantages of Injections

Injectable drug forms

- Produce effects faster than oral forms (but the effects of injectable medications may not last as long)
- May be necessary if the patient is mentally incapacitated, unconscious, or physically unable to swallow or ingest oral medications
- Eliminate the risks of losing the drug due to vomiting or gastric activity and of the drug's becoming inactivated by the digestive tract
- Can be used to slow absorption by the use of dosage forms that contain additives (this is advantageous when prolonged drug effects are desired)

Routes for Administration

Various routes and sites may be selected for drugs administered by injection (Table 15–9). Site selection depends on

- Specific route (ID, SC, IM etc.)
- Type of drug
- Amount of medication to be injected
- Length and size of available needles
- Size of the patient (infant, child, adult, emaciated, or obese)
- Muscle or tissue mass of the site selected
- Physical condition of the skin at the selected site

Intradermal Medications

Intradermal medications are placed into the skin layers (Figure 15–9).

- This route has the slowest absorption rate.
- Only small volumes (0.01–0.2 ml) can be administered.
- The most common sites are the volar surface of the forearm, the upper thorax, or the scapular area (Figure 15–10).
- The most common use of the intradermal injec-

TABLE 15-9

TYPES OF INJECTIONS

Method	Drug amount	Sites	Examples
IM	Adult, 1-2 cc	Deltoid	Adrenalin (epinephrine)
	Adult, 2-5 cc	Vastus lateralis	Penicillin
		Dorsogluteal, ventrogluteal	Demerol (meperidine)
	Child 1-2 cc	Vastus lateralis, ventrogluteal	Penicillin
IM, Z	As above	Dorsogluteal	Irritating drugs
		Ventrogluteal	
SC	Adult, 0.1-2.0 cc	Deltoid	Insulin
		Thigh	Vaccines
		Abdomen	Toxoids
	Child, 0.5 cc	Deltoid	Vaccines
		Thigh, abdomen	Toxoids
ID	Adult and child, 0.1-0.5 cc	Forearm	Tuberculin test, skin tests

Reprinted from Kinn M, Derge E: *The Medical Assistant: Administrative and Clinical,* 6th ed. Philadelphia: W.B. Saunders, 1988, p. 503.

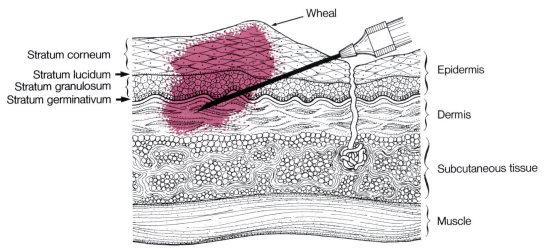

FIGURE 15-9

The intradermal injection is administered just under the epidermis. Because the drug is dispersed into an area rich with nerves, it causes momentary burning or stinging. Minute amounts of medication are injected. This method is used to test for allergies, drug sensitivities, and susceptibility to some diseases. (Reproduced from Kinn M, Derge E: *The Medical Assistant: Administrative and Clinical,* 6th ed. Philadelphia: W. B. Saunders, 1988, p. 514.)

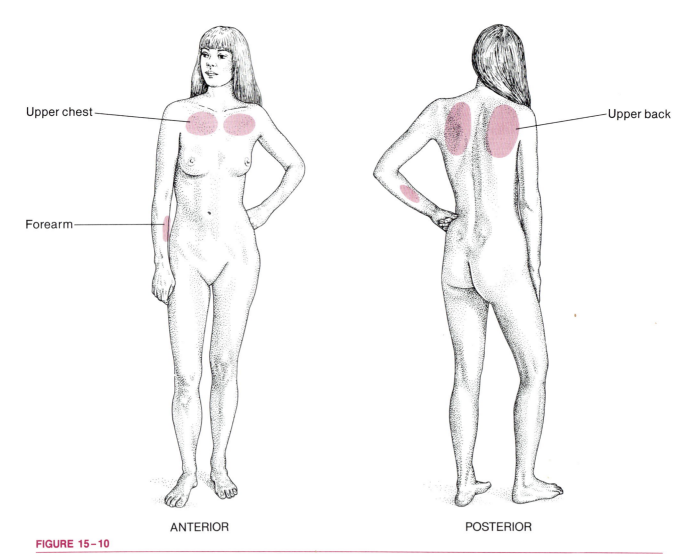

FIGURE 15–10

Sites recommended for intradermal injections. (Reproduced from Kinn M, Derge E: *The Medical Assistant: Administrative and Clinical,* 6th ed. Philadelphia: W. B. Saunders, 1988, p. 515.)

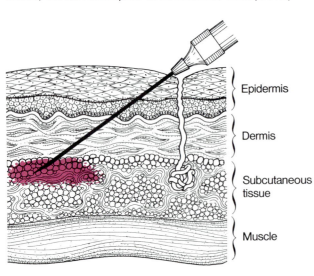

FIGURE 15–11

The subcutaneous injection is administered with a needle smaller and shorter than that used for the intramuscular injection. This method is used for small amounts of nonirritating medications in aqueous solution. It is injected at a 45° angle (90° angle for insulin and heparin). The most common site is the deltoid region of the upper arm. (Reproduced from Kinn M, Derge E: *The Medical Assistant: Administrative and Clinical,* 6th ed. Philadelphia: W. B. Saunders, 1988, p. 512.)

tion is the administration of a tuberculin test or testing with allergy extracts.
- Diluted concentrations of medications may be injected intradermally to test for drug allergy.
- Some vaccinations (e.g., smallpox) are administered intradermally.

Subcutaneous Medications

Subcutaneous medications are injected into the fatty layer beneath the skin (Figure 15–11).

- The blood supply in subcutaneous tissues is minimal, so absorption is slow.
- Volumes of 0.5–1.5 ml may be given into the subcutaneous tissues.
- Many body sites may be used, as long as the underlying tissue is free of large blood vessels and nerves and the site is not located over a bony prominence (Figure 15–12).
- The subcutaneous route is used for medications that are isotonic, nonirritating, and water soluble and are most effective when deposited into subcutaneous tissues.

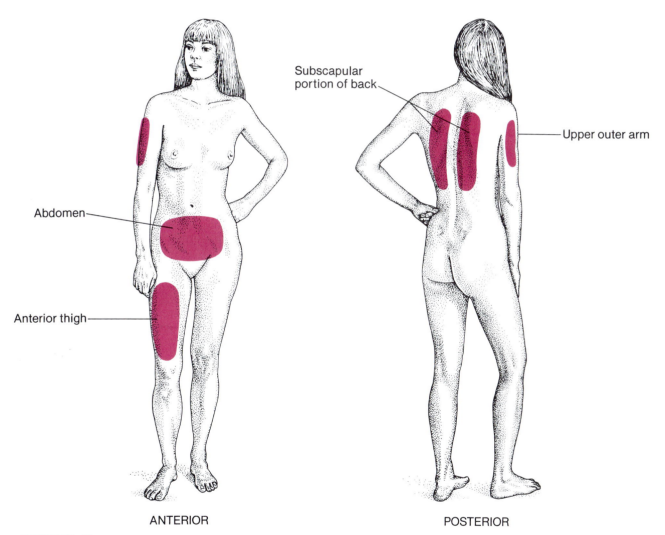

FIGURE 15–12
Areas of the body commonly used for subcutaneous injections. (Reproduced from Kinn M, Derge E: *The Medical Assistant: Administrative and Clinical,* 6th ed. Philadelphia: W. B. Saunders, 1988, p. 512.)

- Heparin, insulin, narcotics, vitamin B_{12}, and some vaccines are administered subcutaneously.

> **SPECIAL HINT**
>
> Heparin is absorbed as quickly subcutaneously as intramuscularly. Histamine release as a result of the trauma of the injection, physical exercise, or anything that affects blood flow to the subcutaneous tissues may increase or decrease absorption rate.

Intramuscular Medications

Intramuscular medications are deposited into the muscle mass (Figure 15–13).

- This injection route is chosen when a more rapid absorption is desired. The absorption time depends on the type of medication, the type of solvent (diluent), and the condition of the muscle.
- Volumes of up to 5.0 ml may be injected into the muscle masses of gluteal or vastus lateralis muscles; 2 1/2–3 ml is considered a more conservative maximum. When large doses are required, medication should be divided into two smaller doses.
- Because muscles have fewer nerve endings, intramuscular injections may be less painful. However, the danger of damage is the greatest using this route: blood vessels may be punctured, resulting in bleeding; medication may be inadvertently deposited into a vessel or joint capsule and cause paralysis and/or abscessing or gangrene; and damage to local nerves can cause pain and temporary or permanent paralysis.
- Intramuscular injections should be contraindicated in undeveloped or atrophied muscles or noninnervated muscles, such as in patients after a stroke or paraplegic or quadriplegic patients.
- The safest sites (Figure 15–14) are the ventrogluteal area, the vastus lateralis muscle (recommended by the American Academy of Pediatrics for infants and children), and the deltoid muscle.
- The dorsogluteal site is no longer recommended, because of the large number of reported injuries to the sciatic nerve and other complications resulting from poor blood flow to the site.

Landmarks

The safe administration of injections requires a knowledge of anatomical landmarks that are both visable and palpable.

Deltoid Muscle

The deltoid muscle is shown in Figure 15–15.

Site. For children and adults, the correct site for injection is one to two inches (two to three fingerbreadths) below the acromium process. The site should be limited to volumes less than 1.0 ml for children and 2.0 ml for adults or to part of a rotation of sites over long periods of time.

Medications. Medications should be of low viscosity, such as vaccines, narcotics, vitamins, and sedatives. Some lipid-type medications may be administered at this site, because the site has greater blood flow and less fatty tissues than other sites which facilitates rapid absorption.

Needle Sizes. Typical needle sizes range from 23 to 25 g and 5/8 to 1 1/2 inches for adults, and from 25 to 27 g and 1/2 to 1 inch for pediatric use.

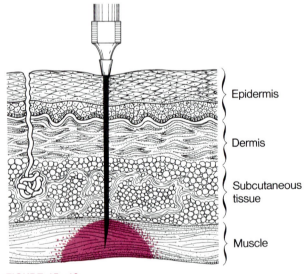

FIGURE 15–13

The intramuscular injection is administered with a needle larger and longer than that used for the subcutaneous injection. This method is used for depositing the medication into the large central part of the muscle. It is Injected at a 90° angle. The most common sites are the deltoid muscle, the vastus lateralis muscle, and the ventrogluteal area. (Reproduced from Kinn M, Derge E: *The Medical Assistant: Administrative and Clinical*, 6th ed. Philadelphia: W. B. Saunders, 1988, p. 502.)

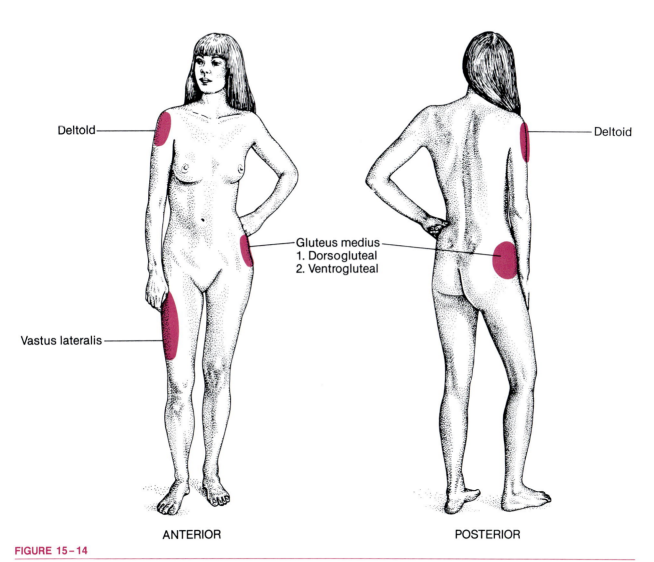

FIGURE 15–14
The muscles commonly used for intramuscular injection. (Reproduced from Kinn M, Derge E: *The Medical Assistant: Administrative and Clinical,* 6th ed. Philadelphia: W. B. Saunders, 1988, p. 503.)

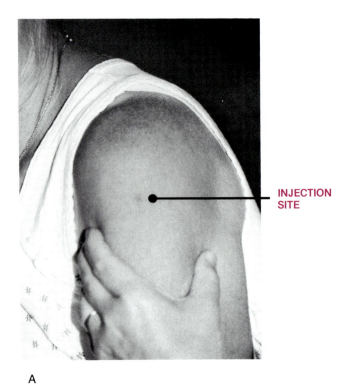

A

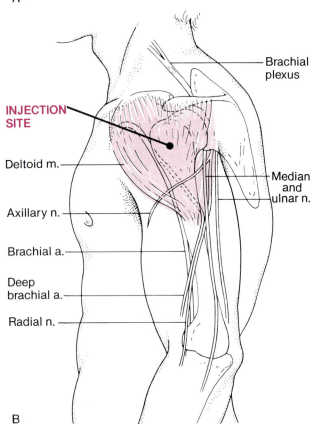

B

FIGURE 15–15

The deltoid muscle site is used for both intramuscular and subcutaneous injections. It is not recommended for infants, because the muscle is not developed until later in childhood, or for adults when the muscle is not well developed. Individual judgment must be used to penetrate but not overshoot the muscle. (Reproduced from Kinn M, Derge E: *The Medical Assistant: Administrative and Clinical,* 6th ed. Philadelphia: W. B. Saunders, 1988, p. 506.)

Administration. The patient should be sitting, prone, or supine. The entire site should be exposed; do not roll up the sleeve. The needle should be inserted at 90° or angled upward.

Vastus Lateralis Muscle

The vastus lateralis muscle is illustrated in Figure 15–16.

Site. For children, the preferred site is the portion of the muscle just below the greater trochanter of the femur, within the upper lateral quadrant of the thigh. For adults, the preferred site is within the middle third of the muscle (one-third the distance between the greater trochanter and the knee joint [one handbreadth below the greater trochanter and one handbreadth above the knee joint]).

This site has a blood flow that is less than the deltoid but greater than the gluteal sites. The site should be limited to volumes less than 1.0 ml for infants, less than 2.0 ml for children, and less than 4.0 ml for adults. Large volumes should be divided into multiple injections at two different sites.

Medications. Most medications, including Z-tract technique, can be administered at this site. For medications that discolor the skin, the ventrogluteal muscle is the better choice.

Needle Size. Typical needle sizes range from 20 g to 23 g and 1 1/4 to 1 1/2 in for adults, and 22 g to 25 g and 5/8 to 1 inch for pediatric use.

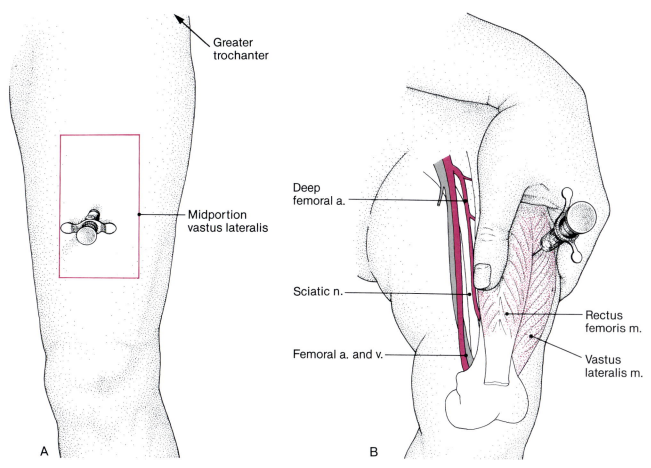

FIGURE 15–16
The vastus lateralis muscle is the preferred site for intramuscular injections in infants and children. **A**, Site selection for adults. **B**, Site selection for infants and children. (Reproduced from Kinn M, Derge E: *The Medical Assistant: Administrative and Clinical,* 6th ed. Philadelphia: W. B. Saunders, 1988, p. 504.)

Administration. The patient should be sitting or lying down. The entire site should be exposed. The needle should be inserted at 90° or angled upward.

Ventrogluteal Site

The ventrogluteal site is shown in Figure 15–17.

Site. The ventrogluteal site is acceptable from birth through adulthood. Medical literature often recommends this site for *all* intramuscular injections. To locate the site, the medical assistant uses his or her hand that is opposite the patient's side. The right palm is placed on the greater trochanter, and the index finger is placed on the anterior superior iliac spine. Fan the middle finger as far out as possible and try to touch the crest of the ilium. The injection is made into the middle of the triangle formed by the index finger and the middle finger at the iliac crest.

This site has a blood flow that is less than the other sites, so absorption will be slow. The site

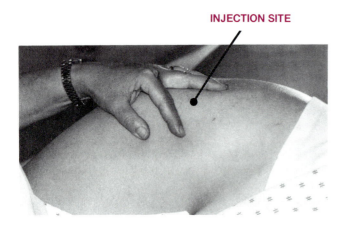

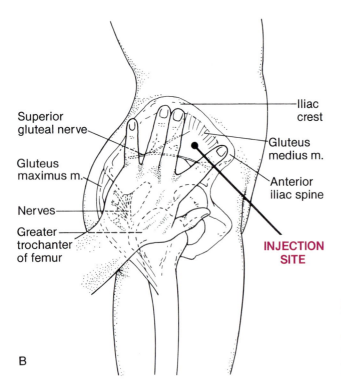

FIGURE 15–17

The ventrogluteal muscle can be used for most intramuscular injections. This technique is preferred over other gluteal area injections. (Reproduced from Kinn M, Derge E: *The Medical Assistant: Administrative and Clinical,* 6th ed. Philadelphia: W. B. Saunders, 1988, p. 506.)

should be limited to volumes less than 1.0 ml for infants, less than 2.0 ml for children, and less than 4.0 ml for adults. Large volumes should be divided into multiple injections at two different sites.

Medications. Most medications, including Z-tract technique, can be administered at this site. For medications that discolor the skin, the ventrogluteal muscle is the site of choice.

Needle Sizes. Typical needle sizes range from 20 to 23 g and 1 1/4 to 1 1/2 inches for adults, and 25 to 27 g and 1/2 to 1 inch for pediatric use.

Administration. The patient should be supine or lateral with appropriate restraint. The entire site should be exposed. The needle should be inserted angled slightly toward the iliac crest.

USING SPECIAL SYRINGE TECHNIQUES

Using Syringe Dead Space and Air Bubbles[1]

Air bubbles may be drawn into a filled syringe for two reasons:

- To prevent irritating medications from escaping into the subcutaneous spaces following intramuscular injections (see also Using the Z-tract Technique).
- To clear any medication that may be sitting in the needle shaft and syringe tip. These are known as "dead space."

Research has mostly concluded that the dead space is not of consequence in most situations. It is generally assumed that the extra medication in the needle and syringe tip before the injection is offset by approximately the same amount remaining in the needle and syringe tip after the plunger has injected the medication.

Therefore, in separate syringe and needle units, most manufacturers do not calculate the dead space (usually 0.002–0.3 ml, depending on the needle size) as a part of the stated dose on the label.

In most single-unit syringes and needles, dead spaces are usually eliminated.

Generally, the ratio of dead space to medication increases as the amount of medication to be administered decreases. However, three situations exist where the existence of dead space may cause problems:

- In infants, some cases of overdose have been attributed to the extra amount of drug in the dead space.
- When the air bubble technique is used, the dead space volume of medication is cleared and added to the medication in the syringe.
- In small dosages of less than 1.0 ml, the ratio of dead space to total medication amount can be significant.

When equipment dead space might cause a significant variation in the amount of the medication delivered, such as in the preceding three situations above, the use of an air bubble is *not recommended*.

Two alternative solutions to the use of the air bubble are:

- The Z-tract technique (see below) for irritating medications
- The smallest calibrated syringe for small doses, especially with infants and children.

Admixing Two Drugs in a Single Syringe[1,2]

Some drugs have chemical properties that are not compatible with the chemical properties of other drugs. Before doing an admixture of two drugs in a single syringe, check the product package insert, the *Physician's Desk Reference*, or special syringe compatibility charts. Drug combinations will be listed as

- Compatible
- Compatible only for a limited period of time, usually 15 minutes
- Incompatible
- Conflicting data
- Data unavailable
- Identical drug

Always consult the physician or a pharmacist if there is any question about syringe compatibility.

If you are mixing medication with a compatible medication, draw 0.2–0.5 ml of air into the syringe and change the needle before drawing out the second medication.

If a single syringe–needle unit is being used,

flick the needle to shake the fluid off the shaft, or wipe the shaft lightly with dry, sterile gauze. Do not use cotton; cotton fibers will adhere to the needle. Do not use alcohol wipes and do not scrub the needle, because heavy wiping could remove the manufacturer's surgical-grade lubricant that coats the needle.

PROCEDURE

DRAWING A MEDICATION INTO A SYRINGE

PURPOSE

The purpose of drawing a medication into a syringe is to prepare a sterile medication for patient injection. Remember to use the first three of four checks and Seven Rights when preparing a sterile medication for injection.

EQUIPMENT AND MATERIALS

Medication in an ampule, vial, or prefilled sterile syringe
Medication package insert
Syringe and needle
Alcohol sponge or other antiseptic
Medication order
Patient medical history

PROCEDURAL STEPS

Preparation

1. Confirm the date and accuracy of the order. Seek answers for any questions about technique.
   RATIONALE: This ensures the right time, technique, and documentation.
2. Compare the name of the patient, the name of the drug, the dose, and the route of administration against the order.
   RATIONALE: This ensures the remaining five of the Seven Rights. This is the first of the four checks.
3. Check the patient's medical history for drug allergies or conditions that may contraindicate the injection.
   RATIONALE: This ensures that the medication is compatible with the patient's history, condition, and other concurrent drug therapies.
4. Reread the accompanying package insert.
   RATIONALE: You will be aware of the properties of the medication and the directions for administration.
5. Wash hands and assemble equipment.
6. Check the expiration date, the name, and the strength of the drug.
7. Inspect the medication for color and appearance. Discard any questionable solutions.
8. Compare the medication once more to the order.
   RATIONALE: This is the second of the four checks.

Performance

9. Draw into the syringe an amount of air equal to the amount of medication to be withdrawn.
   RATIONALE: Too little air will make withdrawal difficult; too much air will increase the air pressure within the vial and blow out the next syringe plunger when inserted into the vial.
10. Cleanse the rubber stopper with an alcohol sponge; allow the alcohol to dry.
    RATIONALE: The needle will "drag" any liquid on the stopper into the vial and contaminate it.
11. Using sterile technique throughout, draw up the amount of medication.
12. Add 0.2 ml of air to the syringe, when appropriate, according to office policy on intramuscular injection and the manufacturer's recommendation.
    RATIONALE: This clears the medication from the needle and prevents seepage of irritating medications into subcutaneous tissues during injection.

Follow-Up

13. Compare the medication once more to the order.
    RATIONALE: This is the third of the four checks.
14. Return the medication to storage, or leave the medication with the filled syringe for the physician to double check.
15. Keep all medications away from patient traffic.

ADMINISTERING PARENTERAL MEDICATIONS

Assessing the Patient Before Injection

1. Carefully review the package insert and compare it to the patient's history for any possible contraindications.
2. Review the patient's age and body size and any special conditions, such as pregnancy, diagnosis, concurrent drug therapy, bleeding disorders, or local circulatory disorders.
3. Palpate the intended injection site for muscle mass, keeping in mind the volume of the dose to be administered.
4. Use good lighting and adequately expose the site for visualization and inspection of injection site landmarks.
5. Visually inspect the injection site for skin lesions, such as inflammation, abrasions, or excoriations.
6. Assess the site for lipodystrophy or lipohypertrophy, because either condition retards medication absorption.
7. Avoid any site that is edematous or has poor perfusion.

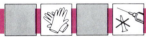

PROCEDURE
ADMINISTERING A PARENTERAL MEDICATION

PURPOSE

To administer a parenteral medication with the knowledge, care, and technique that maximizes a drug's effectiveness and protects the patient from unnecessary anxiety, pain, or injury.

EQUIPMENT AND MATERIALS

Medication in sterile syringe
Alcohol sponge or other antiseptic
Medication order
Patient medical history

 MEDICAL ASSISTING ALERT

If iodophors (povidone–iodine) is being used as an antiseptic, first ask the patient if he or she is allergic to iodine.

PROCEDURAL STEPS

Preparation

1. Ask the patient to state his or her name.
   RATIONALE: If you simply call out a name, children, the elderly, or confused patients may respond to someone else's name.
2. Check the patient's chart to ensure the patient is the right patient.
   RATIONALE: This is the fourth of the four checks.
3. Provide privacy.
   RATIONALE: This allows for the site to be completely exposed.
4. Explain that the patient is to receive an injection and provide a short explanation of what the medication is intended to do.
   RATIONALE: Explanations help to reduce patient anxiety.
5. When administering antibiotics or analgesics, ask the patient about any allergies to these drugs.

RATIONALE: The patient may have forgotten to give this information during the history interview or may have experienced an allergy since the time the history was recorded.

6. Choose the best site and place the patient in the correct position.
   RATIONALE: Correct positioning is important when identifying landmarks.
7. Completely expose the site and assess it by palpation and visualization.
   RATIONALE: This makes sure that the skin and muscle at the site are free from conditions that would contraindicate the area as a site for injection, and makes sure you chose the needle length appropriate for the site.

Procedure

8. Cleanse the site using friction and circular motion from the center outward.
9. Allow the site to dry.
   RATIONALE: Wet antiseptic will be forced into the tissue with the needle.
10. Remove the needle sheath and check the syringe for any excess air that may have been drawn into the syringe.
    RATIONALE: The syringe should be free of air, or hold only 0.2 ml of air if the air bubble technique is being used.
11. Gently stretch the skin taut and/or grasp the muscle at the site.
    RATIONALE: Spreading and grasping the skin make needle insertion smoother and displace subcutaneous tissue.
12. Hold the syringe between the thumb and forefinger and insert the needle with a quick thrust at the angle required for the route and site.
    RATIONALE: A quick, single thrust reduces pain. Correct angles are important for depositing the medication into the correct tissue layer.
13. Leave approximately 1/8 inch of the needle shaft visible.
    RATIONALE: The exposed shaft will allow removal of the needle should it break off during the injection.
14. Aspirate by pulling back on the plunger for 2-3 seconds and watch the barrel for any signs of discoloration (blood).
    RATIONALE: Waiting allows time for blood to travel up the needle and into the syringe.
15. If discoloration appears, withdraw the needle and apply pressure to the site. Discard the syringe and prepare a new medication. Explain what happened to the patient.
    RATIONALE: The medication is contaminated with blood. Blood must not be injected free into the tissues.
16. Hold the needle steady.
    RATIONALE: Avoids further trauma and entry into a blood vessel after aspiration.
17. Inject the medication slowly.
    RATIONALE: Forcing medication into the tissues can cause tissue injury and pain. If the air bubble method is used, the air bubble will be the last to be injected and will seal in the medication.
18. Withdraw the needle rapidly and in a straight line to the angle of insertion.
    RATIONALE: To reduce further tissue injury.
19. Apply pressure with dry, sterile gauze or cotton and gently massage in a circular motion.
    RATIONALE: Massage increases absorption and distributes the medication. *Do not massage* if slow absorption is desired, following an injection of heparin, or if the medication is irritating to the skin or subcutaneous tissues.
20. Inspect the site for bleeding or bruising.
    RATIONALE: If bleeding occurs, further pressure should be applied; for bruising, a cold or ice compress should be applied.
21. Assist the patient into a comfortable position.
22. Inform the patient about any side effects.
23. Give the patient an opportunity to ask any questions about the medication received.

Follow-Up

24. Do not recap or in any way touch the needle of the syringe.
    RATIONALE: This prevents injury after the procedure.
25. Dispose of as a single unit in a rigid sharps disposal container.
    RATIONALE: Used needles should not be placed in pockets, bags, or wastebaskets that would in any way endanger personnel.
26. Wash hands.
27. Observe the patient for any adverse effects from the medication or the injection.
28. Document the medication administration, ensuring that the record includes the date, time (if applicable), drug, dose, route, site, and how the patient tolerated the procedure. Complete the entry with your initials or name.

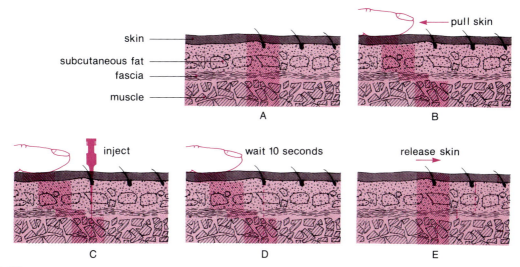

FIGURE 15-18

The Z-tract method of intramuscular injection is used when medications are irritating to subcutaneous tissues. This technique helps prevent the medication from leaking back into the subcutaneous tissues. (Reproduced from Kinn M, Derge E: *The Medical Assistant: Administrative and Clinical,* 6th ed. Philadelphia: W. B. Saunders, 1988, p. 510.)

Using the Z-tract Technique

The Z-tract technique (Figure 15-18) is used to reduce irritation to the subcutaneous tissues or skin discoloration when certain medications are administered intramuscularly. The Z-tract technique prevents medication from seeping into subcutaneous tissues during its absorption in the muscle spaces.

The preferred sites are the ventrogluteal and vastus lateralis. Some literature includes the use of the dorsogluteal; office policy determines whether this site is included. For medications that discolor the skin, the ventrogluteal site is preferred over the vastus lateralis.

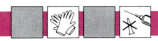

PROCEDURE

ADMINISTERING A Z-TRACT MEDICATION

PURPOSE

To reduce skin discoloration and/or irritation to the subcutaneous tissues.

EQUIPMENT AND MATERIALS

Medication in sterile syringe
Alcohol sponge or other antiseptic
Medication order
Patient medical history

PROCEDURE

Preparation

Follow the steps in the previous procedure for administering a parenteral medication, adding the following additional techniques:

1. Depending on office policy, withdraw the medication with an additional 0.2–0.5 ml of air.

2. Replace the needle with a new needle for injection.

Performance

3. Pull the skin away from the chosen injection site and cleanse the skin with antiseptic. Dry the site with sterile gauze.
4. Insert the needle and aspirate.
5. If no discoloration appears in the syringe, inject the medication slowly followed by an air bubble, if ordered.
6. Wait 10 seconds.
7. Withdraw the needle while releasing the pulled skin. If the needle is thin, release the needle first, then the skin, to prevent bending of the needle shaft during release.
8. Apply light pressure with a dry, sterile gauze or cotton, but do not massage. Massage will force medication into the subcutaneous tissues.

Follow-Up

9. For repeat injections, alternate sites.
10. Advise the patient not to apply pressure to the site and to avoid exercise.

Steps to Reducing Injection Pain[1]

1. Use the best equipment possible.
2. Use the smallest needle size that will allow the medication to flow easily through the needle. Too small a lumen will force the fluid through the needle, tear the tissues, and cause more pain.
3. Change needles after withdrawing irritating medications into the syringe.
4. Use the Z-tract method and/or the air bubble method for irritating drugs.
5. Warm refrigerated drugs to room temperature.
6. Allow skin antiseptics to dry before injection.
7. Avoid pushing the plunger while inserting the needle through the tissues.
8. Do not inject more medication than the site can absorb. Divide the medication between two sites.
9. Inject medication into relaxed muscles.
10. Insert the needle swiftly and with a single motion.
11. Inject medications slowly.
12. Apply pressure and massage after injection to increase absorption.
13. Rotate injection sites.
14. If the patient complains of severe pain, discontinue the injection immediately and seek immediate evaluation from the physician.

TUBERCULIN TESTING[3]

The methods currently in use to test for skin sensitivity to tuberculin are the needle and syringe single injection (Mantoux test) and the multiple-puncture, tine-type intradermal application (tine test). Although frequent and routine in its administration, tuberculin testing must be performed with utmost care, read with timely deliberation, and interpreted with careful discrimination.

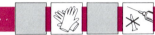

PROCEDURE

ADMINISTERING THE MANTOUX TEST

PURPOSE

To inject 0.1 ml of tuberculin purified protein derivative (PPD) intradermally in such a manner as to form a wheal.

EQUIPMENT AND MATERIALS

Tuberculin syringe
27-g, 1/2-inch bluntly beveled needle
Intermediate-strength PPD (5 tuberculin units per 0.1 ml of tuberculin PPD)
Acetone antiseptic and dry, sterile gauze
Millimeter rule

 MEDICAL ASSISTING ALERT

False-negative results may occur for as long as 4–6 weeks in patients who are concurrently receiving or have recently received immunization with measles or influenza vaccines; patients who have had rubella, influenza, mumps, or other viral infections; and patients who are receiving steroid therapy or immunosuppressive drugs.

PROCEDURAL STEPS

Performance

1. Cleanse the skin of the volar surface of the forearms, about 4 inches below the elbow, with acetone. Allow the surface to dry.
2. Cleanse the rubber stopper and allow the stopper to dry.
3. Withdraw 0.1 ml of PPD into the syringe.
4. Insert the needle, bevel upward, just beneath the surface of the skin and slowly inject the solution.
5. A wheal 6–10 millimeter (mm) diameter should form as the solution is injected.
6. Withdraw the syringe unit and dispose of in a proper container.
7. *Do not* massage the site.
8. The wheal will disappear within minutes; no dressing is required.

Reading the Procedure

9. Read in 48–72 hours.
10. Not looking at the site, gently stroke the area with fingers to determine the existence of induration.
11. With the tip of the index finger, gently determine the limits of the induration.
12. Place the forearm under good light and measure the diameter of induration transversely to the long axis of the forearm.
13. Record the reading in millimeters.

Interpreting the Reaction

Induration 10 mm or More in Diameter

- Positive for past or present infection with *Mycobacterium tuberculosis*.
- Test does not have to be repeated, unless the validity of the test is in question.

Induration of 5–9 mm

- Classified as doubtful, unless the patient has a close contact with an individual known to be positive for *M. tuberculosis*.
- In the presence of positive radiographic or clinical evidence of a disease resembling tuberculosis, the reaction should be read as possibly positive.
- Repeat testing is indicated.

Induration of Less than 5 mm

- Negative reaction
- No repeat test necessary, unless there is clinical suspicion of tuberculosis

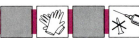

PROCEDURE

ADMINISTERING THE TUBERCULIN TINE TEST

PURPOSE

To deposit a premeasured dose of Old Tuberculin intradermally.

 MEDICAL ASSISTING ALERT

Although rare, using this test in patients with active tuberculosis could activate quiescent lesions. Use with caution in patients allergic to acacia (adhesives, inks, and gum arabic products). Reactions may be suppressed in patients who are receiving corticosteroids or immunosuppressive agents or who have recently received vaccinations with live virus vaccines.

EQUIPMENT AND MATERIALS

Tuberculin, Old, Tine Test or
 Tuberculin PPD
Acetone antiseptic and dry, sterile gauze
Millimeter ruler

PROCEDURAL STEPS

Performance

1. Cleanse the skin of the volar surface of the forearms, about 4 inches below the elbow, with acetone. Allow the surface to dry.
2. Pull the tine test from its protective, plastic cap.
3. Grasp the patient's forearm from behind the site and, with the fingers, stretch the volar surface tightly.
 RATIONALE: A firm grasp keeps the arm in position should the patient flinch.
4. Apply the test unit and press for 1 second after the tines pierce the skin.
 RATIONALE: Pressure should be sufficient to produce four puncture marks and a circular impression from the plastic base of the test device.
5. Release the stretching action.
 RATIONALE: Releasing the stretch before the unit is withdrawn decreases the chance of bleeding in the area and allows the tine material to be "rubbed off" onto the skin.
6. Withdraw the tine test unit.
7. Dispose of in a rigid, sharps container.
8. Instruct the patient that some bleeding may occur at the test site and is of no significance.

Reading the Procedure

9. Read in 48–72 hours.
10. Place the forearm under good light with the forearm slightly flexed.
11. Inspect the four-point pattern for the extent of induration.
 RATIONALE: The size of induration should be determined by visual inspection and gentle palpation.
12. Measure in millimeters the diameter of the largest single reaction (induration) around any one of the puncture sites (Figure 15–19).
 RATIONALE: Separate areas of induration should not be added together, unless they coalesce into one.
13. Record the reading in millimeters.
14. Complete the individual's permanent tine test record (see Figure 15–19).
15. Instruct the patient that pain at the test site is relieved by cold packs, and itching can be relieved by applying glucocorticoid ointment or cream.

Interpreting the Reaction

Negative: Less than 2 mm of induration.
Doubtful: Slightly indurated lesions 2–4 mm in diameter. Follow up with the Mantoux method.
Positive: One or more papules 5 mm or more in diameter. Further clinical testing (x-ray of the chest, microbiolic examination of sputum, and Mantoux testing) is indicated.
Positive: Two or more papules that have fused at the base or are completely fused. Further clinical testing (x-ray of the chest, microbiologic examination of sputum, and Mantoux testing) is indicated.

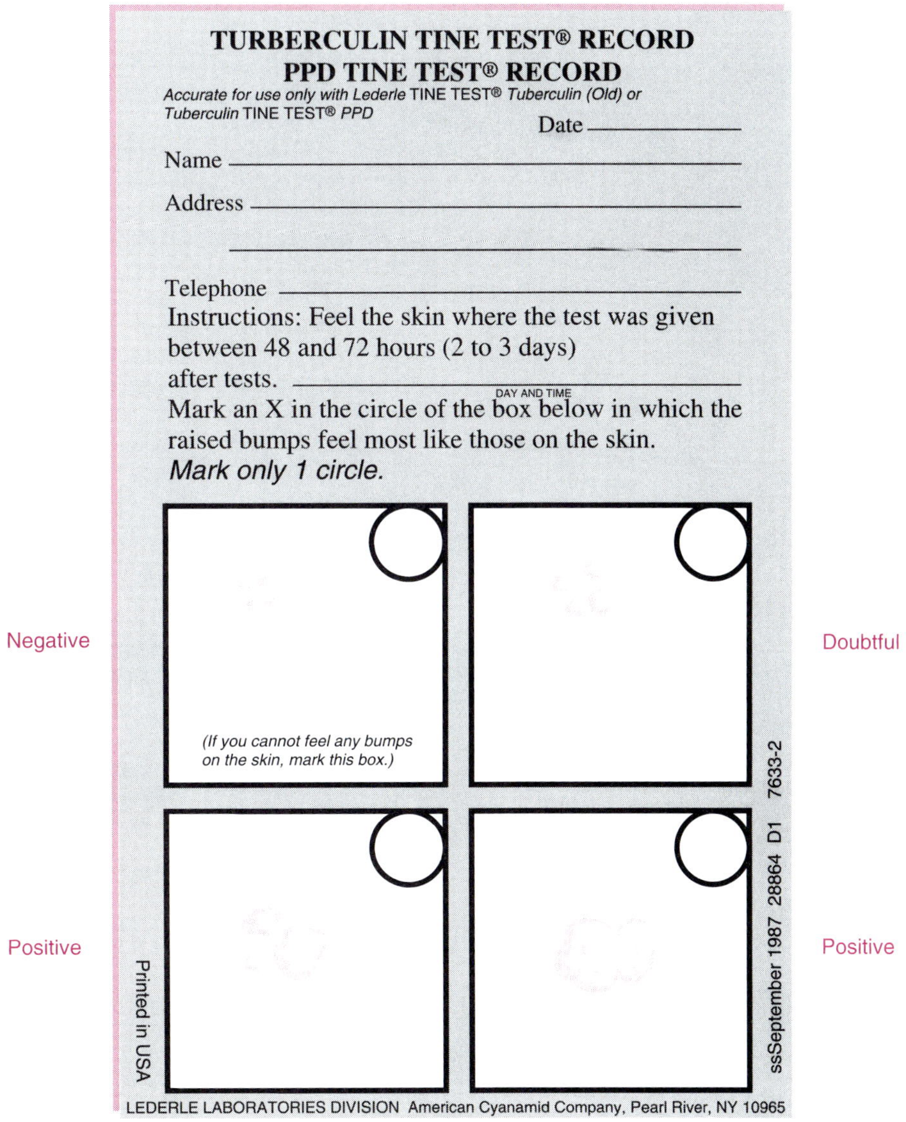

FIGURE 15–19

A recording card that facilitates Tine Test readings and provides permanent patient records of test reactions. (Courtesy of Lederle Laboratories, Pearl River, NY.)

RECOGNIZING POTENTIAL ADVERSE EFFECTS

Emotional Complications of Injections

The most common emotional complication of parenteral therapy is fear. Adults and children alike fear injections. Allow patients to talk about their fears and give patients the reasons for injections.

In addition, children may interpret the pain from an injection as a form of punishment for being "bad." Be brief but truthful with children.

- Tell them the benefits of the injection.
- Tell them there will be a sting.
- Tell them it is okay to cry or otherwise express discomfort.
- Reward them with praise; hold and comfort whenever necessary.
- Solicit help to restrain the uncooperative child.

Physical Complications of Injections

Physical complications include but are not limited to

- The formation of cysts or scar tissue, caused by not properly rotating repeated injections
- Injury to nerves, caused by needle injury or a medication's being deposited into or around a nerve branch
- Injection of a medication into a blood vessel or joint capsule, cause by failure to aspirate before injecting a medication
- Bacterial infections, caused by a break in sterile technique or patient preparation
- Skin pigmentation, cellulitis, localized tissue atrophy, and tissue necrosis or gangrene
- Bone damage
- Injury from broken needle.

Management of Drug Emergencies[2]

Allergy or Unusual Side Effects

- Discontinue suspected medications, if possible
- Make available oral antihistamines
- Keep the patient quiet and monitor for at least 1/2 hour

- Document the incident in the patient's medical history.

Anaphylactic Reactions

- Discontinue suspected medication (stop administration and tourniquet the injection site).
- Maintain airway
- Make available 0.2–0.5 milligram (mg) of epinephrine for intramuscular or subcutaneous injection (for children 0.01 mg/kg body weight). May be repeated every 10–15 minutes (for children, repeat every 15 minutes for two doses, then every 4 hours as required).
- Make available a 10–50-mg intramuscular dose of Benadryl. If additional antihistamine is needed, up to 100 mg of Benadryl may be administered, not to exceed 400 mg/day. Advise the patient not to take oral antihistamines for 24–48 hours.
- Additional emergency drugs to make available are vasopressors (to support blood pressure) and glucocorticoids (to decrease the reaction intensity).
- Document the incident in the patient's medical history and inform the patient or the patient's family to carry medical alert identification.

References

1. Hughes WT, Wong DL: *Intramuscular Injections: A Guide to Sites and Technique*. Philadelphia: Wyeth-Ayerst Laboratories, 1989.
2. Deglin J, Vallerand A, Russin M: *Davis's Drug Guide for Nurses*, 2nd ed. Philadelphia: F. A. Davis, 1991.
3. *Tuberculin, Old, Tine Test and Tuberculin, Purified Protein Derivative, Tine Test PPD*. Pearl River, NY: American Cyanamid Company, 1980.

Bibliography

Bonewit K: *Clinical Procedures for Medical Assistants*, 3rd ed. Philadelphia: W. B. Saunders, 1990.

Cornett E, Blume D: *Dosages and Solutions: A Programmed Approach to Meds and Math*, 5th ed. Philadelphia: F. A. Davis, 1991.

Frew MA, Frew DR: *Clinical Procedures for Medical Assistants*. Philadelphia: F. A. Davis, 1990.

Kinn M, Derge E: *The Medical Assistant: Administrative and Clinical*, 6th ed. Philadelphia: W. B. Saunders, 1990.

Rodman MJ, et al: *Pharmacology and Drug Therapy in Nursing*, 3rd ed. Philadelphia: J. B. Lippincott, 1985.

Chapter 16

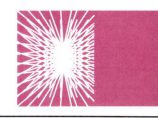

SURGICAL AND REHABILITATIVE PROCEDURES

JUNE M. FRANCIS

SURGICAL PROCEDURES
Surgical Instruments
Procedures

TYPES OF BANDAGES
Elastic Bandage
Cling Bandage
Gauze Roller Bandage

REHABILITATIVE PROCEDURES

SURGICAL PROCEDURES

Surgical Instruments

The medical assistant needs to be familiar with the variety of surgical instruments used in the office for minor office surgery. Some of the more common instruments used are illustrated in Figure 16–1.

Scissors. Scissors are cutting instruments with either straight or curved blades. Both blades may be sharp, or both may be blunt, or one blade may be sharp and the other blade blunt.

- **Suture scissors:** These have a hook on the tip to aid in getting under the suture and a blunt end to prevent injuring the tissue.
- **Bandage scissors:** These have a flat, blunt prow to insert under the dressing or bandage to cut before removing it.
- **Dissecting scissors:** These have a fine cutting edge and are used to divide tissue.

Forceps. Forceps are two-pronged instruments for grasping and squeezing.

- **Thumb forceps:** These have serrated tips and are used to pick up or hold tissue.
- **Tissue forceps:** These have teeth and are used to grasp tissue.
- **Splinter forceps:** These have sharp points to help remove foreign bodies from tissue.
- **Dressing forceps:** These have a blunt end with coarse cross-striations used for grasping.

Hemostatic forceps: These have serrated tips and are used to clamp off blood vessels.

Sponge forceps: These have large serrated rings on the tips for holding sponges.

Needle holders. Needle holders are used to grasp a curved needle firmly.

Towel clamps. Towel clamps have two sharp points to hold the edges of a sterile towel in place.

Retractors. Retractors are used to hold tissues aside to expose the operative area.

Probes. Probes are long, slender instruments used to explore wounds or body cavities.

Sutures. Sutures are either absorbable or nonabsorbable thread used in sewing tissue together. Usually a needle is already attached (Figure 16–2A).

- **Curved-cutting-edge needle:** This needle is used for closing skin where a sharp point is needed to get through tough tissue.

Blades. Blades are placed on a scalpel for surgical use (see Figures 16–1 and 16–2B).

- **# 15 blade:** This blade is used for making skin incisions.
- **# 11 blade:** This blade is used when a point is needed, such as in debridement of necrotic tissue.

Text continued on page 378

372 *Chapter 16:* SURGICAL AND REHABILITATIVE PROCEDURES

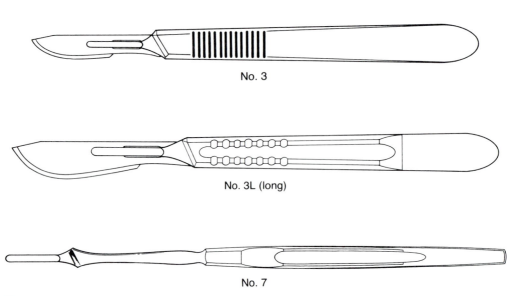

FIGURE 16-1
Instruments commonly used in minor office surgery. (Courtesy of Dittmar and Penn Corporation, Cheltenham, Pennsylvania.)

Chapter 16: SURGICAL AND REHABILITATIVE PROCEDURES

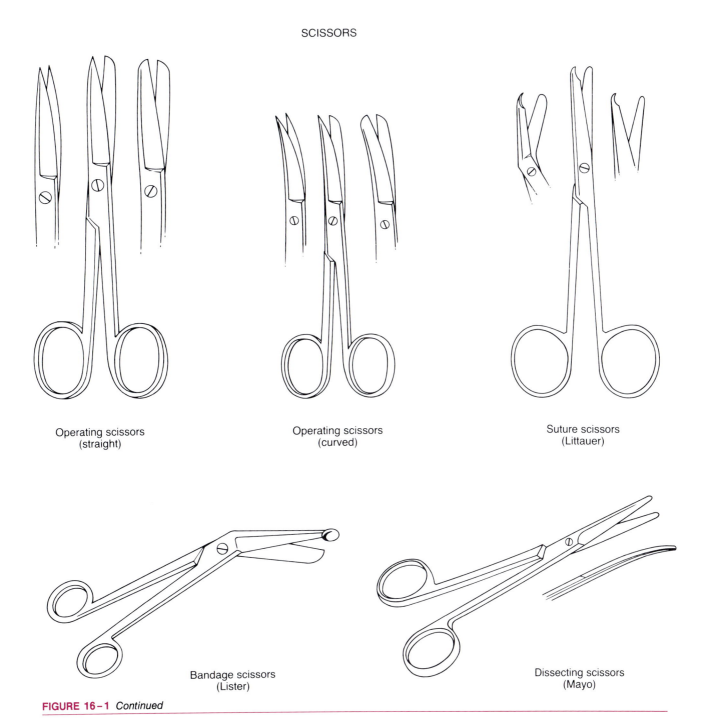

FIGURE 16-1 Continued

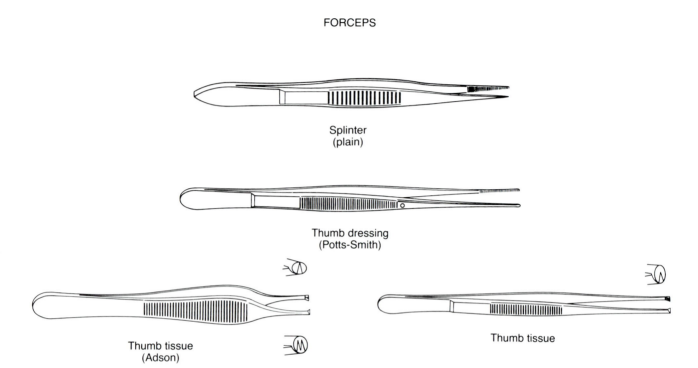
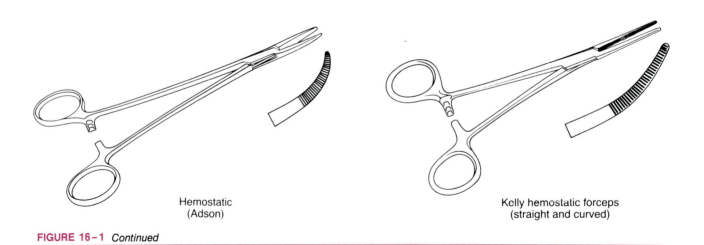

FIGURE 16-1 Continued

Chapter 16: SURGICAL AND REHABILITATIVE PROCEDURES **375**

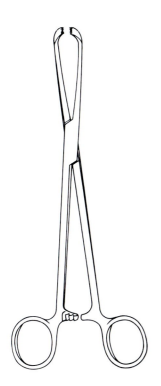
Allis tissue forceps

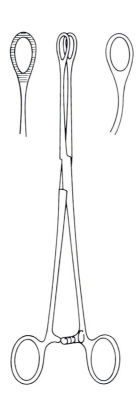
Foerster sponge forceps

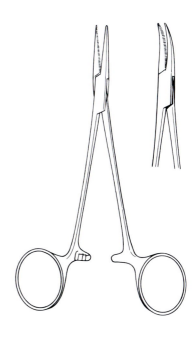
Halstead mosquito hemostatic forceps (straight and curved)

FIGURE 16-1 *Continued*

RETRACTORS

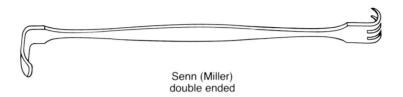

Senn (Miller)
double ended

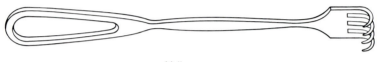

Volkmann

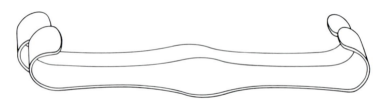

Parker

DIRECTORS AND PROBES

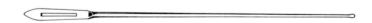

Probe with eye

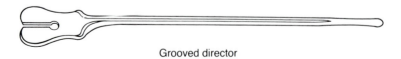

Grooved director

FIGURE 16-1 *Continued*

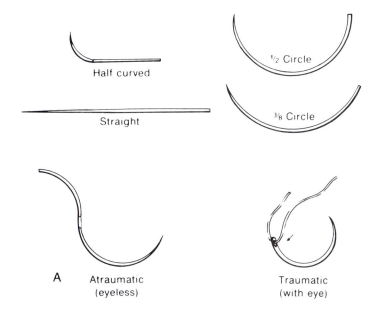

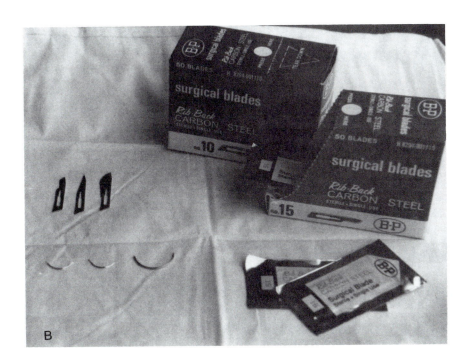

FIGURE 16-2

A, Suture needle shapes and types. **B**, Disposable blade sizes (*top, left to right*, No. 15, No. 11, and No. 10) and disposable suture needles (*bottom*). (**A** from Kinn ME, Derge EF: *The Medical Assistant: Administrative and Clinical*, 6th ed. Philadelphia: W.B. Saunders, 1988, p. 589.)

PROCEDURE

CLEANING SURGICAL INSTRUMENTS

PURPOSE

To clean instruments properly to prolong their use.

EQUIPMENT AND MATERIALS

Basin or pan
Cleaning agent
Soft brush
Gloves

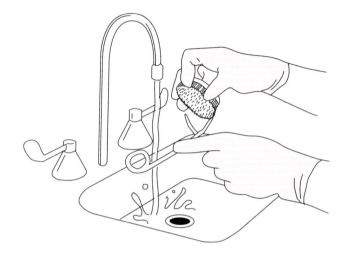

PROCEDURAL STEPS

1. Place instruments in clean water (preferably sterile distilled water) to soak off soil.
   RATIONALE: This prevents blood and tissue fragments from drying on the instruments.
2. Remove instruments from the water and wipe them off to dislodge any particles.
3. Place instruments in a low-suds detergent with a neutral PH and a free-rinsing agent. The detergent should not contain phosphates or chlorides.
   RATIONALE: Breakdown of the protective layer on the instruments is prevented.
4. Scrub instruments thoroughly with a soft brush and the low-suds detergent to remove all foreign matter.
   RATIONALE: This eliminates baked-on soil, which can corrode metal.
5. Rinse and dry well to prevent any corrosion. Do not use oil to lubricate the instruments. Use only a water-soluble lubricant.
   RATIONALE: Steam may not penetrate under oil, leaving an area on the instruments unsterilized.
6. Repackage to autoclave.

PROCEDURE

TRANSFERRING STERILE ARTICLES

PURPOSE

To transport articles from one sterile area to another sterile area without contaminating them.

 MEDICAL ASSISTING ALERT

There should be enough solution in the container to cover approximately two-thirds of the transfer forceps. Change solution according to manufacturer's recommendation.

EQUIPMENT AND MATERIALS

Pronged forceps
Forcep container
Disinfectant solution (for example, Cidex or Zephiran)

PROCEDURAL STEPS

1. *Do not* allow the prongs to touch any part of the container. Allow the excess to drip back

into the container by tapping the prongs together.

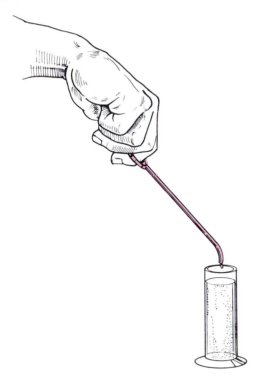

RATIONALE: The outside of the container and the part of the container above the disinfectant solution line are considered contaminated.

2. Hold the lid in your hand with the inside of the lid facing downward, or place the lid on a solid surface with the inside facing up.

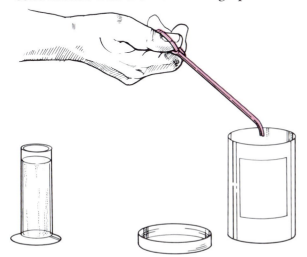

RATIONALE: The inside of the lid must be held downward to prevent microorganisms in the air from settling on it, resulting in contamination. Placing a lid upward on a solid surface keeps the inside of the lid from coming in contact with an unsterile surface.

3. Keeping the prongs of the transfer forceps pointed downward, pick up the sterile article without touching the outside of the cannister (see figure next to step 2). Replace the lid of the cannister as soon as possible.

RATIONALE: This prevents microorganisms in the air from settling on the contents in the cannister, resulting in contamination.

4. Do not let forceps touch the sterile field while dropping the article onto the sterile field.

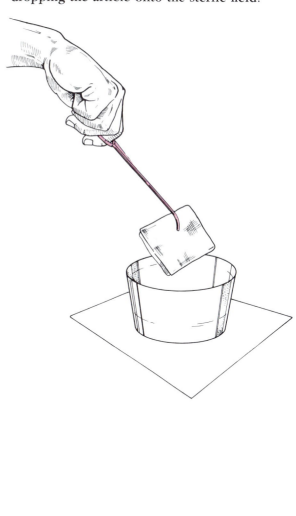

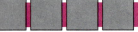 **PROCEDURE**

OPENING A STERILE PACKAGE

PURPOSE

To transfer sterile instruments or supplies to a sterile field without contaminating.

 MEDICAL ASSISTING ALERT

Check the sterilization indicator and the expiration date on the wrapped package to make sure contents are still sterile.

EQUIPMENT AND MATERIALS

Clean surface or tray
Sterile package

PROCEDURAL STEPS

1. Assemble equipment, including a tray (such as a Mayo tray) or other flat, clean surface on which to open the package.
2. Place the wrapped package in your hand or on a flat surface so that the top flap of the wrapper opens away from you.
   RATIONALE: The contents of small opened packages in the hand can be dropped directly onto a sterile field.
3. Remove the fastener on the wrapped package.
4. Handle only the outside of the wrapper while opening the package.
5. Do not cross hands over the sterile field while opening the package.

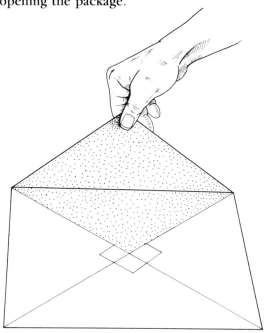

RATIONALE: This prevents dust or lint from unsterile clothing falling onto the sterile field and causing contamination.

6. Touch only the outside of the wrapper while opening the last flap.

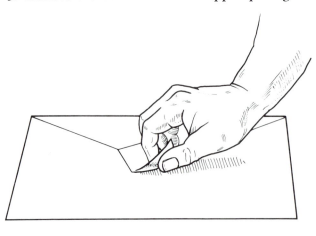

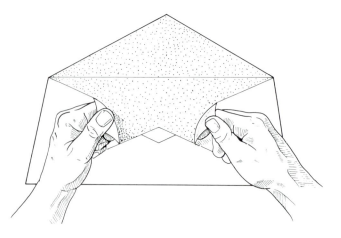

7. Transfer the contents of the package to the sterile field, using sterile gloves or forceps, or use the package itself as a sterile setup.

NOTE: Commercially prepared disposable packages are commonly used in most offices. To open, follow directions stated on the outside of the package.

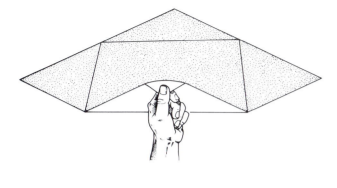
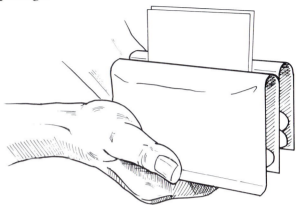

PROCEDURE

TRANSPORTING SPECIMENS

PURPOSE

To transport them to the laboratory in the correct medium and to identify a specimen's source with the correct patient's name.

 MEDICAL ASSISTING ALERT

The ratio of liquid medium (such as 10% formalyn, or normal saline) to specimen is ideally 20:1.

EQUIPMENT AND MATERIALS

Container with transport medium
Laboratory requisition slip
Label for transport medium container
Container or bag for transporting the specimen container and laboratory slip to the laboratory.

PROCEDURAL STEPS

1. Label the specimen container as specified by the laboratory's requirements.
   RATIONALE: This ensures proper processing and reporting.
2. Fill out the proper laboratory requisition slip with patient information and specimen information. Make sure the tissue is properly described on the requisition form. Ask the physician.
   RATIONALE: This ensures proper processing and reporting.

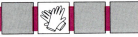

PROCEDURE

PREPARING THE PATIENT FOR A MINOR SURGICAL PROCEDURE

PURPOSE

To make the patient comfortable, adequately expose the surgical site, and cleanse the skin of microorganisms at the surgical site.

 MEDICAL ASSISTING ALERT

If you are using an iodine-based antiseptic for cleansing, ask the patient if he or she has had any allergic reactions to iodine.

EQUIPMENT AND MATERIALS

Patient drape, if indicated
Armboard, if indicated
Skin antiseptic
Razor, if indicated
Wide tape, if indicated

PROCEDURAL STEPS

Patient Preparation

1. Position and drape the patient comfortably, according to the procedure to be performed. Use an armboard, if available, for an upper extremity.

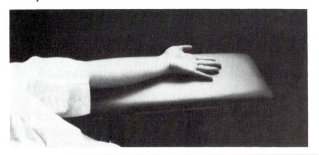

RATIONALE: An uncomfortable position may cause the patient to move during the procedure, or cause a cramping of a muscle in the patient.

2. Adjust the lighting source adequately over the surgical site.

Performance

3. Shave the area if necessary, with a sharp safety razor, keeping the skin taut.
RATIONALE: Hair is a source of microorganisms and can contaminate the wound.
4. Remove small cut hairs from the skin by touching the shaved area with wide tape.

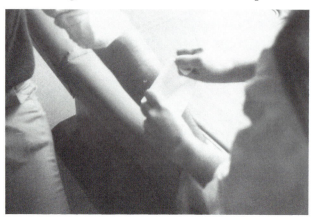

Chapter 16: SURGICAL AND REHABILITATIVE PROCEDURES **383**

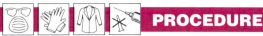

PROCEDURE

SUTURING FOR SIMPLE WOUND CLOSURE

PURPOSE

To close a small wound using absorbable and/or nonabsorbable sutures.

EQUIPMENT AND MATERIALS

Sterile gloves
Sterile syringe with needle
Local anesthesia
Sterile suture set:
    Drape with aperture
    Needle holder for curved needle
    Toothed forceps
    Scissors to cut suture
    Dressings
Sterile saline to cleanse suture line

PROCEDURAL STEPS

Patient Preparation

1. Position and drape the patient comfortably. Use an armboard for upper extremity, if available.

Performance

2. Shave the area if necessary, with a sharp safety razor, keeping the skin taut.
   RATIONALE: Hair is a source of microorganisms and can contaminate the wound.
3. Remove small cut hairs from the skin by touching the area with wide tape (see illustration in previous procedure).
4. Put on gloves.
5. Thoroughly cleanse small wound using detergent–germicidal soap.
   RATIONALE: Foreign bodies, debris, and crusted blood are removed. Also, the possibility of contamination is minimized.

Follow-Through

6. After the procedure, remain with the patient for safety precautions (that is, to prevent accidental falls or injuries).
7. Make sure the patient understands the physician's postoperative instructions.

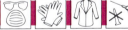

PROCEDURE

EXCISING A LESION FROM UNDER THE SKIN AND TOPICALLY

PURPOSE

To remove a lesion under surgical asepsis.

MEDICAL ASSISTING ALERT

Note that a 1-inch border around the sterile field on a sterile tray is considered unsterile, because this area may have become contaminated while you were setting up the tray.

EQUIPMENT AND MATERIALS

Sterile gloves (two pairs)
Local anesthesia
Sterile syringe with needle
Sterile drape with aperture
Sterile lesion removal set:
    Scalpel
    #15 blade
    Operating scissors
    Needle holder

384 *Chapter 16: SURGICAL AND REHABILITATIVE PROCEDURES*

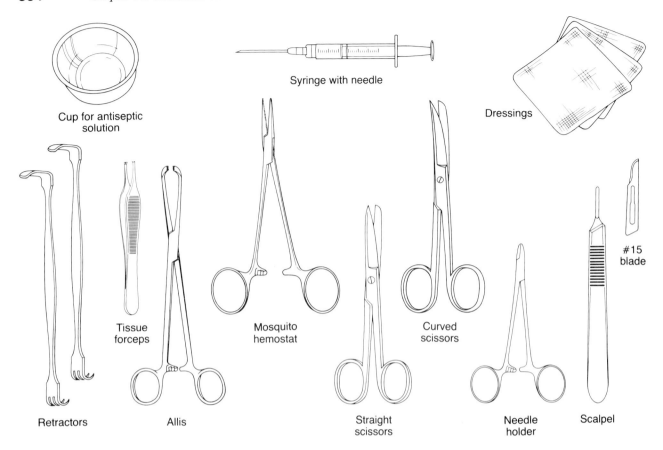
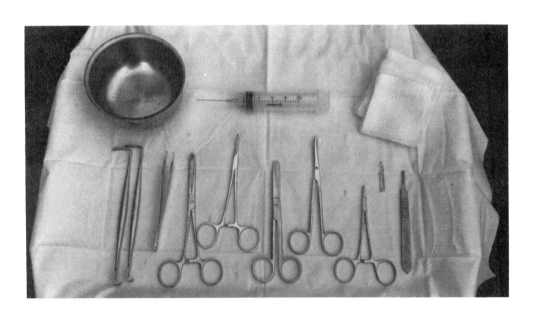

Tissue forceps
Allis forceps
Curved or straight hemostat
Small basin or cup
Suture material with curved cutting needle
Dressings
Specimen container

PROCEDURAL STEPS

Patient Preparation

1. Position and drape the patient comfortably. Use an armboard, if available, for an upper extremity.
   RATIONALE: An uncomfortable position may cause the patient to move during the procedure or cause cramping of a muscle in the patient.
2. Adjust the lighting source adequately over the surgical site.

Performance

3. Shave the area if necessary, with a sharp safety razor, keeping the skin taut.
4. Remove small cut hairs from the skin by touching the shaved area with wide tape.
   RATIONALE: Hair is a source of microorganisms and can contaminate the wound.
5. Cleanse the operative site area with the appropriate antiseptic.
   RATIONALE: This reduces the number of microorganisms present.
6. Put on sterile gloves and place a fenestrated drape over the cleansed lesion.

Follow-Through

7. After the procedure, remain with the patient for safety precautions (that is, to prevent accidental falls or injuries).
8. Make sure the patient understands the physician's postoperative instructions.
9. Prepare the specimen to be sent to the laboratory.

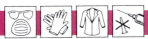 **PROCEDURE**

INCISING AND DRAINING

PURPOSE

To drain an infected cyst, boil, or carbuncle and promote healing.

 MEDICAL ASSISTING ALERT

Carefully dispose of and/or clean the used contaminated articles and instruments according to the office policy.
RATIONALE: This prevents possible spreading of infectious pathogens from purulent drainage to surfaces in the minor surgery room, to the staff, and to other patients.

EQUIPMENT AND MATERIALS

Sterile gloves (two pairs)
Sterile syringe with needle
Local anesthesia
Large irrigating syringe
Sterile saline solution for irrigating
Iodoform gauze for packing wound
Sterile incision and drainage set:
   Scalpel
   #15 blade
   Tissue forceps
   Curved or straight hemostat
   Drape with aperture
   Dressings
Culture swab

PROCEDURAL STEPS

Patient Preparation

1. Position and drape the patient comfortably. Use an armboard, if available, for an upper extremity.
2. Adjust the lighting adequately over the incision and drainage site.

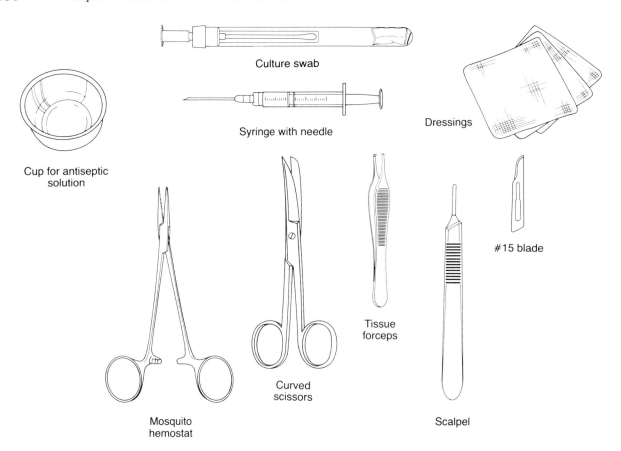
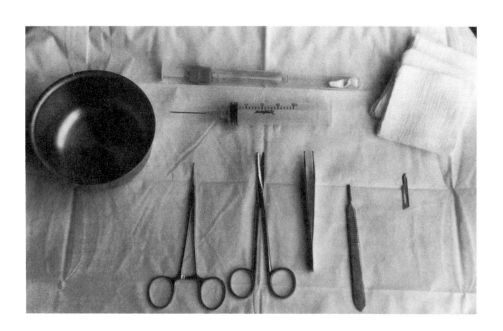

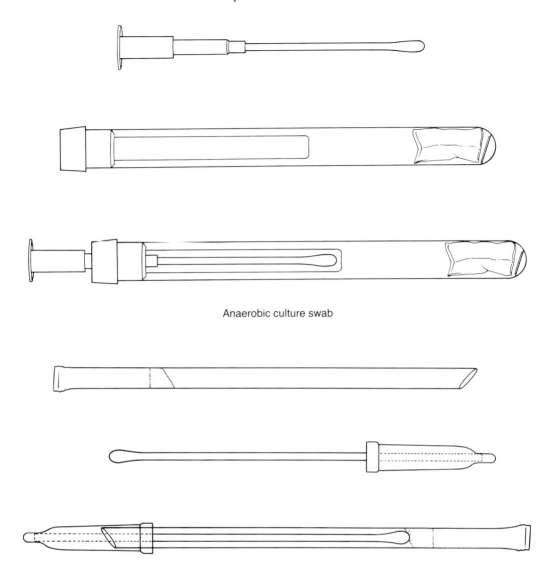

Anaerobic culture swab

Aerobic culture swab

Performance

3. Put on gloves.
4. Cleanse the area with the appropriate antiseptic.

Follow-Through

5. After the procedure, remain with the patient for safety precautions (that is, to prevent accidental falls or injuries).
6. Make sure the patient understands the physician's postoperative instructions.
7. Dispose of articles, and clean reusables according to office policy.
8. Prepare the culture swab to be sent to the laboratory.

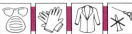

PROCEDURE

USING THE CO₂ LASER UNIT

PURPOSE

To cauterize tissue as a surgical procedure is being performed, to lessen actual surgery time, to lessen chances of infection, and to quicken healing time.

 MEDICAL ASSISTING ALERT

Do not use paper products for a barrier on the patient. Laser-beam flash fire on the paper could burn the patient's skin.

EQUIPMENT AND MATERIALS

Hat
Sterile gloves (two pairs)
Sterile cloth aperture drape
Sterile procedure set and sterile supplies pertaining to the procedure being done

PROCEDURAL STEPS

Patient Preparation

1. Position and drape the patient according to the operative site. Use an armboard, if available, for the upper extremity.
2. Position the lighting source over the operative site.

Performance

3. Put on gloves.
4. Clean the operative site with antiseptic.
5. Rewash the operative site with sterile water.
   RATIONALE: This prevents iodine-based antiseptic from leaving "tattoo" marks on the patient's skin. Alcohol can cause flash fire from the laser beam, burning the patient's skin.
6. Place the aperture drape over the cleansed operative site.

Follow-Through

7. After the procedure, remain with the patient for safety precautions (that is, to prevent accidental falls or injuries).
8. Make sure the patient understands the physicians's postoperative instructions.
9. Prepare any specimen to be sent to the laboratory.

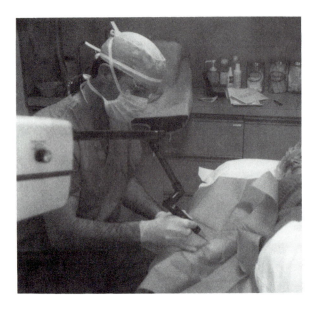

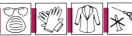

PROCEDURE

REMOVING SMALL MOLES AND WARTS WITH THE ELECTROSURGERY UNIT OR HYFRECATOR

PURPOSE

To achieve rapid and effective destruction of these abnormal growths without loss of blood.

 MEDICAL ASSISTING ALERT

If the unit is to be used with a patient grounding plate, make sure the patient's bare skin is flat against the plate. Grounding the patient prevents any accidental burns to the patient from the electrosurgery current.

EQUIPMENT AND MATERIALS

Electrosurgery unit or hyfrecator
Sterile gloves (two pairs)
Sterile aperture drape
Local anesthesia
Sterile syringe with needle
Sterile forceps
Antiseptic dressing

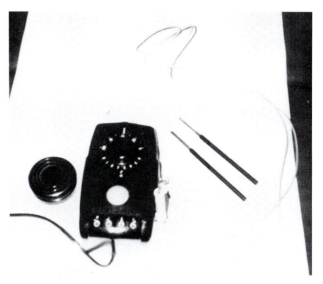

Wall-mounted hyfrecator

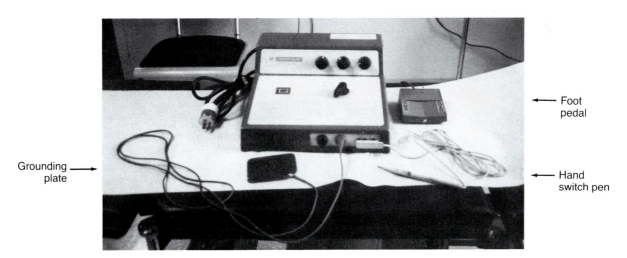

Electrosurgical unit

PROCEDURAL STEPS

Patient Preparation

1. Position and drape the patient according to the minor surgical site. Use an armboard, if available, for an upper extremity.
2. Position the lighting source over the minor surgical site.

Performance

3. Cleanse the operative site with antiseptic.
   NOTE: When using alcohol, which is flammable, be certain that the solution has completely evaporated.

Follow-Through

4. After the procedure, remain with the patient for safety precautions (that is, to prevent accidental falls or injuries).
5. Make sure the patient understands the physician's postoperative instructions.
6. Prepare the specimen to be sent to the laboratory.

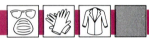

PROCEDURE

CHANGING A STERILE DRESSING

PURPOSE

To protect the wound from contamination, absorb drainage, and restrict motion that may interfere with healing.

EQUIPMENT AND MATERIALS

Clean gloves
Sterile gloves
Sterile forceps
Antiseptic solution
Container for antiseptic solution
Sterile cotton balls or gauze
Sterile dressings
Plastic waste bag

PROCEDURAL STEPS

Patient Preparation

1. Position patient comfortably and drape patient appropriately if necessary.
2. Explain the procedure to the patient.
3. Instruct patient not to move during the procedure and to not talk, laugh, cough, or reach over the sterile field.
   RATIONALE: This prevents the patient from contaminating the field by touching it or transferring microorganisms in water vapors from the nose, mouth, or lungs.

Performance

4. Remove the old dressing with clean gloves or forceps. Place in plastic waste bag.
5. Inspect the wound for progress in the healing. Look for any signs of infection, amount of any drainage, and the type of drainage.
   RATIONALE: This reveals whether drainage is serous (containing serum), sanguineous (containing serum and blood), or purulent (containing pus, usually thick and unpleasant smelling).
6. Discard gloves or forceps without touching yourself.
   RATIONALE: This prevents you from contaminating yourself.
7. Put on a pair of sterile gloves.
8. Moisten a cotton ball with antiseptic. Holding the cotton ball with sterile forceps, cleanse wound from top to the bottom and from the center outward. Use a new cotton ball for each cleansing motion. Discard the used ones in the plastic waste bag.
9. Drop sterile dressing over the wound using sterile forceps or sterile gloves. Hold in place with tape or bandage, as specified by the physician.

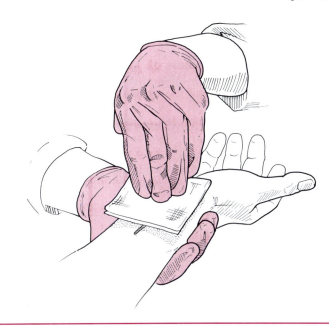

RATIONALE: Dropping the dressing reduces the possibility of transferring microorganisms from the skin to the wound.
10. Remove gloves and place them into the plastic bag.
11. Wash your hands.

Follow-Through

12. Dispose of and clean the contaminated articles per office policy.
13. Record in the patient's chart the wound's appearance, any drainage, and any problems the patient may have experienced.

PROCEDURE

DRESSING A DRAINING WOUND

PURPOSE

To prevent contamination of a clean wound, prevent further contamination of a dirty wound, and prevent transmission of pathogens to clean areas.

 MEDICAL ASSISTING ALERT

Use aseptic technique.

EQUIPMENT AND MATERIALS

Sterile gloves
Clean gloves
Sterile forceps
Antiseptic solution in sterile container
Sterile dressings
Adhesive tape
Plastic waste bag

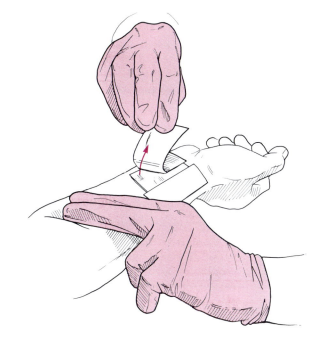

PROCEDURAL STEPS

Patient Preparation

1. Position and drape patient appropriately.
2. Explain the procedure to the patient.
3. Wash your hands and put on clean gloves.
4. Remove old tape and dressing carefully, pulling tape toward wound and peeling the edges by holding skin taut and pushing away from tape.
   RATIONALE: Pushing the skin away from the tape is less traumatic than to pull tape from the skin.
5. Moisten the dressing with sterile saline if it adheres. Withdraw dressing slowly.
   RATIONALE: Moistening the dressing loosens any dried blood or drainage from the dressing, making it easier to remove from the wound.
6. Note amount of drainage on the dressing, its color, and its odor.
   RATIONALE: These are reported to the physician.
7. Discard soiled dressings and gloves in plastic waste bag.
   RATIONALE: This prevents transmission of pathogenic organisms.

Performance

8. Select proper size and type of adhesive for securing the dressing.
   RATIONALE: Hypoallergenic tape is best used when dressing is changed often.
9. Put on sterile gloves.
10. Cleanse wound with antiseptic using sterile forceps and gauze or cotton balls.
11. Apply dressing and secure with tape. A thin layer of liquid protectant, such as tincture of benzoin or Mastisol, may be applied to the skin.
    RATIONALE: This enhances sticking of the tape and helps protect the skin.
12. A Montgomery strap dressing may be used for a dressing that is changed several times a day.

Follow-Through

13. Make sure the patient understands the physician's instructions.
14. Dispose of the soiled dressings in waste bag. Discard the disposable items and clean the equipment that is to be reused.
    RATIONALE: This prevents transmission of pathogenic organisms.
15. Wash your hands.
16. Make notes in the patient's chart.

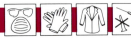

PROCEDURE

ASPIRATING FLUIDS

PURPOSE

To suction fluid from a cavity to relieve pressure and to promote healing.

MEDICAL ASSISTING ALERT

Preserve the aspirated fluid for laboratory analysis, unless directed otherwise by the physician.

EQUIPMENT AND MATERIALS

Antiseptic solution or swab
Sterile gloves (two pairs)
Local anesthesia
Sterile setup:
    Syringe and needle for local anesthesia
    Syringe and needle for aspirating
    Sterile drape with aperture
    Dressings
    Sterile container for fluid

PROCEDURAL STEPS

Patient Preparation

1. Position and drape the patient comfortably. Use an armboard, if available, for an upper extremity.

Performance

2. Put on gloves.
3. Cleanse the area to be aspirated with antiseptic.
4. Place aperture drape over cleansed area to be aspirated.

Follow-Through

5. After the procedure, remain with the patient for safety precautions (that is, to prevent accidental falls or injuries).
6. Make sure the patient understands the physician's postprocedure instructions.
7. If directed to do so by the physician, prepare aspirated fluid for transporting to the laboratory.

 PROCEDURE

REMOVING SUTURES

PURPOSE

To remove sutures after a predetermined number of days before they can act as wicks carrying pathogenic organisms from the skin into the wound.

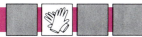 **MEDICAL ASSISTING ALERT**

Observe the wound for any signs of infection or swelling.

EQUIPMENT AND MATERIALS

Clean gloves
Antiseptic
Suture-removal scissors
Smooth forceps
Dressings

PROCEDURAL STEPS

Patient Preparation

1. Position patient comfortably and drape if necessary.
2. Explain the procedure to the patient.

Performance

3. Put on gloves.
4. Cleanse the wound with antiseptic.
   RATIONALE: Stitches provide a pathway for microorganisms.
5. Remove any dried blood encrustations with hydrogen peroxide.
6. *Do not* allow any segment of the stitch that is on the surface of the skin to be drawn below the skin surface.
   RATIONALE: This prevents skin surface contamination from becoming subcutaneous, risking infection.

Interrupted Sutures

1. Lift the knot with thumb forceps.

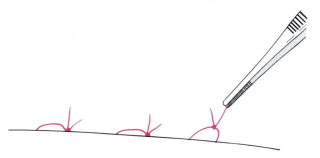

2. Cut the suture close to the skin with suture scissors.

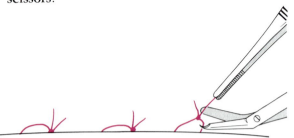

3. Remove suture, pulling the short end under the skin.

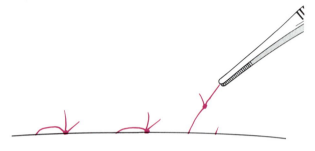

Continuous Sutures

1. Cut every other suture.

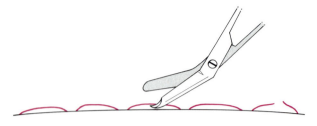

2. Lift the middle of the uncut suture and pull the suture upward.

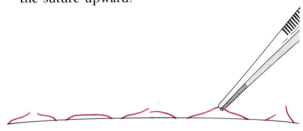

Follow-Through

7. Record in the patient's chart the suture removal and condition of the wound.

TYPES OF BANDAGES

Elastic Bandage

Elastic bandages can be stretched and molded around a body part. These bandages can be removed, rewound, and used again for the same patient (Figure 16–3).

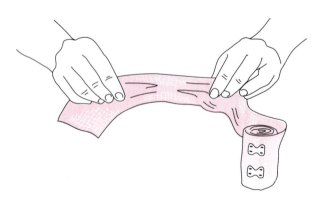

FIGURE 16–3
Elastic bandage.

PROCEDURE

APPLYING AN ELASTIC BANDAGE

PURPOSE

To apply gentle, even pressure to a body part; hold a dressing in place over a wound; and provide immobilization of an injured part.

> **MEDICAL ASSISTING ALERT**
>
> Before wrapping the bandage, inspect the skin for any discoloration, chafing, or edema. Look carefully at bony prominences.

EQUIPMENT AND MATERIALS

Appropriate-width bandage (Table 16–1)
Tape, pins, or clips

PROCEDURAL STEPS

Patient Preparation

1. Place patient in comfortable position with affected body part in good alignment.
   RATIONALE: This avoids having the extremity dangle. Have the body part to be bandaged in a normal functioning position to promote circulation and prevent deformity and discomfort.
2. Explain the procedure to the patient.

3. When possible, elevate the affected extremity 15 minutes before applying an elastic bandage.
   RATIONALE: This aids in venous blood flow.

Performance

4. Hold the roll of elastic bandage in your dominant hand and use other hand to lightly hold beginning of bandage at distal body part. Continue transferring to dominant hand as bandage is wrapped. Hold the roll close to the part being bandaged. Unroll and *slightly* stretch bandage.
   RATIONALE: This ensures even tension and pressure and avoids restriction of circulation.
5. Unroll the bandage as you wrap the body part. Never unroll the entire bandage and then wrap.
   RATIONALE: This prevents uneven pressure, which interferes with blood circulation.
6. Overlap each layer of bandage by one-half to one-third the width of the strip. Avoid leaving gaps in bandage layers or skin surfaces exposed.
   RATIONALE: This prevents uneven pressure on the body part.

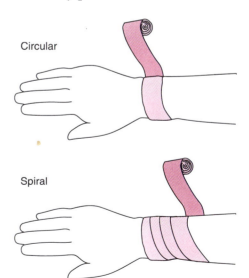

TABLE 16–1

APPROPRIATE LENGTHS AND WIDTHS NEEDED FOR BANDAGING DIFFERENT BODY PARTS

Type	Length	Width
Head bandaging	6 yards	2 inch
Body bandaging	10 yards	3–6 inch
Leg bandaging	9 yards	2–4 inch
Foot bandaging	4 yards	1½–3 inch
Arm bandaging	7–9 yards	2–2½ inch
Hand bandaging	3 yards	1–2 inch
Finger bandaging	1–3 yards	½–1 inch

(Reprinted from Rambo BJ, and Wood LA: *Nursing Skills for Clinical Practice*, 3rd ed. Philadelphia: W. B. Saunders, 1982.)

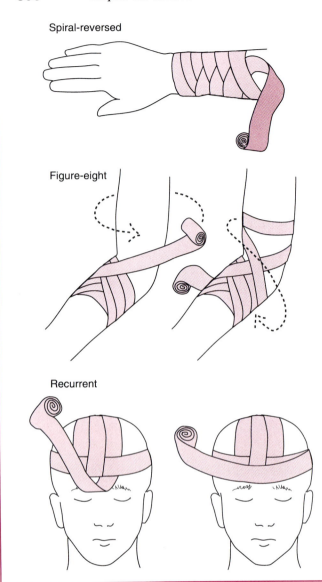

7. As you wrap, ask the patient to tell you whether the bandage feels comfortable. If the patient complains of tingling, itching, numbness, or pain, loosen the bandage.
8. When wrapping an extremity, anchor the bandage initially by circling the distal body part twice. Do not wrap the toes or fingers.
RATIONALE: This permits detection of impaired circulation in the distal extremity.
9. When finished wrapping, secure the end of the bandage with tape, pins, or clips.
10. Check distal extremity after the bandage is in place.
RATIONALE: Paleness or cyanosis, swelling, coolness, or pain in the distal extremity indicates impaired circulation.

Follow-Through

11. Make sure patient understands the physician's instructions.
12. Record in patient's chart the size of bandage used and the patient's response.

Redrawn by permission from Potter P, Perry A: *Fundamentals of Nursing*, 2nd ed. St. Louis, 1989, The C.V. Mosby Co.

Cling Bandage

The Cling bandage stretches but is not elastic. It molds around irregular and hard-to-bandage areas and is often used for holding dressings in place on the head or the stump of an amputated limb.

Gauze Roller Bandage

The Gauze roller bandage is used less frequently for bandaging the arm or leg when there is a difference in the size of the limb. Other bandages that have more elastic or clinging ability provide a firmer wrapping that stays in place and provides better support.

REHABILITATIVE PROCEDURES

Applications of heat or cold to the skin surface are used in treating infectious and traumatic conditions. The physician orders the treatment on the basis of the related and opposing effects produced elsewhere in the body. The order must state the frequency and length of time for the ordered treatment application.

Heat provides general comfort and speeds up the healing process by

- Causing dilation of blood vessels and increasing blood supply to the area
- Stimulating metabolism and growth of new cells and tissues
- Decreasing inflammation and promoting the formation of pus (suppuration)

Cold prevents or reduces swelling by

- Causing contraction of blood vessels and decreasing blood supply to the area
- Retarding metabolism and decreasing cell activity or growth
- Retarding bleeding and decreasing suppuration

PROCEDURE

APPLYING A HOT MOIST PACK

PURPOSE

To promote suppuration, decrease inflammation, reduce pain, and accelerate the healing process in an area by increasing the blood supply.

 MEDICAL ASSISTING ALERT

Young children, elderly patients, and patients with circulatory problems tend to be more sensitive to heat.

EQUIPMENT AND MATERIALS

Solution
Bath thermometer
Gauze or wash cloth
Basin

PROCEDURAL STEPS

Patient Preparation

1. Position and drape the patient comfortably.
2. Explain the procedure to the patient.

Performance

3. Check the solution temperature with the bath thermometer (Table 16–2).
   RATIONALE: The temperature for adults and older children should be 105–110° F (41–44° C).
4. Squeeze the excess solution out of the compress and apply lightly at first to the affected area.
   RATIONALE: This allows the patient to gradually become used to the heat.
5. A waterproof cover may be put over the compress to maintain the heat for a longer period of time.
   RATIONALE: The number of times the compress needs to be changed is reduced.
6. Ask the patient how the temperature feels.

TABLE 16–2

WATER TEMPERATURES FOR HOT MOIST PACKS

Warm	93 to 98° F (34 to 37° C)
Hot	98 to 105° F (37 to 41° C)
Very Hot	105 to 115° F (41 to 46° C)

(Reprinted from Rambo BJ, Wood LA: *Nursing Skills for Clinical Practice*, 3rd ed. Philadelphia: W. B. Saunders, 1982.)

The compress should be as hot as the patient can comfortably tolerate.
7. Repeat the compress application every 2–3 minutes for the duration the physician has specified, usually 15–20 minutes.
8. Check the patient's skin periodically for signs of increased redness or swelling.
9. Check the water temperature periodically and add more if needed.
10. Thoroughly dry the affected area.

Follow-Through

11. Clean and properly care for the equipment.
12. Record in patient's chart the treatment and results.

PROCEDURE

APPLYING A HOT-WATER BOTTLE

PURPOSE

To relieve pain, congestion, muscle spasms, and inflammation in an area by increasing the blood supply.

MEDICAL ASSISTING ALERT

1. Young children, elderly patients, and patients with circulatory problems tend to be more sensitive to heat.
2. Covered skin areas, such as the chest, back, and abdomen, tend to be more sensitive to heat.
3. Broken skin is more sensitive to heat.

EQUIPMENT AND MATERIALS

Hot-water bag
Protective covering, such as a flannel cover, towel, or pillowcase
Pitcher to hold water
Bath thermometer

TABLE 16-3

WATER TEMPERATURE FOR HOT-WATER BOTTLE

115 to 125° F (46 to 52° C) for adults and older children.
105 to 115° F (41 to 46° C) for babies, toddlers and elderly patients.

(Reprinted from Rambo BJ, Wood LA: *Nursing Skills for Clinical Practice*, 3rd ed. Philadelphia: W. B. Saunders, 1982.)

PROCEDURAL STEPS

Patient Preparation

1. Position and drape the patient comfortably.
2. Explain the procedure to the patient.

Performance

3. Check the temperature of the water with the bath thermometer (Table 16-3). Temperature should not exceed 125° F (52° C), which will produce the desired effects.

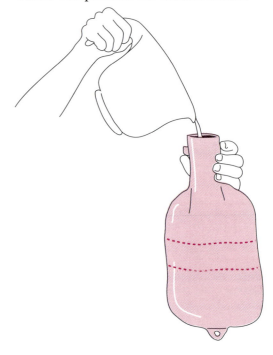

RATIONALE: This prevents burns of the skin.
4. Partially (one-half to two-thirds) fill the hot water bottle.
RATIONALE: This keeps it lightweight and flexible enough to mold to the treatment area.
5. Expel excess air by laying the bag on the table or holding it upright.
RATIONALE: Air is a poor conductor of heat and also makes the bag harder to mold around the body area.

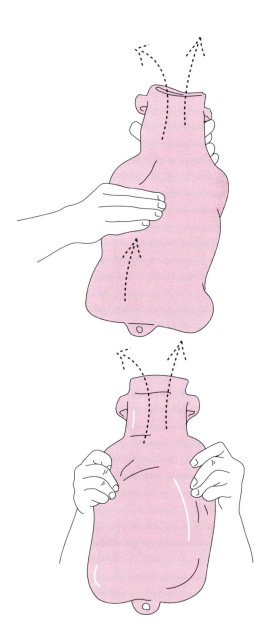

6. Cap the top and wipe the bottle dry. Check for leaks.

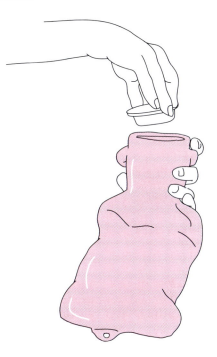

7. Place bottle in a protective covering to help absorb any perspiration and to reduce the danger of burns to the skin.
8. Place the bag on the patient's affected area and ask the patient how it feels. The temperature should feel warm, not hot.
RATIONALE: Individuals vary in their tolerance to heat.

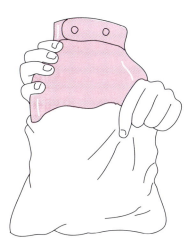

9. Administer the treatment for the length of time specified by the physician, usually 15–20 minutes. Check the patient's skin periodically for signs of increase or decrease in skin redness or swelling.
10. Refill the bag as necessary with hot water to maintain the proper temperature.

Follow-Through

11. Cleanse the hot-water bag with warm detergent solution, rinse well and dry by hanging upside down with the top open. Store bag with top closed, leaving air inside to prevent the sides of the bag from sticking together.
12. Record in the patient's chart the treatment, results, and patient's tolerance.

NOTE: The disposable hot pack can be used in place of the hot-water bottle. The temperature range is 101–114° F (38.3–45.6° C), and the pack lasts 20–60 minutes, depending on its size.

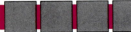

PROCEDURE

APPLYING AN ICE BAG

PURPOSE

To decrease blood supply to the area, prevent or reduce swelling, stop bleeding, decrease suppuration, and reduce pain.

 MEDICAL ASSISTING ALERT

Young children, elderly patients, and patients with circulatory problems tend to be more sensitive to cold.

EQUIPMENT AND MATERIALS

Ice bag
Small ice-cubes or ice chips
Protective covering, such as a flannel cover or towel

PROCEDURAL STEPS

Patient Preparation

1. Position and drape the patient comfortably.
2. Explain the procedure to the patient.

Performance

3. Check the bag for leaks.
   RATIONALE: A leaking bag will get the patient wet and cause chilling.

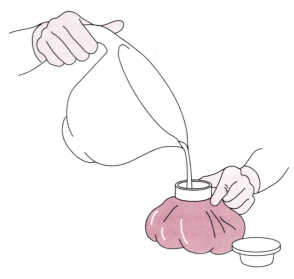

4. Fill the ice bag half full with small pieces of ice.
   RATIONALE: Small pieces of ice reduce the amount of air spaces in the bag, resulting in

better conduction of cold, and allow the bag to mold to the body part.
5. Express air from the bag and replace cap.

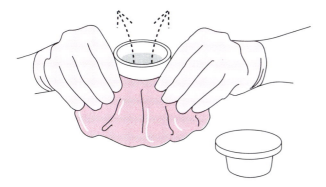

6. Thoroughly dry the ice bag and place into protective covering.
RATIONALE: This prevents tissue trauma and absorbs condensation.

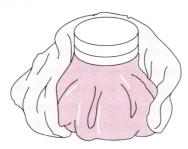

7. Place the bag on the patient's affected area. Ask the patient how it feels. It may feel uncomfortable, but most patients tolerate it if they know the benefits of the cold pack.
RATIONALE: Individuals vary in their tolerance to cold.
8. Administer the treatment for the length of time specified by the physician, usually 20–30 minutes. Check the patient's skin periodically for signs of increase or decrease in redness and swelling. Remove the bag if there is extreme paleness and numbness or a mottled blue appearance at the application site; notify the physician.
9. Refill the bag with ice when necessary.

Follow-Through

10. Cleanse the bag with warm detergent solution, rinse well, and dry by hanging upside down with the top off. Store the bag with the top closed, leaving air inside to prevent the sides of the bag from sticking together.
11. Record in the patient's chart the treatment, results, and patient's tolerance.

NOTE: Single-use cold packs are available for applications of dry cold. These lightweight plastic packs contain a chemical that, when activated, produces a controlled temperature of 50–80° F (10–26.7° C). Most of the packs are designed to be applied directly to the skin surface. The outer covering of the pack is a special material that absorbs condensation and prevents the cold, damp feeling of plastic.

Bibliography

Bonier P: Wound care forum, an unusual alternative. *American Journal of Nursing,* 85:418, 1985.
Bonewit K: *Clinical Procedures for Medical Assistants,* 3rd ed. Philadelphia: W. B. Saunders, 1990.
Brunner LS, Suddarth DS: *Manual of Nursing Practice,* 4th ed. Philadelphia: J. B. Lippincott, 1986.
Ethicon, Inc: *Suture Use Manual.* Somerville, NJ: Ethicon, Inc., 1966.
Hamilton HK, Rose MB: *Procedures. Nurses Reference Library. Nursing 83 Books* Springhouse, PA: Intermed Communications, Inc.
Johnson A: Toward rapid tissue healing. *Nursing Times,* p. 39, 1984.
Nealon T: *Fundamental Skills in Surgery,* 3rd ed. Philadelphia: W. B. Saunders, 1979.
Potter PA: *Fundamental of Nursing: Concepts, Process and Practice,* 2nd ed. St. Louis: C. V. Mosby, 1989.
Rambo BJ, Wood LA: *Nursing Skills for Clinical Practice,* 3rd ed. Philadelphia: W. B. Saunders, 1982.
Wood LA, Rambo BJ: *Nursing Skills for Allied Health Services,* vols. 1 and 2, 2nd ed. Philadelphia: W. B. Saunders, 1977.
Wood LA, Rambo BJ: *Nursing Skills for Allied Health Services,* vol. 3, 2nd ed. Philadelphia: W. B. Saunders, 1980.

Chapter 17

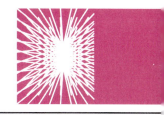

PEDIATRIC PROCEDURES

JUANITA BLOCKER

NEWBORN EVALUATION AND CARE
Instructing Parents on the Care of the Newborn
Assessment of Problems by Telephone
Common Problems of Newborns

GROWTH AND DEVELOPMENT
Head and Chest Circumferences
Weight
Height (Length)
Growth Charts

IMMUNIZATION SCHEDULES

WELL-BABY EXAMINATIONS
Vital Signs

COMMON CHILDHOOD PROBLEMS AND COMMUNICABLE DISEASES
Immunity- and Allergy-Related Conditions
Viral Conditions
Bacterial Conditions
Other Conditions
Parasitic Conditions

BATTERED CHILD SYNDROME

NEWBORN EVALUATION AND CARE

Instructing Parents on the Care of the Newborn

Breast Feeding

The mother should find a comfortable area, preferably one that is free from other distractions. The baby should be held in a gentle, yet strong, supportive manner. Feeding is one of the most pleasant experiences for the infant. Feeding ensures the infant's growth and development to be healthy and strong.

Before breast feeding, the mother should

- Cleanse the nipple area with plain water,
- Dry thoroughly,
- Place two fingers on either side of the nipple and press slightly to prevent the breast from interfering with the baby's breathing.

Each breast should be nursed at each feeding to ensure adequate milk flow. The breast used last during the previous feeding should be the first one used for the present feeding.

Supplemental Feedings. If the baby does not completely empty both breasts at a feeding, the mother should use a breast pump, either a hand or mechanical pump. Caution should be exercised so the breast is not injured. This milk can be stored in the refrigerator or freezer for later use.

Formula Feeding

Table 17-1 lists infant formulas.

When feeding the baby, the mother should find a comfortable, quiet area. The baby should be held in a gentle, yet supportive manner. Instruct the mother to

- Hold the bottle so the neck of the bottle and the nipple are always filled with formula to diminish the chance of air being swallowed.
- Have the formula at body temperature.

TABLE 17-1
INFANT FORMULAS

	Form[2]	A IU	D IU	E IU	C mg	B₁ mg	B₂ mg	B₃ mg	B₆ mg	B₁₂ μg	FA μg	BT μg	PA mg	Ca mg	P mg	Mg mg	Fe mg	Zn mg	Cu mg	I μg	Mn mg	K mg	Na mg	Cl mg	Other Ingredients
USRDA for Infants	—	1,500	400	5	35	0.5	0.6	8	0.4	2	100	150	3	600	500	70	15	5	0.6	45	—	—	—	—	—
ADVANCE (Ross) *OTC* **Protein:** 18.8 g **Fat:** 25.4 g **Carbohydrate:** 51.9 g **Cal:** 508	Conc	1,887	380	18.8	51	0.6	0.9	6.6	0.4	1.5	96.3	2.2	2.9	477	366	39	9.1	4.6	0.6	92	0.03	745	179	449	Choline (81.6 mg), inositol (24 mg)
ENFAMIL (Mead Johnson) *OTC* **Protein:** 14.4 g **Fat:** 36 g **Carbohydrate:** 66 g **Cal:** 640	Conc Pwdr Nurs	2,000	400	20	52	0.5	1	8	0.4	1.5	100	15	3	440	300	50	1	5	0.6	65	0.1	690	175	400	Vit K₁ (55 μg), choline (100 mg), inositol (30 mg)
ENFAMIL Human Milk Fortifier (Mead Johnson) *OTC* **Protein:** 0.7 g **Fat:** 0.05 g **Carbohydrate:** 2.7 g **Cal:** 567	Pwdr[4]	780	260	3.4	24	0.2	0.3	—	0.2	0.21	23	0.8	0.79	60	33	—	—	0.3	0.1	—	9	15.6	7	17.7	Vit K (9.1 μg)
ENFAMIL with Iron (Mead Johnson) *OTC* **Protein:** 14.4 g **Fat:** 36 g **Carbohydrate:** 66 g **Cal:** 640	Conc Pwdr Nurs	2,000	400	20	52	0.5	1	8	0.4	1.5	100	15	3	440	300	50	12	5	0.6	65	0.1	690	175	400	Vit K₁ (55 μg), choline (100 mg), inositol (30 mg)
ENFAMIL Premature Formula (Mead Johnson) *OTC* **Protein:** 19.1 g **Fat:** 32 g **Carbohydrate:** 70 g **Cal:** 640	Nurs	7,700	2,100	29	220	1.6	2.2	26	1.6	1.9	220	12.8	7.7	750	380	32	1.6	6.4	1	51	0.8	710	250	540	Vit K₁ (83 μg), choline (48 mg), inositol (30 mg)
ISOMIL (Ross) *OTC* **Protein:** 17 g **Fat:** 34.6 g **Carbohydrate:** 64.6 g **Cal:** 640	Conc Pwdr Nurs	1,920	384	19.2	57.6	0.4	0.6	9	0.4	3	96	28.8	4.8	672	480	48	11.5	4.8	0.5	96	0.2	691	282	397	Vit K₁ (96 μg), choline (51 mg), inositol (32 mg)
ISOMIL SF (Ross) *OTC* **Protein:** 17.0 g **Fat:** 34.9 g **Carbohydrate:** 64.6 g **Cal:** 640	Conc Nurs	1,920	384	19.2	57.6	0.4	0.6	9	0.4	3	96	28.8	4.8	672	480	48	11.5	4.8	0.5	96	0.2	691	282	397	Vit K₁ (96 μg), choline (51 mg), inositol (32 mg)
I-SOYALAC (Loma Linda) *OTC* **Protein:** 20 g **Fat:** 35 g **Carbohydrate:** 65 g **Cal:** 640	Conc Nurs	2,000	400	15	75	0.6	0.6	8	0.6	2	150	50	3	650	450	70	12	5	0.8	50	0.3	750	270	500	Vit K (50 μg), choline (125 mg), inositol (110 mg)
LOFENALAC (Mead Johnson) *OTC* **Protein:** 21 g **Fat:** 25 g **Carbohydrate:** 83 g **Cal:** 640	Pwdr	2,000	400	20	52	0.5	0.6	8	0.4	2	100	50	3	600	450	70	12	5	0.6	45	0.2	650	300	450	Vit K₁ (100 μg), choline (85 mg), inositol (30 mg)
Low Methionine Diet Powder (Mead Johnson) *OTC* **Protein:** 19.2 g **Fat:** 34 g **Carbohydrate:** 64 g **Cal:** 640	Pwdr	2,000	400	20	52	0.5	0.6	8	0.4	2	100	50	3	600	475	70	12	5	0.6	65	0.16	780	230	530	Vit K (100 μg), choline (50 mg), inositol (30 mg)

Vitamins[1] / Minerals

Formula	Form																		Vit K, choline, inositol
NURSOY (Wyeth-Ayerst) *OTC* Protein: 20.2 g **Fat:** 34.6 g Carbohydrate: 66 g **Cal:** 640	Conc Nurs	2,500	400	9	55	0.67	1	9.5	0.4	2	50	35	3	600	420	65	12	3.5	0.45	65	0.2	700	190	355	Vit K$_1$ (100 μg), choline (85 mg), inositol (26 mg)
NUTRAMIGEN (Mead Johnson) *OTC* Protein: 18 g **Fat:** 25 g Carbohydrate: 86 g **Cal:** 640	Conc Pwdr Nurs	2,000	400	20	52	0.5	0.6	8	0.4	2	100	50	3	600	400	70	12	5	0.6	45	0.2	700	300	550	Vit K$_1$ (100 μg), choline (85 mg), inositol (30 mg)
PORTAGEN (Mead Johnson) *OTC* Protein: 22 g **Fat:** 30 g Carbohydrate: 74 g **Cal:** 640	Pwdr	5,000	500	20	52	1	1.2	13	1.3	4	100	50	6.7	600	450	130	12	6	1	45	0.8	800	350	550	Vit K$_1$ (100 μg), choline (85 mg), inositol (30 mg)
PREGESTIMIL (Mead Johnson) *OTC* Protein: 18 g **Fat:** 26 g Carbohydrate: 86 g **Cal:** 640	Pwdr	2,000	400	15	52	0.5	0.6	8	0.4	2	100	50	3	600	400	70	12	4	0.6	45	0.2	700	300	550	Vit K$_1$ (100 μg), choline (85 mg), inositol (30 mg)
PROSOBEE (Mead Johnson) *OTC* Protein: 19.2 g **Fat:** 34 g Carbohydrate: 64 g **Cal:** 640	Conc Pwdr Nurs	2,000	400	20	52	0.5	0.6	8	0.4	2	100	50	3	600	475	70	12	5	0.6	65	0.2	780	230	530	Vit K$_1$ (100 μg), choline (50 mg), inositol (30 mg)
RCF (Ross) *OTC* Protein: 18.9 g **Fat:** 33.9 g Carbohydrate:[3] **Cal:**[3]	Conc	1,920	384	19.2	57.6	0.4	0.6	9	0.4	3	96	28.8	5	672	480	4.8	1.4	5	0.5	96	0.2	691	282	397	Vit K$_1$ (96 μg), choline (51 mg), inositol (32 mg)
SIMILAC (Ross) *OTC* Protein: 14.2 g **Fat:** 34.4 g Carbohydrate: 68.5 g **Cal:** 600	Conc Pwdr Nurs	1,920	384	19.2	58	0.6	1	6.7	0.4	1.6	96	28	2.9	480	371	38.4	1.4	4.8	0.6	96	0.03	691	179	422	Vit K$_1$ (51 μg), choline (102 mg), inositol (30 mg)
SIMILAC PM 60/40 (Ross) *OTC* Protein: 14.2 g **Fat:** 35.8 g Carbohydrate: 65.3 g **Cal:** 600	Pwdr Nurs	1,920	384	16	58	0.6	1	6.7	0.4	1.6	96	29	2.9	358	179	38.4	1.4	4.8	0.6	38.4	0.03	550	154	378	Vit K$_1$ (51 μg), choline (77 mg), inositol (153 mg)
SIMILAC Special Care with Iron 24 (Ross) Protein: 43.7 g **Fat:** 41.7 g Carbohydrate: 81.4 g **Cal:** 812	Nurs	5,222	1,152	31	284	1.9	4.8	38.4	1.9	4.2	284	284	14.6	1382	691	92	13.8	11.5	1.9	46	0.1	991	330	622	Vit K (92 mg), choline (77 mg), inositol (42 mg)
SIMILAC with Iron (Ross) *OTC* Protein: 14.2 g **Fat:** 34.4 g Carbohydrate: 68.5 g **Cal:** 600	Conc Pwdr Nurs	1,920	384	19.2	58	0.6	1	6.7	0.4	1.6	96	28	2.9	480	371	38.4	11.5	4.8	0.6	96	0.03	691	179	422	Vit K$_1$ (51 μg), choline (102 mg), inositol (30 mg)
SMA (Wyeth-Ayerst) *OTC* Protein: 14.4 g **Fat:** 34.6 g Carbohydrate: 69.1 g **Cal:** 640	Conc Pwdr Nurs	2,500	400	9	55	0.7	1	9.5	0.4	1	50	14	2	420	312	50	12	3.5	0.45	65	0.2	530	142	355	Vit K$_1$ (55 μg), choline (100 mg)
SOYALAC (Loma Linda) *OTC* Protein: 29 g **Fat:** 35 g Carbohydrate: 65 g **Cal:** 640	Conc Pwdr Nurs	2,000	400	15	75	0.5	0.6	8	0.45	2	150	60	3	600	350	75	12	5	0.5	50	1	750	280	420	Vit K (50 μg), choline (100 mg), inositol (100 mg)

[1] B$_3$ = niacin; FA = folic acid; BT = biotin; PA = pantothenic acid or calcium pantothenate.
[2] Values given are amounts per quart (standard dilution).
[3] Varies depending upon the quantity of carbohydrate and water added; if no carbohydrate is used, a 1:1 dilution with water provides approximately 12 kcal/fl oz.
[4] Values given are amounts supplied when 4 packets are added to 100 mL of preterm, human milk.

From the *Compendium of Drug Therapy*, CORE Publishing Division, Excerpta Medica, Inc.

Burping

Whichever method of feeding is chosen for the baby, burping is a very important part of the process. Some infants require frequent burping as they nurse; others need to burp only after finishing.

Instruct the mother to

- Place the infant upright against her chest and pat the infant gently on the back. Or the mother may hold the infant in an upright position, supporting the infant's chest with one hand and patting him or her gently on the back.

Bathing

Instruct the parents to

- Bathe the infant no more than once a day.
- Use a mild soap and warm water.
- Use caution when cleansing the eyelids, wiping from nose to ear side.
- Shampoo the hair and scalp at least twice a week.
- Use a moist (not wet) cotton-tipped applicator or cotton ball to cleanse the nose and ears.
- Do not attempt to cleanse the inside of the mouth!
- Closely trim infant's fingernails two or three times a week.

Hygiene

Some babies develop a slight skin rash over the first few months, which usually lasts only 3–4 days at a time. The diaper area is more prone to rashes than any other area of the body. The diaper should be changed promptly after each bowel movement or wetting.

Females may develop a slight vaginal discharge that may appear to be bloody for the first 1–2 weeks. This is called *pseudomenstruation* and may be due to the absorption of maternal hormones. It is usually not observed after the first month. A white discharge is normal. If the discharge becomes yellow, it is an indication of a pathological condition and should be reported to the physician.

For circumcised males, the parents should be cautioned to

- Watch for bleeding or swelling.
- Apply a thin layer of petroleum jelly until circumcision is healed to prevent the site from adhering to the diaper.
- Notify the physician if bleeding occurs.

For uncircumcised males, the parents should be cautioned to

- Use gentle retraction of the foreskin when cleansing. (The foreskin cannot be completely retracted until the child has reached the age of 3–4.)

Umbilical Care

Instruct the parents the following about caring for the navel:

- The navel should be kept clean and dry.
- Cleanse with a cotton-tipped applicator that has been dipped in alcohol.
- It is not unusual for a small drop of blood to be present after the cord drops off. This is not a cause for alarm.

Umbilical Hernia. Most small umbilical hernias disappear without any treatment. Larger ones may require surgical repair. There are many opinions about whether strapping or taping of the hernia is effective, and this is a decision to be made in each individual case.

Dressing

The baby probably does not require any more clothing than an adult and, often, requires even less. Instruct the parents to

- Not overdress or overcover.
- Dress infant according to the weather.
- Watch for rashes that seem to develop after contact with particular types of fabric.
- Use a mild detergent and rinse clothing well.

Assessment of Problems by Telephone

The following flow charts are samples of telephone decision guidelines that list specific questions the medical assistant should ask when assessing whether the patient should be seen immediately, the same day, or as a future appointment, or if advice can be given for treatment at home.

TELEPHONE DECISION FLOW CHARTS

Decision Guideline	To See the Doctor Immediately If . . .
Abdominal Pain How old is the child?	Child is under 3 years of age or if child appears unusually ill
Is a fever present? If so, how high?	Over 103° F or if present longer than 24 hours
Is there a history of abdominal pain or disturbances in bowel functions?	If present more than 3 days
Is the pain colicky and intermittent?	The pain is constant or if the child is breathing hard and fast or if the child is jackknifing knees to chest with severe cramps
Is diarrhea present?	There have been more than 5–6 watery stools within a 12 hour period in an infant, or blood in the stool, or dehydration
Is nausea and vomiting present?	There is vomiting with right-sided pain
Is there increasing severity of pain and tenderness in the right lower quadrant?	Yes
Is the pain severe, persistent, and of sudden onset?	Yes
Has there been any trauma or accident?	Yes
Headaches When does the headache occur?	If headaches are daily and the frequency and degree of pain are becoming worse
Is a stiff neck present?	Yes
Any cold symptoms, congestion, or fever?	If fever over 103° F or if present longer than 24 hours
Any nausea, vomiting, or diarrhea?	Yes
Any visual disturbance?	Yes
Any change in mental status?	Yes
Any drowsiness?	Yes
Any known drug allergy?	
Head Injury Any evidence of other injury? Laceration? Abdominal pain? Failure to use an arm or leg?	Yes
How did the accident happen?	A high fall, automobile accident, strong blow, or suspicion of child abuse
Any loss of consciousness? Any convulsing?	If convulsing has occurred or if the child has been unconscious for more than a few seconds, an ambulance should be called
Any visual disturbance?	Yes
Any mental status changes? Headache?	Yes
Any discharge of blood or fluid from any body opening?	Yes

Common Problems of Newborns

Burping

See page 406 for a discussion of burping.

Colic

Colic is a symptom that usually occurs in infants under the age of 3 months. The characteristic symptoms are

- Drawing legs up to abdomen, with crying
- Tightly clenching hands
- Cold feet

There does not seem to be an apparent cause of colic; however, some activities seem to make the symptoms worse. These include

- Underfeeding
- Overfeeding
- Failure to burp
- Allergies
- Emotional problems with either parent
- Excessive carbohydrate fermentation

The bright side is that usually by the age of 3 months, the child improves and the family can adjust to each other. Many causes of colic are resolved by simply changing the formula.

In the most severe cases, it may be necessary for the physician to prescribe a mild sedative for the infant and/or mother. In prolonged attacks, a short period of hospitalization may be indicated, often with nothing more than separation from the mother. This is highly debatable among physicians and not a hard and fast rule.

Constipation

Constipation is a common problem that is present from time to time. It may be related to

- Type of formula

- Frequency and amount of water used to supplement formula
- Amount of sugar or karo added to water supplement

NOTE: Enemas should NEVER be given to infants without specific orders from the physician. A glycerine (pediatric) suppository may be used occasionally, but not as a routine practice.

Crying

Crying is a baby's way of stating his or her opinion. The baby may be

- Thirsty
- Wet
- Bored
- Wanting to be turned over
- Hot
- Cold
- Wanting to be covered or uncovered

Parents soon learn to recognize the cries and to respond appropriately. It is important to stress to the parents that *all* babies cry.

Gas (Flatus)

It is very common for babies to pass gas. This is related to their diet. For breastfed babies, the mother's diet has a direct influence on this. If she eats foods that produce gas, the baby is affected. She should be told to avoid foods such as chocolate, nuts, spicy foods, and any others that are particularly prone to producing gas in her.

Hiccoughs

Most babies get hiccoughs periodically. This is not a cause for alarm unless they persist for a long period of time.

Spitting Up

It is probably safe to say that all babies spit up, some more than others. It may be due to inadequate burping or a sensitivity to the formula. If the spitting up is excessive, the infant may need to be tested by the physician.

Diaper Rash

Most diaper rashes are due to the irritation to the skin caused by a wet diaper, combined with the infant's warm body temperature. The diaper should be changed as soon as possible following stooling or wetting. Instruct the parents to

- Cleanse with warm water
- Apply petroleum jelly to the affected area

Thrush

Thrush is characterized by a white, patchy coating of the inside of the infant's mouth and tongue. The parents should be cautioned not to attempt to wipe these lesions off. This is a yeast infection and may require the physician to prescribe a specific medication to relieve the symptoms.

TABLE 17-2

GROWTH AND DEVELOPMENT

Indicator	Average	Range
Birth		
Head circumference	13"	12–14"
Chest circumference		
Weight (males)	7 lb	6–8½ lb
Height (males)	20"	18–21"
Weight (females)	7 lb	5–8½ lb
Height (females)	19½"	17–20"
3–6 Months		
Head circumference	16"	15–17"
Chest circumference		
Weight (males)	14½ lb	11–18 lb
Height (males)	25½ lb	24–27"
Weight (females)	14 lb	11–17 lb
Height (females)	24½"	23–25"
9–12 Months		
Head circumference	17"	16–18"
Chest circumference		
Weight (males)	21 lb	18–26 lb
Height (males)	29"	27–31"
Weight (females)	20 lb	16–24 lb
Height (females)	28"	26–30"
15–18 Months		
Head circumference	18"	17—19"
Chest circumference		
Weight (males)	24 lb	20–29 lb
Height (males)	31"	29–33"
Weight (females)	23 lb	19–27 lb
Height (females)	31"	28–33"
18 Months–3 years		
Head circumference	19"	17–20"
Chest circumference		
Weight (males)	29 lb	24–34 lb
Height (males)	35"	33–37"
Weight (females)	25 lb	20–30 lb
Height (females)	35"	33–37"

Frequent Stooling

Some babies have more frequent stools than others. This may be related to:

- Formula versus breast milk
- Concentration of glucose water and frequency of use

It is not unusual for one infant to have 8–10 stools a day, and another infant to have only 1. The habits of the child emerge within a week or so and the parents will then be able to determine whether the child has developed an abnormal bowel problem.

GROWTH AND DEVELOPMENT

The average weight of infants varies according to socioeconomic groups, variations of their heredity, and the influence of their environments (Table 17-2). Poor weight gain is usually first documented on the growth chart. Weight less than the 10th percentile for the infant's age may indicate nutritional risk factors. Weight for length or height must also be evaluated. Again, a plot less than the 10th percentile raises concern and requires further assessment.

At each visit, the length, weight, and head and chest circumferences are measured and plotted on growth charts. (See instructions under growth charts) Temperature is recorded. If the infant is afebrile and asymptomatic, the first immunizations (diphtheria, tetanus and pertussis [DTP] and trivalent oral polio vaccine [TOPV]) are administered at the 5–9 weeks' visit (see immunization schedules in Tables 17-4–6).

Head and Chest Circumferences

Regularly obtained growth information gives the physician an accurate indicator of nutritional status, growth and development, and brain growth (see Table 17-2). Deviations from the normal range of head circumference may indicate congenital anomalies, hydrocephalus, or underdevelopment.

It is important to note that the equipment does not have to be fancy to provide accurate growth information. One of the easiest and most inexpensive tools with which to measure the infant's head and chest is the measuring tape. Disposable tape measures are available and should be used when possible to avoid cross-contamination.

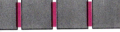

PROCEDURE
MEASURING THE INFANT'S HEAD CIRCUMFERENCE

PURPOSE

To determine brain growth and any deviations from normal brain development.

EQUIPMENT AND MATERIAL

Measuring tape, disposable

PROCEDURAL STEPS

1. Place the child in the supine position.
2. Place the measuring tape at the greatest circumference.
3. Check the position of the tape to ensure it is anteriorly over the lower forehead above the supraorbital ridge.
4. Check the position of the tape to ensure it is posteriorly over the occipital bone.
5. Plot readings on the growth chart.

PROCEDURE

MEASURING THE INFANT'S CHEST CIRCUMFERENCE

PURPOSE

To determine chest growth and any deviations from normal heart and lung development.

EQUIPMENT

Measuring tape, disposable

PROCEDURAL STEPS

1. Place the child in a supine position.
2. Gently slip the measuring tape under the chest and back, checking to ensure it is around the chest at its greatest circumference and across the nipple line.
3. Plot readings on the growth chart.

Regularly obtained growth information provides important facts for the physician about the infant's growth and development. A deviation from the normal range could indicate heart/lung enlargement or underdevelopment. It could also indicate rib-cartilage calcification (see Table 17–2).

Weight

Growth is one of the best indicators of an infant's health. Therefore, measurements are taken at each office visit. Growth charts are often used to plot the growth and to determine whether it is in a normal range. Growth charts compare a child's growth rate with that of other children of the same age to obtain a normal value.

The weight of an infant is very important since it is often the basis for medication dosage. Infant formulas may also be adjusted depending on the growth pattern of the infant.

Infants and young children are weighed recumbent on a table scale with a tray, using a beam balance with nondetachable weights. A platform scale is used for older children. (Spring-type bathroom scales are not recommended.)

Children should wear minimal clothing and no shoes. Consider the location of the clinic scale when asking the child to disrobe.

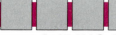

PROCEDURE

MEASURING THE INFANT'S WEIGHT

PURPOSE

To determine height and weight correlation on the growth chart as an indicator of normal growth and development or significant deviation.

EQUIPMENT

Table scale with a tray, using a beam balance (Figure 17-1)

PROCEDURAL STEPS

1. Weigh infant nude.
2. Place clean paper sheet on scale and balance the scale to zero.
3. Place the infant in the center of the scale.
4. Take the reading from the scale once the weight has been moved along the balance bar until it is balanced.
5. Plot reading on growth chart.

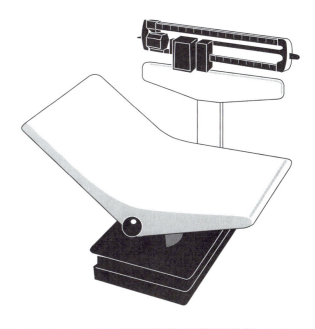

FIGURE 17-1
Infant scale.

PROCEDURE

WEIGHING OLDER CHILDREN

PURPOSE

To determine height and weight correlation on the growth chart as an indicator of normal growth and development or significant deviation.

EQUIPMENT

Beam balance scale with nondetachable weights (Figure 17-2)

PROCEDURAL STEPS

1. Instruct child to wear minimal clothing.
   RATIONALE: To get an accurate measurement.
2. Ask child to remove shoes.
3. Have child stand in the center of the platform with arms hanging naturally at the side.
   To discourage child from holding to scale, provide a small, lightweight, plastic hand puppet to hold, or ask the child to hold his or her shirt down.
   A child who is upset and refuses to step on scale can be weighed easily by having the parent hold the child and step on the platform. Weigh them both and then the parent alone and subtract the parent's weight from the total.
4. Plot reading on growth chart.

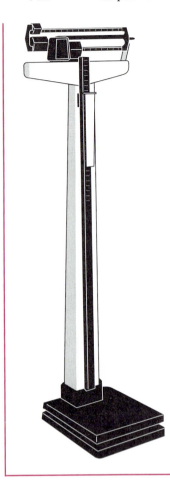

FIGURE 17-2

Beam balance scale with height measuring rod (stadiometer).

Height (Length)

The tools described below are the most accurate length/weight measurement devices. Both are portable and can be made or purchased.

Infants

Use a *length measuring board* to determine length of a child under 3 and unable or unwilling to stand. This board has a rigid, fixed headpiece and a movable footboard at a right angle. A flat metal measuring tape or high-quality measuring rule marked in ⅛-inch increments should be attached to the board. Do not use cloth, paper, fiberglass, or plastic tapes, which can stretch or tear. The tape or guide should be attached to prevent shifting during measurement.

PROCEDURE

MEASURING THE INFANT'S HEIGHT/LENGTH

PURPOSE

To determine height and weight correlation on the growth chart as an indicator of normal growth and development or significant deviation.

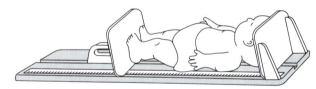

FIGURE 17-3

Length board (horizontal stadiometer).

EQUIPMENT AND MATERIALS

Length board or stadiometer (Figure 17-3)

PROCEDURAL STEPS

1. Remove any clothing, including booties, shoes, and hat.
2. Two people are needed for the measurement. One person holds the child's head against the fixed headpiece while the other checks to make sure the child's head, body, and feet are in a straight line before bringing the footboard up against the heels and taking the reading.
3. Have the child stand upright with head, back, and heels in contact with the instrument; carefully lower the headboard down until contact with head is made.
4. Plot reading on growth chart.

Children up to 24 months of age should be measured lying down. Those 24-36 months old should be able to stand. If so, they should be switched to the growth chart for 2-18 years old, which is based on standing heights (see Table 17-2).

Older Children

Use a *stadiometer* or a *flat wall-mounted metal tape,* with headboard to measure an older child's height.

The stadiometer uses a movable head block to measure height (Figure 17-4). A built-in counter or flat metal rule marked in ⅛-inch or 0.5-cm increments is used.

If a flat metal tape secured to a wall is used, it should not be stretched over a baseboard or be placed above a carpeted floor because this will distort the measurement. A headblock is brought down on the child's head to take the measurement. During the child's measurement, the heels, buttocks, shoulders, and head should contact the wall. A headboard design is pictured in Figure 17-5.

Measurements of Physically Handicapped Children

Some children with handicaps may be difficult to measure because of contractures or the inability to stand.

Armspan length may be used for children with spina bifida. The measurement can be taken with an anthropometer. The measurement compares to height or length in a 1:1 ratio. Tibial length may also be used to estimate length/height in children who have arm contractures.

Growth Charts

There are many growth grids/charts available. The charts included in this chapter (Figures 17-6 through 17-13) are provided by Ross Laboratories. These charts are a measuring record that can help to separate normal growth patterns from abnormal ones. Information from these charts is only as good as the accuracy of measurements and determination of the infant's or child's age for plotting.

Text continued on page 423

414 *Chapter 17: PEDIATRIC PROCEDURES*

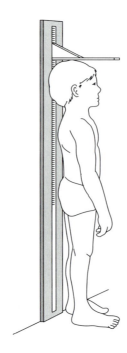

FIGURE 17-4
Upright stadiometer (length board).

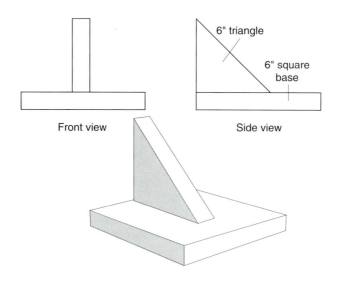

FIGURE 17-5
Flat wall-mounted metal tape with headboard for measuring the height of older children.

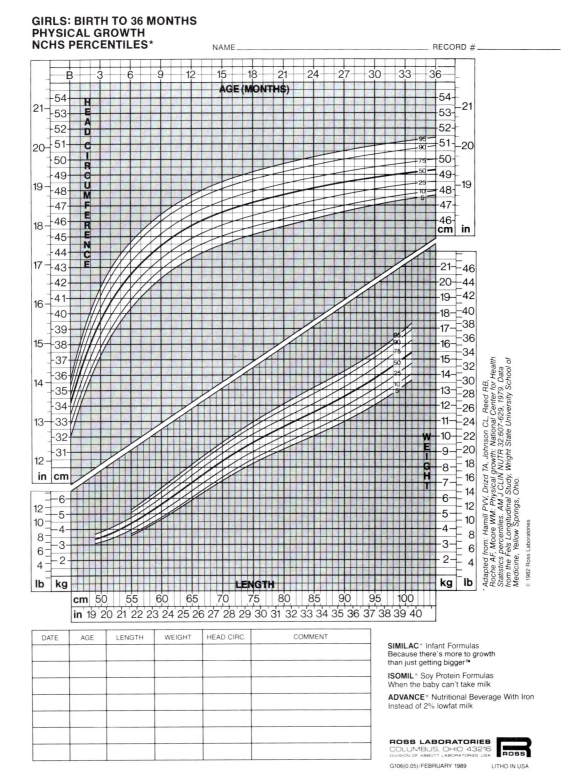

FIGURE 17-6

Growth and head circumference chart for girls: Birth to 36 months. (Used and reprinted with permission of Ross Laboratories, Columbus, OH 43216, from NCHS Growth Charts, © 1976, Ross Laboratories.)

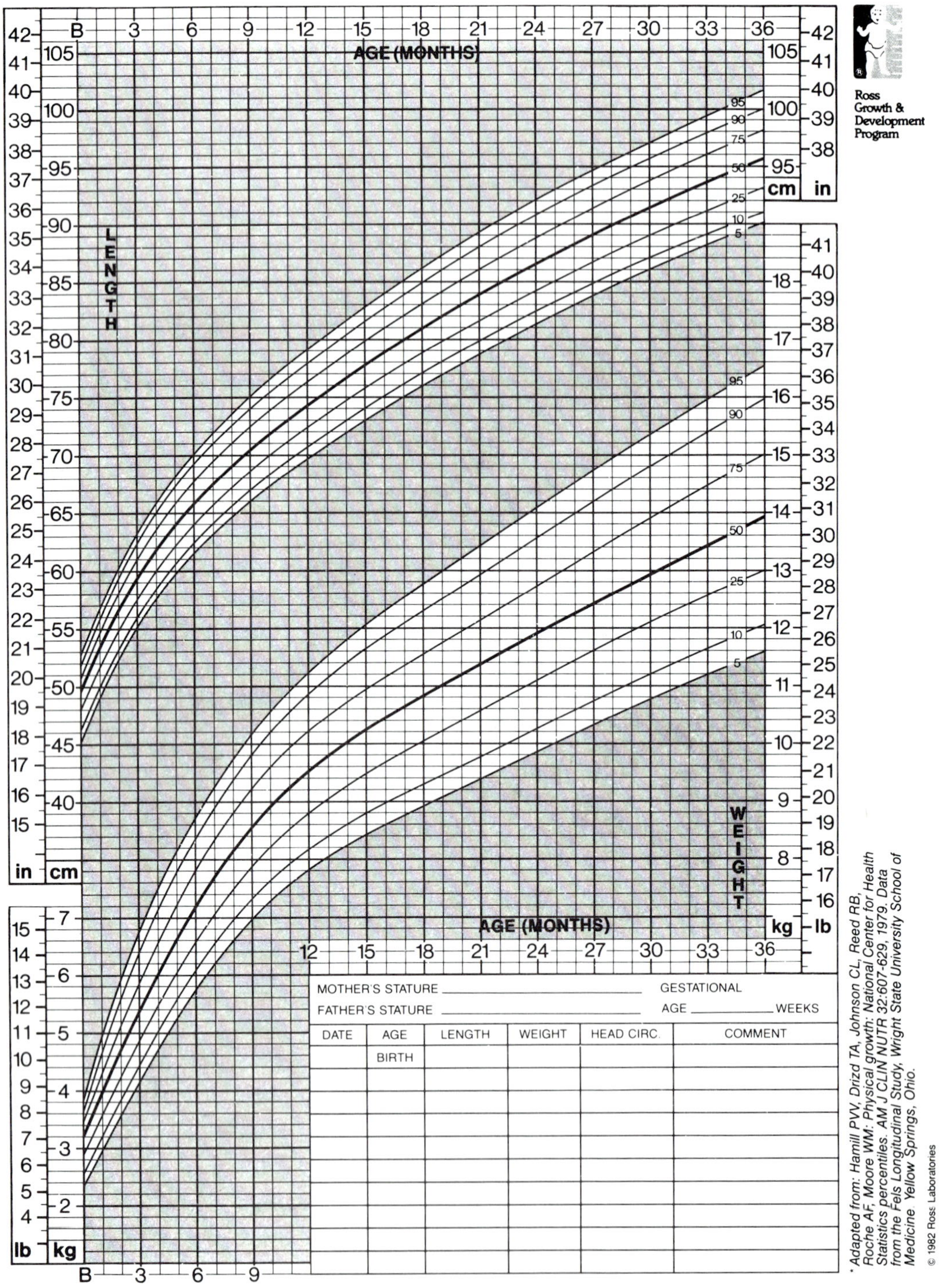

FIGURE 17-7

Growth chart for girls: Birth to 36 months. (Used and reprinted with permission of Ross Laboratories, Columbus, OH 43216, from NCHS Growth Charts, © 1976, Ross Laboratories.)

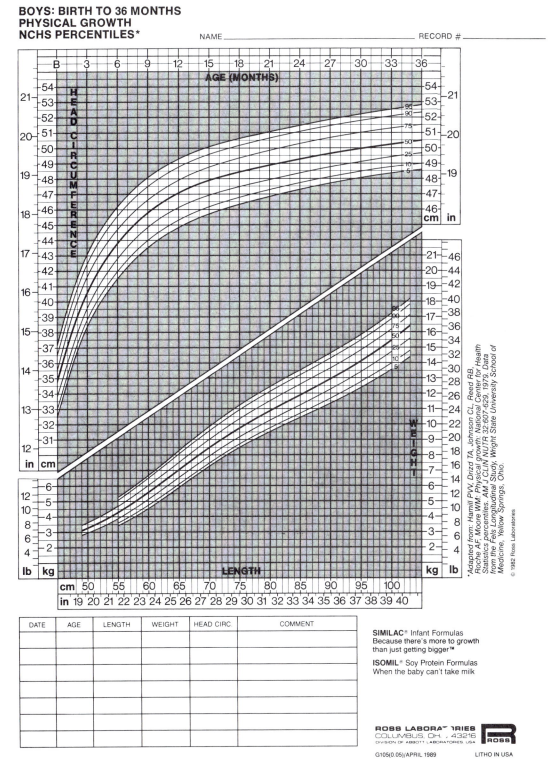

FIGURE 17-8

Growth and head circumference chart for boys: Birth to 36 months. (Used and reprinted with permission of Ross Laboratories, Columbus, OH 43216, from NCHS Growth Charts, © 1976, Ross Laboratories.)

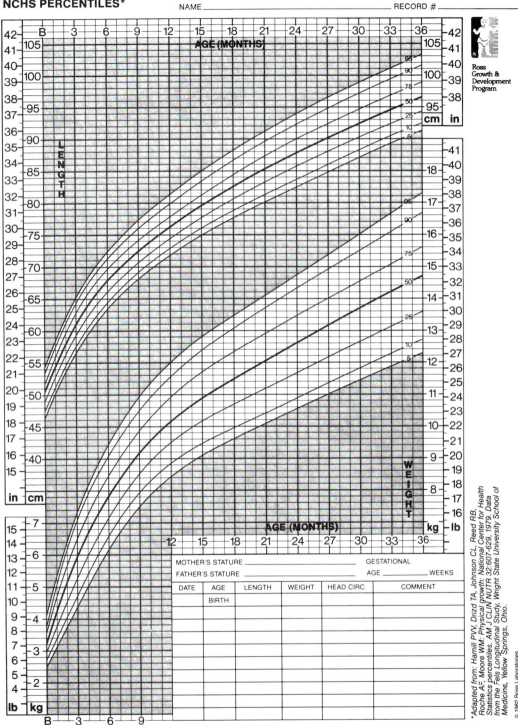

FIGURE 17-9

Growth chart for boys: Birth to 36 months. (Used and reprinted with permission of Ross Laboratories, Columbus, OH 43216, from NCHS Growth Charts, © 1976, Ross Laboratories.)

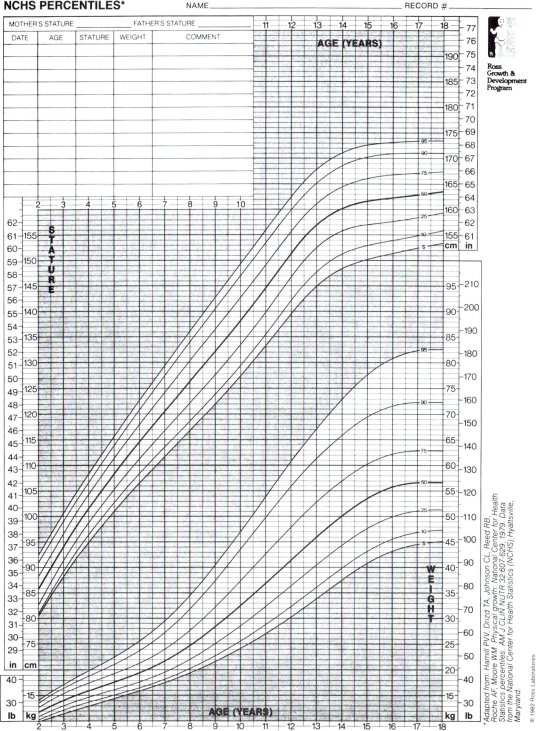

FIGURE 17-10

Growth chart for girls: 2–18 years. (Used and reprinted with permission of Ross Laboratories, Columbus, OH 43216, from NCHS Growth Charts, © 1976, Ross Laboratories.)

420 *Chapter 17: PEDIATRIC PROCEDURES*

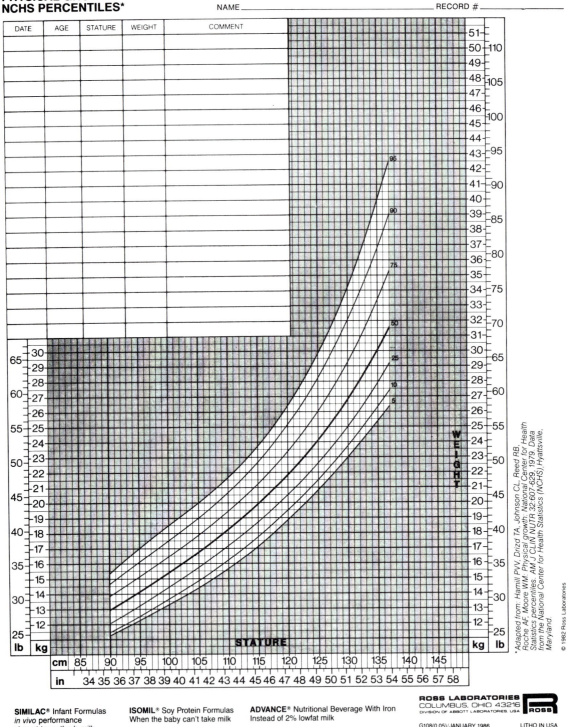

FIGURE 17-11
Growth chart for prepubescent girls. (Used and reprinted with permission of Ross Laboratories, Columbus, OH 43216, from NCHS Growth Charts, © 1976, Ross Laboratories.)

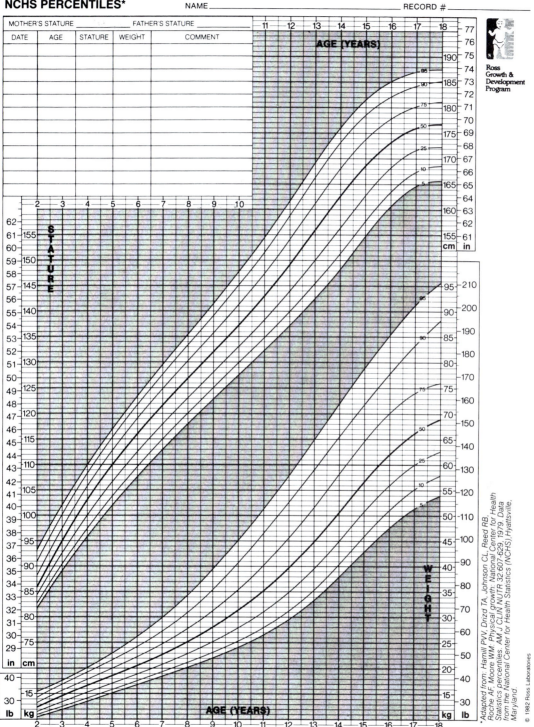

FIGURE 17-12

Growth chart for boys: 2–18 years. (Used and reprinted with permission of Ross Laboratories, Columbus, OH 43216, from NCHS Growth Charts, © 1976, Ross Laboratories.)

422 Chapter 17: PEDIATRIC PROCEDURES

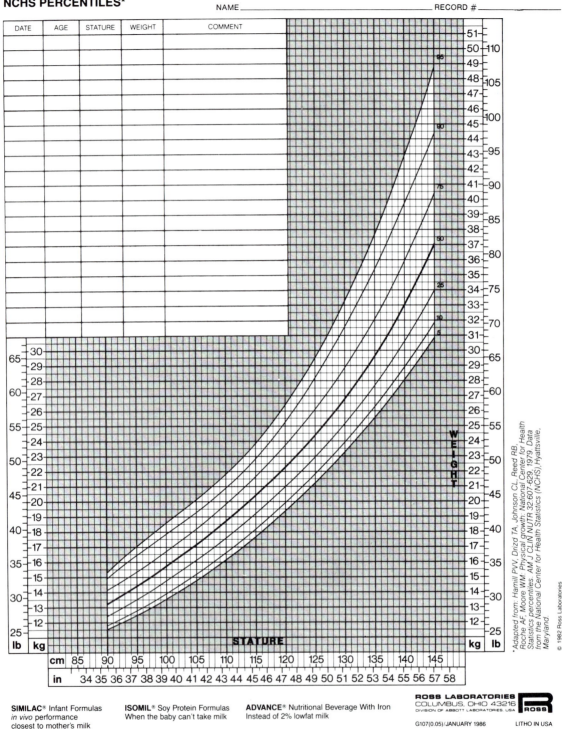

FIGURE 17-13

Growth chart for prepubescent boys. (Used and reprinted with permission of Ross Laboratories, Columbus, OH 43216, from NCHS Growth Charts, © 1976, Ross Laboratories.)

PROCEDURE

PLOTTING A CHILD'S GROWTH

PURPOSE

To chart the growth rate using height and weight measurements.

EQUIPMENT AND MATERIALS

An infant growth chart
Height and weight measurements from the medical history

PROCEDURAL STEPS

Weight

1. Locate the child's weight in kilograms or pounds on the right vertical column.
2. Locate the child's age on the bottom horizontal plane.
3. Locate the site at which these two lines intersect on the graph.
4. Mark an *x* at this site.
5. From the *x*, follow the curved percentile line upward to the percentile numbers at the right side of the chart.
6. Read and record the weight/growth pattern percentile.

Height

1. Locate the child's height in centimeters or inches on the left vertical column.
2. Locate the child's age on the top horizontal plane.
3. Locate the site at which these two lines intersect on the graph.
4. Mark an *x* at this site.
5. From the *x*, follow the curved percentile line upward to the percentile numbers at the right side of the chart.
6. Read and record the height/growth pattern percentile.

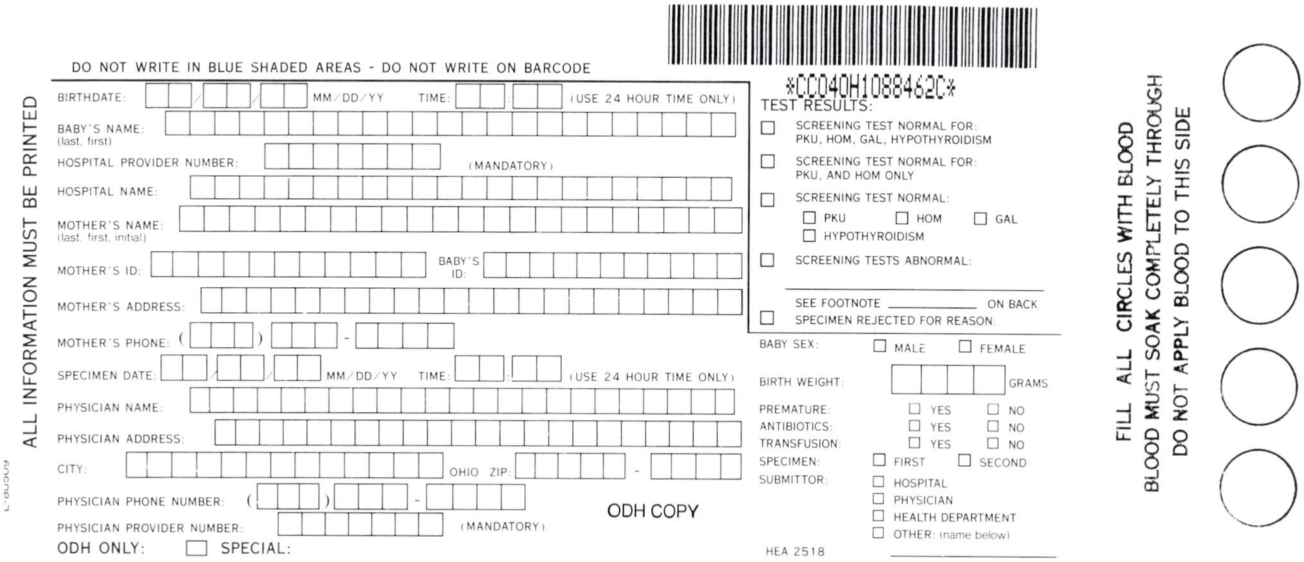

FIGURE 17-14

Newborn PKU and thyroid testing kit. (From Bonewit K: *Clinical Procedures for Medical Assistants,* 3rd ed. Philadelphia: W. B. Saunders, 1990, p. 512.)

IMMUNIZATION SCHEDULES

Phenylketonuria (PKU) and thyroid tests are usually done at the 2–4 weeks' visit. These are usually sent to the state laboratory for processing (Figure 17–14).

Immunizations are usually started at the 5–6 weeks' visit. This may vary from practice to practice. The immunization schedules in Tables 17–3 through 17–5 can serve as guides.

TABLE 17–3

VACCINES AVAILABLE IN THE UNITED STATES, BY TYPE AND RECOMMENDED ROUTES OF ADMINISTRATION

Vaccine	Type	Route
BCG (Bacillus of Calmette and Guérin)	Live bacteria	Intradermal or subcutaneous
Cholera	Inactivated bacteria	Subcutaneous or intradermal*
DTP	Toxoids and inactivated bacteria	Intramuscular
(D = Diphtheria)		
(T = Tetanus)		
(P = Pertussis)		
HB (Hepatitis B)	Inactive viral antigen	Intramuscular
Haemophilus influenzae b		
—Polysaccharide (HbPV)	Bacterial polysaccharide	Subcutaneous or intramuscular†
—or Conjugate (HbCV)	or Polysaccharide conjugated to protein	Intramuscular
Influenza	Inactivated virus or viral components	Intramuscular
IPV (Inactivated Poliovirus Vaccine)	Inactivated viruses of all 3 serotypes	Subcutaneous
Measles	Live virus	Subcutaneous
Meningococcal	Bacterial polysaccharides of serotypes A/C/Y/W-135	Subcutaneous
MMR	Live viruses	Subcutaneous
(M = Measles)		
(M = Mumps)		
(R = Rubella)		
Mumps	Live virus	Subcutaneous
OPV (Oral Poliovirus Vaccine)	Live viruses of all 3 serotypes	Oral
Plague	Inactivated bacteria	Intramuscular
Pneumococcal	Bacterial polysaccharides of 23 pneumococcal types	Intramuscular or subcutaneous
Rabies	Inactivated virus	Subcutaneous or intradermal§
Rubella	Live virus	Subcutaneous
Tetanus	Inactivated toxin (toxoid)	Intramuscular¶
Td or DT**	Inactivated toxins (toxoids)	Intramuscular¶
(T = Tetanus)		
(D or d = Diphtheria)		
Typhoid	Inactivated bacteria	Subcutaneous††
Yellow fever	Live virus	Subcutaneous

* The intradermal dose is lower.
† Route depends on the manufacturer; consult package insert for recommendation for specific product used.
§ Intradermal dose is lower and used only for preexposure vaccination.
¶ Preparations with adjuvants should be given intramuscularly.
** DT = tetanus and diphtheria toxoids for use in children aged <7 years. Td = tetanus and diphtheria toxoids for use in persons aged ≥7 years. Td contains the same amount of tetanus toxoid as DTP or DT but a reduced dose of diphtheria toxoid.
†† Boosters may be given intradermally unless acetone-killed and dried vaccine is used. Reprinted from Recommendations of the Immunization Practices Advisory Committee. *Morbidity and Mortality Weekly Report* 38(13):205–214, 219–227, 1989.

TABLE 17-4

RECOMMENDED SCHEDULE FOR ACTIVE IMMUNIZATION OF NORMAL INFANTS AND CHILDREN*

Recommended Age†	Vaccine(s)§	Comments
2 mos	DTP#1¶, OPV#1**	OPV and DTP can be given earlier in areas of high endemicity
4 mos	DTP#2, OPV#2	6-wk to 2-mo interval desired between OPV doses
6 mos	DTP#3	An additional dose of OPV at this time is optional in areas with a high risk of poliovirus exposure
15 mos††	MMR§§, DTP#4, OPV#3	Completion of primary series of DTP and OPV
18 mos	HbCV¶¶	Conjugate preferred over polysaccharide vaccine***
4–6 yrs	DTP#5†††, OPV#4	At or before school entry
14–16 yrs	Td§§§	Repeat every 10 yrs throughout life

* See Table 17-5 for the recommended immunization schedules for infants and children up to their seventh birthday not immunized at the recommended times.

† These recommended ages should not be construed as absolute, e.g., 2 months can be 6–10 weeks. However, MMR should not be given to children <12 months of age. If exposure to measles disease is considered likely, then children 6 through 11 months old may be immunized with single-antigen measles vaccine. These children should be reimmunized with MMR when they are approximately 15 months of age.

§ For all products used, consult the manufacturers' package enclosures for instructions regarding storage, handling, dosage, and administration. Immunobiologics prepared by different manufacturers can vary, and those of the same manufacturer can change from time to time. The package inserts are useful references for specific products, but they may not always be consistent with current ACIP and American Academy of Pediatrics Immunization schedules.

¶ DTP = Diphtheria and Tetanus Toxoide and Pertussis Vaccine, Adsorbed. DTP may be used up to the seventh birthday. The first dose can be given at 6 weeks of age and the second and third doses given 4–8 weeks after the preceding dose.

** OPV = Poliovirus Vaccine Live Oral, Trivalent; contains poliovirus types 1, 2, and 3.

†† Provided at least 6 months have elapsed since DTP #3 or, if fewer than 3 doses of DTP have been received, at least 6 weeks since the last previous dose of DTP or OPV. MMR vaccine should not be delayed to allow simultaneous administration with DTP and OPV. Administering MMR at 15 months and DTP #4 and OPV #3 at 18 months continues to be an acceptable alternative.

§§ MMR = Measles, Mumps, and Rubella Virus Vaccine, Live. Counties that report >5 cases of measles among preschool children during each of the last 5 years should implement a routine 2-dose measles vaccination schedule for preschoolers. The first dose should be administered at 9 months or the first health-care contact thereafter. Infants vaccinated before their first birthday should receive a second dose at about 15 months of age. Single-antigen measles vaccine should be used for children aged <1 year and MMR for children vaccinated on or after their first birthday. If resources do not allow a routine 2-dose schedule, an acceptable alternative is to lower the routine age for MMR vaccination to 12 months.

¶¶ HbCV = Vaccine composed of *Haemophilus influenzae* b polysaccharide antigen conjugated to a protein carrier. Children <5 years of age previously vaccinated with polysaccharide vaccine between the ages of 18 and 23 months should be revaccinated with a single dose of conjugate vaccine if at least 2 months have elapsed since the receipt of the polysaccharide vaccine.

*** If HbCV is not available, an acceptable alternative is to give *Haemophilus influenzae* b polysaccharide vaccine (HbPV) at age >24 months. Children at high risk for *Haemophilus influenzae* type b disease where conjugate vaccine is not available may be vaccinated with HbPV at 18 months of age and revaccinated at 24 months.

††† Up to the seventh birthday.

§§§ Td = Tetanus and Diphtheria Toxoids, Adsorbed (for use in persons aged ≥7 years): contains the same amount of tetanus toxoid as DTP or DT but a reduced dose of diphtheria toxoid.

Reprinted from Recommedations of the Immunization Practices Advisory Committee. *Morbidity and Mortality Weekly Report* 38(13):205–214, 219–227, 1989.

TABLE 17-5

RECOMMENDED IMMUNIZATION SCHEDULE FOR INFANTS AND CHILDREN UP TO THE SEVENTH BIRTHDAY NOT IMMUNIZED AT THE RECOMMENDED TIME IN EARLY INFANCY*
(See individual ACIP recommendations for details)

Timing	Vaccine(s)	Comments
First visit	DTP#1†, OPV#1§, MMR¶ if child is aged ≥15 mos and HbCV** if child is aged ≥18 mos	DTP, OPV, and MMR should be administered simultaneously to children aged ≥15 mos, if appropriate. DTP, OPV, MMR, and HbCV may be given simultaneously to children aged 18 mos–5 yrs.
2 mos after DTP#1, OPV#1	DTP#2††, OPV#2	
2 mos after DTP#2	DTP#3††	An additional dose of OPV at this time is optional in areas with a high risk of poliovirus exposure.
6–12 mos after DTP#3	DTP#4, OPV#3	
Preschool§§ (4–6 yrs)	DTP#5, OPV#4	Preferably at or before school entry.
14–16 yrs	Td¶¶	Repeat every 10 yrs throughout life.

* If initiated in the first year, give DTP #1, 2, and 3 and OPV #1 and 2 according to this schedule; give MMR when the child becomes 15 months old.

† DTP = Diphtheria and Tetanus Toxoids and Pertussis Vaccine, Adsorbed. DTP can be used up to the seventh birthday.

§ OPV = Poliovirus Vaccine Live Oral, Trivalent; contains poliovirus types 1, 2, and 3.

¶ MMR = Measles, Mumps, and Rubella Virus Vaccine, Live (see text for discussion of single vaccines versus combination).

** HbCV = Vaccine composed of *Haemophilus influenzae* b polysaccharide antigen conjugated to a protein carrier. If HbCV is not available, an acceptable alternative is to give *Haemophilus influenzae* b polysaccharide vaccine (HbPV) at 24 months of age. If HbCV is unavailable and if the child is at high risk for *Haemophilus influenzae* type b disease, HbPV may be given at 18 months of age with a second dose at 24 months. Children aged <5 years who were previously vaccinated with HbPV between 18 and 23 months of age should be revaccinated with a single dose of HbCV at least 2 months after the initial dose of HbPV. Either HbCV or HbPV can be administered up to the fifth birthday. However, they are not generally recommended for persons >5 years of age.

†† The second and third doses of DTP can be given 4–8 weeks after the preceding dose.

§§ The preschool doses are not necessary if the fourth dose of DTP and third dose of OPV are administered after the fourth birthday.

¶¶ Td = Tetanus and Diphtheria Toxoids, Adsorbed (for use in persons aged ≥7 years): contains same dose of tetanus toxoid as DTP or DT and a reduced dose of diphtheria toxoid.

Reprinted from Recommedations of the Immunization Practices Advisory Committee. *Morbidity and Mortality Weekly Report* 38(13):205–214, 219–227, 1989.

PROCEDURE

FILTER-PAPER BLOOD SPOT COLLECTION

PURPOSE

To provide a sample to the state laboratory for PKU and thyroid testing.

EQUIPMENT AND MATERIALS

Soap and water
Gauze swabs soaked with 70% isopropyl alcohol
Dry, sterile gauze pads
A sterile lancet with a point not more than 2.5 mm in depth
Filter paper newborn screening kit with protective mailing envelope (see Figure 17–14)

PROCEDURAL STEPS

1. Thoroughly wash the puncture site with soap and water.
   NOTE: The preferred puncture site is indicated by the shaded area on the heel (Figure 17–15). The least hazardous sites for heel puncture are medial to a line drawn posteriorly from the middle of the big toe to the heel or a similar line drawn on the other side, extending from between the fourth and fifth toes to the heel.
2. Disinfect the skin with 70% isopropyl alcohol and allow to air dry. Vigorous rubbing during this step stimulates blood flow in the area.
3. Puncture the skin in one continuous motion using a sterile lancet with a 2.5-mm tip. Longer tips may damage the heel bone.
4. Wipe away and discard the first drop of blood because it may be contaminated by disinfectant or tissue fluid.
5. Allow the second drop to form by the spontaneous free flow of blood.

Preparing the Blood Spots

1. Touch the back of the circle, as close to the center as possible, to the drop of blood. While observing from the opposite side, allow the blood spot to enlarge until the circle is exactly filled. Fill the circle, front to back, with a *single* application of the filter paper to the heel.
2. Once the blood collection is complete, and while the patient's foot is held above the heart level, press a sterile gauze pad to the puncture site until the bleeding has stopped.
3. Dry the blood spots on a level, nonabsorptive surface, away from direct sunlight and at room temperature for at least 4 hours.
4. After the blood spots are completely dry, place

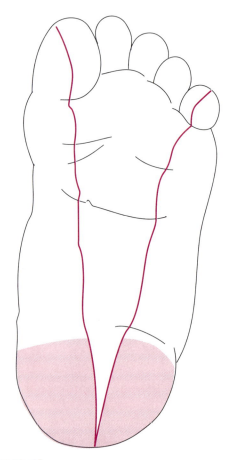

FIGURE 17–15

Skin puncture sites of the infant's heel for blood collection.

them in the protective envelope and ship to the test facility.

NOTE: Improperly prepared blood spots constitute a major problem for the testing laboratories. Radioimmunoassays for hypothyroidism place a greater demand for accurately prepared samples than do other test procedures. Good blood spot preparation ensures prompt and accurate testing of newborns for these serious, but treatable conditions.

WELL-BABY EXAMINATIONS

Vital Signs

Vital signs for the infant include temperature, pulse, respiration, and, if indicated, blood pressure. The temperature should be the last procedure because it will probably cause crying, which would alter the pulse and respirations.

Most physicians prefer that an axillary temperature be taken rather than a rectal, because of the danger of damage to the sensitive mucous membranes of the rectum. Electronic thermometers work very well with infants and are the instrument of choice. Disposable covers are readily available and should be used.

Temperature readings may be expressed in either centigrade or Fahrenheit degrees according to the policy of the practice. To convert centigrade readings to Fahrenheit, multiply by 1.8 and add 32. To convert Fahrenheit readings to centigrade, subtract 32 and divide by 1.8 (see Table 17–7).

The normal pulse and respiratory rates for children are shown in Figures 7–16 and 7–17.

The blood pressure is taken only if ordered by the physician. It is difficult to obtain an accurate blood pressure on an infant or small child, and one must be careful to use the correct-size equipment. An error could be made if a cuff of inappropriate width is used. The cuff should be about the same width in proportion to the arm circumference as that used for an adult, or it should cover approximately two thirds of the upper arm. Table 17–8 lists normal blood pressure readings for children.

Text continued on page 438

TABLE 17–6

EQUIVALENT TEMPERATURE READINGS (CELSIUS AND FAHRENHEIT)*

C	F	C	F	C	F	C	F
0	32.0	37.2	99	39.2	102.6	41.2	106.2
20	68.0	37.4	99.3	39.4	102.9	41.4	106.5
30	86.0	37.6	99.7	39.6	103.3	41.6	106.9
31	87.8	37.8	100.1	39.8	103.7	41.8	107.2
32	89.6	38.0	100.4	40.0	104	42	107.6
33	91.4	38.2	100.8	40.2	104.4	43	109.4
34	93.2	38.4	101.2	40.4	104.7	44	111.2
35	95.0	38.6	101.5	40.6	105.1	100	212
36	96.8	38.8	101.8	40.8	105.4		
37	98.6	39.0	102.2	41.0	105.8		

* To convert Celsius (centigrade) readings to Fahrenheit, multiply by 1.8 and add 32. To convert Fahrenheit readings to Celsius, subtract 32 and divide by 1.8.
Reprinted from Behrman RE: *Nelson Textbook of Pediatrics*, 14th ed. Philadelphia: W. B. Saunders, 1992, p. 1845.

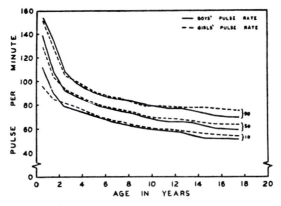

FIGURE 17-16

Pulse rates in infants and children.

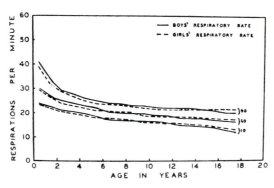

FIGURE 17-17

Respiratory rates in infants and children.

TABLE 17-7

THE AVERAGE NORMAL BLOOD PRESSURE READINGS FOR CHILDREN

Age	Systolic	Diastolic
Birth	40	—
1 month	80	—
4 years	85	60
8 years	95	62
12 years	108	67
16 years (boys)	118	75
20 years (boys)	120	75

Reprinted from Nelson WE: *Textbook of Pediatrics,* 9th ed. Philadelphia: W. B. Saunders, 1969, p. 38.

COMMON CHILDHOOD PROBLEMS AND COMMUNICABLE DISEASES

Immunity- and Allergy-Related Conditions

Allergies

Incubation Period	Contagious Period	Mode of Transmission	Vaccine	Signs and Symptoms	Precautions/Complications
N/A	N/A	Airborne allergen, food, or contact	Hypo-sensitization may be indicated, after the specific allergen is identified.	Asthma, atopic dermatitis, allergic rhinitis, uticaria and angioedema, gastroenteritis	Once allergen is identified, items that contain it should be avoided.

Acquired Immune Deficiency Syndrome (AIDS)

Incubation Period	Contagious Period	Mode of Transmission	Vaccine	Signs and Symptoms	Precautions/Complications
3 months–5 years	May be contracted from blood or other body fluids at any time.	Body fluids (i.e., blood, semen, or saliva). Most infants with AIDS are born to mothers who have risk factors, such as intravenous drug abusers.	Not available	Small for gestational age, failure to thrive, hepatosplenomegaly, lymphoadenopathy, chronic pneumonia, recurrent otitis, media, chronic sinopulmonary infection, *Candida* infection of the mucous membranes, and chronic diarrhea	Infants and children with AIDS should be protected from other infectious diseases because their immunity is diminished. Routine immunizations may be contraindicated.

Viral Conditions

Chickenpox

Incubation Period	Contagious Period	Mode of Transmission	Vaccine	Signs and Symptoms	Precautions/Complications
14–16 days; range is 10–21 days	May be transmitted for 1 day before the onset of rash and until all vesicles have become crusted. Period of infection ranges from 5 to 10 days, depending on the severity of the individual case.	Airborne droplet infection, direct or indirect contact. Dry scabs are not infective.	Not available	Low-grade fever, malaise, and the appearance of the rash. A prodromal period of several days may precede the eruption in adults. The lesions pass rapidly through macule, papule, vesicle, and crust stages, often in 6–8 hours.	Secondary bacterial infection. Encephalitis occurs in less than 1 in 1000 cases and generally is milder than postmeasles encephalitis. Chicken pox encephalitis may, however, be overwhelming, even fatal. Fulminating, often fatal chicken pox occurs in children who received cortisone before contracting the disease!!

COMMON CHILDHOOD PROBLEMS AND COMMUNICABLE DISEASES Continued

Infectious Hepatitis A

Incubation Period	Contagious Period	Mode of Transmission	Vaccine	Signs and Symptoms	Precautions
15–40 days	Isolating the patient during the acute phase of illness (up to 2 weeks after onset of illness) is an effective way of preventing further spread. Rigorous personal hygiene is also necessary.	Contaminated food and water; however, the most important mode of transmission is the fecal–oral route.	Gamma-globulin	Usually the onset is sudden, with fever, fatigue, anorexia, gastrointestinal disturbance, right quadrant tenderness, and varying degrees of icterus.	Enteric precautions; emphasize personal hygiene.

Infectious Mononucleosis

Incubation Period	Contagious Period	Mode of Transmission	Vaccine	Signs and Symptoms	Precautions/Complications
30–50 days	Unknown	Intimate exposure is needed to transfer the disease, i.e., the exchange of saliva from child to child (often in day care centers) or during kissing in young adults.	Not available	Sore throat, malaise, fatigue, headache, nausea, abdominal pain, and fever	The most feared complication is splenic rupture. Swelling of tonsils and pharynx may be so severe it causes respiratory occlusion. Convulsions, ataxia, meningitis, Bell's palsy, encephalitis, Guillain-Barré syndrome, myocarditis, interstitial pneumonia, and hepatitis

Influenza

Incubation Period	Contagious Period	Mode of Transmission	Vaccine	Signs and Symptoms	Precautions/Complications
2–3 days	Not known, possibly during early febrile stages	Directly from person to person by the airborne route or fomites. A fomite is a book, wooden object, or an article of clothing that itself is not corrupted, but is able to harbor pathogenic microorganisms.	Yes	Fever, cough, headache, sore throat, nasal stuffiness, diarrhea, dizziness, vomiting, and myalgia	Pneumonia, encephalitis, myocarditis, myositis, parotitis, severe croup, otitis media, and purulent sinusitis

Mumps

Incubation Period	Contagious Period	Mode of Transmission	Vaccine	Signs and Symptoms	Precautions/Complications
14–21 days	1–6 days before first symptoms appear until swelling disappears	Direct or indirect contact with salivary secretions of infected person	Yes	One or both parotid glands are involved. Submaxillary and sublingual glands may be involved. Parotid mumps is frequently ushered in by fever, headache, and malaise. The child may complain of an earache on the affected side before the onset of swelling.	Epididymo-orchitis is a relative manifestation. Meningoencephalitis occurs in at least 10% of cases. Pancreatitis, thyroiditis, mastitis, dacryoadenitis, and bartholinitis are rare manifestations of mumps.

COMMON CHILDHOOD PROBLEMS AND COMMUNICABLE DISEASES *Continued*

Roseola

Incubation Period	Contagious Period	Mode of Transmission	Vaccine	Signs and Symptoms	Precautions/Complications
Difficult to determine because contact is rarely known. Information available indicates a range of 9–15 days.	Unknown	Unknown	Not available	Fever is high and continuous, often lasting 3–4 days. Typically the fever falls abruptly to normal levels after this period. Generally, the rash develops at the time of disappearance of fever. However, it may appear just before the drop in temperature or up to 24 hours after the temperature reaches normal. The rash is composed of rose-pink maculopapular lesions that tend to remain discreet. It characteristically appears on the trunk and may be spread to the extremities, neck, and face. It may disappear after a few hours or may persist for 2–3 days.	Convulsive seizures that appear to parallel the incidence of other forms of febrile convulsions. Prognosis is uniformly excellent. The often unexplained period of marked elevation of temperature in a small infant is of great concern to both parents and physician. The appearance of the rash is therefore of great comfort.

Rubella (German Measles or 3-Day Measles)

Incubation Period	Contagious Period	Mode of Transmission	Vaccine	Signs and Symptoms	Precautions/Complications
Usually 16–18 days, with a range of 14–21 days	The maximal period of communicability extends from 7 days before to 5 days after onset of the rash.	Direct contact or by contaminated particles in air; from secretions of nose and throat of infected person	Yes	The first symptom is usually the rash. In adolescents and young adults, the rash is usually preceded by a 1–5-day prodromal period characterized by low-grade fever, headache, malaise, anorexia, mild conjunctivitis, sore throat, cough, and lymphadenopathy.	Complications are unusual in rubella. Arthritis is common in adolescents and young adults, especially females. It has rarely been described in young children. The arthritis usually develops just as the rash is fading and may be associated with return of fever, transient joint pain, or massive effusion in one or more joints. The chief danger of the disease is its damaging effect on fetus if mother contracts infection during the first trimester of pregnancy.

Shingles (Herpes Zoster)

Incubation Period	Contagious Period	Mode of Transmission	Vaccine	Signs and Symptoms	Precautions/Complications
Unknown	5–7 days after the vesicles appear	Direct contact with infected vesicle fluid	No	Pain along the involved dermatone, malaise and fever. Within a few days the first vesicles will develop. These painful crops of vesicles are characterized by their distribution being confined to one of the spinal or cranial sensory nerves.	Susceptible individuals may develop chicken pox.

COMMON CHILDHOOD PROBLEMS AND COMMUNICABLE DISEASES Continued

Bacterial Conditions

Diphtheria

Incubation Period	Contagious Period	Mode of Transmission	Vaccine	Signs and Symptoms	Precautions/Complications
2–4 days	2–4 weeks	Either by contact with a carrier or a person with the disease	Yes	Nasal diphtheria is characterized by an excoriating serosanguinous discharge that may obscure the white membrane. Tonsillar and pharyngeal diphtheria is characterized by the presence of a dirty-white membrane on the tonsils and/or pharyngeal wall and possibly extending up to the uvula and soft palate. The membrane varies in color from white to gray to black, and if forcibly removed, will result in bleeding.	Myocarditis is the most frequent complication. It usually occurs during the 2nd week of the disease, but may occur as early as the 1st week and as late as the 6th week. Neuritis, the most frequent being paralysis of the soft palate, may also result in ocular palsy, diaphragmatic paralysis, and a widespread generalized paralysis indistinguishable from Guillain-Barré syndrome. Location of paralysis varies from soft palate during the 3rd week to limb paralysis as late as the 10–12th weeks.

Escherichia coli ("Traveler's Diarrhea")

Incubation Period	Contagious Period	Mode of Transmission	Vaccine	Signs and Symptoms	Precautions/Complications
18–24 hours	Enteric precautions should be used for duration of illness	Contaminated water and food sources	No	Watery diarrhea with low-grade fever and no other systemic symptoms. Stools may contain mucus but usually not blood. The patient may have 10–20 stools/day, and the gastroenteritis usually resolves in 3–7 days.	Vomiting, dehydration, and electrolyte disturbances with acidosis may occur. Severe cases may present with acute onset of diarrhea, urgency, and bloody stools. Nausea, abdominal pain, myalgia, chills, and headache may occur.

Impetigo

Incubation Period	Contagious Period	Mode of Transmission	Vaccine	Signs and Symptoms	Precautions/Complications
2–10 days	Until all lesions have healed	Direct contact with infected persons or by insects	No	Discolored spots of various sizes and shapes. Small vesicles form and break, spreading germ-laden fluid to the surrounding area. These lesions form yellow or honey-colored seropurulent crusts and scabs; the tissue around them is red.	Acute glomerulonephritis may follow if the strain of streptococcus is nephritogenic.

COMMON CHILDHOOD PROBLEMS AND COMMUNICABLE DISEASES Continued

Meningitis Aseptic

Incubation Period	Contagious Period	Mode of Transmission	Vaccine	Signs and Symptoms	Precautions/Complications
3–5 days or longer	Not really known; probably 2–3 days before to several days after onset	Direct contact, via fecal–oral and pharyngeal–oropharyngeal routes	No	Onset is fairly acute. Infants are irritable. Older children have headaches and hyperesthesia. Fever, nausea, and vomiting are common; convulsions are rare. Meningitis aseptic is a mild, self-limited disease. Nuchal–spinal fluid contains many cells. No organisms are seen on direct smears, usually.	Not usually any complications

Meningitis Haemophilus

Incubation Period	Contagious Period	Mode of Transmission	Vaccine	Signs and Symptoms	Precautions/Complications
1–7 days	As long as pathogen is present in nasopharynx; no more than 24 hours after beginning effective microbial therapy	Direct contact or inhalation of infected droplets	Yes	Sudden onset, fever, headaches, chills, convulsions, irritability, stiff neck, and vomiting	Serious neurological and mental sequelea

Meningitis Meningococcal

Incubation Period	Contagious Period	Mode of Transmission	Vaccine	Signs and Symptoms	Precautions/Complications
2–10 days	Until meningococci are no longer present in mouth and nasal discharge	Direct contact or droplet spread from infected person	No	Sudden onset, fever, headache, chills, convulsions, stiff neck, and vomiting. Petechial and purpuric areas are seen in skin and mucous membranes. General muscular rigidity and opisthotonos are seen. Delerium, stupor, or coma may occur. Spinal fluid is cloudy and purulent.	Otitis media, ophthalmia, or pneumonia may occur. Infection may extend to ventricles and cause obstructive hydrocephalus. Subdural collections of fluids may occur. Headache may persist. Intellectual faculties may be impaired. Paralysis, spasticity, and contractures of the lower extremities may result from meningeal irritation.

Meningitis Pneumococcal

Incubation Period	Contagious Period	Mode of Transmission	Vaccine	Signs and Symptoms	Precautions/Complications
1–7 days	As long as the pathogen is present in the nasopharynx	Direct contact or inhalation of infected droplets	No	Same as hemophilus influenza	Serious neurological and mental sequelea

COMMON CHILDHOOD PROBLEMS AND COMMUNICABLE DISEASES Continued

Pertussis (Whooping Cough)

Incubation Period	Contagious Period	Mode of Transmission	Vaccine	Signs and Symptoms	Precautions/Complications
7–10 days	From 7 days after exposure to 3 weeks after the onset of the paroxysmal cough. The disease is more often spread by the patient before the whoops have occurred and before the disease has been diagnosed. Highly contagious during the catarrhal period.	Direct contact or droplet spread from infected person	Yes	The catarrhal or prodromal stage manifests itself by nonspecific upper respiratory symptoms associated with a hacking cough, which gradually becomes more severe. The paroxysmal stage lasts 4–6 weeks, but may be prolonged to 10–12 weeks. It is characterized by the classic series of expiratory coughs climaxed by an inspiratory whoop and often vomiting. Infants under 6 months of age and modified cases may be without the whoop.	Pneumonia, otitis media, or convulsions may occur secondary to gastric tetany, hypoxia, or hemorrhage. Often all these factors contribute to a diffuse encephalopathy with cerebral edema and subsequent cortical atrophy. Hemorrhage may occur in other areas, i.e., conjunctivitis, epistaxis, skin petechiae, or ecchymosis. Other complications include prolapsed rectum, nutritional disturbance, and hernias.

Rheumatic Fever

Incubation Period	Contagious Period	Mode of Transmission	Vaccine	Signs and Symptoms	Precautions/Complications
Usually begins within 1–5 weeks after an upper respiratory illness. Bears an etiological relationship with certain strains of group A Streptococci.	Rheumatic fever is not contagious; the strep infection is.		No	Fever, arthralgia, epistaxis, and rheumatic pneumonia	Bed rest until the major manifestations of the disease (i.e., edema, hematuria, and hypertension) subside. This period usually lasts for 3–4 weeks.

Tuberculosis

Incubation Period	Contagious Period	Mode of Transmission	Vaccine	Signs and Symptoms	Precautions/Complications
3–6 weeks		Droplet infection or by contact with infected human beings; drinking contaminated milk; virus can be adherent to fomites.	No	Cervical adenitis, pneumonic process, meningitis, fever of unknown origin, cough and expectoration, hemoptysis, weight loss, and night sweats	Isolation, bed rest, adequate diet (high in protein, calcium, and vitamins, particularly B, C, and D), fresh air and sunshine

Salmonella

Incubation Period	Contagious Period	Mode of Transmission	Vaccine	Signs and Symptoms	Precautions/Complications
8–48 hours	Enteric precautions should be used for the duration of the illness.	Meat and poultry products, eggs, reptiles (especially turtles). Humans are carriers, and cross-contamination may occur by means of contaminated fingers, clothes, or aerosols.	No	Gastroenteritis	Septicemia, pneumonia, empyema, abscesses, osteomyelitis, septic arthritis, pyelonephritis, and meningitis

COMMON CHILDHOOD PROBLEMS AND COMMUNICABLE DISEASES Continued

Shigellosis (Bacillary Dysentery)

Incubation Period	Contagious Period	Mode of Transmission	Vaccine	Signs and Symptoms	Precautions/Complications
36–72 hours after ingestion	Enteric precautions should be used for duration of illness.	Fecal–oral route	No	Fever, crampy abdominal pain, and loose diarrhea stools that may contain mucus, pus, and blood.	May mimic central nervous system infections such as meningitis and encephalitis. Seizures may occur. Headaches, delerium, nuchal rigidity, fainting, and lethargy.

Staphylococcus aureus

Incubation Period	Contagious Period	Mode of Transmission	Vaccine	Signs and Symptoms	Precautions/Complications
Ranges from a few days to weeks or even months.	Onset to recovery.	Highly contagious, direct contact with infected person or fomites (i.e., a book, wooden object, or an article of clothing, that is not in itself corrupted but is able to harbor pathogenic micro-organisms which may by that means be transmitted to others.)	No	The primary infection is usually, but not always of the skin. It may be an infection of the nasopharynx or of the cord stump of the infant.	Pneumonia, septicemia, enteritis, meningitis, or osteomyelitis.

Hemolytic–Streptococcal Infection (Streptococcal sore throat and scarlet fever)*

Incubation Period	Contagious Period	Mode of Transmission	Vaccine	Signs and Symptoms	Precautions/Complications
2–5 days	From onset to recovery	Droplet infection or direct or indirect transmission may occur.	No	Sore throat, headache, fever, rapid pulse, thirst, vomiting, and swollen glands	Pneumonia, glomerulonephritis, or rheumatic fever

* Many strains of streptococcal bacteria are identified; hemolytic-streptococcal infection is only one.

Other Conditions

Fever, Undetermined Origin

Incubation Period	Contagious Period	Mode of Transmission	Vaccine	Signs and Symptoms	Precautions/Complications
Unknown	Unknown	Unknown	No	Fever must be persistent or frequently recurrent and over 101° F rectally or 102° F orally. An obvious cause must be lacking after at least a preliminary evaluation has been made. It should be remembered the fever must persist for at least 10 days before it is labeled as "fever of unknown origin."	Care should be taken to control fever.

COMMON CHILDHOOD PROBLEMS AND COMMUNICABLE DISEASES Continued

Kawasaki Disease (Mucocutaneous Lymph Node Syndrome)

Incubation Period	Contagious Period	Mode of Transmission	Vaccine	Signs and Symptoms	Precautions/Complications
Unknown	Unknown	Unknown	No	Usually found in children under 5 years of age. Originally found in Japanese children, but now has worldwide distribution among many races. Kawasaki disease is characterized by various combinations of several of the following: prolonged, high, often spiking fevers; usually bulbar conjunctivitis; dry erythematous lips; strawberry tongue and inflamed oropharyngeal mucosa; nonpurulent primary cervical lymphadenopathy; and skin rashes, arthritis (common), uveitis, irritability, cranial nerve palsies, encephalopathy, ataxia, hypertension, pulmonary infiltrates, gallbladder hydrops, ileus, hepatomegaly, and splenomegaly.	Pulmonary, otitis media, obstructive laryngitis, acute encephalitis, purpura, thrombocytopenic and nonthrombocytopenic varieties, appendicitis, and subacute sclerosing panencephalitis

Lyme Disease

Incubation Period	Contagious Period	Mode of Transmission	Vaccine	Signs and Symptoms	Precautions/Complications
3–32 days	Cannot be transmitted to others	Tick-borne illness	No	An erythematous macule or papule, usually following a tick bite. Conjunctivitis, lethargy, fatigue, headaches, fever, chills, migrating musculoskeletal pains, lymphadenopathy, meningismus, encephalopathy, splenomegaly, hepatomegaly, and testicular swelling. Late manifestations may involve the central nervous system, the cardiovascular system and/or musculoskeletal system.	Prevention of tick bites

Otitis Media

Incubation Period	Contagious Period	Mode of Transmission	Vaccine	Signs and Symptoms	Precautions/Complications
None	Usually a noninfectious condition with an accumulation of fluid in the middle ear	Usually caused by an allergy, nasopharyngeal inflammation, or barotrauma (rapid descent in a nonpressurized aircraft cabin).	No	Nasal congestion, cough, and irritability are often the only presenting symptoms. Fever may be absent. Difficulty in hearing, vomiting, and diarrhea may be present.	Chronic serous otitis media, hearing loss, mastoiditis, meningitis.

Parasitic Conditions

Amebic Dysentery (Amebiasis)

Incubation Period	Contagious Period	Mode of Transmission	Vaccine	Signs and Symptoms	Precautions/Complications
A few days	Usually not transmitted to others	Ingestion of contaminated material	No	Diarrhea and blood-streaked stool	Usually occurs in subtropic regions, where sanitation is poor

COMMON CHILDHOOD PROBLEMS AND COMMUNICABLE DISEASES *Continued*

Pinworms (Enterobiasis)

Incubation Period	Contagious Period	Mode of Transmission	Vaccine	Signs and Symptoms	Precautions/Complications
The infection cycle is 3–6 weeks, from egg to adult worm	As long as parasite is present	Contaminated hand to mouth	No	Rectal pruritus, irritability	Teach methods of personal cleanliness: Cut finger-nails short, wash hands with soap and water after using toilet and before meals, etc.

Round Worm (Ascariasis)

Incubation Period	Contagious Period	Mode of Transmission	Vaccine	Signs and Symptoms	Precautions/Complications
Ova hatch in small intestine. Larvae penetrate bowel wall, enter portal system, migrate to the liver and eventually the lungs. From the lungs they ascend to the oropharynx and are swallowed. Thus, the adult worm inhabits the jejunum.	As long as parasite is present	Ingestion of ova contained in soil contaminated with human feces via dirt, food, water.	No	Colicky abdominal pain, poor nutrition, irritability, fatigue, esonophilia.	Pneumonia from invasion of lungs by large numbers of larvae. Invasion of gastrointestinal tract by masses of worms causes gastrointestinal upset, severe abdominal pain, and vomiting.

Scabies

Incubation Period	Contagious Period	Mode of Transmission	Vaccine	Signs and Symptoms	Precautions/Complications
1 week	As long as parasite is present	Clothing, bedding, and human contact	No	The rash appears as a fine, wavy line and may vary from a few millimeters to a centimeter in length. Parasites are barely visible to the naked eye and are pink to grey in color. Itching, the main symptom, is more prevalent at night.	Avoid contact with infected persons.

Toxoplasmosis

Incubation Period	Contagious Period	Mode of Transmission	Vaccine	Signs and Symptoms	Precautions/Complications
Unknown	Not limited to humans. This organism has been found in chickens, ducks, dogs, cats, and horses.	May be contracted by eating raw or uncooked meats. Can be transmitted to an infant through the placenta during primary maternal infection.	No	Rash, lymphoadenopathy	Avoid undercooked meats, and contact with patients with known disease. Take extra precautions when handling cats and their litter boxes.

BATTERED CHILD SYNDROME

In all 50 states, there are three main responsibilities the physician and office personnel have toward abused children:

- Detection
- Reporting
- Prevention

The phone number of the local child protection agency should be posted, along with all other emergency numbers, where it can be easily found. Reluctance to report abuse could lead to further injury or even death of the child.

Abusers are usually family members or friends of the family. Abusers are found in all ethnic, geographical, religious, educational, occupational, and socioeconomic groups. Abusive parents tend to be lonely, unhappy, angry individuals who are currently stressed by the loss of a job, eviction, marital strife, birth of a child, or just physical exhaustion.

Signs of abuse to look for are

- Bruises
- Welts
- Lacerations
- Scars

Bruises that are confined to the buttocks and lower back are most likely related to physical punishment. Thumb or fingerprints are usually found on the arms where the child has been grabbed. Hard pinching leaves two circular or curvilinear bruises. Slap marks most often leave a bruise on the cheek with two or three parallel lines running through it. Forced feeding in an attempt to quiet a screaming child causes bruising of the upper lip and frenulum. Human bite marks are distinctive, paired, crescent-shaped bruises facing each other.

If a blunt instrument has been used in punishment, a bruise or welt most often takes the shape of the instrument. If you suspect a rope or cord has been used, look for loop marks or scars on the skin. Lash marks can be seen after the child has been beaten with a belt, tree branch, or ruler. You may even see choke marks on the neck and circumferential tie marks around the ankles.

The most common sites for accidental bruises are over the forehead, anterior tibia, and bony prominences.

Burns account for approximately 10% of the physical abuse. Hot solid burns are the easiest to recognize. These burns take the shape of the instrument used; for instance, if the child is held against an electric hotplate. A cigarette burn will appear as a circular, punched-out lesion of the uniform size. (Bullous impetigo can be mistaken for these.)

Hot-water burns are the most common types of burns to be inflicted on children. Look for a burn involving only the buttocks and perineum; this may be caused by the parent's or caretaker's holding the child's thighs against the abdomen and placing his or her buttocks into scalding water as a punishment for enuresis or resistance to toilet training. The fact the hands and feet are spared indicates that the child did not fall into a hot tub or turn the hot water on while in the tub. If there is a burn extending well above the wrist and ankle, then there is cause to suspect child abuse.

An extremely dangerous inflicted injury is subdural hematoma, which often leads to death or serious sequelae. Of course the most serious and classic cause of subdural hematoma is the direct blow to the head, resulting in a skull fracture. Others include the 50% of subdural hematomas that occur with no skull fracture, but are the result of a violent, whiplash-type shaking that leads to the tearing of the cerebral veins. In these cases, retinal hemorrhages are almost always present and aid in the diagnosis. Look for grab-mark bruises along the upper extremities and shoulder to support this theory.

The second most common cause of death in abused children is intraabdominal injuries. The most frequent is a ruptured liver or spleen. Others may include intestinal perforation, traumatic pancreatitis, and ruptured blood vessels.

If there is any suspicion that the injury is the result of abuse, the physician and office personnel should take the appropriate steps to

- Ensure the child is treated for the injuries
- Hospitalize selected cases
- Inform the parents of the diagnosis and the need to report it
- Make a telephone call to the child protective agency, immediately
- Complete an official written report within 48 hours

- Request a social worker consultation
- Maintain a helping approach towards the parents
- Examine all siblings within 12 hours
- Provide medical testimony for court cases

The most important thing a physician and the office personnel can do is to work toward the prevention of child abuse. Watch for signs in families that show potential to become abusive. These may include the following:

- Unwanted pregnancies
- A newborn in a family with a history of child abuse
- Drug addiction
- Serious psychiatric illness
- Comments of a derogatory nature about the child
- Lack of maternal attachment
- Infrequent visits to see the newborn in cases of delay of discharge from the hospital.

Persons in any of these groups should be referred to the public health nurse, telephone hotlines, church, and civic support groups.

Bibliography

Practical Points in Pediatrics, Second Edition: Allen, Gururaj, Russo Medical Examination Publishing Company, Inc.
Handbook of Pediatric Primary Care, Chow, Durand, Feldman, Mills, John Wiley & Sons
Nelson Textbook of Pediatrics, Thirteenth Edition, Behrman & Vaughan, W. B. Saunders & Company
Ross Laboratories Growth Charts
Public Health Department Immunization Schedules
Guidelines for Health Supervision, American Academy of Pediatrics
Textbook of Pediatric Nursing, Marlow, Fourth Edition, W. B. Saunders & Company
Comprehensive Pediatric Nursing, Scipien, Barnard, Chard, Howe, Phillips, McGraw-Hill
Telephone Manual of Pediatric Care, Harvey P. Katz, John Wiley & Sons
Growth & Development of Children, Seventh Edition, G. H. Lowery, Yearbook Medical Publishers
Ambulatory Pediatrics, Green & Haggerty, W. B. Saunders & Company
The Lippincott Manual of Nursing Practice, J. B. Lippincott Company
Compendium of Drug Therapy, CORE Publishing Division, Excerpta Medical, Inc.

Chapter 18

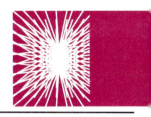

GYNECOLOGICAL AND OBSTETRICAL PROCEDURES

MIDGE NOEL RAY

GYNECOLOGY
Terminology
Gynecological History
Routine Gynecological Examination
Physician's Implementation of Pelvic Examination
Medical Conditions
Contraception

OBSTETRICS
Terminology
Evidence of Pregnancy
Routine Prenatal Care
Disorders
Diagnostic Procedures
Postpartum Care
Infertility

GYNECOLOGY

Terminology

Amenorrhea: Absence of menstruation
Climacteric: Premenopausal period in which the reproductive functions begin to diminish
Coitus: Sexual intercourse
Dysmenorrhea: Painful menstruation
Dilatation and curettage (D & C): Procedure in which the cervical os is dilated and the endometrium is scraped of diseased tissue or uterine contents
Dyspareunia: Painful intercourse
Endometriosis: Occurrence of endometrial tissue abnormally located in the pelvic cavity
Menarche: Onset of the first menstrual period
Menopause: Cessation of menstruation
Menorrhagia: Excessive bleeding during the menses
Menses: Monthly flow of blood; menstrual period

Metrorrhagia: Uterine bleeding occurring between the normal menses
Oligomenorrhea: Scanty or small amount of menstrual flow

Gynecological History

A detailed and comprehensive medical history is vital to quality patient care. An atmosphere must be established that is conducive to ascertaining personal and private information from the patient. Often, a questionnaire may be used to obtain basic information. However, this should be supplemented with an interview by the medical assistant, nurse, or physician.

Routine Gynecological Examination

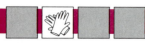

PROCEDURE

ASSISTING WITH THE GYNECOLOGICAL EXAMINATION WITH PAP SMEAR

PURPOSE

To provide a third person of the client's sex present during the examining of the genitalia, to assist in the comfort of the patient, and to assist the physician in the organization of the examination.

 MEDICAL ASSISTING ALERT

Instruct patient not to douche, use vaginal medication, or have sexual intercourse within 24 hours of examination. Determine the purpose of the examination and whether it is the patient's first pelvic examination.

EQUIPMENT AND MATERIALS

Gynecological Examination

Patient drapes (breast towel, full drape)
Lubricant, water soluble
Vaginal speculum, correct size
Uterine sponge forcep
Cotton applicators (two)
Disposable gloves
Light source
Cleansing tissues
Gloves and blood and body fluid protection barriers

Pap Smear

Cervical spatula (wooden or plastic)
Microscopic slides
Fixative spray and container for prepared slides or specimen container with 10% formalin
Laboratory request form
Label for specimen identification

PROCEDURAL STEPS

Patient Preparation

1. Identify patient and explain examination. Offer to answer any questions.
   RATIONALE: Explaining procedure helps establish rapport with patient and reduces the patient's apprehension.
2. Have patient empty bladder and rectum, saving urine specimen if necessary.
   RATIONALE: An empty bladder (within the past half-hour) and rectum facilitate palpation of abdominopelvic structures. Patient is more comfortable.
3. Provide privacy and instruct patient to completely disrobe and drape with sheet or patient gown.
   RATIONALE: A drape sheet allows a patient to feel somewhat covered, which aids in patient relaxation. Adequate privacy should be provided unless patient requires assistance.

Performance

4. Prepare room, equipment, and supplies for pelvic examination.
   RATIONALE: Properly functioning equipment and instruments facilitate examination and promote a professional image.
5. Instruct and position patient for specific area to be examined.
   RATIONALE: Proper positioning facilitates a thorough examination, and explanations aid in decreasing patient anxiety.

   - Position patient in upright or Fowler's position for thoracic, back, breast, head, and neck examination. Patient should be provided a small drape to cover breasts as necessary.
   - Position patient in dorsal recumbent position for examination of breasts, axillae, and abdominopelvic cavity.
   - Position patient in dorsal lithotomy for examination of external genitalia, vagina, cervix, and rectum.

6. Assist physician with gloving and gowning.
7. Focus the light on the female external genitalia.
8. Assist physician as necessary, including handing him or her appropriate instruments and supplies at the appropriate time.

9. Warm the vaginal speculum and moisten it with warm water.
   RATIONALE: Water warms the metal and provides a lubricant that does not interfere with the Pap studies.
10. Assist physician in obtaining vaginal and cervical smears:
    - Label and date slide
    - Hold microscopic slide while physician applies cells and secretions to the slide, or take applicator and make smear
    - Spray slide with fixative solution, following the manufacturer's directions, or submerse the slide into the specimen jar with 10% formalin.
    - Label package for transporting to lab

 MEDICAL ASSISTING ALERT

If a spray cytology fixative is used, do not spray the fixative too close to the slide because this may damage the specimen.

11. Apply water-soluble lubricant across two fingers of physician's hand for the bimanual and rectal examinations.
    RATIONALE: A water-soluble lubricant makes the digital examination easier for the patient.

Follow-Through

12. Instruct the patient to wipe perineum from anterior to posterior with cleansing tissue.
    RATIONALE: This discourages vaginal contamination from the rectum and removes excess lubricant and body fluids.
13. Assist patient to an upright position, being sure to have patient slide up on examination table before removing legs from stirrups.
14. Initiate the sanitization procedure for contaminated instruments.
15. Instruct patient to dress.
16. Reinforce the physician's instructions and allow time for patient to ask questions.
    RATIONALE: Reinforcement and answering patient questions enhance patient cooperation and compliance to treatment plan.
17. Record information on the patient's chart as instructed by the physician and initial.
18. Prepare room for next patient examination.

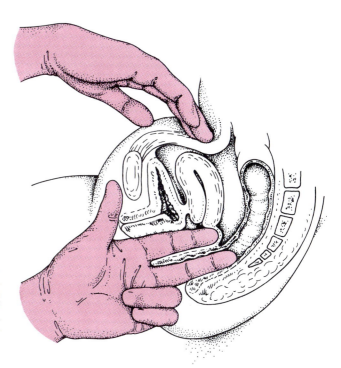

FIGURE 18-1

Bimanual pelvic examination. The hand on the abdomen brings more of the pelvic contents into contact with the inserted fingers. This technique provides a more adequate palpation of the pelvic viscera than can be accomplished by vaginal examination alone. (Reproduced from Kinn ME, Derge EF: *The Medical Assistant: Administrative and Clinical*, 6th ed. Philadelphia: W. B. Saunders, 1988, p. 551.)

Physician's Implementation of Pelvic Examination

1. External genitalia are inspected for hair distribution, symmetry, color, clitoral size, position of urethra, vagina, and rectum. Any lesions, scars, discolorations, unusual discharge, or odors should be noted.
2. Internal genitalia are examined with a vaginal speculum that is warmed and lubricated with warm water. Once speculum is inserted, the cervix and vaginal walls are inspected for discoloration, lesions, discharge, dryness, etc. A Pap smear for cytology and smears for culture are obtained.
3. Palpation of the internal genitalia is performed in a bimanual manner, with physician inserting two fingers of physician's secondary hand into the vagina (Figure 18–1). The uterus and adnexa can then be palpated through the abdominal wall. The uterus is palpated for size, shape, position, (Figure 18–2) and consistency. At this time the physician may detect and locate pain, tenderness, and other abnormalities.
4. A rectovaginal or digital rectal examination, especially in women age 40 and older, concludes the pelvic examination. The physician palpates the uterosacral ligaments, posterior uterus, cervix, cul-de-sac, and rectum. Rectal lesions such as fissures, hemorrhoids, or polyps or rectal bleeding may be detected.

MEDICAL ASSISTING ALERT

- The speculum is warmed by storing on heating pad or rinsing in warm water; a warm-water rinse lubricates the speculum, yet does not interfere with results of the smears.
- Allot ample time to establish rapport with patient; additional time is required for patients scheduled for their first pelvic examination and for those with special needs (handicapped, elderly, and adolescent individuals).
- Remain in the room during examination to reassure patient and provide legal protection to physician.

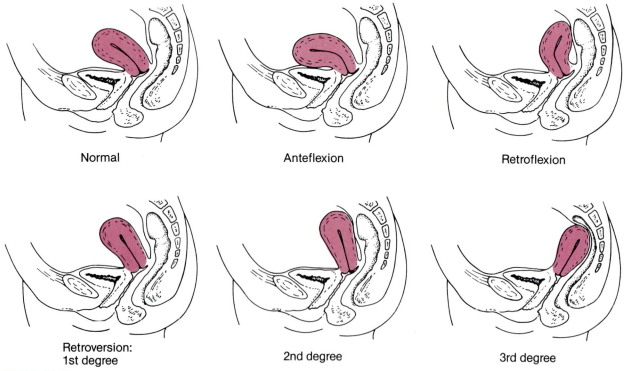

FIGURE 18–2

Positions of the uterus in the sagittal section. (Reproduced from Kinn ME, Derge EF: *The Medical Assistant: Administrative and Clinical,* 6th ed. Philadelphia: W. B. Saunders, 1988, p. 551.)

- The lithotomy position may be difficult for elderly and some handicapped persons to maintain. If necessary, the examination may be conducted while patient is in an alternative position, such as the Sims. Consult with physician if in doubt.
- During examination, advise the patient of each step, especially the insertion of the speculum.
- Allow elderly or special-needs patients additional time in sitting position.
- Provide patient with extra cleansing tissue, sanitary pads, or tampons as necessary.

Guidelines for Selecting the Appropriate-Size Vaginal Speculum

- Because plastic speculums do break, avoid using them on obese or restless women.
- For children, use a small Graves speculum.
- For women who have not become sexually active, use a narrow Pederson speculum or a small Graves speculum.
- For most women, use a medium Graves speculum.
- For obese or grand multiparous women, use a large speculum.
- For women who are very anxious, use the smallest speculum that provides adequate visibility.

Medical Conditions

Vulvovaginitis

Vulvovaginitis is inflammation of the vulva and vagina; inflammation may involve the urethra. Table 18–1 describes various types of vulvovaginitis.

Wet Preparations/KOH Preparations*

Purpose. In physicians' offices, wet (saline) preparations or KOH preparations are usually done on swabs of vaginal discharge to detect

- *T. vaginalis*
- yeast (primarily *Candida albicans*)
- clue cells that indicate infection with *G. vaginalis*

---
* Section provided by Linda Jeff (see also Chapter 23).

Clinical Considerations

Trichomoniasis

- Trichomoniasis is characterized in women by a frothy greenish-gray vaginal discharge.
- Most men who are infected are asymptomatic.
- *T. vaginalis,* the causative agent, is a protozoan parasite that moves by means of four anterior flagella and an undulating membrane.
- The infection is usually diagnosed by the detection of the motile organism in a wet preparation of vaginal secretions (or occasionally in urine).

Candidiasis

- Candidiasis, or infection with *Candida* sp., is characterized by an erythematous and edematous vulva and a thick white discharge.
- Sexual partners may develop balanitis or cutaneous lesions on the penis.
- *C. albicans,* the most common species involved, is a yeast, a unicellular fungus that reproduces by budding.
- Occasionally, other yeasts may cause infections.
- Diagnosis of yeast infection is made by observing budding yeasts or pseudohyphae (tubular structures made of chains of attached buds) on a wet preparation or KOH preparation of vaginal secretions.

Bacterial Vaginosis

- Bacterial vaginosis, previously referred to as "nonspecific vaginitis," has been associated with infection with *G. vaginalis,* a small Gram-negative bacillus or coccobacillus.
- It is believed that *G. vaginalis* works synergistically with a number of anaerobic organisms to cause the condition.
- Characteristic symptoms of the infection include

  Frothy, gray, malodorous vaginal exudate
  Vaginal pH > 4.7
  Production of a strong fish-like odor when 10% KOH is added to secretions
  The presence of clue cells on a wet preparation or Gram stain of vaginal secretions

Methodology

- Vaginal swabs for wet preparations or KOH preparations should be examined within 30 minutes of collection.
- Wet preparations and KOH preparations are performed in the same manner, except that saline is used as the sole wetting agent in the former and KOH is added for the latter.

TABLE 18-1
TYPES OF VULVOVAGINITIS

TYPE AND ETIOLOGY	CHARACTERISTICS	DIAGNOSIS	TREATMENT
Simple Poor hygiene, irritation, or microorganisms	Erythema, itching, burning, edema, and increased discharge	Physical examination; sometimes preparation of discharge using normal saline	Vinegar (1 T. white vinegar to 1 qt H_2O) douche; improve hygiene; avoid irritants
Moniliasis (yeast infection) *Candida albicans*	Thick, curdlike discharge, dyspareunia, dysuria, erythema, itching, and edema; white patches appear on vaginal wall	Wet-mount preparation of discharge using 10% potassium hydroxide	Nystatin; Monistat (miconazole 2%); Mycelex (clotrimazole 1%)
Trichomoniasis *Trichomonas vaginalis*	Profuse, frothy, green discharge with foul odor, dysuria, itching, possibly cervical/vaginal strawberry spots (hemorrhages)	Slide of discharge using normal saline or placing swab with discharge into test tube of normal saline	Metronidazole (Flagyl)
Bacterial vaginosis Gardnerella and other bacteria	Thin gray discharge with foul "fishy" odor that intensifies with alkalinity (after coitus, washing with soap); vulvar itching and irritation	pH of discharge >4.5, appearance and odor of discharge, wet-mount preparation using 10% KOH	Metronidazole (Flagyl)
Atrophic vaginitis Low levels of estrogen	Itching; thinning of vaginal mucosa, which bleeds easily; vulvar irritation; dyspareunia	Physical examination; sometimes a wet-mount preparation to rule out growth of microbes	Estrogen (Premarin)

- A wet preparation and a KOH preparation can be performed on the same slide, increasing the likelihood of finding organisms (see the following procedure).

MEDICAL ASSISTING ALERT

- For moniliasis or bacterial vaginosis, a wet-mount preparation of potassium hydroxide should be used; for trichomoniasis, normal saline should be used.
- If the vaginitis has been sexually transmitted (see Table 18-2), encourage patient to advise her partner to come in for treatment.

- If the patient has simple vaginitis, advise her to avoid tight-fitting pants and undergarments, to always wipe from front to back, and to wear cotton underwear.
- Oral contraceptives predispose to candidiasis and may have to be temporarily discontinued. Antibiotic therapy is also a predisposing factor to candidiasis, and patient may need prophylaxis with antibiotic therapy.
- Patient education regarding the transmission of the disease is important with vaginitis, especially recurrent vaginitis.

TABLE 18-2

SEXUALLY TRANSMITTED DISEASES (STD)

Disease and Etiology	Manifestation in Female	Guidelines for Medical Assistant
Syphilis *Treponema pallidum*	May be asymptomatic. Primary: chancre on cervix, vulva, perineum, or other sites; regional lymphedema. Secondary: transitory or persistent skin rash; lymphedema; condylomata; uveitis and inflammation of other tissues; fever, malaise, weight loss, anorexia. Latent: asymptomatic or mucocutaneous lesions. Tertiary: Presence of chronic granulomatous lesion (gumma) on cutaneous and submucosal tissue causing necrosis and scarring.	Diagnosed by Venereal Disease Research Laboratory (VDRL) test or rapid plasma reagin; Treated with aqueous procaine penicillin G or benzathine penicillin. Encourage sexual partners to come in for treatment.
Gonorrhea *Neisseria gonorrhea*	Asymptomatic; or dysuria, urinary frequency, mucopurulent or purulent discharge, cervicitis. Rectal exposure: symptomless, or perianal irritation and discharge. Orogenital exposure: pharyngitis.	Diagnosed by Gram stain of exudate from cervix or urethra; culture should be performed when Gram stain is positive. Treatment involves a loading dose of penicillin or ceftriaxone with a follow-up of tetracycline or erythromycin.
Genital herpes *Herpes simplex,* type 2	Initially, itching and soreness of genitalia, followed by erythema and vesiculation that ulcerates and is painful. Heals with scarring in about 10 days. Recurrence: malaise, muscular aches, and fever.	Diagnosed clinically by appearance of the vesicles with ulceration and confirmed with tissue culture. Patients are at increased risk for cervical cancer and should be monitored with Pap smears and colposcopy. Acyclovir is helpful in reducing the frequency and length of outbreak. There is NO CURE. Advise patient to abstain from genital or oral contact when lesions exist.
Trichomoniasis *Trichomonas vaginalis*	Asymptomatic. Or vaginitis with burning, itching, and frothy, copious greenish-yellow discharge, erythema and edema of external genitalia. Strawberry spots may appear on vaginal wall and cervix.	Diagnosed by microscopic examination. Treated with metronidazole (Flagyl).
Nongonococcal urethritis *Ureaplasma urealyticum, Chlamydia trachomatis,* and other organisms	Asymptomatic. Or urethritis (dysuria, urinary frequency); pelvic pain; dyspareunia; and cervicitis with yellow, mucopurulent discharge.	Diagnosed by culturing exudate with cellular material from the cervix and urethra. Treated with tetracycline or erythromycin.
Condylomata acuminata (genital warts) Human *papillomavirus*	Groups of soft, pink or red growths on vulva, vagina, cervix or perineum, "cauliflower appearance."	Diagnosed by microscopic examination by colposcopy. Treated with laser, electrocautery, and cryotherapy. Treated with 25% podophyllin in tincture of benzoin.
Pediculosis pubis *Phthirus pubis*	Vulvovaginal papules, itching, erythema, visible lice and nits in pubic area.	Diagnosed by physical examination. Treated with 1% lindane lotion, cream, or shampoo, 0.5% malathion lotion, or 1% permethrin cream rinse.
Acquired immune deficiency syndrome Human immunodeficiency virus	Fatigue, malaise, weight loss, lymphadenopathy, malnutrition, night sweats.	Detected by enzyme-linked immunosorbent assay (ELISA) and confirmed by Western Blot test. Treatment is symptomatic; there is NO CURE. Centers for Disease Control suggests all women at risk who are pregnant or who desire pregnancy be offered testing.

PROCEDURE

PERFORMING A WET PREPARATION/KOH PREPARATION*

PURPOSE

To detect motile forms of *T. vaginalis*, detect yeast cells, and detect clue cells that indicate infection with *G. vaginalis*.

EQUIPMENT AND MATERIALS

Vaginal swab in saline
Glass microscopic slides (3″ × 1″)
Cover slips (22 mm × 22 mm)
10% KOH in dropper bottle
Cotton swabs
Gloves and protective wear for CDC Universal Precautions

PROCEDURAL STEPS

Performance

1. Using a felt tip marker or wax pencil, label the end of a slide with the patient's name or accession number.
2. Touch the tip of the vaginal swab to each end of the slide to deposit a drop of the vaginal exudate–saline mixture.
3. Place a coverslip over the drop on the left. A cotton swab may be used to remove excess liquid from around the coverslip.
4. Add a drop of KOH to the drop on the right side of the slide. Note whether a strong fishy odor is present.
   RATIONALE: A strong fishy odor is characteristic of bacterial vaginosis.
5. Coverslip the drop on the right. Use a cotton swab to remove excess liquid from around the coverslip if necessary.
6. Let the slide sit at room temperature for 5–15 minutes.
   RATIONALE: This allows the KOH to dissolve proteinaceous material in the specimen, making it easier to identify the yeast.
7. Observe the saline preparation (left side). Scan the entire coverslipped area under the X10 objective of the microscope with the condenser down and using low light intensity. Look for possible motile forms of *T. vaginalis*, yeast cells, or clue cells.
8. Switch to high-power objective to better visualize and identify any suspicious structures. If no organisms or clue cells are seen, examine at least 10 fields under the high power.
   RATIONALE: Organisms may be better seen and differentiated from cellular material under high power.
9. Observe the KOH preparation (right side of the slide) in the same manner.

Interpretation

T. Vaginalis. The organism is oval or pear shaped and demonstrates a jerky motility. A flagellum moving back and forth at one end or the undulating membrane extending half the length of the body on one side may be seen (Figure 18–3).

> ### MEDICAL ASSISTING ALERT
> Nonmotile forms of the organism are easily confused with white blood cells.

Yeast. Yeast cells are round to oval or oblong, smooth-walled cells, 2–8 μ in diameter. Budding cells and pseudohyphae may be seen (Figure 18–4).

> ### MEDICAL ASSISTING ALERT
> Yeast cannot be specifically identified on the basis of its microscopic morphology. Just report, "Yeast seen."

Clue Cells. Clue cells are vaginal epithelial cells covered with tiny bacilli or coccobacilli, which are *G. vaginalis*. The bacteria give the cells a characteristic speckled appearance and make cell margins indistinct (Figure 18–5).

---

* Procedure provided by Linda Jeff (see also Chapter 23).

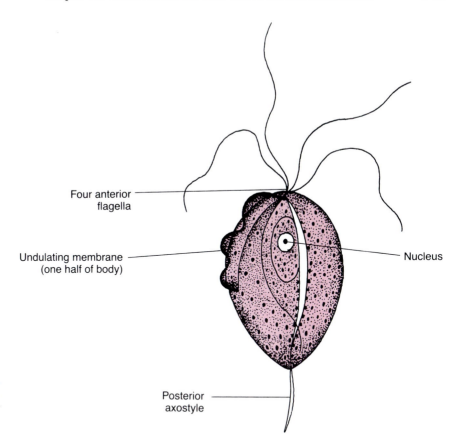

FIGURE 18-3

Diagram of *Trichomonas vaginalis*. (Reproduced from Leventhal R, Cheadle RF: *Medical Parasitology,* 3rd ed. Philadelphia: F. A. Davis, 1989.)

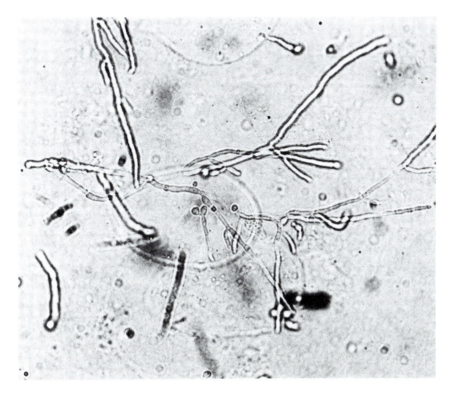

FIGURE 18-4

Candida pseudohyphae in KOH preparation as viewed under high-power objective. (Reproduced from Addison LA, Fischer PM: *The Office Laboratory,* 2nd ed. Norwalk, CT: Appleton and Lange, 1990.)

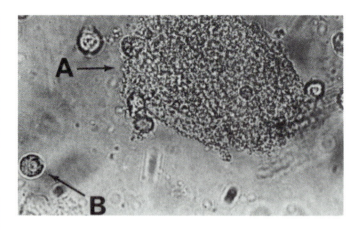

FIGURE 18-5

A, Clue cell in vaginal wet preparation. **B**. White blood cell, viewed under high-power objective. (Reproduced from Addison LA, Fischer PM: *The Office Laboratory*, 2nd ed. Norwalk, CT: Appleton and Lange, 1990.)

Follow-Through

10. Have slide examined by a laboratory professional or the physician.
11. Discard slide in a biohazard container with disinfectant.

PROCEDURE

OBTAINING A VAGINAL DISCHARGE SPECIMEN FOR TRANSPORT TO A LABORATORY

PURPOSE

To obtain a vaginal discharge specimen for the diagnosis of vulvovaginitis.

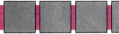 **MEDICAL ASSISTING ALERT**

Instruct the patient not to douche before collection of specimen.

EQUIPMENT AND MATERIALS

Equipment and materials for pelvic examination (see ASSISTING WITH GYNECOLOGICAL EXAMINATION WITH PAP SMEAR procedure)
Completed labels
Commercial kit that contains the culture tubes with swabs and ampules of media.

PROCEDURAL STEPS

Patient Preparation

1. Identify the patient and explain procedure.
2. Have the patient empty bladder and rectum, saving urine specimen if necessary.
   RATIONALE: The physician may request urinalysis to assess involvement.
3. Have the patient disrobe from waist down and drape herself with sheet.

Performance

4. Obtain all necessary equipment and materials.
5. Label the container(s) with patient's name, date, and source of specimen
6. Position the patient in dorsal lithotomy position.
7. Focus light on the vaginal orifice.
8. Assist the physician in obtaining vaginal smear.

- Crush the ampule containing medium by squeezing; the applicator with specimen is then pushed into the tube, submerging in the medium.
- Transport to laboratory (see Chapter 20).

Follow-Through

9. Assist the patient into upright position.
10. Initiate sanitization process.
11. Provide the patient with cleansing tissues and, if necessary, sanitary napkins (minipad or panty liner).
12. Reinforce the physician's instructions regarding medication, personal hygiene, and prevention of recurrence.

Dysfunctional Uterine Bleeding

Dysfunctional uterine bleeding (DUB), one of the most common gynecological problems, is irregular or excessive uterine bleeding. Initially, a pelvic examination is done, but diagnosis is by endometrial biopsy (see ASSISTING WITH COLPOSCOPY procedure) and D & C. The etiology is usually endocrine or organic.

Treatment. The usual treatment is hormone therapy. A D & C is used often, especially with hypovolemia and in women over age 35. Hysterectomy is a last resort.

Pelvic Inflammatory Disease

Pelvic inflammatory disease (PID) is an inflammation of a part or all of the upper part of the genital tract that may include ovaries, fallopian tubes, uterine serosa, endometrium, myometrium, and broad ligaments.

Etiology. PID may be caused by any number of microorganisms, including *Neisseria gonorrhoeae* and *Chlamydia trachomatis*.

Risk Factors. Risk factors include age (young females are at increased risk), multiple sex partners, history of PID, and use of intrauterine device.

Signs and Symptoms. The patient may be asymptomatic or have abdominal tenderness, cervical and uterine tenderness with motion, purulent vaginal discharge, or vaginal bleeding.

Diagnosis. A diagnosis can usually be based on clinical history and physical examination, but a laparoscopy is more definitive. Culdocentesis may be used in diagnosis, if purulent peritoneal fluid is aspirated and found to have an elevated white blood cell count.

Treatment. The usual treatment is antibiotic therapy for both the female and male sexual partner.

Endometriosis

Endometriosis is an abnormal condition in which endometrial tissue is growing outside of the uterus. The endometrial tissue may be found at the ovaries, fallopian tubes, uterosacral ligaments, cul-de-sac, cervix, and, less often, distant sites such as the lungs and nasal mucosa.

Etiology. The cause is unknown, but it is thought to be an autoimmune disease.

Signs and Symptoms. Patient complains of dysmenorrhea, dyspareunia, infertility, abnormal uterine bleeding, and rectal and pelvic pain.

Diagnosis. In mild endometriosis, results of a pelvic examination may be normal. In moderate to advanced endometriosis, examination may reveal vulval and cervical lesions; endometriomas; nodularity along uterosacral ligament and rectovaginal septum; an ovarian "chocolate" cyst, caused by the endometrial tissue that bleeds during menses; pelvic adhesions; and retroverted and/or fixed uterus. Often, laparoscopy may be necessary to determine the degree of involvement.

Treatment. Therapy is individualized and depends on the degree of tissue involvement, patient age, desire for pregnancy, and patient discomfort. For women who desire pregnancy and whose endometriosis is mild, hormonal therapy may be used to relieve symptoms and reduce the endometrial implants. The hormone (Danazol) is administered to suppress ovarian function, which helps relieve symptoms, prevent proliferation, and reduce the size of the endometrial implants.

In cases of severe cyclic pain, surgical intervention to remove the implanted endometrial tissue may be necessary. Preservation of the uterus and ovaries depends on the patient's desire for pregnancy. The removal of the abnormal tissue (endometriomas, adhesions, and cysts) for those who desire pregnancy may be accomplished by laparoscopy, laparotomy, and laser surgery. In patients for whom pregnancy is of no concern and symptoms are severe, a hysterectomy and bilateral salpingo-oophorectomy followed by hormone therapy is the treatment of choice.

Guidelines for Patient Education

- Prepare patient for hormonal therapy by advising her of side effects, instructing her on drug administration, and discussing with her the desired effects versus undesired effects.
- Prepare patient for surgery by arranging admission to hospital, reinforcing physician's instructions, and providing instructions regarding preoperative planning (preliminary tests, anesthesia, diet, etc.) and recovery period (activities, restrictions, and wound care).

Acute Mastitis and Breast Abscess

Mastitis is inflammation of the breast tissue and is often associated with lactation. Mammary abscess may occur.

MEDICAL ASSISTING ALERT

Advise the patient to continue to breastfeed or empty breast with breast pump. Encourage thorough handwashing before breastfeeding.

Etiology. Most often acute mastitis and breast abscess are caused by *Staphylococcus aureus*.

Signs and Symptoms. Localized areas of inflammation are characterized by redness, heat, and tenderness. The patient may have a slight increase in body temperature with chills.

Diagnosis. Diagnosis is based on patient complaints and physical examination. If an abscess is present, the white blood cell count will be elevated and there may be drainage from the nipple.

Treatment. Mastitis should be treated with antibiotic therapy, and the patient should continue to empty breast of milk by breastfeeding or breast pump. If symptoms continue, an abscess may have developed that must be incised and drained using sterile technique. Any discharge from nipple should be cultured (Figure 18-6).

Guidelines for Patient Education

- If an abscess has occurred, instruct the patient to apply warm compresses to affected breast, which will ease the pain and facilitate drainage.
- The patient may find breastfeeding painful if a fissure has occurred on the nipple. If so, advise the patient to continue to empty the breast with a pump until breastfeeding can be resumed.
- Advise the patient to rest and drink additional fluids.

Fibrocystic Breast Disease

This is a benign disease of the breast that occurs in about 50% of premenopausal women. The dysplasia of the breast is characterized by increased fibrous tissue and hyperplasia of epithelial cells resulting in cysts, usually bilaterally.

MEDICAL ASSISTING ALERT

Encourage follow-up visits and breast self-examination, because these patients are at increased risk of developing breast cancer.

Etiology. Not clearly understood; condition is thought to be related to hormone changes.

Signs and Symptoms. The patient may be asymptomatic or have breast pain (mastodynia), premenstrual breast tenderness, and lumpy breasts.

Diagnosis. Physical examination reveals irregular thickening in the upper outer quadrant, and sometimes the breast tissue has a nodular consistency. Cystic fluid may be aspirated and should be excised for cytological study if it reoccurs. A baseline mammogram is advisable.

Treatment. There is no specific treatment for fibrocystic breast disease, but some physicians suggest dietary restrictions on methylxanthine products such as coffee, chocolate, tea, and colas. Some physicians may prescribe vitamin E. Cysts may be aspirated for fluid and/or excised for cytological study.

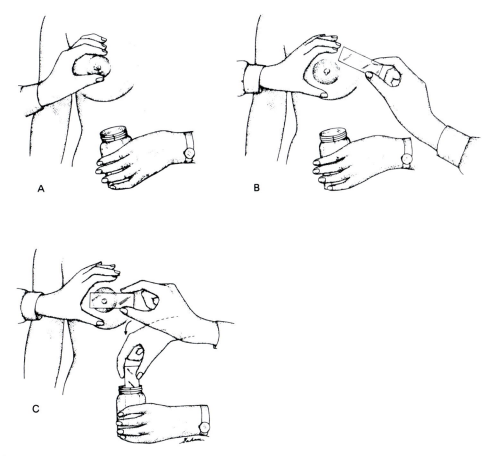

FIGURE 18-6

Obtaining nipple discharge specimen for cytological examination.
1. Wash nipple gently with cotton pledget; pat dry.
2. Gently strip duct and express fluid only until a small, pea-sized drop appears on nipple.
3. Obtain assistance of the patient in holding container of fixative solution near breast to receive prepared slide.
4. Stabilize breast with fingers and thumb of one hand (**A**).
5. Gently place one end of slide on nipple (**B**). Rapidly draw slide across nipple and immediately drop into fixative solution (**C**).
6. This may be repeated to secure additional specimens if necessary.

NOTE: Positive results are significant. Negative results may be falsely negative. This test is never used alone, but in conjunction with other diagnostic tests.
(Reproduced from Brunner LS, Suddarth DS: *The Lippincott Manual of Nursing Practice,* 4th ed. Philadelphia: J. B. Lippincott, 1986, p. 592.)

TABLE 18-3

CANCER IN WOMEN

Warning Signals	Risk Factors	Direction and Diagnosis
Breast		
Persistent breast changes: swelling, lumps, irritation, nipple retraction, pain, thickening, distortion, tenderness, scaling, dimpling, or discharge.	>50 years of age, personal or family history of breast cancer, 1st child born after age 30, or never having children.	Monthly breast self-exam. Professional breast exam every 3 years for ages 20–40 and annually for ages >40. Mammograms for asymptomatic women: baseline for ages 35–39, every 1–2 years for ages 40–49 and annually for ages >50. Diagnosed by fluid aspiration, needle biospy, and/or lumpectomy for cytology.
Uterine		
Bleeding between normal menstrual flow; vaginal discharge occurring after menopause.	Cervical cancers: Coitus at early age, numerous sex partners, cigarette smoking, certain STDs, poor genital hygiene.	Annual Pap smear with pelvic exam for sexually active women and/or women age 18 or older. After three successive, normal smears, physician may perform smear less frequently. Cervical biopsy to confirm diagnosis.
	Endometrial cancer: Long-term estrogen therapy, obesity, ovulation failure, and infertility.	Menopausal women at risk for endometrial cancer need an assessment of endometrial tissue. Diagnosed by endometrial biopsy; fractional curettage is most accurate.
Ovarian		
Often "silent," enlargement of abdomen, vague but persistent gastrointestinal complaints: stomach discomfort, distention, bloating, constipation, gas.	Advancing age, especially >60; nulliparous women; personal history of breast or endometrial cancer; family history of ovarian cancer; obesity. Other interrelated factors.	Periodic, thorough pelvic exam. Women age 40+ need annual cancer-related checkup. Women at risk need a CA 125 drawn. Laparoscopy or laparotomy to obtain tissue for cytology.

Guideline for Patient Follow-up

- Patients who have a family history for breast cancer should be followed more closely.

Cancer

All patients should be routinely checked for and educated about cancer. Patient education should include prevention, incidence, risk factors, early warning signs, and early detection measures (Table 18–3). Both verbal and written information should be provided to every patient. Patients who are at risk should be identified and advised accordingly. Treatment of malignant carcinomas usually involves surgery, radiation therapy, chemotherapy, or, more often, a combination of these. Treatment of benign neoplasms may involve excision of the neoplasm. In carcinoma-in-situ, precancerous stage, the treatment may involve cryotherapy, electrocauterization, or surgery.

MEDICAL ASSISTING ALERT

Early detection of cancer significantly improves the survival rate. Therefore, patient education about breast examination (Figure 18–7), early warning signs (see Table 18–3), and regular gynecological examinations is of utmost importancc.

4. Move around the breast in a set way. You can choose either the circle (A), the up and down line (B), or the wedge (C). Do it the same way every time. It will help you to make sure that you've gone over the entire breast area, and to remember how your breast feels each month.

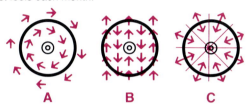

5. Now examine your left breast using right hand finger pads.

You might want to check your breasts while standing in front of a mirror right after you do your BSE each month. You might also want to do an extra BSE while you're in the shower. Your soapy hands will glide over the wet skin, making it easy to check how your breasts feel.

How To Do BSE

1. Lie down and put a pillow under your right shoulder. Place your right arm behind your head.
2. Use the finger pads of the three middle fingers on your left hand to feel for lumps or thickening. Your fingers pads are the top third of each finger.

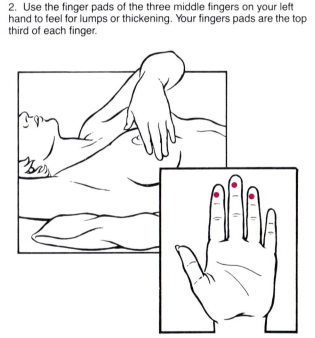

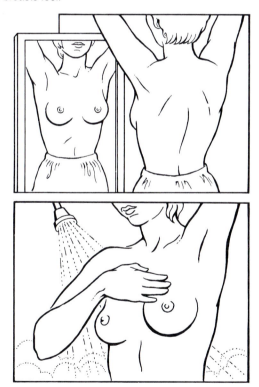

3. Press hard enough to know how your breast feels. If you're not sure how hard to press, ask your health care provider. Or try to copy the way your health care provider uses the finger pads during a breast exam. Learn what your breast feels like most of the time. A firm ridge in the lower curve of each breast is normal.

FIGURE 18–7

Breast self-examination. (Courtesy of the American Cancer Society.)

PROCEDURE

ASSISTING WITH COLPOSCOPY

PURPOSES

To locate source of abnormal cells; to select area for cervical, endocervical, and/or endometrial biopsy; and to evaluate tissue in the presence of cervical lesion, atypical Pap smear, or history of cervical dysplasia or cervical cancer.

MEDICAL ASSISTING ALERT

Colposcopy is the visual inspection of the cervix using a stereoscopic microscope that can magnify 6–40 times. If a biopsy is to be obtained, be sure that an informed consent has been received.

EQUIPMENT AND MATERIALS

Setup for pelvic examination
Long cotton applicators, sterile
Normal saline solution
3% acetic acid
Silver nitrate sticks or ferric subsulfate (Monsel's solution)
Biopsy forcep, sterile
Colposcope
The following, depending on location of biopsy:
    Uterine curette, sterile
    Uterine tenaculum, sterile
    Uterine sound, sterile
    Paracervical block for endocervical or endometrial biopsy
    Specimen container with preservative (10% formalin)
    Sterile gloves
    Sterile towel
    Sterile 4 × 4 gauze
    Povidone-iodine (Betadine)
    Sanitary napkin, minipad (panty liner), or tampon

PROCEDURAL STEPS

Patient Preparation

1. Be sure that the consent form has been filled out completely.
RATIONALE: Colposcopy with biopsy is an invasive procedure that requires a written consent.
2. Prepare the patient in same manner as in gynecological examination.
3. Caution the patient that there may be a sharp cramp at the time of biopsy.

Performance

4. Prepare room, equipment, and supplies for procedure.
NOTE: Be sure colposcope light is functioning properly.
5. Position the patient in the dorsal lithotomy position.
6. Assist the physician as necessary with gloving and materials.

  - Hand the physician an applicator saturated with normal saline, followed by an applicator saturated with acetic acid
  RATIONALE: Acetic acid swabbed on area improves visualization and aids in identifying suspicious tissue
  - After visual inspection with the colposcope, hand the physician an applicator saturated with Betadine
  RATIONALE: Area to be biopsied is prepared by swabbing with antiseptic solution to prevent pathogens from invading
  - The physician obtains biopsies at this time

7. Be prepared to receive the tissue specimen.
NOTE: The specimen should be immediately immersed in 10% formalin to preserve the tissue.
8. Label the specimen container with the patient's name, date, identification number, and site from which biopsy was obtained.
NOTE: Several areas may be biopsied; be sure to correctly identify the site from which each biopsy was obtained.
9. Prepare for specimen transport to the laboratory.

Follow-Through

10. If tampon is inserted, instruct the patient to remove the tampon in 5–6 hours.
11. Reinforce the physician's instructions.

Contraception

Considerations

Decisions regarding contraception may be made individually by the male or the female, or the couple may decide on a contraceptive method together. The role of the physician and/or medical assistant is to educate the patient about the various forms of contraception as part of health care management. The patient's religious, cultural, and personal beliefs and health history should be of utmost importance in counseling the patient about birth control.

MEDICAL ASSISTING ALERT

The medical assistant should be prepared to answer patient questions and reinforce the physician's instructions regarding various forms of contraception.

Oral Contraceptive (Birth Control Pill)

MEDICAL ASSISTING ALERT

Women who smoke cigarettes should be advised not to smoke while taking an oral contraceptive. Cigarette smoking (15 cigarettes/day or more) while taking an oral contraceptive increases the risk of severe cardiovascular side effects, especially in women 35 years or older.

The birth control pill (BCP) is a synthetic combination of various amounts of estrogen and progestin. The lowest dose that provides the desired effect is advised. A second type of BCP is available that contains only progesterone; it is often used when estrogen is contraindicated.

Preprescription Examination. Before the BCP is prescribed, the patient needs an initial breast and pelvic examination, including palpation of the liver and measurement of weight and blood pressure. The patient should be evaluated again in 3 months, and thereafter annually.

Contraindications. Contraindications for the BCP include known or suspected pregnancy, history of thrombophlebitis or thromboembolic disorders, cerebrovascular or coronary artery disease, undiagnosed genital bleeding, liver disease or impaired function, and known or suspected breast cancer or estrogen dependent neoplasia. The BCP should be discontinued immediately if patient has symptoms of thromboembolic or thrombotic disorders, pulmonary embolism, coronary or cerebral thrombosis, or liver dysfunction.

Side Effects. Side effects due to the estrogen in the BCP include breakthrough bleeding, nausea, vomiting, breast tenderness, fluid retention, increased blood pressure, and depression. The progesterone may cause amenorrhea, weight gain, acne, and nervousness. These side effects may be alleviated by changing the combination in the BCP.

Advantages. Advantages of the BCP include easy use, high rate of efficacy, and the fact that no special preparation is needed before coitus.

Guidelines for Instructing the Patient on Taking the Birth Control Pill

- The 21-day BCP should be taken at the same time each day, beginning on day 5 of menses and continuing for 21 consecutive days. Following the 21 days, the patient discontinues taking the BCP for 7 days; menses should occur within 1–4 days. The patient resumes taking the BCP after being off it 7 days.
- The 28-day BCP has seven placebos that are taken during the menses. With the 28-day BCP, the woman continues taking a pill (a placebo) each day through the menses. The 28-day BCP keeps the woman in the habit of taking a pill every day.
- If the patient resumes taking the BCP *after* the 8th day, she should use an additional form of contraception until the BCP has been taken for 7 consecutive days.
- Advise patient that if she is having breakthrough bleeding or spotting, she should use an additional form of birth control until the bleeding subsides.
- Advise patient that if one or two tablets are missed, she must take the missed tablet(s) as soon as she remembers and take the next tablet at the regularly scheduled time; an additional form of contraception should be used until the BCP has been taken for 7 consecutive days.
- Instruct the patient that if she misses 3 or more tablets, she should discard the rest of the prescription and use an alternative form of birth control.

Levonorgestrel Implants

An implant system is comprised of capsules that contain a synthetic hormone called levonorgestrel (a progestin), which is slowly and continuously released into the body. The Norplant System, manufactured by Wyeth Laboratories, Inc., a Wyeth-Ayerst Company, became available for consumer use in 1991 and at this writing is the only implant available for contraception. Pregnancy is prevented by a combination of factors, which include inhibiting ovulation and thickening of the cervical mucus.

The desired contraception is achieved within 24 hours of insertion. The implants may be removed at any time that fertility is desired. At 5 years, the Norplant System begins to lose its effectiveness and should be removed prior to the fifth anniversary of the insertion date.

Informed Consent. The subdermal placement of the capsules is a minor surgical procedure in which the capsules are positioned in the midportion of the upper arm; and as with all surgical procedures, an informed consent must be obtained prior to the insertion.

Patient Information. The manufacturer provides a product insert that informs patient of effectiveness, contraindications, risks, side effects, and warning signs of the implant system.

Advantages. The advantages of the levonorgestrel implants include their annual pregnancy rate (less than 1%), reversibility, and convenience. The Norplant System is effective for 5 years, and, once removed, each patient's ability to conceive will return.

Contraindications. The levonorgestrel implants are contraindicated in patients with acute liver disease, benign or malignant liver tumors, unexplained vaginal bleeding, breast cancer, thrombophlebitis, pulmonary embolism, or thrombosis of the eye.

Risks. The levonorgestrel implants do increase the risk of irregular menstrual bleeding, delayed or disappearance of follicles, and ectopic pregnancies (risk for ectopic pregnancy is no greater than risk with IUD or users of no method). At this writing it is unknown whether the implant will have similar risks as the oral contraceptives.

Side Effects. The most often reported side effect is menstrual cycle irregularities such as prolonged bleeding, spotting, and no bleeding for several months. The patient should be instructed to contact her physician if heavy bleeding occurs. Also, if the patient experiences normal menstrual cycles and misses a period, she should be evaluated for possible pregnancy. Other side effects include headache, nervousness, nausea, dizziness, ovarian and/or fallopian tube enlargement, dermatitis, acne, appetite change, mastalgia, weight gain, hirsutism, alopecia, and discoloration of skin at the site of implantation.

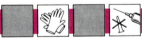

PROCEDURE

INSERTION OF LEVONORGESTREL IMPLANTS

PURPOSE

To prevent pregnancy.

 MEDICAL ASSISTING ALERT

The patient should schedule insertion within 7 days of the onset of menses.

EQUIPMENT AND MATERIALS

Norplant system kit, which contains trocar, scalpel, forceps, syringe, needles, skin closures, sterile gauze sponges and bandage, sterile drapes, and six levonorgestrel implants
Antiseptic solution with container
Sterile gloves
Local anesthetic with 22-gauge × 1½-inch needle and 5-ml syringe
Sterile gauze, extra
Light source
Sterile dressing forcep

PROCEDURAL STEPS

Patient Preparation

1. Ascertain that the patient has read and signed the consent form.

2. Advise the patient what to expect before each step.
   RATIONALE: Explanations aid in alleviating anxiety and enhance patient cooperation.
3. Position patient in supine position.

Performance

4. Prepare room, equipment, and supplies for implant insertion.
5. Assist physician as necessary, including gloving and gowning.
6. Assemble materials on sterile field:

   - Pour antiseptic solution into sterile container
   - Open syringe package and drop contents onto sterile field

7. Open Norplant system kit with sterile technique and either drop contents onto sterile field or allow physician to grasp contents with his or her sterile, gloved hand.
8. Adjust light source over area.
9. At this time, the physician applies antiseptic, administers anesthetic, accomplishes insertion, and closes the skin.
10. Apply sterile, dry compress over insertion site.
11. Wrap patient's arm with sterile gauze to maintain hemostasis.

Follow-Through

12. Observe patient for syncope and/or bleeding from insertion site.
13. Reinforce physician's instructions and answer any questions. Instruct patient that

    - Gauze wrap may be removed after 24 hours
    - Insertion site must be kept dry for 2 days
    - Skin closures should remain in place until healing has occurred (usually 3 days)
    - Tenderness, swelling, bruising, and some discoloration at insertion site can be expected
    - She must notify office of expulsion of implant; arm pain, bleeding, or pus at insertion site; severe lower abdominal pain; heavy vaginal bleeding; or migraines that are new or more frequent or more severe
    - Insertion site should be examined annually

14. Provide patient with written instructions about the date of insertion, date that implants must be removed, location of implants, and the name and location of the health care provider.
15. Initiate sanitization process for contaminants.

NOTE: Handle materials and instruments according to the Centers for Disease Control (CDC) Universal Precautions for blood and body fluid.

PROCEDURE

REMOVAL OF LEVONORGESTREL IMPLANTS

PURPOSE

To discontinue contraception or to change implants and continue same level of contraception.

MEDICAL ASSISTING ALERT

Patient should schedule the removal before the fifth anniversary of the date of insertion. If the patient desires to continue using Norplant, new implants can be inserted at the time of the removal. More time should be allotted for removal than for insertion.

EQUIPMENT AND MATERIALS

Antiseptic solution with container
Sterile drapes
Sterile gloves
Anesthetic with 5-ml syringe and 22-gauge × 1½-inch needle
#11 scalpel
Straight and curved mosquito forceps
Plain tissue and dressing forceps
Skin closures, sterile gauze, and compresses

PROCEDURAL STEPS

Patient Preparation

Same as for insertion.

Performance

1. Prepare room, equipment, and supplies for implant removal.
2. Assist physician as necessary, including gloving and gowning.
3. Assemble materials on sterile field:

   - Pour antiseptic solution into sterile container
   - Open syringe package and drop contents onto sterile field

4. Adjust light source over area.
5. At this time, physician applies antiseptic, administers anesthetic, excises capsules, and closes skin.
6. Apply sterile, dry compress over site.
7. Wrap arm with sterile gauze to maintain hemostasis.

Follow-Through

8. Observe patient for syncope and/or bleeding from site.
9. Reinforce the physician's instructions and answer any questions. Instruct patient that

   - Gauze wrap may be removed after 24 hours
   - Site must be kept clean and dry for 2 days
   - Skin closures should remain in place until healing has occurred (usually 3 days)
   - Tenderness, swelling, bruising, and some discoloration at site can be expected
   - She must notify office of arm pain or bleeding or pus at the insertion site

10. Initiate sanitization process for contaminants.

NOTE: Handle materials and instruments according to the CDC Universal Precautions for blood and body fluid.

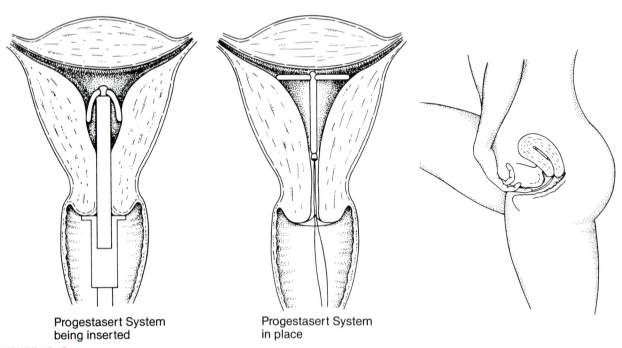

FIGURE 18-8

Insertion of intrauterine device. (Reproduced from Kinn ME, Derge EF: *The Medical Assistant: Administrative and Clinical*, 6th ed. Philadelphia: W. B. Saunders, 1988, p. 559.)

Intrauterine Device

The Intrauterine device (IUD) is a sterile metal or plastic device that is inserted into the uterine cavity for the purpose of preventing pregnancy (Figure 18-8). Currently the U.S. Food and Drug Administration has approved two IUDs for consumer use: the Progestasert and the ParaGard.

The IUD is indicated in women who are in monogamous relationships, are multiparous, and have no history of PID.

Informed Consent. The IUD is inserted under sterile conditions and like all surgical procedures requires an informed written consent. The manufacturers of IUDs provide a product insert that informs patient of risks, alternatives, and efficacy of the IUD that is to be read and signed by the patient. This document should then be retained in the patient's medical record and a copy provided to the patient.

Preprescription Examination. A gynecological examination with Pap smear and appropriate cultures should be conducted before insertion is scheduled. Pregnancy must be ruled out. Patient should be reexamined after first menses postinsertion.

Insertion. The procedure is usually performed during menses to ensure that patient is most likely not pregnant and because insertion may be easier. Also the cramping and slight bleeding that may accompany the insertion will not falsely alarm the patient.

IUDs must be changed at intervals specified by the manufacturer and patient should be informed of that date. The Progestasert is changed at 12-month intervals and the Paragard must be changed within eight years.

Contraindications. Contraindications include history or risk of ectopic pregnancy, multiple sexual partners, pregnancy or suspicion of pregnancy, abnormalities of the uterus causing distortion of cavity, history or risk of PID, known or suspected uterine or cervical malignancy, increased susceptibility to infections, history or presence of a sexually transmitted disease (STD), postpartum endometritis or infected abortion within 3 months, undiagnosed genital bleeding, genital actinomycosis, intravenous drug abuse, and presence of an IUD previously inserted.

Side Effects. Adverse reactions include increased bleeding and pain during menses and increased risk of PID and ectopic pregnancy.

Advantages. The advantages of the IUD include its high rate of effectiveness, no need for preparation before coitus, and the fact that the contraceptive effect is local and long-lasting.

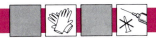

PROCEDURE

INSERTION OF INTRAUTERINE DEVICE

PURPOSE

To prevent pregnancy.

 MEDICAL ASSISTING ALERT

Advise the patient to notify the office if she bleeds between periods; has missed a period; experiences heavy bleeding, severe cramping, unusual vaginal discharge, or lower abdominal pain; has unexplained fever or chills; or is unable to locate string or string feels longer.

EQUIPMENT AND MATERIALS

Vaginal speculum, appropriate size
Sterile uterine sponge forcep
Sterile uterine tenaculum
Sterile uterine sound
Sterile towels
Scissors
Antiseptic solution with container
Sterile gauze (4 × 4)
IUD with insertion kit
Sterile gloves
Light source
Sanitary pad and cleansing tissues
CDC Universal Precautions barriers
Anesthetic, optional

PROCEDURAL STEPS

Patient Preparation

1. Ascertain that the patient has read and signed the consent form.
   RATIONALE: Federal regulations require an informed consent for IUD insertion, meaning that patient must be given product information and counseling about the safety and efficacy of the IUD.
2. Advise the patient of what to expect prior to each step.
   RATIONALE: Explanations aid in alleviating anxiety and enhance patient cooperation.
3. Prepare patient in same manner as for a gynecological examination (see page 442).

Performance

4. Prepare room, equipment, and supplies for IUD insertion.
5. Maintain sterile technique in setting up field.
6. Pour antiseptic solution into sterile container on field.

   NOTE: Some physicians prefer to have a package of sterile 4 × 4 gauzes opened and antiseptic poured directly onto gauze; this should not be done until the physician is ready to prepare the cervix.

7. Assist the physician as necessary, including gloving and gowning.
8. Focus light source on vaginal orifice.
9. Open IUD insertion kit with sterile technique and either drop contents onto sterile field or allow the physician to grasp contents with his or her sterile, gloved hand.
10. Insertion of IUD is accomplished at this time.

Follow-Through

11. Wipe perineum from anterior to posterior with cleansing tissue.
    RATIONALE: Wiping from anterior to posterior avoids vaginal contamination from rectum and removes excess antiseptic solution and body fluids.
12. Instruct the patient on the frequency of checking and how to check for correct placement of IUD.
13. Have the patient demonstrate how to check for correct placement of IUD nylon string (see Figure 18–5).
    RATIONALE: Correct placement of the nylon string indicates that the IUD remains properly positioned.
14. Offer patient a sanitary pad (minipad or panty liner) and cleansing tissue.
    RATIONALE: There will most likely be some spotting from the procedure, and patient may be menstruating.
15. Reinforce the physician's instructions and answer any questions.
16. Initiate sanitization process for contaminants.

NOTE: Handle insertion device and instruments according to the CDC Universal Precautions for blood and body fluid.

Diaphragm

The diaphragm is a dome-shaped rubber cup that fits snugly over the cervix and serves as a barrier to sperm. The inside and rim of diaphragm should be covered with about 1½ teaspoons of spermicide before each use.

The diaphragm is indicated for women who prefer not to use the BCP or IUD or are not suited for these methods because of patient history and existing conditions.

The diaphragm is individually sized for the patient by a health professional, and periodically a new size must be prescribed. The size of the diaphragm is related to weight fluctuations and gravidity.

The diaphragm must be inserted immediately before sexual intercourse and left in place 6–8 hours after intercourse (Figure 18–9). Continuous wearing of the diaphragm may increase the risk of infection. Therefore, it should not be left in place for more than 24 hours.

Instruct the patient to routinely check diaphragm for holes or tears by holding up to light.

1 INSERTING THE DIAPHRAGM

The diaphragm can be inserted while standing with one leg on a low chair or stool, lying down, squatting, or sitting forward on the edge of a chair. Remember, however, that the position of the cervix and vaginal vault changes with each position that you take, so always be certain that the cervix is completely covered.

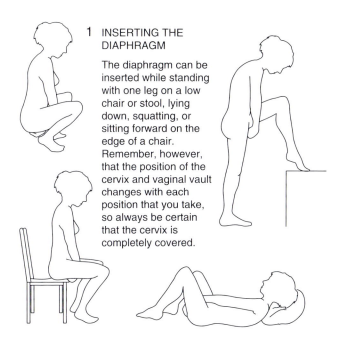

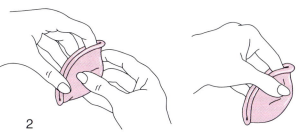

2

Holding the diaphragm with the dome down, *press the two notches in the diaphragm lip together.* Now spread the lips of the vagina with one hand and with the other hand gently insert the diaphragm (dome down) into the vagina along the rear wall as far as it will comfortably go. Your index finger can guide the diaphragm as you gently push it into place. *Do not pinch the diaphragm.*

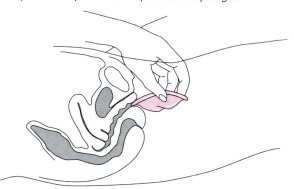

3

POSITIONING THE DIAPHRAGM

Tuck the front rim of the diaphragm up into the pubic notch so it is pressed against the front wall of the vagina.

4

As an added precaution, feel the cervix through the silicone-rubber shield (it is shaped like the tip of a dented nose) to make certain that the diaphragm is securely in place and that the entire cervix is covered.

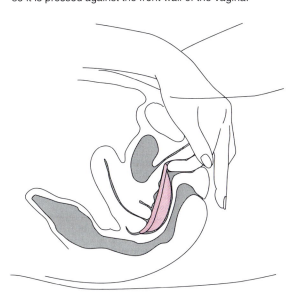

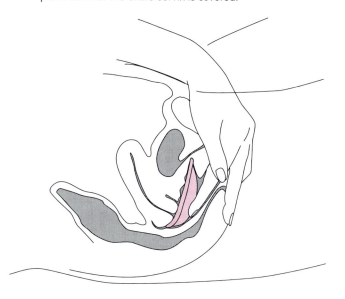

FIGURE 18-9

Insertion and removal of diaphragm. (Courtesy of Milex Products, Inc. Chicago, IL.)

Illustration continued on following page

5

Do not douche or remove the diaphragm for at least six hours after intercourse. Diaphragm should be removed as soon after this as possible. Additional gel should be applied if you desire to have intercourse again.

Diaphragm should never be left in place continuously, over 24 hours.

To reapply, tear open a new gel pak and squeeze contents on one or two fingers.

6

Insert digitally as shown to deposit gel in vagina and at the same time make sure the diaphragm silicone covers the cervix. This added precaution should be followed in all gel paks or tube applications of spermicide.

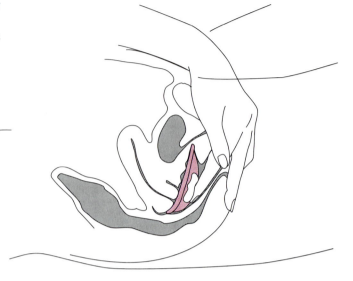

7

REMOVING THE DIAPHRAGM

To remove the diaphragm, insert your index finger behind the front rim to break the suction. With your finger under the rim pull the diaphragm down and withdraw it, but be careful not to puncture the silicone dome with your finger nail. *Do not pinch the diaphragm*–simply pull it gently with your finger.

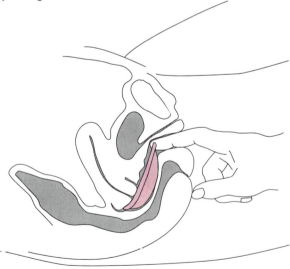

8

CARE OF THE DIAPHRAGM

After removal, wash the diaphragm in mild soap and lukewarm water, rinse in clear water and dry carefully. Mild soap should be the only soap used. When it is thoroughly dried, dust it with cornstarch (do not use talc, baby powder, etc.) and place the diaphragm in its original container. Do not use cold cream, petroleum jelly, or any other product that is not specifically intended for use with a diaphragm. Do not place the diaphragm on varnished or painted surface. Before each use, hold the diaphragm up to a bright light to check for cracks or holes.

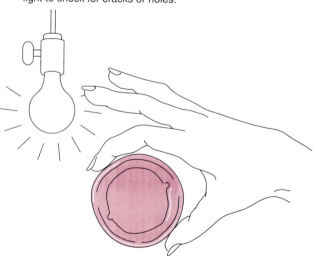

FIGURE 18–9 *Continued*

PROCEDURE

SIZING OF DIAPHRAGM

PURPOSE

Making sure diaphragm is of the correct size is to prevent pregnancy.

MEDICAL ASSISTING ALERT

Inform the patient that if her weight changes by 15 pounds or more after each pregnancy, she will need to have the diaphragm resized.

EQUIPMENT AND MATERIALS

Gloves
Diaphragm-sizing kit
Lubricant, water soluble
Cleansing tissue
Light source

PROCEDURAL STEPS

Patient Preparation

1. Counsel the patient regarding the various methods of contraception before the visit.
2. Prepare patient in same manner as for gynecological examination, described at the beginning of this chapter.

Performance

3. Prepare room, equipment, and supplies for diaphragm sizing.
4. Position the patient in the dorsal lithotomy position.
5. Assist the physician with gloving and materials as necessary.
6. Focus light on vaginal orifice.

NOTE: The physician determines appropriate size for diaphragm at this time.

Follow-Through

7. Instruct the patient on manual insertion and removal of diaphragm.

   - Use lubricant to demonstrate how to cover diaphragm with spermicide

8. Have patient demonstrate the insertion.
9. Reinforce patient instruction and allow for questions.

NOTE: Manufacturers of the diaphragm, such as Milex Products, Inc., have excellent materials available to assist with patient instruction.

Cervical Cap

The cervical cap is similar to the diaphragm but is smaller and is held in place by suction; the degree of suction depends on the fit. The cervical cap must be sized by a health professional; the procedure for sizing is similar to that for the diaphragm. Spermicidals should be used in conjunction with the cap.

Advantage. The advantage of the cervical cap is that it may be inserted for up to 72 hours and not just prior to intercourse. Because of the increased risk of infection, it is advisable to limit wearing to 24 hours.

Vaginal Foams, Creams, Suppositories, and Sponges

These medicated agents contain spermicide and must be inserted into the vaginal orifice just before sexual intercourse. Unlike the foams, creams, and suppositories, the contraceptive sponge remains effective for 24 hours. The patient should be directed to read manufacturers' directions for the contraceptive product chosen.

Condoms

The condom is a penile sheath that serves as a barrier to sperm and, if used properly, discourages the transmission of STDs. The use of a spermicide enhances the effectiveness of the condom.

MEDICAL ASSISTING ALERT

The condom is also advisable for prevention of STDs. Patients who have multiple sexual partners should be advised accordingly.

The condom is a good choice for patients who have multiple sexual partners or who are exposed to STDs. There are a wide variety of condoms on the market, and patients should be advised to read manufacturers' directions for use. Advise patients to never use a condom that is more than 2 years old.

Rhythm Method

MEDICAL ASSISTING ALERT

Women who have irregular menstrual cycles should be advised to not use this method of contraception.

The rhythm method is based on abstinence during the fertile period and is appropriate only for women who have normal, regular periods. To calculate the fertile period, it is necessary to keep a record of menstrual cycles for 8–12 months.

The fertile period is from 3 days before to 7 days after ovulation. It is also possible to determine when ovulation takes place by daily readings of body temperature, since the temperature is elevated after ovulation takes place.

Ovulation Method

The patient's fertile period may be determined by charting her basal body temperature, the quantity of cervical mucus, or a combination of these two parameters (the symptothermal method). This is based on the fact that a unique "fertile mucus" appears in the vaginal area at the time of ovulation. The mucus usually appears 3 days prior to ovulation. It is cloudy at first, then becomes clear, similar in appearance and consistency to the white of an uncooked egg. Ovulation occurs within 24–48 hours of the peak of the wetness. Abstinence is recommended from the first appearance of the fertile mucus through the peak of wetness and then for another 72 hours. The advantage of this method is that it can be used by women with irregular menstrual cycles and does not rely on extensive keeping of accurate records of menstrual cycles.

NOTE: The medical assistant should have available temperature charts for patient use and should be prepared to answer questions regarding this method of contraception.

Efficacy of Methods of Contraception

Method	Efficacy
Levonorgestrel implant	99%
Oral contraceptive	98%
Intrauterine device	95%
Condom	90%
Contraceptive sponge	85%
Vaginal foam, cream, suppository	82%
Cervical cap	82%
Diaphragm	81%

The rates of efficacy are based on compliance with recommended use. Data on cervical cap and implants are from patient labeling, Norplant system (Pl 4069-1). Philadelphia: Wyeth Laboratories, a Wyeth-Ayerst Company, 1990. All other data are from Ladewig PW, London ML, Olds SB: *Essentials of Maternal-Newborn Nursing*, 2nd ed. Redwood City, CA: Benjamin/Cummings Publishing Company, 1990.

OBSTETRICS

Terminology

Abortus: Fetal death before 20 weeks' gestation
Abortion: Loss of pregnancy before 20 weeks' gestation; may be induced or spontaneous
Antepartum: Time before onset of labor
Braxton-Hicks sign: Painless, intermittent uterine contractions, usually occurring in last trimester
Chadwick's sign: Color of vagina and cervix becomes bluish to purple, indicating pregnancy
Ectopic pregnancy: Pregnancy located outside the uterine cavity

Expected date of confinement (EDC): Approximate date birth is expected

Gestation: Length of time from conception to birth; period of intrauterine growth

Gestational weeks: Periods by which pregnancies are usually dated, based on the first day of the last menstrual period

Goodell's sign: Softening of the cervix, which indicates pregnancy

Gravid: Pregnant

Gravida: A pregnant woman

Hegar's sign: Softening of the lower third of the uterus, occurring at about 6–8 weeks after last menstrual period.

Human chorionic gonadotropin (hCG): Hormone produced by placenta to maintain pregnancy; detection of hCG is used to diagnose pregnancy

Intrauterine pregnancy (IUP): Pregnancy located in the uterus

Last menstrual period (LMP): First day of last menstrual period

Multigravida: Woman who has been pregnant more than once

Multipara: Woman who has produced more than one viable offspring

Nagele's rule: Formula for estimating the duration of pregnancy: To get the EDC add 7 days to the first day of the last normal menstrual period; subtract 3 months and add 1 year

Nulligravida: Woman who has never been pregnant

Nullipara: Woman who has not produced a viable offspring, regardless of number of pregnancies

Parity: Pregnancies that resulted in a viable birth ("para") (see Table 18–4)

Primigravida: Woman who is pregnant for the first time

Primipara: Woman delivering first child after 20 weeks' gestation

Quickening: First movements of fetus, occurring at about 16 weeks in multipara women and 18 weeks in primigravida women

Presumptive Evidence of Pregnancy

Patient Symptoms

- Absence of expected menses (>1 week)
- Breast engorgement and tenderness
- Nipples become more pigmented and larger
- Nausea and occasional vomiting
- Fatigue
- Possible abdominal bloating
- Urinary frequency

Physician's Findings

- Positive Hegar's sign
- Softened cervix (Goodell's sign)
- Positive Chadwick's sign
- Fresh reddish striae on abdomen and breasts
- Enlargement of uterus

Confirmation of Pregnancy

- Presence of fetal heart tones detected by physician or Doppler ultrasound device
- Detection of fetal movements by physician
- Ultrasound detection of amniotic sac with fetus
- Visualization of fetus via x-ray (not recommended today)
- Elevated (hCG) levels

Routine Prenatal Care

Initial Visit

Obtain complete health history from the patient, including family medical history, patient's medical history, and present medical condition (Figure 18–10). The present obstetrical condition must be detailed and complete. Data include the following:

- LMP with menstrual history
- Gravidity and parity with history of past pregnancies
- EDC
- Symptoms
- Medications used since LMP and those currently used
- Social habits: consumption of nicotine, alcohol, caffeine, and recreational drugs
- Activity and/or habits: sleep patterns and exercise (type, duration, and frequency)
- Employment: screen for occupational hazards

TABLE 18–4

EXAMPLES OF GRAVIDITY AND PARITY

Patient Situation	Gravida	Para	Abortus
Never been pregnant	0	0	0
Pregnant for the first time	1	0	0
Third pregnancy, two viable births	3	2	0
Three abortions, no viable births	3	0	3
Fourth pregnancy, two viable births, one abortion	4	2	1
Two pregnancies, two abortions	2	0	2

SAMPLE PRENATAL HISTORY

DATE _____ HOSPITAL FOR DELIVERY _____ REFERRED BY _____

NAME _____ ADDRESS _____

OCCUPATION _____ PHONE _____ CONTACT FOR EMERGENCY _____

AGE _____ RACE _____ GRAVIDA _____ PARA _____ ABORTUS _____ CONTRACEPTION _____

ABO _____ Rh _____ PCV _____ EDC _____ ALLERGIES _____

LMP _____ AGE AT MENARCHE _____ REGULARITY OF MENSTRUATION _____

PREVIOUS PREGNANCIES

No	DOB	Gestation	WT	Sex	Hrs Labor	EPIS	Hosp/Phys	ANES	Comment

Sexually transmitted diseases: SYPHILIS _____ HERPES _____ GONORRHEA _____ OTHER _____

MEDICATIONS & DRUGS _____

EXERCISE: YES ___ NO ___ TYPE & FREQUENCY _____

SMOKES: YES ___ NO ___ PPD ___ ALCOHOL: ___ NEVER ___ OCCASIONALLY ___ DAILY, quantity _____

DIETARY HISTORY _____

SURGERIES _____

FAMILY MEDICAL HISTORY: HEART ___ HYPERT ___ DIAB ___ KIDNEY ___ CANCER ___ THYROID ___ SEIZURES ___

OTHER _____

PRENATAL MEDICAL HISTORY _____

PHYSICAL: BP ___ HT ___ WT ___ GLUCOSE SCREEN: DATE/RESULTS _____

ULTRASOUND: date/findings _____ AFP: date/level _____

PELVIC _____

CERVIX _____

BREAST _____ PRENATAL VIT _____ IRON _____

FIGURE 18-10
Sample prenatal history and physical form. (Modified from the prenatal history and physical form of the Henderson and Walton Women's Center, P.C., Birmingham, AL.)

ABDOMEN _____ HEART _____ LUNGS _____

BREAST FEEDING _____ BOTTLE FEEDING _____ PEDIATRICIAN _____ ANES _____

PAP SMEAR CLASS _____ VDRL _____ RUB _____ CMV _____

Date	WT	Urine	PCV	BP	FUNDUS	FHT	FM	Gestation	Comments/Procedures

FIGURE 18–10 Continued

- Diet history: weight fluctuation, meals per day, food likes and dislikes, special diets
- Psychosocial concerns: reaction to pregnancy, family support, significant other
- Risk factors: factors that increase the chances of a poor fetal and/or maternal outcome, such as maternal age, height and weight, disease, socioeconomic status, and genetic history

A complete physical examination includes a complete examination of all body systems, specifically:

- Weight and height
- Blood pressure
- Pelvic examination with a Pap smear
- Pelvimetry
- Listening for fetal heart tones
- Palpation of fundal height
- Breast and nipple examination

Equipment and materials for the initial physical examination include

- Patient drapes (breast towel, full drape)
- Disposable gloves
- Vaginal speculum
- Microscopic slides
- Fixative spray
- Laboratory request form
- Label for specimen identification
- Uterine dressing forceps
- Uterine sponge forceps
- Lubricant, water soluble
- Cotton applicators
- Cervical spatula
- Cleansing tissues
- Blood and body fluid protection barriers
- External fetalscope
- Measuring tape

Obstetrical Disorders

MEDICAL ASSISTING ALERT

Obstetrical patients who encounter any problems with the pregnancy are usually very anxious about the safety of their baby and need a lot of reassurance about the positive aspects without false reassurance. The medical assistant needs to allot extra time to listen to these patients, explain procedures, and answer questions.

Spontaneous Abortion

MEDICAL ASSISTING ALERT

Because the medical assistant often relays information to the physician, he or she needs to know the early signs of impending abortion and septic abortion to alert the physician and advise patient. The medical assistant may need to make arrangements for admission to hospital or for diagnostic and therapeutic procedures.

Spontaneous abortion occurs when the pregnancy terminates before the 20th week of gestation. The abortion is due to a fetal or maternal condition and not to any instrumentation.

Spontaneous abortion may be classified and treated as follows:

- **Threatened:** Bleeding and/or cramping occur within the first 20 weeks of pregnancy. Treatment is usually bed rest and avoidance of coitus until symptoms subside.
- **Inevitable:** Patient feels intolerable pain with bleeding and/or rupture of membranes, and, upon examination, the internal cervical os is dilated. There is no fetal survival with inevitable abortion. Treatment is D & C of the uterine cavity.
- **Incomplete:** Part of the products of conception have passed through the cervical canal. Treatment is D & C.
- **Complete:** All of the products of conception have been expelled from the uterine cavity; pain and bleeding will subside. Treatment may be simply watching the patient for further bleeding or infection or may include D & C.

Missed Abortion

Missed abortion is when the fetus dies and is retained for a minimum of 4 weeks in the uterine cavity. Diagnosis is confirmed by ultrasound, and treatment is usually either induction of labor with oxytocin or dilatation and evacuation of the dead fetus. Maternal infection is a major concern.

Septic Abortion

Septic abortion, whether induced or spontaneous, refers to an abortion that results in maternal infection. This is characterized by chills, fever, uterine tenderness, and abdominal pain. If treatment is delayed, the condition progresses to septicemia and septic shock. Treatment includes complete evacuation of products of conception and antibiotic therapy.

Hyperemesis Gravidarum

With this condition, there is unrelenting nausea and vomiting that causes fluid and electrolyte imbalance, and dehydration. The patient fails to gain weight and may even lose weight. She is hospitalized for intravenous fluid therapy to correct the fluid and electrolyte imbalance; antiemetics and sedatives are administered as necessary.

Supine Hypotension

Supine hypotension occurs when patient near term lies in a supine position. The patient's arte-

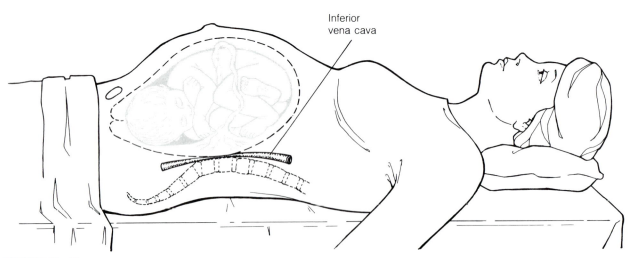

FIGURE 18-11

Vena caval syndrome. The gravid uterus compresses the vena cava when the woman is supine. This reduces the blood flow returning to the heart and may cause maternal hypotension. (Reproduced from Ladewig P, London ML, Olds SB: *Essentials of Maternal–Newborn Nursing*, 2nd ed. Menlo Park, CA: Addison-Wesley Nursing, a division of the Benjamin/Cummings Publishing Company, 1990, p. 164.)

rial blood pressure drops due to the fetal pressure on the abdominal aorta (Figure 18–11).

MEDICAL ASSISTING ALERT

Avoid leaving a third-trimester patient in supine position as this may cause hypotension and fetal distress. Advise patients near term to sleep/rest on their sides and avoid lying flat on their backs.

Signs and Symptoms

- Light-headedness
- Nausea and vomiting
- Bradycardia
- Hypotension
- Fetal distress (fetal bradycardia)

Treatment. Turn the patient onto her left side and monitor fetal heart rate and maternal blood pressure, heart rate, and respiratory rate; advise the physician immediately. Be prepared to administer oxygen.

Preeclampsia (Toxemia)

This condition is also known as pregnancy-induced hypertension. Preeclampsia is characterized by proteinuria, generalized edema, and increased blood pressure. Symptoms usually occur in primigravida and after the 20th gestational week. Treatment includes monitoring fetal growth by ultrasound, increasing frequency of prenatal visits, ordering renal function studies and possibly administering antihypertensive drugs. Preeclampsia requires very close monitoring by the physician and staff, because it can progress very rapidly to eclampsia.

MEDICAL ASSISTING ALERT

Patients with preeclampsia are frequently placed on complete bed rest, and if condition remains unimproved, patients must be hospitalized. While on bed rest, patients are advised to rest on their left side and increase their water intake.

Eclampsia

Eclampsia is preeclampsia characterized by convulsion and/or coma. The progression from preeclampsia to eclampsia may be quite sudden and constitutes an emergency situation. Treatment is similar to that for preeclampsia, but is more progressive. Seizures must be controlled, and delivery of the infant must be accomplished once patient is responsive and oriented.

Abruptio Placentae

Abruptio placentae is a premature separation of the placenta from the uterus. The symptoms and severity depend on the degree of separation. Symptoms include pain, uterine tenderness, fetal distress or even death, bleeding, and signs of impending shock. The bleeding that occurs may be obscured because the bleed is retroplacental and accumulating in the amniotic fluid, or it may be seen as dark blood from the cervix. Diagnosis is based on symptoms and ultrasound. If bleeding is minimal and fetal heart rate is normal, the patient may be treated with bed rest and close observation. If bleeding persists and/or maternal or fetal condition changes for the worse, immediate delivery is necessary.

Placenta Previa

In this condition, the placenta is implanted partially or completely over the internal cervical os, which makes delivery of fetus before delivery of the placenta difficult. Placenta previa is described according to how near the os the placenta is or how much of the os is covered.

Signs of placenta previa include painless, vaginal bleeding with sudden onset. Ultrasound is used to diagnose the condition and differentiate it from abruptio placentae. Patients who have minimum bleeding and are not near term are confined to bed rest until symptoms subside. Patients near term or those with heavy or recurrent bleeding need immediate delivery.

Ectopic Pregnancy

An ectopic pregnancy occurs when implantation is outside the uterine cavity; most often, implantation occurs in the fallopian tube. Ectopic pregnancy is characterized by spotting of blood and cramping pain beginning soon after the missed period. Bleeding may be gradual, causing pain and tenderness, or hemorrhage with shock may occur. When ectopic pregnancy is suspected, a hCG level is obtained. If the hCG is positive for pregnancy, then the diagnosis should be confirmed with an ultrasound. If intraperitoneal pregnancy, then the diagnosis should be confirmed with ultrasound. If intraperitoneal bleeding is suspected, then a culdocentesis may be performed to confirm a rupture. Treatment is surgical removal of the products of conception and preservation of the tube, which is accomplished by laparoscopy or laparotomy.

Obstetrical Diagnostic Procedures

MEDICAL ASSISTING ALERT

The medical assistant may be responsible for ordering or scheduling the diagnostic procedures and providing the initial patient instructions about the procedure. The hospital or diagnostic facility should be contacted about any special patient instructions. The medical assistant needs to include the facility name, address, and phone number; diagnostic tests; and special instructions and information from the office procedure manual. The patient should be given oral and written information about location, date, and time and special instructions about the procedure.

Fetal Monitoring

Fetal monitoring may be accomplished by either internal or external method. External monitoring by auscultation using a fetoscope or by an electronic fetal monitoring device is appropriate for normal, routine obstetrical examinations. Internal monitoring requires hospitalization and is usually reserved for the high-risk patient whose membranes are ruptured. The electronic device is proving to be more reliable when assessing the fetal heart rate.

Non-Stress Test

The non-stress test (NST) is used to evaluate the fetal heart rate compared to the fetal activity and spontaneous uterine contractions. Because contractions are not induced in the NST, it is a noninvasive procedure. The recording is usually continued for 20–30 minutes and requires no prior patient preparation.

Oxytocin Challenge Test

The oxytocin challenge test (OCT), a contraction stress test, is used to determine how well a fetus will tolerate labor and delivery. The OCT is indicated for postterm pregnancies, nonreactive NST, intrauterine growth retardation, and other medical conditions. Contractions are induced in the OCT by administering oxytocin intravenously or by nipple stimulation to induce a minimum of three contractions within 10 minutes. Like the NST, the fetal heart rate in response to the uterine contractions is evaluated; fetal activity is also monitored. The OCT is usually performed in the hospital (outpatient unit) since the patient is at risk of going into labor.

MEDICAL ASSISTING ALERT

Because the patient may go into active labor and require anesthesia, the medical assistant should instruct her to not eat within 6 hours of the test.

Ultrasonography

Ultrasonography is the use of high-frequency sound waves to produce an image of internal structures, abnormal and normal. In obstetrics, the ultrasound is used to assess the size, age, and sometimes sex of the fetus. In addition, the ultrasound can diagnose multiple fetuses and some abnormal maternal and fetal conditions. Some conditions that are often identified on ultrasound are placenta previa, abruptio placentae, neurotube defects, and anatomical defects. Some physicians request ultrasounds on all obstetrical patients, and others request the test only if indicated.

Alpha-Fetoprotein

Alpha-fetoprotein (AFP) is a product of the fetal liver and can be found in the maternal serum; the level in the maternal serum slowly increases as the pregnancy progresses. Abnormally high levels in the maternal serum increase the risk of open neurotube defect in fetus, other fetal abnormalities, and multiple fetuses. The maternal serum is drawn between the 15th and 19th weeks of gestation. Ultrasound is indicated for elevated AFPs to rule out open neurotube defect or multiple births or to reevaluate the fetal age.

MEDICAL ASSISTING ALERT

The normal level of AFP varies with the week of gestation; therefore, the laboratory request must include as accurate a statement of gestation weeks as possible.

Postpartum Care

Postpartum care after the patient is discharged from the hospital depends on whether the patient delivered vaginally or by cesarean section and what, if any, complications occurred during pregnancy.

First Postpartum Visit

1. The medical assistant obtains the patient's weight, vital signs, hematocrit, and hemoglobin levels.
2. The physician performs a complete gynecological examination with particular attention to the breasts, uterine size, vaginal discharge (lochia), surgical wounds (episiotomy, abdominal incision), and healing of lacerations.
3. The physician along with medical assistant assesses the patient's adjustment to parenting, including infant care, attachment to infant, and family planning (contraception).
4. The medical assistant prepares the examination room and patient in same manner as for a gynecological examination (discussed at the beginning of this chapter).

> **MEDICAL ASSISTING ALERT**
>
> Often, patients who are breastfeeding may call the office because their nipples are sore or cracked. The medical assistant may reinforce instructions on the care of nipples while breastfeeding. If nipples are cracked or there are signs of infection, patient should be scheduled for appointment.

Guidelines for Treating Nipple Soreness or Cracked Nipples

- Be sure the infant has as much areola, not just the nipple, in his or her mouth as possible.
- Encourage patient to clean milk from nipples with water and apply breast cream or A & D ointment around nipple (not over the duct).
- Patient should allow nipples to air dry.
- Instruct patient to change breast pads frequently.
- Suggest alternate breastfeeding positions, for example, from side-lying to upright with infant cradled, to upright with infant tucked under arm on same side infant is nursing, or other positions.
- Instruct patient to break suction between infant and nipple by inserting her finger into the infant's mouth.
- If nipple is cracked, instruct patient to discontinue feeding on that side; however, the affected breast must be emptied on same schedule by pumping manually or with breast pump. She may resume breastfeeding on that side as soon as possible, usually 2–3 days.
- The patient may find that a nipple shield helps.

Infertility

Infertility is defined as the inability of a couple to either conceive or produce a living child. The etiologies of infertility are numerous and include ovulation failure, cervical mucus that is hostile to sperm, low sperm count, occluded fallopian tubes, and/or endometriosis.

Alternatives for couples who cannot conceive include in vitro and in vivo fertilization managed by a fertility specialist.

> **MEDICAL ASSISTING ALERT**
>
> Some patients may be uncomfortable talking about infertility and the diagnostic procedures. The medical assistant must be direct and matter-of-fact when instructing patient about procedures. Encourage questions by letting patient know that the testing may be unpleasant but is important in identifying problems causing infertility.

Diagnostic Procedures for Infertility

Basal Body Temperature (BBT) Charting. Charting the BBT aids the physician in identifying ovulation problems. The patient must be instructed on how to complete the chart; when to take the BBT; and to note changes such as stress, gastrointestinal problems, headaches, and medications.

The medical assistant should reinforce the physician's instructions:

- The patient should use only the BBT thermometer that measures the degrees in tenths, which will show slight changes in the body temperature.
- The patient should take her temperature before getting out of the bed each morning, at the same time.

- The patient should consistently use the same site for measuring the body temperature — axillary, oral, or rectal.
- Specify the time that the thermometer should be left in place, depending on the anatomical site the patient is using.
- Be sure patient shakes thermometer down immediately after recording the temperature.

MEDICAL ASSISTING ALERT

Any activity may cause the body temperature to rise slightly, which interferes in accurately identifying the process of ovulation. Instruct the patient that the temperature must be obtained *before* any activity.

Cervical Mucus Test. This is a test for elasticity (Spinnbarkeit) and ferning of the mucus. The time at which cervical mucus can be drawn to the maximum length usually precedes or coincides with the time of ovulation (see Ovulation Method of Contraception, above). Ferning is the appearance of a fern-like pattern in a dried cervical mucus specimen, an indication of the presence of estrogen. The medical assistant prepares the patient in manner similar to that for a gynecological examination (discussed at the beginning of this chapter). In addition to the gynecological setup, the medical assistant needs to obtain two microscopic slides for the test for elasticity, one of which will be used for the ferning. The physician tests for elasticity by placing cervical mucus on one slide and using the second slide to stretch the mucus. The mucus should stretch about 5–6 cm. Once the cervical mucus is allowed to air dry, the physician will observe the ferning under a microscope.

Postcoital Test. The postcoital test is used to evaluate the number and motility of the sperm with the cervical mucus. The couple is asked to have intercourse on an expected date of ovulation, and examination of the female occurs within 2–6 hours of intercourse. In addition to the gynecological setup, the medical assistant should obtain microscopic slides and a rubber catheter with a 5–10-ml syringe attached. The syringe is used to aspirate the specimen from the cervical os.

Hysterosalpingogram (HSG). This is a radiographic procedure used to determine tubal patency. The procedure requires a contrast media (radiopaque) to be injected through the cervical os and into the fallopian tubes. The medical assistant is responsible for scheduling this invasive procedure.

Semen Analysis. Semen analysis evaluates numerous characteristics, including the sperm count and the pH, motility, and volume of semen. The male is provided a sterile specimen container and instructed to provide a specimen of semen by masturbating or by interrupting coitus and ejaculating into cup. The specimen must be delivered to the office within 2 hours of collection. Instruct patient to not use a condom when collecting the specimen because of the sometimes spermicidal effect.

Bibliography

Benson RC, et al: *Current Obstetric and Gynecologic Diagnosis and Treatment,* 7th ed. Los Altos: Lange Medical Publications, 1991.

Berkow R (Ed): *The Merck Manual* (15th ed.). Rahway, NJ: Merck Sharp and Dohme Research Laboratories, Division of Merck & Company, Inc., 1987.

Brunner LS: *The Lippincott Manual of Nursing Practice,* 4th ed. Philadelphia: J. B. Lippincott, 1986.

Cancer Facts and Figures—1990. Atlanta, GA: American Cancer Society, Inc.

Danforth DN, Scott JR: *Obstetrics and Gynecology,* 6th ed. Philadelphia: J. B. Lippincott, 1990.

Deitch KV, Smith JE: Symptoms of chronic vaginal infection & microscopic condyloma in women. *Journal of Obstetrics, Gynecology and Neonatal Nursing* 19(2):133–40, 1990.

Dorland's Pocket Medical Dictionary, 24th ed. Philadelphia: W. B. Saunders, 1989.

Droegemueller W, Herbst AL, Mishell DR, Stenchever MA: *Comprehensive Gynecology,* 1st ed. St. Louis: C. V. Mosby, 1987.

Frew MA, Frew DR: *Comprehensive Medical Assisting: Administrative and Clinical Procedures,* 2nd ed. Philadelphia: F. A. Davis, 1988.

Greene CS: *Handbook of Adult Primary Care.* New York: John Wiley & Sons, 1987.

Kinn ME, Derge EF: *Medical Assisting: Administrative and Clinical,* 6th ed. Philadelphia: W. B. Saunders, 1988.

Ladewig PW, London ML, Olds SB: *Essentials of Maternal–Newborn Nursing,* 2nd ed. Redwood City, CA: Addison-Wesley Nursing, 1990.

Nettles-Carlson B: Early detection of breast cancer. *Journal of Obstetric, Gynecologic and Neonatal Nursing* 18(5):373–381, 1989.

Norplant system, product insert—C1 4064-1. Philadelphia: Wyeth Laboratories, a Wyeth-Ayerst Company, December 1990.

Norwood SL: Fibrocystic breast disease: An update and review. *Journal of Obstetric, Gynecologic and Neonatal Nursing* 19(2):116–121, 1990.

Physicians Desk Reference, 44th ed. Oradell, NJ: Medical Economics, 1990.

Perry AG, Potter PA: *Clinical Nursing Skills and Techniques,* 2nd ed. St. Louis: C. V. Mosby, 1990.

Thompson JM, McFarland JE, Hirsch JE, Tucker SM, Bowers AC: *Mosby's Manual of Clinical Nursing.* St. Louis: C. V. Mosby, 1990.

Whitley N: *A Manual of Clinical Obstetrics.* Philadelphia: J. B. Lippincott, 1985.

Chapter 19

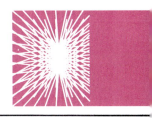

DIAGNOSTIC PROCEDURES

WALTER R. FRANK, III
GARY M. MUNSON
DALE DAVIS
BETTY BATES TEMPKIN

RADIOGRAPHY
Safety
Making a Radiograph (General Guidelines)
Abdomen (AP)
Ankle (AP)
Ankle (oblique)
Ankle (lateral)
Cervical Spine (AP)
Cervical Spine (lateral)
Chest (PA)
Chest (lateral)
Elbow (AP)
Elbow (lateral)
Femur (AP)
Femur (lateral)
Foot (AP)
Foot (oblique)
Foot (lateral)
Forearm (AP)
Forearm (lateral)
Hand (PA)
Hand (oblique)
Hand (lateral)
Hip (AP)
Hip (lateral)
Humerus (AP)
Humerus (lateral)
Knee (AP)
Knee (lateral)
Lumbar Spine (AP)
Lumbar Spine (lateral)
Pelvis (AP)
Shoulder (AP, external rotation)
Shoulder (lateral, internal rotation)
Skull (PA)
Skull (Chamberlain-Towne)
Skull (lateral)
Sinuses (Caldwell)
Sinuses (Waters)
Sinuses (lateral)
Thoracic Spine (AP)
Thoracic Spine (lateral)
Tibia and Fibula (AP)
Tibia and Fibula (lateral)
Wrist (PA)
Wrist (oblique)
Wrist (lateral)

ELECTROCARDIOGRAM AND ARRHYTHMIA INTERPRETATION
Electrocardiography
Arrhythmias
Cardiac Diagnostic Tests

SONOGRAPHY
How Sonography Is Performed
Sonography Examinations

RADIOGRAPHY

Safety

For almost 100 years, radiography has been a powerful diagnostic tool. The x-ray beam penetrates flesh, revealing structures previously unseen without surgery and thus enabling the physician to diagnose many disorders quickly and safely. However, radiography is not without risk to both the patient and the medical assistant.

X-rays are a form of ionizing radiation; that is, they can electrically charge neutral atoms or molecules. When charged, an atom or molecule is called an *ion*. Ionizing radiation may also split molecules to form free radicals. Ions and free radicals produced in the body are very reactive and may disrupt cellular activity.

Effects of Radiation

The effects of ionizing radiation can be classified as *acute* (short term) or *chronic* (long term). Acute effects manifest themselves within 60 days of exposure and only occur after exposure to extreme doses of ionizing radiation. Such high radiation levels do not occur in a clinical setting and need not be discussed further.

The medical assistant must consider the chronic effects of ionizing radiation. Chronic effects may develop 1 or more years after exposure. Alteration of the genetic code is responsible. Encoded in the genes of each cell is the information required for the cell to survive and reproduce. When a cell is exposed to ionizing radiation, subtle changes may occur in its genes, thereby distorting part of the encoded message. If such a change takes place in a germ cell, a mutation results. A *mutation* is a change in the genetic code that may pass from one generation to another. A mutation may not express itself for several generations, but when it does, it is usually lethal or debilitating. If the change occurs in a somatic cell, the cell may die. On the other hand, if the change occurs in the section of the gene responsible for limiting the cell's reproduction rate, uncontrolled cell growth takes place. This is cancer.

Cells that reproduce most rapidly, such as bone marrow and germ cells, are most susceptible to radiation. Cells that reproduce slowly or not at all, such as nerve and muscle cells, are much less susceptible. During pregnancy, mitotic activity is most rapid in the first trimester; thus, fetuses are most vulnerable at this stage.

> **SPECIAL HINT**
>
> The medical assistant must realize that there is no safe dose of ionizing radiation below which chronic effects will not occur. Moreover, because long-term risk rises with increased exposure, limiting the amount of radiation received by the patient and the medical assistant to the lowest possible dose is essential.

Three ways to reduce exposure to the patient are

- Proper collimation
- Proper shielding
- Preventing the need for repeat studies

To prevent irradiation of body parts not under study, the primary x-ray beam must be collimated so that it does not exceed the film borders. Lead shielding of the gonads should be used whenever possible. For children, shield the arms, thighs, and sternum to reduce exposure to the underlying bone marrow. Do not use shielding if it will obstruct the part being examined.

The most significant way to reduce patient exposure is to produce a quality study on the first attempt.

- Make sure that artifact-producing objects (jewelry, clothing, dentures, hair pieces, eyeglasses, etc.) are removed if they will obstruct the part being examined.
- Double check the request form to make sure that the examination being performed is the one requested.
- To avoid mix-ups, properly identify each radiograph with the patient's name, the date the radiograph was taken, and the proper *L* and *R* markers.
- Measure each part being examined and carefully select the proper technical factors on the control panel to ensure adequate penetration of the part.
- Finally, recheck the letter marker, the focal distance, and the control panel *before* making the exposure.

Three basic factors for protecting yourself from radiation are

- Time
- Distance
- Shielding.

These factors are especially important if you are asked to hold a patient being radiographed or are using a portable x-ray machine. It is obvious that the less time you are exposed to radiation, the less exposure you receive. Distance is also effective in reducing exposure. On the basis of the *inverse square law*, if you double your distance from a radiation source, you receive only one-fourth of the radiation. During portable radiography, the operator must stand at least 6 feet away from the patient. Shielding is also a very effective way to reduce exposure. Any substance placed between you and the source of the x-rays absorbs some of the radiation. When holding a patient or using a portable machine, you must wear a lead apron and gloves to reduce your exposure.

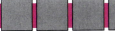

PROCEDURE
MAKING A RADIOGRAPH (GENERAL GUIDELINES)

PURPOSE

To describe procedures common for all radiographs.

EQUIPMENT AND MATERIALS

Calipers
Lead shielding

PROCEDURAL STEPS

Patient Preparation

1. Have the patient remove artifacts (jewelry, hair pieces, dentures, clothing, etc.) that may obscure the part being studied).

Performance

2. Measure the part to be studied.
3. Consult the technique chart for the required exposure factors.
4. Set the control panel, milliamperes (ma) and time first; kilovolt peak (kvp) second.
5. Place the proper right (*R*) or left (*L*) letter marker on the cassette.
6. Move the cassette to the proper work area (a Bucky tray or tabletop).
7. Angle the central ray as required and set the focal distance.
8. Position the part being studied.
9. Immobilize the part if necessary.
10. Place gonadal shielding if necessary.
11. Adjust the collimator so the primary beam does not extend beyond the film borders.
12. Recheck the letter marker, focal distance, and exposure factors.
13. Give the patient final instructions.
14. Make the exposure.

Follow-Through

15. Tell the patient to breathe and relax.

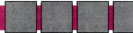

PROCEDURE

RADIOGRAPHING THE ABDOMEN (ANTEROPOSTERIOR [AP] PROJECTION)

PURPOSE

To demonstrate the kidneys, ureters, bladder, liver, spleen, stomach, and intestines using the anteroposterior projection.

EQUIPMENT AND MATERIALS

14″ × 17″ cassette

PROCEDURAL STEPS

Patient Preparation

1. Have the patient remove clothing and dress in a gown.

Performance

2. Place the cassette in the table Bucky lengthwise.
3. Have the patient lie supine with the legs extended and the median plane centered to the table.
4. Position the film so the tops of the iliac crests are even with the center of the film.
5. Direct the central ray vertically to the center of the film.
6. Instruct the patient to stop breathing after expelling a breath.
   RATIONALE: This raises the diaphragm and immobilizes the patient.

Follow-Through

7. Tell the patient to breathe and relax.

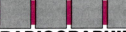

PROCEDURE

RADIOGRAPHING THE ANKLE (AP PROJECTION)

PURPOSE

To demonstrate the distal tibia and fibula, the ankle joint, and the talus using the anteroposterior projection.

EQUIPMENT AND MATERIALS

10″ × 12″ cassette
Lead shielding

PROCEDURAL STEPS

Patient Preparation

1. Have the patient remove shoes and socks.

Performance

2. Place the cassette on the table crosswise (with respect to the leg) and mask either lateral half of the cassette with lead shielding.
   RATIONALE: AP and oblique projections are taken on one film.
3. Have the patient fully extend the leg and place the patient's heel on the film.
4. Flex the ankle so that the foot and leg form a 90° angle.
5. Rotate the leg so that the plantar surface of the foot is perpendicular to the film.
6. Position the midpoint of the malleoli to the center of the film.
7. Direct the central ray vertically to the center of the film.

Chapter 19: DIAGNOSTIC PROCEDURES **479**

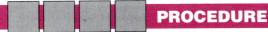 **PROCEDURE**

RADIOGRAPHING THE ANKLE (OBLIQUE PROJECTION)

PURPOSE

To demonstrate the distal tibia and fibula, the ankle joint, and the talus using the oblique projection.

EQUIPMENT AND MATERIALS

10″ × 12″ cassette
Lead shielding

PROCEDURAL STEPS

Performance

1. Place the cassette on the table crosswise and mask the lateral half that was used for the AP projection.
2. Have the patient fully extend the leg and place the heel on the film.
3. Flex the ankle so that the foot and leg form a 90° angle.
4. Rotate the leg medially so that the plantar surface of the foot forms a 45° angle with the film.
5. Position the midpoint of the malleoli to the center of the film.
6. Direct the central ray vertically to the center of the film.

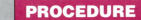 **PROCEDURE**

RADIOGRAPHING THE ANKLE (LATERAL PROJECTION)

PURPOSE

To demonstrate the distal tibia and fibula, the talus, and the tarsals using the lateral projection.

EQUIPMENT AND MATERIALS

8″ × 10″ cassette

PROCEDURAL STEPS

Performance

1. Place the cassette on the table lengthwise (with respect to the leg).
2. Have the patient lie on the affected side and place the lateral aspect of the ankle on the film.
3. Flex the ankle so that the foot and leg form a 90° angle.
4. Center the lateral malleolus to the film.
5. Direct the central ray vertically to the center of the film.

PROCEDURE

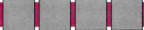

RADIOGRAPHING THE CERVICAL SPINE (AP PROJECTION)

PURPOSE

To demonstrate the lower five cervical vertebrae using the anteroposterior projection.

EQUIPMENT AND MATERIALS

10″ × 12″ cassette

PROCEDURAL STEPS

Patient Preparation

1. Have the patient remove clothing from the waist up, as well as necklaces, earrings, dentures, eyeglasses, and hair pieces. Have females dress in gowns.

Performance

2. Place the film lengthwise in the table Bucky tray.
3. Have the patient lie supine on the table with the median plane centered to the table.
4. Position the patient's head so that the acanthomeatal line is perpendicular to the table.
5. Direct the central ray 15° cephalad to project the midpoint of the thyroid cartilage to the center of the film.
6. Instruct the patient to stop breathing.
   RATIONALE: This helps immobilize the patient.

Follow-Through

7. Tell the patient to breathe and relax.

PROCEDURE

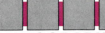

RADIOGRAPHING THE CERVICAL SPINE (LATERAL PROJECTION)

PURPOSE

To demonstrate all seven cervical vertebrae using the lateral projection.

EQUIPMENT AND MATERIALS

10″ × 12″ cassette
Two 5-lb sandbags

PROCEDURAL STEPS

Performance

1. Place the cassette lengthwise in the vertical film holder.
2. Seat the patient in a chair and place the left shoulder against the film holder so that the median plane is perpendicular to the film.
3. Position the head so the acanthomeatal line is parallel to the floor.
4. Center the neck to the film at the level of the thyroid cartilage.
5. Place a sandbag in each hand.
   RATIONALE: This brings the shoulders down to allow C-7 to be unobstructed.
6. Direct the central ray horizontally to the center of the film.
7. Instruct the patient to stop breathing.

Follow-Through

8. Tell the patient to breathe and relax.

PROCEDURE

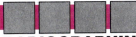

RADIOGRAPHING THE CHEST (POSTEROANTERIOR [PA] PROJECTION)

PURPOSE

To demonstrate the heart, lungs, and aorta using the posteroanterior projection.

EQUIPMENT AND MATERIALS

14" × 17" cassette

PROCEDURAL STEPS

Patient Preparation

1. Have the patient remove clothing and jewelry from the waist up. Females are dressed in gowns.

Performance

2. Place the cassette lengthwise (with respect to the body) in the vertical film holder.
3. Stand the patient erect with the anterior aspect of the chest against the film and the median plane perpendicular and centered to the film.
4. Place the hands on the patient's hips and rotate the shoulders forward to remove the scapula from the lung fields.
5. Position the cassette so the tops of the shoulders are 3 inches below the upper film border.
6. Direct the central ray horizontally to the center of the film.
7. Instruct the patient to stop breathing after taking a deep breath.
RATIONALE: This lowers and immobilizes the diaphragm.

Follow-Through

8. Tell the patient to breathe and relax.
9. If a lateral view is ordered, change cassettes.

PROCEDURE

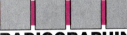

RADIOGRAPHING THE CHEST (LATERAL PROJECTION)

PURPOSE

To demonstrate the heart, lungs, and aorta using the lateral projection.

EQUIPMENT AND MATERIALS

14" × 17" cassette

PROCEDURAL STEPS

Performance

1. Place the cassette lengthwise in the vertical film holder.

> **SPECIAL HINT**
>
> It is not necessary to readjust the height of the film holder after the PA projection is taken.

2. Stand the patient erect with the arms above the head, the lateral side of the chest against the film, and the frontal plane through the shoulders perpendicular and centered to the film.
3. Direct the central ray horizontally to the center of the film.
4. Instruct the patient to take a deep breath and then stop breathing.

Follow-Through

5. Tell the patient to breathe and relax.

PROCEDURE
RADIOGRAPHING THE ELBOW (AP PROJECTION)

PURPOSE

To demonstrate the distal humerus, the proximal radius and ulna, and the elbow joint using the anteroposterior projection.

EQUIPMENT AND MATERIALS

10" × 12" cassette
Lead shielding

PROCEDURAL STEPS

Patient Preparation

1. Have the patient remove clothing and jewelry that may obstruct the elbow.

Performance

2. Place the film on the table crosswise (with respect to the arm) and mask one lateral half of the cassette.
3. Fully extend the elbow with the palm facing up and the plane through the epicondyles parallel to the film.
4. Center the midpoint of the epicondyles to the film.
5. Direct the central ray vertically to the center of the film.

PROCEDURE
RADIOGRAPHING THE ELBOW (LATERAL PROJECTION)

PURPOSE

To demonstrate the distal humerus, the proximal radius and ulna, and the elbow joint using the lateral projection.

EQUIPMENT AND MATERIALS

10" × 12" cassette
Lead shielding

PROCEDURAL STEPS

Performance

1. Place the cassette on the table crosswise and mask the lateral half used for the AP projection.
2. Position the patient so the shoulder is level with the film and the elbow is flexed 90°.
3. Rotate the forearm to bring the plane through the epicondyles and styloid processes perpendicular to the table.
   RATIONALE: To prevent the proximal radius from overlapping the proximal ulna.
4. Center the epicondyles to the film.
5. Direct the central ray vertically to the center of the film.

PROCEDURE

RADIOGRAPHING THE FEMUR (AP PROJECTION)

PURPOSE

To demonstrate the proximal two-thirds of the femur and the hip joint or the distal two-thirds of the femur and the knee using the anteroposterior projection.

MEDICAL ASSISTING ALERT

Use gonadal shielding.

EQUIPMENT AND MATERIALS

14″ × 17″ cassette

PROCEDURAL STEPS

Patient Preparation

1. Clothing is removed from the waist down and the patient is dressed in a gown.

Performance

2. Place the cassette lengthwise in the table Bucky.
3. Have the patient lie supine with the knee fully extended and the plane through the epicondyles parallel to the table.
4. Center the plane through the anterior superior iliac spine (ASIS) and the midpoint of the epicondyles to the table.
5. To demonstrate the proximal two-thirds of the femur, position the film so that the ASIS is 3 inches below the upper film border. To demonstrate the distal two-thirds, position the film so the apex of the patella is 3 inches above the lower film border.
6. Direct the central ray vertically to the center of the film.

PROCEDURE

RADIOGRAPHING THE FEMUR (LATERAL PROJECTION)

PURPOSE

To demonstrate the proximal two-thirds of the femur and the hip joint or the distal two-thirds of the femur and the knee using the lateral projection.

EQUIPMENT AND MATERIALS

14″ × 17″ cassette

PROCEDURAL STEPS

Performance

1. Place the cassette lengthwise in the table Bucky.
2. Have the patient lie on the affected side with the knee flexed and the plane through the epicondyles perpendicular to the table.
3. Move the unaffected leg backward to avoid superimposition of femur images.
4. Center the plane through the greater trochanter and the epicondyles to the table.
5. To demonstrate the proximal two-thirds of the femur, position the film so the anterior superior iliac spine is 3 inches below the upper film border. To demonstrate the distal two-thirds of the femur, position the film so the apex of the patella is 3 inches above the lower film border.
6. Direct the central ray vertically to the center of the film.

PROCEDURE
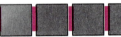

RADIOGRAPHING THE FOOT (AP PROJECTION)

PURPOSE

To demonstrate the distal tarsals, the metatarsals, and the phalanges using the anteroposterior projection.

EQUIPMENT AND MATERIALS

10″ × 12″ cassette
Lead shielding

PROCEDURAL STEPS

Patient Preparation

1. Have the patient remove the shoe and sock of the affected foot.

Performance

2. Place the cassette lengthwise on the table top and mask either lateral side.

> **SPECIAL HINT**
>
> To prevent the cassette from sliding, place a sandbag on the distal border of the cassette.

3. Place the plantar surface of the foot on the film so that the great toe is 1 inch below the upper film border.
4. Direct the central ray 15° cephalad to the center of the film.

PROCEDURE
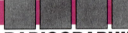

RADIOGRAPHING THE FOOT (OBLIQUE PROJECTION)

PURPOSE

To demonstrate the tarsals, metatarsals, and phalanges using the oblique projection.

EQUIPMENT AND MATERIALS

10″ × 12″ cassette
Lead shielding

PROCEDURAL STEPS

Performance

1. Place the cassette lengthwise on the table top and mask the side used for the AP projection.
2. Place the foot on the film so that the great toe is 1 inch below the upper film border.
3. Rotate the foot medially until the plantar surface is 45° from the film.
4. Direct the central ray vertically to the center of the film.

PROCEDURE

RADIOGRAPHING THE FOOT (LATERAL PROJECTION)

PURPOSE

To demonstrate the tarsals and metatarsals using the lateral projection.

EQUIPMENT AND MATERIALS

10″ × 12″ cassette

PROCEDURAL STEPS

Performance

1. Place the cassette lengthwise (with respect to the foot) on the table.
2. Have the patient lie on the affected side with the knee flexed and the plantar surface of the foot perpendicular to the film.
3. Center the foot to the film.
4. Direct the central ray vertically to the center of the film.

PROCEDURE

RADIOGRAPHING THE FOREARM (AP PROJECTION)

PURPOSE

To demonstrate the proximal two-thirds of the radius and ulna, including the elbow, or the distal two-thirds of the radius and ulna, including the wrist, using the anteroposterior projection.

EQUIPMENT AND MATERIALS

10″ × 12″ cassette
Lead shielding

PROCEDURAL STEPS

Patient Preparation

1. Have patient remove clothing and jewelry from the forearm.

Performance

2. Place the cassette lengthwise on the table and mask either lateral half.
3. Fully extend the arm with the palm up and center the shaft of the forearm to the film.
4. To include the elbow, position the epicondyles 2 inches below the upper film border. To include the wrist, position the styloids 2 inches above the lower film border. Be sure to include the joint closest to the injury.
5. Direct the central ray vertically to the center of the film.

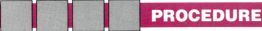

RADIOGRAPHING THE FOREARM (LATERAL PROJECTION)

PURPOSE

To demonstrate the proximal two-thirds of the radius and ulna, including the elbow, or the distal two-thirds of the radius and ulna, including the wrist, using the lateral projection.

EQUIPMENT AND MATERIALS

10″ × 12″ cassette
Lead shielding

PROCEDURAL STEPS

Performance

1. Place the cassette on the table lengthwise (with respect to the forearm) and mask the side used for the AP projection.
2. Position the patient so the shoulder is level with the film and the elbow is flexed 90°.
3. Rotate the forearm externally until the palm is perpendicular to the table and center the shaft of the forearm to the film.
4. To include the elbow, position the epicondyles 2 inches below the upper film border. To include the wrist, position the styloids 2 inches above the lower film border.
5. Direct the central ray vertically to the center of the film.

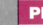

RADIOGRAPHING THE HAND (PA PROJECTION)

PURPOSE

To demonstrate the carpals, metacarpals, and phalanges using the posteroanterior projection.

EQUIPMENT AND MATERIALS

10″ × 12″ cassette
Lead shielding

PROCEDURAL STEPS

Patient Preparation

1. Have the patient remove jewelry from wrist and fingers.

Performance

2. Place the cassette crosswise on the table and mask either lateral half.
3. Place the hand palm down on the cassette with the fingers extended and equally separated.
4. Center the head of the third metacarpal to the film.
5. Direct the central ray vertically to the center of the film.

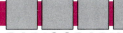
PROCEDURE
RADIOGRAPHING THE HAND (OBLIQUE PROJECTION)

PURPOSE

To demonstrate the carpals, metacarpals, and phalanges using the oblique projection.

EQUIPMENT AND MATERIALS

10″ × 12″ cassette
Lead shielding

PROCEDURAL STEPS

Performance

1. Place the cassette on the table crosswise and mask the side used for the PA projection.
2. Place the hand on the cassette palm down with the fingers extended and equally separated.
3. Rotate the hand externally until the metacarpal plane forms a 45° angle with the film.
4. Center the head of the third metacarpal to the film.
5. Direct the central ray vertically to the center of the film.

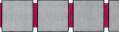
PROCEDURE
RADIOGRAPHING THE HAND (LATERAL PROJECTION)

PURPOSE

To demonstrate the carpals, metacarpals, and phalanges using the lateral projection.

EQUIPMENT AND MATERIALS

8″ × 10″ cassette

PROCEDURAL STEPS

Performance

1. Place the cassette on the table lengthwise.
2. Place the medial aspect of the hand on the cassette so that the palm is perpendicular to the film.
3. Extend the fingers and position the thumb beside the palm parallel to the fingers.
4. Center the head of the second metacarpal to the center of the film.
5. Direct the central ray vertically to the center of the film.

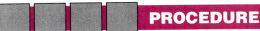
PROCEDURE

RADIOGRAPHING THE HIP (AP PROJECTION)

PURPOSE

To demonstrate the head and neck of the femur and the hip joint using the anteroposterior projection.

MEDICAL ASSISTING ALERT

Use gonadal shielding.

EQUIPMENT AND MATERIALS

10" × 12" cassette

PROCEDURAL STEPS

Patient Preparation

1. Have the patient remove clothing from the waist down and dress in a gown.

Performance

2. Place the cassette lengthwise in the table Bucky.
3. Have the patient lie supine on the table with the legs fully extended.
4. Center the plane through the midpoint of the epicondyles and the anterior superior iliac spine (ASIS) to the midline of the table.
5. Position the patient so that the intersection of sagittal plane through the ASIS and the transverse plane through the greater trochanter is centered to the film.
6. Rotate the foot and lower leg 15° medially. RATIONALE: This brings the femoral neck parallel to the film.
7. Direct the central ray vertically to the center of the film.

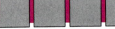
PROCEDURE

RADIOGRAPHING THE HIP (LATERAL PROJECTION)

PURPOSE

To demonstrate the head and neck of the femur and the hip joint using the lateral projection.

MEDICAL ASSISTING ALERT

Use gonadal shielding.

EQUIPMENT AND MATERIALS

10" × 12" cassette

PROCEDURAL STEPS

Performance

1. Place the cassette crosswise with respect to the long axis of the body in the table Bucky.
2. Have the patient lie on the affected side and move the unaffected leg backward to avoid superimposition.
3. Center the plane through the epicondyles and the greater trochanter to the midline of the table.
4. Center the point midway between the anterior superior iliac spine and the symphysis pubis to the film.

SPECIAL HINT

The centering point can also be found by palpating the femoral pulse.

5. Direct the central ray vertically to the center of the film.

PROCEDURE

RADIOGRAPHING THE HUMERUS (AP PROJECTION)

PURPOSE

To demonstrate the entire humerus with the elbow and shoulder joints using the anteroposterior projection.

EQUIPMENT AND MATERIALS

14" × 17" cassette
Lead shielding

PROCEDURAL STEPS

Patient Preparation

1. Remove clothing or jewelry that may obstruct humerus.
2. Females are dressed in a gown, opening in the back.

Procedure

3. Place the cassette lengthwise on the table and mask either lateral half.
4. Have the patient lie supine on the table.
5. With the patient's elbow fully extended and the palm up, center the shaft of the humerus to the film.
6. Position the cassette so the acromion processes are 2 inches below the upper film border.
7. Direct the central ray vertically to the center of the film.
8. Instruct the patient to stop breathing.
   RATIONALE: This immobilizes the humerus.

Follow-Through

9. Tell the patient to breathe and relax.

PROCEDURE

RADIOGRAPHING THE HUMERUS (LATERAL PROJECTION)

PURPOSE

To demonstrate the entire humerus with the elbow and shoulder joints using the lateral projection.

EQUIPMENT AND MATERIALS

14" × 17" cassette
Lead shielding

PROCEDURAL STEPS

Performance

1. Place the cassette lengthwise on the table and mask the lateral half used for the AP projection.
2. Have the patient lie supine on the table.
3. With the patient's elbow flexed and the palm down, center the shaft of the humerus to the film.
4. Position the cassette so the acromion process is 2 inches below the upper film border.
5. Direct the central ray vertically to the center of the film.
6. Instruct the patient to expel a breath and then stop breathing.

Follow-Through

7. Tell the patient to breathe and relax.

PROCEDURE

RADIOGRAPHING THE KNEE (AP PROJECTION)

PURPOSE

To demonstrate the distal femur, the proximal tibia and fibula, and the knee joint using the anteroposterior projection.

EQUIPMENT AND MATERIALS

8" × 10" cassette

PROCEDURAL STEPS

Patient Preparation

1. Have the patient remove outer clothing from the waist down.
2. Dress in gown, opening in the back.

Procedure

3. Place the cassette lengthwise on the table.
4. Have the patient sit on the table and fully extend the knee.
5. Rotate the leg until the plane through the epicondyles is parallel to the film.
6. Center the apex of the patella to the film.
7. Direct the central ray vertically to the center of the film.

PROCEDURE

RADIOGRAPHING THE KNEE (LATERAL PROJECTION)

PURPOSE

To demonstrate the distal femur, the proximal tibia and fibula, the knee joint, and the patella using the lateral projection.

EQUIPMENT AND MATERIALS

8" × 10" cassette

PROCEDURAL STEPS

Performance

1. Place the cassette lengthwise on the table.
2. Have the patient lie on the affected side with the knee flexed and the unaffected leg moved backward to avoid superimposition.
3. Rotate the leg until the plane through the epicondyles is perpendicular to the film.
4. Center the knee to the film at the level of the apex of the patella.
5. Direct the central ray 5° cephalad to the center of the film.

PROCEDURE

RADIOGRAPHING THE LUMBAR SPINE (AP PROJECTION)

PURPOSE

To demonstrate the lumbar vertebral bodies and the interspaces using the anteroposterior projection.

> **MEDICAL ASSISTING ALERT**
> Use gonadal shielding.

EQUIPMENT AND MATERIALS

14" × 17" cassette

PROCEDURAL STEPS

Patient Preparation

1. Have the patient remove clothing and dress in a gown.

Performance

2. Place the cassette lengthwise in the table Bucky.
3. Have the patient lie supine with the median plane centered to the midline of the table.
4. Flex the knees and place the feet flat on the table.
   RATIONALE: This reduces the lordotic curvature.
5. Position the cassette so the iliac crests are 1 inch below the center of the film.
6. Direct the central ray vertically to the center of the film.
7. Instruct the patient to stop breathing.
   RATIONALE: This helps immobilize the patient.

Follow-Through

8. Tell the patient to breathe and relax.

PROCEDURE

RADIOGRAPHING THE LUMBAR SPINE (LATERAL PROJECTION)

PURPOSE

To demonstrate the lumbar vertebral bodies and the interspaces using the lateral projection.

EQUIPMENT AND MATERIALS

14" × 17" cassette

PROCEDURAL STEPS

Performance

1. Place the cassette lengthwise in the table Bucky.
2. Have the patient lie laterally recumbent with knees flexed and the coronal plane perpendicular and centered to the midline of the table.
3. Position the cassette so the iliac crests are 1 inch below the center of the film.
4. Direct the central ray vertically to the center of the film.
5. Instruct the patient to stop breathing.

Follow-Through

6. Tell the patient to breathe and relax.

PROCEDURE

RADIOGRAPHING THE PELVIS (AP PROJECTION)

PURPOSE

To demonstrate the pelvis and both hips using the anteroposterior projection.

EQUIPMENT AND MATERIALS

14" × 17" cassette

PROCEDURAL STEPS

Patient Preparation

1. Have the patient remove clothing and dress in a gown.

Performance

2. Place the cassette crosswise in the table Bucky.
3. Have the patient lie supine on the table with the median plane centered to the midline of the table.
4. Fully extend the knees and rotate both feet and lower legs 15° medially.
   RATIONALE: This brings the femoral necks parallel to the film.
5. Position the cassette so the iliac crests are 3 inches below the upper film border.
6. Direct the central ray vertically to the center of the film.

PROCEDURE

RADIOGRAPHING THE SHOULDER (AP PROJECTION, EXTERNAL ROTATION)

PURPOSE

To demonstrate the proximal humerus and the structures of the externally rotated shoulder using the anteroposterior projection.

EQUIPMENT AND MATERIALS

10" × 12" cassette

PROCEDURAL STEPS

Patient Preparation

1. Have the patient remove clothing from the waist up and dress in a gown.

Performance

2. Place the cassette crosswise in the table Bucky.
3. Have the patient lie supine on the table with the elbow fully extended and the palm up.
4. Center the coracoid process to the film.
5. Direct the central ray vertically to the center of the film.
6. Instruct the patient to expel a breath and then stop breathing.

Follow-Through

7. Tell the patient to breathe and relax.

PROCEDURE

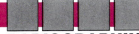

RADIOGRAPHING THE SHOULDER (LATERAL PROJECTION, INTERNAL ROTATION)

PURPOSE

To demonstrate the proximal humerus and the structures of the internally rotated shoulder using the lateral projection.

EQUIPMENT AND MATERIALS

10" × 12" cassette

PROCEDURAL STEPS

Performance

1. Place the cassette crosswise in the table Bucky.
2. Have the patient lie supine on the table with the elbow flexed and the palm down.
3. Center the coracoid process to the film.
4. Direct the central ray vertically to the center of the film.
5. Instruct the patient to expel a breath and then stop breathing.

Follow-Through

6. Tell the patient to breathe and relax.

PROCEDURE

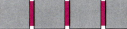

RADIOGRAPHING THE SKULL (PA PROJECTION)

PURPOSE

To demonstrate the frontal bone, orbits, and petrous ridges using the posteroanterior projection.

EQUIPMENT AND MATERIALS

10" × 12" cassette

PROCEDURAL STEPS

Patient Preparation

1. Have the patient remove necklaces, earrings, eyeglasses, hair piece, and dentures.

Performance

2. Place the cassette lengthwise in the table Bucky.
3. Have the patient lie prone with the nose and forehead on the table.
4. Position the head so the median plane is centered to the midline of the table and the acanthomeatal line is perpendicular to the film.
5. Center the nasion to the film.
6. Direct the central ray vertically to the center of the film.
7. Instruct the patient to stop breathing.
   RATIONALE: This helps immobilize the patient.

Follow-Through

8. Tell the patient to breathe and relax.

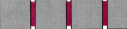

PROCEDURE

RADIOGRAPHING THE SKULL (CHAMBERLAIN–TOWNE PROJECTION)

PURPOSE

To demonstrate the occipital bone and the foramen magnum using the Chamberlain–Towne projection.

EQUIPMENT AND MATERIALS

10″ × 12″ cassette

PROCEDURAL STEPS

Performance

1. Place the cassette lengthwise in the table Bucky.
2. Have the patient lie supine with the median plane centered to the midline of the table.
3. Position the head so the orbitomeatal line is perpendicular to the film.
4. Move the cassette so the cranial vertex is even with the upper film border.
5. Direct the central ray 30° caudad to the center of the film.

> **SPECIAL HINT**
>
> If the neck cannot be flexed enough for the orbitomeatal line to be perpendicular to the table, position the head so that the infraorbital meatal line is perpendicular to the table and direct the central ray 37° caudad.

6. Instruct the patient to stop breathing.

Follow-Through

7. Tell the patient to breathe and relax.

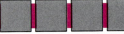

PROCEDURE

RADIOGRAPHING THE SKULL (LATERAL PROJECTION)

PURPOSE

To demonstrate the frontal, parietal, and occipital bones and the sella turcica using the lateral projection.

EQUIPMENT AND MATERIALS

10″ × 12″ cassette

PROCEDURAL STEPS

Performance

1. Place the cassette crosswise in the table Bucky.
2. Have the patient lie prone with the lateral aspect of the head on the table and the chin supported with one hand.
3. Position the head so the median plane is parallel to the table and the infraorbital-meatal line is parallel to the lower film border.
4. Center the point 3/4 of an inch superior and 3/4 of an inch anterior to the external auditory meatus to the film.
5. Direct the central ray vertically to the center of the film.
6. Instruct the patient to stop breathing.

Follow-Through

7. Tell the patient to breathe and relax.

PROCEDURE

RADIOGRAPHING THE SINUSES (CALDWELL PROJECTION)

PURPOSE

To demonstrate the frontal and ethmoid sinuses using the Caldwell projection.

EQUIPMENT AND MATERIALS

8" × 10" cassette

PROCEDURAL STEPS

Patient Preparation

1. Have the patient remove necklaces, earrings, eyeglasses, hair piece, and dentures.

Performance

2. Place the cassette lengthwise in the vertical Bucky.

   RATIONALE: The patient is erect to allow the presence of fluid levels in the sinuses to be visualized on the radiograph.
3. Have the patient sit in a chair and place the nose and forehead on the film holder.
4. Position the head so the median plane is centered to the midline of the film holder and the orbitomeatal line is parallel to the floor.
5. Center the nasion to the film.
6. Direct the central ray 15° caudad to the center of the film.
7. Instruct the patient to stop breathing.
   RATIONALE: This helps immobilize the patient.

Follow-Through

8. Tell the patient to breathe and relax.

PROCEDURE

RADIOGRAPHING THE SINUSES (WATERS PROJECTION)

PURPOSE

To demonstrate the maxillary, frontal, and ethmoid sinuses using the Waters projection.

EQUIPMENT AND MATERIALS

8" × 10" cassette

PROCEDURAL STEPS

Patient Preparation

See Radiographing the Sinuses (Caldwell Projection)

Performance

1. Place the cassette lengthwise in the vertical Bucky.
2. Have the patient sit in a chair and place the chin on the film holder.
3. Position the head so the median plane is centered to the midline of the film holder and the orbitomeatal line is elevated 37° from the horizontal.
4. Center the acanthion to the film.
5. Direct the central ray horizontally to the center of the film.
6. Instruct the patient to stop breathing.

Follow-Through

7. Tell the patient to breathe and relax.

PROCEDURE

RADIOGRAPHING THE SINUSES (LATERAL PROJECTION)

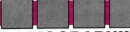

PURPOSE

To demonstrate the frontal, ethmoid, maxillary, and sphenoid sinuses using the lateral projection.

EQUIPMENT AND MATERIALS

8" × 10" cassette

PROCEDURAL STEPS

Patient Preparation

See Radiographing the Sinuses (Caldwell Projection).

Performance

1. Place the cassette lengthwise in the vertical Bucky.
2. Have the patient sit in a chair with the lateral aspect of the head against the film holder.
3. Position the head so the median plane is parallel to the film and the orbitomeatal line is parallel to the floor.
4. Center the lateral canthus to the film.
5. Direct the central ray horizontally to the center of the film.
6. Instruct the patient to stop breathing.

Follow-Through

7. Tell the patient to breathe and relax.

PROCEDURE

RADIOGRAPHING THE THORACIC SPINE (AP PROJECTION)

PURPOSE

To demonstrate the thoracic vertebrae and the interspaces using the anteroposterior projection.

EQUIPMENT AND MATERIALS

14" × 17" cassette

PROCEDURAL STEPS

Patient Preparation

1. Have the patient remove clothing from the waist up and dress in a gown.

Performance

2. Place the cassette lengthwise in the table Bucky.
3. Have the patient lie supine and center the median plane to the midline of the table.
4. Position the film so the acromion processes are 3 inches below the upper film border.
5. Direct the central ray vertically to the center of the film.
6. Instruct the patient to stop breathing after expelling a breath.

Follow-Through

7. Tell the patient to breathe and relax.

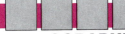

PROCEDURE

RADIOGRAPHING THE THORACIC SPINE (LATERAL PROJECTION)

PURPOSE

To demonstrate the thoracic vertebrae and the interspaces using the lateral projection.

EQUIPMENT AND MATERIALS

14" × 17" cassette

PROCEDURAL STEPS

Performance

1. Place the cassette lengthwise in the table Bucky.
2. Have the patient lie laterally recumbent with the knees flexed and the hands under the head and the coronal plane perpendicular and centered to the midline of the table.
3. Position the film so the acromion processes are 2 inches below the upper film border.
4. Direct the central ray vertically to the center of the film.
5. Instruct the patient to take a breath and then stop breathing.

Follow-Through

6. Tell the patient to breathe and relax.

PROCEDURE

RADIOGRAPHING THE TIBIA AND FIBULA (AP PROJECTION)

PURPOSE

To demonstrate the proximal two-thirds of the tibia and fibula, including the knee, or the distal two-thirds of the tibia and fibula, including the ankle, using the anteroposterior projection.

EQUIPMENT AND MATERIALS

14" × 17" cassette
Lead shielding

PROCEDURAL STEPS

Patient Preparation

1. Have the patient remove outer clothing from the waist down.
2. Dress in gown, opening in back.

Performance

3. Place the film lengthwise on the table and mask either lateral half.
4. With the patient's knee fully extended and the ankle flexed 90°, center the shaft of the leg to the film.
5. Rotate the leg so the plane through the epicondyles is parallel to the film.
6. To include the knee, position the apex of the patella 3 inches below the upper film border. To include the ankle, position the malleoli 3 inches above the lower film border.
7. Direct the central ray vertically to the center of the film.

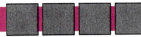

PROCEDURE

RADIOGRAPHING THE TIBIA AND FIBULA (LATERAL PROJECTION)

PURPOSE

To demonstrate the proximal two-thirds of the tibia and fibula, including the knee, or the distal two-thirds of the tibia and fibula, including the ankle using the lateral projection.

EQUIPMENT AND MATERIALS

14" × 17" cassette
Lead shielding

PROCEDURAL STEPS

Performance

1. Place the cassette lengthwise on the table and mask the lateral half used for the AP projection.
2. Have the patient lie on the affected side with the knee flexed and the shaft of the leg centered to the film.
3. Rotate the leg so the plane through the epicondyles is perpendicular to the table.
4. To include the knee, position the apex of the patella 3 inches below the upper film border. To include the ankle, position the malleoli 3 inches above the lower film border.
5. Direct the central ray vertically to the center of the film.

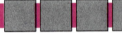

PROCEDURE

RADIOGRAPHING THE WRIST (PA PROJECTION)

PURPOSE

To demonstrate the distal radius and ulna, the carpals, and the wrist joint using the posteroanterior projection.

EQUIPMENT AND MATERIALS

8" × 10" cassette
Lead shielding

PROCEDURAL STEPS

Patient Preparation

1. Have the patient remove watch and bracelets from the affected wrist.

Performance

2. Place the cassette on the table crosswise and mask either lateral half.
3. Place the anterior aspect of the wrist on the cassette and flex the fingers to form a loose fist.
4. Center the midpoint of the styloid processes to the film.
5. Direct the central ray vertically to the center of the film.

PROCEDURE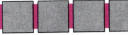

RADIOGRAPHING THE WRIST (OBLIQUE PROJECTION)

PURPOSE

To demonstrate the distal radius and ulna, the carpals, and the wrist joint using the oblique projection.

EQUIPMENT AND MATERIALS

8" × 10" cassette
Lead shielding

PROCEDURAL STEPS

Performance

1. Place the cassette on the table crosswise and mask the lateral half used for the PA projection.
2. Place the anterior aspect of the wrist on the cassette and then rotate the wrist externally 45°.
3. Center the midpoint of the styloid processes to the center of the film.
4. Direct the central ray vertically to the center of the film.

PROCEDURE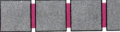

RADIOGRAPHING THE WRIST (LATERAL PROJECTION)

PURPOSE

To demonstrate the distal radius and ulna, the carpals, and the wrist joint using the lateral projection.

EQUIPMENT AND MATERIALS

8" × 10" cassette

PROCEDURAL STEPS

1. Place the cassette on the table lengthwise.
2. Place the medial aspect of the wrist on the cassette so that the plane through the styloid processes is perpendicular to the film.

SPECIAL HINT

Slightly supinating the hand ensures that the wrist is in true lateral alignment.

3. Center the styloid processes to the film.
4. Direct the central ray vertically to the center of the film.

ELECTROCARDIOGRAM AND ARRHYTHMIA INTERPRETATION

Electrocardiography

Electrocardiogram

An electrocardiogram (ECG) records the electrical activity of the heart from 12 different positions. Each position represents an ECG lead:

Standard Leads	Augmented Leads	Chest Leads
I	aVR	V_1 V_4
II	aVL	V_2 V_5
III	aVF	V_3 V_6

With electrodes placed on the patient's arms, legs, and six positions on the chest, a 12-lead ECG can be recorded.

PROCEDURE

HOOKING UP AN ECG

PURPOSE

To record the heart's electrical activity from 12 different positions.

EQUIPMENT AND MATERIALS

ECG machine
Electrode pads and electrode gel

PROCEDURAL STEPS

Patient Preparation

1. Patient should lie comfortably in the supine position on a bed or examining table. If the patient is unable to lie down, an ECG can be recorded with the patient on his or her side or sitting up.

Performance

2. Place electrodes on both wrists and ankles as indicated in Figure 19–1, and insert an electrode pad or gel between the electrode and the patient's skin.

   - White lead wire and electrode attached to left wrist
   - Black lead wire and electrode attached to right wrist
   - Red lead wire and electrode attached to left ankle
   - Green lead wire and electrode attached to right ankle

3. Place six electrodes on the chest (see Figure 19–1), and place electrode gel between the electrode and the patient's skin.

   - V_1 — 4th intercostal space immediately to the right of the sternum
   - V_2 — 4th intercostal space immediately to the left of the sternum
   - V_3 — Directly between V_2 and V_4

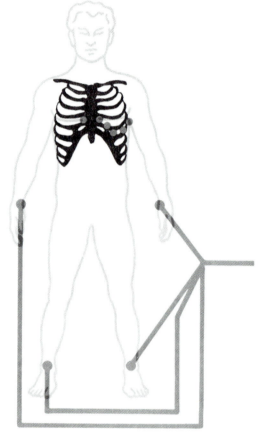

FIGURE 19–1

Twelve-lead electrocardiogram. (Reproduced from Davis D: *Differential Diagnosis of Arrhythmias*. Philadelphia: W. B. Saunders, 1992, p. 11.)

   - V_4 — 5th intercostal space, left midclavicular line
   - V_5 — 5th intercostal space, left anterior axillary line
   - V_6 — 5th intercostal space, left midaxillary line

4. Patient should remain relaxed and immobile during running of ECG.

Follow-Through

5. Remove remaining electrode gel and/or pads from the patient's body.

Electrical Conduction System

Depolarization and Repolarization. The electrical signals generated in the heart originate from the passage of ions inside and across cardiac cell membranes. Each cardiac cell becomes excited. This cell excitation is called *depolarization*. The return of the depolarized cell to its resting state is termed *repolarization*.

Electrical Conduction System. The electrical conduction system is composed of specialized conduction tissue that transfers the electricity throughout the heart (Figure 19–2).

The electrical impulse initiating depolarization begins in the sinoatrial (SA) node, called the "pacemaker" of the heart. The SA node is located in the wall of the right atrium. The SA node transfers the electrical activity to both atria by way of the internodal tracts, and the atrial cells depolarize. The depolarization wave travels to the atrioventricular (AV) node, bundle of His, right bundle branch, left bundle branch (which divides into the left anterior and left posterior fascicles), and the purkinje fibers located in the walls of the ventricles.

Waves and Intervals. The P, QRS, and T waves represent the depolarization and repolarization and of the cardiac cells during an ECG recording (Figure 19–3).

- The *baseline* or *isoelectric line* precedes the P wave on an ECG.
- The *P wave* represents atrial depolarization and should appear upright and slightly rounded.
- The *PR interval* represents the time from the beginning of the P wave to the first wave of the QRS complex.
- The *QRS complex* represents ventricular depolarization and is measured from the beginning of the first wave of the QRS to the end of the last wave of the QRS.

  Q wave is a negative wave, preceding an R wave
  R wave is a positive wave
  S wave is a negative wave, following an R wave

- The QRS complex can be composed of only one of the waves or various combinations.
- The *ST segment* is the line between the last wave of the QRS complex and the beginning of the T wave and is an indicator of myocardial ischemia.

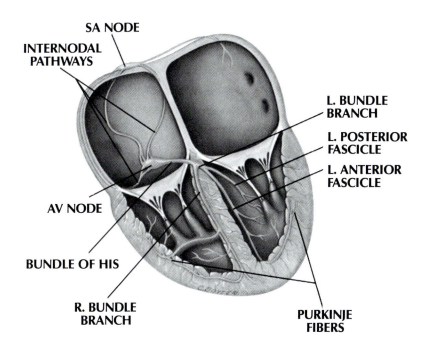

FIGURE 19–2

Electrical conduction system of the heart. (Reproduced from Davis D: *Differential Diagnosis of Arrhythymias*. Philadelphia: W. B. Saunders, 1992, p. 9.)

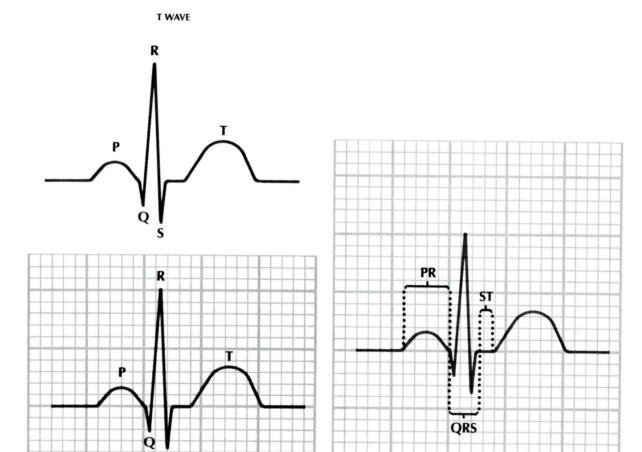

FIGURE 19-3

Waves and intervals on an electrocardiogram. (Reproduced from Davis D: *Differential Diagnosis of Arrhythmias*. Philadelphia: W. B. Saunders, 1992, pp. 15-16.)

- The *T wave* represents ventricular repolarization and should be upright and rounded.

Electrocardiogram Graph Paper and Measurements

ECG graph paper is divided into 1-mm squares by the light lines and 5-mm squares by the dark lines.

Voltage. Voltage is measured on the vertical axis in millimeters. The height of R waves, depth of S waves, and ST elevation and depression are calculated from the baseline (Figure 19-4).

Time. Time is measured on the horizontal axis in seconds. Each small box represents .04 second (See Figure 19-4).

Heart Rate. Heart rate can be calculated using the 300-150-100-75-60-50 method. Find an R wave that falls on or near a heavy black line on the graph paper. Count the heavy black lines to the right using 300 for the first line, 150 for the second line, 100 for the third line, 75 for the fourth line etc., until the next R wave occurs. If the next R wave falls on the fourth line, the heart rate is 75 beats per minute (Figure 19-5).

Sinus Rhythms. Sinus rhythm is a heart rhythm beginning in the SA node. The atrial (P-P) rate and the ventricular (R-R) rate are exactly the same and the PR interval remains constant.

The sinus rhythms are differentiated by rate (Figure 19-6):

Sinus rhythm: 60-100 beats per minute

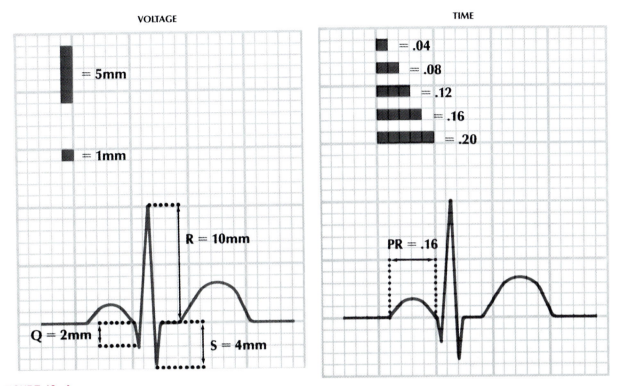

FIGURE 19-4

Graphic measurements of voltage and time. (Reproduced from Davis D: *Differential Diagnosis of Arrhythmias.* Philadelphia: W. B. Saunders, 1992, pp. 18-19.)

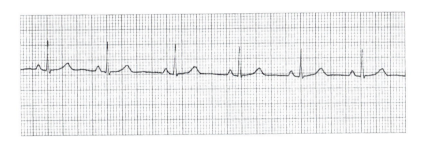

FIGURE 19-5

The heart rate is approximately 75 beats per minute.

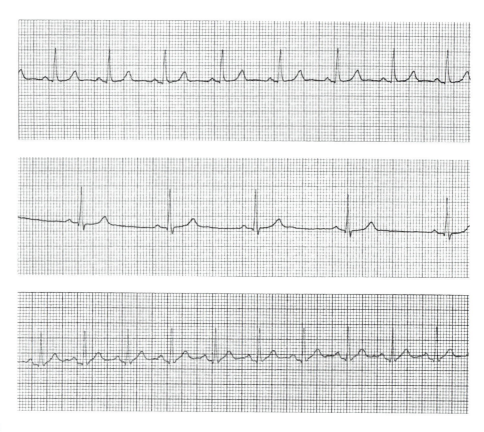

FIGURE 19-6

First electrocardiogram (ECG): Sinus rhythm at approximately 80 beats per minute (bpm). Second ECG: Sinus bradycardia at approximately 50 bpm. Third ECG: Sinus tachycardia at slightly over 100 bpm.

Sinus bradycardia: Below 60 beats per minute
Sinus tachycardia: Over 60 beats per minute

Normal Electrocardiogram Patterns

1. The P wave should be upright in lead I and inverted in lead aVR.
2. The PR interval should remain constant and should measure between .12 and .20 second. A PR greater than .20 second demonstrates first-degree atrioventricular (AV) block.
3. The QRS interval should measure between .04 and .11 second. A QRS interval of .12 second or greater signifies a bundle branch block.
4. Sinus rhythm should be present.
5. Chest leads V_1-V_6 should conform to a standard format in order to be considered normal. The QRS in V_1 should have a small R wave and a larger S wave. As the leads move across the chest from V_1 to V_6, the R wave should increase in height and the S wave should decrease in depth. This is called normal R-wave progression.

Electrocardiogram Interpretation

Bundle Branch Block. Bundle branch block represents a delay or blockage in either the right or left bundle branch. Because of the delay, the QRS complex is widened to .12 second or greater on an ECG. Right bundle branch block can be seen in healthy individuals, but left bundle branch block occurs only in heart disease.

Right bundle branch block: QRS .12 second or greater and QRS predominantly positive in V_1 (Figure 19–7)
Left bundle branch block: QRS .12 second or greater and QRS predominantly negative in V_1 (Figure 19–8)

Myocardial Infarction. The coronary arteries

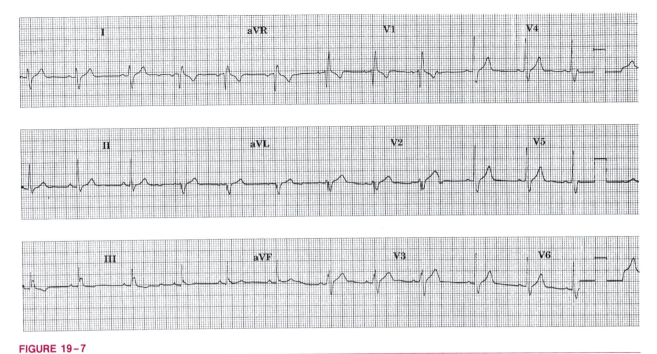

FIGURE 19-7
Right bundle branch block.

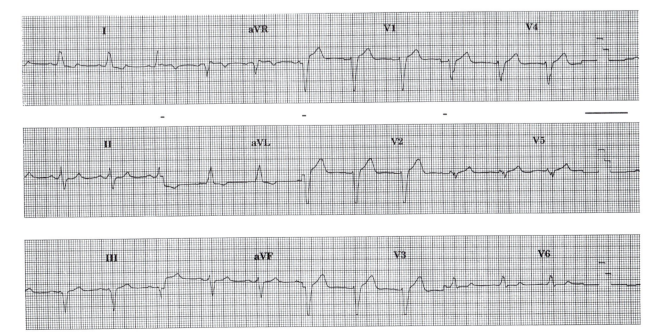

FIGURE 19-8
Left bundle branch block.

nourish the heart muscle with blood. If they become narrowed or blocked, an area in the left ventricle fed by the artery becomes either temporarily or permanently deprived of its blood supply.

If the lack of blood supply is of short duration, such as during a burst of exercise when the blood needs increase, *myocardial ischemia* occurs. ST segment depression or symmetrical T-wave inversion is seen on the ECG in the leads over the area of ischemia. No permanent damage to the ventricular muscle occurs and ST segment depression or T-wave inversion will return to baseline with cessation of exercise and time.

If the deprivation of coronary blood flow continues, *myocardial injury* takes place. ST segment elevation is seen on the ECG in the leads that lie over the injured area in the left ventricle. The myocardium is not permanently damaged, and the ST elevation gradually returns to baseline.

If the lack of blood supply is of longer duration or a coronary artery becomes totally blocked, a death of a portion of the ventricular myocardium occurs called *myocardial infarction*. An infarction is recognized on an ECG by the presence of significant Q waves. To be significant, a Q-wave's voltage must be one-third that of the R wave or at least .04 second wide. An infarction is diagnosed on the ECG by the presence of two or more significant Q waves in an infarction location within the left ventricle.

Infarction Location	ECG Leads to Check
Anterior	V_1, V_2, V_3, V_4 (Figure 19-9)
Lateral	I, aVL, V_5, V_6 (Figure 19-10)
Inferior	II, III, aVF (Figure 19-11)

The posterior wall of the left ventricle has no ECG leads lying directly over it, as do the other left ventricular walls. An infarction in this location is recognized by tall R waves in V_1 and V_2 accompanying an inferior infarction (Figure 19-12).

The age of the infarction is calculated by reviewing the ECG leads where the significant Q waves are seen. If the infarction is acute, the ST segments will be elevated. As the infarction evolves, the ST segments return to baseline and the T waves invert and the exact age of the infarction is indeterminate. An old infarction is recognized by significant Q waves and no ST- or T-wave abnormalities.

Hypertrophy. Enlargement of the muscular wall of the atria or ventricles constitutes hyper-

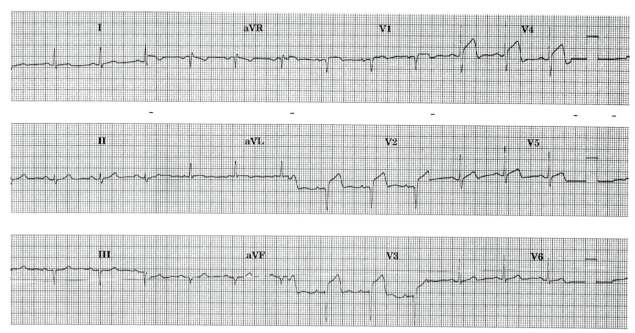

FIGURE 19-9

Acute anterior infarction.

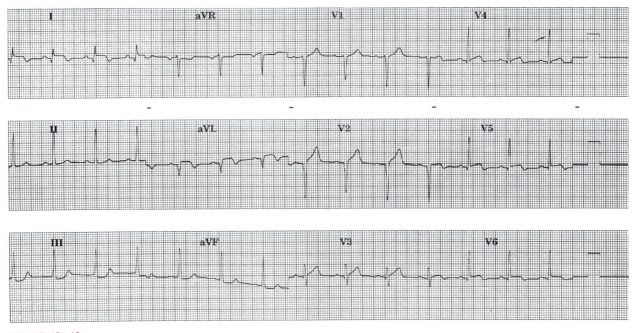

FIGURE 19-10
Acute lateral infarction.

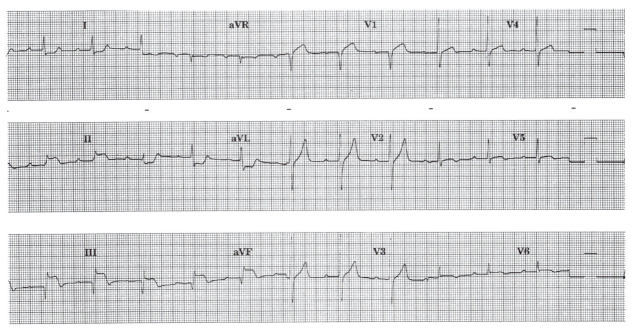

FIGURE 19-11
Acute inferior infarction.

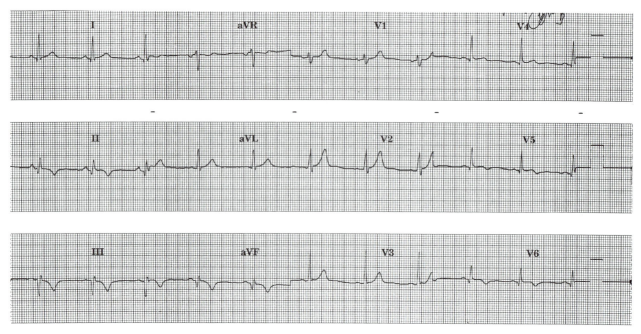

FIGURE 19-12
Inferior and posterior infarction, age indeterminate.

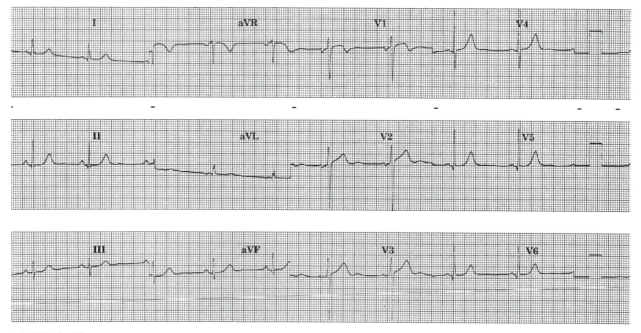

FIGURE 19-13
Left atrial hypertrophy.

trophy. Hypertrophy is associated with heart disease or congenital abnormalities.

- Left atrial hypertrophy is recognized when the terminal portion of the P wave in lead V_1 inverts more than -1 mm (Figure 19-13).
- Right atrial hypertrophy is demonstrated by a P wave in lead II that is 2.5 mm or greater (Figure 19-14).
- Left ventricular hypertrophy is diagnosed when the voltages of the S wave in lead V_1 and the R wave in lead V_5 are equal to or greater than 35 mm (Figure 19-15).
- Right ventricular hypertrophy is diagnosed when the R wave is equal to or larger than the S wave in lead V_1 accompanied by a right-axis deviation. A right axis can be recognized by a QRS complex that is either predominantly negative in lead I or the R wave and the S wave have approximately equal voltages (Figure 19-16).

Arrhythmias

Premature Contractions

Although the sinus node is the pacemaker of the heart, other areas or foci in the atria, AV junction, and ventricles are capable of initiating electrical activity. If the premature contractions originate from the same focus in an area of the heart, they are called *unifocal beats* and resemble one another in configuration. If they arise from multiple foci they are called *multifocal beats* and vary in their configurations. Premature contractions may occur in normal individuals or may be associated with heart disease.

Atrial Premature Contraction. An atrial premature contraction (APC) is a beat that arrives early in the cardiac cycle, begins in an area of the atria other than the SA node, and records a P wave that is different from the sinus P wave. The QRS complex resembles that of the normal cardiac rhythm (Figure 19-17).

A nonconducted APC is recognized by a P wave that arrives extremely early in the cardiac cycle, usually deforming the T wave of the previous beat, and is not followed by a QRS complex (Figure 19-18).

Junctional Premature Contraction. A junctional premature contraction (JPC) is a beat that arrives early in the cardiac cycle, begins in the area around the AV junction, and records an inverted P wave that precedes the normal QRS

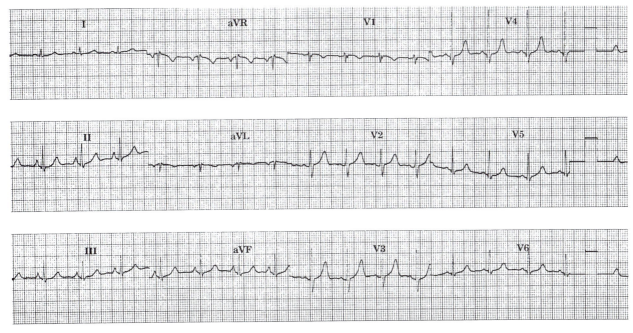

FIGURE 19-14

Right atrial hypertrophy.

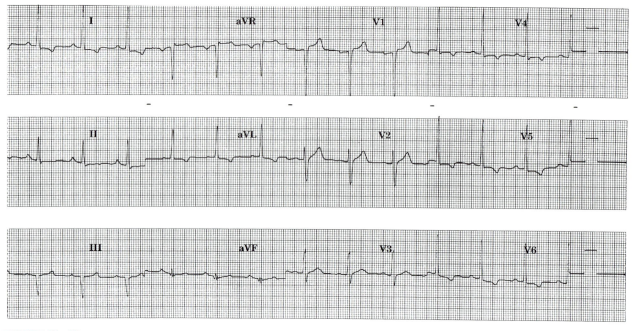

FIGURE 19-15
Left ventricular hypertrophy.

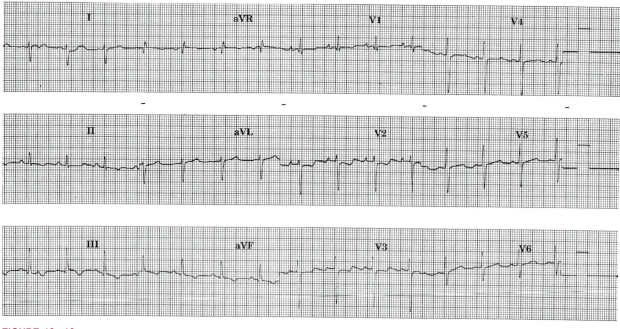

FIGURE 19-16
Right ventricular hypertrophy.

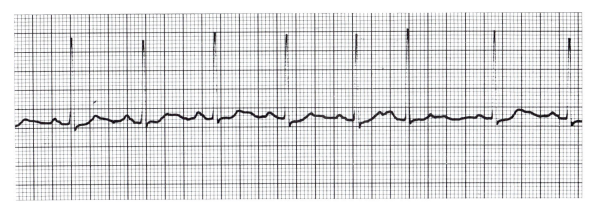

FIGURE 19–17
Sinus rhythm with one isolated atrial premature contraction.

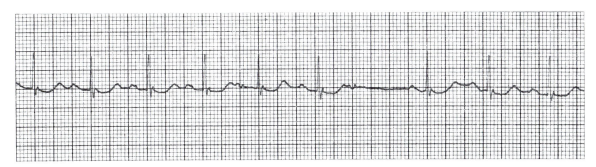

FIGURE 19–18
Sinus rhythm with one nonconducted atrial premature contraction.

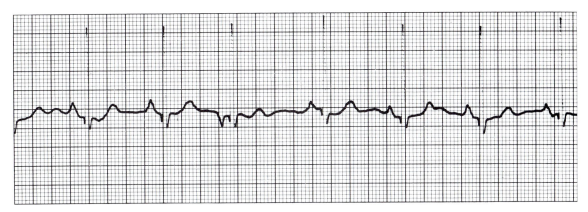

FIGURE 19–19
Sinus rhythm with one isolated junctional premature contraction.

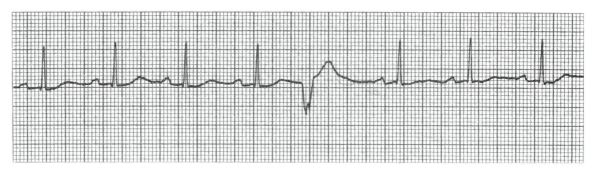

FIGURE 19-20

Sinus rhythm with one isolated ventricular premature contraction.

complex, is buried within it, or follows it (Figure 19-19).

Ventricular Premature Contraction. A ventricular premature contraction (VPC) is a beat that arrives early in the cardiac cycle, has no P wave of its own, and displays a wide and bizarre QRS complex (Figure 19-20).

Atrial Rhythms

Atrial rhythms may occur in healthy hearts although atrial flutter and fibrillation are usually associated with heart disease. The rapid rates of these arrhythmias are usually not tolerated well in diseased hearts.

Atrial Tachycardia. Atrial tachycardia is a run of four or more APCs in a row at a rate of 140-220 beats per minute and is usually a transient arrhythmia (Figure 19-21).

Atrial Flutter. Atrial flutter arises when one focus in the atria fires 220-350 beats per minute and flutter waves replace P waves. There can be one, two, three, four, etc. flutter waves for each QRS complex (Figure 19-22).

Atrial Fibrillation. Atrial fibrillation occurs when two or more foci in the atria fire 350-650 beats per minute in random fashion and fibrillatory waves replace P waves. The QRS complexes respond in a totally random fashion to the fibrillatory waves recording varying R-R cycles (Figure 19-23).

Junctional Rhythms

Junctional tachycardia is a run of four or more JPCs in a row and usually occurs in the presence of heart disease or digitalis toxicity (Figure 19-24).

Ventricular Rhythms

All rapid ventricular rhythms create emergency situations and are usually associated with heart disease.

Ventricular Tachycardia. Ventricular tachycardia is a run of four or more VPCs in a row. If ventricular tachycardia is left untreated, it often degenerates into ventricular flutter or fibrillation (Figure 19-25).

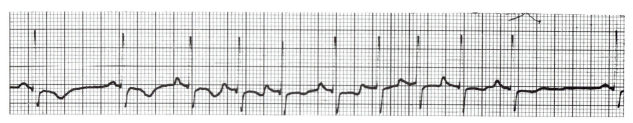

FIGURE 19-21

Atrial tachycardia often begins and ends quite suddenly and is termed paroxysmal atrial tachycardia (PAT). Normal sinus rhythm at 61 minutes, with a burst of PAT.

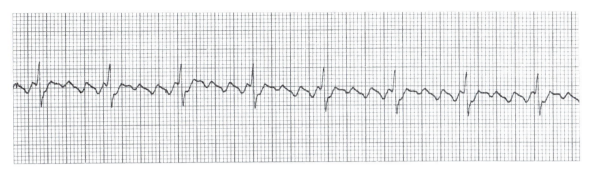

FIGURE 19-22
Atrial flutter at 300 beats per minute with the ventricles responding to every fourth flutter wave (atrial flutter with 4:1 conduction).

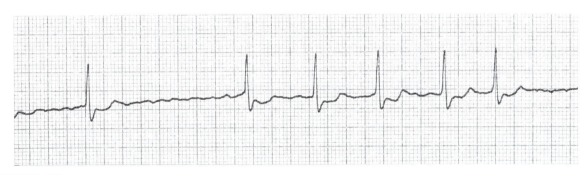

FIGURE 19-23
Atrial fibrillation.

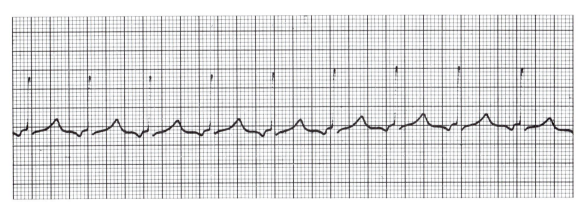

FIGURE 19-24
Junctional tachycardia.

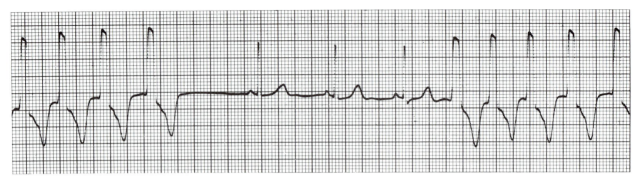

FIGURE 19-25

Sinus rhythm with two short bursts of ventricular tachycardia.

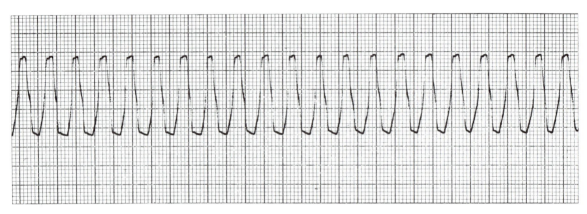

FIGURE 19-26

Ventricular flutter.

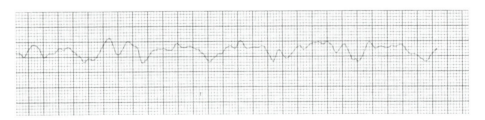

FIGURE 19-27

Ventricular fibrillation.

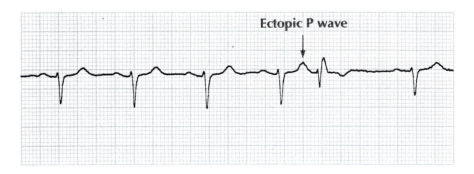

FIGURE 19–28
Sinus rhythm with an isolated atrial premature contraction. (Reproduced from Davis D: *Differential Diagnosis of Arrhythmias.* Philadelphia: W. B. Saunders, 1992, p. 152.)

Ventricular Flutter. Ventricular flutter occurs when one focus in the ventricles fires at a rate of 150–300 beats per minute. The QRS complexes appear to run into one another, and no atrial activity can be seen (Figure 19–26).

Ventricular Fibrillation. Ventricular fibrillation is the random and rapid firing of multifocal foci at a rate of 150–500 beats per minute. No atrial or ventricular activity is seen. Death occurs if no corrective action is taken (Figure 19–27).

Aberration

Aberration occurs when one of the bundle branches is temporarily unable to conduct an electrical impulse and the resulting QRS becomes wide and bizarre. It has no more significance than either an APC or a JPC.

An APC with aberration records an early upright different-looking P wave followed by a wide and bizarre QRS complex (Figure 19–28).

A JPC with aberration records an early inverted P wave either preceding or following a wide and bizarre QRS complex (Figure 19–29).

Atrioventricular Block

First- and second-degree AV block Wenckebach can occur in normal hearts but are often associated with heart disease. Second-degree AV block Mobitz and complete AV block require pacemaker insertion.

First-Degree AV Block. First-degree AV block occurs when the PR interval exceeds .20 second in duration (Figure 19–30).

Second-Degree AV Block. Second-degree AV block Wenckebach is diagnosed when the PR interval progressively lengthens from beat to beat until a P wave occurs without a QRS complex following it and a ventricular pause occurs (Figure 19–31).

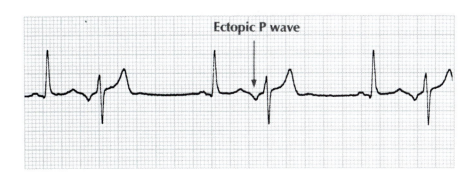

FIGURE 19–29
Sinus rhythm with three isolated junctional premature contractions with aberration. (Reproduced from Davis D: *Differential Diagnosis of Arrhythmias.* Philadelphia: W. B. Saunders, 1992, p. 154.)

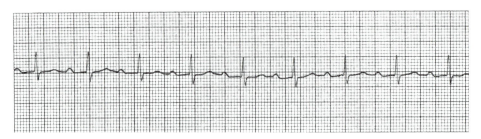

FIGURE 19-30

Sinus rhythm with first-degree atrioventricular block.

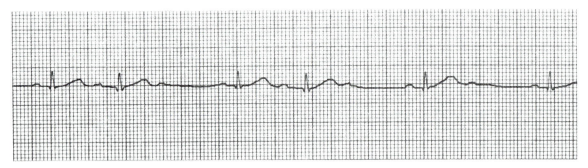

FIGURE 19-31

Sinus rhythm with second-degree atrioventricular block Wenckebach.

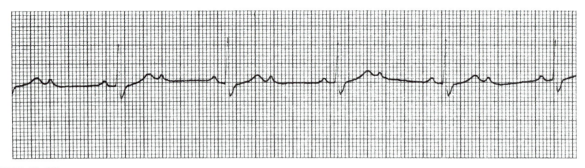

FIGURE 19-32

Sinus rhythm with second-degree atrioventricular block Mobitz.

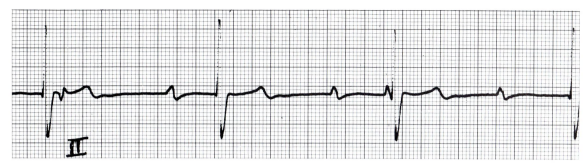

FIGURE 19-33
Complete atrioventricular block.

Second-degree AV block Mobitz is recognized when the PR interval is constant, sinus P wave occurs without a QRS complex following it, and a ventricular pause occurs (Figure 19-32).

Complete AV Block. Complete AV block represents a complete lack of conduction between the atria and ventricles. The atria and ventricles are each under the control of separate pacemaking foci. The ventricular rate is generally much slower than the atrial rate, and the PR interval varies (Figure 19-33).

Sinoatrial Block

SA block is associated with heart disease and does not usually require pacemaker insertion.

SA block is diagnosed when the SA node's electrical impulse fails to reach the atrial musculature. Ventricular pauses occur with no P wave or QRS complex present (Figure 19-34). Be sure to rule out the presence of a nonconducted APC, which can be seen deforming the previous T wave.

Cardiac Diagnostic Tests

Holter Monitor

The Holter monitor is a small portable tape recorder that allows 12-24-hour ambulatory heart rhythm monitoring for arrhythmia detection. Indications for monitoring include

- Irregular heart beat
- Syncope
- Postmyocardial infarction
- Postpacemaker insertion
- Monitoring medical therapy

Procedure. Electrodes are placed on designated areas on the torso and chest to monitor either one or two lead ECG recordings. The patient's skin should be cleansed with alcohol and slightly abraded with gauze. Male patients should be shaven at the electrode site to ensure quality tracings. Securing the electrodes with adhesive tape or a bandage will help prevent artifact caused by excessive electrode movement.

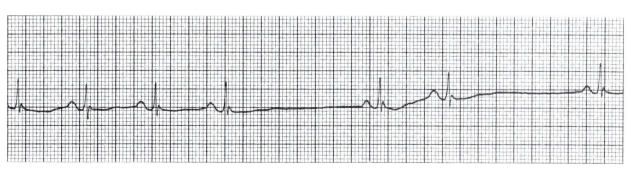

FIGURE 19-34
Sinus rhythm with two episodes of sinoatrial block.

Exercise Stress Test

An exercise stress test is an exercise electrocardiogram that increases the heart rate to a maximal level by the use of a treadmill or bicycle ergometer in order to evaluate cardiac fitness. The stress test is used primarily to make or remove a diagnosis of coronary artery disease.

Indications for exercise stress testing include

- Detection of coronary artery disease
- Assessment of exercise capability
- Evaluation of medical or surgical treatment
- Postmyocardial infarction
- Assessment of arrhythmias
- Induction into exercise program over the age of 40

Procedure. The patient's skin should be cleansed with alcohol and slightly abraded with gauze. Male patients should be shaven at the electrode site to ensure quality tracings. Securing the electrodes with adhesive tape or a bandage will help prevent artifact caused by excessive electrode movement. Electrodes are attached in a 12-lead ECG format, usually with the leg and arm electrodes moved to the lower torso and upper chest, respectively, in order to minimize artifact while exercising.

Echocardiography

Echocardiography is a noninvasive diagnostic test that uses ultrasound to image internal cardiac structures. Chamber size, valvular function, cardiac muscle function, and general anatomical orientation are assessed.

Procedure. The patient is required to lie comfortably on an examining table and an ECG should be hooked up to the patient's limbs as in a 12-lead ECG, minus the chest leads.

SONOGRAPHY

Sonography (also known as ultrasonography and ultrasound) is a noninvasive, diagnostic medical procedure that uses sound waves to evaluate internal organs, blood vessels, and pregnancies. Physicians request an ultrasound to rule out or diagnose various diseases of internal organs (Figure 19–35).

Sonography personnel include sonologists and sonographers. *Sonologists* are physicians with specialized training in performing and interpreting ultrasound images. Sonologists are generally radiologists, but obstetricians and cardiologists may also be skilled in sonography. *Sonographers* are professionally registered individuals that are specially trained to perform the ultrasound examination. They have 1–2 years of training and supervised experience in sonography.

How Sonography Is Performed

Sonography does not involve the use of x-rays and is considered to be a safe procedure. Sonography involves the use of highly technical equipment. The procedure is painless and simple. A handheld transducer that acts as a transmitter and receiver of high-frequency sound waves is placed against the body and moved over the area of interest. Sound waves pass through the skin and strike internal structures, sending back reflections or echoes to the transducer. Different structures produce different echoes that are analyzed by the transducer and a computer and converted into a cross-sectional, gray scale image. Particular echoes may also be converted into the form of wavy lines that represent pulse tracing of blood flow. The study is documented by films and or photographs accompanied by a formal report by the physician (Figure 19–36**A** and **B**).

Sonography Examinations

Abdominal Organ Examinations

Liver (Figure 19–37)
Gallbladder and biliary tract
Pancreas
Kidneys
Spleen
Adrenal glands

Patient Preparation. Fasting for 8–12 hours before the examination. Although a specific organ is ordered as the area of interest, most abdominal studies include the evaluation of all the abdominal organs and vasculature. Fasting ensures dilatation of the normal gallbladder and biliary tract and may help reduce bowel gas.

RADIOLOGY REQUISITION

FORM # 724-8AS (Rev. 2/89)

PLATE

SPECIAL NEEDS: ☐ WHEELCHAIR ☐ IV ☐ STRETCHER ☐ O₂ ☐ IVAC

PATIENT'S NAME

PREGNANT
☐ YES
☐ NO
IF NO, LAST MENS.
DATE _____

VOUCHER PREPARED BY	EXAMINATION REQUESTED	DEPT.	PROCEDURE NO.	QUAN.	PRICE
SIGNATURE					
TIME _____ A/P	BILIARY SYSTEM				
_____ A/P ARRIVAL TIME					
DATE TO BE DONE	PREVIOUS X-RAY EXAMINATION ☐ YES ☐ NO WHERE:	TECHNICIAN		NO. OF FILMS	

CLINICAL DIAGNOSIS -
AND
REASON FOR THIS STUDY: R/O Cholelithiasis
RUQ Pain

REQUESTED BY DR. _____
MEDICAL IMAGING

FIGURE 19–35

Sample of an ultrasound requisition form.

Referring Physician _____   Patient Name _____

Date _____

X-RAY EXAMINATION:

ULTRASOUND OF THE GALLBLADDER

Realtime ultrasonography of the gallbladder was performed in transverse and longitudinal planes. Numerous echogenic foci are seen within lumen of gallbladder which move within lumen of gallbladder with changes in patient positioning. There is distal acoustic shadowing produced. The gallbladder wall is normal for size, shape and echo texture. No pericholecystic fluid collections are seen and no abnormal echoes are present. There is no intrahepatic or extrahepatic biliary duct dilatation. The liver is normal for size, shape, and echo texture. The subhepatic and subdiaphragmatic spaces are normal and there is no subcapsular fluid. Porta hepatis region is unremarkable. No pancreatic masses or textural abnormalities are seen. No abnormal echoes emanate from pancreas.

IMPRESSION:

Cholelithiasis.

7/91-1706   _____ M.D.

FIGURE 19-36

A and **B**, Samples of ultrasound report, giving results and diagnosis.

Referring Physician _____   Patient Name _____

Date _____

X-RAY EXAMINATION:

ULTRASOUND EXAMINATION OF THE BILIARY SYSTEM

Real time images of right upper quadrant were obtained in transverse and longitudinal planes. The gallbladder is normal for size, shape, and contour. No intraluminal echogenic focci are seen, and there is no distal acoustic shadowing present. Liver texture is normal, and there are no hypo or hyperechoic mass lesions within liver. There is no intrahepatic or extrahepatic biliary duct dilatations present. Pancreas is normal for size, shape and echo texture. Peripancreatic regions are normal.

IMPRESSION:

Normal ultrasound of the biliary system.

FIGURE 19-36 Continued

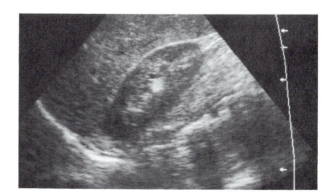

FIGURE 19-37
Sonogram of the liver and right kidney.

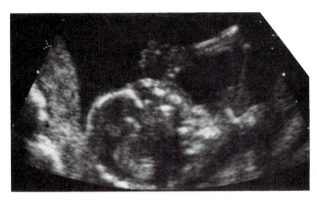

FIGURE 19-38
Sonogram of fetus sucking its thumb.

Abdominal Vasculature Examinations

Aorta
Inferior vena cava

Patient Preparation. Fasting for 8-12 hours before the examination.

Obstetrics/Gynecology Examinations

Uterus and ovaries
Urinary bladder
Early pregnancy
First-, second-, and third-trimester pregnancy (Figure 19-38)
Amniocentesis (needle-guided sampling of amniotic fluid)

Patient Preparation. A full urinary bladder is required; 32-40 oz of clear fluid should be ingested 1 hour before the examination and finished within 15-20 minutes. If for any reason the patient cannot have fluids, sterile water can be used to fill the bladder through a Foley catheter at the examination site. NOTE: In some cases, an endovaginal study may accompany the transpelvic study, and the patient will be asked to empty bladder.

Breast Examination

Usually the composition of an isolated lesion, but possibly whole breast evaluation

Patient Preparation. None.

Chest Examination

Usually an isolated area

Patient Preparation. None.

Echocardiography

The heart

Patient Preparation. None

Intraoperative Sonography

Brain and spinal cord
Abdominopelvic organs
Vasculature

Male Pelvis Examinations

Prostate gland
Urethra
Bladder

Patient Preparation. A full urinary bladder is required; 32-40 oz of clear fluid should be ingested 1 hour before the examination and finished within 15-20 minutes. If for any reason the patient cannot have fluids, sterile water can be used to fill the bladder through a Foley catheter at the examination site. NOTE: In some cases, and endovaginal study may accompany the transpelvic study, and the patient will be asked to empty the bladder.

Needle-Guided Biopsies or Fluid Aspirations

Organ lesions
Isolated fluid collections

Patient Preparation. None.

Neurosonography

Infant brain and ventricular system

Patient Preparation. None.

Ophthalmology Sonography

The eye

Patient Preparation. None.

Salivary Glands Examination

Patient Preparation. None.

Scrotum Examination

Patient Preparation. None.

Thyroid Examination

Patient Preparation. None.

Vascular Examinations

Carotid arteries
Femoral arteries
Popliteal arteries and veins

Patient Preparation. None

Bibliography

Radiography

Ballinger PW: *Merrill's Atlas of Radiographic Positions and Radiologic Procedures,* 3 vols., 5th ed. St. Louis: C. V. Mosby, 1982.
Jucius RA: *Radiation Safety and You.* Milwaukee, WI: General Electric, 1972.
Radiologic Technology. Washington, DC: Departments of the Air Force, the Army, and the Navy, 1983.
Sanders RC: *Clinical Sonography,* 1st ed. Boston: Little, Brown, 1984.

Electrocardiography

Bronson L: *Textbook of Cardiovascular Technology.* Philadelphia: J. B. Lippincott, 1987.
Chung E: *Electrocardiography,* 2nd ed. New York: Harper & Row, 1980.
Davis D: *Differential Diagnosis of Arrhythmias.* Philadelphia: W. B. Saunders, 1992.
Goldman MJ: *Principles of Clinical Electrocardiography,* 11th ed. Los Altos, CA: Lange, 1982.
Mangiola S, Ritota M: *Cardiac Arrhythmias.* Philadelphia: J. B. Lippincott, 1974.
Marriot H: *Practical Electrocardiography,* 7th ed. Baltimore: Williams & Wilkins, 1983.

Sonography

Callen PW: *Ultrasonography in Obstetrics and Gynecology,* 2nd ed. Philadelphia: W. B. Saunders, 1988.
Hagen-Ansert SL: *Textbook of Diagnostic Ultrasonography,* 3rd ed. St. Louis: C. V. Mosby, 1989.
Mittelstaedt CA: *Abdominal Ultrasound,* New York: Churchill Livingstone, 1987.
Sanders RC: *Clinical Sonography,* Boston: Little, Brown, 1984.

Chapter 20

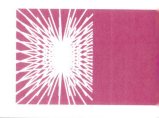

SPECIMEN COLLECTION AND PROCESSING

PATRICIA S. HURLBUT

TERMINOLOGY
LABORATORY REQUEST FORMS
CATEGORIES OF LABORATORY TESTS
PANELS AND PROFILES
PATIENT INSTRUCTION TECHNIQUES
　Fasting
　Medications
　Patient Instructions
COLLECTION EQUIPMENT AND SUPPLIES
　Appropriate Containers
　Correct Preservatives
　Collection Time Factors
　Labeling
　Centers for Disease Control Universal Precautions for Blood and Body Fluids
TYPES AND METHODS OF SPECIMEN COLLECTION
　Blood
　Urine
　Stool
　Sputum
　Semen
　Throat Specimens
　Genital Tract Specimens
SPECIMEN PREPARATION
　Preservation Techniques
METHODS OF DELIVERY OF SPECIMENS
　In Person
　Mail Service
　Pick-Up Service
　Chain of Custody
PROCEDURES FOR DISPOSAL
　Labeling of Waste
　Occupational Safety and Health Act Regulations
　Health and Safety of the Community
QUALITY CONTROL
　Reagent Management
　Control Requirements
　Instrument Calibration
　Instrument and Testing Logbooks/Worksheets
　Preventive Maintenance of Equipment

TERMINOLOGY

Aliquot: A small sampling of a specimen.
Anticoagulant: Chemical used to prevent blood from clotting.
Biohazard: May be harmful to human life.
Calibration: Checking the accuracy of the equipment using standards (known values).
Culture: Living microorganisms growing on media for identification.

Plasma: The liquid part of the blood that contains all the nutrients and chemicals and clotting factors outside of the blood cells.
Preservative: Chemical used to prevent the breakdown of a specimen before testing.
Quality control: Methods of testing to ensure that results are reliable and accurate and that all errors are eliminated.

525

Reference laboratory: Centralized laboratory that can service many physicians in a cost-effective manner in a short time.

Serum: The liquid part of the blood that remains after a blood specimen has been allowed to clot.

Specimen: A small sample of something taken to show the nature of the whole.

LABORATORY REQUEST FORMS

Tests need to be ordered in a manner that will ensure that the specimen will be tested correctly. Incorrect paperwork often causes the testing to be delayed. Some tests need to be run immediately, and the results may be altered by delay.

PROCEDURE
COMPLETING LABORATORY REQUEST FORMS

PURPOSE

To ensure correct collection, testing, and reporting of laboratory results within the time limits required of the test.

EQUIPMENT AND MATERIALS

Physician's order for laboratory tests
Laboratory form
Patient's chart

PROCEDURAL STEPS

1. Carefully read the physician's orders for laboratory tests.
   RATIONALE: Because many laboratory tests have similar names, accuracy is necessary to ensure the proper tests are performed. Using the patient's chart, complete the specimen request form as completely as possible. Refer to Figure 20–1 for a sample form.
2. Fill in the space for the physician's name with the name of the physician requesting the tests.
   RATIONALE: This ensures that the results return to the proper physician.
3. Complete the patient's personal information, including patient name, address, date of birth, sex, and identification number (often the social security number).
   RATIONALE: Many laboratory results vary with the age or sex of the patients. With this information, the laboratory can more accurately evaluate the results obtained from testing.
4. Complete the billing information.
   RATIONALE: Like all physicians, laboratories are reimbursed by insurance companies. By supplying the laboratory with the proper information, you enable them to submit their fees directly to the insurance company in a timely manner and for the convenience of the patient.
5. Have the *patient* complete the authorization to release and assign benefits (Figure 20–2).
   RATIONALE: The patient must give permission to release the tests ordered so the insurance company has the information it needs for billing.
6. Complete the specimen collection information, including reporting status, specimen type, and collection date and time.
   RATIONALE: Laboratories are more efficient when they know the proper priority of specimens. The integrity of some specimens will deteriorate with time, and thus certain tests need to be run first in the laboratory. By knowing this information about each specimen, the laboratory can organize and test the most critical specimens quickly.
7. Complete the test request information.
   RATIONALE: The tests listed are the most commonly ordered tests. Marking tests ordered on preprinted forms enables you to save time and avoid possible errors from confusing abbreviations.

IMAGING & LABORATORY DIAGNOSTIC CENTER (ILDC)
2500 W. Layton Ave., Milwaukee, WI 53221   Phone: (414) 282-5314

BILL: ☐ INSURANCE   ☐ PATIENT   ☐ ACCOUNT   Accession #

DATE	PHYSICIAN	PRIMARY INSURANCE CO.	SECONDARY INSURANCE CO.
PATIENT NAME – LAST, FIRST, MI		PRIMARY INSURANCE CO. ADDRESS	SECONDARY INSURANCE CO. ADDRESS
PATIENT STREET ADDRESS			
CITY STATE ZIP CODE		PRIMARY INSURANCE NO(S)	SECONDARY INSURANCE NO(S)
DATE OF BIRTH / /	SEX PHONE	PRIMARY SUBSCRIBER NAME	SECONDARY SUBSCRIBER NAME
SOCIAL SECURITY NO.		PRIMARY SUBSCRIBER ADDRESS	SECONDARY SUBSCRIBER ADDRESS
EMPLOYER NAME – RESP. PARTY		CITY STATE ZIP CODE	CITY STATE ZIP CODE
EMPLOYER ADDRESS		RELATIONSHIP TO PATIENT	RELATIONSHIP TO PATIENT
CITY STATE ZIP CODE		DIAGNOSIS	

SPECIMEN INFORMATION   ☐ ROUTINE ☐ ASAP ☐ STAT ☐ CALL RESULTS
TYPE OF SPECIMEN   ☐ SERUM ☐ URINE 24 HR. VOL. ___ ml ☐ PLASMA
☐ FASTING ☐ NON-FAST   TIME COLLECTED ☐ AM ☐ PM

Collection Fee	100	Cholesterol	10	Lithium	35	UAR-REFLEX	200
Handling-Send out	98 or 99	HDL	24	Phenobarbital	29	Urinalysis-Routine	201
DIAGNOSTIC PROFILES		CPK	11	Primidone	32	**SEROLOGY**	
BCL Panel	403			Procainamide/NAPA	36/37	ABO & Rh(D) (L & R)	163
Lipid Panel	437	Creatinine	7	Prolactin	66	Antibody Screen (L & R)	165
Cardiac Risk Panel #1	407	GGTP	16	Pros. Acid Phos.	26	ANA-REFLEX	156
Cardiac Risk Panel #2	408	Glucose-Fasting	6	PSA	62	CMV-IgG	158
Chem 12 Panel	404	Glucose-2 Hr. PP	6	Quinidine	30	HIV Antibody	157
Chem 24 Panel +	/405	Glucose-Random	6	Theophylline	27	Mono Screen	153
Chem 25	24/405	Glucose-Tol-3 Hr.	67/68/69	TSH	57	RA Screen	151
Diabetic Profile #1 (L & R)	6/43	Lipase	60	Free-T4	56	Lymes Disease AB.	175
Electrolytes	406	LDH	12	T4	53	RPR	150
Health Screen I (L & R)	(423)	Magnesium	25	T3 Uptake	54	RSV-IgG	159
Health Screen II (L & R)	(424)	Phosphorus	22	FTI (T7)	55	Rubella Index	161
Health Screen III (L & R)	(425)	Potassium	2	T3-Total	58	STD Profile	(422)
SIMBA Panel #1 (L & R)	(443)	SGOT (AST)	13	**HEMATOLOGY**		TORCH Screen	421
Liver Profile	417	SGPT (ALT)	14	CBC w/Plat.-REFLEX (L)	429/130	Toxoplasma-IgG	160
Mini Panel #1	400	Sodium	1	Cell Ct.-Body Fluid	124	**MICROBIOLOGY-REFLEX MIC**	
Mini Panel #2	401	T. Protein	20	Eos. Ct. (L)	119	C. Difficile Toxin	332
Mini Panel #3	402	Triglycerides	9	Hemogram (L)	431	Chlamydia Culture	335
OB Profile #1 (L & R)	413	Uric Acid	8	HGB & HCT (L)	103/104	Chlamydia Rapid Screen	334
OB Profile #2 (L & R)	414	**SPECIAL CHEMISTRIES**		Platelet Ct. & MPV (L)	109/110	GC Culture	336
Prostatic Profile	17/26/62	AFP	63	Protime (B)	121	Herpes Culture	337
Renal Profile	418	B-12 & Folate	42/41	PTT (B)	122	Mycoplasma Culture	339
Thyroid-REFLEX	410	Carbamazepine	33	Retic Ct.	118	Ova & Parasites	333
Thyroid Profile #1	(411)	CEA	45	Sed Rate (L)	117	Pinworm Prep	329
Thyroid Profile #2	(412)	Digoxin	31	Synovial Fluid Anal.	125	Strep Screen-Rapid	302
ROUTINE CHEMISTRIES		Dilantin	28	WBC Ct. (L)	101	Strep Culture	303
ALK PHOS	17	Ferritin	46	WBC & Diff (L)	430	Throat Culture	301
Albumin	21	Fructosamine	44	**URINALYSIS**		Trich Screen	330
Amylase	15	LH/FSH	65/64	Creat. Clear.-24 Hr.	7/48/70	Urine Culture	300
Bilirubin Direct	19	Glycohemoglobin (L)	43	HCG-Urine Qual.	205	Other Culture (State Source)	
Bilirubin Total	18	HCG-Serum Qual.	171	Occult Blood-Feces	206		
BUN	5	HCG-Serum Quant.	171	Protein-Qual.	202		
Calcium	23	Iron & TIBC	38/39	Protein-24 Hr.-Quant.	203		

OTHER TESTS:

CYTOLOGY EXAMINATION

# SLIDES	GYNECOLOGIC SPECIMEN SOURCE	NON GYNECOLOGIC SPECIMEN SOURCE
1 2 3		
☐ VCE 250	☐ MATURATION INDEX 251	☐ SPUTUM
☐ CERVICAL		☐ BRONCHIAL WASHINGS LOBE ___
☐ VAGINAL		
PERTINENT INFORMATION		☐ GASTRIC ___
☐ HORMONE Rx ☐ DISCHARGE		☐ PLEURAL FLUID
☐ NOW PREGNANT ☐ MENOPAUSE		☐ PERITONEAL FLUID
☐ POST PARTUM ☐ HYSTERECTOMY		☐ URINE
☐ BLEEDING ☐		☐ OTHER
FDLNMP	DATE OF LAST PAP	**PERTINENT INFORMATION**
		☐ INFLAMMATORY
		☐ TUMOR ☐ OTHER

TISSUE EXAMINATION

SPECIMEN DESCRIPTION: (If biopsy, describe lesion & give exact location)

CLINICAL DIAGNOSIS:

SYMPTOMS/HISTORY

FIRST OBSERVED

FORM ILDC-5882

FIGURE 20–1

Sample Laboratory Request form. (Courtesy of Imaging and Laboratory Diagnostic Center, Milwaukee, WI.)

To Our Patient:

To provide you with the most efficient service possible, please complete this information and sign the authorization below **prior** to arriving at our facility. Present this form with your Medicare and/or insurance cards to our receptionist as soon as you arrive.

Thank you for your cooperation!

(PLEASE PRINT)

Patient Name _____ Birthdate _____

Home Address _____ Phone No. _____

City/State/Zip _____ Work No. _____

Social Security No. _____

AUTHORIZATION TO RELEASE AND ASSIGN INSURANCE BENEFITS

I authorize release of all information required to act on insurance claims and permit a photographic or other facsimile reproduction of this authorization to be used in place of the original assignment. I hereby assign to _____ the medical and/or surgical benefits I am entitled from my insurance company for services the partnership has provided for a period of one year from date of signature.

I further acknowledge that I am responsible for payment in full of any amounts not covered by insurance benefits (including amounts above usual and customary charges). _____ accepts assignment from Medicare, Medicaid, and SIMBA IPA.

Patient or Subscriber _____
(Signature)   (Date)

(Signature of Parent or Guardian if under 14 years of age)

FIGURE 20-2

Sample Authorization to Release and Assign Insurance Benefits form. (Courtesy of Imaging and Laboratory Diagnostic Center, Milwaukee, WI.)

CATEGORIES OF LABORATORY TESTS

Laboratories are generally divided into smaller departments by the types of tests run in order to better organize their workloads. The following is a list of the basic departments and the types of testing each department performs:

Blood Bank: Study of grouping, typing, and preparation of blood specimens for compatible transfusions. Tests ordered by the physician's office for this laboratory would be ABO, Rh factors, and crossmatches for presurgery patients.

Chemistry: Study of body fluids. Tests included in this area are serum tests checking specific levels of chemicals, such as electrolytes, glucose, proteins, or drugs.

Coagulation: Study of the factors involved in the blood clotting process. Tests ordered may include tests run to monitor anticoagulant therapy and effectiveness of the body's ability to clot.

Hematology: Study of the actual blood cells. This department includes testing of white blood cells (WBCs), red blood cells (RBCs), and platelets, and observation of their sizes, shapes, and functions.

Microbiology: Study of bacteria, fungi, parasites, and viruses. Tests included are cultures and sensitivity of microorganisms.

Serology/Immunology: Study of the body's immune responses by detection of antibodies in the serum and enzymes from the white blood cells. Tests prepared in this department would be tests for immunization status or exposure to specific pathogens.

Urinalysis: Study of physical, chemical, and microscopic structures of urine. Tests ordered most often for this department are routine urinalysis (UA), drug screening, glucose, or pregnancy tests.

PANELS AND PROFILES

Tests are often ordered in groups, called "panels" or "screens." A panel is useful when the physician needs a general overview of how well the body is functioning. Usually it includes

TABLE 20-1

CHEMISTRY PANELS AND PROFILES

Full panel
  Glucose
  Electrolytes (sodium [Na], potassium [K], chloride [Cl], carbon dioxide [CO_2])
  Blood urea nitrogen (BUN)
  Creatinine
  Uric acid
  Creatine kinase (CK)
  Lactate dehydrogenase (LD)
  Total protein
  Albumin
  Albumin: globulin ratio
  Total bilirubin
  Direct bilirubin
  Cholesterol
  Triglyceride
  Calcium (C)
  Phosphorus (P)
  Iron (Fe)
  Serum glutamic-oxaloacetic transaminase (SGOT)
  Serum glutamic-pyruvic transaminase (SGPT)
  Gamma-glutamyl transpeptidase (GGTP)

Mini-panel
  Glucose
  Electrolytes (Na, K)
  Creatinine

Electrolytic panel
  Na
  K
  Cl
  HCO_3

Lipid panel
  Triglycerides
  Cholesterol
  High-density lipoprotein (HDL)
  Calculated low-density lipoprotein (LDL)

OB profile
  Blood group and type (ABO, Rh)
  Antibody Screen
  Rubella
  Rapid plasma reagin (RPR)
  Chlamydia
  Toxoplasma

Thyroid panel
  Triiodothyrine (T3) uptake
  Thyroxine (T_4)
  Calculated T7
  Thyroid-stimulating hormone (TSH)

at least one test to detect any abnormalities from each of the 12 body systems. If an abnormality is found, the physician can then follow up with more specific tests in that area. Table 20-1 is a brief listing of tests commonly run in panels. Panels can be run to gain the maximum information about a patient's condition using a very small amount of blood.

PATIENT INSTRUCTION TECHNIQUES

Laboratory results are only as good as the integrity of the specimen collected. If care is not taken to obtain a good specimen, results may be inaccurate. It is very important that the patient understands any special conditions he or she must prepare for a specimen. It is the medical assistant's responsibility to explain to the patient any special requirements, such as fasting, timing before or after taking medications, or cleansing techniques.

Fasting

A fasting specimen is preferred for tests run on the digestive system. Fasting is abstaining from food, smoking, gum, and liquids (except small sips of water) for a specific amount of time. Usually fasting is done overnight and the specimen collected early in the morning, so that fasting is less of an inconvenience to the patient.

When a patient is fasting, he or she should abstain from drinking liquids such as coffee and tea, because the use of sugar or creamer can stimulate the digestive system and alter the results.

Caffeine and nicotine may inhibit the processes of the digestive system and alter the results.

Medications

The patient needs to be told whether or not to take normal medications before laboratory testing. An insulin-dependent diabetic should refrain from taking medications or eating until after the fasting specimen is collected. (If the patient takes insulin but does not eat soon afterward due to a delay in the specimen collection, he or she may face severe side effects of the medication.)

Tests for medications (such as Vancomycin) may need to be taken at "peak" or "trough" levels to give the physician the most valuable information for evaluating the progress of the treatment. Peak levels are drawn 1/2–1 hour *after* the patient has taken the medication. This is when the medicine should be at the highest level in the bloodstream. Trough levels are taken 1/2 to 1 hour *before* the next dose of medicine, when the medicine should be at the lowest level in the bloodstream.

Patient Instructions

Often a preprinted sheet explaining the preparations for testing is given to the patient. Some of these instructions may be complicated, and it is helpful for patients to have a copy to refer to once they are at home.

- A preprinted sheet is especially useful for long or detailed diet restrictions. Patients may take this sheet home and refer to it as they prepare meals.
- It is a good practice to read these preprinted instructions to patients before they leave the office. Although it may require additional time, it gives patients an opportunity to ask questions about any of the instructions.
- Any questions regarding the specimen collection should be answered before collection. The laboratory personnel may be called for more specific details.

COLLECTION EQUIPMENT AND SUPPLIES

Appropriate Containers

When collecting specimens, it is important to use the proper containers to avoid contamination or deterioration of a specimen.

Lid. All specimens collected must have a tightly fitting lid. It is important to remember that the specimen collected may contain the pathogens that are causing the patient's illness. A tight lid prevents accidental spills and transmis-

TABLE 20-2

VACUTAINER TUBES, CONTENTS, AND THEIR USES

Stopper Color	Contents (Anticoagulant)	Uses*
Red	None	Serum for chemistry, serologic tests, typing and crossmatching
Royal blue	Chemically clean	Trace metals (iron, lead); serum for chemistry
Black/red mottled (serum separation tube)†	Serum-separator gel	Serum for most chemistries, serologic tests
Black/yellow mottled (chlormerodrin accumulation test) (CAT)†	Clot activator, separator gel	STAT serum collections
Light blue†	Citrate	Coagulation studies, some hematology tests
Lavender†	EDTA	Hematology tests, some chemistries
Black†	Balanced oxalate	Coagulation
Green†	Heparin	Plasma for some chemistries, especially STATs
Gray†	Fluoride	STAT glucose tests, alcohol levels, drug screening

* Specimen requirements vary, depending on the method used in testing. Always check the laboratory specimen requirements manual before collecting a specimen.
† Denotes tubes that must be thoroughly mixed by gentle inversion after the blood is collected.
Reprinted from Kinn ME, Derge EF: *The Medical Assistant: Administrative and Clinical*, 6th ed. Philadelphia: W. B. Saunders, 1988, p. 722.

sion of the disease to the medical assistant or laboratory personnel.

Vacutainers. Vacutainer systems are used for the collection of blood specimens according to the specific requirement of the tests ordered. Table 20-2 summarizes the color coding used for blood collection.

Sterile Versus Nonsterile Collection Cup. Collection cups may be sterile or nonsterile. Sterile cups are needed whenever a specimen is collected to estimate the quantity of pathogens involved in a disease. Nonsterile cups may be used whenever a physician needs to know simply if a pathogen is present. A general rule is that if you are unsure of what the physician wishes to know, use a sterile cup.

Culture Swabs. Culture swabs may be used to collect a specimen from the specific area affected. Swabs should be polyester (not cotton) to prevent excessive absorption into the swab by the organisms. A swab is only a transport method until the organisms can be transferred to a media plate (culture plate) where they can grow for further testing.

Stool Specimens. Parasites found in stool specimens are generally collected in a container with preservatives. Stool cultures, however, are collected in a nonsterile collection cup, as discussed above.

Correct Preservatives

Preservatives are used to help prevent deterioration of a specimen over time. Always refer to the specific test requirements to make sure the proper method of preservation is being used.

Refrigeration

Refrigeration of the specimen until testing can be performed is the most common form of preservation. A few specimens may be damaged or destroyed by cold temperatures, however, so it is important to check the requirements of each test before collection of the specimen.

Chemical Preservatives

Preservatives, such as hydrochloric acid (HCl) and boric acid, are used for collection of 24-hour urine samples. Because the nature of the specimen requires that the specimen be collected over a longer period of time, it is important that the earliest collected portion be of the same quality when the laboratory receives it.

Preservatives such as formaldehyde or formalin are used whenever a tissue or a parasite is being collected.

Collection Time Factors

Timing of the collection of a specimen may be important whenever the body's level of chemicals fluctuates.

Fasting

Fasting before collection of a specimen obtains results at the body's minimum concentrations. These values are useful for comparison to previous results to indicate when the body's minimum requirements for a chemical or medication have changed.

Timed Tolerances

A glucose tolerance test (GTT) must be carefully timed. The purpose of this test is to monitor levels of blood glucose at specific times after the intake of a known level of glucose. Because a healthy body can quickly restore its normal levels of glucose, it is important to time the GTT carefully and draw blood at the exact times requested.

Medication Levels

As previously mentioned, some medications require peak and trough levels. Refer to Patient Instruction Techniques for further discussion of collection requirements.

First Morning

Urine generally has the highest chemical concentrations after an extended period of sleeping. The first morning specimen also yields higher bacterial colony counts. For these reasons, a first morning specimen is usually the specimen of choice. It is important to remember, however, that if a person generally sleeps through the day (as with a third-shift job), it may be desirable to bring in the first specimen after he or she awakens.

Labeling

A specimen must have enough information on its label that there can be no mix-up of specimens once the patient has left.

Items to be included on a label are generally

- the patient's name
- the patient's identification number (often the social security number)
- tests ordered
- date and time of collection
- the patient's birthdate
- the physician's name
- the medical assistant's initials

The date and time of the specimen collection should be included as part of the label to avoid confusions between timed specimens or recheck specimens on the same patient.

The label of the specimen needs to match the information given on the specimen test request form. Any discrepancies *must* be corrected before any testing is performed.

Centers for Disease Control Universal Precautions for Blood and Body Fluids

The Centers for Disease Control have issued Universal Precautions for Blood and Body Fluids to protect medical personnel and the public from the spread of infectious diseases. These precautions treat *every* patient as potentially infectious. If you use these guidelines, there is no need to take further measures against specific diseases.

Barrier Protection

Gloves. Gloves should be changed after contact with each patient and after the handling of specimens. Gloves should be worn when

- Touching a patient's blood and body fluids, mucous membranes, or skin that is not intact.
- Handling items and surfaces contaminated with blood and body fluids.
- Performing venipuncture and other vascular access procedures.
- Performing any invasive procedure. If a glove is torn or an injury occurs, the glove should be removed and replaced with a new glove as soon as safety permits. The instrument involved in the incident should be removed from the sterile field to a safe container.
- Changing dressing. Enclose small dressings inside the glove as you remove it, by grasping the dressing as you pull the glove off inside out.
- Handling and processing all specimens of blood and body fluids.
- Cleaning and decontaminating spills of blood or other body fluids.
- Disposing of bulk blood, suctioned fluids, excretions, and secretions down a drain connected to a sanitary sewer.

Gowns and Aprons. Cover gowns or disposable plastic aprons should be worn when

- It is probable that your clothing will be soiled with body substances.
- Procedures are likely to generate splashes of blood or other body fluids.
- Assisting in invasive procedures that are likely to splash blood or other body fluids.
- Cleaning and decontaminating spills of blood or other body fluids.

Masks, Glasses, and Goggles. Protect your eyes and oral and nasal mucous membranes from contamination by shielding your face. Use disposable masks. Reusable goggles should be on hand for each physician and assistant and should be washed after each use. Eyeglasses are considered an effective barrier. Use masks and protective eyewear when

- Procedures are likely to generate droplets of blood or body fluids.
- Mucous membrane contact with blood or body fluids is anticipated during the handling of blood or body fluid specimens.
- High-speed suctioning or evacuation equipment is likely to generate aerosol contamination.
- Laboratory procedures have a high potential for generating droplets (for example, blending, ultrasonic procedures, centrifugation, and vigorous mixing).

Hands and Skin Surfaces

If you have exudative lesions or weeping dermatitis, you should not perform any duties involving direct patient care. In addition, you should not handle any equipment used in patient care until the condition resolves. Hands and skin surfaces should be washed

- Immediately after gloves are removed.
- Immediately and thoroughly after any accidental contact with blood or other body fluids.
- Immediately after the completion of any specimen processing.
- After completing daily clinical or laboratory activities and before leaving the office.

Needles and Sharp Instruments

Special care must be taken to prevent injuries caused by needles and sharp instruments during procedures, when cleaning used instruments, and during the disposal of instruments. The following precautions should be followed

- Do not recap used needles and scalpel blades.
- Do not bend or break needles and scalpel blades.
- Do not remove used needles from syringes.
- Do not otherwise manipulate used needles by hand.
- Do not remove used scalpel blades from handles by hand. Use a hemostat to remove the blade.
- Immediately after use, place reusable sharp materials in a puncture-resistant container for transport to the reprocessing room.
- If a needle cap must be replaced during work with specimens, recap with only one hand. Place the cap on a clean surface, and insert the needle into it.

Laboratory Specimens

All blood and other body fluids from every patient should be considered infective. The following precautions should be followed when handling specimens

- Place all specimens in well-constructed containers with secure lids. Place these in a second container, such as an impervious bag, for transport. Check the bag for cracks or leaks.
- Avoid contaminating the outside of the container or the label with the specimen substance. If the outside is contaminated, the container should be disinfected, for example, with 1:10 dilution of 5.25% sodium hypochlorite (household chlorine bleach and water), and placed in an impervious bag for transport.
- Biological safety cabinets should be used if procedures are performed that generate droplets or spattering.
- Mouth pipetting must not be done.
- Laboratory work surfaces must be immediately decontaminated with a disinfectant (such as 10% bleach) after accidental spills of blood or body fluids, and at the end of each procedure.
- Contaminated test materials should be decontaminated before being repaired in the office or transported to the manufacturer.

TYPES AND METHODS OF SPECIMEN COLLECTION

Blood

Vacuum Tube System

The vacuum tube system is a quick, efficient method of collection of blood. In addition, because the blood enters the tube directly instead of being manually pipetted, this method reduces the risk of transmission of infections.

The needles used for this technique have two sharp ends. The first is used for entering the vein

TABLE 20-3

COLLECTION REQUIREMENTS OF COMMONLY ORDERED TESTS

Red top tubes
  Chemistry panels
  Drug levels (therapeutic or abusive)
  Blood urea nitrogen (BUN)
  Creatinine
  Uric acid
  Cholesterol
  High-density lipoprotein (HDL)

Green tubes
  Electrolyte panels
  Sodium (Na)
  Potassium (K)
  Chloride (Cl)
  Carbon dioxide (CO_2)

Grey tubes
  Glucose, fasting
    2-hour postprandial
    tolerance testing

Lavender tubes
  Complete blood count (with or without differential)
  Hemoglobin (Hgb)
  Hematocrit (Hct)
  Erythrocyte sedimentation rates (ESR)
  Platelet studies

Light blue tubes
  Prothrombin time (PT)
  Partial thromboplastin time (PTT)
  ESR

---

of the patient, and the second is used for entering the rubber stopper. Extreme care must be used when handling these needles.

Multiple tubes may be collected using this method without having to restick the patient. Different tests have different anticoagulant requirements. The ability to change tubes allows for several types of specimen to be collected at the same time. Table 20-3 is a brief listing of the different types of tubes and tests.

Procedure. The patient should be seated in a sturdy, comfortable chair. The medical assistant must always be prepared for the occasional patient who may faint.

When possible, ask the patient if there is a preference of arms. Often the patient will remember which arm has been successfully drawn in the past.

Anchoring above and slightly below the puncture site serves two purposes: It holds the vein in place as you enter with the needle, and it lessens the pain the patient may feel when the skin is held taut.

In the event that blood does not begin flowing immediately, try to gently relocate the vein. If you have entered too deeply or too shallowly, reanchor and gently insert or withdraw the needle. If you feel that the vein is off to either side of the needle, discontinue the procedure. Moving the needle sideways in the arm causes much discomfort and possible tissue and nerve damage in the area.

Syringe Methods

The syringe method of blood collection is the method of choice when the patient's veins cannot withstand the vacutainer method; for examples, the veins are very weak or small enough that the vacuum from the tube would cause them to collapse under pressure.

Because a syringe draw involves the transfer of blood products from the syringe into another container, wearing gloves is recommended.

Prime the syringe before beginning the procedure to make sure the plunger moves easily. This is done by simply moving the plunger up and down once to make sure that it does not stick.

A syringe draw must be performed very quickly. Because blood begins clotting as soon as it leaves the body, so it must be added to the anticoagulant as soon as possible.

Capillary Puncture Methods

The capillary puncture is ideal for when only a small amount of blood is required.

Appropriate Sites. The most common sites for collection are the ring and great fingers. The earlobe, the sides of the great toe of a nonwalking infant, and the heel are also acceptable sites (Figure 20-3).

Inappropriate Sites. Avoid areas of callouses, such as the feet of toddlers or the fingers of patients who work extensively with their hands. A callous may become hardened enough to prevent penetration of the lancet into the capillary bed underneath.

Avoid areas of cyanosis. This condition is a sign of poor blood circulation to the area, making collection of blood in this area difficult.

Avoid areas of edema. Edema is an accumulation of tissue fluids between the layers of skin. A puncture of this area deep enough to reach the capillary bed may be difficult and the excess fluids can also compromise the integrity of the blood specimen.

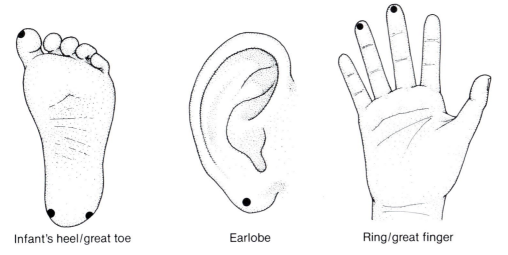

Infant's heel/great toe   Earlobe   Ring/great finger

FIGURE 20-3

Skin puncture sites. (Reproduced from Kinn ME, Derge EF: *The Medical Assistant: Administrative and Clinical,* 6th ed. Philadelphia: W. B. Saunders, 1988, p. 730.)

Patients Ideally Suited for Capillary Puncture. A capillary puncture may be the best collection technique for patients with very tiny veins and weak, surface veins. Often a patient is able to tell you if he or she has had difficulty collecting blood by venipuncture in the past.

Capillary puncture is also an ideal method of collection for self-monitoring testing by patients, as in the case of a diabetic patient checking his or her blood glucose levels daily. It must be emphasized to the patient that poor collection of a specimen may alter the laboratory results and therefore it is very important that proper techniques be used.

Administering a Capillary Puncture to a Child or Fearful Patient. When handling a child or fearful patient, explain what is going to happen in terms the patient understands before the procedure begins. This helps build the patient's confidence and cooperation. A child should not be told that the puncture will not hurt. Even with excellent technique there is minimal discomfort. Saying it will not hurt could break down the patient's trust in you and other health care workers.

SPECIAL HINT

Platelets begin forming a clot over the puncture site as soon as possible. If the blood flow begins to slow, it is often helpful to wipe the puncture site briskly with a sterile gauze to slow the clotting process.

536 Chapter 20: SPECIMEN COLLECTION AND PROCESSING

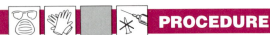

PROCEDURE

COLLECTING A VENOUS BLOOD SPECIMEN USING A SYRINGE OR VACUUM TUBE SYSTEM

PURPOSE

To obtain a venous blood specimen suitable for testing.

EQUIPMENT AND MATERIALS

Nonsterile gloves
Needle, syringe, or Vacutainer needle, adapter, and tube(s)
70% alcohol
Sterile gauze pads
Tourniquet
Bandages
Needle container for disposal of used needles

PROCEDURAL STEPS

1. Wash and dry your hands. Follow the CDC Universal Precautions. Glove yourself with nonsterile gloves.
2. Check the physician's requisition for tests ordered and specimen requirements. Gather the materials needed.
3. Identify the patient and explain the procedure.
   RATIONALE: Patient identity is ascertained, and explanations help gain the patient's cooperation.
4. Instruct the patient to sit with the arm well supported in a downward position (Figure 20-4).
   RATIONALE: The veins are more easily located when the elbow is straight.
5. Assemble equipment. Attach the needle to the syringe or the Vacutainer holder. Keep the cover on the needle at this time (Figure 20-5).
6. Apply the tourniquet around the patient's arm approximately 3-4 inches above the elbow. The tourniquet should be taut, but not so tight that it restricts blood flow in the artery (Figure 20-6).
   RATIONALE: The tourniquet is used to make the veins more prominent by restricting venous flow (but not arterial flow), causing a slight back pressure of blood in the veins.

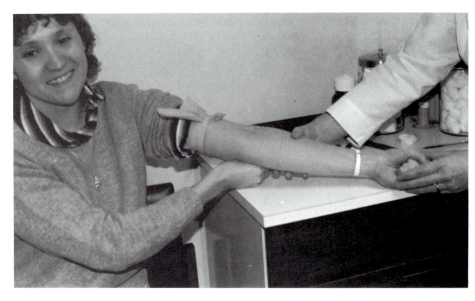

FIGURE 20-4

(Reproduced from Kinn ME, Derge EF: *The Medical Assistant: Administrative and Clinical,* 6th ed. Philadelphia: W. B. Saunders, 1988, p. 725.)

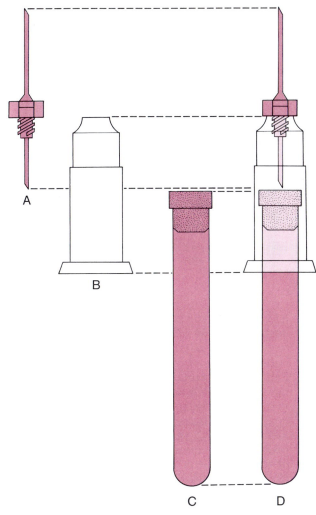

FIGURE 20-5

(Reproduced from Kinn ME, Derge EF: *The Medical Assistant: Administrative and Clinical,* 6th ed. Philadelphia: W. B. Saunders, 1988, p. 660.)

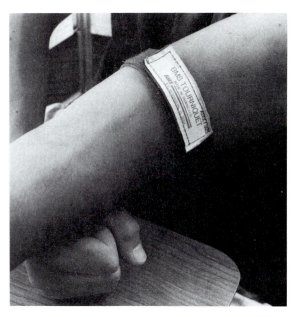

FIGURE 20-6

(Reproduced from Bonewit K: *Clinical Procedures for Medical Assistants,* 3rd ed. Philadelphia: W. B. Saunders, 1990, p. 338.)

RATIONALE: This prevents recontamination of the area just cleansed.

9. Dry the site with a sterile gauze.
    RATIONALE: Puncturing a wet area stings and can cause hemolysis of the sample.

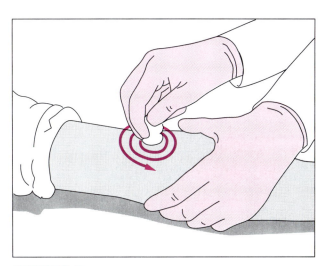

FIGURE 20-7

(Redrawn from Kinn ME, Derge EF: *The Medical Assistant: Administrative and Clinical*, 6th ed. Philadelphia: W. B. Saunders, 1988, p. 726.)

7. Select the venipuncture site by palpating the antecubital space, and use your index finger to trace the path of the vein and to judge its depth. The vein most often used is the median cephalic, which lies in the middle of the elbow.
    RATIONALE: The index finger is most sensitive for palpating. Do not use the thumb, as it has a pulse of its own, which may confuse you.
8. Cleanse the site, starting in the center of the area and working outward in a circular pattern (Figure 20-7).

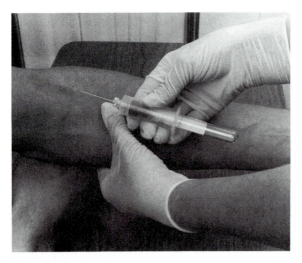

FIGURE 20-8

(Reproduced from Bonewit K: *Clinical Procedures for Medical Assistants*, 3rd ed. Philadelphia: W. B. Saunders, 1990, p. 339.)

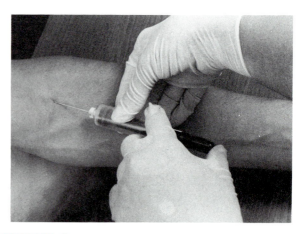

FIGURE 20-9

(Reproduced from Bonewit K: *Clinical Procedures for Medical Assistants*, 3rd ed. Philadelphia: W. B. Saunders, 1990, p. 339.)

10. Remove the needle sheath.
11. Hold the syringe or Vacutainer assembly in your dominant hand. Your thumb should be on top and your fingers underneath the adaptor (Figure 20-8).
12. Touch the index finger that you used to palpate the vein to the alcohol swab, and then repalpate the vein.
    RATIONALE: This affirms your location of the vein just before the puncture.
13. Anchor the vein by rolling your index finger slightly above the point you have chosen to puncture and placing your thumb firmly on the vein slightly below the chosen puncture site (see Figure 20-8).
    RATIONALE: Anchoring the vein ensures that the vein will not move when puncturing and causes less pain to the patient when the skin is held taut.
14. Insert the needle through the skin and into the vein with the bevel of the needle up, aligned parallel to the vein, at a 15°-angle, rapidly and smoothly.
    RATIONALE: The sharpest point of the needle is inserted first.
15. Slowly pull back the plunger of the syringe with the nondominant hand, or place two fingers on the holder and, with the thumb, push the tube onto the needle inside the holder (Figure 20-9). Make sure that you do not move the needle after entering the vein. Allow the syringe or tube to fill to optimum capacity (Figure 20-10).

    RATIONALE: The tubes are made to allow the correct amount of blood to mix with the anticoagulant. Variation in the amount of blood collected may alter some test results.
16. Remove the vacuum tube from the adapter before removing the needle from the vein. As you remove the tubes, gently invert the anticoagulated tubes several times.
    RATIONALE: A nontraumatic venipuncture produces the most reliable results. Removal of the tube from the holder before removal from the vein prevents any excess blood from dripping from the tip of the needle onto the patient. Inverting the tubes will mix the

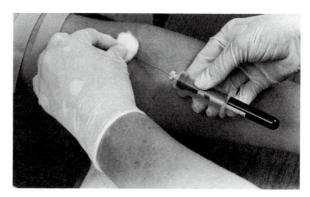

FIGURE 20-10

(Reproduced from Bonewit K: *Clinical Procedures for Medical Assistants*, 3rd ed. Philadelphia: W. B. Saunders, 1990, p. 340.)

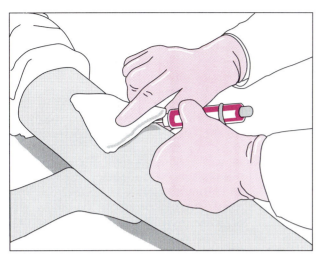

FIGURE 20–11

(Redrawn from Kinn ME, Derge EF: *The Medical Assistant: Administrative and Clinical*, 6th ed. Philadelphia: W. B. Saunders, 1988, p. 728.)

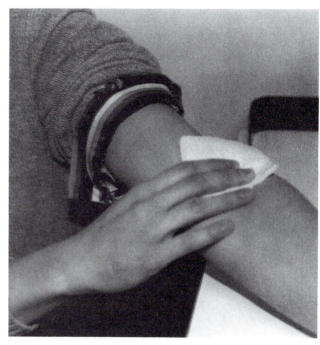

FIGURE 20–12

(From Kinn ME, Derge EF: *The Medical Assistant: Administrative and Clinical,* 6th ed. Philadelphia: W. B. Saunders, 1988, p. 728.)

blood with the anticoagulants completely and best prevent clotting in the tubes.

17. You may release the tourniquet as soon as blood starts to flow (see Figure 20–10). It must be released before the needle is removed from the arm.
    RATIONALE: Removal of the tourniquet releases pressure on the vein and helps prevent blood from getting into adjacent tissues and causing a hematoma.
18. Place a sterile gauze pad over the puncture site and withdraw the needle (Figure 20–11).
19. Apply direct pressure over the site. The patient may elevate the arm (Figure 20–12).
    RATIONALE: Direct pressure is the best method to stop bleeding. Elevating the arm above the heart also stops bleeding.
20. Transfer the blood to a tube if using a syringe. Open the top of the tube and gently let the blood flow down the inside of the tube.
    RATIONALE: Vigorous pressure may cause hemolysis of the cells.
21. Label the tubes. Labels should include at least the patient's name, the patient's identification number, time and date of collection, and the tests ordered.
22. Check the puncture site for bleeding and apply a bandage if indicated.
23. Dispose of the needle in a needle container. Allow it to drop directly into the disposal unit without touching it with your fingers. Do not recap used needles.
    RATIONALE: Most accidental needle sticks occur when a needle is being recapped. Report any accidents to your supervisor or the physician.
24. Clean the work area, using CDC Universal Precautions.
25. Remove your gloves and wash your hands.

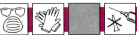

PROCEDURE

COLLECTING A CAPILLARY BLOOD SPECIMEN USING FINGERTIP PUNCTURE

PURPOSE

To obtain a capillary blood specimen suitable for testing.

EQUIPMENT AND MATERIALS

Nonsterile gloves
Sterile disposable lancet or Autolet lancet (Ames)
70% alcohol
Sterile gauze pads
Bandage
Supplies for requested test (for example, pipettes, Unopettes, slides, capillary tubes)
Needle container for disposal of lancet

PROCEDURAL STEPS

1. Wash and dry your hands. Follow the CDC Universal Precautions. Glove yourself with nonsterile gloves.
2. Greet and identify the patient.
3. Explain the procedure.
   RATIONALE: Explanations help gain the patient's cooperation.
4. Assemble the needed materials, based upon the physician's requisition.
   RATIONALE: Once the skin has been punctured, the collection must proceed as rapidly as possible so the blood does not clot before the entire specimen has been collected.
5. Select a puncture site (side of middle finger of nondominant hand, outer edge of earlobe, or medial or lateral curved surface of the heel or the great toe for an infant).
   RATIONALE: The nondominant hand may have fewer callouses. The side of the finger is less sensitive and the skin is usually not as thick.
6. "Milk" (very gently rub) the finger along the sides.
   RATIONALE: This promotes circulation. If the finger is very cold, you may immerse it in warm water or moisten it with warm towels.
7. Clean the site with alcohol, and dry it with sterile gauze.
   RATIONALE: Puncturing wet skin is painful and can hemolyze the specimen. Alcohol increases blood circulation to that area.
8. Have the patient place his or her elbow on the table with their hand raised near their shoulder. Squeeze the finger tightly to minimize pain the patient may feel and to keep the skin taut when it is punctured.
   RATIONALE: Having the elbow braced on the table prevents the patient from jumping and ensures a good puncture.
9. Hold the lancet at a right angle to the patient's finger, and make a rapid, deep puncture on the patient's fingertip (Figure 20–13).
   RATIONALE: Lancets are designed to puncture at a depth of 3–4 mm, which is sufficient to obtain the required drops of blood.
10. Wipe away the first drop of blood.

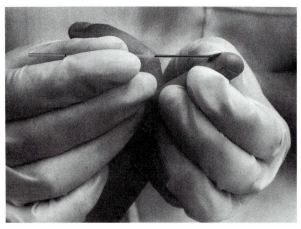

FIGURE 20–13

(Reproduced from Bonewit K: *Clinical Procedures for Medical Assistants,* 3rd ed. Philadelphia: W. B. Saunders, 1990, p. 374.)

RATIONALE: The first drop of blood contains tissue fluid.
11. Apply *gentle* pressure to cause the blood to flow freely.
RATIONALE: Squeezing liberates tissue that dilutes the blood and causes inaccurate results.
12. Collect blood samples:

- Express a large, rounded drop of blood, and fill capillary tubes or pipettes. When filling tubes for a hematocrit, place one end of the tube into a clay tray to prevent blood from leaving the tube.
- Wipe the finger with a clean sterile gauze pad, and place a fresh drop of blood on a slide for a smear. Immediately make the smear, using the two-slide method.

13. Apply pressure to the site with clean sterile gauze.
14. Label all samples and requisitions correctly and forward to the laboratory for testing. Because capillary tubes are so small and cannot be labeled easily, it is best to label a second, larger container and place the tubes into the container. The label should include the patient's name, the patient's identification number, the time and date drawn, and the tests requested.
15. Check the patient for bleeding and apply a bandage if indicated.
16. Dismiss the patient.
17. Clean the work area. Follow the CDC Universal Precautions for proper disposal of all materials.
18. Remove your gloves and wash your hands.

Urine

See Chapter 21.

Stool

The procedure for collection of stool specimens depends on what type of problem is suspected. The two most common types of specimens collected are for bacterial cultures or for ova and parasites testing.

Bacterial Cultures

Have the patient collect a stool specimen in an 8–12-oz water-resistant container. It is helpful to first collect the specimen by wrapping the back half of the toilet with plastic kitchen wrap and then transfer the stool to the smaller container. Make sure that the container has a tight-fitting lid. The specimen container only needs to be filled about halfway to avoid possible contamination or spillage in transport. The specimen may be refrigerated for up to 48 hours before it is cultured.

Ova and Parasite Testing

Obtain a prepared collection kit containing 10% formalin and 10% polyvinyl alcohol (PVA) fixative. Begin by collecting the specimen in the same manner as the bacterial culture to avoid any dilution from water from the toilet. The lid of this kit has a spoon-like attachment that can be used to collect enough stool to make a 1:3 ratio of stool to preservative. A line on the label of the kit also indicates how full the vial should be to meet this ratio. Once the specimen is collected it should be tightly closed, well mixed, and kept either at room temperature or refrigerated until it can be tested in the reference laboratory. Only the preserved specimen then needs to be sent to the laboratory.

 MEDICAL ASSISTING ALERT

Any stool collected by or from the patient may harbor pathogens that are **immediately** infective.

Collection from Infants and Small Children

Specimens may be obtained for culture by collecting rectal swabs. To do this, first moisten the tips of two cotton-tipped applicators with water. Insert the moistened swabs one at a time into the rectum 1–1 1/2 inches, rotating gently. Refrigerate swabs immediately and transport to the laboratory within 48 hours.

Sputum

Sputum is the deep lung secretion produced by the bronchioles.

- Have the patient gargle with water before beginning collection. This reduces the amount of upper respiratory (mouth and throat) flora that may contaminate the deep lung specimen.
- Generally a first morning specimen is the specimen of choice. After the body has been at rest for several hours, the secretions have been allowed to accumulate and the best results are received.
- If possible, collect the specimen before the administration of antibiotics. If the antibiotics are effective, no bacteria is recovered after their exposure to the medication.
- It is important that patients understand that they need to cough "from the lungs." This is not the same as having patients clear their throat—this technique would collect saliva rather than sputum.

Semen

Semen is generally collected for fertility studies and as a follow-up test to ensure that a vasectomy was effective.

- Semen may be collected by masturbation or coitus interruptus, as long as a semen collection kit is used. A condom should not be used, because condoms often contain a spermicide and could alter the test results.
- Because of the frailty of spermatozoa, the specimen must be collected and analyzed as soon as possible. Ideally, the specimen should be tested within a half-hour from the time of collection, to prevent deterioration and possible inaccurate results.

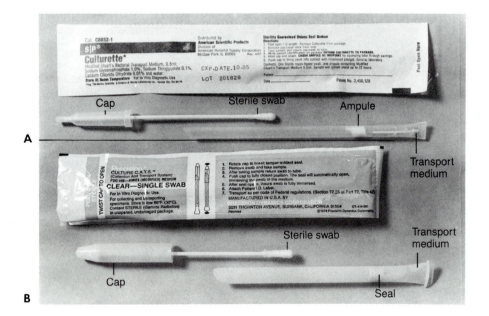

FIGURE 20–14

Two examples of collection and transport systems: **A**, Culterette and **B**, Precision Culture CATS. A collection and transport system is packaged in a peel-apart envelope and consists of a plastic tube containing a sterile swab and transport medium. Once the swab has been used to collect the specimen, the cap/swab unit is then placed in the transport medium. This prevents drying of the specimen and preserves it until it reaches the laboratory. (Reproduced from Bonewit K: *Clinical Procedures for Medical Assistants*, 3rd ed. Philadelphia: W. B. Saunders, 1990, p. 424.)

Throat Specimens*

Purpose

Throat specimens are collected to

- Perform rapid screening tests to detect the presence of group A beta-hemolytic streptococci (see Chapter 23).
- Culture to confirm the presence or absence of group A beta-hemolytic streptococci (see Chapter 23).

Collection Devices

Sterile cotton-, dacron-, or calcium-alginate-tipped swabs are satisfactory to use for the collection of throat specimens.

Collection Method

An adequate specimen must be obtained in order to isolate group A beta-hemolytic streptococci (see COLLECTING A THROAT SPECIMEN procedure, Chapter 23).

---

* Section provided by Linda Jeff (see also Chapter 23).

Specimen Handling

- Throat swabs should be processed within 2–3 hours of collection or a swab-transport media system should be used.
- Examples of swab-transport media systems include the Culturette (Marion Scientific Corporation), Culture C.A.T.S. (Precision Dynamics Corporation), Transwab (Microdiagnostics), and Culture swab (Difco) (Figure 20–14).

  Most systems are available with one or two swabs.
  Two-swab systems should be used if throat cultures are done to follow-up negative screening tests.

- Some reference laboratories recommend putting swab tips in a drying agent, such as silica gel, when the recovery of only group A beta-hemolytic streptococcus is desired. The drying agent suppresses the survival of contaminants and allows the recovery of the more resistant group A beta-hemolytic streptococci.[3]
- Swabs in transport media should be processed within 24 hours of collection.

PROCEDURE

COLLECTING A THROAT SPECIMEN†

PURPOSE

To provide an adequate, noncontaminated specimen to screen or culture for group A beta-hemolytic streptococci.

EQUIPMENT AND MATERIALS

Sterile swab or swab-transport media device
Tongue blade
Gloves and protective wear for universal precautions

---

† Procedure provided by Linda Jeff (see also Chapter 23).

PROCEDURAL STEPS

1. Position the patient so that the pharynx is clearly visible.
2. Remove the sterile swab from the container, being careful not to let the tip touch anything. Use two swabs if a screening test is to be performed.
   RATIONALE: One swab is used for the screening test and the second is cultured, if the screening test is negative.
3. Instruct the patient to open his or her mouth while saying "ah-h." Depress the tongue with the tongue blade.
4. Extend the swab into the posterior pharynx,

avoiding contact with the tongue, teeth, uvula, or internal surfaces of the mouth.
5. Vigorously rub the swab back and forth across the posterior pharynx touching any lesions, white patches, or inflamed areas. Also, swab the tonsillar areas.
6. Remove the swab, again avoiding contact with the inside of the mouth.
7. Remove the tongue blade and discard in a biohazard container.
8. Return the swab to its paper envelope or insert it into a transport medium.

MEDICAL ASSISTING ALERT

Follow the manufacturer's directions for using swab-transport media devices. Some require that an ampule be broken, after inserting the swab into the device, in order to release the transport medium.

9. Label the container that holds the swab as instructed.

Genital Tract Specimens*

Purpose

Genital tract specimens are collected to

- Perform wet preparations/potassium hydroxide (KOH) preparations to identify *Trichomonas vaginalis,* yeast, or *Gardnerella vaginalis* (see Chapter 18)
- Prepare Gram-stained smears to screen for *Neisseria gonorrhoeae* (see Chapter 23)
- Culture for *N. gonorrhoeae* (see Chapter 23)
- Culture or perform direct antigen tests for *Chlamydia trachomatis*

Collection Devices

- Swabs composed of nontoxic synthetic material, such as calcium alginate or dacron, or cotton treated with charcoal are recommended for collecting endocervical or urethral specimens.

MEDICAL ASSISTING ALERT

Untreated cotton-tipped swabs should not be used because cotton may contain substances toxic to *N. gonorrhoeae*.

- Sterile cotton-tipped swabs are used for the collection of vaginal specimens for wet preparations/KOH preparations.

---

* Section provided by Linda Jeff (see also Chapter 23).

Collection Methods

Endocervical Specimens

- The endocervical canal is the best site from which to collect specimens from females when gonorrhea or chlamydial infection is suspected.
- Specimens are collected by the physician during a gynecological examination.

Urethral Specimens

- In men, urethral discharge is the specimen of choice on which to perform diagnostic tests for *N. gonorrhoeae* or *C. trachomatis*.
- Urethral specimens are collected from women in some cases of urinary frequency or dysuria yielding negative urine cultures, or in women in whom endocervical specimens cannot be collected.
- Specimens of urethral discharge are collected by the physician using a swab.
- If there is no discharge, a calcium alginate urethral or nasopharyngeal swab may be inserted into the urethra to obtain a specimen.

Vaginal Specimens

- Vaginal discharge is collected with a swab by the physician during the gynecological examination.

Specimen Handling

N. gonorrhoeae

- Specimens in which *N. gonorrhoeae* is suspected should be immediately inoculated to selective media such as MTM (see the PREPARING SMEARS FOR STAINING procedure, Chapter 23) or put into transport media.

The organism is very sensitive to extremes in temperature and drying.

In many cases, only small numbers of the organism are present in clinical specimens.

- Commercial swab-transport media devices such as those described for throat specimens may be used.

  Systems with two swabs are recommended when both Gram stain and culture are requested.

  Swabs in transport media should be processed within 24 hours, optimally within 6 hours, of collection.

  Swabs in transport media should be held at room temperature, never refrigerated, until processed.

- When prolonged delays in processing are expected, such as when specimens are collected and sent to reference laboratories, nutritive agar plate transport systems should be used.

  These systems consist of a plate of selective medium in a plastic, zip-lock bag which contains a CO_2 generating tablet. Manufacturers' instructions should be followed when using these systems.

  Examples of such systems include the JEMBEC plate (Ames Company), the Bio-Bag (Marion Laboratories), and Gono-Pak (BBL Microbiology Systems).

  For maximum recovery of *N. gonorrhoeae*, it is recommended that nutritive transport systems be incubated 18–24 hours at 35° C before the specimen is transported to a reference laboratory.

SPECIAL HINT

Nutritive systems may also be used in house instead of using the conventional culture technique.

C. trachomatis

- Specimens for culture must be put into special transport media, for example, Chlamydia Transwab (Microdiagnostics), or frozen and shipped at 70° C to a reference laboratory.
- If direct antigen tests such as Microtrak (Syva) or Chlamydiazyme (Abbott) are done, the manufacturer's directions or guidelines furnished by the reference laboratory performing the test should be followed.

Vaginal Swabs for Wet Preparations/KOH Preparations

- Vaginal swabs should be placed in a tube of 0.5 ml of sterile saline immediately after collection and transported to the laboratory as soon as possible.
- The specimen should be kept at room temperature until processed.
- Wet preparations/KOH preparations should be performed within 30 minutes of specimen collection (see Chapter 23).

SPECIMEN PREPARATION

Preservation Techniques

Because it is impractical to perform every laboratory test immediately upon specimen collection, most specimens need to be preserved until the tests can be performed.

Whenever there is a question about specimen preservation, it is best to contact the laboratory and check before the specimen is collected. If improper preservation techniques damage the specimen, a second specimen may have to be collected.

Table 20–4 is a generalized chart listing the most common types of specimens and their preservation requirements. Table 20–5 is a chart listing the media requirements for various types of cultures.

TABLE 20–4

PRESERVATION REQUIREMENTS OF SPECIMENS

Type of Specimen	Preservation Requirements
Throat culture swab	Refrigeration
Wound swab	Refrigeration
Urine culture	Refrigeration
Genital culture	Room temperature (or incubation, if possible)
Viral culture	Room temperature (or incubation, if possible)
Whole blood specimens	Refrigeration
Serum specimens	Frozen (check with laboratory first—a few tests deteriorate if frozen)

TABLE 20-5
MEDIA REQUIREMENTS FOR VARIOUS TYPES OF CULTURES

Specimen	Loop Discs	Loop BAP	Eosin-methylene blue	Chocolate	Thayer-Martin	Thioglycolate	Gram stain	Hektoen	XLD	Mannitol salt	Miscellaneous
Urine	Calibrated	✓	✓								1 ml pour plate/antibiotic
Sputum	OPT⊛	✓⊛	✓	✓							
Throat	BAC, OPT⊛	✓⊛	✓	✓							
Nasal	BAC, OPT⊛	✓⊛	✓	✓							
Eye/ear		✓	✓	✓		✓	✓				
Cerebrospinal fluid		✓	✓	✓		✓	✓				India ink
Urethral/vaginal (any genital site)		✓	✓	✓	✓	✓	✓				
Fluids (pleura, synovial, peritoneal)		✓	✓	✓		✓	✓				Consult supervisor for current method
Tissue/biopsy		✓	✓	✓		✓	✓				Tissue grinder
Suprapubic aspirate		✓	✓	✓							*
Transtracheal aspirate	OPT⊛	✓⊛	✓	✓		✓					*
Decubitis		✓	✓	✓		✓	✓				*
Feces/rectal swab			✓					✓	✓		GN broth
Rectal swab (for gonorrhea)				✓	✓		✓				
Miscellaneous wounds		✓	✓	✓		✓	✓				
Anaerobe setup	Place in Gas Pak jar	*Brucella* blood A.	K-V laked blood A.	THIO							

*These specimens should have the anaerobe setup described above in addition to aerobic setup.
⊛ Disc on BAP.
BAP = blood agar plate; XLD = xylose lysine desoxycholate; OPT = optochin; BAC = Bacitracin; GN = Gram-negative.
Loops and discs are "special instructions," ie., calibrated loops are required for urine samples, and BAC or OPT discs are used on all plates indicated. When placing discs on a plate, they should be placed on the blood agar plate (BAP) because it is a nonselective media and will grow all types of bacteria.

METHODS OF DELIVERY OF SPECIMENS

In Person

Advantages

- By having a patient deliver his or her own specimens the delivery is made directly to the appropriate testing areas.
- In-person delivery is usually the fastest method of delivery. Because the laboratory is usually close, specimen testing may begin sooner than with other methods of delivery.

Disadvantage

- A medical assistant may sometimes be responsible for delivering the specimens to the laboratory, and it is sometimes difficult to leave other office duties.

Mail Service

- Although generally adequate, this method of specimen transport is not preferred by most offices.
- There is a risk to mail handlers if a package is damaged in the postal process and the handler is unaware of CDC Universal Precautions. All packages must be labeled with a "Biomedical" label to notify the handlers of this possible risk.

Advantage

- The travel expenses of a specimen are lower when a carrier (in person) is not required.

Disadvantages

- The mail service cannot guarantee the specimen requirements are met (for example, refrigeration or incubation), and this may alter the test results.
- Specimens must be well packed to avoid breakage or spills and possible contamination of the mail service personnel.
- The time it takes to reach the laboratory is generally several days, which would be unacceptable for a STAT specimen.

Pick-Up Service

Generally this is the most convenient method of specimen transport from a physician's office.

Advantages

- The laboratory personnel (carrier) assumes responsibility for the specimen as soon as the pick-up occurs.
- These persons are trained in proper handling and preservation of specimens; therefore the integrity of the specimen is better maintained.
- Usually the same person will bring the laboratory results from completed work at the time of the pick-up of the next specimens, providing prompt delivery of results to the office.
- A pick-up service usually can arrange special trips for STAT specimens or specimens with special handling instructions.

Disadvantages

- The carrier usually makes only one pick-up per day, so early specimens may sit in the office for an extra length of time.
- If a specimen is collected after the pick-up time, it may have to remain in the office until the following pick-up. This is particularly a problem if the storage time is over a weekend, because many tests are valid only for the first 24 hours after collection.

Chain of Custody

All persons involved in specimen handling are responsible in part for the preservation of that specimen. If any of the paperwork or procedures are incomplete, the chain of custody is invalidated.

The purpose of a chain of custody is to ensure that there is no mix-up or tampering of a specimen. A chain of custody form is a written document to verify that proper protocols were used by everyone involved. This written form may then be used in a court of law as evidence of the identity and integrity of the specimen throughout the collecting and testing process.

As the first person in the chain of custody, it is the medical assistant's job to

- Observe the specimen actually being collected from the patient.
- Carefully and completely label the specimen and complete the paperwork.
- Sign and date the form for verification of correct procedures.
- Have the participant (patient) also initial the form verifying that this is his or her specimen.

The chain of custody form has a minimum of three pages:

1. The original is placed directly in the clear plastic bag with the specimen and is securely sealed in place. (The original is not signed again once the bag is sealed.)
2. The first copy is attached to the bag, and is signed by every person handling the specimen.
3. The second copy is kept by the office for their files.

MEDICAL ASSISTING ALERT

When completed paperwork is put into the specimen bag, it is important that the name of the patient can be read through the bag. This is done by folding the paper with the printed side facing outward. If the paper is placed so that the name could not be read, the bag would have to be opened, which would invalidate the chain of custody.

PROCEDURES FOR DISPOSAL

Labeling of Waste

Waste products fall into three general classifications

- Nonhazardous
- Hazardous
- Hazardous-sharps

Table 20-6 is a basic guideline for types of waste products in each category.

All hazardous waste should be clearly labeled with the biohazardous waste symbol shown in Figure 20-15. In addition to labeling specimens and contaminated materials as hazardous, all health and physical hazards must have a hazard label (Figure 20-16). The term "health hazard" includes chemicals that are carcinogens, toxic or highly toxic agents, reproductive toxins, irritants, corrosives, sensitizers, hepatotoxins, nephrotoxins, neurotoxins, and agents that damage the lungs, skin, eyes, or mucous membranes. "Physical hazards" include any chemical that is considered combustible, explosive, flammable, or otherwise unstable or water-reactive.

Hazardous-sharps should be disposed of in a nonbreakable sealable box. It is recommended that these boxes not be completely filled. Pushing an item into a box may lead to an accidental puncture. If a sharp object does not fall easily into the container, it should be sealed and prepared for disposal according to the manufacturer's instructions.

Occupational Safety and Health Act Regulations

The Occupational Safety and Health Act (OSHA) was designed to protect workers from hazards in the workplace. OSHA is also the enforcement arm for the CDC. OSHA has developed a list of recommendations to protect health care workers known

TABLE 20-6

CLASSIFICATIONS OF WASTE MATERIALS

Nonhazardous	Hazardous	Hazardous-Sharps
Gowns	Table paper soaked with body fluids	Needles
Table paper not soaked with body fluids	Gauze pads soaked with body fluids	Syringes with needles
Paper towels	Tubes of blood	Scalpel blades
Tissues	Used specimen collection containers	Broken or very thin glass
Paper sheaths of disposable supplies	Disposable pipette tips	Lancets
	Used specimen collection swabs	
	Used gloves	
	Dressings	
	Test tubes	
	Microbiology specimens (once testing is completed)	

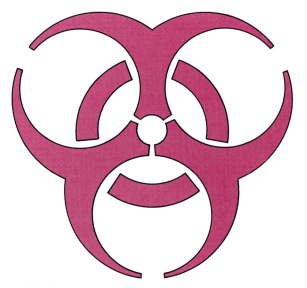

FIGURE 20-15

Hazard warning symbol.

as the Hazard Communication Standard (CFR 1910.1200), which became effective in the non-manufacturing sector in September, 1988.

These standards provide the guidelines for the management of hazards in the workplace, hazard labeling, employee information and training, medical waste disposal, Standard Operating Procedures (SOPs) for Universal Blood and Body Fluid Precautions, and accident reporting. These standards may be obtained from:

> OSHA
> Health Standards
> 200 Constitution Avenue
> Washington, DC 20210

Health and Safety of the Community

The best precaution in the medical office to prevent the spread of infection is frequent handwashing. Hands should be washed not only to protect each patient, but also to prevent the medical assistant from receiving any infectious pathogens.

Good hygiene practices by the medical assistant is vital to prevention of the spread of infection. By washing hands in the examination rooms, the medical assistant also demonstrates a positive example to patients.

Keeping the work areas and patient rooms clean after each patient visit can also help prevent the spread of pathogens.

Finally, proper disposal of biohazardous wastes helps prevent the spread of infection once the materials have left the physician's office.

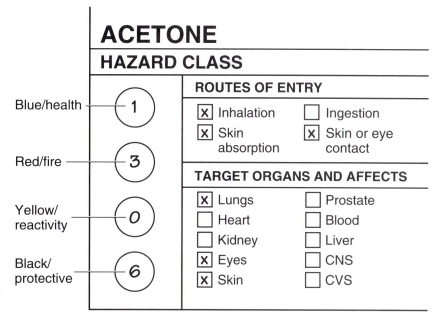

FIGURE 20-16

Hazard label displayed on or affixed to containers of hazardous chemicals.

QUALITY CONTROL

Reagent Management

All reagents are given two printed numbers. The first is a lot number and the second is an expiration date. These numbers are to be recorded in a quality-control manual with the date the reagents were received and the date they were opened. Many reagents will remain stable and usable for only a short period of time once they are opened. The literature accompanying the reagents always states the shelf life or stability of the reagent. Reagents should never be used past their expiration date.

Lot numbers are recorded so that in the event that a manufacturer discovers a problem with a reagent, the medical assistant can quickly tell whether this problem will affect the current office stock. Likewise, if results in the office are questionable, the medical assistant can contact the manufacturer with this lot number, and the manufacturer can further investigate the integrity of the reagents.

If reagents are stored improperly, their shelf life may be shortened considerably and they should be replaced.

Control Requirements

Every time a laboratory test is performed, controls must be run to make sure that the test has been run correctly and that the reagents are good.

A *control* is manufactured to be like a patient specimen. For example, if a test requires whole blood, the control to be used will resemble whole blood; if the test requires serum, the control will resemble serum. When the medical assistant needs to run a laboratory test, the control should be used as if it were another patient specimen.

Controls are shipped with a list of expected values or ranges of values. The ranges allow for slight variations of timings and techniques. However, *if the control results do not fall within the expected range, no patient results may be given out*. This is an indication of a problem with either the technique or the reagents. The problem must be resolved before patient results can be considered reliable.

If controls and patients are run and the results of the control are within the expected range of values, the technique is good and the reagents are reliable. The patient results can also be considered reliable and may be reported.

Every time a new lot of reagents is opened, the medical assistant should run a complete set of controls to make sure the reagents are good and have not been altered in shipping.

Controls often come as sets of normal and abnormal results. This is a way of testing different values run with the same reagents. If even one control does not work, there is a problem and *no* patient results should be given out until the problem is solved.

Instrument Calibration

Because laboratory instruments are very sensitive, many variables can alter their performance. Some of these variables include the electrical current (or battery power), the type of light used, time required for the instrument to warm up, or repeated use. Calibration is a method of eliminating many of these variables before a test is run.

TABLE 20-7

REAGENT LOGBOOK SAMPLE

Date Opened	Tech Initials	Reagent	Lot Number	Expiration Date	Stable Until	Checked Standards/Controls	Notes
1/3/91	PSH	Glucose	XT4617	6/14/91	6/14/91	OK	
1/6/91	PSH	BUN	BR305T	6/1/91	1/7/91	OK	stable 1 week
1/7/91	PSH	Urine Sticks	4077151	3/92	3/92	OK	
1/10/91	PSH	Glucose	XT4617	6/14/91	6/14/91	OK	
1/10/91	PSH	BUN	BR305T	6/1/91	1/17/91	OK	stable 1 week

TABLE 20-8

QUALITY-CONTROL LOGBOOK FOR GLUCOSE

Date Run	Normal Control			Abnormal Control			Comments/ Initials
	Expected	Result	OK?	Expected	Result	OK?	
1/3/91	88 - 106 mg/dl	91	yes	210 - 243 mg/dl	227	yes	PSH
1/4/91	' '	88	yes	' '	230	yes	PSH
1/5/91	' '	84	no	' '	212	yes	re-run controls PSH
1/5/91	' '	95	yes	' '	228	yes	OK PSH

Tests cannot be performed accurately if the instrument itself is not accurate.

It is desirable to have the instruments work exactly the same for each patient test. To eliminate any variations that may occur in the instruments, it is important to make sure that the instrument is calibrated before each use.

Calibration is done with a set of standards. A standard is generally a chemical with an exact value. Because the standard is very stable, the machine can then be set to read this exact amount before the controls or patient specimens are tested.

Unlike controls, standards may or may not appear like the specimens. Often they are liquids in sealed containers, so that nothing can interfere with their exact values. Also unlike controls, standards are run *before* the patient specimens and may not need to be run every time a patient specimen is tested. The calibration of an instrument can be run any time a control fails to fall within the expected range to check that the instrument is functioning properly.

Every time a new lot of reagents is opened, the medical assistant should run a complete set of standards to make sure the reagents are good and have not been altered in shipping.

Instrument and Testing Logbooks/ Worksheets

Every time a control or standard is run, it should be documented in the laboratory. When a control or standard fails, this is also documented. In addition, there should be room for notes on what corrective actions were taken before standards and controls were rerun. Tables 20-7 and 20-8 show examples of quality control logbooks properly completed.

Preventive Maintenance of Equipment

Maintenance is broken down into the categories of yearly, monthly, weekly and daily maintenance. All categories are necessary for the longevity of the instrument, but they are only guidelines for a minimum amount of maintenance.

Any maintenance performed should be recorded at the time of service, whether it was scheduled to be done at this time or not. Good maintenance records help eliminate many possible causes of breakdown of the instruments and aid in troubleshooting new problems.

Maintenance guidelines are provided with each instrument at the time of purchase. Extra copies of the guidelines can be provided by the manufacturer upon request. Often, the manufacturer representatives can also help by providing basic training in general maintenance procedures for the entire staff.

Bibliography

Bonewit K: *Clinical Procedures for Medical Assistants,* 3rd ed. Philadelphia: W. B. Saunders, 1990.
Condensed Chemical Dictionary, New York, NY: Van Nostrand Reinhold Co. (latest edition should be used).
Frew MA, Frew DR: *Comprehensive Medical Assisting: Administrative and Clinical Procedures.* Philadelphia: F. A. Davis, 1982.
Henry JB: *Clinical Diagnosis and Management by Laboratory Methods,* 16th ed. Philadelphia: W. B. Saunders, 1979.
Kinn ME, Derge E: *Medical Assisting: Administrative and Clinical,* 6th ed. Philadelphia: W. B. Saunders, 1988.
Koneman EW, Allen SD, Dowell VR Jr, Sommers HM: *Color Atlas and Textbook of Diagnostic Microbiology,* 2nd ed. Philadelphia: J. B. Lippincott, 1983.
The Merck Index: An Encyclopedia of Chemicals and Drugs. Rahway, NJ: Merck and Company, Inc. (latest edition should be used).
Shea MA, Zakus SM: *Fundamentals of Medical Assisting: Administrative and Clinical Theory and Technique.* St. Louis: C. V. Mosby, 1984.

Chapter 21

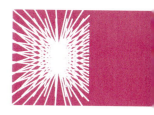

URINALYSIS

LORETTA HATLESTAD

CLINICAL CONSIDERATIONS
Quality Control
Safety
Recording the Urinalysis
Mailing
COLLECTION METHODS
Fundamentals
Catheterized Specimen
Specimen for Drug Screening
First Morning Specimen
Infant Specimen
Random, Clean-Catch Specimen
Timed (24-Hour) Specimen
Two-Glass Specimen
URINE TESTS
Physical Examination
Chemical Examination
Microscopic Examination

Urinalysis is one of the most useful diagnostic tools available, and more than 100 tests can now be performed on urine. Urine tests can help the physician diagnose diseases of the kidney, bladder, and liver, as well as disorders of the metabolic and endocrine systems. Besides in the offices of specialists such as urologists and nephrologists, medical assistants frequently perform urinalyses in family practice, internal medicine, pediatrics, gynecology, gerontology, and general practice.

The urinary system consists of the kidneys, ureters, bladder, and urethra. Blood enters the kidneys, where it passes through microscopic filters, called *glomeruli,* that filter out blood cells and protein while allowing the serum to pass through to the ureters. The blood cells and protein are then reabsorbed into the blood and passed on to other parts of the body through the circulatory system. The serum passes down the ureters into the bladder, where it is collected until the bladder becomes full and then is excreted through the urethra as urine. If there is damage or disease to any part of this system, the urine is usually abnormal.[1]

CLINICAL CONSIDERATIONS

Quality Control

Maintaining a high level of accuracy in performing urinalyses is vital in an office laboratory.

- Supplies should be stored according to the manufacturer's directions.
- All equipment should be kept clean and in good working order.
- Make sure specimens are adequately labeled and there is no possibility of mixing up patients' names and samples.
- Check clinical accuracy on a regular basis by sending a sample to an outside laboratory to see

URINALYSIS

Leukocytes _____ Ketones _____ MICRO _____

Nitrites _____ Urobilinogen _____ WBC/Hpf _____

pH _____ Bilirubin _____ RBC/Hpf _____

Protein _____ Blood _____ Bacteria _____

Glucose _____   Casts _____

FIGURE 21–1

Sample urinalysis form. (Courtesy of Dr. Robert J. Towers.)

that identical results for the same sample are obtained by both laboratories.

Safety

All urine specimens should be handled as if they are infected, and the Centers for Disease Control (CDC) Guidelines for Universal Precautions should be carefully observed. Gloves should be worn when handling urine. Supplies that have come into contact with urine must be properly disposed of, and cleanliness of all equipment and the area must be maintained.

Recording the Urinalysis

It is important that there be a uniform method of reporting test results in each laboratory. Although vocabulary and method of recording may differ from laboratory to laboratory, it is important that universal terminology be used.

- Red blood cells (RBCs), white blood cells (WBCs), and casts are counted and the number seen per field reported. For example, if 5, 10, and 8 RBCs are seen in three different fields, the number reported on the form would be 5–10. Generally, these are reported by actual count as 1–2, 5–10, 40–50, etc.
- Bacteria and epithelial cells are usually reported as "occasional," "few," "moderate," or "too numerous to count" (or "packed field") (Figure 21–1).

Mailing

Sometimes the physician wants the patient to collect a urine sample to be mailed to an outside laboratory for testing. This is often done for cytology testing in the case of tumors. It may also be the method used by some insurance companies during a routine physical on a potential client. The outside laboratory provides a container (usually glass) into which a preservative has been measured. The bottle should be labeled and the patient instructed to obtain a sample in a cup and then carefully transfer the urine into the bottle. This should be sealed with tape and then mailed to the outside laboratory, which patients often can do themselves without having to bring the sample into the office, because laboratories usually provide postage-paid, preaddressed bottles ready for mailing.[2]

COLLECTION METHODS

Fundamentals

Different forms of specimen collection are used depending on what the physician is testing for. Proper collection of specimens is vital (Table 21–1). Although there are cases in which a first morning specimen or other timed specimen is needed, as a general rule the best specimen for an office laboratory is a freshly voided specimen. The sample should be analyzed as soon as possible after the patient has obtained it and never longer than 20 minutes later, because urine decomposes quickly, causing both physical and chemical changes (Figure 21–2). If, for some reason, there will be a delay of more than 20 minutes in testing the urine, the specimen should

TABLE 21–1

TYPES OF SPECIMENS USED FOR URINE TESTS

Random	Catheterized	24-Hour	First Morning
Bilirubin	Bacteria	Aldosterone	HCG (pregnancy)
Blood		Creatinine clearance	Nitrates
Color		Glucose	
Glucose		Ketones	
Human chorionic gonadotropin (HCG) (pregnancy)		Lead	
Ketones		Protein	
Leukocytes		Sodium	
Odor		Toxicology	
pH		Uric acid	
Protein			
Specific gravity			
Toxicology			

Adapted from *Urinalysis Today,* Indianapolis, Boehringer Mannheim Diagnostics, 1986.

- Red blood cells undergo hemolysis
- White blood cells degenerate
- Protein could become positive due to changes in higher pH values
- Casts disappear
- Bacteria multiply
- pH fluctuates due to carbon dioxide loss and reduction of urea to ammonia
- Urine becomes cloudy due to solute precipitates
- Glucose level is reduced since glucose is metabolized by bacteria and cells
- Ketone level is reduced because of bacterial effect
- Bilirubin level is reduced due to light sensitivity
- Urobilinogen level is reduced since urobilinogen is converted to urobilin
- Nitrite appears as bacteria grow
- Ascorbic acid level is reduced
- Ammonia level increases because of bacterial effect
- Color darkens
- Odor becomes foul

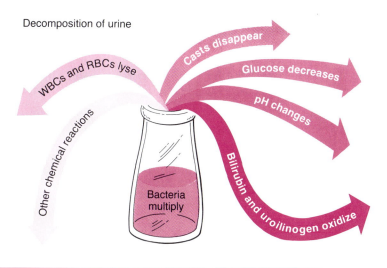

FIGURE 21–2

Common changes in decomposed or old urine. (Redrawn from *Urinalysis Today,* Indianapolis, Boehringer Mannheim Diagnostics, 1986.)

be refrigerated until it can be examined. This may also be done by a patient who needs to bring in a sample obtained at home but cannot get it to the laboratory within the 20-minute period.[1]

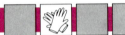
SPECIAL HINTS

- Disposable plastic cups are the best specimen containers.
- Do not have the patient bring a specimen in an empty pill bottle, particularly one that contained antibiotics, because residue from the medication can retard bacteria growth.
- Soaps or other chemical residues may also alter results.
- If the urine must be transported any distance from the bathroom to the laboratory, the cup should have a screw-on cover.

PROCEDURE

COLLECTING A URINE SAMPLE

PURPOSE

To obtain the urine sample most appropriate for the test.

EQUIPMENT AND MATERIALS

Private toilet area
Urine cup
Gloves and protective wear for CDC Universal Precautions

PROCEDURAL STEPS

1. For most urinalyses done in the office laboratory, a random, clean-catch sample is best.
   RATIONALE: The sample is fresh, proper handling of the specimen is ensured, and results can be available to the physician within a few minutes.
2. First morning specimens are preferred when concentrated specimens are needed, such as for pregnancy tests (human chorionic gonadotropin) (see Chapter 18) or nitrate level determinations (see Chapter 23).
3. Twenty-four-hour urine samples are commonly obtained when checking for the presence of a specific substance, such as protein or calcium. For a 24-hour sample, all of the urine produced during a 24-hour period must be collected and brought to the laboratory.
4. At times, it may be necessary to obtain a catheterized specimen, for example, when the patient is unable to urinate normally or a non-contaminated specimen cannot be obtained from voiding.
5. If a patient needs to bring a sample from a long distance, ask him or her to transport the specimen in a plastic bag filled with ice cubes.

Catheterized Specimen

Some patients, particularly females, consistently show bacteria in their urine samples, regardless of how carefully they clean themselves or obtain their specimen. A catheterized specimen from such patients confirms urinary tract infection rather than vaginal contamination. The specimen container should be labeled with the patient's name and annotated as a "catheterized specimen."

MEDICAL ASSISTING ALERT

Occasionally it is necessary to catheterize a female infant. Because this can be a difficult procedure, it is usually done by the physician. Catheterization of males is generally done by the physician or office personnel who have specialized training in this area. Personnel who do not have specific training should *not* perform this procedure.

PROCEDURE

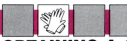

OBTAINING A CATHETERIZED SPECIMEN FROM A FEMALE PATIENT

PURPOSE

To collect a urine specimen directly from the bladder of a female patient.

 MEDICAL ASSISTING ALERT

This procedure requires specific training or is performed by a physician.

EQUIPMENT AND MATERIALS

Glass catheters (sterilized or in Zephiran solution)
K-Y jelly
Zephiran Chloride Aqueous Solution 1:1000 (22 ml of Zephiran Chloride 17% q.s. ad. 1 gallon of distilled water)
Labeled specimen container
Gloves and protective wear for CDC Universal Precautions

PROCEDURAL STEPS

Patient Preparation

1. Ask patient to undress from the waist down and lie prone on an examining table.
2. Position the patient's legs comfortably in the stirrups.

Performance

3. Place a small amount of K-Y jelly on a paper towel.
4. Spread the labia, using slight upward motion to expose urethral orifice (Figure 21-3).
5. Dip cotton balls into Zephiran solution and clean urethral orifice by using a downward motion, wiping once with each cotton ball and then discarding it. Repeat two more times, always wiping from front to back.
6. Holding the catheter by the end, lubricate the rounded tip with K-Y jelly.
7. Insert the catheter slowly into the urethra until urine starts to drain. Drain urine into a container.
8. If a postvoid residual is desired, leave the catheter in the bladder until the bladder is completely empty and no more urine is flowing out of the catheter. A large, calibrated container should be used to collect and measure the urine obtained.
9. Slowly remove the catheter.

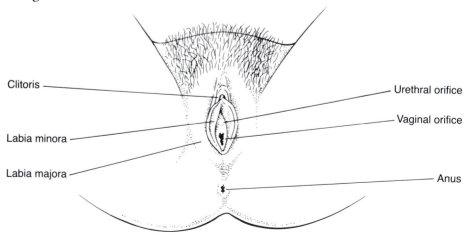

FIGURE 21-3

Female anatomy. (Courtesy of Dr. Robert J. Towers.)

Specimen for Drug Screening

Patients may be tested for the presence of drugs or other toxic substances in their urine. Generally, the urine is obtained at the medical office and then sent to an outside laboratory for chemical analysis. Patients may be screened as part of a routine physical examination or employment physical examination, or to rule out suspected abuse or contact with toxins. Whether this is a routine screening or testing of suspected misuse or contact, it is vital that the specimen be handled in such a way as to ensure accurate identification, collection, and transport of the specimen.[3]

 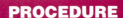

OBTAINING A URINE SPECIMEN FOR DRUG SCREENING

PURPOSE

To collect the urine sample and ensure that it is accurately identified and transported to the laboratory.

EQUIPMENT AND MATERIALS

Toilet area
Urine cup labeled with patient's name
Patient consent form
Container bottle for shipment
Shipping container
Chain-of-custody form
Tamper-proof tape
Specimen label with patient identification information
Gloves and protective wear for CDC Universal Precautions

PROCEDURAL STEPS

Patient Preparation

1. Verify patient's identity by asking him or her to produce a pictured identification card.
2. Ask patient to sign a preprinted consent for drug screening form on which he or she lists any drugs or alcohol ingested over the last 10 days. Sign the form as a witness.
3. Ask the patient to provide a urine sample of at least 60 ml into the labeled urine cup. If the patient's behavior is suspicious, ask the physician to witness the voiding.

Performance

 MEDICAL ASSISTING ALERT

Complete all the remaining steps in view of the patient.

4. Take the labeled sample from the patient.
5. Transfer the urine sample from the cup to the urine container bottle for shipment.
6. Securely cap the shipping bottle and seal the bottle with the patient identification label and tamper-proof tape.
7. Complete the chain-of-custody form (Figure 21–4).
8. Place original of chain-of-custody form into the shipping container, along with the sealed and labeled bottle.
9. Seal the shipping container.
10. Dismiss the patient and file the remaining copies of the chain-of-custody form.

FIGURE 21-4

Chain of custody. (Reproduced from CompuChem Laboratories, Western Division, Sacramento, CA.)

First Morning Specimen

The first morning specimen voided by the patient is generally the most concentrated specimen of the day. In the past, it was necessary to obtain the first morning specimen to determine pregnancy; now, however, sophisticated commercial test kits enable random samples to be tested for pregnancy. When checking for the presence of nitrates, which indicate urinary tract infections, the first morning specimen is best, because urine needs to remain in the bladder from 4 to 6 hours for nitrates to form. Occasionally the physician may be looking for some other substance in the concentrated urine that will require the first morning specimen.

If the first morning specimen needs to be brought into the office for examination later in the day, it should be refrigerated until it can be transported.

Infant Specimen

Collecting a noncontaminated urine sample from an infant presents special challenges, particularly getting the infant to urinate when you want him or her to and preventing the sample from becoming contaminated. Commercially available pediatric urine collection bags are available to help in this process.

SPECIAL HINT

Placing the infant's feet in cold water may help stimulate urination.

 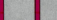

PROCEDURE
OBTAINING A URINE SAMPLE FROM AN INFANT

PURPOSE

To collect a noncontaminated urine sample from the infant.

EQUIPMENT AND MATERIALS

Soap
Water
Cotton balls
Pediatric urine collection bag
Container
Gloves and protective wear for CDC Universal Precautions

PROCEDURAL STEPS

1. Cleanse the infant's genital area thoroughly.
2. Tape the sterile collection bag over the genitals.
3. Ask a parent or other adult to remain with the infant until the specimen is obtained.
4. Drain the collected specimen from the collection bag into a clean container.

Random, Clean-Catch Specimen

For most routine urinalyses, a random, clean catch is an easy and adequate method of obtaining acceptable urine samples. The medical assistant should explain to the patient how to obtain the sample and provide the patient with a clean specimen container labeled with his or her name. Although some physicians prefer to have the patient clean the area around the urethra before voiding, this usually is not necessary, because wiping the area with a cleaning solution often smears any bacteria present around the area and thus does not ensure an uncontaminated specimen. However, if the physician prefers this technique, instruct the patient to cleanse the area before voiding.[2]

PROCEDURE

INSTRUCTING A PATIENT TO OBTAIN A RANDOM, CLEAN-CATCH URINE SAMPLE

PURPOSE

To enable the patient to obtain a sample that is not contaminated.

EQUIPMENT AND MATERIAL

Private toilet area
Labeled specimen container

PROCEDURAL STEPS

Males

1. Instruct the patient to begin urinating forcibly into the toilet and, about half-way through his void, collect about 2 inches of urine in the container provided.
RATIONALE: By voiding first into the toilet, the patient flushes away any bacteria and other contaminates, and the midstream sample will provide an accurate urinalysis.

Females

1. Instruct the patient to stand astride the toilet bowl and separate the labia, begin urinating forcibly into the toilet, and, about half-way through her void, collect about 2 inches of urine in the container provided.
RATIONALE: By voiding first into the toilet, the patient flushes away any bacteria and other contaminates, and the midstream sample will provide an accurate urinalysis.

Timed (24-Hour) Specimen

Timed collections of urine specimens require the patient to collect all the urine he or she produces within a 24-hour period. There are many tests that require a 24-hour sample; most of these tests are done not in the physician's laboratory but in an outside laboratory (Table 21–2). However, the medical assistant needs to instruct patients in the proper method of obtaining a 24-hour specimen. It is helpful to have written instructions available for the patient to refer to when he or she gets home.

TABLE 21–2

COMMON 24-HOUR URINE TESTS

Test	Definition	Normal Value	Pathology
Aldosterone	A hormone produced by the adrenal glands that influences fluid balance and blood pressure	2–25 μg/24 hr	High levels may indicate adrenal tumor (Conn's syndrome), excessive secretion by the adrenal gland, kidney disease, liver disease, or congestive heart failure. Low levels may indicate decreased function of the adrenal gland (Addison's disease), salt-losing syndrome, or diabetes.
Calcium	Influences maintenance and repair of bones and teeth, transmission of nerve stimuli, muscle contraction, heart function, and blood clotting	100–240 mg/24 hr	High levels may indicate excess of parathyroid hormone, cancer, excessive intake of vitamin D or calcium, prolonged bed rest, or kidney disease. Low levels may indicate low levels of serum protein, decreased parathyroid gland function, low dietary intake or absorption of calcium or vitamin D, bone disorders, certain kidney diseases, or pregnancy.

TABLE 21–2

COMMON 24-HOUR URINE TESTS *Continued*

Test	Definition	Normal Value	Pathology
Creatinine clearance	Creatinine is a waste product filtered by the kidneys and excreted in the urine. The creatinine clearance represents the volume of blood cleared of creatinine per minute.	Male: 107–135 ml/min Female: 87–107 ml/min	High levels may indicate kidney disease. Low levels may indicate kidney damage caused by decreased blood flow to the kidneys, urinary tract obstruction, or inflammation of the kidneys.
Glucose	The primary energy source for all body tissues	None	High levels may indicate diabetes, pregnancy, hypertension, hyperthyroidism, excessive pituitary function, excessive adrenal function, obesity, thiazide therapy, carbon monoxide poisoning, infectious disease, or disease of the central nervous system. Low levels may indicate hypoglycemia, cold exposure, liver disease, excessive insulin levels, underactive adrenal glands, underactive pituitary gland, hypothyroidism, prolonged vomiting, prolonged fever, poor nutrition, severe exercise, or von Gierke's disease.
Ketones	Waste products of fat breakdown	None	High levels may indicate uncontrolled diabetes, starvation, low carbohydrate diet, prolonged vomiting or diarrhea, or severe distress.
Lead	A nonessential mineral that is present in small amounts in many patients without doing apparent harm	0–199 μg/24 hr	High levels may indicate lead poisoning.
Protein	Normally filtered through the kidneys and then reabsorbed into the bloodstream	0–150 mg/24 hr	High levels may indicate glomerulonephritis, polycystic kidneys, renal tubular disorders, urinary tract infections, cancer of the kidneys, lupus erythematosus, venous congestion of the kidney, heart failure, toxemia of pregnancy, anemia, leukemia, multiple myeloma, or mercury/lead/opiate poisoning.
Sodium	One of the body's principal electrolytes (electronically charged minerals dissolved in body fluids)	75–200 mEq/l	High levels may indicate dehydration, excessive salt intake, inadequate adrenal gland function, kidney disease, or severe diabetes. Low levels may indicate excessive adrenal gland activity, congestive heart failure, severe lung disease, or very low salt intake.
Toxic screening	Measures the presence of such substances as narcotics, acetaminophens, barbiturates, tranquilizers, antidepressants, antipsychotic medications, alcohol, amphetamines, hallucinogens, or other substances	None	High levels may indicate recent contact with the substances.
Uric acid	A by-product of metabolism of purine-rich foods, such as liver, kidneys, and sweetbreads	250–750 mg/24 hr	High levels may indicate gout, leukemia, multiple myeloma, chemotherapy or radiation therapy, or toxemia of pregnancy.

Data are from Sobel DS, Ferguson T: *The People's Book of Medical Tests.* New York: Summit Books, 1985.

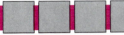

PROCEDURE

INSTRUCTING A PATIENT TO OBTAIN A 24-HOUR URINE SAMPLE

PURPOSE

To enable the patient to obtain an accurate 24-hour collection.

EQUIPMENT AND MATERIALS

Large plastic urine collection bottle (available commercially or from your outside laboratory)
Instruction sheet

PROCEDURAL STEPS

1. Instruct the patient to empty his or her bladder upon awakening in the morning and not to collect this urine.
   RATIONALE: Only one morning void is collected, because an exact 24-hour collection is desired.
2. Instruct the patient that from this point on, he or she is to collect all the urine he or she passes during the day and night, including the urine the patient voids the first thing the next morning.
3. Instruct the patient to keep the collected urine in the container provided and keep it refrigerated.
   RATIONALE: Refrigeration will retard decomposition of urine and growth of bacteria.
4. Instruct the patient that as soon as possible after the collection is finished, he or she is to bring the sample into the laboratory.
5. Emphasize that if the patient is collecting a 24-hour sample for a creatinine clearance or any other test that requires a blood sample be taken, the *patient* must come in with the urine sample so that a blood sample may be drawn at the same time.
6. Instruct the patient to drink either the same amount of liquid as usual, or more, during the collection period. The patient is not to drink any alcoholic beverages and should stay on his or her regular diet.
   RATIONALE: The 24-hour specimen should reflect the patient's normal eating and drinking pattern.

Two-Glass Specimen

Some physicians wish to obtain two-glass urinalyses from male patients in an attempt to pinpoint the source of an infection in the urinary tract system. If the first specimen shows signs of infection, the source is likely to be lower in the urinary tract than if both samples or only the second sample is infected. The medical assistant examining the two-glass urine sample treats them as two separate specimens, checking both specimens with Chemstrips and examining them microscopically.

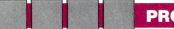

PROCEDURE

INSTRUCTING A PATIENT TO OBTAIN A TWO-GLASS URINE SPECIMEN

PURPOSE

To enable the patient to obtain this specimen.

EQUIPMENT AND MATERIALS

Private toilet area
Labeled specimen containers

PROCEDURAL STEPS

1. Give the patient two cups, labeled 1 and 2.
2. Instruct the patient to void the first part of his specimen into cup 1, collecting about 1 inch of urine.
3. Have the patient void into the toilet until he feels his bladder is about half empty. At this point, the patient should collect about 1 inch of urine into cup 2.
4. The patient can then continue voiding into the toilet.

URINE TESTS

Physical Examination

General Appearance

The general appearance of the urine sample includes color, clarity (transparency), and odor. Abnormal observations of the general appearance of the urine are always recorded on the urinalysis report. Causes of change in color and appearance of urine are listed in Table 21–3. When the appearance of the urine is normal, it is often not mentioned. It is important to follow consistently the established office policies when recording the general appearance of the sample.

Volume

The volume of urine is generally measured over a 24-hour period. A normal adult produces 750–2000 ml in 24 hours. Excessive urine production, called *polyuria,* is common in diabetes and kidney disorders. *Oliguria,* insufficient urine production, may be caused by dehydration, shock, or renal disease.

The volume of a urine sample run in the medical laboratory generally is not of concern, except in cases where the sample is too small to obtain accurate readings.

Specific Gravity

Specific gravity is a ratio of the weight of the urine compared with the weight of an equal volume of water. Although not performed in all office laboratories, determination of specific gravity is an easy test to perform and can indicate to the physician the presence of a concentrated or diluted urine sample. Specific gravity of normal urine is between 1.002 and 1.030.

Specific gravity may be checked by using a Chemstrip or dipstick, which indicates specific gravity after being dipped in the urine sample for 1 minute (see Chemical Examination). Another method is to use a calibrated urinometer, which is inserted into a cylindrical container filled with urine.[2]

TABLE 21-3
CAUSES OF CHANGES IN COLOR AND APPEARANCE OF URINE

Nearly Colorless	Dark or Bright Yellow	Orange	Red-Orange, Pink, or Red	Green or Blue-Green	Brown or Brown-Black	Cloudy	Foamy
Large fluid intake	Concentrated urine (dehydration, fever, exercise, etc.)	Carotene (found in carrots and spinach)	Beets	Urate crystals	Rhubarb	Crystals (urate, uric acid, carbonates, phosphates)	Bilirubin
Alcohol ingestion	Vitamin B-complex (especially riboflavin)	Phenazopyridine (Pyridium) (urinary anesthetic)	Blackberries	Methylene blue	Cascara (laxative)	Bacteria	
Nervousness	Yeast concentrate	Sulfonamides (antibiotics)	Food coloring	Amitriptyline (Elavil) (antidepressant)	Chloroquine (Aralen) (antimalarial)	Pus (WBCs)	
Diuretic therapy	Food coloring	Bilirubin	Phenolphthalein laxatives (Ex-Lax, Mondane, Senekot)	Triamterene (Dyrenium) (diuretic)	Phenacetin (pain medication)	Blood (RBCs)	
Uncontrolled diabetes mellitus	Quinacrine (Atabrine, antimalarial drug)		Dioctyl sodium sulfosuccinate laxative (Doxidan)	Indomethacin (Indocin) (antiinflammatory)	Sulfonamides (antibiotic)	Mucus	
Diabetes insipidus			Cascara (laxative)	*Pseudomonas* urinary tract infection	Nitrofurantoin (anibiotic)	Prostatic fluid	
Chronic kidney disease			Senna (laxative)		Metronidazole (Flagyl) (antibiotic)	Sperm	
			Phenothiazine tranquilizers (Thorazine, Mellaril, Haldol)		Quinine iron preparations (injectable)		
			Phenazopyridine (Pyridium) (urinary anesthetic)		Levodopa (L-dopa) (antiparkinsonism medication)		
			Methyldopa (Aldomet) (antihypertensive)		Lysol poisoning		
			Phenytoin (Dilantin) (anticonvulsant)		Blood or hemoglobin		
			Sulfasalazine (Azulfidine) (antibiotic)		Bilirubin		
			Iron preparations (injectable)		Porphyrins		
			Pyruvinium parmoate (Povan) (antiworm medication)		Alkaptonuria		
			Aniline dyes		Melanin		
			Blood and hemoglobin				

Adapted from Sobel DS, Ferguson T: *The People's Book of Medical Tests.* New York: Summit Books, 1985, pp. 113–114.

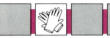

PROCEDURE

PERFORMING A PHYSICAL EXAMINATION OF A URINE SAMPLE

PURPOSE

To determine its general appearance, volume, and specific gravity.

EQUIPMENT AND MATERIALS

Specimen container with urine sample
Urinalysis form
Urinometer (if using urinometer for specific gravity determination)
Cylindrical container (if using urinometer for specific gravity determination)
Refractometer (if using refractometer for specific gravity determination)
Gloves and protective wear for universal precautions

PROCEDURAL STEPS

 MEDICAL ASSISTING ALERT

All physical examinations of urine must be done on a specimen that has not been spun in a centrifuge.

1. Observe the urine for color and record abnormal observations.
   RATIONALE: The color of normal urine is a pale yellow or straw color. Other colors may include pink, red, black-red, orange, or a greenish tinge. A frequent cause of abnormal color in the urine is the presence of blood. This can range from a light pink tinge, through various shades of red, to a black-red appearance in the case of massive blood and clots. A specimen that contains large amounts of blood is called "grossly bloody."

 MEDICAL ASSISTING ALERT

Ask the patient if he or she is taking any drugs (such as Pyridium) or, if the patient is a woman, if she is menstruating, because these can alter the color of urine.

2. Observe the urine for clarity or transparency and record abnormal findings.
   RATIONALE: Normal urine is clear or transparent. Abnormal samples may range from slightly cloudy to completely opaque, which is common when the urine is infected with bacteria or if RBCs or WBCs are present. Occasionally, urine appears abnormally clear, almost water-like in clarity. This is usually caused by the patient's having consumed large amounts of water before giving the sample and is called a "dilute" sample.

3. Observe the urine for odor and record abnormal observations.
   RATIONALE: Normal urine has a slight but not unpleasant odor. Urine that is infected with bacteria usually has a strong, ammonia odor and may be unpleasantly overpowering.

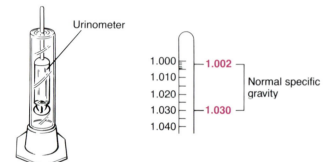

FIGURE 21-5

Obtaining specific gravity by use of a urinometer. (Redrawn from *Urinalysis Today*, Indianapolis, Boehringer Mannheim Diagnostics, 1986.)

Urine can also have a sweet, fruity odor, which may indicate the presence of diabetes.

4. Measure the volume of the specimen and record findings. Specimens that contain 80–100 ml are adequate for most urinalyses.

MEDICAL ASSISTING ALERT

If the sample contains less than 20 ml the medical assistant should alert the physician and ask if the urinalysis should still be performed.

5. Determine specific gravity.
   a. Chemstrip method: See Chemical Examination.
   b. Urinometric method:
      - Fill the cylindrical container about three-quarters full of urine.
      - Insert the calibrated urinometer into the urine, using a spinning motion, so that it floats freely.
      - Read the specific gravity at eye level and record the findings (Figure 21–5).
   c. Refractometer method:
      - Fill refractometer with one drop of fresh or slightly agitated urine.
      - Close the hinged lid.
      - Read the specific gravity by holding the instrument near a light source and focusing the rotating ring on the eyepiece. Record the findings.[2]

Chemical Examination

Chemical examination of urine is done by dipping plastic strips that contain specially treated paper patches, called *Chemstrips* or *dipsticks*, into the urine. A wide range of substances can be tested in this manner, depending on the interests of the physician. Usually from eight to nine substances are screened in the office laboratory; however, Chemstrips or dipsticks that test for only one chemical, such as glucose, are also available.

Common substances that may be checked by the use of Chemstrips or dipsticks are

- Leukocytes
- Nitrates
- Ketones
- Urobilinogen
- Bilirubin
- Glucose
- Protein
- Blood

In addition, pH and specific gravity may also be determined by Chemstrips or dipsticks.

Chemstrips and Dipsticks

- Chemstrips or dipsticks come in aluminum or glass containers.
- Store in a cool, dry area protected from temperatures over 30° C (86° F) and under freezing.
- Check the expiration date frequently. *Note:* Never use outdated Chemstrips or dipsticks.
- Until the container is opened, it should be stored on a dry shelf.
- Once the container is opened, it should be kept where urine and other liquids cannot leak into it.
- When the container is not in use, it should be tightly covered to protect the unused strips from contamination.[4]

PROCEDURE
PERFORMING A CHEMICAL EXAMINATION OF URINE

PURPOSE
To determine pH, specific gravity, and the presence of eight chemicals.

EQUIPMENT AND MATERIALS
Specimen container with urine sample
Chemstrips or dipsticks

568 *Chapter 21: URINALYSIS*

Chemstrip or dipstick container guide
Timer
Urinalysis form
Gloves and protective wear for CDC Universal Precautions

PROCEDURAL STEPS

 MEDICAL ASSISTING ALERT

All chemical examinations of urine must be done on a specimen that has not been spun in a centrifuge.

Preparation

1. Check that the specimen is properly labeled and is fresh.
   RATIONALE: Urine should be examined chemically within 20 minutes after it is obtained, because it decomposes rapidly after 20 minutes (see Figure 21–2).
2. If the sample has been refrigerated, allow it to come to room temperature.
   RATIONALE: Chemstrips or dipsticks may not react accurately on cold specimens.
3. Check that the Chemstrips or dipsticks have not expired and are not contaminated.

Performance

4. Take a Chemstrip or dipstick by the top edge, which does not contain patches, and dip it briefly into the urine. Make sure all the patches are moistened but do not leave the strip in the urine more than 1 second.

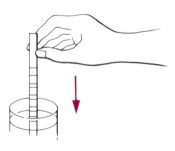

Redrawn from *Urinalysis Today*, Indianapolis, Boehringer Mannheim Diagnostics, 1986, 43.

5. With a sharp tap, shake off the excess urine so that the liquid does not leak from one patch to another.

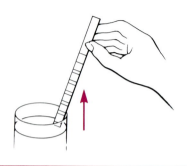

Redrawn from *Urinalysis Today*, Indianapolis, Boehringer Mannheim Diagnostics, 1986, 44.

6. Holding the strip with the patches down, match the patches to the color guide on the outside of the container, which will be labeled. Wait the appropriate time for what you are testing and then immediately read the test results, matching the individual chemical test with the color indicated on the strip.
   RATIONALE: The reagent patches are treated to change colors when they come in contact with the chemical being tested.

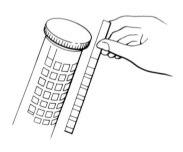

Redrawn from *Urinalysis Today*, Indianapolis, Boehringer Mannheim Diagnostics, 1986, 44.

 MEDICAL ASSISTING ALERT

Any color changes that occur more than 2 minutes after the Chemstrip has been dipped are invalid and should not be recorded.

7. Record the results on a urinalysis form.

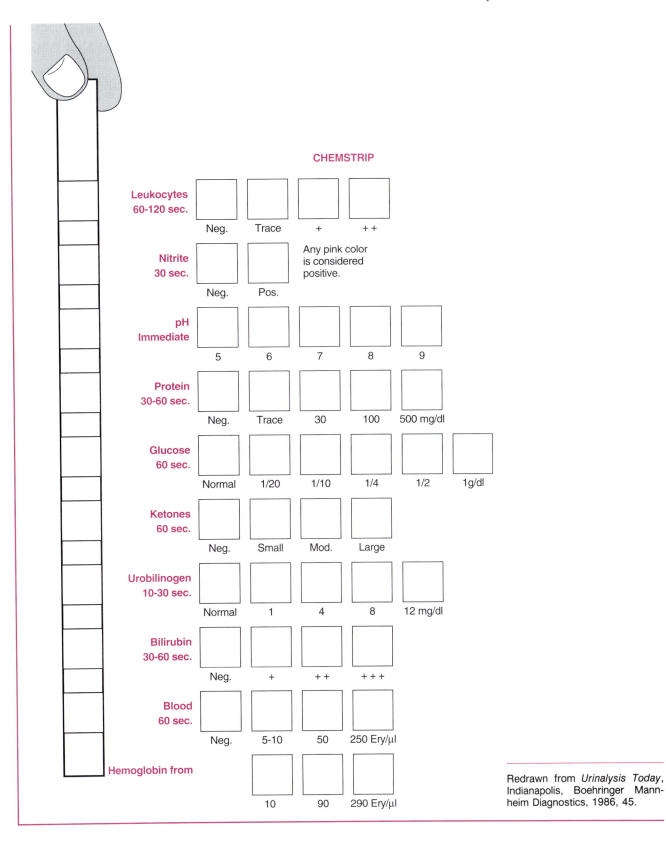

Redrawn from *Urinalysis Today*, Indianapolis, Boehringer Mannheim Diagnostics, 1986, 45.

Microscopic Examination

In the microscopic examination of urine, the specimen is first spun for 5 minutes in a centrifuge to allow the heavier particles in the urine to become concentrated in the bottom of the test tube. These few drops at the bottom of the tube are examined under the microscope, using both the low- and high-power lenses. Ten to fifteen low-power fields and ten to fifteen high-power fields should be scanned. A field is the area that can be seen at one time. Casts, WBCs, and RBCs are counted, totaled, and averaged. Epithelial cells are counted, averaged, and reported as 0, occasional (1–3), few (3–6), moderate (6–12), or many (>12). The remaining elements are reported as occasional (not seen in every field), few (seen in less than one-fourth of the field), moderate (covering one-half of the field), or many (covering most or the entire field).

A variety of particles may be visible in urine under the microscope. Those of major importance to the physician are

- Casts
- Cells
- Crystals
- Microorganisms

Urine may also contain cells and artifacts that are normal and of no clinical interest to the physician (Table 21–4).

TABLE 21–4

CELLS AND PARTICLES FOUND IN URINE

	Normal	Abnormal
Casts		
Hyaline casts	X	X
Granular casts	X	X
RBC casts		X
WBC casts		X
Renal tubular epithelial cell casts		X
Waxy casts		X
Cells		
RBCs		X
WBCs		X
Renal tubular epithelial cells		X
Transitional epithelial cells	X	
Squamous epithelial cells	X	
Oval fat bodies		X
Phosphates	X	
Crystals	X	X
Microorganisms		
Bacteria		X
Yeast		X
Sperm	X	
Other artifacts		
Threads and fibers	X	

Casts

Casts are cylindrical tubular forms that represent accumulations of protein that were formed in

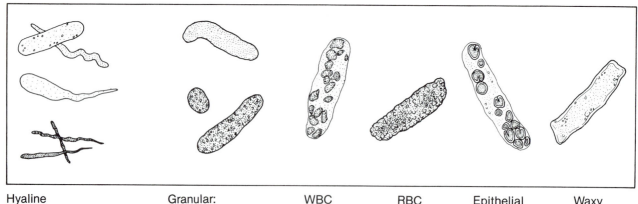

Casts: 100×   450× (to identify cells)

Hyaline / Cylindroid / Mucus (not a cast)   Granular: • Fine (top) • Coarse (bottom)   WBC   RBC   Epithelial   Waxy (broad)

FIGURE 21–6

Urine casts. (Reproduced from Kinn ME, Derge EF: *The Medical Assistant: Administrative and Clinical*, 6th ed. Philadelphia: W.B. Saunders, 1988, p. 706.)

the tubules of the kidney. They are located using the low-power lens; however, it is usually necessary to move to the high-power lens to identify the type of cast (Figure 21–6).

Hyaline Casts. Hyaline casts are cylindrical forms with long, parallel sides and rounded ends. They are pale and are best viewed by creating a shadow by darkening the microscope base light. They may be present in the urine of patients with kidney disease but are also present in normal urine.

Granular Casts. Granular casts appear similar in shape to the hyaline cast but have a granular or grainy appearance, which may be either fine or coarse. They are present after exercise but may indicate renal disease if numerous.

RBC Casts. RBC casts are hyaline casts that are filled with RBCs and thus may have a slightly brownish color. RBC casts are diagnostic of glomerulonephritis.

WBC Casts. WBC casts are hyaline casts that contain WBCs. The cells usually have a nucleus, are slightly larger than RBC casts, and are not so tightly packed. WBC casts are associated with pyelonephritis.

Renal Tubular Epithelial Cell Casts. Renal tubular epithelial cell casts are hyaline casts filled with renal tubular epithelial cells, which closely resemble WBCs. These casts are rare but when found indicate renal damage, particularly from shock or poisoning.

Waxy Casts. Waxy casts are smooth, glassy casts that appear to have cracks and broken ends. These are rarely seen and are associated with severe renal damage.

Cells

Cells commonly found in urine include WBCs, RBCs, and epithelial cells. RBCs and WBCs are of major diagnostic interest to the physician (Figure 21–7).

RBCs. RBCs appear as pale, round, small circular cells. They are nongranular and have a distinct, round, black edge with no nucleus. In dilute urine they may swell or burst, and in concentrated urine they may crenate and wrinkle. A few RBCs (one or two per high-power field) are present in normal urine, but more than that indicates the presence of inflammation or injury.

WBCs. WBCs are larger than RBCs and have a less definite edge. They have a granular texture and may contain a nucleus. Normal urine contains a few WBCs, but more than five WBCs per high-power field indicates an inflammatory process is going on.

Renal Tubular Epithelial Cells. Renal tubular epithelial cells are larger than WBCs, are round or oval in shape, and may contain a large, oval nucleus. If present in large numbers, these may indicate renal damage.

Transitional Epithelial Cells. Transitional ep-

Cells: 450×

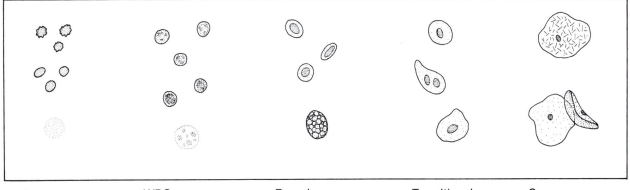

RBC:
- Crenated (top)
- Normal
- Swollen (bottom)

WBC:
- Glitter (bottom)

Round:
- Oval fat body (bottom)

Transitional

Squamous:
- Clue cell (top)
- Folded (bottom)

FIGURE 21–7
Red and white blood cells in urine. (Reproduced from Kinn ME, Derge EF: *The Medical Assistant: Administrative and Clinical,* 6th ed. Philadelphia: W. B. Saunders, 1988, p. 707.)

Crystals of Urine

Nonpathologic Acid pH	Crystal	Description and Occurrence
	Calcium oxalate	Clear, colorless, bipyramidal or envelope-shaped. Occasionally, shaped like dumbbell or safety pin. Very common
	Uric acid*	Pleomorphic, clear to yellow-brown, flattened, often four-sided, football-shaped, often in rosettes. Quite common
	Hippuric acid	Elongated, six-sided, colorless to yellow-brown, often in clusters
	Amorphous urates	Seen as salmon-pink precipitate in the centrifuge tube. Microscopically: shapeless, sand-like; brownish in color if heavy. Can be dispersed by warming tube prior to centrifugation. Very common
	Sodium urate	Colorless to yellow, long, thin, blunt-ended needles, often in rosettes or clumps
Alkaline pH		
	Triple phosphate	Colorless "coffin lid" six-sided prisms, often very large. Common in alkaline urines
	Amorphous phosphate	Seen in centrifuge tube as a white precipitate. Microscopically, shapeless, whitish, granular "sand." Can be dispersed by adding acetic acid to the sediment. Fairly common
	Calcium phosphate	Flat plates; long, thin needles or prisms; stars, crosses, or rosettes. Not very common
	Ammonium biurate	Brown "thorn apples" or greasy brown spherules. Rare
Pathologic All Found at an Acid pH		
	Tyrosine needles	Colorless to yellow, fine, silky needles in sheaves, rosettes. Found in severe liver damage, often with leucine
	Leucine spheres	Yellow, radially or concentrically striated spheres. Seen in liver disease
	Bilirubin	Brownish cubes, rhombic plates, or needles in pompom ball arrangement. Free bilirubin stains sediment brown
	Cholesterol plates	Colorless, flat plates with parallel sides and a characteristic notched corner. Seen in some renal diseases
	Cystine	Clear, colorless, hexagonal plates. Seen in the congenital disorder cystinosis

*May be pathologic.

FIGURE 21–8

Crystals of urine. (Reproduced from Kinn ME, Derge EF: *The Medical Assistant: Administrative and Clinical*, 6th ed. Philadelphia: W. B. Saunders, 1988, p. 708.)

Illustration continued on opposite page

Crystals of Urine

Nonpathologic ACID pH	Crystal	Description and Occurrence
OTHER		
	Radiocontrast dyes	Colorless, long, thin rhombic crystals. Specific gravity may be very high (often greater than 1.050). History will reveal recent x-ray studies
	Sulfa	Clear to brown sheaves of needles with eccentric, central constriction. History of sulfa medication

FIGURE 21–8 Continued

ithelial cells vary in size and may be round to oval in shape. Occasionally they may have a tail. They may have one or two nuclei and resemble poached eggs in appearance. These are present in normal urine, although larger numbers may be a sign of disease.

Squamous Epithelial Cells. Squamous epithelial cells are large, flat, irregularly shaped cells. They have small, round nuclei and may be folded over on themselves. They are similar to fried eggs in appearance. Large numbers of these cells indicate vaginal contamination of the urine specimen.

Oval Fat Bodies. Oval fat bodies are oval structures that are formed when a renal tubular epithelial cell accumulates droplets of fats. These are larger than WBCs and are found in the urine of patients with nephrotic syndrome.

Phosphates. Phosphates are black, dot-like structures that appear in the urine of children and adults after exercise. These usually appear in cluster-like formations and are not clinically significant.

Crystals

Crystals are clear, geometrically shaped forms that can look almost rock-like under the microscope (Figure 21–8). They generally are not of great clinical value; however, they may be an in-

Miscellaneous: 450×

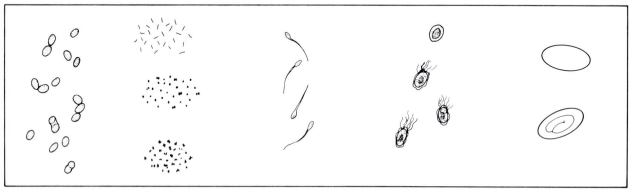

Yeast Bacteria:
• Bacilli (top)
• Cocci (middle)
• Amorphous crystals (bottom)

Sperm • Round epithelial cell (top)
• *Trichomonas* (bottom)

Pin worm eggs:
• Empty shell (top)
• Egg with embryonic worm (bottom)

FIGURE 21–9

Microorganisms and other structures found in urine. (Reproduced from Kinn ME, Derge EF: *The Medical Assistant: Administrative and Clinical*, 6th ed. Philadelphia: W. B. Saunders, 1988, p. 709.)

dication of kidney stones or the result of drug or medication use. Crystals sometimes have a colored tinge and may be quite beautiful in form.

Microorganisms

Microorganisms and other structures commonly found in urine are illustrated in Figure 21-9.

Bacteria. Bacteria in the urine are usually found in two forms. Most common are rods, which look like a cluster of thin, black lines resembling tiny pieces of fine hair. A few rods may be found in normal urine; however, if more than an occasional rod is present, the urine is probably infected. Other bacteria may appear as round or spiral-shaped cells; these are cocci. These are smaller than RBCs or WBCs and do not have the distinct outer edges or nuclei.

Yeast. Yeast is primarily found in the urine of females, although it may appear in males on occasion. Yeast is easy to confuse with RBCs, because they are round and about the same size. Yeast is often seen to "bud" (reproduce) under the microscope.

Sperm. It is not uncommon to find sperm present in the urine of both males and females. Sperm have small, pointed heads and long, hair-like tails. They may be alive and actively swimming about, although they usually will be nonmotile.

Other Artifacts

Other artifacts and structures may also be observed microscopically in urine. Thread-like artifacts and other harmless objects may frequently appear in urine and are not of interest to the physician.[1]

Urine Cultures

See Chapter 23.

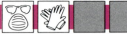

PROCEDURE

PERFORMING A MICROSCOPIC EXAMINATION OF URINE

PURPOSE

To determine the presence of casts, cells, crystals, microorganisms, and other artifacts.

EQUIPMENT AND MATERIALS

Microscope
Centrifuge
Glass slides
Glass slide covers
Centrifuge test tubes
Sink
Specimen container with urine sample
Timer
Urinalysis form
Gloves and protective wear for CDC Universal Precautions

PROCEDURAL STEPS

1. Pour 10 ml of urine into a centrifuge tube labeled with the patient's name. Place the tube into one of the centrifuge slots.
2. Place 10 ml of water into a centrifuge tube and place it into the centrifuge slot opposite the tube filled with urine.
   RATIONALE: The centrifuge must be balanced to spin properly.
3. Allow the urine to spin for 5 minutes. It is helpful to have a timer with a bell available to make sure the urine is spun the proper length of time.
4. After 5 minutes, turn off the centrifuge and remove the tube full of urine. Discard all of the spun urine into a sink except for the few drops that will cling to the bottom of the tube.
   RATIONALE: The heavier sediment and cells will have accumulated at the bottom of the tube during the centrifuge process.

5. Sharply tap the bottom of the centrifuge tube with the finger several times to mix the remaining drops of urine.
6. Place a glass microscope slide on the stage of the microscope, carefully shake out one or two drops of the urine sediment onto the slide, and place a glass slide cover over the urine.
7. Using the low-power lens, focus on an area of the slide edge, using the coarse adjustment, until the edge appears as a sharp, distinct line. At this point, move the lens into the center of the slide and examine 5–10 fields for the presence of casts or other artifacts.
8. Keeping the slide focused for the low-power lens, move to the high-power lens without changing the coarse adjustment. When the high-power lens has been snapped firmly in place, focus gently by turning the fine adjustment. At this point, any sediment in the urine sample should begin to come into focus. It is occasionally necessary to move back and repeat step 7 to get a clear view of the urine sediment.
9. After the slide has been focused clearly, carefully examine 5–10 fields. This is done by moving the slide but not changing the focus or the lens. Check the slide for the presence of casts, cells, crystals, microorganisms, and other artifacts.
10. After careful observation of several fields, record the results on the urinalysis form.

References

1. *Urinalysis Today.* Indianapolis, Boehringer Mannheim Diagnostics, 1986.
2. Kinn ME, Derge EF: *The Medical Assistant: Administrative and Clinical,* 6th ed. Philadelphia: W. B. Saunders, 1988.
3. Instruction sheet, CompuChem Laboratories, Western Division, Sacramento, CA.
4. Package insert from Chemstrips, Boehringer Mannheim Diagnostics, P.O. Box 50100, Indianapolis, IN 46250.

Bibliography

Johnson DF: *Total Patient Care: Foundations and Practice.* St. Louis: C. V. Mosby, 1972.
Morrison Treseler K: *Clinical Laboratory and Diagnostic Tests: Significance and Nursing Implications,* 2nd ed. Englewood Cliffs, NJ: Appleton and Lange, 1988.
Sobel DS, Ferguson T: *The People's Book of Medical Tests.* New York: Summit Books, 1985.
Thompson JM, McFarland GK, Hirsch JE, Tucker SM, Bowers AC: *Clinical Nursing.* St. Louis: C. V. Mosby, 1986.

Chapter 22

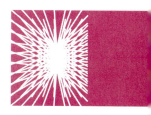

HEMATOLOGY AND BLOOD CHEMISTRY

JEANNETTE R. BELL
PATRICIA S. HURLBUT

HEMATOLOGY
Guidelines for Performing a Hematocrit
Sources of Error
Guidelines for Performing a Hemoglobin Concentration
Sources of Error
Guidelines for Performing an Erythrocyte Sedimentation Rate
Sources of Error
Guidelines for Performing a Manual Leukocyte Count
Sources of Error
Guidelines for Performing a Peripheral Blood Smear Examination
Sources of Error

Guidelines for Electronic Blood Cell Counting
Sources of Error
Guidelines for Performing a Prothrombin Time
Sources of Error

BLOOD CHEMISTRY
Purpose and Significance of Routine Blood Chemistries
Specimen Integrity
Use and Care of Laboratory Equipment
Quality Control
Accurate Reporting Procedures
Testing and Reporting Cholesterol Levels

HEMATOLOGY

Hematology is the study of the formed elements in the blood, which are erythrocytes (red blood corpuscles), leukocytes (white blood cells), and thrombocytes (platelets). The primary function of the red blood cells is to deliver oxygen from the lungs to the cells throughout the body and to transport carbon dioxide from the cells to the lungs to be exhaled. The primary function of the white blood cells is to defend the human body against infectious agents such as bacteria and viruses. The primary function of the platelets is to assist in blood clot formation, which prevents the escape of blood from the vascular system. The study of hemostasis, keeping the blood circulating in the blood vessels, is also included in the field of hematology.

When performing laboratory tests, it is essential that good quality assurance practices be maintained, from the collection and handling of the specimens, through the analytical procedures, to the final reporting of results to the physician. This ensures that the reported information reflects as closely as possible the true condition of the patient. It is most important to follow directed protocols exactly in collecting and handling specimens. Manufacturers' instructions must be followed completely when using test kits, preparing reagents, and performing test procedures. When

TABLE 22-1
REFERENCE RANGES FOR HEMATOLOGY PROCEDURES

Hematocrit
Adult male: 0.365–0.52
Adult female: 0.330–0.470
Birth: 0.40–0.644
1 month: 0.256–0.427
1 year: 0.270–0.450
10 years: 0.331–0.484

Hemoglobin
Adult male: 13.0–18.2 g/dl
Adult female: 11.0–16.3 g/dl
Birth: 13.6–19.6 g/dl
1 month: 9.5–12.5 g/dl
1 year: 11.0–13.0 g/dl
10 years: 11.5–14.8 g/dl

Erythrocyte Sedimentation Rate
Westergren method:
Male: 0–10 mm fall in 1 hour
Female: 0–20 mm fall in 1 hour

White Blood Cell Count
Adult: $3.9–10.9 \times 10^9/l$
Birth: $10.0–25.0 \times 10^9/l$
1 month: $7.0–15.0 \times 10^9/l$
1 year: $6.0–15.0 \times 10^9/l$
10 years: $4.5–12.0 \times 10^9/l$

Red Blood Cell Count
Adult male: $4.20–6.10 \times 10^{12}/l$
Adult female: $3.70–5.50 \times 10^{12}/l$
Birth: $4.00–5.60 \times 10^{12}/l$
1 month: $3.20–4.50 \times 10^{12}/l$
1 year: $3.60–5.20 \times 10^{12}/l$
10 years: $4.20–5.20 \times 10^{12}/l$

Platelet Count
$150–450 \times 10^9/l$

Differential Leukocyte Count
Adults: manual method
Neutrophils: 50–75% ($2.5–7.5 \times 10^9/l$)
Bands: 2–6% ($0.1–0.6 \times 10^9/l$)
Eosinophils: 1–5% ($0.05–0.40 \times 10^9/l$)
Basophils: 0–2% ($0–0.2 \times 10^9/l$)
Monocytes: 2–9% ($0.1–0.9 \times 10^9/l$)
Lymphocytes: 20–40% ($1.0–4.0 \times 10^9/l$)
Infants:
Neutrophils: 21–81% ($2.1–20.3 \times 10^9/l$)
Eosinophils: 0–5% ($0–1.3 \times 10^9/l$)
Basophils: 0–1% ($0–0.3 \times 10^9/l$)
Monocytes: 0–6% ($0–1.5 \times 10^9/l$)
Lymphocytes: 8–38% ($0.8–9.4 \times 10^9/l$)
Children:
Neutrophils: 33–45% ($1.5–6.5 \times 10^9/l$)
Eosinophils: 0–5% ($0–0.6 \times 10^9/l$)
Basophils: 0–2% ($0–0.2 \times 10^9/l$)
Monocytes: 0–7% ($0–0.8 \times 10^9/l$)
Lymphocytes: 33–45% ($1.5–6.5 \times 10^9/l$)

Prothrombin Time
10–13 seconds

Modified from Simmons A: *Hematology: A Combined Theoretical and Technical Approach.* Philadelphia: W. B. Saunders, 1989.

---

using instrumentation, proper installation and calibration must be performed. It is strongly recommended that these be done in conjunction with the manufacturer or distributor and with a certified medical technologist as a consultant. Preventive maintenance procedures must be properly performed, and operators' manuals must be strictly followed. All laboratory data should be reviewed for correctness and completeness. The results should be compared with the reference ranges as listed in Table 22–1 and correlated with the patient's condition. Control samples should be tested with patient samples, and records should be kept of the control values. All quality assurance practices should be accurately and completely documented. Patient and control values should be verified periodically by an accredited clinical laboratory.

Guidelines for Performing a Hematocrit

- Blood must be freshly collected, well-mixed, anticoagulated, unclotted, and unhemolyzed.
- Venous blood may be collected into disodium ethylenediaminetetraacetic acid (Na_2EDTA), 1.5–1.8 mg/ml of blood, or free-flowing blood from a skin puncture may be collected directly into a heparinized microhematocrit capillary tube.
- One whole blood control sample of known value, obtained commercially, should be run with each set of patient blood samples.

- Hematocrit values may be expressed either as a decimal fraction (for example, 0.42) or as a percentage (42%).
- For venous blood that has been drawn into Na₂EDTA, gently invert tube 12 times to ensure homogeneous mixing of the blood sample. Cover the stopper with a gauze square and gently wedge it out to prevent splattering of blood. Place it on a disposable tissue to keep the blood from contaminating the workspace. Take two wooden applicator sticks and rim the inside of the tube to check for clots. If no clots are present, process the sample as directed in the procedure.

Sources of Error

- Leaving the tourniquet fastened for longer than 2 minutes
- Probing for the vein more than twice
- Hemolysis

MEDICAL ASSISTING ALERT

Visible hemolysis (pink to red color in the plasma layer) while reading the test must be noted on the report.

- Inadequate mixing with anticoagulant
- Inadequate skin puncture
- Overfilling the capillary tubes
- Inadequately sealing the capillary tubes

MEDICAL ASSISTING ALERT

Affix a piece of white tape to the inside of the centrifuge. If leakage occurs, a band of blood will be visible on the tape. If this happens, the centrifuge must be decontaminated by wiping with a 10% solution of household bleach.

PROCEDURE

DETERMINING A HEMATOCRIT USING THE MICROHEMATOCRIT METHOD

PURPOSES

To detect anemia and evaluate treatment of anemia using the microhematocrit method.

EQUIPMENT AND MATERIALS

Apparel for Centers for Disease Control (CDC) Universal Precautions
Centrifuge (Figure 22–1) that meets the following specifications:
   Radius is greater than 8.0 cm
   Maximum speed is reached within 30 seconds
   A relative centrifugal field (RCF) of 10,000–15,000 × g_n is sustained at the periphery for 5 minutes without exceeding a temperature of 45° C
   Automatic timer calibrated in 30-second intervals from 0 to 5 minutes is included[1]
Microhematocrit reader (Figure 22–2)

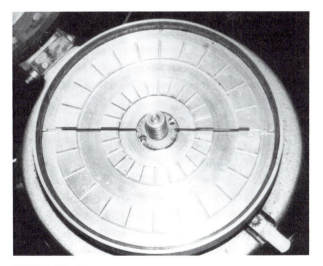

FIGURE 22–1

Microhematocrit centrifuge. (Reproduced from Kinn ME, Derge EF: *The Medical Assistant: Administrative and Clinical,* 6th ed. Philadelphia: W. B. Saunders, 1988, p. 734.)

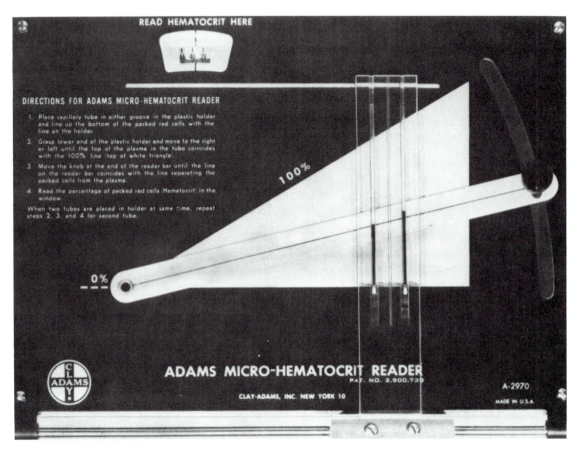

FIGURE 22-2

Microhematocrit reader. (Reproduced from Simmons A: *Hematology: A Combined Theoretical and Technical Approach.* Philadelphia: W. B. Saunders, 1989.)

Microhematocrit capillary tubes
> 75 mm in length with an internal diameter of 1.155 mm
>
> Plain, for EDTA anticoagulated blood, or heparinized, for blood specimen from skin puncture

Clay-like capillary sealing compound
Gauze or tissues
Note paper
Tape

PROCEDURAL STEPS

1. Fill a microhematocrit capillary tube approximately 3/4 full of blood.
2. Remove the capillary tube from the blood sample and allow the blood to flow an additional 0.5 cm toward the clean end of the capillary tube.
   RATIONALE: This allows the capillary to be plugged with sealing clay without causing blood to escape from the tip of the capillary.
3. Clean the outside of the tube with gauze or tissue and insert the capillary tube into a flat, smooth surface of sealing clay. Rotate the capillary slightly and remove it from the sealing compound.

 MEDICAL ASSISTING ALERT

Hold the capillary tube near the clean end that is being inserted into the clay to prevent breaking the tube, which could cause a cut and injection with potentially contaminated blood. Hold the container of sealing compound vertically and insert the clean end of the capillary tube horizontally at a 90° angle. Make sure none of the sample is forced out of the end of the microhematocrit capillary tube during this process.

4. Fill and seal a second capillary with the patient sample.
5. Fill and seal two capillary tubes with a control sample.

 MEDICAL ASSISTING ALERT

Keep the patient and control samples separated by taping them to a sheet of note paper that is properly labeled.

6. Place the two patient capillaries in the radial grooves of the centrifuge head and place the control capillaries in the opposite grooves. Record the groove number for each sample in the centrifuge.

 MEDICAL ASSISTING ALERT

Ensure that the clay seals in each capillary tube are touching the outer rubber gasket to prevent the samples from spinning out of the tubes.

7. Secure the inner lid firmly without cracking the tubes, and then lower the outer lid and securely fasten the latch. Turn on the centrifuge, and set the timer for 5 minutes.
8. When the centrifuge has stopped rotating, read the results in the microhematocrit capillary reader. Duplicate samples should be within ±0.02 (2%). Control values should be within the manufacturer's specified range.

 MEDICAL ASSISTING ALERT

Stopping the centrifuge with your hand invalidates the results by causing the red cells to flow back into the plasma. Results must be read within 10 minutes after the centrifuge has stopped, because leaving the capillary tubes in a horizontal position will invalidate the results by causing a slant in the cells/plasma interface. When taking readings, ensure that the bottom of the packed red cell column is lined up to the zero mark and that the "buffy coat" (grayish-creamy colored layer of white cells and platelets) is not included in the red cell column measurement. Avoid errors due to parallax which can be caused by changing the position of the head.

Guidelines for Performing a Hemoglobin Concentration

- Blood must be well mixed and unclotted. It may be collected from a free-flowing skin puncture into a pipette and measured directly into the cyanmethemoglobin reagent or venous blood may be collected into Na_2EDTA, 1.5–1.8 mg/ml. It may be stored at room temperature for up to 24 hours.
- One whole blood control sample of known value, obtained commercially, should be run with each set of patients.
- For venous blood that has been drawn into Na_2EDTA, gently invert tube 12 times to ensure homogeneous mixing of the blood sample. Cover the stopper with a gauze square and gently wedge it out to prevent splattering of blood. Place it on a disposable tissue to keep the blood from contaminating the workspace. Take two wooden applicator sticks and rim the inside of the tube to check for clots. If no clots are present, process the sample as directed in the following procedure.

Sources of Error

- Excessive exposure of reagent to light
- Insufficient mixing of blood sample
- Inaccurate pipettes and pipetting
- Contaminated reagents and glassware
- Insufficient mixing of sample and reagent
- Insufficient time for color development
- Improper operation of spectrophotometer
- Improper calibration of spectrophotometer
- Errors in reading and recording results

MEDICAL ASSISTING ALERT

Precautions with cyanmethemoglobin reagent include

- washing hands thoroughly immediately after handling the reagent
- using safety bulbs to pipette the reagent
- flushing with copious amounts of water in case of contact with skin or eyes
- seeking medical attention if eyes are contacted
- avoiding mixture with acids and breathing fumes
- emptying reagent directly into the drain of a sink with a lot of water running before, during, and after the disposal to completely eliminate the danger of cyanide fumes

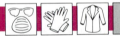
PROCEDURE

DETERMINING A HEMOGLOBIN CONCENTRATION USING THE CYANMETHEMOGLOBIN METHOD

PURPOSES

To detect anemia and evaluate treatment of anemia using the cyanmethemoglobin method.

EQUIPMENT AND MATERIALS

Apparel for CDC Universal Precautions
Cyanmethemoglobin reagent, obtained commercially, that contains potassium cyanide and potassium ferricyanide
Cyanmethemoglobin standard concentrate, obtained commercially, that contains 80 mg/dl of cyanmethemoglobin, equivalent to 20 g/dl of hemoglobin
Pipettes, 0.02 ml and 5.0 ml
Safety bulb or autodilutor
Test tubes, 13 mm × 100 mm
Gauze or tissues
Parafilm
Spectrophotometer capable of measuring absorbance at a wavelength of 540 nm

PROCEDURAL STEPS

1. Prepare the spectrophotometer for use and set the wavelength at 540 nm according to the manufacturer's instructions.
2. Label clean 13 mm × 100 mm test tubes for each reagent blank, control, and patient sam-

ple to be tested, and dispense 5.0 ml of cyanmethemoglobin reagent into each tube.
3. Prepare a standard solution of cyanmethemoglobin, which is equivalent to 10 g/dl of hemoglobin, by labeling a clean 13 mm × 100 mm test tube for the standard, adding exactly 2.5 ml of reagent and exactly 2.5 ml of the standard to the tube. Cover the tube with parafilm and invert five times to mix well.

SPECIAL HINT

Instead of the preceding procedure, a standard curve may be used. Follow the directions received with the standard reagent.

4. Draw blood into a 0.02-ml pipette. Remove blood from the outside of the pipette with a clean gauze or tissue, without touching the bore of the pipette. Adjust the amount of blood in the pipette to the 0.02-ml calibration mark.
5. Add the blood to the cyanmethemoglobin reagent and rinse the pipette in the reagent four times. Cover the test tube with parafilm and mix by inversion five to six times. Repeat this procedure for each control and patient sample to be tested.
6. Allow the tubes to stand at room temperature for at least 5 minutes.

MEDICAL ASSISTING ALERT

The resulting solutions are stable; however, they should be kept out of direct sunlight. If the tests cannot be read within 30 minutes, they may be covered and stored in the refrigerator in the dark for up to 6 hours.

7. Visually inspect each tube for clarity. All solutions must be crystal clear.

MEDICAL ASSISTING ALERT

Turbidity causes erroneous results, and the procedure must be repeated. If turbidity is present only in a patient tube, the blood sample should be sent to a reference laboratory for special processing.

8. Transfer the contents of the test tubes to an identically labeled matching set of cuvettes. Wipe the outside of each cuvette to remove fingerprints and moisture.

MEDICAL ASSISTING ALERT

Lint-free material should be used to clean the outside of the cuvettes. Scratching the cuvettes causes erroneous results.

9. Set the wavelength on the spectrophotometer at 540 nm. Read and record the absorbance of each test, standard, and control against the reagent blank.
10. Calculate the concentration of each patient sample and control using the following formula[2],[*]:

Concentration of hemoglobin (g/dL) in the sample =

$$\frac{\text{Absorbance of sample}}{\text{Absorbance of standard}} \times \text{Concentration of standard}$$

11. Check calculations for accuracy.
12. Ensure that the control is in range.
13. Report the hemoglobin concentration in g/dL.

---

[*] Reprinted with permission from Turgen M: *Clinical Hematology: Theory and Procedures.* Little, Brown and Company, copyright 1988.

Guidelines for Performing an Erythrocyte Sedimentation Rate

- Collect venous whole blood into an evacuated vacuum tube containing tripotassium ethylenediaminetetraacetic acid (K_3EDTA) at a concentration of 1.4–1.6 mg/ml of blood.

 MEDICAL ASSISTING ALERT

The test must be set up within 2 hours if the blood is left at room temperature, or within 6 hours if the blood is kept at 4° C.[3] The sample must be at room temperature when the test is set up. The blood must be well mixed, unclotted, and unhemolyzed.

- For venous blood that has been drawn into K_3EDTA, gently invert tube 12 times to ensure homogeneous mixing of the blood sample. Cover the stopper with a gauze square and gently wedge it out to prevent splattering of blood. Remove the stopper and place it on a disposable tissue to keep the blood from contaminating the workspace. Take two wooden applicator sticks and rim the inside of the tube to check for clots. If no clots are present, process the sample as directed in the procedure.
- Erythrocyte sedimentation rate values are expressed in millimeters/hour.

Sources of Error

- Incorrect blood:anticoagulant ratio
- Room temperature sample over 2 hours old or refrigerated sample over 6 hours old
- Sample not at room temperature when test is performed (18–25° C)
- Blood:diluent errors
- Bubbles in the blood column
- Faulty Westergren tubes or reservoirs
- Westergren racks not leveled

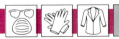 **PROCEDURE**

DETERMINING AN ERYTHROCYTE SEDIMENTATION RATE USING THE WESTERGREN METHOD

PURPOSE

To assist in diagnosing and monitoring inflammatory or infectious states.

EQUIPMENT AND MATERIALS

Apparel for CDC Universal Precautions
Applicator sticks
Westergren tubes, commercially available, which must be clean, dry, easily readable, and guaranteed by the manufacturer to provide results comparable to those of standard glass Westergren tubes[4]
Westergren rack or stand equipped with an accurate leveling bubble device

PROCEDURAL STEPS

1. Place the Westergren rack as follows:
   - at room temperature (18–25° C)
   - out of direct sunlight
   - out of direct range of heating/cooling vents
   - in an area where there is no vibration
2. Adjust the leveling bubble device.
3. Add blood to the prefilled diluent in the reservoir as specified by the manufacturer and mix well.
4. Insert the Westergren tube into the mixture in the reservoir as directed by the manufacturer.
5. Ensure that the top of the column of blood rests exactly at the zero mark on the Westergren tube and that no leakage of blood can occur.
6. Insert the Westergren tube and reservoir into the Westergren rack and set the timer for 60 minutes.
7. At 60 ±1 minutes, read directly from the tube the distance in millimeters from the bottom of the plasma meniscus to the top of the column of sedimented erythrocytes.

 MEDICAL ASSISTING ALERT

Do not include any leukocytes (buffy coat) with the erythrocyte column.

8. Record the results in millimeters/hour.

Guidelines for Performing a Manual Leukocyte Count[5]

- Blood must be well mixed and unclotted. It may be collected from a free-flowing skin puncture into a capillary pipette and measured directly into the Unopette reservoir, or venous blood may be collected into Na_2EDTA, 1.5–1.8 mg/ml. It may be stored *in the refrigerator* for up to 24 hours prior to testing.
- A manual leukocyte count should also be performed on a whole blood control of known value, obtained commercially.
- For venous blood that has been drawn into Na_2EDTA, gently invert tube 12 times to ensure homogeneous mixing of the blood sample. Cover the stopper with a gauze square and gently wedge it out of the tube to prevent splattering of blood. Place the stopper on a disposable tissue to keep the blood from contaminating the workspace. Take two wooden applicator sticks and rim the inside of the tube to check for clots. If no clots are present, process the sample as directed in the following procedure.

Sources of Error

- Inadequate mixing of sample
- Incorrect pipetting
- Inadequate mixing of reservoir before filling hemacytometer
- Irregular filling of hemacytometer
- Trapped air bubbles under cover glass
- Dust, oil, or scratches on surface of hemacytometer and/or cover glass
- Errors in counting cells
- Transcription errors
- Using dilutions or counting areas other than those prescribed without changing the calculation factor

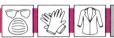

PROCEDURE

PERFORMING A MANUAL LEUKOCYTE COUNT USING THE UNOPETTE METHOD[6]

PURPOSE

To detect diseases, follow the course of diseases, and monitor therapy.

EQUIPMENT AND MATERIALS

Apparel for CDC Universal Precautions
Hemacytometer with improved Neubauer ruling and cover glass that meet the specifications of National Bureau of Standards Form 80[7]; cover glass must be plane on both sides within 0.002 mm.
Prefilled reservoirs containing 3% acetic acid to provide a 1:20 dilution when 25 μl of blood is added
Capillary pipettes, 25-μl capacity
Gauze or tissue
Hand tally
70% alcohol
Lens paper
Petri dish
5% sodium hypochlorite solution
Microscope
Interval timer

PROCEDURAL STEPS

1. Puncture the diaphragm of the test reservoir using the protective shield on the capillary pipette (Figure 22–3).

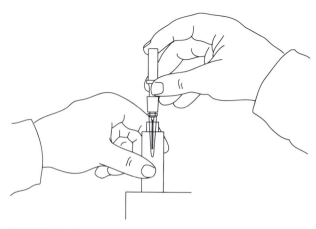

FIGURE 22–3

Puncture diaphragm. (Redrawn from Unopette Test 5877, Rutherford, NJ: Becton-Dickinson and Company, 1974.)

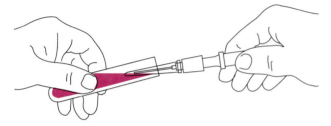

FIGURE 22-4
Fill capillary. (Redrawn from Unopette Test 5877, Rutherford, NJ: Becton-Dickinson and Company, 1974.)

2. Fill a 25-μl capillary tube with blood sample to be tested and remove blood from the outside of the capillary with a clean gauze or tissue, without touching the tip of the capillary (Figure 22-4).
3. Transfer the sample to the properly labeled test reservoir (Figure 22-5).

 MEDICAL ASSISTING ALERT

Squeeze reservoir to force out air without expelling diluent. Maintain pressure on reservoir. Cover capillary overflow chamber with index finger and seat pipette securely in reservoir neck. Release pressure on reservoir then remove finger from overflow chamber, allowing blood to flow into the diluent. Rinse capillary three times without expelling reservoir contents through the top of the overflow chamber.

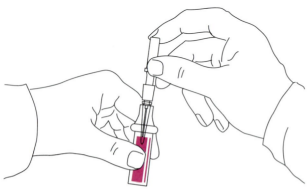

FIGURE 22-5
Transfer sample. (Redrawn from Unopette Test 5877, Rutherford, NJ: Becton-Dickinson and Company, 1974.)

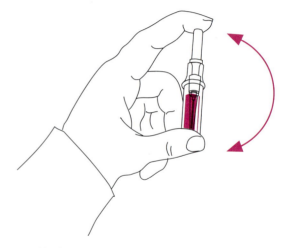

FIGURE 22-6
Invert to mix. (Redrawn from Unopette Test 5877, Rutherford, NJ: Becton-Dickinson and Company, 1974.)

4. Place index finger over sample opening and gently invert several times to mix sample with diluent (Figure 22-6).
5. Let stand for 10 minutes to allow red cells to hemolyze.

 MEDICAL ASSISTING ALERT

Diluted sample is stable for 3 hours. If the count cannot be completed after 10 minutes of standing, the capillary should be withdrawn and reseated securely in the reverse position. Cover the capillary tip with the capillary shield during the storage period.

6. Clean and dry the hemacytometer and cover glass with 95% ethanol and lens paper folded flat.

 MEDICAL ASSISTING ALERT

Using lens paper, wipe alcohol from the hemacytometer surface before evaporation to avoid a residue that will destroy blood cells. After cleaning, avoid getting fingerprints or other debris on the surfaces of the coverglass or hemacytometer, because these will interfere with blood cell distribution.

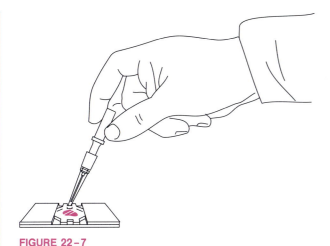

FIGURE 22-7

Fill hemacytometer. (Redrawn from Unopette Test 5877, Rutherford, NJ: Becton-Dickinson and Company, 1974.)

7. Check surface of the hemacytometer and cover glass for scratches, which will render the cell count inaccurate.
8. Mix diluted blood thoroughly by inverting reservoir to resuspend cells immediately prior to actual count and fill both sides of the hemacytometer (Figure 22-7).

 MEDICAL ASSISTING ALERT

Convert to dropper assembly by withdrawing pipette from reservoir and reseating securely in reverse position. Invert reservoir, gently squeeze sides, and discard first 3 or 4 drops. Carefully fill Neubauer hemacytometer with diluted blood by gently squeezing sides of reservoir to expel contents until chamber is properly filled. Allow the fluid to seep under the cover glass evenly and quickly. Any unevenness or slowness in filling greatly affects the cell distribution. Avoid flooding the hemacytometer. The cover glass must not be allowed to shift or move during any portion of the filling or counting procedure.

9. Allow the filled hemacytometer to sit for approximately 1 minute and then proceed to count the cells without delay.

 MEDICAL ASSISTING ALERT

If the fluid in the hemacytometer begins to evaporate, the blood cell count will be inaccurate.

10. Lift the hemacytometer, keeping it in a horizontal position at all times, and place it on the microscope stage.
11. With the low power (×10) objective, locate the large upper left square on the hemacytometer surface (the large corner square marked "1") (Figure 22-8).
12. Count all of the white blood cells in square 1, focusing the fine adjustment as necessary to see all the cells. Keep a count of the cells with the hand tally and record the total number.

 MEDICAL ASSISTING ALERT

Count all cells that touch the top and left hand boundaries of each large square and do not count any cells that touch the bottom or right hand boundaries (Figure 22-9). This provides an accurate cell count.

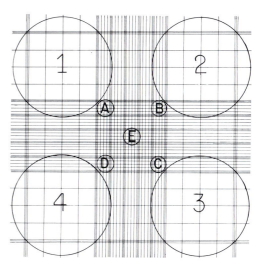

FIGURE 22-8

Hemacytometer surface. (Reproduced from Bonewit K: *Clinical Procedures for Medical Assistants*, 3rd ed. Philadelphia: W. B. Saunders, 1990, p. 376.)

588 Chapter 22: HEMATOLOGY AND BLOOD CHEMISTRY

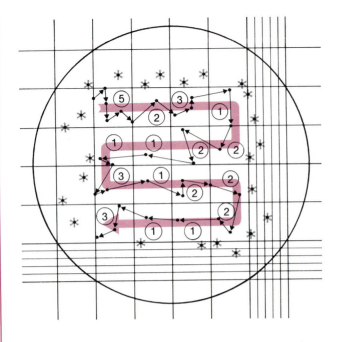

← The eye following the field
✻ Not counted into total
◯ Number counted into each square

FIGURE 22-9

Counting. Begin counting cells in the upper left-hand corner. Proceed across the top row, counting cells, including those that touch the top and left sides of each square. Continue to count the remainder of cells in the same fashion. Count in the direction of the arrows. The number of cells in each square is indicated in a circle. (Reproduced from Kinn ME, Derge EF: *The Medical Assistant: Administrative and Clinical,* 6th ed. Philadelphia: W. B. Saunders, 1988, p. 739.)

13. Count the cells in squares 2, 3, and 4 and record the total of each square. These totals should agree within 15 cells of each other.

MEDICAL ASSISTING ALERT

If the totals of each of the four squares do not agree within 15 cells of each other, the cell distribution is uneven, and the cell count will be inaccurate. The hemacytometer should be cleaned and filled again and the cell count repeated.

14. Add the number of cells counted in the four squares and multiply the total by 50 to obtain the total number of white blood cells/microliter.

MEDICAL ASSISTING ALERT

This formula is valid only when this procedure is followed EXACTLY. If a different dilution or counting area is needed, the blood sample should be sent to an accredited clinical laboratory for analysis.

15. Repeat steps 11–14 on the other side of the hemacytometer. The duplicate sides should agree within 1,000 cells/μl.

MEDICAL ASSISTING ALERT

If the duplicates do not agree within 1,000 cells, there is an error and the procedure should be repeated.

16. Average the acceptable duplicate results and report the results to the nearest 100 cells/μl.
17. Disinfect the hemacytometer and cover glass by immersing them in a solution of 5% bleach for 10 minutes, then rinse with tap water and dry using lens paper on the cover glass and on the surface of the hemacytometer.

Guidelines for Performing a Peripheral Blood Smear Examination

- Blood must be well mixed and unclotted. It may be collected from a free-flowing skin puncture with immediate smear preparation, or venous blood may be collected into K_3EDTA, 1.5 mg/ml, in liquid or power form. The anticoagulated blood may be stored at room temperature for 1 hour.
- Reference values are listed in Table 22–1.
- For venous blood that has been drawn into

K₃EDTA, gently invert tube 12 times to assure homogeneous mixing of the blood sample. Cover the stopper with a gauze square and gently wedge it out to prevent splattering of blood. Place the stopper on a disposable tissue to keep the blood from contaminating the workspace. Take two wooden applicator sticks and rim the inside of the tube to check for clots. If no clots are present, process the sample as directed in the following procedure.

Sources of Error

- Using blood stored longer than 1 hour after collection
- Delay in spreading blood following application to slide
- Dirty or poor quality slides
- Inappropriate size of drop of blood
- Improper angle of pusher slide
- Improper speed of pushing
- Improper pressure on pusher slide
- High humidity in testing environment
- Failure to allow smear to dry thoroughly before staining
- Deteriorated stain reagents
- Improper timing with staining reagents
- Infrequent changing of rinse water
- Examining improper area of smear
- Misidentification of blood cells

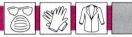

PROCEDURE

PERFORMING A PERIPHERAL BLOOD SMEAR EXAMINATION

PURPOSES

To estimate white cell and platelet numbers, evaluate red cell morphology, and assess relative white cell distribution.

EQUIPMENT AND MATERIALS

Apparel for CDC Universal Precautions
Clean glass slides with frosted ends
Transfer pipettes
Gauze or tissue
Pencil
Coplin staining jars (two)
Forceps
Flexible rinsing bottle
Stopwatch
Slide drying rack
Sink or basin
Fresh deionized water
Wright stain, commercially available
Microscope equipped with ×10 (low-power), ×40 (high-power), and either ×50 or ×100 (oil immersion) objectives
Immersion oil
Lens paper
Hand tally
Differential counter
Ethanol

PROCEDURAL STEPS

1. Place a slide on a flat surface with frosted end on the right (reverse, if you are left-handed).
2. With the transfer pipette, place a small drop of blood in the center of the slide near the frosted end.
3. Place another, pusher, slide in front of the drop of blood at a 30–45° angle, as illustrated in Figure 22–10, and quickly draw the pusher back into the drop of blood. Allow the blood to spread only 3/4 of the way across the bevel of the slide.

 MEDICAL ASSISTING ALERT

If blood spreads to the edges of the slide, the side margins of the blood smear, where the larger cells are pushed, cannot be examined under the microscope.

4. Quickly push the slide forward (away from the drop).

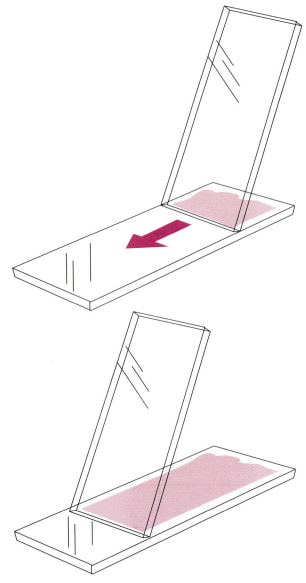

FIGURE 22-10

Blood smear preparation. (Redrawn from Simmons A: *Hematology: A Combined Theoretical and Technical Approach.* Philadelphia: W. B. Saunders, 1989.)

 MEDICAL ASSISTING ALERT

This forward move must be smooth and continue to the end of the slide.

5. Allow the smear to air-dry for 15 minutes before staining.
6. With a pencil, label slide on the frosted end.
7. Dispense staining reagents as directed in reagent kit.
8. Holding the blood smear with forceps, immerse it in the stain for 15 seconds or as directed by the manufacturer.
9. Remove the slide from the stain and immerse it in deionized water for 30 seconds or as directed by the manufacturer.
10. Remove the slide from deionized water and rinse thoroughly with deionized water in flexible bottle.
11. With gauze and methanol, remove stain from back of the slide and stand the slide in the rack to dry.
12. Examine the blood smear on low ($\times 10$) power to evaluate the stain quality and blood cell distribution.

 MEDICAL ASSISTING ALERT

The red cells should be evenly stained a light buff color and be free of precipitated stain. The white cells should show a prominent distinction between the nucleus and the cytoplasm. The red cells should be evenly distributed without streaks. The white blood cells should be evenly distributed and not clumped along the periphery. There should not be more than 5 times the number of white cells at the feathered edge than at the examining area of the smear. Platelets should not be clumped along the periphery or at the feathered edge. There should be at least 10 low-power fields in which the red cells are lying side by side but not overlapping. This assures that there is an adequate area for performing a white blood cell differential.

13. Move the blood smear to a viewing area that contains at least 50% of the red cells overlapping and lock the high ($\times 40$) power objective in place to estimate the number of white blood cells.

 MEDICAL ASSISTING ALERT

Count the number of white cells in 10 fields, divide by 10 to obtain the average, and multiply this average by 2000. The value obtained should be within 20% of the total white count.

14. Move the blood smear to a viewing area where the red blood cells are lying side by side but not overlapping. Move the high-power objective aside, add a drop of immersion oil to the slide, and lock the oil immersion objective into place.
15. Evaluate the red blood cell morphology.

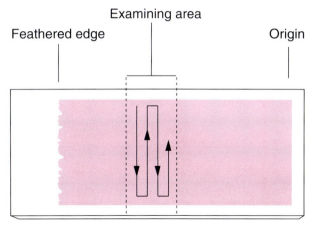

FIGURE 22-11

Blood smear examination.

> **MEDICAL ASSISTING ALERT**
>
> The red cells should be uniform in size, shape, and color and free of inclusions and precipitated stain. The area of central pallor should occupy 30-40% of the red cell. Any abnormalities should be noted on the report.

16. Estimate and evaluate the platelets.

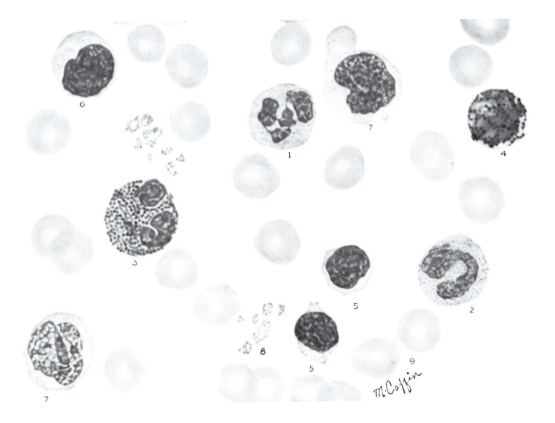

FIGURE 22-12

Types of human blood cells: **1-7,** White cells (or leukocytes) stained as they are in the laboratory to show the many different types. They play the active role in immune response, that is, defense against disease. (**1,** neutrophil; **2,** neutrophilic band; **3,** eosinophil; **4,** basophil; **5,** lymphocyte; **6,** large lymphocyte; **7,** monocyte.) **8,** Platelets (thrombocytes). They are responsible for clotting. Red blood cells (erythrocytes). They carry oxygen. (Reproduced from Custer RP: *An Atlas of the Blood and Bone Marrow,* 2nd ed. Philadelphia: W. B. Saunders, 1974.)

MEDICAL ASSISTING ALERT

There should be an average number of 10–20 platelets per oil immersion field. They should stain lilac in color with multicolored central granules and a fuzzy periphery. They should be 1/4–1/3 the size of red cells. Any abnormalities should be noted on the report.

17. Perform a white cell differential. Begin at the top of the smear in the examining area and move the smear downward, over one field, and back up, as illustrated in Figure 22–11. As each white cell comes into view, identify it and tabulate it on a differential white cell counter until 100 white cells have been identified.

MEDICAL ASSISTING ALERT

Assistance in identifying blood cells can be obtained from the illustration in Figure 22–12, from commercially available illustrated atlases of blood cell morphology, and from the descriptive criteria outlined in the chart below.

18. Record the number of cells in each category on the report form and verify that the total equals 100.

Guidelines for Electronic Blood Cell Counting

- Blood must be well mixed and unclotted. Venous blood should be collected and mixed in the correct proportion with a salt of EDTA. It may be stored at room temperature for up to 4 hours if a platelet count is required. If a platelet count is not required, the sample can be stored in the refrigerator for up to 24 hours prior to testing.

SEGMENTED NEUTROPHILS

Cytoplasm: Pink with granules pink to lavender in color
Nucleus: Lobulated with thin connecting filaments; dark, dense blocks of purple chromatin separated by lighter purple bands

BAND NEUTROPHILS

Cytoplasm: Similar to that in segmented neutrophil
Nucleus: Curved or sausage-shaped, with parallel sides; lobes may be connected by wide bands instead of filaments (when in doubt, classify as segmented neutrophil)

LYMPHOCYTES

Cytoplasm: Abundant to sparse, pale to bright blue in color
Nucleus: Usually round, but may be kidney-shaped; chromatin is arranged in densely staining compact blocks separated by lighter tones without demarcation

MONOCYTES

Cytoplasm: Abundant, round; may have blunt protrusions; stains gray-blue; and contains many small dust-like granules, sometimes vacuolated
Nucleus: Variable in shape; may be folded or convoluted; chromatin stains light purple and is usually fine and lacy

EOSINOPHILS

Cytoplasm: Contains many large, spherical granules that stain bright orange-red
Nucleus: Usually segmented into two or three purple-staining lobes

BASOPHILS

Cytoplasm: Contains dark purple-black granules, variable in size and unevenly distributed
Nucleus: Deeply indented or segmented, often obscured by granules

- For venous blood that has been drawn into EDTA, gently invert tube 12 times to ensure homogeneous mixing of the blood sample. Cover the stopper with a gauze square and gently wedge it out of the tube to prevent splattering of blood. Place the stopper on a disposable tissue to keep the blood from contaminating the workspace. Take two wooden applicator sticks and rim the inside of the tube to check for clots. If no clots are present, process the sample as directed in the procedure.

Sources of Error

- Incorrect blood:anticoagulant ratio
- Insufficient mixing of sample
- Failure to detect clots or hemolysis
- Contaminated reagents
- Improper instrument calibration
- Inattention to instrument quality control checks
- Inattention to whole blood control data
- Inattention to instrument error codes
- Inattention to data review

PROCEDURE

ELECTRONIC BLOOD CELL COUNTING USING THE COULTER COUNTER MODEL $T_5 40$[8]

PURPOSE

To quantitatively measure white blood cells, red blood cells, hemoglobin, hematocrit, and platelets in the peripheral blood using the Coulter Counter.

EQUIPMENT AND MATERIALS

Apparel for CDC Universal Precautions
Coulter Counter Model $T_5 40$ equipped with roll printer (see Figure 22–13)
Coulter Unit-T-Pak reagent system

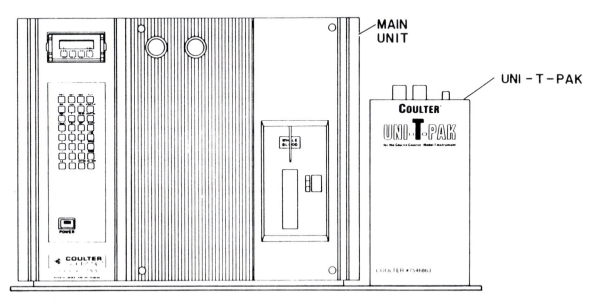

FIGURE 22–13

Coulter Counter Model T Series Instrument. (Reproduced from *Coulter Counter Models $T_5 40$, $T_6 60$ and $T_8 90$ Product Reference Manual*, Hialeah, FL: Coulter Corporation, 1986.)

Gauze
Wooden applicator sticks
Lint-free tissues

PROCEDURAL STEPS

1. Press the POWER button on the main unit and allow to warm up for 30 minutes before running patient samples or controls.

 MEDICAL ASSISTING ALERT

It is recommended that the power in the main unit be left on during shutdown periods to maintain the stability of the electronic components.

2. Set date and test number on the unit.
3. Check that the power supply gauges indicate the appropriate values.
4. Verify that the top of the red indicating light in the electronic manometer is within the green operating range.
5. Press STARTUP on the keyboard and observe the automatic startup cycle assuring that all systems are functioning properly.
6. Prime the instrument by cycling a normal whole blood sample as follows:

   - Hold the mixed primary sample to the aspirator tip with the tip submerged in the sample.
   - Press the WHOLE BLOOD button and hold the sample in position until the display changes from ASPIRATING to WIPE TIP.
   - With a clean, lint-free tissue, wipe the aspirator tip vertically, taking care not to bend it.

7. Observe the diluter during the rest of the cycle.
8. Perform step 6 on each control and patient sample.

 MEDICAL ASSISTING ALERT

Verify that all control sample results are within the established range.

9. Review printed patient data. Verify that data are *not* printed with result codes.

 MEDICAL ASSISTING ALERT

Any data printed with result codes must have corrective action before results are reported.

NOTES: The identification number on the printed results must correspond to patient identification system.
The results must be within the established reference ranges.
The results must be compatible with those observed on the peripheral blood smear.
The results must be physiologically possible and correspond to the patient's clinical data.

10. Repeat the procedure for any abnormal results and send a sample to a reference clinical laboratory for verification.
11. At the end of each day of use, perform instrument shutdown procedures.

Guidelines for Performing a Prothrombin Time

- Blood should be collected by a clean, untraumatic venipuncture and mixed with the dihydrate form of trisodium citrate ($Na_3C_6H_5O_7 \cdot 2H_2O$) in a ratio of nine parts blood to one part anticoagulant. The blood and anticoagulant must be well mixed, unclotted, and unhemolyzed.
- To obtain a plasma sample, the capped specimen is centrifuged at $2500 \times g$ for 15 minutes. To transfer plasma, a clean, nonwettable pipette is used and the sample is transferred to a clean container with a nonwettable surface. The allowable time interval between obtaining the specimen and testing of the sample will depend on the temperature maintained during transport and storage of the sample using the following guidelines: 22–24° C = 2 hours; 2–4° C = 4 hours. If the testing has not been completed within 4 hours, plasma samples must be frozen.[9]
- Manufacturers' instructions for reagents and equipment must be carefully read prior to per-

formance of the prothrombin time and strictly followed.
- A coefficient of variation of less than 5% should be obtained on vials of thromboplastin-calcium reagent within the same lot, and the same variance limits should be obtained from lot to lot of thromboplastin-calcium reagent.
- The instrument used must give a coefficient of variation of less than 5% for the mean of the replicates of an abnormally prolonged prothrombin time, that is, longer than 30 seconds.
- The delivery systems of reagents and plasmas must be accurate to within ±5% of the stated volume.
- Use type I reagent grade water when preparing and reconstituting reagents and controls.
- Collection tubes, storage tubes, plastic ware, pipettes, and delivery system must be scrupulously clean in performing prothrombin times.
- All tests must be performed at 37° ± 1° C.
- The pH of the reaction mixture must be 7.2–7.4.
- Reagents and aliquots of plasma must be prewarmed to 37° C prior to performance of the test. The plasma should not be warmed for longer than 10 minutes before testing. The manufacturers' inserts must be followed in regard to preparation and handling of individual thromboplastin.
- One normal and one abnormal plasma control of known value, obtained commercially, should be run with each set of patient samples.

Sources of Error

- Incorrect anticoagulant
- Improperly filled tubes
- Clotted, hemolyzed, icteric, or lipemic blood specimens
- Contaminated collection or storage tubes
- Improper treatment of sample prior to testing
- Improperly diluted thromboplastin
- Contaminated samples or reagents
- Incorrect incubation time, temperature, pH, volumes, or instrumentation procedures

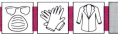

PROCEDURE

PERFORMING A PROTHROMBIN TIME PHOTO-OPTICAL END-POINT DETECTION USING MLA ELECTRA 750[10]

PURPOSE

To detect disorders of coagulation factors I, II, V, VII, and X, and to monitor oral coumarin anticoagulant therapy.

EQUIPMENT AND MATERIALS

Apparel for CDC Universal Precautions
MLA Electra 750 (see Figure 22–14)
0.2-ml instrument pipette
0.1-ml pipette—MLA # 1055
Pipette tips—MLA # 9620
Test cuvettes—MLA # 9005
Stopwatch
Test tube rack
Thromboplastin reagent, obtained commercially

PROCEDURAL STEPS

1. Turn on Electra 750 and allow to warm for 5 minutes or until AT TEMP lights, whichever is later. Perform abbreviated operator confidence test as follows:

- Set LAMP LEVEL switch to B and MODE SELECT switch to PT.
- Place an empty cuvette and instrument pipette in place at test station and press the pipette plunger. Check that the OFF SCALE indicator remains extinguished for at least 10 seconds, as indicated on TIME display.
- Remove and reinsert the empty cuvette, replace the instrument pipette, set LAMP LEVEL switch to A, and press the pipette plunger. Check that OFF SCALE indicator lights after approximately 7 seconds, and TIME indicator automatically sets to 0 after the count.
- Check that workstation thermometer indicates 37° ± 0.5° C.

2. Set LAMP LEVEL switch to B.
3. Reconstitute reagents and controls per manufacturer's instruction.
4. Prewarm thromboplastin in REAGENT reser-

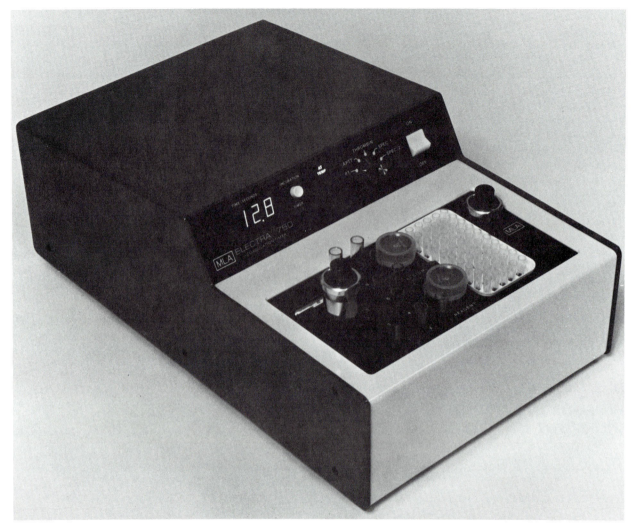

FIGURE 22–14
MLA Electra 750. (Reproduced from *MLA Instruction Manual.* Pleasantville, NY: Medical Laboratory Automation, Inc., 1990.)

voir. Use magnetic stirring bar for reagents that require agitation.
5. Set MODE SELECT switch to PT.
6. Pipette 0.1 ml of control or patient plasma, in duplicate, into the bottom of MLA test cuvettes and place in rack.
7. Place first sample in incubation station 1 and start stopwatch.
8. After 30 seconds, place next sample in incubation station 2.
9. Continue in this manner, adding the next tube every 30 seconds.
10. After 180 seconds (3 minutes), take the sample from incubation station 1 and place it in test station.
11. Using a 0.2-ml (red top) instrument pipette, aspirate 0.2 ml of warm thromboplastin and align the pipette over the test station. Firmly push the pipette plunger and hold it down for one second to start test.
12. When the timer stops, record clot time. If, during the test, the OFF SCALE indicator lights, the specimen under testing is outside the instrument range. Refer to operator manual for further instructions.
13. Continue in this manner, adding a new sam-

ple to the heating block and starting a test every 30 seconds.
14. Use a clean pipette tip on the instrument pipette for each test to prevent carryover contamination.
15. Assure that duplicate values for both patient and control samples are within ±0.6 second. If not, the tests should be repeated.
16. Report the average of acceptable duplicates to the nearest 0.1 second. Both patient and control values should be reported.
17. Patient values should be within the normal range, except for patients on anticoagulant therapy. In this case, values 2–2 1/2 times longer than normal are expected.

BLOOD CHEMISTRY

Purpose and Significance of Routine Blood Chemistries

Blood chemistry tests measure the chemicals dissolved in the blood that circulate to and from all organs of the body.

Chemistry tests are often ordered in "panels." A panel is a group of chemistry tests that evaluate several of the 12 body systems. By screening for a particular chemical or chemicals produced or used by each body system, the doctor can obtain a good overview of the general health of the patient. If any one test is abnormal, the physician can further investigate that particular body system.

Panels generally require a very small amount of blood for multiple results.

Normal Values, Standard Abbreviations, and Significance of Results

Table 22–2 gives an overview of commonly ordered blood chemistry tests, their common abbreviations, their normal values, and several possible causes of abnormalities.

Different laboratories may use different instruments. There also may be slight variations in different populations of patients. Therefore, it is recommended to use the normal ranges given by the laboratory that ran the testing when analyzing specific patient data.

Related Terminology

Concentration: The amount of chemical found in a specific amount of serum, control, or standard
Fasting: Abstaining from food or fluids for a specific time before testing
Hemolysis: The breakdown of red blood cells (RBCs), resulting in a red tint to the serum
Integrity: The quality of a specimen collection
Lipemia: Increase in lipids (fats) in the blood, which may cause turbidity
Panel/profile: A group of tests that evaluate several of the body systems
Postprandial: After eating
Turbidity: Cloudiness of the specimen

Specimen Integrity

A laboratory result is only as good as the specimen the laboratory receives. Some of the chemicals to be tested may continue to break down even after a specimen is collected. Therefore, it is of the utmost importance to follow *all* of the guidelines below for collecting and preserving specimens.

Choice of Tubes

- Special preservatives are added to blood collection tubes for maintaining the best specimen integrity. Because each preservative acts very specifically on different parts of the chemical structures, tests often cannot be run if the samples are collected in the wrong type of collection tube.
- Combining preservatives is not recommended. The collection of multiple tubes is the preferred method of collection when multiple tests are ordered.
- Table 22–3 displays the various anticoagulants and the general types of tests run from each tube.

Proper Specimen Handling

- If there is a question of how to preserve a specimen, contact the laboratory before collection to avoid possible mistreatment of the specimen.

TABLE 22-2

COMMON BLOOD CHEMISTRY TESTS

Name of Test and Specimen Requirement	Abbreviation	Purpose	Normal Range	Increased with	Decreased with
Alkaline phosphate (serum)	ALP	Assists in the diagnosis of liver and bone diseases.	30–115 mU/ml	Liver disease Bone disease Hyperparathyroidism Infectious mononucleosis	Hypophosphatasia Malnutrition Hypothyroidism Chronic nephritis
Blood urea nitrogen (serum)	BUN	Used as a screening test to detect renal disease, especially glomerular dysfunction.	8–25 mg/dl	Kidney disease Urinary obstruction Dehydration Gastrointestinal bleeding	Liver failure Malnutrition Impaired absorption
Calcium (serum)	Ca	Used to assess parathyroid functioning and calcium metabolism, and to evaluate for malignancies.	8.5–10.5 mg/dl	**Hypercalcemia** Hyperparathyroidism Bone metastases Multiple myeloma Hodgkin's disease Addison's disease Hyperthyroidism	**Hypocalcemia** Hypoparathryoidism Acute pancreatitis Renal failure
Chloride (serum)	Cl	Assists in diagnosing disorders of acid-base and water balance.	96–110 mEq/L	Dehydration Cushing's syndrome Hyperventilation Eclampsia Anemia	Severe vomiting Severe diarrhea Ulcerative colitis Pyloric obstruction Severe burns Heat exhaustion

Cholesterol (serum)	CH
	Chol
		Used to screen for the presence of atherosclerosis related to coronary artery disease. Also used as a secondary aid in the study of thyroid and liver functioning.	**Total cholesterol**
			120–200 mg/dl (An upper range of 200 mg/dl is usually now preferred by most physicians to reduce the risk of coronary artery disease.)
			LDL cholesterol
			  0–19 yr 50–170 mg/dl
			  20–29 yr 60–170 mg/dl
			  30–39 yr 70–190 mg/dl
			  40–49 yr 80–190 mg/dl
			  50–59 yr 80–210 mg/dl
			HDL cholesterol
			Male
			  0–19 yr 30–65 mg/dl
			  20–29 yr 35–70 mg/dl
			  30–39 yr 30–65 mg/dl
			  40–49 yr 30–65 mg/dl
			  50–59 yr 30–65 mg/dl
			Female
			  0–19 yr 30–70 mg/dl
			  20–29 yr 35–75 mg/dl
			  30–39 yr 35–85 mg/dl
			  40–49 yr 40–95 mg/dl
			  50–59 yr 35–85 mg/dl
				Atherosclerosis
				Cardiovascular disease
				Obstructive jaundice
				Hypothyroidism
				Nephrosis
					Malabsorption
					Liver disease
					Hyperthyroidism
					Anemia

Creatinine (serum)	creat	Used as a screening test of renal functioning.	0.4–1.5 mg/dl	Impaired renal function Chronic nephritis Obstruction of the urinary tract Muscle disease	Muscular dystrophy

TABLE 22-2

COMMON BLOOD CHEMISTRY TESTS Continued

Name of Test and Specimen Requirement	Abbreviation	Purpose	Normal Range	Increased with	Decreased with
Globulin (serum)	glob	Used to identify abnormalities in the rate of protein synthesis and removal.	1.0–3.5 g/dl	Brucellosis Chronic infections Rheumatoid arthritis Dehydration Hepatic carcinoma Hodgkin's disease	Agammaglobulinemia Severe burns

Glucose
  Fasting blood sugar
  Two-hour postprandial
  Glucose tolerance test
(serum)
	FBS
	2-hr PPBS
	GTT
		Used to detect disorders of glucose metabolism.	FBS: 70–110 mg/100 ml
			2-hr PPBS: < 140 mg/dl
			
			GTT (mg/100 ml)
			        Normal Diabetic
			FBS 70–110 >120
			30 min 120–170 >200
			1 hr 120–170 >200
			2 hr 100–140 >140
			3 hr <125 >140
				Hyperglycemia
				Diabetes mellitus
				Hepatic disease
				Brain damage
				Cushing's syndrome
					Hypoglycemia
					Excess insulin
					Addison's disease
					Bacterial sepsis
					Carcinoma of the pancreas
					Hepatic necrosis
					Hypothyroidism

Lactic acid dehydrogenase (serum)	LDH LD	Used to assist in confirming a myocardial or pulmonary infarction. Also used in the differential diagnosis of muscular dystrophy and pernicious anemia.	100–225 mU/ml	Acute myocardial infarction Acute leukemia Muscular dystrophy Pernicious anemia Hemolytic anemia Hepatic disease Extensive cancer	
Phosphorus (serum)	P	Assists in the proper evaluation and interpretation of calcium levels. Used to detect disorders of the endocrine system, bone diseases, and kidney dysfunction.	2.5–4.5 mg/dl	**Hyperphosphatemia** Renal insufficiency Severe nephritis Hypoparathyroidism Hypocalcemia Addison's disease	**Hypophosphatemia** Hyperparathyroidism Rickets and osteomalacia Diabetic coma Hyperinsulinism
Potassium (serum)	K	Used to diagnose disorders of acid-base and water balance in the body.	3.5–5.5 mEq/L	**Hyperkalemia** Renal failure Cell damage Acidosis Addison's disease Internal bleeding	**Hypokalemia** Diarrhea Pyloric obstruction Starvation Malabsorption Severe vomiting Severe burns Diuretic administration Chronic stress Liver disease with ascites
Serum glutamic-oxaloacetic transaminase (serum)	SGOT (AST)	Used to detect tissue damage.	0–41 mU/ml	Myocardial infarction Liver disease Acute pancreatitis Acute hemolytic anemia	Beriberi Uncontrolled diabetes mellitus with acidosis
Serum glutamic-pyruvic transaminase (serum)	SGPT (ALT)	Used to detect liver disease.	0–45 mU/ml	Hepatocellular disease Active cirrhosis Metastatic liver tumor Obstructive jaundice Pancreatitis	

Table continued on following page

TABLE 22-2

COMMON BLOOD CHEMISTRY TESTS *Continued*

Name of Test and Specimen Requirement	Abbreviation	Purpose	Normal Range	Increased with	Decreased with
Sodium (serum)	Na	Used to detect changes in water and salt balance in the body.	135–145 mEq/L	**Hypernatremia** Dehydration Conn's syndrome Primary aldosteronism Coma Cushing's disease Diabetes insipidus	**Hyponatremia** Severe burns Severe diarrhea Vomiting Addison's disease Severe nephritis Pyloric obstruction
Free thyroxine T$_4$ (serum)	FT$_4$ T$_4$	Used to assess thyroid functioning and to evaluate thyroid replacement therapy.	1–2.3 mg/dl	Hyperthyroidism Grave's disease Thyrotoxicosis Thyroiditis	Hypothyroidism Cretinism Goiter Myxedema Hypoproteinemia
Total bilirubin (serum)	TBrli	Used to evaluate liver function and to detect hemolytic anemia.	0.1–1.2 mg/dl	Liver disease Obstruction of the common bile or hepatic duct Hemolytic anemia	
Total protein (serum)	TP	Used as a screening test for diseases which alter the protein balance and to assess the state of body hydration.	6.0–8.0 g/dl	Dehydration (vomiting, diarrhea) Chronic infections Acute liver disease Multiple myeloma Lupus erythematosus	Severe hemorrhaging Hodgkin's disease Severe liver disease Malabsorption
Triglycerides (serum)	Trig	Used to evaluate patients with suspected atherosclerosis. (Elevated triglyercides along with elevated cholesterol are risk factors for atherosclerosis.)	40–170 mg/dl	Risk factor for atherosclerosis Liver disease Nephrotic syndrome Hypothyroidism Poorly controlled diabetes Pancreatitis	Malnutrition Congenital lipoproteinemia
Uric acid (serum)	UA	Used to evaluate patients for renal failure, gout, and leukemia.	2.2–9.0 mg/dl	Renal failure Gout Leukemia Severe eclampsia Lymphomas	Patients undergoing treatment with uricosuric drugs

Reproduced from Bonewit K: *Clinical Procedures for Medical Assistants*, 3rd ed. Philadelphia: W. B. Saunders, 1990, pp. 390–392.

TABLE 22-3

ANTICOAGULANTS IN VACUUM COLLECTION TUBES

Color of Tube	Anticoagulant	Action on Blood	Common Tests
Green	Heparin	Inhibits clotting	STAT tests, electrolytes
Light blue	Sodium citrate	Interferes with calcium in clotting	Prothrombin time, partial prothrombin time, coagulation
Lavender	EDTA*	Preserves cell membranes	Hematology, complete blood count, cell counts
Gray	Sodium fluoride	Stops glycolysis	Glucose
Any speckled	(Whatever color applies)	Physically separates red blood cells from plasma or serum	(Whatever color applies)

* Ethylenediaminetetraacetic acid.

- Hemolysis is a problem laboratories commonly encounter. Hemolysis is often caused by poor collection techniques and may result in incorrect laboratory results.
- Lipemia is the buildup of lipids (fats) in the bloodstream. Special care and dilutions must be used in analyzing lipemic specimens. These techniques and calculations are best done by trained laboratory personnel.
- Speckled-top tubes contain a physical barrier to separate RBCs from serum. This prevents any further metabolism of the chemicals. If a speckled-top tube is unavailable, serum should be removed from the cells and placed in a separate tube for storage.
- If the specimen handling requirements are to freeze the serum, it is very important to place the serum in a separate, labeled tube. Freezing RBCs causes them to rupture, which results in a hemolyzed specimen. Hemolysis could interfere with the readings of laboratory test results.
- Refrigeration and freezing of specimens slow the metabolism and deterioration of specimens. Preparing the specimens as soon as possible after collection best preserves the conditions the patient had at the time of collection and give the most accurate results.

Use and Care of Laboratory Equipment

Kit Methods

- Kits are used most for self-monitoring of blood levels by the patient. Kits usually require little maintenance and are simple to use.
- Reagent strips can give a visual color comparison to a chart and need little or no maintenance. Although this method cannot give specific numerical values, it is often enough information for the patient to know whether immediate follow-up care by a physician is required.
- Reagents should be allowed to warm to room temperature before performing testing. Chemical reactions involve heat transfer and may not be able to work to completion if the reagents or specimens are too cold.

Chemistry Analyzers

- Chemistry analyzers vary greatly. Things to consider when purchasing an analyzer are the ease of use, cost, number of tests the analyzer can perform compared with the number of tests the office needs to run, cost of reagents, and any special conditions that the instrument or office may require (for example, humidity control or portable size).
- Most chemistry tests are run using a photometer (light source). Many photometers are calibrated for specific brands of reagents and often are not interchangeable.
- All instrumentation can vary slightly with repeated use and should be calibrated according to the manufacturer's recommendations prior to any testing.

Quality Control

Importance of Controls

Controls should be run with any test to make sure the technique and reagents are good. If controls do not fall within the expected range of results, *no* patient results may be given. The controls run should have similar results to the patient results. This ensures that the reagents work well for all possible levels of the chemical in the blood.

Error Recognition

A control's not falling within the expected range is an indication of either technique error or poor reagents. Some general troubleshooting guidelines are

1. Check the expiration date of the reagents. Never use reagents that have expired.
2. Check that the amounts of specimen and reagent were the proper amounts to be used.
3. Check for instrument problems (for example, burned-out light source or power failure).
4. Recalibrate the instrument.
5. Rerun the tests with controls.

If a problem persists, or if there is still a question of the accuracy of the test, send the specimen to a reference laboratory. (An old saying in laboratories is "when in doubt, send it out.") It is in the patient's best interest to wait a bit longer for an accurate result than to give out an incorrect value.

Accurate Reporting Procedures

- Avoid rewriting laboratory results whenever possible. Transcription errors are the main source of error in laboratories.
- When reporting out numerical values, always report out the units of measure (for example,

15 mg/dl and 5.3IU/l). Different laboratories may use different testing methods, and the units of measure often indicate which method was used.
- Always initial your laboratory results. This confirms that the testing was performed by trained personnel if a question of the result's integrity occurs.
- Always record laboratory results in ink.
- Make sure that decimal points are very clear. When reporting a value less than 1, use the format "0._" so that the decimal is not overlooked, for example, 0.5 mg/dl, not .5 mg/dl)
- Always double-check your results before reporting them to the physician.

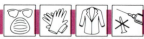

PROCEDURE

MEASURING AND REPORTING GLUCOSE FASTING BLOOD SAMPLE (FBS) LEVEL ON ACCUCHECK II GLUCOSE METER

PURPOSE

To quickly verify abnormalities of carbohydrate metabolism, such as occurs in diabetes mellitus, hypoglycemia, and liver and adrenocortical dysfunction.

EQUIPMENT AND MATERIALS

Accucheck II glucose meter and reagent strips
Lancet
Cotton balls
Alcohol preparation pad
Bandage

PROCEDURAL STEPS

1. Assemble the equipment. Check the expiration date on the container of reagent strips.
   RATIONALE: Outdated reagent strips can cause falsely low test results.
2. Wash the patient's hands thoroughly to remove any interfering substances.
3. Place the glucose meter on a flat surface and turn it on by pressing the ON/OFF button.
4. Ensure that the glucose meter is properly calibrated by viewing the screen. A properly calibrated glucose meter exhibits information as follows: The digits 888 appear on the display screen, followed by a three-digit code that corresponds to the code on the container of test strips currently in use. If the meter is not calibrated, perform this operation as outlined at the end of the procedure.
   RATIONALE: The glucose meter must be calibrated to ensure accurate and reliable test results.
5. Remove a Chemstrip bG reagent strip from the container and place it on a clean, dry surface with the reagent pad facing up. Do not touch the reagent pad with the fingers. Promptly replace the lid of the container.
   RATIONALE: The reagent pads are moisture sensitive and could be affected by environmental moisture or moisture present on the fingers, leading to inaccurate test results. In addition, oil from the skin may clog the reagent coating, interfering with a proper chemical reaction.
6. Identify the patient and explain the procedure. If a fasting blood specimen is required, ask the patient if he or she has had anything to eat or drink for the past 12 hours.
   RATIONALE: Do not begin testing if the patient has not followed the preparations required by the test. Glucose levels change quickly upon eating.
7. Cleanse the puncture site with an alcohol preparation pad and allow it to dry. Apply gloves and perform a capillary puncture.
   RATIONALE: The alcohol must be allowed to evaporate to prevent it from reacting with the chemicals on the reagent pad and leading to inaccurate test results. Gloves are a CDC Universal Precaution that provides a barrier against contaminated blood.
8. Once the puncture has been made, wipe away the first drop of blood with a cotton ball. Place the hand with the palm facing downward, and gently squeeze the finger

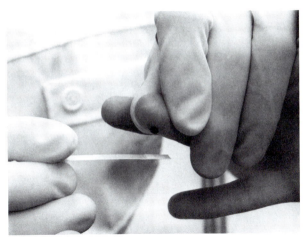

FIGURE 22-15
Procedures for proper collection and performance of the Accu-chek glucose testing. (Reproduced from Bonewit K: *Clinical Procedures for Medical Assistants*, 3rd ed. Philadelphia: W. B. Saunders, 1990.)

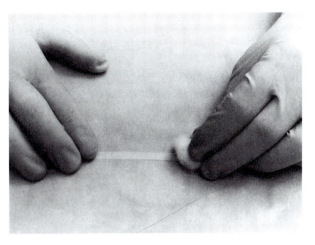

FIGURE 22-16
Removal of all excess blood from reagent strip. (Reproduced from Bonewit K: *Clinical Procedures for Medical Assistants*, 3rd ed. Philadelphia: W. B. Saunders, 1990, p. 398.)

around the puncture site until a large drop of blood forms (Figure 22-15).
RATIONALE: The first drop of blood contains a large amount of serum, which dilutes the specimen and leads to inaccurate test results. A large drop of blood is needed to completely cover the reagent pad.

9. Hold the plastic strip in a horizontal position with the reagent pad facing upward. Bring the test strip to the finger, and allow the reagent pad to contact the drop of blood. Completely cover both test zones of the reagent area with the blood specimen.
RATIONALE: If the reagent pad is not completely covered with blood, test results may be falsely low.

10. Immediately press the TIME button on the glucose meter, until a beep is heard. The timing button activates and monitors a 60-second reaction period. The liquid crystal diode (LCD) screen shows the elapsed seconds. Be sure to maintain the strip in a horizontal position during the timing period to prevent the blood from spilling off the reagent pad.
RATIONALE: The timing period allows the blood to react with the chemicals on the reagent pad, resulting in a blue color.

11. Apply pressure to the patient's finger with a cotton ball to control blood flow.

12. When the screen displays 57, 58, 59, and 60 (seconds), the glucose meter emits three high beeping sounds and one low sound. As soon as the monitor displays 60 and emits the low beep, remove the excess blood from the reagent pad by blotting with a cotton ball and moderate pressure (Figure 22-16).
RATIONALE: All of the excess blood residue must be wiped from the reagent pad.

13. Turn the reagent strip on its side with reagent pad facing the ON/OFF button. Insert the reacted reagent pad into the strip adapter

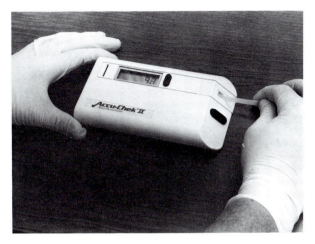

FIGURE 22-17
Proper insertion of reagent strips. (Reproduced from Bonewit K: *Clinical Procedures for Medical Assistants*, 3rd ed. Philadelphia: W. B. Saunders, 1990, p. 398.)

located on the side of the glucose meter (Figure 22-17). The reagent pad must be inserted before the LCD screen displays 120 (seconds).
14. When the display reads 120, a high beep automatically sounds, and the glucose value is displayed in milligrams per deciliter (mg/dl). If the glucose value is higher or lower than expected or if the screen displays something other than the glucose value, refer to the manufacturer's operation manual to correct any problems.
15. Remove the reacted reagent pad from the glucose meter and properly dispose of it in a hazardous waste container.
16. Remove the gloves and wash hands. Record the results. Include the patient's name, the date and time, when the patient last ate (for example, "FBS, 2 hr pp"), and the glucose test result. Also record the last time the patient has taken any hypoglycemic medications (such as insulin).
17. Turn off the instrument and properly store it.

PROCEDURE

CALIBRATING THE ACCUCHEK II GLUCOSE METER

PURPOSE

To determine the accuracy of the glucose meter, by measurement of its variation from a standard, to ascertain necessary correction factors.

EQUIPMENT AND MATERIALS

Accuchek glucose meter
Calibration strip
Chemstrip bG reagent strip

PROCEDURAL STEPS

1. Place the glucose meter on a flat surface.
2. Insert the pointed end of the calibration strip into the calibration compartment located at the left of the display screen.
3. Continue inserting the strip until it touches the flat surface on which it lies (Figure 22-18).
4. Press the ON/OFF button to turn on the glucose meter.
5. The following symbol will appear on the LCD screen: ∣∥∣
6. Pick up the glucose meter and grasp the end of the calibration strip that extends from the back of the calibration compartment.
7. Using a slow and steady motion, pull the calibration strip through the compartment. (Figure 22-19).
8. Proper calibration of the glucose meter results in a beeping sound and a display of the letters CCC on the LCD screen.
9. Position an unused Chemstrip bG reagent strip on its side with the reagent pad facing *away* from the ON/OFF button (Figure 22-20). (The strip is inserted in this position for calibration only.)
10. Insert the reagent strip into the test strip adapter until it reaches the end of the chamber.

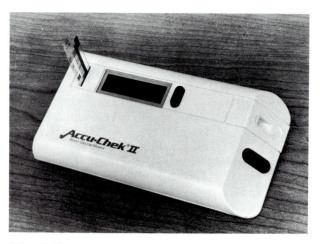

FIGURE 22-18

Insertion of calibration strip. (Reproduced from Bonewit K: *Clinical Procedures for Medical Assistants*, 3rd ed. Philadelphia: W. B. Saunders, 1990, p. 398.)

Chapter 22: HEMATOLOGY AND BLOOD CHEMISTRY

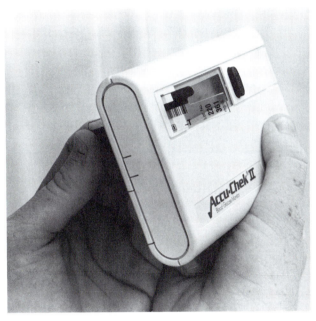

FIGURE 22-19
Pull the calibration strip through the monitor completely. (Reproduced from Bonewit K: *Clinical Procedures for Medical Assistants,* 3rd ed. Philadelphia: W. B. Saunders, 1990, p. 398.)

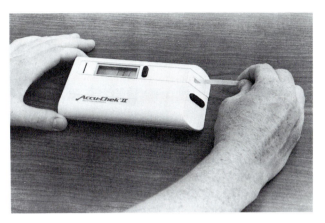

FIGURE 22-20
Proper positioning of the reagent strip for calibration of each lot of reagents. (Reproduced from Bonewit K: *Clinical Procedures for Medical Assistants,* 3rd ed. Philadelphia: W. B. Saunders, 1990, p. 399.)

11. Press the TIME button until a beep is heard. The numbers 888 will appear on the display screen, followed by a three-digit code, which corresponds to the code printed on the label of the Chemstrip vial.
12. Remove the test strip from the test strip adapter and turn off the glucose meter.

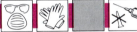 **PROCEDURE**

COLLECTING SPECIMENS FOR A GLUCOSE TOLERANCE TEST

PURPOSE

To measure glucose metabolism.

EQUIPMENT AND MATERIALS

CDC Universal Precautions barriers as necessary
Nonsterile gloves
Blood collection supplies
Sterile gauze pads
Bandages
Needle container for disposal of used needles
Urine specimen collection cups

PROCEDURAL STEPS

1. Prior to testing, the patient should be told to consume a high-carbohydrate diet for 3 days.
   RATIONALE: This saturates the body's glucose needs prior to testing.
2. The patient to then fast for a minimum of 6 hours.
   RATIONALE: This assures that the patient's body will have metabolized all previous meals.

3. Collect a fasting blood specimen and a urine specimen from the patient.

MEDICAL ASSISTING ALERT

If these results are elevated, do not continue the testing and contact the physician immediately.

RATIONALE: It is important to make sure that the patient does not already have an elevated glucose level before giving the patient the high glucose load required for testing.

4. Have the patient consume a known high level (load) of glucose (100 g is the normal adult dose) within 10 minutes. Upon consumption of the glucose, begin timing.
NOTE: No other food or fluids (except water), smoking, or physical activity is allowed during the testing, as any of these factors may also alter metabolism rates.
5. Collect specimens of blood and urine at 30 minutes, 1 hour, 2 hour, and 3 hours. Watch the patient closely for severe adverse effects such as fainting, vomiting, headaches, and excessive sweating.

MEDICAL ASSISTING ALERT

If severe effects are seen, contact the physician immediately.

RATIONALE: Timing of collections is very important. If a specimen is collected too early or late, the peak levels may not be detected.
NOTE: Normal results will show a sharp increase in blood glucose levels at 1/2–1 hour, but blood levels will be near fasting again by 2–3 hours postprandially. Table 22–2 shows a normal glucose tolerance test.
6. Encourage the patient to drink water to help obtain the urine specimens.
7. After the study, encourage the patient to eat and drink normally. Insulin or oral hypoglycemics may be administered, if ordered, after the study.

Testing and Reporting Cholesterol Levels

Cholesterol is a combination of several types of blood lipids (fats). The body needs a certain level of these lipids, but in excessive amounts, they can block the arteries by attaching to the inner arterial walls. The general formula used to show the relationship of all of these lipids is:

$$\text{Cholesterol} = \frac{\text{Triglycerides}}{5} + \text{HDL} + \text{LDL} + \text{VLDL}$$

where HDLs are high-density lipoproteins, LDLs are low-density lipoproteins, and VLDLs are the very-low-density lipoproteins.

A guideline used for the evaluation of overall health is the ratio of cholesterol to HDL. HDLs provide the most efficient storage of lipids in the body.

When the ratio is <5, the patient has low risk of atherosclerosis.
When the ratio is 5–6, the patient's risk factor is twice that of the average person.
When the ratio is 6–7, the patient's risk factor is three times that of the average person.
When the ratio is 7–8, the patient's risk factor is four times that of the average person.
When the ratio is 8–9, the patient's risk factor is five times that of the average person.

Most physicians feel that this ratio is a better indicator in the cases of poor health than just the cholesterol value. A cholesterol value alone may be sufficient when there are few physical factors suggesting an elevated level.

PROCEDURE
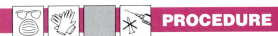

COLLECTING SPECIMENS FOR SERUM LIPID STUDIES

PURPOSE

To aid in the diagnosis of atherosclerotic disease and to help determine the dietary treatment of a patient with atherosclerosis.

EQUIPMENT AND MATERIALS

CDC Universal Precautions barriers as necessary
Nonsterile gloves
Blood collection supplies (including one red-top and one lavender-top Vacutainer tube)
Sterile gauze pads
Bandages
Needle container for disposal of used needles

PROCEDURAL STEPS

1. Prior to testing, the patient should be instructed to take nothing by mouth, except water, for 12 hours before the test.
2. The physician may order the discontinuance of thyroid medications, steroidal contraceptives, and lipid-lowering drugs for at least 3 weeks before the test.
3. Following standard venipuncture procedure, draw two tubes of blood.
4. Apply pressure and a bandage to the puncture site.
5. Observe the site for bleeding
6. Prepare the specimens for transport to the laboratory. Table 22–2 shows normal lipid study values.

References

1. National Committee for Clinical Laboratory Standards: *Procedure for Determining Packed Cell Volume by the Microhematocrit Method; Approved Standard* (NCCLS Document H7-A). Villanova, PA: NCCLS, 1985.
2. Turgeon ML: *Clinical Hematology.* Boston: Little, Brown, 1988.
3. National Committee for Clinical Laboratory Standards: *Procedure for the Erythrocyte Sedimentation Rate (ESR) Test; Approved Standard* (NCCLS Document H2-A). Villanova, PA: NCCLS, 1988.
4. National Committee for Clinical Laboratory Standards: *Reference Procedure for the Erythrocyte Sedimentation Rate (ESR) Test; Approved Standard* (NCCLS Document H2-A). Villanova, PA: NCCLS, 1988.
5. National Committee for Clinical Laboratory Standards. *Leukocyte Differential Counting; Tentative Standard* (NCCLS Document H20-T). Villanova, PA: NCCLS, 1984.
6. Becton Dickinson, Division of Becton-Dickinson and Company. Rutherford, NJ. Product information, Unopette Test 5877, 1974.
7. Miale JB: *Laboratory Medicine Hematology* (6th ed.). St. Louis: C. V. Mosby, 1982.
8. *Product Reference Manual, Coulter Counter Models T_540, T_660, and T_890.* Hialeah, FL: Coulter Electronics, Inc., 1987.
9. National Committee for Clinical Laboratory Standards: *Collection, Transport, and Processing of Blood Specimens for Coagulation Testing and Performance of Coagulation Assays (2nd ed.); Approved Guideline* (NCCLS Document H21-A2). Villanova, PA: NCCLS, 1991, pp. 3–4.
10. *Instruction Manual, MLA Electra 750.* Pleasantville, NY: Medical Laboratory Automation, Inc., 1990.

Bibliography

Bonewit K: *Clinical Procedures for Medical Assistants,* 3rd ed. Philadelphia: W. B. Saunders, 1990.
Brown BA: *Hematology: Principles and Procedures,* 5th ed. Philadelphia: Lea & Febiger, 1988.
Diggs LW, Sturm D, Bell A: *The Morphology of Human Blood Cells,* 5th ed. Abbott Park, IL: Abbott Laboratories, 1985.
Henry JB: *Clinical Diagnosis and Management by Laboratory Methods,* 18th ed. Philadelphia: W. B. Saunders, 1991.
Kinn ME, Derge E: *Medical Assisting: Administrative and Clinical,* 6th ed. Philadelphia: W. B. Saunders, 1988.
Miale JB: *Laboratory Medicine Hematology,* 6th ed. St. Louis: C. V. Mosby, 1982.
Pittiglio DH: *Clinical Hematology and Fundamentals of Hemostasis.* Philadelphia: F. A. Davis, 1987.
Shea MA, Zakus SM: *Fundamentals of Medical Assisting: Administrative and Clinical Theory and Technique.* St. Louis: C. V. Mosby, 1984.
Simmons A: *Hematology: A Combined Theoretical and Technical Approach.* Philadelphia: W. B. Saunders, 1989.
Turgeon ML. *Clinical Hematology.* Boston: Little, Brown, 1988.

Chapter 23

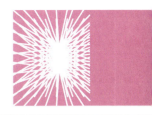

MICROBIOLOGY, SEROLOGY, AND IMMUNOLOGY

LINDA JEFF
MARGARET GIDDENS FRITSMA

MICROBIOLOGY
Special Hints for Equipment and Supplies
Safety in the Work Area
Specimen Collection and Handling
Urine Specimens
Microscopic Procedures
Screening Procedures
Culture Techniques

SEROLOGY
General Guidelines

C-Reactive Protein Tests
Human Immunodeficiency Antibody Tests
Infectious Mononucleosis Antibody Tests
Pregnancy Tests
Rheumatoid Factor Tests
Rapid Plasma Reagin Tests for Syphilis
Rubella Antibody Tests
Streptococcal Antibody Tests

MICROBIOLOGY

The main functions of clinical microbiology laboratories are to isolate microorganisms, which are involved in infections, from specimens; to identify and perform susceptibility tests on potential pathogens; and to provide this information to the physician as soon as possible so that patients can be appropriately treated. Culturing—growing bacteria on solid media—is still the mainstay in clinical microbiology testing. The Gram stain and other rapid tests are used to presumptively identify potential pathogens in or isolated from clinical specimens. Susceptibility testing is usually not performed in physicians' office laboratories. Currently, techniques are available to detect the presence of microorganisms directly in clinical specimens. These methods are much faster than traditional tests, resulting in more rapid and cost-effective treatment of patients.

Special Hints for Equipment and Supplies

Incubator

- The temperature of the incubator should be 35° (±1°) C. Temperature measurements should be taken and recorded daily, using a calibrated thermometer immersed in a tube or flask of water inside the incubator.
- Humidity should be maintained at 70–80%. If the incubator does not have built-in water reservoirs, a pan filled with sterile deionized water should be placed on the shelves to provide moisture through evaporation.
- The temperature and humidity of the incubator should be monitored daily. Figure 23–1 shows an example of a quality-control form that can be used for this purpose.

Month _____ Year _____

INCUBATOR

Unit No. _____

Temperature, Humidity, CO_2 Record

Date	Range 34–36 Temp °C	Range 30%–50% Humidity	H_2O Level*	Range 4%–6% CO_2	Init.	Corrective action
1						
2						
3						
4						
5						
6						
7						
8						
9						
10						
11						
12						
13						
14						
15						
16						
17						
18						
19						
20						
21						
22						
23						
24						
25						
26						
27						
28						
29						
30						
31						

* Water level adequate in humidity pan (fill with sterile deionized water)

FIGURE 23–1
Sample quality control form for incubators. (Reprinted from Howard B, et al: *Clinical and Pathogenic Microbiology*. St. Louis: C. V. Mosby, 1987, p. 36.)

Refrigerators

- Temperatures of refrigerators should likewise be monitored daily and fall within a range of 2–8° C.
- Two separate refrigerators should be available, one in which to store uninoculated media and reagents and the second to hold specimens and media on which bacteria are growing.

MEDICAL ASSISTING ALERT

OSHA regulations prohibit food or drinks in laboratory refrigerators.

Electric Loop Incinerator or Bunsen Burner

- An electric loop incinerator is preferred to a Bunsen burner for the sterilization of microbiology loops because it eliminates the hazards of working with an open flame and prevents the production of aerosols.

MEDICAL ASSISTING ALERT

Do not leave a loop "parked" in the incinerator. The end of the loop will become extremely hot.

Heat Block

- Smears of clinical material may be fixed prior to staining by placing on a 55–65° C heat block for 10 minutes. This method not only fixes the material to the slides, but also kills any bacteria present.
- If a heat block is not available, an electric loop incinerator or Bunsen burner may be used to fix slides; however, bacteria may not be killed.

Inoculating Loops

- Loops made of tungsten or nickel-chromium wire with plastic or metal handles are suitable for streaking out most types of specimens or bacterial colonies onto culture media.
- Plastic disposable loops are also available.
- Platinum loops calibrated to hold 0.01 or 0.001 ml of liquid are used to perform urine colony counts.

Loop Holders

- When not in use, loops should be put in holders, handle ends down, to keep them readily accessible and prevent bending of the wire.
- Loop holders may be purchased or made by drilling holes in wooden blocks.
- Test tubes taped to the wall may be used to hold loops.
- Many of the electric loop incinerators have built-in holders.

Staining Rack

- A staining rack should be used over a laboratory sink or basin to hold slides while they are being stained.
- Racks can be bought or made from two pieces of glass tubing, each slightly longer than the sink. The pieces of tubing are placed parallel to each other and connected at the ends with rubber tubing.

Petri Dish Holders

- Metal or plastic holders should be used to store uninoculated plated media or inoculated plates that are being incubated.
- Holders prevent dropping or knocking over the plates.

Media

- The manufacturer's instructions for storage and handling of media should always be followed. Most media are stored in the dark in sealed plastic bags at 4–8° C.
- The expiration date is put on media by the manufacturer. Media should not be used after this date.
- Upon their arrival and before use, media should be inspected for

  Cracked petri dishes or agar
  Unequal filling of plates
  Hemolysis (sheep blood agar)
  Discoloration
  Freezing
  Excess of bubbles
  Contamination

- If any deficiencies are noticed, the media should not be used and the manufacturer should be notified.
- Samples of each medium used should be inocu-

lated with known organisms to test the medium's ability to support or inhibit growth and to demonstrate growth characteristics or biochemical reactions for which it is intended.
- Most commercially prepared ready-to-use media do not need to be retested by purchasers, provided the media are obtained from commercial sources that employ quality-control criteria recommended by the National Committee for Clinical Laboratory Standards and assure the purchaser that the criteria have been met.
- Some media have to be retested by the user because they display higher than acceptable failure rates on quality-control tests. Such media must be tested in the office or by a reference laboratory before use. Modified Thayer Martin (MTM) medium falls in this category.
- Records should be maintained on all media (Figure 23–2, Table 23–1). (See also Chapter 20, Table 20–5.)

Reagents and Stains

- All reagents and stains bought from a commercial source should be checked upon receipt and before use for:

    Cracked bottles or containers
    Differences in color compared to previous lots
    Cloudiness
    Leaking bottles or containers
    Presence of precipitation

- Reagents and stains should be stored and handled according to the manufacturer's instructions.
- Reagents and stains should be dated upon receipt and when opened. They should not be used after the expiration date.
- Performance checks on reagents and stains should be done when a new lot is received and then each day they are used thereafter.
- Table 23–2 lists organisms that may be used for performance checks on reagents and stains and expected results. A sample quality-control worksheet for use with stains and reagents is shown in Figure 23–3.

Test Kits

- Test kits should be stored according to the manufacturer's instructions.
- Kits should not be used after the indicated expiration date.
- Quality-control checks for test kits should be performed according to the manufacturer's instructions.

I. Identification
   A. Name: D. Date rec'd:
   B. Lot no.:   E. Expir. date:
   C. Source: F. Storage conditions:

II. Appearance of medium
   A. Packaging damage?
   B. Medium color?
           clarity?
           excess moisture or drying?
   C. Visible contamination?
   D. Date checked: By:

III. Performance test
    Test organism   Expected result   Observed result

    Date checked: By:

IV. Corrective action:
V. Final action:

FIGURE 23–2

Quality-control worksheet for media. If medium does not need to be retested, write, "medium has been tested by the manufacturer" under part III. (Reprinted from Howard B, et al: *Clinical and Pathogenic Microbiology.* St. Louis: C. V. Mosby, 1987, p. 39.)

TABLE 23-1

PRIMARY ISOLATION MEDIA

Media	Main Ingredients	Purpose	*Specimen
Sheep blood agar (SBA)	Trypticase soy agar 5% sheep blood	Cultivation of most common pathogens; Visualization of hemolytic reactions	Urine
Eosin methylene blue (EMB)	Peptone Agar Lactose Sucrose Eosin Y Methylene blue	Cultivation of Gram-negative bacilli; differentiation of lactose fermenters from nonfermenters	Urine
Modified Thayer Martin (MTM)	Gonococcus agar base Hemoglobin Isovitalex Vancomycin Colistin Nystatin Trimethoprim lactate	Isolation of *Neisseria gonorrhoeae*; inhibits normal flora	Genital tract
Group A-selective streptococcus agar (ssA)	Trypticase soy agar 5% sheep blood Crystal violet Colistin Trimethoprim-sulfamethoxazole	Isolation of group A streptococci; inhibits normal flora	Throat

* Type of specimen with which each medium is used.

I. Identification
   A. Name: D. Date rec'd:
   B. Lot no.:   E. Expir. date:
   C. Source: F. Storage conditions:

II. Appearance of medium
   A. Packaging damage?
   B. Reagent color?
        clarity?
   C. Visible contamination:
   D. Date checked: By:

III. Performance test
    Test organism   Expected result   Observed result

    Date checked: By:

IV. Corrective action:
V. Final action:

FIGURE 23-3

Quality-control worksheet for reagents. (Reprinted from Howard B, et al: *Clinical and Pathogenic Microbiology.* St. Louis: C. V. Mosby, 1987, p. 60.)

TABLE 23-2

QUALITY CONTROL FOR STAINS AND REAGENTS

Stain/Reagent	Organisms	Expected Results
Gram stain	*Escherichia coli*	Gram-negative bacilli
	Staphylococcus aureus	Gram-positive cocci
3% H_2O_2 (catalase)	*S. aureus*	Positive (bubbles)
	Enterococcus sp.	Negative (no bubbles)
Spot indole reagent	*E. coli*	Positive (red to purple color)
	Proteus mirabilis	Negative (no color change)
Oxidase reagent	*Pseudomonas aeruginosa*	Positive (violet to purple color)
	E. coli	Negative (no color change)

Safety in the Work Area

Prepare and Organize Work Area

1. Disinfect the countertop before beginning work each day.
   - Pour a generous amount of disinfectant in the center of the countertop.
   - With paper towels, wipe the entire area thoroughly.
   - Discard used towels in a biohazard container.
2. Cover the workspace with a large, white, plastic-coated absorbent towel.
3. Organize materials in the work area.
   - Place the electric incinerator or Bunsen burner, loop holder with inoculating loops, and biohazard containers to one side of the paper covering (on the same side as the writing hand).
   - Arrange small utensils and equipment such as slides and pencil in the middle (toward the top edge) of the paper covering.
   - Set up the microscope on the side opposite the writing hand (close to but not on the paper covering).
   - Store other items in a nearby drawer readily accessible to work area.
   - Keep all clinical specimens and perform all tests on the middle area of the paper covering.

Disinfect the Work Area at the End of the Day

1. Discard the paper covering in the biohazard container.
2. Pour disinfectant onto the countertop.
3. Wearing gloves, wipe the area with paper towels.
4. Discard the towels and gloves in a biohazard container.

Avoid Risks of Fires or Burns Due to Incinerators or Bunsen Burners

1. Keep burners and incinerators away from other items on the desk.
2. Avoid reaching across burners or incinerators.
3. Tie back long hair to keep it out of the Bunsen burner flame.
4. Turn off incinerators or burners as soon as possible after use.

Do Not Create Microbial Aerosols

1. Cool incinerated or flamed loops by holding them still in the air for 10–15 seconds.
2. Do not wave loops in the air or plunge hot loops into culture media to cool.
3. Be careful not to spill clinical specimens or drop inoculated media.

Properly Clean Spilled Specimens or Cultures

1. Pour disinfectant over the contaminated area, cover with paper towels, and allow to sit for 15 minutes.
2. Wearing gloves, wipe up the area with paper towels.
3. Add more disinfectant to the area and wipe again.
4. Dispose of towels and gloves in a biohazard container.

Specimen Collection and Handling

An improperly collected specimen may result in failure to isolate the etiologic agent of an infectious process or improper therapy due to the presence of contaminating organisms. (See also Chapter 20, Specimen Collection and Handling.)

General Considerations

1. Collect specimens prior to administering antibiotics.

   - The presence of antibiotics in the specimen may inhibit the growth of pathogenic bacteria.
   - If the patient has already received antibiotics, the name of the medication and the time administered should be noted on the laboratory request form.

2. Give patients complete and clear instructions.

   - Give instructions both orally and in writing using terms that are readily understood.
   - Patients should be allowed to ask questions about collection procedures prior to obtaining specimens.

3. Avoid contamination of specimens.

   - When collecting a throat specimen, avoid touching the swab to the inside of the mouth.
   - The clean-catch midstream method of collecting urine avoids contamination of the specimen by organisms found normally in the urethra and on the external genitalia.

4. Use appropriate collection devices and specimen containers.

   - Only sterile swabs and containers that have been specified for use in the collection of microbiological specimens are recommended.

5. Obtain a sufficient quantity of specimen.

   - 2–3 ml of urine is needed to perform a urine screen and culture.
   - Two swabs should be collected to do a throat screen and culture.
   - Two swabs are preferred when both Gram stain and culture of a genital tract specimen are ordered.

6. Properly label specimen containers (see Chapter 20).

7. Promptly process specimens or handle appropriately (see Chapter 20).

Urine Specimens

Purpose

Urine specimens are collected to

- Perform screening tests for bacteriuria.
- Culture to determine colony counts and isolate and identify bacteria involved in urinary tract infections.

Collection Device

A sterile, wide-mouthed plastic cup with a screw cap is used to collect urine for microbiological tests.

Collection Methods

The clean-catch midstream technique is the method most commonly used to collect urine specimens (see Chapter 21). Urine may also be collected by catheterization or suprapubic aspiration.

Specimen Handling

- Urine is an excellent culture medium, and bacteria present in voided urine multiply rapidly at room temperature.
- Urine specimens should be processed as soon as possible, preferably within 30 minutes, but at least within 2 hours of collection.
- Specimens that cannot be processed within 2 hours should be refrigerated or put in a preservative.

  Bacteria colony counts in refrigerated urine have been shown to remain relatively constant for 24 hours or longer.[1]

  Transport systems containing preservatives are available from various commercial sources. The Vacutainer Brand Urine Collection Kit (Becton-Dickinson and Company) has been found to be equivalent to refrigeration for maintaining constant urine colony counts for at least 24 hours.[2]

TABLE 23-3

GRAM-STAIN MORPHOLOGY OF FREQUENTLY ENCOUNTERED BACTERIA

Organism	Morphology
A. Gram-Positive Cocci	
Streptococcus	Occur in short or long chains, occasionally in pairs
Staphylococcus	Occur in irregular "grapelike" clusters; may appear singly, in pairs, short chains, or tetrads
S. pneumoniae	Diplococcus, lancet-shape, oval; distal ends pointed; usually encapsulated.
B. Gram-Negative Cocci or Coccobacillus	
Neisseria	Diplococcus with adjacent sides flattened giving a "kidney bean" appearance; longer in width than length
Acinetobacter Moraxella	Coccobacillus; may be pleomorphic; appear almost spherical; longer in length than width
C. Gram-Negative Rods	
Enterics E. coli Klebsiella	Occur singly, in pairs, short chains; stain darker at ends; may be pleomorphic; barrel shape
Pseudomonas	Occur singly, in pairs, short chains; rods are straight, more slender, less pleomorphic than enterics; stain evenly
Haemophilus	Small coccobacillus; occur singly, in pairs, short chains; pleomorphic; stain faintly.
D. Gram-Positive Rods	
Clostridium	Fat boxy rod with blunt ends; occur singly, in pairs; may be encapsulated
Bacillus	Large rod; occur singly, pairs, short chains; ends may be rounded
Corynebacterium (Diphtheroids)	Small rod; occur singly, pairs, short chains; pleomorphic, rounded or club-shaped ends; may occur in clumps

Reprinted from Belsey RE, Baer DM, Statland BE, Sewell DL: *The Physician's Office Laboratory*. Oradell, NJ: Practice Management Information Corporation, 1986.

Microscopic Procedures

Gram Stain

Purpose. The Gram stain is used to

- Enable bacteria to be visualized microscopically.
- Categorize bacteria into two groups, Gram-positive and Gram-negative, on the basis of their color after application of the reagents.
- Make presumptive identifications of bacteria based on Gram stain reaction and shape and arrangement of cells (Table 23-3).

Methodology. Performing a Gram stain can be divided into three steps:

1. Preparing smears,
2. Staining smears,
3. Examining Gram-stained smears.

These are described in the following three procedures.

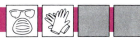 **PROCEDURE**

PREPARING SMEARS FOR GRAM STAINING

PURPOSE

To prepare a smear from a clinical specimen or cultured bacteria to observe microscopically for the presence of pathogens or as preparation for Gram staining.

EQUIPMENT AND MATERIALS

Clinical specimen or bacteria growing on media
Frosted-edge microscopic slides (3″ × 1″)
Pencil
Inoculating loop
Bunsen burner or incinerator
Heat block (optional)
Sterile saline or water (if preparing smear from colonies)
Gloves and protective wear for universal precautions

PROCEDURAL STEPS

1. Use a pencil to label a 3″ × 1″ frosted-edge microscopic slide with the patient's name, accession number, source of specimen, and date.
2. With a wax pencil, draw an oval around the specimen area (approximately 2/3 of the slide).
   RATIONALE: This enables the specimen to be found more easily and acts as well to minimize the amount of stain that needs to be used.

   - If the specimen is liquid,

     Mix the specimen.
     Flame or incinerate the inoculating loop. Let the loop cool by holding it in the air for 10–15 seconds.
     Remove the top of the specimen container. Withdraw a loopful of the specimen.
     Deposit the specimen in the middle of the slide and spread the liquid within the oval.
     Flame or incinerate the loop.
     Replace the top on the specimen container. Discard the specimen in a biohazard container.

   - If the specimen is on a swab,

     Remove the swab from its container, being careful not to touch it to any surfaces.
     Roll the swab on the slide in the oval so that all surfaces of the swab come in contact with the slide (Figure 23–4).
     RATIONALE: Rolling the swab allows white blood cells and bacteria in the specimen to adhere to the slide in layers, making the smear easier to read and interpret.
     Return the swab to its holder and discard in a biohazard container.

 MEDICAL ASSISTING ALERT

Inoculate culture medium first if only one swab is collected for Gram stain and culture. Once the swab has touched the nonsterile slide, it becomes contaminated.

   If colonies of bacteria are used,

     Place a drop of sterile saline or water in the center of the slide.
     Flame or incinerate the inoculating loop. Cool.
     Touch the loop to the center of a single colony of bacteria to obtain a small portion of growth.

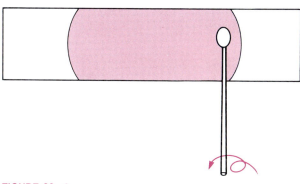

FIGURE 23–4

Preparation of a fixed smear.

Emulsify the bacteria on the loop in the drop of liquid on the slide spreading to fill the oval.

3. Place prepared smear on a slide warmer at 55–65° C for 10 minutes to dry and fix. If a slide warmer is not available, allow slide to air dry. Then, holding slide with forceps, heat-fix by passing it, smear slide away from heat, through the blue flame of a bunsen burner or passing it in front of the opening of an incinerator three or four times.

MEDICAL ASSISTING ALERT

Treat slides as potentially infectious unless they are heat-fixed using a heat block.

4. Let slides cool prior to staining.

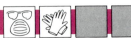 **PROCEDURE**

STAINING SMEARS USING GRAM STAIN METHOD

PURPOSE

To stain bacteria so they can be visualized microscopically and categorized on the basis of their reaction to the stain and their characteristic shape and arrangement.

EQUIPMENT AND MATERIALS

Gram stain reagents
    Crystal violet
    Gram's iodine
    Acetone alcohol
    Safranin

Sink or basin
Rubber tubing or squeeze bottle of water
Staining rack
Forceps
Bibulous paper
Gloves and protective wear for CDC Universal Precautions

PROCEDURAL STEPS

1. Place the slide, specimen side up, on the staining rack over a laboratory sink or basin.
2. Flood the slide with crystal violet and allow it to stand on the slide for 1 minute.
RATIONALE: The crystal violet is the primary stain, staining all bacteria purple.
3. Pick up the slide with forceps, hold it at a 45° angle, and rinse it with a gentle stream of tap water. Flexible rubber tubing may be attached to the faucet to provide a gentle stream or a squirt bottle may be used to apply the water to the slide.
4. Replace the slide on the staining rack. Flood the slide with Gram's iodine and allow it to stand for 1 minute.
RATIONALE: The Gram's iodine functions as a mordant forming a complex with crystal violet. The complex becomes firmly attached to the cell wall of Gram-positive organisms. All bacteria are purple after this step.
5. Rinse the slide as previously described.
6. Holding the slide at a 45° angle, rinse with acetone alcohol just until the fluid dripping from the slide has changed from purple to colorless. This usually takes around 5 seconds. Thicker smears may require more decolorizing.
RATIONALE: The acetone alcohol decolorizes Gram-negative organisms by changing the permeability of their cell walls, allowing the crystal violet–Gram's iodine complex to wash out. Thus, Gram-negative organisms appear clear after this step. Gram-positive organisms are resistant to decolorization and remain purple.

MEDICAL ASSISTING ALERT

Be careful not to overdecolorize (apply too much acetone alcohol) or underdecolorize (apply too little acetone alcohol).

7. Immediately rinse the slide with water, as previously described.
8. Flood the slide with safranin and allow it to stand for 30 seconds.
   RATIONALE: The safranin is the counterstain staining the Gram-negative organisms pink or red so that they can be visualized. The Gram-positive bacteria remain purple.
9. Rinse the slide with water, as previously described.
10. Stand the slide on its end on paper towels and allow it to air dry or gently blot slide with bibulous paper.

 MEDICAL ASSISTING ALERT

Blotting must be done gently to avoid rubbing off the smear with the paper. Clean sheets of bibulous paper must be used to prevent carry over of bacteria from one slide to another.

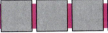 **PROCEDURE**

EXAMINING GRAM-STAINED SMEARS

PURPOSE

To note the staining reaction and morphology of bacteria in order to make preliminary identifications.

EQUIPMENT AND MATERIALS

Stained smear
Bright-field microscope
Oil immersion
Lens paper

PROCEDURAL STEPS

Performance

1. Place a drop of immersion oil on the slide in the center of the oval area.
2. Focus the microscope on the slide using the oil immersion objective with the condenser up and the diaphragm open.

SPECIAL HINT

The microscope can first be focused on the line made with the wax pencil.

3. Observe the color of cells and background material. They should stain pink or red.
   RATIONALE: This assures that the slide was stained correctly. If cells and background material are purple, the slide was not decolorized enough.
4. Examine the slide, observing the Gram reaction and morphology (shape and arrangement) of any bacteria present. Also note the presence of white blood cells, epithelial cells, or yeast.

Interpretation

Gram Reaction of Bacteria

Gram-Positive Organisms. Purple-stained cells.

Gram-Negative Organisms. Pink- to red-stained cells.

Morphology of Bacteria. The main morphologies of bacteria are coccus, bacillus, and spirillum.

Cocci. Cocci are circular or sphere shaped. They are usually arranged in characteristic patterns. The most common patterns are pairs (diplococci), chains (streptococci), or grape-like clusters (staphylococci).

Bacilli. The bacilli are rod-shaped organisms commonly referred to as "rods." They may be long or short, fat or thin, and rounded or pointed at the ends. Some organisms are described as being "coccobacilli," which means their shape is between a coccus and a bacillus.

Spirilla. The spirilla or spiral forms are corkscrew or comma shaped. These are rarely seen in outpatient specimens.

Other Structures

White Blood Cells. Note the presence of white blood cells. An increased number indicates an infection. If bacteria are found within the cells, this should be noted.

Epithelial Cells. Note the presence of epithelial cells. An increased number of epithelial cells usually indicates a contaminated specimen.

Yeast Cells. Report the presence of yeast cells. Indicate whether budding cells or pseudohyphae are present.

Follow-Through

1. Save all Gram-stained smears for review by the physician or a trained laboratory professional.
2. Remove the oil from the slide by blotting gently with lens paper or a Kimwipe (a few drops of xylene may be added). File the slide in a slide box. If slides are not to be kept, discard in a biohazard container containing disinfectant.

Cellophane Tape Preparation

Purpose. The cellophane tape (cellulose tape, Scotch tape, and pinworm) preparation is the most common technique used to detect the presence of *Enterobius vermicularis,* the pinworm.

Clinical Considerations

- Enterobiasis, infection with *E. vermicularis,* is the most common intestinal roundworm infection in the United States.
- Pinworm infection is especially common in children.
- The infection is acquired by ingesting infective eggs, usually by hand-to-mouth transport.
- Symptoms associated with infection may include perianal itching, restlessness, irritability, mild nausea or vomiting, slight irritation to intestinal mucosa, and, in girls, vaginitis.
- At least one-third of all cases are asymptomatic.
- The adult worms live in the cecum but migrate to the perianal region, usually at night, to lay eggs.
- The infection is diagnosed by detecting the characteristic eggs in a Scotch tape preparation of perianal material.

Methodology

Specimen Collection

- Optimally, specimens should be collected in the morning before bathing, urinating, or defecating.
- In young children, it is best to collect specimens early in the morning before they awaken.
- Pinworm collecting kits are available from commercial sources. Alternatively, a collection device may be made using clear cellophane tape (not frosted or opaque), a microscopic slide, and a tongue depressor (Figure 23–5).
- Kits may be sent home with parents for specimen collection from children. The kits should be returned to the office as soon as possible.

Examining the Preparation

- Preparations should be examined as soon as possible after collection

MEDICAL ASSISTING ALERT

In cases of light infections, 3-5 early morning specimens may be necessary to demonstrate the presence of eggs.

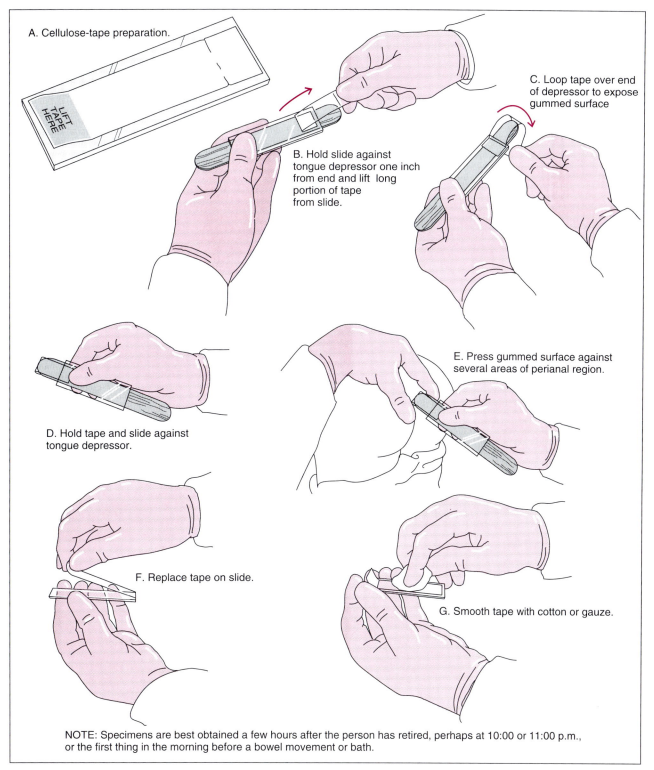

FIGURE 23-5

Collection of a cellulose tape preparation for the diagnosis of pinworm infection. (Reproduced from Melvin DM, Brooke MM: *Laboratory Procedures for the Diagnosis of Intestinal Parasites* (U.S. Department of Health, Education, and Welfare Publication No. (CDC) 82-8282), 3rd ed. Atlanta: Centers for Disease Control, 1982.)

PROCEDURE
EXAMINING A CELLOPHANE TAPE PREPARATION

PURPOSE

To detect the eggs of the pinworm, *E. vermicularis*.

EQUIPMENT AND MATERIALS

Specimen (cellophane tape preparation)
Xylene or toluene in dropper bottle
Gloves and protective wear for CDC Universal Precautions

PROCEDURAL STEPS

Performance

1. Use forceps to peel back the sticky portion of the tape from the microscopic slide. Add 1-2 drops of xylene or toluene to the slide.
   RATIONALE: This clears away fecal material so the eggs are easier to see.
2. Replace the tape on the slide. Use a gauze to press the tape down-removing air bubbles.
3. Examine the entire area under the tape, including the edges, using the low-power objective with the condenser down and the light reduced.
4. Switch to high power if any suspicious objects are seen. If no eggs are found, examine at least 10 fields using the high-power objective.

Interpretation

The eggs of *E. vermicularis* are oval and flattened on one side with a thick colorless shell. They are $50-60\mu$ long $\times$ $20-40\mu$ wide. The inside of the egg may appear granular or may contain a tadpole-like larva form (Figure 23-6).

Follow-Through

5. Let the slide be examined by a trained laboratory professional or the physician.
6. Discard the slide in a biohazard container with disinfectant.

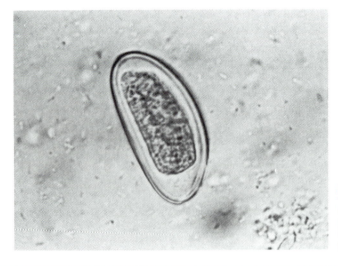

FIGURE 23-6

Egg of *Enterobius vermicularis* as viewed in a cellophane tape preparation. (Reproduced from Howard B, et al: *Clinical and Pathogenic Microbiology*. St. Louis: C. V. Mosby, 1987, p. 659.)

Screening Procedures

Rapid Identification Tests for Group A Beta-Hemolytic Streptococci

Purpose. Laboratory tests that detect the presence of group A beta-hemolytic streptococci directly in throat specimens are used to rapidly confirm a diagnosis of streptococcal pharyngitis.

Clinical Considerations

- *Streptococcus pyogenes,* group A beta-hemolytic *Streptococcus,* is the primary cause of bacterial pharyngitis in the United States.
- Children ages 3–12 are most often infected with the organism.
- Transmission usually results from direct contact with a patient or carrier.
- Typical symptoms of streptococcal pharyngitis ("strept" throat) include

  Fever
  Headache
  Sore throat
  Painful swallowing
  Beefy red pharyngeal tissue and tonsils
  Edema of uvula
  Exudate covering tonsils and throat
  Enlargement of cervical lymph nodes

- Adequate therapy, usually with penicillin, is necessary to

  Decrease the severity of the disease
  Prevent suppurative complications such as peritonsillar abscesses, otitis media, and sinusitis
  Prevent nonsuppurative sequelae of rheumatic fever and acute glomerulonephritis
  Control the spread of the organism to other susceptible persons

- There is an overlap between the clinical symptoms of streptococcal pharyngitis and pharyngitis due to other agents, predominantly viruses. Therefore, reliable laboratory tests are needed to confirm a diagnosis of strept throat.
- The standard method for detecting the presence of group A beta-hemolytic streptococci is the throat culture.
- Many diagnostic test kits are now available for the rapid detection of group A beta-hemolytic streptococci directly from throat swabs.
- Most rapid screening tests may be performed in 10–15 minutes, compared with the 24–48 hours needed for the traditional culture technique. Thus, screening tests may be performed while the patient waits and antimicrobial therapy may be promptly initiated if needed.

Methodology

- Most of the commercially available streptococcus test kits are based on serological detection, using latex agglutination or enzyme immunoassay, of the group A specific carbohydrate (antigen) after it is extracted, by chemicals or enzymes, from the cell wall of the organism.
- In general, enzyme tests are easier to interpret because a positive reaction is indicated by a visible color change.
- Examples of rapid identification kits for group A streptococci include Abbott Testpack Strept A (Abbott Laboratories), Concise Strept A (Hybritech Incorporated), Culturette Brand 10-Minute Group A Strept ID (Marion Scientific), Directigen 1-2-3 Group A Strept Test (Becton Dickinson Microbiology Systems), Tandem Icon Strept A (Hybritech Incorporated) and Ventrescreen Strept A (Ventrex Laboratories). Studies comparing the Abbott Testpack Strept A with culture reported sensitivities (percentage of positive results in patients with streptococcal infection) of 77%,[4] 73.3%,[5] and 90.0%.[6] Specificities (percentage of negative results obtained in patients who do not have streptococcal infection) for the test have been reported as 98%,[4] 94.8%,[5] and 97.4%.[6]

PROCEDURE

SCREENING THROAT SPECIMENS FOR GROUP A STREPTOCOCCI USING THE BBL DIRECTIGEN 1-2-3™ GROUP A STREP TEST[7]

PURPOSE

To rapidly detect group A streptococci in throat swabs.

EQUIPMENT AND MATERIALS

BBL Directigen 1-2-3 Testpack
    Reagent 1 — acetic acid
    Reagent 2 — sodium nitrite
    Reagent 3 — TRIS buffer
    Reagent 4 — anti-strept A
    Reagent 5 — guanidine hydrochloride wash
    DispensTube
    Pipettes
    Reaction discs

Throat specimen
Swabs
Clock or watch
Gloves and protective wear for CDC Universal Precautions

 MEDICAL ASSISTING ALERT

A dry swab or swabs in transport systems containing 1 ml or less of liquid may be used. Do not use calcium alginate swabs or systems containing semisolid transport media. Two swabs should be collected in case a follow-up culture is necessary.

PROCEDURAL STEPS

Performance

1. Add reagent 1 to a DispensTube. Rotate the swab for several seconds to saturate.

 MEDICAL ASSISTING ALERT

All reagents should be brought to room temperature before beginning the assay. All bottles should be held vertically so that all reagents are dispensed as free-falling drops.

2. Add reagent 2 to the same tube.
3. Place the specimen swab in the tube, twirl swab to mix, and then let stand for 2 to 30 minutes. The solution should be yellow.
   RATIONALE: The chemicals in reagents 1 and 2 extract the group A-specific carbohydrate from the cell wall of the bacteria.
4. Add 3 drops of reagent 3 to the same tube. Twirl swab to mix. The solution should turn light pink.
   RATIONALE: Reagent 3 is a buffer that stops the action of the chemicals.
5. Express the liquid from the swab by pressing and rotating the fiber portion against the tube wall. Discard the swab in a biohazard container.
6. Remove a reaction disc from its pouch. Do not remove the purple filter.
7. Dispense 3 drops from the tube into the center of the filter. Allow the specimen to soak through the filter.
   RATIONALE: Any group A carbohydrate (antigen) present in the sample attaches to antibodies to group A streptococci bound to the filter.
8. Add 3 drops of reagent 4. Wait 1 minute.
   RATIONALE: Reagent 4 contains antibodies to group A streptococci attached to an enzyme, alkaline phosphatase. The antibodies attach to any group A carbohydrate (antigen) present on the filter.
9. Add 3 drops of reagent 5 and allow to completely absorb.

10. Add 3 drops of reagent C to the reaction disc. Wait 2 minutes.
RATIONALE: Reagent C is the substrate for the enzyme. Reaction of the enzyme with its substrate will result in the production of a colored product.
11. Wash by filling the reagent D dropper to the white line with the reagent and adding it to the reaction disc. Allow the solution to flow through completely.
RATIONALE: Washing removes any excess substrate.

Interpretation

Pink Triangle of Any Intensity with a Simultaneous Pink Dot in the Center. This indicates that the specimen contains group A streptococci. The background area should be white to light pink.

No Pink Triangle Visible, But a Pink Dot Appears. This indicates the specimen is negative for group A streptococci according to this technique.

Neither a Pink Dot nor a Triangle. This indicates improper addition of reagents or deterioration of reagents. Quality-control procedures should be performed and the patient retested.

SPECIAL HINT

More than one test may be run at a time. Each step must be completed for all reaction discs before proceeding to the next step. The test may also be used to confirm the identification of group A streptococci using colonies on a sheep blood agar plate. One to five suspect colonies should be picked with a sterile swab. The swab is then handled in the same manner as a throat swab.

Follow-Through

13. If the screening test is negative on a patient with symptoms suggestive of streptococcal pharyngitis, a throat culture should be performed.
RATIONALE: The throat screen may not be sensitive enough to pick up small numbers of streptococci that may be present in the specimen.

LIMITATIONS

- The test should be used only with throat swabs or colonies taken directly from a plate.
- The test does not differentiate between a carrier state and true infection.
- Pharyngitis may occasionally be caused by other groups of streptococci that are not detected by this test.

QUALITY CONTROL

- Positive and negative control organisms should be tested with the first run from each new kit and then once each day that the test is run.
- Stock cultures of group A streptococcus and group B streptococcus on sheep blood agar plates should be used as positive and negative controls, respectively. The stock cultures should be less than 72 hours old.

Urine Screening Tests

Purpose. Screening tests are performed on urine specimens to detect the presence of bacteria and/or white cells, either of which might indicate an infection. Screening tests may be requested on

- Patients with symptoms of urinary tract infection (UTI)
- Asymptomatic high-risk patients.

Clinical Considerations

- UTIs are among the most common infections of humans.
- Most UTIs occur in married females with the incidence increasing with age.[8]
- The risk of developing UTI may be higher because of the presence of congenital or acquired structural abnormalities of the urinary tract, conditions such as pregnancy, tumors, or foreign bodies such as indwelling catheters or stones.[9]
- Common etiological agents of UTIs include *Escherichia coli, Proteus mirabilis,* other Enterobacteriaceae, *Enterococcus* sp., and *Staphylococcus saprophyticus.*[8]
- The most common symptomatic UTIs are cystitis, acute urethral syndrome, and pyelonephritis. *Cystitis,* infection of the bladder, is characterized by urgency, frequency, dysuria, and suprapubic discomfort. *Acute urethral syndrome* is the name given to the infection found primarily in young, sexually active females with symptoms of acute dysuria, urgency, and frequency whose urine cultures yield fewer than 10^5 colony-forming units (CFUs)/ml.[10] *Pyelonephritis,* infection of the kidney, is characterized by mild to severe costovertebral tenderness and pain, chills, fever, nausea, and sometimes vomiting.
- Symptomatic UTIs are usually diagnosed by culturing a single organism from the urine specimen, most often in numbers exceeding 10^5 CFUs/ml.[8]
- Asymptomatic UTIs, colony counts $> 10^5$ CFUs/ml obtained on patients without overt symptoms, may also occur.
- Several screening tests have been developed for the rapid detection of bacteriuria and/or pyuria, which might indicate the presence of UTI.
- Specimens that have negative screens may be reported immediately with no additional processing done. This eliminates the cost of culturing negative specimen and reduces the workload of office personnel.
- Most screening tests are reliable for detecting bacteriuria at levels $> 10^5$ CFUs/ml; however, they may fail to identify bacteriuria in a significant number of symptomatic patients with lower numbers of bacteria in their urine.

Methodology

- Screening methods available for the detection of bacteriuria and/or pyuria include chemical, colorimetric, automated, and culture kit methods.
- One of the most commonly used screening tests is the combination nitrite/leukocyte esterase dipstick (Boehringer Mannheim Diagnostics) (see the following procedure).

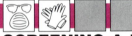

PROCEDURE
SCREENING A URINE SPECIMEN USING A CHEMSTRIP 2 LN STRIP[11]

PURPOSE

To determine the presence of leukocytes and/or nitrite in the urine, which may indicate the presence of white blood cells and/or bacteria that may be associated with an infection.

EQUIPMENT AND MATERIALS

Urine specimen
Chemstrip 2 LN (Boehringer Mannheim Diagnostics)
Stopwatch or timer
Gloves and protective wear for CDC Universal Precautions

PROCEDURAL STEPS

Performance

1. If the specimen has been refrigerated, allow it to warm to room temperature.
2. Gently swirl the specimen in the cup to mix.
3. Remove the top from the urine container. Briefly (no longer than 1 second) dip test strip into urine. Ensure that the chemically impregnated patches on the test strip are totally immersed.
4. Draw the edge of the strip along the rim of the specimen container to remove excess urine.
5. After 30 seconds, hold the strip so that the nitrite patch is aligned with the nitrite color blocks on the vial label.
6. Compare the color on the strip with the color scale printed on the vial label.
   RATIONALE: Nitrite, if present in the specimen, reacts with the aromatic amine 3-hydroxy-1,2,3,4-tetrahydro-7, 8-benzoquinoline on the test strip to give a diazonium salt, which couples with sulfanilamide (on the strip) to yield a red-violet azo dye.
7. After 60–120 seconds, hold the strip so that the leukocyte esterase patch is aligned with the appropriate color blocks on the vial label.
8. Compare the color on the strip with the color scale printed on the vial label.
   RATIONALE: Esterase, present in granulocytic leukocytes, catalyzes the hydrolysis of an indoxylcarbonic acid ester, in the strip, to indoxyl. The indoxyl reacts with the diazonium salt in the strip to produce a purple color.

SPECIAL HINT

For convenience, all values on the strip may be read between 1 and 2 minutes after immersion in urine. Color changes that occur after 2 minutes should be ignored.

Interpretation

Nitrite

No Color Change. Test is negative. Nitrite is not present.

Red-Violet or Pink Color. Test is positive. Nitrite is present.

Leukocyte Esterase

No Color Change. Test is negative. Leukocytes are not present.

Light Purple Color or Trace Result. Situation is borderline. The test should be repeated on a fresh urine sample from the same patient.

Moderate Purple Color (+) or a Dark Purple Color (++). Both are positive and indicate the presence of increasing amounts of clinically significant numbers of leukocytes.

Follow-Through

9. If the strip is negative for both leukocyte esterase and nitrite, the specimen should not be cultured unless the patient is symptomatic or the physician requests that a culture be done.
   RATIONALE: A culture should be done on urine from a symptomatic patient even though the urine screen is negative. The concentration of bacteria in the urine may be $<10^5$ CFUs/ml, which is below the sensitivity of the test.
10. If the strip is positive for leukocyte esterase and/or nitrite, the specimen should be cultured.
    RATIONALE: Positive tests indicate the presence of white blood cells and/or bacteria that reduce nitrate to nitrite, either of which may be indicative of a urinary tract infection. The specimen must be cultured to isolate and identify the etiologic agent.

LIMITATIONS

Leukocyte Esterase Test

- Specimens should not be collected in containers that have been cleaned with strong oxidizing agents. Do not use formaldehyde preservatives.
- The drugs cephalexin and gentamicin have been found to interfere with the test. In addition, nitrofurantoin colors the urine, and this interferes with visual interpretation of the test strip.
- High levels of ascorbic acid or albumin in the urine may result in false-positive tests.[3]
- Most false-negative results occur in the urine when blood cell counts are in the marginal range of 5–10/high-power field.[3]

Nitrite Test

- A large amount of ascorbic acid in the urine decreases the sensitivity of the test.
- False-positive readings may be produced by medication that colors the urine red or which turns red in an acid medium.
- False-positive findings may occur if the specimen has been delayed in transit and overgrown with nitrate reducing bacteria.[3]
- False-negative results are encountered if the organism causing the infection does not reduce nitrates, the patient was on a vegetable-free diet (loss of an important source of nitrate), or the urine was collected too soon after previous voiding (within 4–6 hours), not providing sufficient time for nitrite concentrations to reach the lower chemical sensitivity of the test.[3]

QUALITY CONTROL

- Strips should be stored at temperatures under 30° C. They should not be frozen.
- The vial must be closed immediately after removal of a strip to avoid exposure to moisture. (The stopper contains a drying agent.)
- Strips should not be used after the expiration date indicated on the vial.

Direct Smear for Neisseria gonorrhoeae

Purpose. Gram-stained smears of urethral discharge or endocervical exudate may be performed to diagnose gonorrhea in males or make a presumptive diagnosis in females.

Clinical Considerations

- Gonorrhea is the most commonly reported bacterial infection in the United States, occurring in an estimated 3 million individuals each year.[12]
- The etiological agent of gonorrhea is *N. gonorrhoeae,* the gonococcus, a Gram-negative, kidney-shaped diplococcus.
- The organism is transmitted between individuals by direct, usually sexual, contact.
- Most infections are genital; however, anorectal and pharyngeal infections may occur.
- In males, the most common manifestation of infection is acute urethritis, characterized by rapid onset of dysuria and a purulent urethral discharge.[12] Ascending infection may result in such complications as epididymitis, prostatitis, and periurethral abscesses. Asymptomatic infections may also occur.
- The primary site of infection in females is the endocervix. The infection may be characterized by a purulent vaginal discharge, menstrual irregularity, lower abdominal pain, and dysuria. The infection may ascend resulting in salpingitis, pelvic peritonitis, or both, complications referred to as pelvic inflammatory disease.[12] A majority of women remain asymptomatic or have minimal symptoms.
- Penicillin has historically been used to treat gonococcal infections; however, resistant strains of *N. gonorrhoeae* have been isolated throughout the United States.

Methodology

- A Gram stain is performed on the genital tract specimen, following the previously given guidelines.
- The microscopic examination of the stained smear should be thorough.
- The Gram stain reaction, morphology, and location (intra- or extracellular) of all organisms seen on the slide should be reported. Also, the presence of polymorphonuclear leukocytes should be noted.
- Gram-stained smears of genital tract discharge from patients with acute gonorrhea typically contain groups of Gram-negative, kidney-shaped diplococci located intracellularly within polymorphonuclear neutrophils (Figure 23–7).
- In males, gonorrhea can be diagnosed with approximately 95% sensitivity and close to 100% specificity by microscopic examination of a Gram stain of urethral exudate by trained laboratory personnel.[11] If the direct smear is negative or equivocal, cultures should be done. The direct smear is not sensitive enough to detect infection in asymptomatic men; a culture must be done.
- The sensitivity of endocervical smears in detecting gonorrhea in symptomatic women is only 60%; thus typical Gram stain results are only considered presumptive evidence of infection.[11] Some bacteria found normally in the female genital tract resemble *N. gonorrhoeae* on a Gram-stained smear. In addition, the number of *N. gonorrhoeae* organisms may be too few to

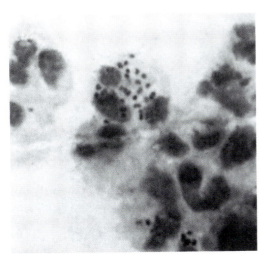

FIGURE 23-7
Gram stain of male urethral exudate showing intracellular Gram-negative diplococci. (Reproduced from Lennette EH (ed): *Manual of Clinical Microbiology,* 4th ed. Washington, DC: American Society for Microbiology, 1985, p. 179.)

be seen on the smear. Cervical cultures should be done on females to confirm or rule out an infection.

Tests for Fecal Occult Blood

Purpose

Tests for fecal occult blood are used as preliminary screening tests to aid in the early detection of colorectal cancer.

Clinical Considerations

- Colorectal cancer is the second most common cause of cancer in the United States, striking approximately 145,000 Americans each year.[12]
- Factors that predispose to colorectal cancer include

  Family history of juvenile polyps, colon cancer, adenoma, or familial polyposis syndromes

  Past history of colon cancer, adenomas, polyps, or female genital or breast cancer

  Associated diseases such as ulcerative colitis, granulomatous colitis, or familial polyposis syndromes.[13]

- Symptoms associated with colorectal cancer are relatively nonspecific but may include changes in normal bowel habits; persistent constipation, diarrhea, or tenesmus; cramping abdominal pain; or symptoms mimicking acute diverticulitis.[14]
- Rectal bleeding, visible or occult, is often associated with colorectal cancer; therefore, tests for fecal occult blood are often used with other techniques to screen for the condition.
- Positive tests for occult blood should be followed up by additional procedures in order to confirm the presence of lesions.

Methodology

- Most of the tests currently used to detect fecal occult blood use the chemical reagent guaiac.
- Hemoccult II (Smith-Kline Diagnostics) is one of the most common methods used for fecal occult blood testing (see the following procedure).
- Other commercially available guaiac-based fecal occult blood tests include ColoScreen (Helena Laboratories), Colo-Rect (Roche Diagnostics), FeCult (Gamma Diagnostics), Hemachek (Miles Laboratories), and Quik-Cult (Laboratory Diagnostics).

PROCEDURE

TESTING FOR FECAL OCCULT BLOOD USING HEMOCCULT II SLIDE TEST[17]

PURPOSE

To detect occult blood in fecal specimens, which may be suggestive of early colorectal cancer.

EQUIPMENT AND MATERIALS

Hemoccult II Patient Collection Kit contains:
    3 Hemoccult II slides
    Applicator sticks
    Mail envelope
    Diet and test instructions
    Developing solution

Gloves and protective wear for CDC Universal Precautions

PROCEDURAL STEPS

Specimen Collection

1. Provide the patient with a collection kit.
2. Instruct the patient to follow the meat-free, high-residue diet outlined on the instruction sheet for 2 days before and during the test period.
   RATIONALE: The diet helps reduce the number of false-positive reactions and provides roughage to uncover silent lesions that may bleed only intermittently.
3. Review with the patient the procedure for collecting and processing three separate fecal specimens.
   RATIONALE: Three specimens are collected because gastrointestinal bleeding tends to be intermittent and false-negative results may be obtained with a single test.
4. Instruct the patient to mail the slides to the office in the provided envelope as soon as possible after the third specimen is collected. Slides may be prepared and stored for up to 14 days at room temperature before developing.

Performance

5. Open the flap in the back of the slide.
6. Apply two drops of hemoccult developer to the guaiac paper directly over each smear.
   RATIONALE: The developer is a stabilized hydrogen peroxide solution. If hemoglobin is present in the specimen, it will catalyze the phenolic oxidation of the guaiac-impregnated paper forming a blue compound.
7. Read results between 30 and 60 seconds.
   RATIONALE: The color reaction may fade after 2–4 minutes.

Interpretation

Any Trace of Blue. Any trace of blue on or at the edge of the smear indicates the test is positive for occult blood.

MEDICAL ASSISTING ALERT

Hemoccult developer may produce a pale blue ring on the test paper. Do not interpret this as a positive reaction.

No Detectable Blue. No blue on or at the edge of the smear indicates the test is negative for occult blood.

LIMITATIONS

- Gastrointestinal bleeding may occur in patients with other conditions such as gastritis, ulcers, gastric cancer, or hiatal hernia.
- False-positive tests may be due to

    Dietary factors such as ingestion of red meat (beef, lamb) or raw fruits and vegetables high in peroxidase, such as horseradish, turnips, melons, and radishes
    Drugs including iron preparations, aspirin,

corticosteroids, indomethacin, anticoagulants, cancer chemotherapeutic drugs, and alcohol in excess[18]

- False-negative tests may be due to

  Neoplasms not bleeding enough to produce positive tests
  Intermittent tumor bleeding
  Irregular distribution of blood in feces
  Ascorbic acid intake of more than 250 mg/day[18]

QUALITY CONTROL

- Apply one drop of Hemoccult developer between the positive and negative "performance monitors." Read results within 10 seconds.
- A blue color will appear in the positive performance monitor, and no blue color will appear in the negative one if the slides and developer are working properly. Neither the intensity nor the shade of the blue from the positive performance monitor should be regarded as an indication of what the blue from a positive fecal specimen should look like.

MEDICAL ASSISTING ALERT

Do not apply developer to performance monitors before interpreting patient test results. Any blue originating from the performance monitors should be ignored in the reading of the patient test results.

- Store test kits at a controlled room temperature (15–30° C) in original packaging. Do not refrigerate. Protect from heat and light.
- Do not use cards or developer after the indicated expiration date.

Culture Techniques

Throat Culture for Group A Beta-Hemolytic Streptococci

Purpose. Throat cultures are performed to isolate and identify group A beta-hemolytic streptococci in order to confirm or rule out a diagnosis of streptococcal pharyngitis. Throat cultures may be ordered on patients who

- Demonstrate symptoms compatible with streptococcal pharyngitis if direct streptococcal tests are negative or not performed
- Have completed treatment for streptococcal pharyngitis to confirm that the organism has been eradicated

Clinical Considerations. See section entitled Rapid Identification Tests for Group A Beta-Hemolytic Streptococci.

Methodology

- Throat cultures remain the gold standard to which new rapid tests for the detection of group A beta-hemolytic streptococci are compared.
- Throat cultures are more sensitive than rapid screening tests; thus, they may detect the presence of small numbers of organisms in specimens that may test negative on screening tests.
- The use of group A streptococcus-selective agar (ssA) (BBL Microbiology Systems) instead of the traditional sheep blood agar has been shown to improve the recovery and rapid identification of group A beta-hemolytic streptococcus (see the following procedure).[19]
- Serological tests are recommended for the confirmation of group A streptococci. Although A disks are still commonly used for the presumptive identification of group A streptococci, an estimated 5–15% of bacitracin (A disk)-sensitive streptococci isolated from clinical specimens belong to groups other than group A.[3] False-negative reactions may also occur.

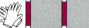 **PROCEDURE**

CULTURING A THROAT SPECIMEN FOR GROUP A STREPTOCOCCUS

PURPOSE

To isolate and identify Group A streptococci from throat specimens

EQUIPMENT AND MATERIALS

Throat swab
ssA (BBL Microbiology Systems)
Inoculating loop
Bunsen burner or incinerator
BioBag environmental chamber, Type C (Marion Scientific) (optional)
Incubator set at 35° C
Gloves and protective wear for CDC Universal Precautions

PROCEDURAL STEPS

Performance

1. Allow the ssA plate to warm to room temperature.
   RATIONALE: The use of cold media may kill the bacteria in the specimen.
2. Using a black marker or wax pencil, label the bottom of the ssA plate (the part with the media) with the patient's name, culture accession number, source of specimen, and date of inoculation. Write small, around the edge of the plate.
3. Inoculate the plate by rolling the swab three or four times over a small area in the upper middle of the plate touching all parts of the swab to the medium (Figure 23–8).
4. Return the swab to the collection holder and discard in a biohazard container.
5. Flame or incinerate inoculating loop and cool by holding it still in the air for 10–15 seconds.
6. Streak the specimen onto the agar plate as follows (Figure 23–8):

   - Starting at the top of the plate, move the loop back and forth through the inoculum, making a series of close but nonoverlapping zigzag lines. The lines should fill approximately half the plate.
   - Turn the plate counterclockwise so that the first streak area is on the left side of the plate. Without flaming the loop, streak the second area of the plate in the same manner overlapping the first only two or three times. Cover approximately half the remaining agar.
   - Turn the plate so that the second streaked area is on the left. Streak the rest of the plate in a similar manner, except spread out the lines more. Again, the streak lines should not overlap the previously streaked area more than two or three times.

   RATIONALE: This technique, known as the "streak-plate" method of isolation, results in the growth of bacteria in isolated or individual colonies. Isolated colonies are necessary to perform identification tests and susceptibility tests when required.

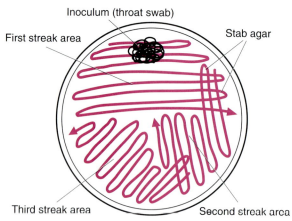

FIGURE 23–8

Streaking pattern for the inoculation of throat specimens. (Modified from Baron EJ, Finegold SM: *Diagnostic Microbiology*, 8th ed. St. Louis: C. V. Mosby, 1990, p. 95.)

> **SPECIAL HINT**
>
> This same pattern of streaking may be used to isolate bacteria that are not isolated on original plates inoculated with clinical specimens. In this situation, however, the loop may be flamed or incinerated between each streaked area to obtain better isolation of colonies.

7. Make several 45°-angle stabs into the medium with the inoculating loop. These should be in the first- and second-streaked areas. Flame or incinerate the loop.
   RATIONALE: The stabs force some of the bacteria below the surface of the agar where relatively anaerobic (lacking oxygen) conditions are present. A small percentage of group A streptococci are only able to produce beta-hemolysis under anaerobic conditions.
8. Incubate the plate in an inverted position (agar side up) at 35° C for 18–24 hours. Alternatively, the plate may be placed in a type C Bio-Bag, which provides a CO_2 environment, prior to incubation. Follow the manufacturer's instructions for using the bag.
   RATIONALE: CO_2 enhances the growth and hemolysis of some strains of group A streptococci.
9. Examine the plate for beta-hemolytic colonies by holding the bottom (medium portion) in front of a light so that the light comes through the underside of the agar. Beta-hemolysis appears as clear zones around colonies because of the complete hemolysis of red blood cells by the organism.

Interpretation

No Beta-Hemolytic Colonies on the Plate. If no beta-hemolytic colonies are seen, reincubate at 35–37° C for an additional 24 hours. If no beta-hemolytic colonies are seen after 48 hours, report the culture "negative for group A beta-hemolytic streptococci."
RATIONALE: A greater yield of group A streptococci may be seen if plates are incubated a total of 48 hours prior to reporting as negative.

Small, Translucent to Opaque, White to Gray Colonies Surrounded by Zones of Beta-Hemolysis. These may be presumptively identified as beta-hemolytic streptococci.

 MEDICAL ASSISTING ALERT

Group B streptococci and occasionally other organisms may grow on the medium.

Follow-Through

10. Serological tests should be performed to confirm that an isolate is group A streptococcus.

   - Commercial kits available for the serological identification of streptococci include Phadebact (Pharmacia Diagnostics), Sero-STAT (Scott Laboratories), Streptex (Wellcome Laboratories), Strept-sec (Organon), and PathoDx (Diagnostic Products Corporation).
   - Many of the rapid screening kits for group A streptococcus may also be used to confirm the identification of isolated colonies (see the Abbott Testpack Strept A procedure).
   - If negative results are obtained when beta-hemolytic colonies are tested by serological methods, the culture should be reported as "negative for group A beta-hemolytic streptococci."

Urine Cultures

Purpose. Urine cultures are performed to

- Confirm or rule out UTIs
- Isolate, semiquantitate, identify, and perform susceptibility tests on etiological agents of UTIs

Urine cultures may be requested on patients who

- Have positive urine screening tests
- Are symptomatic, regardless of the results of screening tests
- Are asymptomatic but at risk of developing UTI
- Have been treated for UTI, to confirm that treatment was effective

Clinical Considerations. See Urine Screening Tests section.

Methodology

Calibrated Loop Method. The conventional and most frequently used technique for isolating and enumerating bacteria from urine specimens is the calibrated loop method (see the following procedure).

- Traditionally, colony counts of $>10^5$ (100,000) CFUs/ml have been associated with UTI, colony counts of $<10^4$ (10,000) CFUs/ml have usually been indicative of urethral or vaginal contamination, and colony counts between 10^4 and 10^5 CFUs/ml have been evaluated on the basis of clinical information.[9]
- Colony counts as low as $10^2 - 10^4$ CFUs/ml have been shown to be significant in certain patient populations:[20]

   Women with acute urethral syndrome
   Infants and children
   Catheterized patients
   Patients who have previously received antibiotic agents
   Patients who consume large amounts of liquid
   Symptomatic patients (usually with pyuria)
   Patients with urinary obstruction
   Patients with pyelonephritis acquired from hematogenous spread

- The physician decides, on the basis of the characteristics of the patient population tested, what size colony count loop to use and what colony count is the cutoff point for performing identification tests and antimicrobial susceptibilities on isolates.

Kits

Several commercial culture kits are available that have been recommended for use in physicians' offices. Kits contain agar-coated slides or paddles, or trays or plates of medium. The device is either dipped in the urine or inoculated with the specimen. After overnight incubation, colonies are counted or growth is compared against pictures provided by the manufacturer to determine approximate colony counts and, in some cases, presumptive identification of isolates.

The advantages of kits are

- They are simple to use.
- They are faster than conventional technique.
- Some show good correlation with the colony count loop method.

The disadvantages of kits are

- There is observer variation in reading results.
- Kits are more expensive than the calibrated loop method.
- They are unable to determine presence of more than one isolate.
- It is difficult to subculture isolates to send to a reference laboratory.

Examples of kits include Bacturcult (Wampole Laboratories), Uricult (Medical Technology Corporation), Clinicult (Smith Kline Diagnostics), Uri-Dip (Scott Laboratories), Dip'N Count (Royal Scientific), and Isocult (Smith Kline Diagnostics).

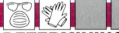

PROCEDURE

DETERMINING URINE COLONY COUNTS USING THE CALIBRATED LOOP METHOD

PURPOSE

To isolate and semiquantitate bacteria present in urine specimens.

EQUIPMENT AND MATERIALS

Urine specimen
Medium
Sheep blood agar plate
Eosin–methylene blue plate

Calibrated loop, 0.001 ml (or 0.01 ml)
Bunsen burner or incinerator
Incubator set at 35° C
Gloves and protective wear for CDC Universal Precautions

PROCEDURAL STEPS

Performance

1. If the specimen has been refrigerated, let it warm to room temperature. Allow the media to warm to room temperature prior to use.
2. Gently mix the urine in the cup or tube.
3. Label the agar plates with the patient's name, culture accession number, specimen source, and date of inoculation.
4. Using a standard 0.001-ml (or 0.01-ml) calibrated platinum loop, inoculate the media with the urine as follows:

   - Hold the heated and cooled loop vertically and immerse just below the surface of the urine specimen to pick up a loopful of urine.
   - Deliver the loopful of urine to the surface of the sheep blood agar plate by making a single streak down the center of the plate (Figure 23–9).
   - Spread the inoculum over the surface of the plate by making a series of streaks at right angles to the original streak (Figure 23–9).

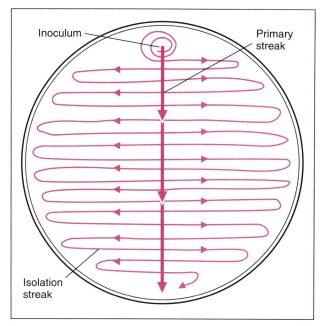

FIGURE 23–9

Method of streaking plates with calibrated loop in order to determine urine colony counts. (Redrawn from Howard B, et al: *Clinical and Pathogenic Microbiology*. St. Louis: C. V. Mosby, 1987, p. 215.)

TABLE 23–4

PRELIMINARY IDENTIFICATION OF COMMON URINE PATHOGENS

Preliminary Identification	Colony Morphology	
	Sheep Blood Agar	*Eosin Methylene Blue*
Escherichia coli	Large, gray, with or without beta-hemolysis	Green to black, metallic sheen
Lactose positive, Gram-negative rod	Large and gray	Pink to purple
Proteus sp.	Flat, gray, swarming (thin film or waves)	Colorless, flat, with or without swarming
Lactose negative, Gram-negative rod	Large and gray	Colorless to slightly pink
Pseudomonas aeruginosa	Flat, feathered edges, rough, gray to green, beta-hemolysis, grapelike odor	Colorless, flat, grapelike odor
Staphylococcus sp.	Medium, white to yellow, opaque, with or without beta-hemolysis	No growth or small colonies
Enterococcus sp. or *Streptococcus* sp.	Small, gray, translucent, shiny; alpha-, beta-, or nonhemolytic	No growth or pinpoint colonies

- Insert the loop into the urine again to obtain a second loopful of urine. Streak the urine onto the surface of the eosin–methylene blue plate in the same manner.
5. Invert plates, put them in a holder, and incubate overnight at 35°C aerobically.

Interpretation

6. Count the number of colonies growing on the sheep blood agar plate and multiply by 1,000 (or 100 if the 0.01-ml loop was used) to determine the number of colonies or CFUs per milliliter of urine.
7. If more than 100 colonies are seen on the plate, report the colony count as >100,000 or 10^5 CFUs/ml.
8. If no growth or only tiny colonies are present on the original plates, the plates should be reincubated for an additional 24 hours. If no growth is present after 48 hours, the culture is reported as "no growth (<1,000 CFUs/ml)" or "no growth (<100 CFUs/ml)."

Follow-Through

9. The presumptive (preliminary) identification of the isolate may be determined by observing its colony morphology on sheep blood agar and eosin–methylene blue (see Table 23–4).
10. The isolate may be sent to a reference laboratory for identification and susceptibility testing, if desired.
11. If two different types of colonies are seen, subculture each one to a fresh sheep blood agar plate, streaking for isolation as previously described. After overnight incubation, send each isolate to a reference laboratory for identification and susceptibility testing, if desired.
12. If more than two types of colonies are present, the culture should be reported as contaminated and no additional testing done unless requested by the physician. A new specimen should be collected, making sure that the patient carefully follows the clean-catch, midstream collection procedure.

Genital Tract Cultures for Neisseria gonorrhoeae

Purpose. Cultures of the genital tract are usually performed to

- Confirm or rule out a diagnosis of gonorrhea in women
- Confirm or rule out gonorrhea in men when direct smears are equivocal
- Detect gonorrhea in contacts of known cases
- Screen asymptomatic females during prenatal examinations
- Follow up patients who have been treated for gonorrhea to ensure that treatment was effective
- Isolate the organism for beta-lactamase and susceptibility testing in patients who do not respond to penicillin therapy.

Clinical Considerations. See Direct Smear for *N. gonorrhoeae* section.

Methodology

- MTM medium is the medium most commonly used for the isolation of *N. gonorrhoeae* from genital tract specimens (see Table 23–1). Moisture and an increased level of CO_2 are required for growth of the organism.
- Specimens received in nonnutritive transport media should be kept at room temperature and processed within 6 hours of collection (see the following procedure).

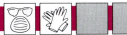

PROCEDURE

CULTURING A GENITAL TRACT SPECIMEN FOR *NEISSERIA GONORRHOEAE*

PURPOSE

To isolate *N. gonorrhoeae* to confirm a diagnosis of gonorrhea or to rule out an infection by failing to isolate the organism.

EQUIPMENT AND MATERIALS

Genital tract specimen
MTM medium
Inoculating loop
Bunsen burner or incinerator
Incubator set at 35° C
BioBag environmental chamber, Type C (Marion Scientific)
Gloves and protective wear for CDC Universal Precautions

PROCEDURAL STEPS

Performance

1. Allow the medium to warm to room temperature.
2. Label the bottom of the plate with the patient's name, laboratory accession number, specimen source, and date of inoculation.
3. Remove the specimen swab from its container. Roll the swab over the surface of the plate in a Z or W pattern. Make sure that all areas of the swab, even the tip, touch the medium.

SPECIAL HINT

The specimen may be inoculated to the medium immediately after collection in the same manner. Take the inoculated plate to the laboratory as soon as possible to complete the procedure. Likewise, the specimen may be inoculated to a nutritive transport system such as a Jembec plate (Figure 23–10).

4. Using a heated and cooled inoculating loop, streak across the inoculum, spreading it over the surface of the plate.
5. Place the plate in a BioBag and activate the CO_2-generating device (follow the manufacturer's directions). If a nutritive transport system is being used, activate the CO_2 according to the manufacturer's instructions.
6. Incubate the plate in the CO_2 environment at 35° C.
7. Examine the plate for colonies exhibiting the typical colonial morphology of *N. gonorrhoeae*.

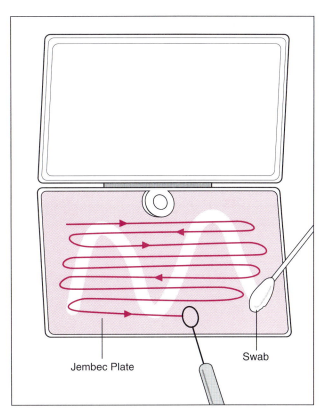

FIGURE 23–10

Method of streaking Jembec plates. The specimen swab is rolled over the plate in a "W" pattern, then the inoculum is streaked over the surface of the agar using an inoculating loop. The same method may be used to streak MTM plates. (Redrawn from Baron EJ, Finegold SM: *Diagnostic Microbiology*, 8th ed. St. Louis: C. V. Mosby, 1990, p. 271.)

MEDICAL ASSISTING ALERT

The growth of most bacteria found normally in the genital tract is inhibited by the antimicrobial agents found in MTM. Occasionally, however, normal flora organisms are resistant to the antimicrobials and grow on the medium.

Interpretation

8. Typical colonies of *N. gonorrhoeae* are small, translucent, grayish, convex, and shiny. Such colonies should be further tested to confirm their identification.
9. If no growth appears after 24 hours, the plate should be reincubated for up to 72 hours. If no colonies are detected after 72 hours, the culture should be reported "negative for *N. gonorrhoeae*."

MEDICAL ASSISTING ALERT

Rarely, strains of *N. gonorrhoeae* are sensitive to the drugs in MTM. If a negative culture is obtained on a patient whose direct smear results were suspicious of gonorrhea, a new specimen should be collected. The specimen should be plated onto chocolate agar, which does not contain antibiotics.

Follow-Through

10. The oxidase test (see the following procedure) should be performed on colonies suggestive of *N. gonorrhoeae*.
    RATIONALE: All *Neisseria* species are oxidase positive.
11. A Gram stain should be performed on any colonies resembling *N. gonorrhoeae*.
    RATIONALE: All *Neisseria* species are Gram-negative diplococci. Other organisms that may occasionally grow on MTM medium may have different Gram reactions and morphologies.
12. Isolates from genital tract specimens that demonstrate the typical colonial morphology on MTM are oxidase positive and appear as Gram-negative diplococci on a colony Gram stain may be reported as "presumptive *N. gonorrhoeae*."
    RATIONALE: Presumptive identification should be made only when the organism is recovered from genital sites, because other species may be more commonly recovered from other sites.
13. Isolates should be sent to a reference laboratory for confirmatory testing and beta-lactamase testing.
    RATIONALE: *Neisseria* species other than *N. gonorrhoeae* may occasionally be recovered from urogenital sites; therefore, confirmatory testing is highly recommended. Because strains of penicillin-resistant *N. gonorrhoeae* are being found in the United States, it is recommended that isolates be tested for the production of beta-lactamase (the enzyme that breaks down penicillin drugs).

PROCEDURE

DETERMINING OXIDASE REACTION USING OXIDASE REAGENT DROPPERS[21]

PURPOSE

To determine the oxidase reaction of an isolate and to aid in the presumptive identification of *N. gonorrhoeae*.

EQUIPMENT AND MATERIALS

Isolate to be tested
Oxidase reagent droppers (Becton Dickinson)
Filter paper (Whatman No. 1 or equivalent)

Plastic disposable petri dish
Applicator stick
Gloves and protective wear for CDC Universal Precautions

PROCEDURAL STEPS

Performance

1. Place a piece of filter paper in the lid of the petri dish.
2. Hold the oxidase dropper upright, pointing the tip away from yourself.
3. Grasp the middle of the dropper with thumb and forefinger and squeeze gently to crush the ampule inside the dropper. Tap bottom on table top a few times.
4. Invert the dropper. Add a few drops of oxidase reagent to the piece of filter paper.
5. Pick several colonies of the isolate to be tested with an applicator stick.
   RATIONALE: Iron-containing inoculating loops cannot be used because iron may give a false-positive reaction.
6. Streak the growth onto the reagent-saturated paper and look for an immediate purple color.
   RATIONALE: Cytochrome oxidase in the presence of atmospheric oxygen oxidizes the phenylenediamine oxidase reagent to form a colored compound, indophenol.

Interpretation

Positive. A violet to purple color appears on the filter paper immediately or within 10–30 seconds.

MEDICAL ASSISTING ALERT

Delayed reactions should be ignored.

Negative. No color change occurs.

MEDICAL ASSISTING ALERT

Viscid colonies may be negative due to poor penetration of the reagent.

Follow-Through

7. Gram-stain all oxidase-positive colonies.
8. If a negative oxidase test is obtained on an isolate whose colonial and microscopic morphologies fit *N. gonorrhoeae*, send the isolate to a reference laboratory for additional testing.

SEROLOGY

Serology tests are used primarily to aid in diagnosis of either infectious or autoimmune diseases. When a patient has an infectious disease, the immune system responds by producing an antibody against the infectious agent. In autoimmune disease, an antibody may be produced that reacts with the patient's own tissue components. In either event, detection and identification of the antibody produced are of diagnostic importance.

Serology tests are laboratory procedures that are based on the interaction of antigen and antibody to produce some type of visible or measurable result. Testing the patient's serum with a known antigen (reagent) can reveal the presence of the corresponding antibody. Conversely, using a known antibody as the reagent allows detection of a particular antigen in the patient's serum.

General Guidelines

- Many reagents are derived from biological sources and should be handled as if capable of transmitting infectious agents.
- Reagents in kits are matched for proper sensitivity and accuracy. Therefore, reagents from different kits must not be interchanged.
- The manufacturer's instructions for the test kit must be strictly followed.
- Follow the procedure in a stepwise manner and add the reagents in the correct order.
- Markedly lipemic, contaminated, or hemolyzed samples may produce false results.
- Store reagents at the appropriate temperature and do not use after the expiration date.
- Bring all reagents and samples to room temperature before testing.

- Exercise care not to contaminate reagents by touching the dropper against slide or fingers.
- When adding reagents with a dropper, hold the dropper high enough to allow a drop to fall freely to ensure that the proper amount is added and avoid contaminating the dropper. Exercise caution to ensure that the drop is free of air bubbles.
- Test positive and negative controls in each test series. It is not necessary to run controls with each individual serum tested, but controls should be performed with every batch of tests. Controls indicate proper performance of the test and appropriate reactivity of reagents. In addition, controls provide a basis for comparison and interpretation of test results. Always read the results of control tests before reading patient test results.
- For slide tests,

    Use a clean slide, free of fingerprints or traces of detergent.

    Mix reactants with a new stirrer for each sample and spread mixture over the entire area of the circle.

    Rotate the slide slowly, using a rotary motion.

    Read reactions within the stated time period. Reaction times longer than those stated may produce false results.

- Technical information regarding the serology tests presented in this chapter is summarized in Table 23–5.

C-Reactive Protein Tests

Purpose

For reasons unknown, C-reactive protein (CRP) forms in the body when inflammation or tissue breakdown occurs. Blood from patients with inflammatory conditions or tissue necrosis gives a positive result with the test. This test is therefore used to diagnose or determine the progress of

TABLE 23–5

SEROLOGY TESTS: QUICK REFERENCE CHART

Test	Specimen/Vacutainer Stopper	Amount Needed	Storage	Positive Test	Quality Control
Latex Agglutination Slide Test for C-reactive protein	Serum/red top	0.1 ml	2–8° C for 72 hours; freeze for longer storage	Agglutination of latex particles	Positive and negative controls with each batch of tests
HIV-1 antibody	Serum or plasma/red or lavender top	1 ml			
Color Slide II Mononucleosis Test	Serum or plasma/red, lavender, or blue top; also fingerstick	0.1 ml	2–8° C for 24 hours; freeze for longer storage	Dark agglutination against a blue-green background	Positive and negative controls with each batch of tests
Tandem ICON II pregnancy test	Urine (first morning specimen preferred)	5 drops	2–8° C for 48 hours; add thimerosal for longer storage	Blue color change in both test and reference zones	Positive and negative controls with each batch of tests
Rheumaton Slide Test for rheumatoid factor	Serum/red top	0.2 ml	2–8° C for 24 hours; freeze for longer storage	Agglutination with undiluted and 1:10 dilution	Positive and negative controls with each batch of tests
Rapid Plasma Reagin Card Test	Serum or plasma/red, lavender, or blue top	0.1 ml	2–8° C for up to 5 days; freeze for longer storage	Clumping of charcoal particles	Nonreactive, reactive and minimally reactive controls with each batch of tests; see text for additional requirements
Rubascan Card Test for rubella	Serum/red top	0.1 ml	2–8° C for 48 hours; freeze for longer storage	Agglutination of latex particles	Nonreactive and low reactive controls with each batch of tests
Streptozyme for streptococcal antibody	Serum or plasma/red or lavender top, fingerstick	0.1 ml	2–8° C for 24 hours; freeze for longer storage	Agglutination of test cells	Positive and negative controls with each batch of tests

such disorders as rheumatoid arthritis, acute rheumatic fever, widespread malignancy, and severe bacterial infections.

Clinical Considerations

- C-reactive protein is an acute-phase protein that is a sensitive and responsive indicator of inflammation and/or necrosis.
- It is normally present in blood and body fluids in very low levels, undetectable by latex agglutination methods.
- In acute inflammatory or necrotic conditions, CRP becomes elevated within 1–2 days of onset.[22]
- CRP levels rise faster than the erythrocyte sedimentation rate in response to inflammation and may be positive before the leukocyte count rises and before culture results can be obtained.[23]
- CRP reaches peak levels within 2–3 days and then subsides to undetectable levels during convalescence.
- The CRP test is not only useful as an indicator of early infection but also helpful in monitoring the course of the disease and its response to treatment.

Types of Tests

- Latex agglutination methods
- Radial immunodiffusion
- Radioimmunoassay
- Capillary precipitation
- Nephelometry
- Fluorescent immunoassay

PROCEDURE

CRP LATEX AGGLUTINATION TEST, GAMMA BIOLOGICALS, INC.[24]

PURPOSE

To detect CRP in the patient's serum by agglutination of latex particles coated with anti-CRP obtained by animal immunization.

 MEDICAL ASSISTING ALERT

Strictly follow the manufacturer's instructions for the test kit in use.

EQUIPMENT AND MATERIALS

CRP Latex Agglutination Test Kit
    CRP latex reagent
    Glycine-saline buffer diluent concentrate
    CRP positive control serum
    CRP negative control serum
    Test slide
Test tubes
Serological pipettes
Applicator sticks
Timer
Light source
Gloves and protective wear for CDC Universal Precautions

PROCEDURAL STEPS

Specimen Collection

No special preparation of the patient is required prior to specimen collection. Blood should be drawn by aseptic technique into a red-stopper tube and the serum separated from the clot as soon as possible. Store the serum at 2–8° C until testing can be performed or freeze the sample if testing cannot be accomplished within 72 hours. Sera that are heavily contaminated or markedly lipemic may give false-positive results. Plasma from anticoagulated blood should not be used for the test because fibrinogen may cause nonspecific aggregation of the latex particles.

Performance

1. Bring all reagents and serum samples to room temperature.

2. Dilute the glycine-saline buffer concentrate 1:20 in distilled water by adding the 10-ml vial to 190 ml of water. Store in refrigerator.
3. Prepare a 1:20 dilution of the patient's serum by adding 0.1 ml of serum to 1.9 ml of working buffer.
4. Place one drop of the diluted serum in one of the circles on the slide.
5. Place one drop each of positive and negative control serum to appropriate sections of the glass slide. (Control sera should not be further diluted.)
6. Mix the vial of CRP latex reagent well to obtain a uniform suspension, expel the contents of the dropper and refill, and add one drop of reagent to each test and control serum.
7. Mix well with separate applicator sticks, spreading the mixture over the entire circle.
8. Tilt and rotate the slide slowly for 2 minutes.
9. Observe for agglutination.

Interpretation

Agglutination. Agglutination of the latex reagent indicates a positive test.

No Agglutination (or Slight Granularity Not Exceeding that Observed in the Negative Control Test). This indicates a negative test.

QUALITY CONTROL

- Positive and negative controls should be run with each batch of tests in order to provide assurance of reagent reactivity and specificity.
- In addition, control tests provide a comparison for interpreting patient results.

Human Immunodeficiency Virus Antibody Tests

Clinical Considerations

- Acquired immune deficiency syndrome (AIDS) is caused by the human immunodeficiency virus (HIV-1), a retrovirus that infects T-helper lymphocytes and other cells and ultimately destroys the immune system.
- HIV-1 is transmitted by infected blood, semen, vaginal fluids, and breast milk.[22]
- Transmission occurs through sexual contact and parenteral exposure to blood (usually through intravenous drug use) and from an infected mother to her fetus or infant.[25]
- Typically, antibody to HIV-1 appears in the blood (seroconversion) about 6–12 weeks after initial infection,[25] although in some cases it takes much longer to appear.
- The mean incubation period from time of infection and appearance of symptoms is 8–11 years.
- Samples that are repeatedly reactive with a screening test, and positive with a confirmatory test, are considered positive for antibody to HIV-1.[25]
- A positive HIV-1 antibody test result indicates that an individual is infected with HIV-1, is considered infected for life, and is potentially infectious to others.[26]
- HIV antibody tests are not usually performed in the physician office setting. Samples to be sent to reference laboratories should be collected using CDC Universal Precautions.

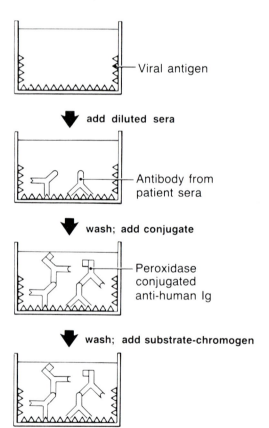

FIGURE 23–11

ELISA test for human immunodeficiency virus antibody. (Reproduced from Hopp JW, Rogers EA: *AIDS and the Allied Health Professions*. Philadelphia: F. A. Davis, 1989, p. 50.)

Types of Tests

Enzyme-linked immunosorbent assays (ELISAs) are currently used as screening tests for HIV-1 infection. Reactive results should be substantiated by specific confirmatory tests, such as the Western Blot or the indirect immunofluorescence assay. A brief description of each test follows.

ELISA Screening Test (Figure 23–11)

1. HIV antigen (either viral lysate or recombinant protein) is attached to a solid phase, such as a bead or the side of a microwell plate.
2. Add the patient's serum, incubate with the antigen, and wash.
   NOTE: If antibody to HIV is present, it will bind to the HIV antigen.
3. Add enzyme-conjugated antihuman globulin and then wash the test system.
   NOTE: The enzyme-labeled antihuman globulin will attach to the HIV antibody bound to the antigen.
4. Addition of enzyme substrate results in a color change proportional to the amount of HIV antibody present in the patient's serum (positive test). If no antibody is present, there is no color change (negative test).

Western Blot Test for HIV-1 Antibody (Figure 23–12)

1. Lyse HIV-1 and separate the protein antigens according to molecular weight by sodium dodecyl sulfate–polyacrilamide gel electrophoresis.
2. By using a blotting technique transfer the separated protein bands to nitrocellulose paper and cut the paper into strips.
3. Add the patient serum to the strips. Each antibody in the serum binds to its protein antigen, resulting in specific bands that can be stained and visualized.
4. The test is considered positive when antibodies to the p24, p31, and gp41 or gp 120/160 proteins are present.[22] Other patterns are classified as indeterminate; the absence of bands constitutes a negative reaction.

Indirect Immunofluorescence Assay

1. Incubate HIV-1 antigen attached to a glass slide or well with the patient's serum, wash the mixture, and stain it with a fluorescent-labeled antihuman globulin.
2. Detection of fluorescence indicates the presence of HIV-1 antibody in the patient's serum.

Infectious Mononucleosis Antibody Tests

Clinical Considerations

- Infectious mononucleosis is an acute infectious disease characterized by fatigue, lymphadenopathy, sore throat, enlarged spleen, fever, headache, and weakness.
- The Epstein-Barr virus (EBV) is the most common cause of infectious mononucleosis, accounting for 90% of the cases.[27]
- EBV is transmitted through oral–pharyngeal secretions and infects B lymphocytes.
- In childhood, most EBV infections are mild or asymptomatic.
- In adolescents and young adults, EBV infections are likely to produce symptoms of infectious mononucleosis.[28]
- Diagnosis of infectious mononucleosis is made on the basis of clinical symptoms and laboratory evidence of disease.

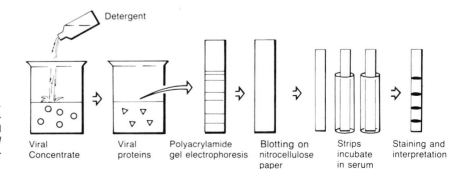

FIGURE 23–12

Western Blot test for human immunodeficiency virus antibody. (Reproduced from Hopp JW, Rogers EA: *AIDS and the Allied Health Professions.* Philadelphia: F. A. Davis, 1989, p. 51.)

- Patients with infectious mononucleosis typically show

    Lymphocytosis
    Atypical lymphocytes
    Slightly abnormal liver function tests
    Positive serological tests for infectious mononucleosis heterophile antibody

- Two types of antibodies are produced by patients with infectious mononucleosis:

    Infectious mononucleosis heterophile antibodies
    Specific EBV antibodies

- The most commonly performed serological tests for infectious mononucleosis detect the infectious mononucleosis heterophile antibody. Performing tests for specific EBV antibody is not usually necessary.
- Infectious mononucleosis heterophile antibodies may become detectable during the first week after appearance of symptoms and usually peak within 2–3 weeks.[29] The antibodies may persist for several months after recovery.
- Antibody titers do not correlate with the severity of the disease,[30] and approximately 5–15% of patients with infectious mononucleosis do not develop infectious mononucleosis heterophile antibodies.[31]

Types of Tests

Methods of testing for infectious mononucleosis heterophile antibodies include hemagglutination slide tests using horse erythrocytes, enzyme immunoassay, agar gel diffusion, immune adherence agglutination, and latex agglutination. Antibodies to EBV are detected using ELISA and indirect fluorescent antibody techniques. An example of an enzyme immunoassay to detect infectious mononucleosis heterophile antibodies follows.

PROCEDURE

TESTING FOR INFECTIOUS MONONUCLEOSIS HETEROPHILE ANTIBODY, COLOR SLIDE II MONONUCLEOSIS TEST, SERADYN, INC.[32]

PURPOSE

To detect the infectious mononucleosis heterophile antibody by differential agglutination of horse erythrocytes.

 MEDICAL ASSISTING ALERT

Strictly follow the manufacturer's instructions for the test kit in use.

Mix all reagents before use by gently swirling.

Reagents and controls contain sodium azide, which may react with lead and copper plumbing to form highly explosive metal azides. If discarded into a sink, flush with a large volume of water to prevent azide buildup.

EQUIPMENT AND MATERIALS

Color Slide II Mononucleosis Test Kit
    Reagent A, guinea pig kidney antigen
    Reagent B, Horse erythrocytes
    Positive control serum
    Negative control serum
    Test cards
    Pipettes
    Bottle droppers
    Optional wooden stirrers
Timer
Light source
Gloves and protective wear for CDC Universal Precautions

Chapter 23: MICROBIOLOGY, SEROLOGY, AND IMMUNOLOGY

PROCEDURAL STEPS

Specimen Collection

No special preparation of the patient is required prior to specimen collection. Either serum (red-stopper tube) or plasma collected into EDTA anticoagulant (lavender-stopper tube), sodium citrate (blue-stopper tube), heparin, or acid citrate dextrose (ACD) may be used for testing. Blood should be drawn by aseptic technique and the serum or plasma removed from the red cells as soon as possible. Avoid using a grossly hemolyzed, turbid, or contaminated sample. The sample should be stored at 2–8° C until testing; if testing cannot be performed within 24 hours of collection, the sample should be frozen.

Fingerstick blood may also be used for testing.

Performance

1. Bring all reagents and samples to room temperature.
2. Determine the number of test circles required (one circle for each patient sample or control to be tested). Tear along test card perforation to remove test circles. Save extra test circles for future testing.
3. Gently shake Reagent A vial (guinea pig kidney antigen) and add one drop to the left side of the test circle on the test card.
4. Invert Reagent B vial (horse erythrocytes) several times to mix. Add one drop of Reagent B to the right side of the test circle.
5. Using a pipette provided, add one drop of the patient or control serum, plasma, or whole blood to Reagent A on the left side of the test circle.
6. Invert the pipette and use the flat end to thoroughly mix Reagent A (clear liquid) and sample (patient or control). Alternatively, the wooden stirrer may be used for mixing.
7. Gradually stir the mixture into Reagent B (reddish-brown liquid) and cover the entire test circle.
8. Rock the card slowly and gently for 1 minute.
9. Observe immediately for agglutination and color change.

Interpretation (Figure 23–13)

Serum/Plasma. Reading with a direct light source is not necessary for test interpretation.

Positive Test. A positive infectious mononucleosis test will show uniform dark agglutination against a blue-green background throughout the test circle.

Negative Test. A negative test will show no agglutination, or a fine granularity, against a brown/tan background. A faint blue-green halo on the periphery of a test circle with no agglutination should be interpreted as negative.

Whole blood. Read with a direct light source.

Positive Test. A positive infectious mononucleosis test is indicated by any agglutination when viewed under a direct light source. NOTE: When using whole blood, the blue-green color background will not be evident.

Negative Test. A negative test will show no agglutination when viewed under a direct light source.

QUALITY CONTROL

- Positive and negative controls should be run with each batch of tests in order to provide assurance of reagent reactivity and specificity.
- In addition, control tests provide a comparison for interpreting patient test results.

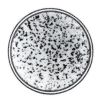
Strong positive result

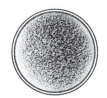
Weak positive result

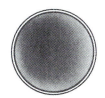
Negative result

FIGURE 23–13

Interpretations of Color Slide II Mononucleosis Test results. (Courtesy of Seradyn, Inc., Indianapolis.)

Pregnancy Tests

Clinical Considerations

- Human chorionic gonadotropin (hCG) is a hormone produced by the placenta about 7–10 days after fertilization.[33]
- In a normal pregnancy, hCG levels increase by 66% every 2 days during the first 6 weeks.[34]
- HCG levels rise rapidly during the first trimester of pregnancy to peak at approximately 100,000 IU/ml, then decline to about 10,000 IU/ml during the second and third trimesters.[33]
- In abnormal pregnancies and ectopic pregnancy, hCG levels are much lower, usually less than 10 IU/ml.
- HCG may also be produced in trophoblastic tumors, hydatidiform mole, chorionic carcinoma, testicular tumors, and some nontrophoblastic tumors.[33] These conditions may produce false-positive results in pregnancy tests.

Types of Tests

Agglutination inhibition tests, both tube and slide, have traditionally been used for routine pregnancy testing, but these are relatively insensitive and subject to false reactions when compared with newer enzyme immunoassay methods. There are many types of kits commercially available that offer ease of performance and interpretation, and a high level of sensitivity. Radioimmunoassay methods are also available, but are not suitable for routine pregnancy testing. An example of an enzyme immunoassay test follows.

PROCEDURE

TANDEM ICON II HCG TEST KIT, HYBRITECH, INC.[35]

PURPOSE

To detect hCG in urine by an enzyme immunoassay method.

MEDICAL ASSISTING ALERT

Strictly follow the manufacturer's instruction for the test kit in use.

Reagents contain sodium azide, which may react with lead and copper plumbing to form highly explosive metal azides. If discarded into a sink, flush with a large volume of water to prevent azide buildup.

EQUIPMENT AND MATERIALS

Tandem ICON II HCG Test Kit
- Test cylinder
- Antibody conjugate (bottle A)
- Substrate reagent (bottle B)
- Wash concentrate (bottle C)
- Transfer pipettes

Positive control urine
Negative control urine
Distilled or deionized water
500-ml plastic squirt bottle or 2.0 ml/repipettor
Gloves and protective wear for CDC Universal Precautions

PROCEDURAL STEPS

Specimen Collection

Any urine specimen is appropriate for hCG testing, but the first morning urine is optimal because it generally contains the highest concentration of hCG. Very turbid urine specimens should be centrifuged prior to use. Specimens containing particulate matter, such as salts that have settled out of solution, should not be shaken or disturbed; samples should be pipetted from the clear supernatant of such specimens.

Urine specimens may be collected in any suitable clean plastic or glass container. If specimens cannot be assayed immediately, they may be stored at 2–8° C for up to 48 hours. For longer storage, thimerosal, an antibacterial preservative, should be added.

Performance

1. Prepare wash solution by mixing sufficient distilled or deionized water with the contents of bottle C (wash concentrate) to make

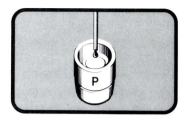

FIGURE 23-14

(Courtesy of Hybritech, Inc., San Diego, CA.)

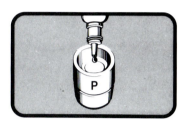

FIGURE 23-15

(Courtesy of Hybritech, Inc., San Diego, CA.)

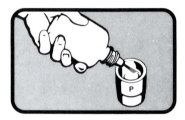

FIGURE 23-16

(Courtesy of Hybritech, Inc., San Diego, CA.)

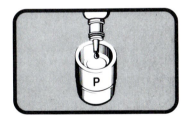

FIGURE 23-17

(Courtesy of Hybritech, Inc., San Diego, CA.)

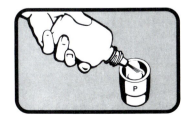

FIGURE 23-18

(Courtesy of Hybritech, Inc., San Diego, CA.)

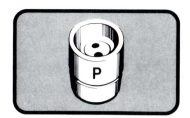

FIGURE 23-19

(Courtesy of Hybritech, Inc., San Diego, CA.)

    500 ml of wash solution. Store at room temperature until expiration of the kit.
2. Dispense 5 drops of urine sample onto the center of the test cylinder membrane (Figure 23-14); dispense sample drop by drop, allowing each drop to absorb into the membrane before adding the next.
3. Dispense 3 drops from bottle A (antibody conjugate) in rapid succession onto the membrane so that the reagent covers the entire surface of the membrane (Figure 23-15). Wait 1 minute.
4. Dispense wash solution by directing the flow toward the inner wall of the test cylinder (Figure 23-16). Fill the cylinder up to the ridged fill line; wait for complete drainage of wash solution (less than 1 minute) before adding the next reagent.
5. Dispense 3 drops from bottle B (substrate reagent) in rapid succession onto the membrane so that reagent covers the entire surface of the membrane (Figure 23-17). Wait 2 minutes.
6. Stop the color development by filling the cylinder up to the fill line with wash solution (Figure 23-18).
7. Facing the indicator mark (P) on the outside of the cylinder, observe the color development at the test zone (center of the membrane) and the positive reference zone (perimeter of the membrane) (Figure 23-19).

Interpretation (Figure 23-20)

Positive Result. There is blue color development in the center test zone (circular blue spot) and blue color development in the peripheral positive reference zone.

Positive Result Approximating or Greater than 50 mIU of hCG/ml. Color development in the center test zone is comparable to or darker than the color development in the positive reference zone.

Positive Result Less than 50 mIU of hCG/ml. Color development in the center test zone is

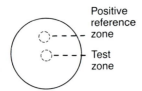

FIGURE 23-20

Interpretation of Tandem ICON II human chorionic gonadotropin results. (Courtesy of Hybritech, Inc., San Diego, CA.)

lighter than the color development in the positive reference zone.

Negative Result. There is no color development (no circular blue spot) in the center test zone, but blue color development in the outside positive reference zone.

Invalid Test

No Color Development at the Positive Reference Zone. This indicates that the reagents were not added correctly or were not performing properly. Repeat the test using a new cylinder.

Light Blue Color Development over the Entire Surface of the Membrane. This indicates inadequate washing. Repeat the test using a new cylinder.

Random Blue Specks on the Membrane. This should not be interpreted as a positive test.

QUALITY CONTROL

- Positive and negative urine specimens should be tested according to the above procedure prior to testing the patient's sample.
- The positive reference zone serves as an internal assay control, because it turns blue only if the reagents are added correctly and are performing properly.

Rheumatoid Factor Tests

Clinical Considerations

- Rheumatoid factor tests are used primarily for the diagnosis of rheumatoid arthritis, an autoimmune disease characterized by inflammation of the joints and destruction of joint tissue, producing joint deformity.
- The disease occurs most frequently in women ages 20–40.[30]
- Rheumatoid factor is a group of autoantibodies that react with the patient's own immunoglobulin (IgG, as well as IgG from animal sources.
- Rheumatoid factor is found in the serum of 75–85% or more of patients with rheumatoid arthritis, but it may also be present at lower

levels in other diseases, such as tuberculosis, bacterial endocarditis, hepatitis, systemic lupus erythematosus, and collagen diseases.

Types of Tests

Many screening test kits are available commercially to detect rheumatoid factor. Most are slide agglutination tests, which use either latex particles or sheep red cells coated with IgG to detect anti-IgG (rheumatoid factor) in the patient's serum. Other tests recently developed include ELISA, radioimmunoassay, solid-phase fluorescent immunoassay, and nephelometric and turbidometric assays.[36] An example of a hemagglutination slide test follows.

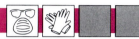

PROCEDURE

TESTING FOR RHEUMATOID FACTOR, RHEUMATON SLIDE TEST, WAMPOLE LABORATORIES[37]*

PURPOSE

To detect rheumatoid factor by agglutination of sheep red cells sensitized with rabbit IgG

 MEDICAL ASSISTING ALERT

Strictly follow the manufacturer's instructions for the test kit in use.

EQUIPMENT AND MATERIALS

Rheumaton Slide Test Kit
    Rheumaton reagent—stabilized sheep red cells sensitized with rabbit IgG
    Positive reaction reference control serum
    Negative reaction reference control serum
    Calibrated capillary tubes with rubber bulbs
    Glass slide
    Disposable card slides
Disposable stirrers
Distilled water or isotonic saline (0.85% sodium chloride)
Timer
Gloves and protective wear for CDC Universal Precautions

PROCEDURAL STEPS

Specimen Collection

No specimen preparation of the patient is required prior to specimen collection. Fresh serum should be used for testing, collected in a red-stopper tube by an aseptic technique and removed from the red cells as soon as possible. If serum cannot be tested within 24 hours of collection, it should be stored frozen.

Performance

1. Bring all reagents and serum samples to room temperature.
2. Fill capillary tube to the mark with the patient's serum and expel the contents into the center of a section of the glass or card slide.
To use the calibrated capillary tube,

- Insert the capillary tube into the bulb far enough to penetrate the thin membrane within bulb.
- Fill the capillary tube to the line with the patient's serum.
- Place finger over the hole in the top of the bulb to stop the capillary action.
- With the finger covering the hole in the bulb, squeeze the bulb to release contents onto the slide.

*Reprinted with permission of Wampole Laboratories Division, Carter-Wallace, Inc., Cranbury, NJ 08512.

3. Place 1 drop of positive reaction reference control serum in the center of another area of the slide.
4. In another section of the slide, place 1 drop of negative reaction reference control serum.
5. Add 1 drop of Rheumaton reagent to each of the patient's serum and control drops.
6. Mix with a disposable stirrer, spreading over the entire section. Use a clean disposable stirrer for each mixture.
7. If card is used, rock it gently with rotary motion for 30 seconds, leave it undisturbed for 90 seconds, and then observe for agglutination immediately afterward.
8. If glass slide is used, rock it gently with rotary motion for 2 minutes and observe immediately for agglutination.
9. If agglutination is observed, dilute the patient's serum 1:10 volumes with distilled water or isotonic saline and repeat the test.

Interpretation

Positive. Agglutination of the undiluted serum and the 1:10 dilution of serum indicates a positive test.

Low Titer. Absence of agglutination of the diluted serum following a positive test with the undiluted specimen indicates a very low titer of rheumatoid factor, such as may exist in a variety of diseases other than rheumatoid arthritis, including lupus erythematosus; endocarditis; tuberculosis; syphilis; sarcoid cancer; viral infections; and diseases affecting the liver, lung, or kidney.

False Positive. High titer heterophile sheep red cell agglutinins found in infectious mononucleosis may also cause agglutination of the Rheumaton reagent by the undiluted serum.

Negative. Absence of agglutination in the undiluted serum indicates a negative test result.

QUALITY CONTROL

- Positive and negative controls should be run with each batch of tests to ensure reagent reactivity and specificity.
- In addition, control tests provide a comparison for interpreting patient test results.

Rapid Plasma Reagin Tests for Syphilis

Clinical Considerations

- Syphilis is a chronic systemic infection caused by the spirochete *Treponema pallidum.*
- Syphilis is transmitted primarily through sexual contact of infectious lesions with skin or mucous membranes.
- The disease may also be transmitted from the infected mother to the developing fetus (congenital syphilis).
- Two types of antibodies are produced by persons who have syphilis:

  A specific antibody against *T. pallidum,* found only in patients with syphilis

  A nonspecific antibody-like substance called *reagin,* which is found in most patients with syphilis but may also be seen in many other diseases.

Types of Tests

- Screening tests, which detect the nonspecific reagin antibody

  Rapid plasma reagin (RPR) card test
  Venereal Disease Research Laboratory (VDRL) test

- Confirmatory tests, which detect a specific anti-*Treponema* antibody

  Fluorescent treponemal antibody absorption (FTA-ABS) test
  T. pallidum hemagglutination (TPHA) test

The screening tests are sensitive, economical, and relatively easy to perform. However, biological false-positive reactions may be seen in diseases such as infectious mononucleosis, viral pneumonia, leprosy, malaria, lupus erythematosus, and many others. Therefore, it is advisable that a positive screening test be verified by a confirmatory test for specific antibodies to *T. pallidum* (the FTA-ABS or the TPHA) in cases where the diagnosis of syphilis is not supported by clinical and/or epidemiological evidence.[38]

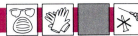

PROCEDURE

MICROSCAN IMMUNOSCAN RPR CARD TEST, MICROSCAN, TRAVENOL LABORATORIES, INC.[39]

PURPOSE

To screen for syphilis by detection of a nonspecific antibody, reagin.

MEDICAL ASSISTING ALERT

Strictly follow the manufacturer's instructions for the test in use.

The controls contain sodium azide, which may react with lead and copper plumbing to form highly explosive metal azides. If discarded into a sink, flush with a large volume of water to prevent azide buildup.

EQUIPMENT AND MATERIALS

MicroScan ImmunoSCAN RPR Card Test Kit
    RPR Card Test antigen suspension
    Antigen-dispensing vial
    Antigen-dispensing needle (20-gauge needle without bevel)
    RPR Card Test controls — reactive, moderate – minimally reactive, nonreactive
    RPR test cards

Dispensing-spreading pipettes
Mechanical rotator set to 100 revolutions per minute
Humidifying cover
Saline, 0.85 – 0.9%
Normal human serum
1-ml syringe (for needle calibration)
Timer
Gloves and protective wear for CDC Universal Precautions

PROCEDURAL STEPS

Specimen Collection

No special preparation of the patient is required. Either fresh serum or plasma collected in EDTA, CPDA-1, or sodium citrate (red-, lavender-, or blue-stopper tube) may be used for testing. Collect sample by aseptic technique and centrifuge to separate serum or plasma. Sample should be tested within 48 hours. If serum cannot be tested within 48 hours of collection, it may be stored at 2 – 8° C for up to 5 days or stored frozen.

Performance

1. Allow antigen to come to room temperature (23 – 29° C). Use of refrigerator temperature antigen may result in decreased sensitivity.
2. Squeeze the disposable dispensing-spreading pipette and draw the test serum into the pipette.
3. Hold the pipette vertically and squeeze to deliver a free-falling drop (0.05 ml) of the test serum or plasma to a circle on the test card. Do not touch the card surface.
4. With the sealed end of the same pipette, spread the specimen to fill the entire surface of the circle.
5. Add nonreactive, reactive, and moderate – minimally reactive control serums in the same manner.
6. Gently shake the antigen dispensing vial sufficiently to give a smooth suspension. Holding the vial in a vertical position, dispense several drops into the cap of the dispensing vial to clear the needle of air. Dispense a free-falling drop of antigen into each of the spread specimens on the test card. Do not touch the needle to serum or plasma. Do not stir the mixture as this is accomplished during the rotation.
7. Rotate card for 8 minutes at 100 rpm on a mechanical rotator. Use humidifying cover with wet sponge to keep card moist during rotation.
8. Read macroscopically under a direct light source. Briefly rotate the card manually to differentiate reactive from nonreactive specimens.

Interpretation

Reactive. Black clumping of charcoal particles, ranging from slight (minimal to moderate) to intense, is reported as reactive.

Nonreactive. Gray homogeneous suspension, no clumping or very slight roughness, is nonreactive.

QUALITY CONTROL

- Calibration of delivery needles

  The calibration of the antigen-delivery needle is important to ensure the proper amount of antigen is added to the test. The needle should deliver 1/60 ml and should be checked daily before use.

  Place the needle on a 1-ml syringe (or pipette).
  Fill the syringe with the antigen suspension.
  Holding the syringe in a vertical position, count the number of drops delivered in the first 0.5 ml. There should be 30 ± 1 drops per 0.5 ml.
  If the needle does not meet this specification, a new needle should be used.

- Rotator

  The rotation speed should be 100 rpm (acceptable range is 95–110 rpm) and should circumscribe a 3/4-inch diameter circle.
  Check the speed of rotation by turning on the rotator, holding a pen next to the rotating platform, and counting the number of times the platform taps the pen during 1 minute.

- Temperature

  The test should be performed at 23–29° C. The RPR antigen and test serum should be at room temperature before testing.

- Controls (Figure 23–21)

  Reactive, moderate–minimally reactive, and nonreactive controls should be run prior to each test series to determine sensitivity of the antigen to ensure proper test performance.
  Expected reactivities are:

  Reactive: Distinct flocculation of the charcoal particles
  Moderate–minimally reactive: Slight but definite flocculation
  Nonreactive: A gray, homogeneous suspension or only slight roughness

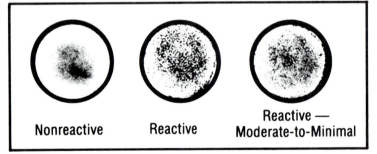

FIGURE 23–21

Expected results of rapid plasma reagin controls. (Courtesy of Baxter Diagnostics, Inc., MicroScan, Sacramento, CA.)

Rubella Antibody Tests

Clinical Considerations

- Rubella, or German measles, is caused by the rubella virus and is generally a mild, self-limiting disease in children and susceptible adults.
- Symptoms, when present, include low fever and rash occurring 10–21 days after initial infection and lasting 3–5 days.[40]
- Although acquired rubella is quite benign, rubella infection during pregnancy can have a profound effect on the developing fetus.
- Congenital rubella can produce stillbirth, mental retardation, cardiovascular defects, cataracts and ocular defects, deafness, enlarged liver and spleen, bone lesions, and other organ defects.
- The earlier in the gestational cycle that maternal infection occurs, the greater the risk of birth defects to the infant.

- In acquired rubella, IgM antibody is detectable a few days after symptoms appear, peaks within 10 days, then gradually diminishes within 4–5 weeks.[40]
- IgG antibodies also appear and persist throughout life.
- Testing for rubella antibody is performed to either determine a patient's immune status (and the need for vaccination) or to diagnose a recent acute rubella infection.
- A single specimen can be used to determine immune status. The presence of any detectable antibody is considered evidence of previous exposure to rubella, and subsequent immunity.
- Diagnosis of active infection following recent exposure to rubella may be accomplished by demonstrating seroconversion, by a fourfold or greater rise in titer with paired specimens, or by testing specifically for IgM antibody.

Types of Tests

The standard reference test to measure total antibody to rubella has been the hemagglutination inhibition test, although newer procedures are widely available. Enzyme immunoassay measures total antibody or can be used to distinguish IgM and IgG antibodies. Latex agglutination methods are fast and easy to perform, and provide both a qualitative and quantitative method of testing.[41] Other methods of testing include fluorescent immunoassay, complement fixation, radioimmunoassay, and passive hemagglutination. An example of a latex agglutination test follows.

PROCEDURE

RUBASCAN CARD TEST, BECTON DICKINSON COMPANY[42]

PURPOSE

To detect rubella antibodies in the patient's serum by agglutination of latex particles sensitized with solubilized rubella virus antigens from disrupted virions.

MEDICAL ASSISTING ALERT

Strictly follow the manufacturer's instructions for the test kit in use.

Reagents contain sodium azide, which may react with lead and copper plumbing to form highly explosive metal azides. If discarded into a sink, flush with a large volume of water to prevent azide buildup.

EQUIPMENT AND MATERIALS

Rubascan Card Test Kit
    Reagent A, Rubascan latex antigen
    Nonreactive control
    High reactive control (for use with quantitative procedure only)
    Low reactive control
    Reagent B, Card dilution buffer
    Test cards
    Plastic stirrers
    Dispensing needle, 21 gauge

Mechanical rotator set to 100 rpm
Humidifying cover
High-intensity incandescent lamp
Micropipettors, 100 and 25 μl delivery
Pipette tips
Gloves and protective wear for CDC Universal Precautions

PROCEDURAL STEPS

Specimen Collection

The manner of specimen collection varies with the testing objectives. Single specimens are required for qualitative antibody level determinations. In suspected clinical infections or exposure, two specimens for quantitative testing should be obtained. The first should be collected within 3 days of the onset of rash or at the time of exposure and tested upon arrival at the laboratory. This specimen should be stored frozen until the second specimen is collected 7–21 days after the onset of the rash or at least 30 days after exposure if no clinical symptoms occur. Both specimens should then be tested simultaneously for antibodies to rubella.

No special preparation of the patient is required. Blood should be drawn by aseptic technique into a red-stopper tube and the serum separated from the clot as soon as possible. Serum may be stored up to 48 hours at 2–8° C. Specimens should be frozen if longer storage is required. The serum should not be heat inactivated. The presence of particulate matter, lipemia, or hemolysis could affect the test.

Performance

Undiluted Specimens

1. Remove the cap from Reagent A and attach the green hub needle to the tapered fitting.
2. Label the card to identify the low reactive and nonreactive controls and all samples to be tested.
3. With a micropipettor, place 25 μl of low reactive control onto the appropriate circle.
4. With the same micropipettor, and a new tip each time, repeat the procedure in step 3, using the nonreactive control and each sample being tested.
5. Using a new plastic stirrer for each circle, spread the serum to fill the entire circle.
6. Hold the bottle cap over the tip of the needle and gently invert the dispensing bottle several times to thoroughly mix the Reagent A.
7. Hold the bottle in a vertical position and dispense several drops of Reagent A into the bottle cap to clear the needle of air. Dispense one free-falling drop of Reagent A (approximately 15 μl) onto each circle containing the serum. Do not touch the needle to the serum. Recover the predropped Reagent A from the bottle cap.
8. Place the card on a rotator and rotate for 8 minutes at 100 rpm under a moistened humidifying cover.
9. Immediately following the mechanical rotation, read the card macroscopically in the wet state under a high-intensity incandescent lamp. Gently tilt the card (three or four back-and-forth motions) to help differentiate weak agglutination from no agglutination. Fluorescent lighting is generally insufficient to distinguish minimally reactive results. Do not use magnification in reading test results.

1:10 Specimen Dilutions

NOTE: This procedure approximates the sensitivity level obtained with hemagglutination inhibition methods and may be used if desired instead of testing undiluted serum.

1. Remove the cap from the Reagent A and attach the needle to the tapered fitting.
2. Label the cards to identify the low reactive and nonreactive controls and each sample being tested.
3. With a micropipettor, add 100 μl of Reagent B to the appropriate squares for each control and sample being tested.
4. With a micropipettor, add 25 μl of Reagent B to the appropriate circles for each control and sample being tested.
5. Using the same micropipettor and a new tip, place 25 μl of low reactive control directly into the buffer in the appropriate square and mix the serum and buffer by drawing up and down with the micropipettor 12 times, avoiding the formation of bubbles. This serum represents a 1:5 dilution.
6. Using the same micropipettor and tip, transfer 25 μl of the 1:5 dilution from the square and place directly into the buffer in the correspondingly numbered circle. Mix by drawing up and down with the micropipettor six times. Withdraw 25 μl from the circle and discard. The serum in the circle is now a 1:10 dilution.
7. Repeat steps 5 and 6 for the nonreactive control and for each sample being tested.
8. Proceed with steps 5–9 for undiluted specimens.

Interpretation

Positive Result. Agglutination of the latex particles is a positive test.

Negative Result. No agglutination of the latex particles is a negative test.

Note: In the evaluation of immune status, the presence of any antibody (either in the undiluted serum or the 1:10 dilution) is an indication of immunity and protection against subsequent infection.

A quantitative procedure is also available with the Rubascan kit to determine a four-fold rise in titer between acute and convalescent specimens as an indication of recent exposure to rubella. Consult the manufacturer's directions for use.

QUALITY CONTROL

- The nonreactive, low reactive, and high reactive (quantitative procedure only) should be run with each test series to provide assurance of reagent reactivity and specificity.
- In addition, control tests provide a comparison for interpreting patient test results.

Streptococcal Antibody Tests

Clinical Considerations

- Group A streptococci are a major cause of acute upper respiratory infections, such as tonsillitis, scarlet fever, pharyngitis, and skin infections (pyoderma, impetigo, and cellulitis). Acute strept throat infections may be diagnosed either by detection of streptococcal antigen from a throat swab or by culture.
- Rheumatic fever and glomerulonephritis are late complications of acute infection.
- These poststreptococcal inflammatory diseases may occur 2–3 weeks after the initial infection and are believed to represent a cross-reactive autoimmune response to group A streptococci.[40]
- In most cases, the organism is undetectable by culture by the time the patient becomes symptomatic.[29] However, antibodies against extracellular antigens of group A streptococcus may be elevated in 7–10 days after the initial infection. Serological tests to detect these antibodies are useful in the diagnosis of rheumatic fever and glomerulonephritis.

Types of Tests

There are many serological tests designed to measure various antibodies to extracellular antigens. The most widely used is the antistreptolysin O titer. Screening tests are available that use particles (latex, treated red cells, or certain bacteria) coated with streptococcal antigen(s) to detect antibody elevation. An example of a hemagglutination test follows.

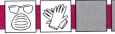

PROCEDURE
STREPTOZYME TEST KIT, WAMPOLE LABORATORIES[43]*

PURPOSE

To detect antibodies against group A streptococcus by agglutination of red cells coated with extracellular streptococcal antigens, including streptolysin O, streptokinase, hyaluronidase, DNase and NADase.

 MEDICAL ASSISTING ALERT

Strictly follow the manufacturer's instructions for the test kit in use.

Reagent and controls contain sodium azide, which may react with lead and copper plumbing to form highly explosive metal azides. If discarded into a sink, flush with a large volume of water to prevent azide buildup.

EQUIPMENT AND MATERIALS

Streptozyme Test Kit
    Streptozyme reagent—sheep cells sensitized with streptococcus A extracellular antigens
    Positive control serum
    Negative control serum
    Calibrated capillary tubes and bulbs
    Mirrored glass slide

Stirrers
Test tubes
Isotonic saline (0.85% sodium chloride)
Pipettes
Timer
Gloves and protective wear for CDC Universal Precautions

---

*Reprinted with permission of Wampole Laboratories Division, Carter-Wallace, Inc., Cranbury, NJ 08512.

PROCEDURAL STEPS

Specimen Collection

No special preparation of the patient is required prior to specimen collection. Fresh or inactivated serum or plasma, collected into a red- or lavender-stopper tube, as well as peripheral blood from fingertip or earlobe may be used. Blood should be collected by an aseptic technique, and, if collected by venipuncture, the serum or plasma should be separated from the red cells as soon as possible. If serum or plasma cannot be tested within 24 hours of collection, it should be stored frozen.

Performance

Serum or Plasma

1. Dilute the sample 1:100 with isotonic saline.
2. Fill capillary tube to the mark (0.05 ml) with the diluted sample and expel onto a section of the slide.
   To use the calibrated capillary tube,

   - Insert capillary tube into the bulb far enough to penetrate the thin membrane within the bulb.
   - Fill the capillary tube to the line with the patient's serum.
   - Place finger over the hole in the top of the bulb to stop capillary action.
   - With the finger covering the hole in the bulb, squeeze the bulb to release contents onto the slide.

3. Fill a clean capillary tube to the mark with positive control serum and deliver to another section of the slide. (Do not dilute the control serums 1:100.)
4. Fill a clean capillary tube to the mark with negative control serum and deliver to separate section of the slide.
5. Add 1 drop of Spectrozyme reagent to each of the patient's serum and control drops.
6. Mix with a disposable stirrer, spreading over the entire section. Use a clean disposable stirrer for each mixture.
7. Rock the mirror slide back and forth gently and evenly for 2 minutes, at a rate of 8–10 times per minute.
8. Place slide on a flat surface and observe for agglutination within 10 seconds.
   NOTE: A direct light source above the slide facilitates reading.

Peripheral Blood

1. Fill capillary tube to the line (0.05 ml) with blood from fingertip, earlobe, or other suitable area.
2. Without allowing blood to clot, squeeze bulb to expel sample into a tube containing 2.5 ml of isotonic saline. On the basis of a 50% hematocrit, this 1:50 blood dilution is equivalent to a 1:100 serum dilution.
3. Proceed with steps 2–8 for serum or plasma.

Interpretation

Agglutination of the Reagent Red Cells. This indicates a positive result.

No Agglutination. Uniformly turbid or slightly granular appearance is a negative result.

QUALITY CONTROL

- Positive and negative controls should be run with each batch of tests in order to provide assurance of reagent reactivity and specificity.
- In addition, control tests provide a comparison for interpreting patient results.

References

1. Mou TW, Feldman HA: The enumeration and presentation of bacteria in urine. *American Journal of Clinical Pathology* 35:572–575, 1961.
2. Hubbard WA, Shales PJ, McClatchey KD: Comparison of the B-D urine collection kit with a standard culture method and with MS-2. *Journal of Clinical Microbiology* 17:327–331, 1983.
3. Koneman EW, Allen SD, Dowell VR Jr, Junda WM, Sommers HM, Winn WC Jr: *Color Atlas and Textbook of Diagnostic Microbiology,* 3rd ed. Philadelphia: J. B. Lippincott, 1988.
4. Yu PK, Germer JJ, Torgerson CA, Anhalt JP: Evaluation of TestPack Strept A for the detection of group A streptococci in throat swabs. *Mayo Clinic Proceedings* 63:33–36, 1988.
5. Kellogg JA, Bankert DA, Levisky JS: Comparison of the TestPack Strept A enzyme immunoassay system with anaerobically incubated cultures for detection of group A streptococci from oropharyngeal swabs. *American Journal of Clinical Pathology* 88:631–634, 1987.
6. Schwabe LD, Small MT, Randall EL: Comparison of TestPack Strept A test kit with culture technique for detection of group A streptococci. *Journal of Clinical Microbiology* 25:309–311, 1987.

7. *Directigen 1-2-3 Group A Strept Test package insert.* Cockeysville, MD: Becton Dickinson Microbiology Systems, 1991.
8. Pezzlo MT, Hibbard JS: *Monograph: Screening for Urinary Tract Infections.* Kansas City, MO: Marion Scientifics, 1984.
9. Clarridge JE, Pezzlo MT, Vosti KL: *Cumitech 2A, Laboratory Diagnosis of Urinary Tract Infections.* Washington, DC: American Society for Microbiology, 1987.
10. Stamm WE, Wagner KF, Amsel R, Alexander ER, Turck M, Counts GW, Holmes KK: Causes of the acute urethral syndrome in women. *New England Journal of Medicine* 303:409–415, 1980.
11. *Chemstrip 2 LN Strip Product Brochure.* Indianapolis, IN: Boehringer Mannheim Diagnostics, 1988.
12. Lennette EH, Balows A, Hausler W Jr, Shadomy HJ (Eds). *Manual of Clinical Microbiology,* 4th ed. Washington DC: American Society for Microbiology, 1985.
13. Kellogg DS, Holmes KK, Hill GA: *Cumitech 4, Laboratory Diagnosis of Gonorrhea.* Washington DC: American Society for Microbiology, 1976.
14. American Cancer Society: Cancer statistics. *Cancer* 36:9–25, 1986.
15. Winawer SJ, Sherlock P: Detecting early colon cancer. *Hospital Practice* 12:49–56, 1977.
16. Fleischer DE, Goldberg SB, Browning TH, Cooper JN, Friedman E, Goldner FH, Keeffe EB, Smith LE: Detection and surveillance of colorectal cancer. *Journal of the American Medical Association* 261:580–585, 1989.
17. *Hemoccult Product Instructions.* San Jose, CA: SmithKline Diagnostics, Inc., 1990.
18. Griffith CDM, Turner DJ, Saunders JH: False-negative results of Hemoccult test in colorectal cancer. *British Medical Journal* 283:472, 1981.
19. Carlson JR, Merz WG, Hansen BE, Ruth S, Moore DG: Improved recovery of group A beta-hemolytic streptococci with a new selective medium. *Journal of Clinical Microbiology* 21:307–309, 1985.
20. Finegold SM, Baron EJ: *Diagnostic Microbiology,* 7th ed. St. Louis: C. V. Mosby, 1986.
21. *Oxidase Reagent Droppers Product Brochure.* Cockeysville, MD: Becton Dickinson Microbiology Systems, 1989.
22. Miller LE, Ludke HR, Peacock JE, Tomar RH: *Manual of Laboratory Immunology,* 2nd ed. Philadelphia: Lea & Febiger, 1990.
23. Ramos CE, Tapia RH: C-reactive protein. *Laboratory Medicine* 15:737–739, 1984.
24. *CRP Latex Test Set Product Brochure.* Houston, TX: Gamma Biologicals, 1990.
25. U.S. Department of Health and Human Services, Public Health Service, Centers for Disease Control: Public health service guidelines for counseling and antibody testing to prevent HIV infection and AIDS. *Morbidity and Mortality Weekly Report* 36:509–515, 1987.
26. National Institutes of Health: The impact of routine HTLV-III antibody testing on public health. *International Journal of Technology Assessment in Health Care* 3:310, 1987.
27. Englund JA: The many faces of Epstein-Barr virus. *Postgraduate Medicine* 83(2):167–170,173,176–179, 1988.
28. Sumayo CV: Infectious mononucleosis and other EBV infections: Diagnostic factors. *Laboratory Management* 23(10):37–46, 1986.
29. Rose NR, Friedman H, Fahey JL. *Manual of Clinical Immunology,* 3rd ed. Washington, DC: American Society for Microbiology, 1986.
30. Bryant NJ: *Laboratory Immunology and Serology,* 2nd ed. Philadelphia: W. B. Saunders, 1986.
31. Lennette ET, Henle W: Epstein-Barr virus infections: Clinical and serologic features. *Laboratory Management* 25:23–28, 1987.
32. *Color Slide II Mononucleosis Test Product Brochure.* Indianapolis: Seradyn, Inc., 1990.
33. Henry JB: *Clinical Diagnosis and Management by Laboratory Methods,* 18th ed. Philadelphia: W. B. Saunders, 1991.
34. Kadar N, Caldwell B, Romero R: A method of screening for ectopic pregnancy and its indications. *Obstetrics & Gynecology* 58:162–165, 1981.
35. *Tandem ICON II HCG Product Brochure.* San Diego, CA: Hybritech, Inc., 1989.
36. Adams LE, Spencer-Green G, Donovan-Brand R, McEnery P, Hayden L, Hurtubise P, Hess EV: Comparison of four rheumatoid factor assays. *Clinical Laboratory Science* 1:362–365, 1988.
37. *Rheumaton Slide Test Product Brochure.* Cranbury, NJ: Wampole Laboratories, 1983.
38. U.S. Department of Health and Human Services, Public Health Service, Centers for Disease Control: *The Laboratory Aspects of Syphilis.* Atlanta, GA: Centers for Disease Control, 1982.
39. *MicroScan ImmunoSCAN RPR Card Test Product Brochure.* Sacramento, CA: Microscan, Baxter Diagnostics, Inc., 1992.
40. Turgeon ML: *Immunology and Serology in Laboratory Medicine.* St. Louis: C. V. Mosby, 1990.
41. Kyriatzis D, Kampa IS, Garner S. Comparison of three diagnostic test kits for rubella. *Laboratory Medicine* 15:199–201, 1984.
42. *Rubascan Card Test Product Brochure.* Cockeysville, MD: Becton Dickinson and Company, 1991.
43. *Streptozyme Product Brochure.* Cranbury, NJ: Wampole Laboratories, 1990.

Bibliography

Addison LA, Fischer PM: *The Office Laboratory,* 2nd ed. Norwalk, CT: Appleton & Lange, 1990.

Bannatyne RM, Clausen C, McCarthy LR. *Cumiteck 10, Laboratory Diagnosis of Upper Respiratory Tract Infections:* Washington, DC: American Society for Microbiology, 1979.

Becan-McBride K, Ross DL: *Essentials for the Small Laboratory and Physician's Office.* Chicago: Year Book Medical Publishers, 1988.

Belsey RE, Baer DM, Statland BE, Sewell DL: *The Physician's Office Laboratory.* Oradell, NJ: Medical Economics Books, 1986.

Bobb H, Brenan K, Ellner PD, Fisher T, Hosmer M: Urine collection and transport for culture and screening tests. *Laboratory Medicine* 19:490–492, 1988.

Bonewit K: *Clinical Procedures for Medical Assistants,* 3rd ed. Philadelphia: W. B. Saunders, 1990.

Facklam RR: Specificity study of kits for detection of group A streptococci directly from throat swabs. *Journal of Clinical Microbiology* 25:504–507, 1987.

Hopp JW, Rogers EA: *AIDS and the Allied Health Professions.* Philadelphia: F. A. Davis, 1989.

Howard BJ, Klaas J II, Rabin SJ, Weissfield AS, Tilton, RC: *Clinical and Pathogenic Microbiology.* St. Louis: C. V. Mosby, 1987.

Isenberg HD, Schoenknecht FD, von Graevenitz A: *Cumitech 9, Collection and Processing of Bacteriological Specimens.* Washington, DC: American Society for Microbiology, 1979.

Kaplan EL: The rapid identification of group A beta-hemolytic streptococci in the upper respiratory tract. *Pediatric Clinics of North America* 35:535–541, 1988.

Kellogg JA, Manzella JP, Shaffer SN, Schwartz BB: Clinical relevance of culture versus screens for the detection of microbial pathogens in urine specimens. *American Journal of Medicine* 83:739–743, 1987.

Knight K, Fielding JE, Battista RN: Occult blood screening for colorectal cancer. *Journal of the American Medical Association* 261:587–592, 1989.

Miller LE, Ludke HR, Peacock JE, Tomar RH. *Manual of Laboratory Immunology*. 2nd ed. Philadelphia: Lea & Febiger, 1990.

Pfaller MA, Kountz FP: Laboratory evaluation of leukocyte esterase and nitrite tests for the detection of bacteriuria. *Journal of Clinical Microbiology* 21:840–842, 1985.

Radetsky M, Wheeler RC, Roe MH, Todd JK: Comparative evaluation of kits for rapid diagnosis of group A streptococcal disease. *Pediatric Infectious Disease* 4(3):274–281, 1985.

Ramsey MK: *Gardnerella vaginalis:* Clinical implications and laboratory identification. *Clinical Laboratory Science* 2:48–51, 1989.

Stamm WE: Protocol for diagnosis of urinary tract infection: Reconsidering the criterion for significant bacteriuria. *Urology* (Suppl) 32(2):6–10, 1988.

Todd JK: Diagnosis of urinary tract infections. *Pediatric Infectious Disease* 1(2):126–131, 1982.

Todd JK: Throat cultures in the office laboratory. *Pediatric Infectious Disease.* 1(4):265–270, 1982.

Turgeon ML: *Immunology and Serology in Laboratory Medicine*. St. Louis: C. V. Mosby, 1990.

Chapter 24

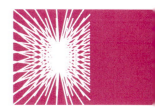

EMERGENCY PROCEDURES

LINDA T. POWELL

SCHEDULING — KEEPING THE OFFICE FUNCTIONAL
Assessment of Office
Steps to Effective Schedule Management

OUTPATIENT EMERGENCY PROCEDURES
Developing an Office Emergency Procedures Guide
Documentation

HANDLING OFFICE EMERGENCIES
General Guide for Handling Office Emergencies

TRIAGE
The Office Triage System
Communications Triage
General Steps of Triage
Patient Assessment Process

CARDIOPULMONARY RESUSCITATION

EMERGENCY TREATMENTS
Medical Emergencies Due to Disease, Illness, or Trauma

SCHEDULING — KEEPING THE OFFICE FUNCTIONAL

A systemic plan for continuation of office functions in the event of a potential or actual emergency is essential in the medical setting. Such policies and procedures should be created and updated on a regular basis. Emergency plans must take into account a detailed assessment of office productivity and schedule progression, patient population, emergency potential, and environmental restraints. Reevaluation of these procedures is indicated after each emergency event, to ensure workability.

Assessment of Office

- Frequently assess the appointment book, be aware of any physician ammendments, and make revisions as needed.
- Initiate schedule changes in the event of an emergency.
- Be aware that some medical specialties have greater emergency potential and may require additional special equipment.
- Use a designated treatment area, keeping emergency equipment and supplies readily available.
- Locate treatment area in an easily accessible place, outside of heavy office traffic.
- Allocate adequate space to provide quick access to equipment and provide an examination table or stretcher.
- Provide appropriate lighting in the treatment area.
- Maintain telephone service to the area to provide quick communications.

Steps to Effective Schedule Management

- Be familiar with the day's schedule and its current success.
- Assess time lost due to the emergency.

659

MEDICAL OFFICE EMERGENCY CHART	
Defibrillator	EKG recorder including patient cable, lead wires and EKG pads Protective defibrillator pads
Oxygen	Tank, including flowmeter, tubing, nasal prongs, mask and wrench for opening tank Airways—oral and nasal in assorted sizes Ambu bag

IV supplies	Angiocaths #16, #18, #20, and #22—three of each size
	Tourniquet
	Betadine
	Alcohol wipes
	Butterfly needles #19 and #21—three of each size
	Tape
	Scissors
	Hemostat
	IV fluids (as specified by the physician)
	    500 ml of D5W
	    500 ml of NS
	    500 ml of D10W
	IV tubing, to include Solusets

Medications	Atropine Lidocaine Instant glucose or glucagon Insulin Diphenydramine (Benadryl) Nitroglycerin (Nitrostat) Ammonia ampules Normal saline Epinephrine
General supplies	Blood pressure cuff, in proper working order Stethoscope Syringes—assorted sizes; insulin Needles—assorted sizes 4 × 4 sponges Kling Gloves—examination and sterile Nasogastric tube Catheter-tip syringe Water-soluble lubricant Paper, pen Penlight Pocket mask

FIGURE 24–1

Medical office emergency chart.

- Survey remaining patients to be seen and identify any patients that could be rescheduled.
- Offer patients who are waiting the opportunity to make necessary phone calls to adjust their schedules.
- Give appropriate information to the waiting patients, explaining the reasons for delay and offer the opportunity to reschedule.
- Consider the physician's appointments and include these in the schedule revision.

OUTPATIENT EMERGENCY PROCEDURES

Administering effective emergency care in an outpatient setting requires careful planning. Using procedural guides for emergency treatment, documentation of treatments, and steps for securing support from the patient, family, office staff, and outside emergency medical services is mandatory.

Developing an Office Emergency Procedures Guide

- Emergency procedures should be documented and accessible to all personnel.
- Emergency treatments, especially those that may occur infrequently, need to be displayed near the emergency treatment area (for example, steps in cardiopulmonary resuscitation [CPR]).
- Current CPR certification is essential for emergency preparedness; annual recertification is required. The Good Samaritan Act protects the health care worker and any person who is trained in first-aid and CPR from any liability incurred during a first aid or emergency situation.
- Keep emergency supply list current.
- Check the emergency cart on a regular basis, preferably weekly, to ensure that all supplies are present and that no dated items have expired (Figure 24–1).

Documentation

In an atmosphere of excitement and energy, documentation of an emergency requires great organization and attention to detail. An emergency flow sheet facilitates the correct documentation of events and provides emergency medical services (EMS) personnel with a concise record of what treatments were done before their arrival (Figure 24–2).

HANDLING OFFICE EMERGENCIES

- The person witnessing the emergency situation immediately alerts the appropriate personnel.
- Those first to the patient immediately begin patient assessment (see Patient Assessment Process).
- If possible, emergent or acutely ill patients are moved to the emergency treatment area. If transfer aggravates the condition, first-aid should begin immediately on site.
- After airway and circulation assessment, access of support personnel is initiated by dialing the telephone emergency number 911.
- One designated person should remain in charge of the situation until EMS personnel or the physician arrives.
- An emergency flow sheet facilitates the correct documentation of events, providing outside EMS with a concise record of what treatments have been rendered.
- Anticipated hospital admission should prompt the receptionist to make copies of any pertinent patient information and have this information ready when the transfer occurs.
- A copy of the emergency documentation checklist should accompany the patient to the hospital.

General Guide for Handling Office Emergencies

Chain of Command

- The person witnessing the emergency situation immediately alerts the appropriate personnel.
- Those first to the patient immediately begin patient assessment (see Patient Assessment Process).
- One designated person should remain in charge

EMERGENCY DOCUMENTATION CHECKLIST

Patient Name: _____

Date: _____

Time: _____

Person Initiating First-Aid: _____

Description or Treatment: _____

_____

_____

CPR Required: Yes _____ No _____

Medications Administered: Yes _____ No _____

    List _____

           _____

           _____

           _____

Oxygen Required: Yes _____ No _____

EKG Monitored: Yes _____ No _____

Defibrillation Required: Yes _____ No _____

EMS Notified: Yes _____ No _____

    By Whom: _____

Family Member Notified: _____

Physician Signature: _____

Transfer to Hospital: Yes _____ No _____

    Location _____

    Departure Time _____

    Accompanied By: _____

    Medical Records Sent: Yes _____ No _____

FIGURE 24-2

Emergency documentation checklist.

of the situation until EMS personnel or the physician arrives.

Accessing Emergency Equipment

- If possible, acutely ill or injured patients are moved to the emergency treatment area. If transfer aggravates the condition, first-aid should begin immediately on site.
- A mobile emergency cart is desirable.

Accessing Support Systems

- After airway and circulation assessment, access of support personnel is initiated by dialing the telephone emergency number 911.
- Emergency situations create an emotional environment in the office that can complicate matters if not recognized. Acknowledging these emotions helps in maintaining some control.
- Even if resuscitation is necessary, allowing a family member to witness these efforts may not be detrimental. Efficiency and human emotions are not necessarily incompatible, as long as the personnel are prepared to provide support and compassion.
- Remaining calm is essential.
- Insisting that a family member or friend leave the area while the loved one is being treated may produce negative results. Studies have shown that family participation in resuscitation efforts does not necessarily have a negative effect.
- Anticipated hospital admission should prompt the receptionist to make copies of any pertinent patient information and have this information ready when the transfer occurs.
- A copy of the emergency documentation checklist should accompany the patient to the hospital.

> **MEDICAL ASSISTING ALERT**
>
> The medical assistant should use the support of all office personnel to facilitate emergency management.

TRIAGE

Triage literally means to sort. Triage of ill patients by office personnel may be necessary, even though these patients are not considered emergencies.

The Office Triage System

Office personnel must be able to recognize immediate and nonimmediate needs. *Immediate needs* include alterations in consciousness or responsiveness, airway problems, breathing difficulties, and circulation disturbances. The office personnel must be prepared to recognize and respond to these events.

Communications Triage

A communications triage may be necessary, meaning the prompt recognition of precisely who

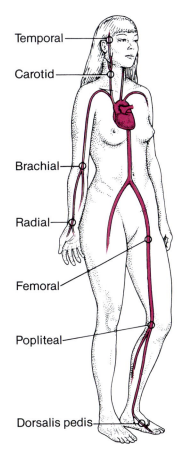

FIGURE 24–3

Locations of pulse. (Reproduced from Kinn M, Derge E: *The Medical Assistant: Administrative and Clinical,* 6th ed. Philadelphia: W. B. Saunders, 1988, p. 441.)

needs to be notified first of the emergency. For example, the designee must be aware if there is a physician present in the office. If not, the designee must then contact emergency medical services, ambulance services, or whatever support persons have been agreed upon at a prior time. One person should perform this notification to prevent duplication and confusion.

A list of emergency numbers such as the ambulance, the hospital emergency room, and any other pertinent numbers should be posted in an area that is easily accessible.

General Steps of Triage

1. Study the situation.
2. Determine the nature of illness or injury.
3. If the patient is able to talk, perform an interview to ascertain the nature of the emergent situation.
4. Administer appropriate first-aid.
5. Notify appropriate authorities and arrange for transportation.

Patient Assessment Process

Assessment of the emergency patient involves precise and organized steps to determine appropriate action.

Life Signs

1. Listen for air passing from nose, mouth, or tracheostomy.
2. Look for rise and fall of chest or abdomen.
3. Observe skin color for bluish tint indicating lack of oxygen.
4. Look for adequate circulation of blood.
5. Check for presence of carotid or radial pulse (Figure 24–3).
6. Note size of pupils (dilated, nonresponsive pupils indicate ineffective circulation).

Evidence of Trauma

1. Check for bleeding, carefully noting back side of supine patient.
2. Check for visible injury such as malalignment of extremities, protruding bone fragments, swelling.
3. Check skin integrity for cuts, abrasions, or discolorations.

CARDIOPULMONARY RESUSCITATION

CPR is the procedure for attempting to restore breathing and circulation to the patient where these processes are impaired or absent.

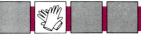

PROCEDURE

CARDIOPULMONARY RESUSCITATION

PURPOSE

To restore breathing and circulation.

PROCEDURAL STEPS

1. Determine unresponsiveness (Figure 24–4).
    Shake patient.
    Shout "Are you okay?"
    RATIONALE: To be sure patient is not conscious.
2. Check for open airway.
    Position patient on back, tilt head back, and lift chin.
    Look for foreign body.
    RATIONALE: Obstructed airway prevents air exchange.
3. Determine breathlessness.
    Look for rising chest or abdomen.
    Listen for passage of air through nose or mouth.
    Feel for air movement by putting cheek close to patient's nose and mouth.
    If breathing is absent, maintain head position, make seal over patient's mouth and nose, and ventilate twice (Figure 24–5).
    Observe for spontaneous respiration.
    Determine circulatory status.
    RATIONALE: The need for ventilatory assistance is determined.
4. Determine pulselessness.

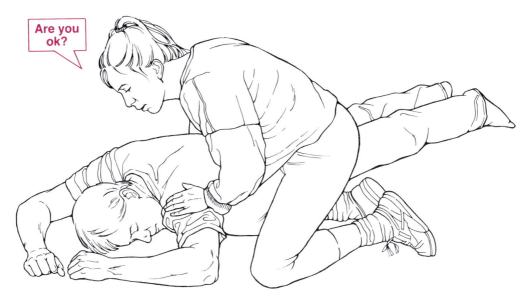

FIGURE 24–4
Check for responsiveness. (Adapted with permission. *Instructor's Manual for Basic Life Support*, 1990. Copyright American Heart Association.)

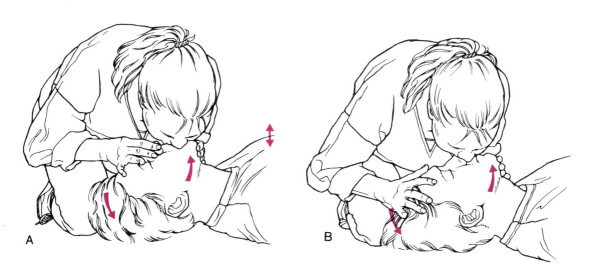

FIGURE 24–5
Maintaining proper head position. (Adapted with permission. *Instructor's Manual for Basic Life Support*, 1990. Copyright American Heart Association.)

666 *Chapter 24: EMERGENCY PROCEDURES*

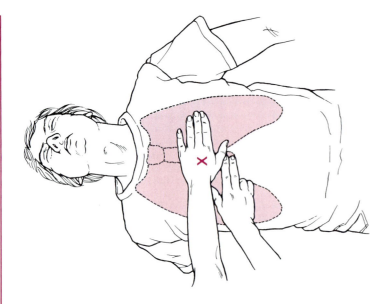

FIGURE 24-6

Proper hand placement for chest compression. (Adapted with permission. *Instructor's Manual for Basic Life Support*, 1990. Copyright American Heart Association.)

Check for the carotid pulse for at least 5 seconds.

If there is no pulse, locate lower half of the sternum and begin external chest compressions at rate of 15 per 11 seconds (80–100 compressions per minute) (Figure 24–6).

Perform compression-ventilation cycles at the rate of 15 compressions to 2 ventilations (Figures 24–7 and 24–8).

Continue for four cycles and reassess for pulse. If there is no pulse, continue CPR.

RATIONALE: This determines absence of heart activity and need for chest compressions.

Adapted with permission. *Instructor's Manual for Basic Life Support*, 1990. Copyright American Heart Association.

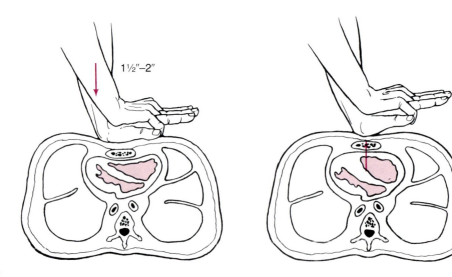

FIGURE 24-7

Depth of compression for the adult chest. (Adapted with permission. *Instructor's Manual for Basic Life Support*, 1990. Copyright American Heart Association.)

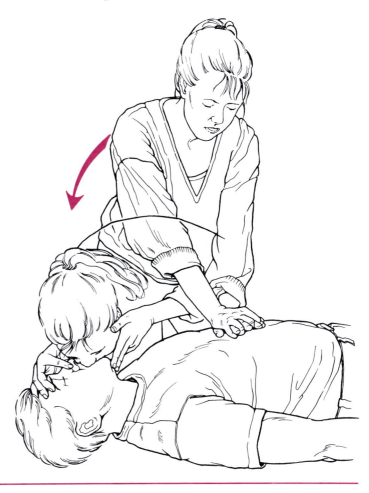

FIGURE 24-8
Positioning for one-rescuer CPR. (Adapted with permission. *Instructor's Manual for Basic Life Support*, 1990. Copyright American Heart Association.)

EMERGENCY TREATMENTS

Medical Emergencies Due to Disease, Illness, or Trauma

Airway Obstruction

Airway obstruction results from the muscular relaxation in the unconscious patient, aspiration of stomach contents, damage due to trauma, or presence of a foreign body.

Clinical Findings

- Inability to speak, grasping the throat, violent coughing, symptoms of air hunger (conscious patient).
- Cyanosis and absence of air movement (unconscious patient).

Immediate Management

1. Determine if airway obstruction is partial or complete. (No air will move through complete obstruction.)
2. If patient is coughing, indicating partial obstruction, initially do not interfere except to remain with the patient.
3. If condition worsens, perform the Heimlich maneuver (Figure 24-9).

    The Heimlich maneuver is performed by wrapping one's arms around the patient from behind, below the ribs, placing a fisted hand in the center of the upper abdomen (above the umbilicus). Use the other hand to grasp the fist and sharply pull up and inward. This movement is intended to push the diaphragm up, forcing

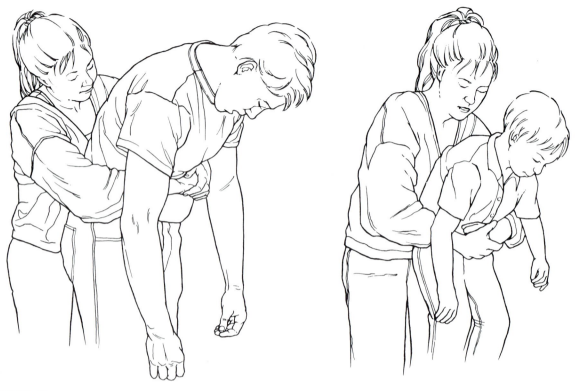

FIGURE 24–9

The Heimlich maneuver. (Adapted with permission. *Instructor's Manual for Basic Life Support*, 1990. Copyright American Heart Association.)

air and the foreign object from the respiratory tract.

Performing the Heimlich maneuver on an unconscious patient (Figure 24–10) is done by kneeling astride the patient's thighs and delivering upward and inward abdominal thrusts with the heel of the hand.

SPECIAL HINT

Always position the head and neck before attempting to dislodge a foreign body. The material will not be able to move past an obstruction by the tongue.

MEDICAL ASSISTING ALERT

Timing is critical. Irreversible brain damage can occur within 4–5 minutes if oxygen is not restored to the cerebral circulation.

Bleeding

Bleeding is produced by the interruption in the integrity of a vessel wall, usually due to trauma or incision.

Clinical Findings

- Obvious blood loss.
- Bruising or formation of hematomas.
- Symptoms of shock following blunt trauma that might indicate internal bleeding.

   Venous bleeding: Blood is dark red and flows from the site.
   Arterial bleeding: Blood is bright red and spurts from the site.
   Capillary bleeding: Blood oozes from the site.

Immediate Management

1. Firmly apply direct pressure to the area. Continue such pressure until a pressure dressing and bandage are applied (Figure 24–11).
2. Locate pressure points and compress to control bleeding (Figure 24–12).

Chapter 24: EMERGENCY PROCEDURES **669**

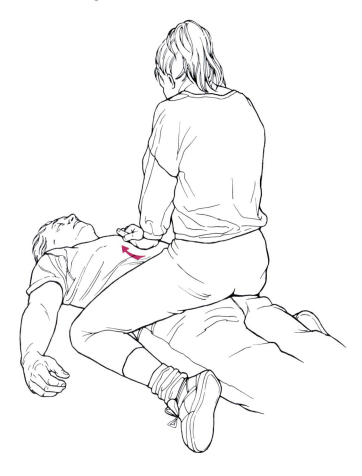

FIGURE 24-10

The Heimlich maneuver performed on the unconscious patient. (Adapted with permission. *Instructor's Manual for Basic Life Support,* 1990. Copyright American Heart Association.)

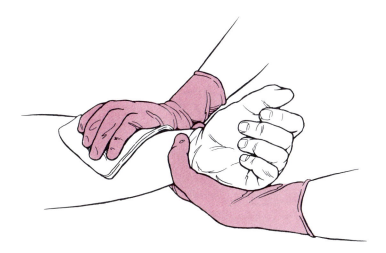

FIGURE 24-11

Application of direct pressure. (Reproduced from Parcel GS: *Basic Emergency Care of the Sick and Injured,* 2nd ed. St. Louis: C. V. Mosby, 1982.)

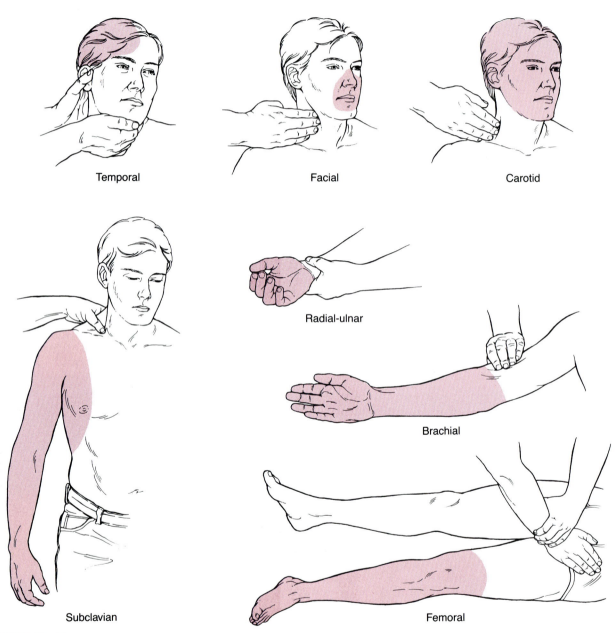

FIGURE 24-12

Location of pressure points. (Reproduced from Parcel GS: *Basic Emergency Care of the Sick and Injured,* 2nd ed. St. Louis: C. V. Mosby, 1982.)

3. Elevate the affected limb to decrease blood flow to the injury.
4. Apply ice to the area if bleeding is not severe.
5. Do not apply a tourniquet unless bleeding is due to injury of a limb, in which case the limb may be sacrificed to save the patient's life.
6. Monitor vital signs. Observe for signs of shock.

Burns

Burns are skin and tissue destruction caused by heat, chemicals, or radiation.

Classification

First degree: Redness of the affected area
Second degree: Destruction of the superficial skin layers and blistering.
Third degree: Destruction of all the epithelium, possibly involving the underlying tissues; pain, usually severe; fluid loss; and shivering.

Immediate Management

1. Apply cold to burns—immerse in ice water or wrap in cold towels.
2. Avoid application of ointment, antiseptic, or any other topical medication.
3. First-degree and small second-degree burns can usually be managed in the office. For all others, prepare for immediate transfer to burn treatment facility.
4. Cover the area with a sterile dressing or clean cloth to minimize contamination and reduce contact with the air.
5. Monitor vital signs. Watch for symptoms of shock.
6. Reassure the patient continuously. Keep the patient at rest.

Cerebrovascular Accidents

Cerebrovascular accident is an interruption of blood flow to the brain, lasting long enough to cause brain damage. There may be a clot in one of the cerebral arteries, a rupture of an artery, or an occlusion of an artery due to the formation of plaque.

Clinical Findings. Symptoms depend on the particular area of the brain affected and on the mechanism that is causing the interruption of blood flow.

- Paralysis (either partial or complete) affecting one side of the body. Rarely are both sides of the body affected at the same time.
- Headache, often severe.
- Difficulty with vision, speech, and movement.
- Seizures.
- Difficulty breathing or swallowing.
- Alterations in consciousness.
- Absence of, or alteration in, facial expression.

Immediate Management

- Assess vital signs, especially noting carefully the breathing as to rate, depth, and character. Blood pressure should be carefully checked. A high blood pressure in combination with a slow pulse may indicate swelling in the brain. Immediate treatment by a physician is essential to prevent permanent damage.
- Carefully assess the patient's neurological status. Make notes on the initial assessment in order to have a baseline assessment reference if mental status should deteriorate.
- Do not give anything by mouth because of the potential for aspiration.
- Position the paralyzed patient carefully, supporting the flaccid side and using the unaffected extremities.
- Prepare the patient for transfer.
- Prepare for deterioration of the condition with airway assistance and oxygen.
- Obtain intravenous access, if possible.

 MEDICAL ASSISTING ALERT

Vital signs can change quickly with a cerebrovascular accident.

Common Fainting

Common fainting occurs when there is a dilation of blood vessels, often produced by a strong emotional response. This vessel dilation is sufficient to cause temporary loss of consciousness.

Clinical Findings

- Loss of consciousness.
- Paleness of skin.

Immediate Management

- Usually the supine position is all that is needed.
- Elevating the lower extremities may help in patients who cannot tolerate lying flat.

- Assess vital signs (usually within normal limits).
- Pass spirits of ammonia under the nose.

Diabetic Coma

Diabetic coma is a condition in which the blood glucose level is high and acid waste products, called *ketones,* build up in the body. It occurs in the diabetic who is not under medical management, the diabetic who has eaten too much without adequate insulin adjustment, or in the well-controlled diabetic who has undergone significant stress or is ill.

Clinical Findings

- Diminished responsiveness.
- Rapid, deep respirations (Kussmaul breathing).
- Hot, dry skin with a deep red tint.
- Weak, thready pulse.
- Fruity (acetone) odor on the breath.

Immediate Management

1. Assess the serum glucose immediately.
2. Obtain intravenous access, if possible.
3. Administer insulin (under physician supervision).
4. Prepare for transfer to the hospital.

Diabetic Insulin Shock

Diabetic insulin shock is a condition in which the patient has taken too much insulin; eaten too little to properly use the insulin dose; or exercised excessively, using up available glucose.

Clinical Findings

- Breathing is usually normal. This is an important finding in determining the difference between insulin shock and diabetic coma.
- Skin is pale, moist, even diaphoretic.
- Patient is dizzy and progresses to fainting, seizure, or coma if there is no intervention.
- Hunger.
- Pulse and blood pressure are normal.
- Agitated behavior.

Immediate Management

1. If the patient is awake and alert, ask the patient if he or she has eaten and has taken his insulin and, if so, how much.
2. Give the patient sugar or a sugary drink, unless he or she is too disoriented and there is risk of aspiration.
3. Assess blood glucose level.
4. If condition does not improve or seems to worsen, prepare the patient for transfer to the hospital.

Drug Overdose and Poisonings

Drug overdosage and poisonings are the intentional or nonintentional ingestion of chemicals, prescription drugs, or nonprescription drugs in large amounts.

Clinical Findings. Findings depend on the material ingested and the time of the event.

Immediate Management

1. Assess vital signs, noting the character of respirations. Many chemicals cause respiratory depression.
2. Determine the history of the event. Knowledge of the agent ingested is essential in determining the course of action. Have another office worker contact the nearest poison control center. The poison control center phone number should be listed with other emergency numbers in the office. The following specific information should be reported when contacting poison control:

- Your location and phone number.
- The type and amount, if known, of the agent ingested.
- Age and weight of the patient.
- Time since poison was taken.
- Whether vomiting has occurred.
- Any treatment that has been given.

3. Inspect the mouth for burns. Drooling may be present if the patient is unable to swallow.
4. Removal of stomach contents is performed only if the ingested material is not corrosive. This is best performed by induction of vomiting, either by stimulating the gag reflex or by giving the patient syrup of ipecac.
5. Specific treatment of drug overdosage or poisoning should be attempted only if the agent is known.
6. Prepare patient for transfer.

Epilepsy

Epilepsy is a condition in which an abnormal focus of electrical activity in the brain produces exaggerated motor activity and changes in consciousness.

Clinical Findings. Clinical findings depend on the type of seizure.

Generalized Seizures

- Are usually preceded by an aura—a vague feeling that something is about to happen.
- Include muscle contractions of most, if not all, muscle groups. This produces rigidity.
- Include muscle spasms, occurring simultaneously with the muscle contractions, producing jerking movements.
- Loss of consciousness.
- Usually followed by a postictal state or period of recovery.

Partial Seizures

- Usually involve one side of the body, one or more extremities.
- Usually consciousness is affected, but not lost (the patient may be foggy or may be behaving in an unusual manner, such as muttering, playing with his or her clothes, chewing, etc.).

Immediate Management

1. Protect the patient. Self-injury is common. Lying down on the ground will lessen the chances of injury.
   Padded tongue blades are usually not necessary, because the risk of injury due to the presence of a foreign body in the mouth may be greater.
2. Keep the airway open with positioning.
3. Position the patient on his or her side to guard against aspiration of saliva or vomitus.
4. Attempt vital signs only after the muscle movement has ended.
5. Remain with the patient. Interfere as little as possible. Transfer to a hospital is usually not necessary unless the patient has another seizure.

 MEDICAL ASSISTING ALERT

Status epilepticus is the situation in which one seizure closely follows another, usually without the patient fully regaining consciousness in between. This constitutes a medical emergency requiring rapid intervention.

Fracture

Fracture is a break or crack in a bone resulting from trauma or disease. See Figure 24-13 for types of fractures.

Clinical Findings

- In *open* fractures, broken skin (broken by the end of the bone).
- In *closed* fractures, intact skin (a radiographic picture of the bone is the only definitive diagnostic tool).
- Swelling at the site of injury.
- Muscle spasm, resulting from the trauma to the adjacent muscle groups.
- Deformities.
- Pain or pressure in the affected area.
- Symptoms of shock.

Immediate Management

1. Make the patient as comfortable as possible.
2. Immobilize the joint above and below the suspected fracture.
3. Control bleeding. If direct pressure is needed, be gentle. Ice is recommended for control of bleeding in fractures.
4. Stabilize the area before transport.

Hypertensive Crisis

Hypertensive crisis is a sudden sustained rise in blood pressure, with a diastolic reading of greater than 120 mm Hg.

Clinical Findings

- Sudden, severe headache.
- Nausea, vomiting.
- Changes in responsiveness.
- Signs of impending stroke.

Immediate Management

1. Reassure the patient.
2. Administer antihypertensive medications as directed by physician.
3. Get immediate medical attention.
4. Obtain intravenous access.
5. Prepare the patient for transfer.
6. Carefully monitor vital signs, especially blood pressure.

Hyperventilation

Hyperventilation is overbreathing, producing a rapid fall in carbon dioxide levels.

Clinical Findings

- Rapid breathing, with a perceived sense of shortness of breath.
- Numbness and tingling of hands and feet.

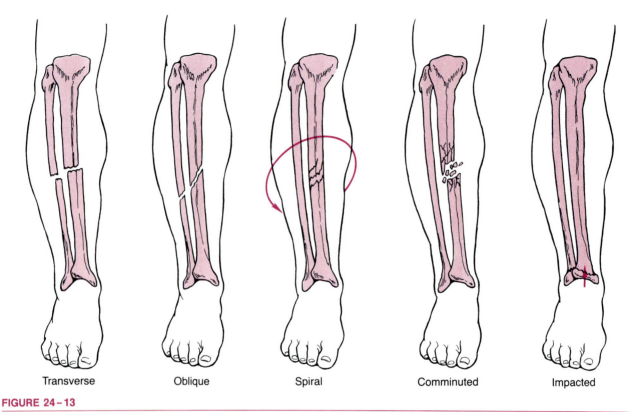

FIGURE 24-13

Types of fractures. (Reproduced from Parcel GS: *Basic Emergency Care of the Sick and Injured,* 2nd ed. St. Louis, 1982, C. V. Mosby.

- Dizziness that may progress to fainting.
- Rapid pulse.

Immediate Management

1. Reassure patient.
2. Have patient breathe into a paper bag.

Myocardial Infarction

Myocardial infarction is an inadequate oxygen supply to myocardium, producing death to that area of the heart muscle.

Clinical Findings

- Chest pain that may be described as crushing or tightness, usually located substernally and radiating down the left arm, both arms, or into the jaw.
- Weakness, sweating.
- Nausea that occurs rather suddenly without an apparent cause.
- Shortness of breath.
- Paleness of skin, progressing to cyanosis.

Immediate Management

1. Reassure the patient. Speak calmly, letting the patient know that care will be provided.
2. Attempt a brief history.
3. Administer nitroglycerin sublingually.
4. Obtain vital signs.
5. Obtain intravenous access.
6. Obtain electrocardiographic monitoring (a continuous-rhythm strip is ideal). Monitor closely for arrhythmias.
7. Arrange patient transfer quickly. If physician is unavailable, call EMS.

Shock

Shock is the condition in which there is lack of sufficient circulation to the body tissues. Shock is produced in several ways, including blood loss, loss of body fluids, loss of the nervous control to the vascular system, loss of adequate cardiac function, severe infection with blood vessel damage, and the common faint.

Clinical Findings

- Patient is very anxious and restless.
- Rapid pulse that is difficult to feel (thready).
- Clammy skin.
- Sweating.
- Thirst.
- Paleness that progresses to cyanosis if shock worsens.
- Nausea that may progress to vomiting.
- Falling blood pressure.
- Diminished responsiveness, progressing to loss of consciousness.
- Shallow, diminished respirations.
- Dilated pupils.

Immediate Management

1. Secure patency of airway. Administer oxygen immediately.
2. Control any bleeding sites with direct pressure.
3. Cover patient with blankets to prevent loss of body heat.
4. Keep patient supine, unless this position interferes with ability to breathe.
5. Measure vital signs frequently, especially pulse and blood pressure (at approximately 5-minute intervals).
6. Do not give the patient anything by mouth, because of the possibility of aspiration.
7. Prepare for transfer.

Wounds

Wounds are described as an interruption in the continuity of the skin or internal tissues caused either intentionally (as in surgery) or accidentally (as in trauma).

Classification

Open: Skin is broken and tissues are exposed.
Closed: Underlying tissues are damaged, as in bruising.
Incised: Wound is caused by clean, cutting instruments.
Lacerated: Wound is caused by a tear to the tissue.
Penetrating: Wound is caused by a sharp object passing through the skin into the underlying tissue.

Immediate Management

1. Control bleeding with pressure.
2. Wash the wound as thoroughly as possible, with an antiseptic solution.
3. Assist the physician with any suturing that is indicated.
4. Apply dressing.

Bibliography

American Academy of Orthopaedic Surgeons: *Emergency Care of the Sick and Injured*. Menasha, WI: George Banta Company, 1987.

Doyle C, Post H, Burney R, Maino J, Rhee K: Family participation during resuscitation: An option. *Annals of Emergency Medicine* 16:673–675, 1987.

Fordney MT, Follis JJ: *Administrative Medical Assisting*. Media, PA: Harwel, 1988.

Instructor's Manual for Basic Life Support. Dallas: American Heart Association, 1990.

Kinn ME, Derge EF: *The Medical Assistant: Administrative and Clinical,* 6th ed. Philadelphia: W. B. Saunders, 1988.

Kitt S, Kaiser J: *Emergency Nursing: A Physiologic and Clinical Perspective*. Philadelphia: W. B. Saunders, 1990.

Parcel GS: *Basic Emergency Care of the Sick and Injured*. St. Louis: C. V. Mosby, 1982.

Brunner, LS, Suddarth, DS, et al. *The Lippincott Manual of Nursing Practice*. Philadelphia: J. B. Lippincott, 1974.

APPENDIX A
GENERAL INFORMATION RESOURCES

A–1	AIDS Information and Resources
A–2	Sources for Patient Education Materials
A–3	Directory of Pharmaceutical Manufacturers
A–4	Poison Control Centers
A–5	Public Health Service Agencies
A–6	Voluntary Health and Welfare Agencies and Associations
A–7	1-800 Telephone Numbers for Health Care Information, Products, and Services

A-1
AIDS INFORMATION AND RESOURCES

Hotlines and Other Telephone Numbers

American Foundation for AIDS Research	212-719-0033
American Red Cross AIDS Education Office	202-737-8300
Centers for Disease Control—Statistics:	
AIDS cases and deaths	404-330-3020
Distribution–categories	404-330-3021
Demographics	404-330-3022
Hearing Impaired AIDS Hotline	800-243-7889
National AIDS Hotline	800-342-AIDS
National AIDS Information Clearing House	800-458-5231
National AIDS Network	202-293-2437
National Gay/Lesbian Crisis Line	800-767-4297
Pediatric and Pregnancy AIDS Hotline	212-340-3333
Project Inform (Drug Information)	800-822-7422
National Sexually Transmitted Diseases Hotline	800-227-8022
Spanish AIDS Hotline	800-344-7432
U.S. Public Health Service	202-245-6867

Regional AIDS Education and Training Centers

New England (excluding Connecticut)

For Maine, Massachusetts, New Hampshire, Rhode Island, and Vermont:
New England AIDS Education and Training Center
Contact Person: Donna Gallagher
506-856-5515

Mid-Atlantic Region (includng Connecticut, Puerto Rico, and Virgin Islands)

For New York City, Long Island, New York, New Jersey, Connecticut, Puerto Rico, and the Virgin Islands:
New York University
AIDS Education and Training Center
Contact Person: Erline McGriff
212-995-3143

For New York State (excluding New York City and Long Island) and Pennsylvania:
University of Pittsburgh
AIDS Education and Training Center
Contact Person: Linda Frank-Hertweek, M.S.N.
412-624-1895

For Maryland, District of Columbia, Virginia, West Virginia, and Delaware:
Mid-Atlantic AIDS Education and Training Center
Contact Person: Moses B. Pounds
301-328-8334

Southeast (including Arkansas and Louisiana)

For Alabama, Florida, Georgia, North Carolina, and South Carolina:
Emory AIDS Training Network
Contact Person: Kathleen R. Miner
404-727-5827

For Arkansas, Louisiana, and Mississippi:
Delta Region AIDS Education and Training Center
Contact Person: Robert L. Marier, M.D.
504-568-3855

Midwest (including Texas and Oklahoma)

For Ohio, Michigan, Kentucky, and Tennessee:
East Central AIDS Education and Training Center
Contact Person: Lawrence L. Gabel
614-293-4318

For Texas and Oklahoma:
University of Texas
AIDS Education and Training Center
Contact Person: Robert Falletti
713-792-4471

For Iowa, Minnesota, Wisconsin, Illinois, Indiana, and Missouri:
Midwest AIDS Training and Education Center
Contact Person: Nathan L. Linsk
312-996-1426

Great Plains and Mountain States

For North Dakota, South Dakota, Utah, Colorado, New Mexico, Nebraska, Kansas, and Wyoming:
Mountain Plains Regional AIDS Education and Training Center
Contact Person: Richard Call
303-270-5885

Pacific Northwest (including Montana and Alaska)

For Washington, Oregon, Montana, Idaho and Alaska:
WAMI AIDS Education and Training Center
Contact Person: Susan Kaetz
206-543-9750

California and Southwest (including Hawaii)

For California (excluding five southern counties), Nevada, Arizona, and Hawaii:
University of California
Davis AIDS Education Center
Contact Person: Charles Gessert, M.D.
209-252-2581

For five counties in Southern California (Los Angeles, Orange, Ventura, Riverside, San Bernardino):
USC AIDS Education and Training Center
Contact Person: Jerry Gates
213-224-7711

From Miller BF, Keane CB: *Encyclopedia and Dictionary of Medicine, Nursing, and Allied Health,* 5th ed. Philadelphia: W.B. Saunders, 1992, p. 1750.

A-2
SOURCES FOR PATIENT EDUCATION MATERIALS

Patient Education is a serious responsibility for health care professionals. Many health care facilities develop their own patient teaching materials. There are also groups, associations, businesses, and agencies that develop patient education materials for dissemination to the lay public. There are many tools that can be used to improve an individual's knowledge about a particular health care problem. These include, but are not limited to, pamphlets, movies, videotapes, audiotapes, and newsletters. The names and addresses identified below are potential sources of information. Local chapters of national organizations may be found in the telephone book and may serve as valuable resources for patient education material and resources.

Abbott Film Service
Abbott Park
N. Chicago, IL 60064

Abbott Laboratories
Professional Services—D383
Abbott Park
N. Chicago, IL 60064

American Cancer Society
1599 Clifton Rd. NE
Atlanta, GA 30329

American Dental Association
211 E. Chicago Ave.
17th Floor
Chicago, IL 60611

American Diabetes Association
National Center
1660 Duke St.
Alexandria, VA 22314

American Liver Foundation
1425 Pompton Ave.
Cedar Grove, NJ 07009

American Lung Association
1740 Broadway
New York, NY 10019

American Red Cross
431 18th St. NW
Washington, DC 20006

Arthritis Foundation
1314 Spring St. NW
Atlanta, GA 30309

Channing L. Bete Co., Inc.
200 State Rd.
South Deerfield, MA 01373

Boehringer Mannheim Corporation
Patient Care Systems Division
9115 Hague Rd.
Indianapolis, IN 46256

Burroughs Wellcome Co.
Public Affairs Department
3030 Cornwallis Rd.
Research Triangle Park, NC 27709

Ciba Pharmaceutical Company
Medical Services Department
556 Morris Ave.
Summit, NJ 07901

Council on Health Information and Education
444 Lincoln Blvd., No. 107
Venice, CA 90291

Cystic Fibrosis Foundation
6931 Arlington Rd.
Bethesda, MD 20814

Health Media Education
1207 De Haro St.
San Francisco, CA 94107

Healthy Mothers, Healthy Babies Coalition
600 Maryland Ave. SE, Suite 300E
Washington, DC 20024-2588

Alfred Higgins Productions, Inc.
6350 Laurel Canyon Blvd., Suite 305
North Hollywood, CA 91606

Johnson and Johnson
The Johnson and Johnson Bldg.
New Brunswick, NJ 08903

Juvenile Diabetes Foundation International
432 Park Ave. South
New York, NY 10016

Eli Lilly and Company
Educational Resources Program
PO Box 100B
Indianapolis, IN 46206

March of Dimes Birth Defects Foundation
1275 Mamaroneck Ave.
White Plains, NY 10605

Maternity Center Association
42 E. 92nd St.
New York, NY 10128

McNeil Laboratories
Consumer Affairs Department
Camp Hill Rd.
Ft. Washington, PA 19034

Merck, Sharpe and Dohme
Professional Services Department
West Point, PA 19486

National Clearinghouse for Alcohol and Drug Information
PO Box 2345
Rockville, MD 20852

National Council on Alcoholism
12 W. 21st St.
New York, NY 10010

Table continued on following page

A-2

SOURCES FOR PATIENT EDUCATION MATERIALS Continued

National Head Injury Foundation
333 Turnpike Rd.
Southborough, MA 01772

National Hydrocephalus Foundation
22427 S. River Rd.
Joliet, IL 60436

National Institute on Drug Abuse (NIDA)
5600 Fishers Ln.
Rockville, MD 20857

National Kidney Foundation
30 E. 33rd St., Suite 1100
New York, NY 10016

National Mental Health Association
1021 Prince St.
Alexandria, VA 22314-2971

National Multiple Sclerosis Society
205 E. 42nd St.
New York, NY 10017

National Safety Council
444 N. Michigan Ave.
Chicago, IL 60611

National Scoliosis Foundation
93 Concord Ave.
PO Box 547
Belmont, MA 02178

National Tay-Sachs and Allied Diseases Association
2001 Beacon St.
Brookline, MA 02146

National Woman's Health Network
1325 G St. NW
Washington, DC 20005

Norwich Eaton Pharmaceuticals
Film Library
1327 Eaton Ave.
Norwich, NY 13815-1709

Novo Nordisk Pharmaceuticals
100 Overlook Center, Suite 200
Princeton, NJ 08540-7810

Nutrition Education Association
PO Box 20301
Houston, TX 77225

Organon Teknika Corporation
100 Akzo Ave.
Durham, NC 27704

Ortho Pharmaceutical Corporation
Raritan, NJ 08869

Parke-Davis
Division of Warner Lambert Company
201 Tabor Rd.
Morris Plains, NJ 07950

Perennial Education, Inc.
930 Pitner Ave.
Evanston, IL 60202

513-751 Pfizer Laboratories
Pfizer, Inc.
235 E. 42nd St.
New York, NY 10017

Phoenix Society (assistance following burn injuries)
11 Rust Hill Rd.
Levittown, PA 19056

Planned Parenthood Federation of America
810 Seventh Ave.
New York, NY 10019

A.H. Robbins Co.
Public Information Department
PO Box 26609
Richmond, VA 23261-6609

Ross Laboratories
Creative Services and Information Department
625 Cleveland Ave.
Columbus, OH 43216

Sandoz Pharmaceuticals
59 Route 10
East Hanover, NJ 07936

W.B. Saunders Co.
The Curtis Center
Independence Square West
Philadelphia, PA 19106-3399

Schering Corporation
Professional Film Library
Galloping Hill Rd.
Kenilworth, NJ 07033

G.D. Searle and Company
Box 5110
Chicago, IL 60680

Skin Cancer Foundation
245 Fifth Ave., Suite 2402
New York, NY 10016

SmithKline Beecham Corporation
regarding prescription medications:
   Pharmaceutical Products Division
   1 Franklin Plaza
   PO Box 7929
   Philadelphia, PA 19102

regarding over the counter medications:
   Consumer Products Division
   100 Beecham Rd.
   Pittsburgh, PA 15205

Spina Bifida Association of America
1700 Rockville Pike, Suite 250
Rockville, MD 20852

A-2
SOURCES FOR PATIENT EDUCATION MATERIALS *Continued*

United Ostomy Association
36 Executive Park, Suite 120
Irvine, CA 92714

Warner Chilcott
201 Tabor Rd.
Morris Plains, NJ 07950

Whittle Communications
333 Main Ave.
Knoxville, TN 37902

Winthrop Pharmaceuticals
90 Park Ave.
New York, NY 10016

Wyeth-Ayerst Laboratories
PO Box 8299
Philadelphia, PA 19101

From Miller BF, Keane CB: *Encyclopedia and Dictionary of Medicine, Nursing, and Allied Health,* 5th ed. Philadelphia: W.B. Saunders, 1992, pp. 1742–1744.

Appendix A: GENERAL INFORMATION RESOURCES

A-3

DIRECTORY OF PHARMACEUTICAL MANUFACTURERS

Key

- BH = Business hours
- N = Nights (after business hours)
- H = Holidays
- W = Weekends
- A = All times (including nights, holidays, and weekends)

Abbott Laboratories, D-355, 1400 Sheridan Road, North Chicago, IL 60064 Tel: 312/937-7069 (8 am–5 pm Mon–Fri), 312/937-7970 (N,H,W)

Adria Laboratories, Division of Erbamont Inc., PO Box 16529, Columbus, OH 43216 Tel: 614/764-8100 (A)

Advanced Care Products, Division of Ortho Pharmaceutical Corporation, Route 202, Raritan, NJ 08869 Tel: 201/524-1305 (8:30 am–4:30 pm Mon–Fri), 201/218-7399 (N,H,W)

Alcon Laboratories, Inc., 6201 South Freeway, Fort Worth, TX 76134 Tel: 817/293-0450 (BH), 817/921-0884 (N,H,W)

Allergan Pharmaceuticals, Inc., 2525 Dupont Drive, Irvine, CA 92715 Tel: 714/752-4500 ext 4281, 4586, or 4959 (BH); 714/752-4335 or 714/752-4244 (N,H,W)

Alza Corporation, 950 Page Mill Road, Palo Alto, CA 94303-0802 Tel: 800/227-9953 (BH) (outside CA), 415/494-5000 (BH), 415/494-5395 James L. Strand, MD (A, emergencies)

American Dermal Corporation, 12-L World's Fair Drive, Somerset, NJ 08873 Tel: 800/526-0199 (BH) (outside NJ), 201/356-5544 (A)

Ames Division, see Miles Inc. Diagnostics Division

Anaquest, Division of BOC Inc., 2005 West Beltline Highway, Madison, WI 53713-2318 Tel: 1-800/ANA-DRUG (BH), 608/273-0019

Apothecon, see Bristol Laboratories

Armour Pharmaceutical Company, 920A Harvest Drive, Suite 200, Blue Bell, PA 19422 Tel: 215/540-8100 (A)

B.F. Ascher & Company, Inc., 15501 West 109th Street, Lenexa, KS 66219 Tel: 913/888-1880 (8 am–4:30 pm Mon–Fri)

Astra Pharmaceutical Products Inc., 50 Otis Street, Westborough, MA 01581-4428 Tel: 617/366-1100 (BH), 1-800/225-4803 (N,H,W) (outside MA), 1-800/451-2512 (N,H,W) (in MA)

Baxter Healthcare Corporation, Route 120 and Wilson Road, Round Lake, IL 60073 Tel: 312/546-6311 ext 2120 (8:30 am–5 pm Mon–Fri)

Beecham Laboratories, Division of Beecham, Inc., 501 Fifth Street, Bristol, TN 37620 Tel: 1-800/251-0271 (8 am–5 pm Mon–Fri) (outside TN), 615/764-5141 (A)

Beecham Products, Division of Beecham, Inc., PO Box 1467, Pittsburgh, PA 15230 Tel: 800/245-1040 (A) (outside PA), 800/242-1718 (A) (in PA)

Berlex Laboratories, Inc., Professional Services, 110 East Hanover Avenue, Cedar Knolls, NJ 07927 Tel: 201/292-3007 (A)

Block Drug Company Inc., 257 Cornelison Avenue, Jersey City, NJ 07302 Tel: 201/434-3000 (A)

Boehringer Ingelheim Pharmaceuticals, Inc., 90 East Ridge, PO Box 368, Ridgefield, CT 06877 Tel: 203/438-0311 (A)

Boehringer Mannheim Diagnostics, A Division of Boehringer Mannheim Corporation, 9115 Hague Road, Indianapolis, IN 46250 Tel: 800/428-5074

Bolar Pharmaceutical Co., Inc., 33 Ralph Avenue, Copiague, NY 11726 Tel: 516/842-8383

Boots Pharmaceuticals, Inc., 8800 Ellerbe Road, PO Box 6750, Shreveport, LA 71136-6750 Tel: 318/861-8200 (8:30 am–4:30 pm Mon–Fri), 318/861-8298 (N,H,W)

Boots-Flint, Inc., 300 Tri-State International Center, Suite 200, Lincolnshire, IL 60015 Tel: 312/405-7400 (7:30 am–4:30 pm Mon–Fri)

Bristol Laboratories, A Bristol-Myers Company, 2404 Pennsylvania Street, Evansville, IN 47721-0001 Tel: 812/429-5000 (A)

Bristol Laboratories Oncology Products, A Bristol-Myers Company, 2404 Pennsylvania Street, Evansville, IN 47721-0001 Tel: 812/429-5000 (A)

Bristol-Myers Products, A Bristol-Myers Company, 1350 Liberty Avenue, Hillside, NJ 07205 Tel: 212/546-4616 (9 am–5 pm Mon–Fri), 212/546-4700 (N,H,W)

The Brown Pharmaceutical Company, Inc., 3300 Hyland Avenue, Costa Mesa, CA 92626 Tel: 800/548-5100 (8 am–5 pm Mon–Fri)

Burroughs Wellcome Company, 3030 Cornwallis Road, Research Triangle Park, NC 27709 Tel: 800/443-6763 (A)

Canaan Laboratories Ltd., 50 Locust Avenue, New Canaan, CT 06840 Tel: 800/222-0830 (9 am–5:30 pm Mon–Fri) (outside CT), 203/966-6700 (9 am–5:30 pm Mon–Fri)

Carnrick Laboratories, Inc., 65 Horse Hill Road, Cedar Knolls, NJ 07927 Tel: 201/267-2670

Central Pharmaceuticals, Inc., 120 East Third Street, Seymour, IN 47274 Tel: 812/522-3915

Chattem Consumer Products, Division of Chattem, Inc., 1715 West 38th Street, Chattanooga, TN 37409 Tel: 615/821-4571 (BH), 615/842-0751 (N,H,W)

CIBA Pharmaceutical Company, Division of CIBA-GEIGY Corporation, 556 Morris Avenue, Summit, NJ 07901 Tel: 201/277-5000 (A), 201/277-5342

Clay Adams, 299 Webro Road, Parsippany, NJ 07054 Tel: 201/887-4800

Colgate-Hoyt Laboratories, Division of Colgate-Palmolive Company, 1 Colgate Way, Canton, MA 02021 Tel: 800/225-3756 (8:30 am–4:15 pm)

Connaught Laboratories, Route 611, Box 187, Swiftwater, PA 18370 Tel: 800/822-2463 (8 am–8 pm Mon–Fri), 717/839-7187 (A)

Danker Laboratories, Inc., 6805 33rd Street East, PO Box 1899, Sarasota, FL 33578 Tel: 800/237-9641 (8:30 am–5:30 pm Mon–Fri) (outside FL), 800/282-9661 (8:30 am–5:30 pm Mon–Fri) (in FL), 813/758-7711 (8:30 am–5:30 pm Mon–Fri) (local)

Dermik Laboratories, Inc., Division of William H. Rorer, Inc., 790 Penllyn Pike, Blue Bell, PA 19422 Tel: 215/283-2000 (8:30 am–4:30 pm Mon–Fri)

Dista Products Company, Division of Eli Lilly and Company, Lilly Corporate Center, Indianapolis, IN 46285 Tel: 317/276-3714 (BH), 317/276-4000 (N,H,W)

Du Pont Critical Care, Subsidiary of E.I. du Pont de Nemours & Co., 1600 Waukegan Road, Waukegan, IL 60085 Tel: 800/323-4980 (A), 312/473-3000 (A)

Du Pont Pharmaceuticals, E.I. du Pont de Nemours & Co., Barley Mill Plaza, Caverly Mill, Building 26, Wilmington, DE 19898 Tel: 1-800/441-8961 (A) (outside DE), 800/441-3273 (A) (in DE)

Elkins-Sinn, Inc., Subsidiary of A.H. Robins Company, Two Esterbrook Lane, Cherry Hill, NJ 08003-4099 Tel: 800/257-8349

Ethitek Pharmaceuticals Company, 8104 North Lawndale Avenue, Skokie,

A-3

DIRECTORY OF PHARMACEUTICAL MANUFACTURERS *Continued*

Key

BH = Business hours
N = Nights (after business hours)
H = Holidays
W = Weekends
A = All times (including nights, holidays, and weekends)

IL 60076 Tel: 312/675-6616 (A)

Fisher Medical Division, Division of Fisher Scientific Group Inc., 526 Route 303, Orangeburg, NY 10962 Tel: 800/431-1861 (8 am-5 pm Mon-Fri) (outside NY), 914/359-9200 (A)

Fisons Corporation, Pharmaceutical Division, Two Preston Court, Bedford, MA 01730 Tel: 617/275-1000 ext 352 (BH), 617/275-3037 (N,H,W), 617/275-1000 ext 341 (emergencies)

C.B. Fleet Company, Inc., 4615 Murray Place, Lynchburg, VA 24506 Tel: 800/446-0991 (8 am-5 pm Mon-Fri) (outside VA), 804/528-4000 (BH)

Forest Pharmaceuticals, Inc., Subsidiary of Forest Laboratories, Inc., 2510 Metro Boulevard, Maryland Heights, MO 63043-9979 Tel: 314/569-3610 (A)

Geigy Pharmaceuticals, Division of CIBA-GEIGY Corporation, 556 Morris Avenue, Summit, NJ 07901 Tel: 201/277-5000 (A)

Genentech, Inc., 460 Point San Bruno Boulevard, South San Francisco, CA 94080 Tel: 800/821-8590 (A)

Glaxo Inc., Five Moore Drive, Research Triangle Park, NC 27709 Tel: 1-800/334-0089 (A), 919/248-2100 (A)

Glenbrook Laboratories, Division of Sterling Drug Inc., 90 Park Avenue, New York, NY 10016 Tel: 1-800/331-4536 (8:30 am-4:30 pm Mon-Fri), 212/907-2764 (BH), 212/907-2000 (BH), 212/734-5976 Earl Lockhart, MD (N,H,W)

Gray Pharmaceutical Co., Affiliate of The Purdue Frederick Company, 100 Connecticut Avenue, Norwalk, CT 06856 Tel: 203/853-0123

Herbert Laboratories, Dermatology Division of Allergan Pharmaceuticals, Inc., 2525 Dupont Drive, Irvine, CA 92715 Tel: 714/752-4500 ext 4281, 4586, or 4959 (BH); 714/752-4335 or 714/752-4244 (N,H,W)

Hermal Pharmaceutical Laboratories, Route 145, Oak Hill, NY 12460 Tel: 518/239-4714 (8 am-4:30 pm Mon-Fri)

Hoechst-Roussel Pharmaceuticals Inc., Route 202-206 North, Somerville, NJ 08876 Tel: 201/231-2611 (8:30 am-5 pm Mon-Fri), 201/231-2000 (A)

Hynson, Westcott & Dunning Products, BBL Microbiology Systems, Division of Becton Dickinson and Company, 250 Schilling Circle, Cockeysville, MD 21030 Tel: 301/584-7177

ICI Pharma, Division of ICI Americas Inc., Concord Pike and New Murphy Road, Wilmington, DE 19897 Tel: 800/456-5678 (8:15 am-4:30 pm Mon-Fri) (outside DE), 302/575-2331 (8:15 am-4:30 pm Mon-Fri), 302/575-3000 (A)

ICN Pharmaceuticals, Inc., 3300 Hyland Avenue, Costa Mesa, CA 92626 Tel: 800/556-1937 (outside CA), 800/331-2331 (in CA), 714/545-0100 (A)

Iolab Pharmaceuticals, Division of Johnson & Johnson Company, 861 South Village Oaks Drive, Covina, CA 91724 Tel: 800/423-1871 (outside CA), 800/352-1891 (in CA), 818/915-7681 (A)

Janssen Pharmaceutica Inc., Division of Johnson & Johnson Company, 40 Kingsbridge Road, Piscataway, NJ 08854-3998 Tel: 201/524-9881 (A)

Kendall McGaw Laboratories, Inc., PO Box 25080, Santa Ana, CA 92799-5080 Tel: 800/854-6851 (7:15 am-3:45 pm Mon-Fri) (outside CA and AK), 714/660-2147 collect (in CA and AK)

Key Pharmaceuticals, Division of Schering-Plough Corporation, Galloping Hill Road, Kenilworth, NJ 07033 Tel: 800/526-4099 (BH) (outside NJ), 201/298-4908 (BH), 201/298-4000 (N,H,W)

Knoll Pharmaceuticals, A Unit of BASF K&F Corporation, c/o Medical Affairs Department, 30 North Jefferson Road, Whippany, NJ 07981 Tel: 800/526-0221 (outside NJ), 201/428-8250 (A)

Kremers Urban Company, PO Box 2038, Milwaukee, WI 53201 Tel: 800/558-5114 (7:30 am-4 pm Mon-Fri) (outside WI), 414/354-4300

Lactaid Inc., 600 Fire Road and Lister Lane, PO Box 111, Pleasantville, NJ 08232-011 Tel: 800/257-8650, 609/653-6100

Lakeside Pharmaceuticals Inc., Division of Merrell Dow Pharmaceuticals Inc., 10123 Alliance Road, Cincinnati, OH 45242-9553 Tel: 513/948-6040 (8:15 am-5 pm), 513/948-9111 (N,H,W, emergencies)

Lederle Laboratories, A Division of American Cyanamid Company, Middletown Road, Pearl River, NY 10965 Tel: 914/732-2815 (A)

Leeming Division, Pfizer Inc., 100 Jefferson Road, Parsippany, NJ 07054 Tel: 201/887-2100

Lemmon Company, 650 Cathill Road, Sellersville, PA 18960 Tel: 800/523-6542 (8 am-12 midnight Mon-Fri) (outside PA), 215/723-5544 (8 am-12 midnight Mon-Fri), 609/779-7417 David Haenick, MD (N,H,W)

Eli Lilly and Company, Lilly Corporate Center, Indianapolis, IN 46285 Tel: 317/276-3714 (BH), 317/276-2000 (N,H,W)

Loma Linda Foods, Inc., 11503 Pierce Street, Riverside, CA 92515 Tel: 1-800/932-5525 (8 am-5 pm Mon-Thurs, 8 am-2 pm Fri) (outside CA), 800/442-4917 (8 am-5 pm Mon-Thurs, 8 am-2 pm Fri) (in CA), 714/687-7800 (8 am-5 pm Mon-Thurs, 8 am-2 pm Fri)

LyphoMed, Inc., 10401 West Touhy, Rosemont, IL 60018 Tel: 312/345-9746 (A)

Marion Laboratories, Inc., Medical Information, HBC #3, PO Box 9627, Kansas City, MO 64134 Tel: 800/821-2130 (A) (outside MO), 816/966-5000 (A)

McNeil Consumer Products Company, Camp Hill Road, Fort Washington, PA 19034 Tel: 215/233-7000

McNeil Pharmaceutical, Welsh Road, Spring House, PA 19477 Tel: 215/628-5000 (A)

Mead Johnson Laboratories, A Bristol-Myers Company, 2404 Pennsylvania Street, Evansville, IN 47721-0001 Tel: 812/429-5000 (A)

Mead Johnson Nutritionals, A Bristol-Myers Company, 2404 Pennsylvania Street, Evansville, IN 47721-0001 Tel: 812/429-5000 (A)

Mead Johnson Oncology Products, A Bristol-Myers Company, 2404 Pennsylvania Street, Evansville, IN 47721-0001 Tel: 812/429-5000 (A)

Mead Johnson Pharmaceuticals, A Bristol-Myers Company, 2404 Pennsylvania Street, Evansville, IN 47721-0001 Tel: 812/429-5000 (A)

Medicone Company, 225 Varick Street, New York, NY 10014 Tel: 212/924-5166

The Mentholatum Company, 1360 Niagara Street, Buffalo, NY 14213 Tel: 800/822-1400 (9 am-5 pm Mon-Fri) (outside NY), 716/882-7660 (A)

Merck Sharp & Dohme, Division of Merck & Co., Inc., West Point, PA 19486 Tel: 215/661-7300 (8:30 am-4:45 pm Mon-Fri), 215/661-5000 (N,H,W, emergencies)

Merrell Dow Pharmaceuticals Inc., Subsidiary of The Dow Chemical Company, 10123 Alliance Road, Cincinnati, OH 45242-9553 Tel: 513/948-6040 (8:15 am-5 pm), 513/948-9111 (N,H,W, emergencies)

Miles Inc. Consumer Healthcare Division, 1127 Myrtle Street, Elkhart, IN 46515 Tel: 219/264-8955 (8 am-5 pm Mon-Fri), 219/264-8111 (N,H,W)

Miles Inc. Diagnostics Division, PO Box 70, Elkhart, IN 46515 Tel: 1-800/348-8100 (BH), 219/264-8781 (N,H,W)

Miles Inc. Pharmaceutical Division, 400 Morgan Lane, West Haven, CT 06516 Tel: 1-800/937-2000 (A)

Monoclonal Antibodies, Inc., 2319 Charleston Road, Mountain View, CA 94043 Tel: 800/227-8855 (outside CA), 415/960-1320

Neutrogena Corporation, 5755 West 96th Street, Los Angeles, CA 90045 Tel: 800/421-6857 (8:30 am-5 pm Mon-Fri) (in CA), 213/642-1150 (8:30 am-5 pm Mon-Fri)

NMS Pharmaceuticals, Inc., 1533 Monrovia Avenue, Newport Beach, CA 92663 Tel: 800/854-3002 (outside CA), 800/367-4200 (in CA), 714/645-2111

Norcliff Thayer Inc., 303 South Broadway, Tarrytown, NY 10591 Tel: 914/631-0033

Nordisk-USA, Affiliate of Nordisk Gentofte, 3202 Monroe Street, Suite 100, Rockville, MD 20852 Tel: 1-800/822-6487 (BH), 301/770-4400 (BH)

Norwich Eaton Pharmaceuticals, Inc., A Procter & Gamble Company, PO Box 231, Norwich, NY 13815-0231 Tel: 607/335-2565 (A)

A-3

DIRECTORY OF PHARMACEUTICAL MANUFACTURERS Continued

Key

BH = Business hours
N = Nights (after business hours)
H = Holidays
W = Weekends
A = All times (including nights, holidays, and weekends)

Organon Inc., 375 Mount Pleasant Avenue, West Orange, NJ 07052 Tel: 800/631-1253 (8 am-5 pm Mon-Fri) (outside NJ), 201/325-4500 (8 am-5 pm Mon-Fri)

Organon Teknika Inc., 800 Capitol Drive, Durham, NC 27713 Tel: 919/361-1995

Ortho Dermatological Division, Ortho Pharmaceutical Corporation, Route 202, PO Box 300, Raritan, NJ 08869-0602 Tel: 201/218-6000

Ortho Diagnostic Systems, Inc., Route 202, Raritan, NJ 08869 Tel: 800/526-3875 (outside NJ), 201/218-8152

Ortho Pharmaceutical Corporation, Route 202, PO Box 300, Raritan, NJ 08869-0602 Tel: 201/218-6000 (BH), 201/524-0400 (N,H,W)

Owen Laboratories, Division of Alcon Laboratories, Inc., 6201 South Freeway, Fort Worth, TX 76134 Tel: 817/293-0450

Parke-Davis, Division of Warner-Lambert Company, 201 Tabor Road, Morris Plains, NJ 07950 Tel: 800/223-0432 (9 am-5 pm Mon-Fri) (outside NJ), 201/540-2000 (A)

Parke-Davis Consumer Health Products Group, Warner-Lambert Company, 201 Tabor Road, Morris Plains, NJ 07950 Tel: 800/524-2624 (outside NJ), 800/338-0326 (in NJ)

Pennwalt Prescription Division, Pennwalt Corporation, 755 Jefferson Road, Rochester, NY 14623 Tel: 716/475-9000 (A)

Pfizer Laboratories Division, Pfizer Inc., 235 East 42nd Street, New York, NY 10017 Tel: 212/573-2422 (A)

Pharmacia Inc., 800 Centennial Avenue, Piscataway, NJ 08854 Tel: 1-800/526-3619 (8:30 am-4:45 pm Mon-Fri) (outside NJ), 201/457-8000 (A)

Pharmacraft Division, Pennwalt Corporation, 755 Jefferson Road, Rochester, NY 14623 Tel: 716/475-9000 ext 2375 (8 am-4:45 pm) (BH), 716/475-9000 (N,H,W)

Plough, Inc., 3030 Jackson Avenue, Memphis, TN 38151-0377 Tel: 901/320-2386 (BH), 901/320-2011 (emergencies)

Polymer Technology Corporation, 100 Research Drive, Wilmington, MA 01887 Tel: 800/343-1445 (A) (outside MA), 617/658-6111 (A)

Poythress Laboratories, Inc., 16 North 22nd Street, Richmond, VA 23261 Tel: 804/644-8591 (8 am-4:30 pm Mon-Fri)

Princeton Pharmaceutical Products, Subsidiary of E.R. Squibb & Sons, Inc., PO Box 4500, Princeton, NJ 08543-4500 Tel: 609/243-6305 (A)

The Procter & Gamble Company, 11511 Reed Hartman Highway, Cincinnati, OH 45241 Tel: 513/530-2154 (BH) (in OH), 513/751-5525 (N,H,W) (call collect)

The Purdue Frederick Company, 100 Connecticut Avenue, Norwalk, CT 06856 Tel: 203/853-0123

Reed & Carnrick Pharmaceuticals, Division of Block Drug Company, One New England Avenue, Piscataway, NJ 08854 Tel: 201/981-0070

Reid-Rowell, 901 Sawyer Road, Marietta, GA 30062 Tel: 800/241-5534, 404/578-9000 (8 am-4:45 pm Mon-Fri)

Richardson-Vicks Inc. Health Care Products Division, One Far Mill Crossing, Shelton, CT 06484 Tel: 203/929-2500 (A)

Richardson-Vicks Inc. Personal Care Products Division, One Far Mill Crossing, Shelton, CT 06484 Tel: 203/929-2500 (8:30 am-4:30 pm Mon-Fri), 301/328-2425 (N,W, emergencies)

Riker Laboratories, Inc., Subsidiary of 3M Company, Building 225-1N-07, 3M Center, St. Paul, MN 55144-1000 Tel: 612/736-4930 (A)

A.H. Robins Company, 1407 Cummings Drive, Richmond, VA 23220 Tel: 804/257-2000 (A), 804/257-7788 (N,H,W)

Roche Diagnostic Systems, Division of Hoffmann-La Roche Inc., 11 Franklin Avenue, Belleville, NJ 07109 Tel: 1-800/526-1247 (BH), 1-201/235-5000 (N,H,W emergencies)

Roche Laboratories, Division of Hoffman-La Roche Inc., Professional Services Department, 340 Kingsland Street, Nutley, NJ 07110 Tel: 201/235-2355 (A)

Roerig, A Division of Pfizer Pharmaceuticals, 235 East 42nd Street, New York, NY 10017 Tel: 212/573-2187 (A)

Rorer Consumer Pharmaceuticals, A Division of Rorer Pharmaceutical Corporation, 500 Virginia Drive, Fort Washington, PA 19034 Tel: 215/628-6159 (8:15 am-4:45 pm Mon-Fri), 215/628-6671 (A), 215/628-6200 (N,H,W)

Rorer Pharmaceuticals, A Division of Rorer Pharmaceutical Corporation, 500 Virginia Drive, Fort Washington, PA 19034 Tel: 215/628-6159 (8:15 am-4:45 pm Mon-Fri), 215/628-6671 (A), 215/628-6200 (N,H,W)

Ross Laboratories, A Division of Abbott Laboratories, 625 Cleveland Avenue, Columbus, OH 43216 Tel: 614/227-3333 (A)

Roxane Laboratories, Inc., PO Box 16532, Columbus, OH 43216 Tel: 800/848-0120 (BH) (outside OH), 614/276-4000 (BH), 614/261-6563 (N,H,W)

Sandoz Consumer Health Care Group, One Upper Pond Road, Parsippany, NJ 07054 Tel: 201/503-7764 (BH), 201/503-7500 (N,H,W)

Sandoz Nutrition Corporation, Clinical Products Division, 5320 West 23rd Street, Minneapolis, MN 55440 Tel: 800/328-7874, 612/925-2100

Sandoz Pharmaceuticals Corporation, 59 Route 10, East Hanover, NJ 07936 Tel: 201/386-7764 (BH), 201/386-7500 (N,H,W)

Savage Laboratories, A Division of Altana Inc., 60 Baylis Road, Melville, NY 11747 Tel: 800/231-0206 (8:45 am-4:45 pm Mon-Fri) (outside NY), 516/454-9071 (8:45 am-4:45 pm Mon-Fri)

Schering Corporation, Galloping Hill Road, Kenilworth, NJ 07033 Tel: 800/526-4099 (BH) (outside NJ), 201/298-4908 (BH), 201/298-4000 (N,H,W)

Schmid Laboratories, Inc., Route 46 West, Little Falls, NJ 07424-0415 Tel: 201/256-5500 (BH)

G.D. Searle & Co., 4901 Searle Parkway, Skokie, IL 60077 Tel: 800/323-4204 (BH) (outside IL), 312/982-7000 (A)

Self Care Systems, Inc., 1527 Monrovia Avenue, Newport Beach, CA 92663 Tel: 800/854-3002 (outside CA), 800/367-4200 (in CA), 714/645-4244

Serono Laboratories, Inc., 280 Pond Street, Randolph, MA 02368 Tel: 800/225-5185 (A) (outside MA), 617/963-8154 (A)

Smith Kline & French Laboratories, Division of SmithKline Beckman Corporation, PO Box 7929, 1500 Spring Garden Street, Philadelphia, PA 19101 Tel: 800/523-4835 (A) (outside PA), 215/751-5231 (8 am-6 pm Mon-Fri) (Medical Affairs), 215/751-4000 (9 am-5 pm Mon-Fri)

SmithKline Consumer Products, A SmithKline Beckman Company, PO Box 8082, Philadelphia, PA 19101 Tel: 215/751-7706 (BH), 215/751-5000 (N,H,W)

SmithKline Diagnostics, Inc., A SmithKline Beckman Company, 485 Potrero Avenue, PO Box 3947, Sunnyvale, CA 94008-3947 Tel: 800/538-1581, 408/732-6000

E.R. Squibb & Sons, Inc., PO Box 4500, Princeton, NJ 08543-4500 Tel: 609/243-6305 (A)

Squibb-Novo, Inc., 211 Carnegie Center, Princeton, NJ 08540-6213 Tel: 609/987-5800 (8:30 am-5 pm), 609/987-5800 (N,H,W)

Stiefel Laboratories, Route 145, Oak Hill, NY 12460 Tel: 518/239-6901 (8:30 am-5 pm Mon-Fri)

Stuart Pharmaceuticals, Division of ICI Americas Inc., Concord Pike and New Murphy Road, Wilmington, DE 19897 Tel: 800/441-7758 (8:15 am-4:30 pm Mon-Fri) (outside DE), 302/575-2231 (8:15 am-4:30 pm Mon-Fri), 302/575-3000 (A)

Syntex Laboratories, Inc., 3401 Hillview Avenue, Palo Alto, CA 94304 Tel: 415/855-5545 or 415/852-1386 (BH), 415/855-5050 (A)

Syntex Medical Diagnostics, 900 Arastradero Road, Palo Alto, CA 94304 Tel: 800/821-1131 (outside CA), 800/367-7633 (in CA), 415/494-1086

Syva Company, 900 Arastradero Road, Palo Alto, CA 94304 Tel: 800/227-8994 (outside CA), 800/982-6006 (in CA)

Tambrands Inc., One Marcus Avenue, Lake Success, NY 11042 Tel: 516/437-8800

TAP Pharmaceuticals, 1400 Sheridan

A-3

DIRECTORY OF PHARMACEUTICAL MANUFACTURERS Continued

Key

- BH = Business hours
- N = Nights (after business hours)
- H = Holidays
- W = Weekends
- A = All times (including nights, holidays, and weekends)

Road, North Chicago, IL 60064 Tel: 1-800/622-2011 (A)

Thompson Medical Company, Inc., 919 Third Avenue, New York, NY 10022 Tel: 212/688-4420 (A)

3M Company, Consumer Specialties Division—Personal Care Products, 3M Center, St. Paul, MN 55144-1000 Tel: 612/733-1110

Travenol Laboratories, Inc., see Baxter Healthcare Corporation

United States Packaging Corporation, 506 Clay Street, La Porte, IN 46350 Tel: 219/362-9782

The Upjohn Company, 7000 Portage Road, Kalamazoo, MI 49001 Tel: 616/323-6615 (A)

Upsher-Smith Laboratories, Inc., 14905 23rd Avenue North, Minneapolis, MN 55447 Tel: 612/473-4412 (8 am-5 pm Mon-Fri)

Wallace Laboratories, Division of Carter-Wallace, Inc., Half Acre Road, Cranbury, NJ 08512 Tel: 609/655-6000 (BH), 609/799-1167 (N,H,W)

Wampole Laboratories, Division of Carter-Wallace, Inc., Half Acre Road, Cranbury, NJ 08512 Tel: 800/257-9525 (outside NJ), 609/655-6000

Warner Chilcott Laboratories, Division of Warner-Lambert Company, 201 Tabor Road, Morris Plains, NJ 07950 Tel: 800/223-0432 (9 am-5 pm Mon-Fri) (outside NJ, AK, and HI), 201/540-2000 (A)

Warner-Lambert Consumer Health Products Group, Warner-Lambert Company, 201 Tabor Road, Morris Plains, NJ 07950 Tel: 800/562-0266 (e.p.t.) (outside NJ), 800/334-3577 (Early Detector) (outside NJ), 800/223-0182 (all other products) (outside NJ), 800/338-0326 (all products) (in NJ)

Webcon Pharmaceuticals, Division of Alcon Laboratories, Inc., 6201 South Freeway, Fort Worth, TX 76134 Tel: 817/293-0450 (BH), 817/921-0884 (N,H,W)

Westwood Pharmaceuticals Inc., 100 Forest Avenue, Buffalo, NY 14213 Tel: 716/887-3400

Whitehall Laboratories, Division of American Home Products Corporation, 685 Third Avenue, New York, NY 10017-4076 Tel: 212/878-5508

Winthrop Consumer Products, Division of Sterling Drug Inc., 90 Park Avenue, New York, NY 10016 Tel: 1-800/331-4536 (8:30 am-4:30 pm Mon-Fri), 212/907-3027 (BH), 212/907-2000 (BH)

Winthrop Pharmaceuticals, Division of Sterling Drug Inc., 90 Park Avenue, New York, NY 10016 Tel: 1-800/446-6267 (9 am-5 pm Mon-Fri), 212/907-2000 (A)

Wyeth-Ayerst Laboratories, Division of American Home Products Corporation, King of Prussia Road and Lancaster Avenue, Radnor, PA 19087 Tel: 215/688-4400 (A)

From *The Family Physician's Compendium of Drug Therapy.* New York: McGraw-Hill Book Company, 1988, pp. 84-87.

POISON CONTROL CENTERS

The poison control centers listed below are certified by the American Association of Poison Control Centers. These centers are supervised by a medical director and are required to have either a registered pharmacist or a nurse available to answer questions from the public. Large databanks that are updated on a quarterly basis are available to certified Poison Control Centers. Each of the certified poison control centers serves a large geographic area as listed below. A certified poison control center offers educational services to both the public and health care professionals. There are often other smaller poison control centers working collaboratively with the certified centers. Health care providers should be aware that the telephone number of a poison control center may change. It is a professional responsibility to be aware of the current number of the poison control center for the area in which patient care is provided and to share this information in patient teaching. A listing of certified poison control centers is updated yearly and published in the *Physician's Desk Reference*.

ALABAMA
Alabama Poison Control Systems, Inc.
809 University Boulevard East
Tuscaloosa, AL 35401
Emergency Numbers:
(800) 462-0800 (AL only); (205) 345-0600

Children's Hospital of Alabama—Regional Poison Control Center
1600 Seventh Avenue, South
Birmingham, AL 35233-1711
Emergency Numbers:
(205) 939-9201; (205) 933-4050; (800) 292-6678

ARIZONA
Arizona Poison & Drug Information Center
Arizona Health Sciences Center, Room 3204K
University of Arizona
Tucson, AZ 85724
Emergency Numbers:
(602) 626-6016; (800) 362-0101 (AZ only)

Samaritan Regional Poison Center
Good Samaritan Medical Center
1130 East McDowell Road, Suite A-5
Phoenix, AZ 85006
Emergency Number:
(602) 253-3334

CALIFORNIA
Fresno Regional Poison Control Center of Fresno Community Hospital and Medical Center
P.O. Box 1232
2823 Fresno Street
Fresno, CA 93715
Emergency Numbers:
(209) 445-1222; (800) 346-5922 (CA only)

Los Angeles County Medical Association Regional Poison Control Center
1925 Wilshire Boulevard
Los Angeles, CA 90057
Emergency Numbers:
(213) 484-5151; (800) 77 POISN

San Diego Regional Poison Center
UCSD Medical Center
225 Dickinson Street
San Diego, CA 92103
Emergency Numbers:
(619) 543-6000; (800) 876-4766

San Francisco Bay Area Regional Poison Control Center
San Francisco General Hospital, Room 1E86
1001 Potrero Avenue
San Francisco, CA 94110
Emergency Numbers:
(415) 476-6600; (800) 523-2222 (415, 707 only)

UCDMC Regional Poison Control Center
2315 Stockton Boulevard
Sacramento, CA 95817
Emergency Number:
(916) 453-3414

COLORADO
Rocky Mountain Poison and Drug Center
645 Bannock Street
Denver, CO 80204-4507
Emergency Numbers:
(303) 629-1123; (800) 332-3073 (CO only)

D.C.
National Capital Poison Center
Georgetown University Hospital
3800 Reservoir Rd., NW
Washington, DC 20007
Emergency Number:
(202) 625-3333

FLORIDA
Florida Poison Information Center at the Tampa General Hospital
P.O. Box 1289
Tampa, FL 33601
Emergency Numbers:
(813) 253-4444; (800) 282-3171 (FL only)

GEORGIA
Georgia Poison Control Center
Grady Memorial Hospital
Box 26066
80 Butler Street, SE
Atlanta, GA 30335-3801
Emergency Numbers:
(404) 589-4400; (800) 282-5846 (GA only);
(404) 525-3323 (TTY)

KENTUCKY
Kentucky Regional Poison Center of Kosair
Children's Hospital
P.O. Box 35070
Louisville, KY 40232-5070
Emergency Numbers:
(502) 589-8222; (800) 722-5725 (KY only)

MARYLAND
Maryland Poison Center
20 North Pine Street
Baltimore, MD 21201
Emergency Numbers:
(301) 528-7701; (800) 492-2414 (MD only)

A-4
POISON CONTROL CENTERS *Continued*

MASSACHUSETTS
Massachusetts Poison Control System
300 Longwood Avenue
Boston, MA 02115
Emergency Numbers:
(617) 232-2120; (800) 682-9211 (MA only)

MICHIGAN
Blodgett Regional Poison Center
1840 Wealthy SE
Grand Rapids, MI 49506
Emergency Numbers:
(800) 832-2727 (MI only); (800) 356-3232 (TTY)

Poison Control Center, Children's Hospital of Michigan
3901 Beaubien Boulevard
Detroit, MI 48201
Emergency Numbers:
(313) 745-5711; (800) 462-6642 (MI only)

MINNESOTA
Hennepin Regional Poison Center
Hennepin County Medical Center
701 Park Avenue
Minneapolis, MN 55415
Emergency Numbers:
(612) 347-3141; (612) 337-7474 (TTY)

Minnesota Regional Poison Center
St. Paul-Ramsey Medical Center
640 Jackson Street
St. Paul, MN 55101
Emergency Numbers:
(612) 221-2113; (800) 222-1222 (MN only)

MISSOURI
Cardinal Glennon Children's Hospital Regional Poison Center
1465 South Grand Boulevard
St. Louis, MO 63104
Emergency Numbers:
(314) 772-5200; (800) 392-9111 (MO only);
(800) 366-8888; (314) 557-5336 (TTY)

MONTANA
Rocky Mountain Poison and Drug Center
645 Bannock Street
Denver, CO 80204-4507
Emergency Number:
(800) 525-5042 (MT only)

NEBRASKA
Mid-Plains Poison Control Center
8301 Dodge Street
Omaha, NE 68114
Emergency Numbers:
(402) 390-5400; (800) 642-9999 (NE only);
(800) 228-9515 (surrounding states)

NEW JERSEY
New Jersey Poison Information and Education System
201 Lyons Avenue
Newark, NJ 07112
Emergency Numbers:
(201) 923-0764; (800) 962-1253 (NJ only)

NEW MEXICO
New Mexico Poison and Drug Information Center
University of New Mexico
Albuquerque, NM 87131
Emergency Numbers:
(505) 843-2551; (800) 432-6866 (NM only)

NEW YORK
Long Island Regional Poison Control Center
Nassau County Medical Center
2201 Hempstead Turnpike
East Meadow, NY 11554
Emergency Number:
(516) 543-2323

New York City Poison Control Center
455 First Avenue, Room 123
New York, NY 10016
Emergency Numbers:
(212) 340-4494; (212) POISONS

OHIO
Central Ohio Poison Center
Columbus Children's Hospital
700 Children's Drive
Columbus, OH 43205
Emergency Numbers:
(614) 228-1323; (800) 682-7625 (OH only);
(614) 228-2272 (TTY)

Cincinnati Drug and Poison Information Center
231 Bethesda Avenue, M.L.
#144
Cincinnati, OH 45267-0144
Emergency Numbers:
(513) 558-5111; (800) 872-5111

OREGON
Oregon Poison Center
Oregon Health Sciences University
3181 SW Sam Jackson Park Road
Portland, OR 97201
Emergency Numbers:
(503) 279-8968 (local); (800) 452-7165 (OR only)

PENNSYLVANIA
Delaware Valley Regional Poison Control Center
One Children's Center
34th & Civic Center Boulevard
Philadelphia, PA 19104
Emergency Number:
(215) 386-2100

Pittsburgh Poison Center
3705 Fifth Avenue at DeSoto Street
Pittsburgh, PA 15213
Emergency Number:
(412) 681-6669

RHODE ISLAND
Rhode Island Poison Center—Rhode Island Hospital
593 Eddy Street
Providence, RI 02902
Emergency Number:
(401) 277-5727

Table continued on following page

A–4
POISON CONTROL CENTERS *Continued*

TEXAS
North Texas Poison Center
P.O. Box 35926
Dallas, TX 75235
Emergency Numbers:
(214) 590-5000; (800) 441-0040 (TX only)

Texas State Poison Center
The University of Texas Medical Branch
Galveston, TX 77550-2780
Emergency Numbers:
(409) 765-1420; (713) 654-1701 (Houston);
(512) 478-4490 (Austin); (800) 392-8548 (TX only)

UTAH
Intermountain Regional Poison Control Center
50 North Medical Drive, Building 428
Salt Lake City, UT 84132
Emergency Numbers:
(801) 581-2151; (800) 456-7707 (UT only)

WEST VIRGINIA
West Virginia Poison Center
West Virginia University Health Sciences Center/
 Charleston Division
3110 MacCorkle Avenue, SE
Charleston, WV 25304
Emergency Numbers:
(304) 348-4211; (800) 642-3625 (WV only)

WYOMING
Rocky Mountain Poison and Drug Center
645 Bannock Street
Denver, CO 80204-4507
Emergency Number:
(800) 442-2702 (WY only)

From Miller BF, Keane CB: *Encyclopedia and Dictionary of Medicine, Nursing and Allied Health,* 5th ed. Philadelphia: W.B. Saunders 1992, pp. 1751–1753.

A-5

PUBLIC HEALTH SERVICE AGENCIES

1. Physical Activity and Fitness .... President's Council on Physical Fitness and Sports
2. Nutrition .... National Institutes of Health and Food and Drug Administration
3. Tobacco .... Centers for Disease Control
4. Alcohol and Other Drugs....................... Alcohol, Drug Abuse, and Mental Health Administration
5. Family Planning .... Office of Population Affairs
6. Mental Health and Mental Disorders .... Alcohol, Drug Abuse, and Mental Health Administration
7. Violent and Abusive Behavior .... Centers for Disease Control
8. Educational and Community-Based Programs ...... Centers for Disease Control and Health Resources and Services Administration
9. Unintentional Injuries .... Centers for Disease Control
10. Occupational Safety and Health .... Centers for Disease Control
11. Environmental Health .... National Institutes of Health and Centers for Disease Control
12. Food and Drug Safety .... Food and Drug Administration
13. Oral Health .... National Institutes of Health and Centers for Disease Control
14. Maternal and Infant Health .... Health Resources and Services Administration
15. Heart Disease and Stroke .... National Institutes of Health
16. Cancer .... National Institutes of Health
17. Diabetes and Chronic Disabling Conditions .... National Institutes of Health and Centers for Disease Control
18. HIV Infection .... National AIDS Program Office
19. Sexually Transmitted Diseases .... Centers for Disease Control
20. Immunization of Infectious Diseases .... Centers for Disease Control
21. Clinical Preventive Services .... Health Resources and Services Administration and Centers for Disease Control
22. Surveillance and Data Systems .... Centers for Disease Control

From Public Health Service, US Department of Health and Human Services, Office of Disease Prevention and Health Promotion, Washington, DC, 1990.

Appendix A: GENERAL INFORMATION RESOURCES

A-6
VOLUNTARY HEALTH AND WELFARE AGENCIES AND ASSOCIATIONS

There are a wide variety of agencies and associations that contribute to the well being of individuals with health care problems. These agencies can be sponsored by governmental agencies or they may be voluntary. A *voluntary agency* is nongovernmental and nonprofit in nature; the term voluntary is used to denote that a major source of support is contributed. Regardless of the nature of the sponsoring group, health and welfare agencies provide many services such as development of educational programs, sponsorship of research, increasing public awareness of a specific disease or disorder, and support services. The agencies listed below will help the physician, nurse, and allied health professional to improve patient care and services. The listing of agencies is current at the time of publication of the *Miller-Keane Encyclopedia and Dictionary of Medicine, Nursing, and Allied Health;* users are cautioned that these addresses change frequently.

ACTION (programs for older adults)
806 Connecticut Ave. NW
Washington, DC 20525
202-254-7310

Administration on Aging
Department of Health and Human Services
200 Independence Ave. SW
Washington, DC 20201
202-245-0724

Alcoholics Anonymous
468 Park Ave. South
New York, NY 10016
212-686-1100

Alzheimer's Disease and Related Disorders
 Association
70 E. Lake St.
Chicago, IL 60601
800-621-0379

American Academy of Allergy and Immunology
611 E. Wells St.
Milwaukee, WI 53202
414-272-6071

American Anorexia/Bulimia Association, Inc.
133 Cedar Ln.
Teaneck, NJ 07666
201-836-1800

American Association on Mental Deficiency
PO Box 96
Willimantic, CT 06226

American Association of Retired Persons (AARP)
1909 K St. NW
Washington, DC 20005

American Burn Association
Shriner's Burn Institute
University of Cincinnati
202 Goodman St.
Cincinnati, OH 45219
513-751-3900

American Cancer Society
1599 Clifton Rd. NE
Atlanta, GA 30329
404-320-3333

American Dental Association
Council on Dental Care Programs
211 E. Chicago Ave.
17th Floor
Chicago, IL 60611
312-440-2500

American Diabetes Association
National Center
1660 Duke St.
Alexandria, VA 22314
800-232-3472

American Foundation for the Blind
15 W. 16th St.
New York, NY 10016
212-620-2000

American Liver Foundation
1425 Pompton Ave.
Cedar Grove, NJ 07009
800-223-0179

American Lung Association
1740 Broadway
New York, NY 10019
215-315-8700

American Pain Society
PO Box 186
Skokie, IL 60076
312-475-7300

American Parkinson's Disease Association, Inc.
116 John St.
New York, NY 10038
212-732-9550

American Speech-Language-Hearing Association
10801 Rockville Pike
Department AP
Rockville, MD 20852
301-897-5700

American Spinal Injury Association
2020 Peachtree Rd. NW
Atlanta, GA 30309

American Tinnitus Association
PO Box 5
Portland, OR 97207
503-248-9985

Arthritis Foundation
1314 Spring St. NW
Atlanta, GA 30309
404-872-7100

Asthma and Allergy Foundation of America
1717 Massachusetts Ave. NW
No. 305
Washington, DC 20036
800-7ASTHMA

A-6
VOLUNTARY HEALTH AND WELFARE AGENCIES AND ASSOCIATIONS Continued

Centers for Disease Control
Department of Health and Human Services
U.S. Public Health Service
Atlanta, GA 30333
404-639-3534

Concern for Dying
250 W. 57th St.
New York, NY 10107
215-246-6962

Cystic Fibrosis Foundation
6931 Arlington Rd.
Bethesda, MD 20814
800-FIGHT-CF

Epilepsy Foundation of America
815 15th St. NW, Suite 528
Washington, DC 20005
202-638-5229

Guide for Infant Survival (sudden infant death syndrome)
PO Box 17432
Irvine, CA 92713-7432

Guillain-Barré Foundation
129 North Carolina Ave. SE
Washington, DC 20003
202-387-2216

HELP (Herpes Resource Center)
PO Box 100
Palo Alto, CA 94302
919-361-2120

La Leche League International
9616 Minneapolis Ave.
Franklin Park, IL 60131
800-LA-LECHE

Leukemia Society of America
31 St. James Ave.
Boston, MA 02116
617-482-2256

Muscular Dystrophy Association
3561 E. Sunrise Ave.
Tucson, AZ 85718
602-529-2000

Myasthenia Gravis Foundation
61 Gramercy Park North
New York, NY 10010
212-533-7005

National Association to Control Epilepsy
22 E. 67th St.
New York, NY 10012

National Association of Patients on Hemodialysis and Transplantation
211 E. 43rd St.
New York, NY 10017
212-867-4486

National Association for Retarded Citizens
2501 Ave. J
Arlington, TX 76011

National Association for Sickle Cell Disease
4221 Wilshire Blvd., Suite 360
Los Angeles, CA 90010
213-936-7205

National Cancer Institute
Office of Cancer Communications
Building 31, Room 10A24
National Institutes of Health
Bethesda, MD 20892
800-4-CANCER

National Center for the American Heart Association
7320 Greenville Ave.
Dallas, TX 75231
214-373-6300

National Easter Seal Society
2023 W. Ogden Ave.
Chicago, IL 60612
312-243-8400

National Foundation for Ileitis and Colitis
444 Park Ave. South
New York, NY 10016
212-685-3440

National Head Injury Foundation
333 Turnpike Rd.
Southborough, MA 01722
508-485-9950

National Hemophilia Foundation
110 Greene St., Suite 406
New York, NY 10012
212-219-8180

National Institute of Allergy and Infectious Diseases
Building 10, National Institutes of Health
Bethesda, MD 20892
301-496-4000

National Institute of Arthritis and Musculoskeletal and Skin Diseases
National Institutes of Health
Bethesda, MD 20892
301-496-4000

National Jewish Center for Immunology and Respiratory Medicine
1400 Jackson St.
Denver, CO 80206
800-222-LUNG

National Kidney Foundation
30 E. 33rd St.
New York, NY 10016
212-889-2210

National Multiple Sclerosis Society
205 E. 42nd St.
New York, NY 10017
212-532-3060

Table continued on following page

VOLUNTARY HEALTH AND WELFARE AGENCIES AND ASSOCIATIONS Continued

National Parkinson's Foundation
1501 NW 9th Ave.
Miami, FL 33136
305-547-6666

National Psoriasis Foundation
6443 Southwest Beaverton Hwy., Suite 210
Portland, OR 97221
503-297-1545

National Safety Council
444 N. Michigan Ave.
Chicago, IL 60611
800-621-7619

National SIDS Alliance (sudden infant death syndrome)
10500 Little Patuxent Pkwy., Suite 420
Columbia, MD 21044
800-221-SIDS

National Society to Prevent Blindness
500 E. Remington Rd.
Schaumburg, IL 60173
312-843-2020

National Spinal Cord Injury Association
600 W. Cumming Park, #3200
Woburn, MA 01801
800-962-9629

Office for Handicapped Individuals
Department of Education
Room 3106, Switzer Building
400 Maryland Ave. SW
Washington, DC 20202
202-245-0080

Osteoporosis Foundation
612 N. Michigan Ave., Suite 510
Chicago, IL 60611

Paget's Disease Foundation
PO Box 2772
Brooklyn, NY 11202
718-596-1043

Parkinson Disease Foundation
Medical Center
William Black Medical Research Bldg.
640 W. 168th St.
New York, NY 10032
212-923-4700

Phoenix Society (assistance following burn injuries)
11 Rust Hill Rd.
Levittown, PA 19056
215-946-BURN
800-888-BURN

Scoliosis Association
PO Box 51353
Raleigh, NC 27609
919-846-2639

Self Help for Hard of Hearing People (Shhh)
4848 Battery Ln.
Department E
Bethesda, MD 20814
301-657-2248

Sex Information and Education Council of the United States (SIECUS)
130 W. 42nd St., Suite 2500
New York, NY 10036
212-819-9770

United Cerebral Palsy Association (UCPA)
1522 K St. NW
Washington, DC 20005
800-872-5827

United Network for Organ Sharing
3001 Hungary Spring Rd.
Richmond, VA 23228
804-289-5380

From Miller BF, Keane CB: *Encyclopedia and Dictionary of Medicine, Nursing, and Allied Health,* 5th ed. Philadelphia: W.B. Saunders, 1992, pp. 1745–1747.

A-7
1-800 TELEPHONE NUMBERS FOR HEALTH CARE INFORMATION, PRODUCTS, AND SERVICES

Alzheimer's Disease and Related Disorders Association	800-621-0379
American Academy of Allergists	800-842-7777
American Association of Occupational Health Nurses	800-241-8014
American Cancer Society	800-ACS-2345
American Diabetes Association	800-232-3472
American Dietetic Association	800-877-1600
American Kidney Fund	800-638-8299
American Liver Foundation	800-223-0179
American Nurses Association	800-274-4ANA
Asthma and Allergy Foundation of America	800-7-ASTHMA
Cystic Fibrosis Foundation	800-FIGHT-CF
Drug Abuse Hotline	800-662-HELP
Georgia Safety Council	800-441-5103
Health Careers Hotline	800-999-4248
Hearing Impaired AIDS Hotline	800-243-7889
Human Growth Foundation (growth disorders)	800-451-6434
Institute for Limb Preservation	800-262-5462
Kraftec (physical therapy products)	800-348-4848
La Leche League International	800-LA-LECHE
The Living Bank International (organ donation)	800-528-2971
Lumex Inc. (equipment)	800-645-5272
Medco Instruments	800-626-3326
MedicAlert	800-ID-ALERT
Medical Express (traveling health professionals)	800-544-7255
National AIDS Hotline	800-342-AIDS
National AIDS Information Clearing House	800-458-5231
National Cancer Institute, Office of Cancer Communications	800-4-CANCER
National Clearinghouse for Alcohol and Drug Information	800-729-6686
National Health Careers Information Hotline	800-999-4248
National Jewish Center for Immunology and Respiratory Medicine	800-222-LUNG
National Resource Center on Child Sexual Abuse	800-543-7006
National Safety Council	800-621-7619
National Sexually Transmitted Diseases Hotline	800-227-8922
National SIDS Alliance	800-221-SIDS
National Spinal Cord Injury Association	800-962-9629
Phoenix Society (for clients following burns)	800-888-BURN
Project Inform (AIDS treatment information)	800-822-7422
Quality Line Health Education Videos	800-356-0986
Simon Foundation for Continence	800-237-4666
SmithKline Beecham Corp. (information on over the counter medications)	800-456-6670
SmithKline Beecham Corp. (information on prescription medications)	800-366-8900
Spanish AIDS Hotline	800-344-7432
Travel Nurse Hotline	800-247-4774
United Cerebral Palsy Foundation	800-872-5827
United Ostomy Association	800-826-0826
Visiting Nurse Associations of America	800-426-2547

From Miller BF, Keane CB: *Encyclopedia and Dictionary of Medicine, Nursing, and Allied Health,* 5th ed. Philadelphia: W.B. Saunders, 1992, p. 1749.

APPENDIX B
ADMINISTRATIVE INFORMATION

B–1 Abbreviations Commonly Used by Hospitals
B–2 Acronyms for Selected Health Care Organizations, Associations, and Agencies
B–3 Alphabet Soup of Heath Care
B–4 Combining Forms in Medical Terminology
B–5 Medicare Physician Payment Reform (PPR)
B–6 Medicare PPR Procedure Codes Subject to the Outpatient Limit
B–7 Medicare PPR Facility-Based Procedures for Which Additional Amount for Supplies May Be Payable if Performed in a Physician's Office
B–8 Medicare PPR Evaluation and Management Codes
B–9 Professional Designations for Health Care Providers
B–10 Specialized Terms Used in Medical Records
B–11 Symbols Commonly Used in Clinical Practice
B–12 Words and Phrases Commonly Misinterpreted

ABBREVIATIONS COMMONLY USED BY HOSPITALS

Most hospitals, community health agencies, and other clinical facilities have a list of approved abbreviations to be used in patient records. The abbreviations listed below are often used when charting and will assist in the interpretation of patient records, but they should not be utilized on the record unless they are on the approved list for the clinical site.

AA	Alcoholics Anonymous
aa	of each
AAROM	active assistive range of motion
abd.	abdomen
a.c.	before meals
ACTH	adrenocorticotropin
AD	right ear
ADA	American Diabetes Association
ADL	activities of daily living
ad lib	as desired
AHA	American Heart Association
AIDS	acquired immune deficiency syndrome
AK	above the knee
ALS	amyotrophic lateral sclerosis
A.M.	morning
AMA	against medical advice
AMI	acute myocardial infarction
ant.	anterior
AODM	adult onset diabetes mellitus
AP	antepartum, anteroposterior
A & P	auscultation and percussion
A-P	anterior-posterior
A/R	apical/radial
AROM	active range of motion; artificial rupture of membranes
ARROM	active resistive range of motion
AS	left ear
ASA	acetylsalicylic acid (aspirin)
ASAP	as soon as possible
ASCVD	arteriosclerotic cardiovascular disease
ASD	atrial septal defect
ASHD	arteriosclerotic heart disease
AU	both ears
AV	atrioventricular
A & W	alive and well
Ba	barium
BC/BS	Blue Cross/Blue Shield
BCP	birth control pill
BE	barium enema
b.i.d.	two times a day
BK	below the knee
BLE	bilateral lower extremity
BM	bowel movement
BMR	basal metabolic rate
BP	blood pressure
BPH	benign prostatic hypertrophy
BR	bathroom
BRP	bathroom privileges
BSE	breast self examination
BUE	bilateral upper extremity
BUN	blood, urea, nitrogen
BVR	Bureau of Vocational Rehabilitation
BW	birth weight
bx.	biopsy
C	Centigrade
C(x)	C followed by a number indicates a specific cervical vertebra
CA	cancer
c̄	with
Ca	calcium, cancer
CAD	coronary artery disease
cap.	capsule
CBC	complete blood count
CC	chief complaint
cc	cubic centimeter
CCU	coronary care unit
CF	cystic fibrosis
CHD	coronary heart disease
CHF	congestive heart failure
CHO	carbohydrate
cm.	centimeter
CMV	cytomegalovirus
CNS	central nervous system
CO	carbon dioxide
C/O	complains of
COPD	chronic obstructive pulmonary disease
CP	cerebral palsy
CPD	cephalopelvic disproportion
CPK	creatine phosphokinase
CPR	cardiopulmonary resusitation
CS	cesarean section
C&S	culture and sensitivity
CSF	cerebrospinal fluid
CV	cardiovascular
CVA	cerebral vascular accident
D&C	dilatation and curettage
d.c.	discontinue
D&E	dilatation and evacuation
DJD	degenerative joint disease
DKA	diabetic ketoacidosis
DM	diabetes mellitus
DOA	dead on arrival
DOB	date of birth
DOE	dyspnea on exertion
DTR	deep tendon reflex
DTs	delirium tremens
Dx.	diagnosis
ECF	extended care facility
ECG	electrocardiogram
ECT	electroconvulsive therapy
EDC	estimated date of confinement
EEG	electroencephalogram
EENT	eyes, ears, nose, and throat
EKG	electrocardiogram
ENT	ears, nose, and throat
EOM	extraocular movement
ER	emergency room
ETOH	ethanol (ethyl alcohol)
F	Fahrenheit
FBS	fasting blood sugar
Fe	iron
FeSO$_4$	ferrous sulfate
FH	family history
FHR	fetal heart rate
FM	fine motor
FTND	full term normal delivery
FUO	fever of unknown origin
FWB	full weight bearing
Fx	fracture
G	gravida
GB	gallbladder
GC	gonococcus
GFR	glomerular filtration rate

B-1
ABBREVIATIONS COMMONLY USED BY HOSPITALS Continued

GG	gamma globulin	LVH	left ventricular hypertrophy
GI	gastrointestinal	L & W	living and well
GM	gross motor	mcg.	microgram
gm.	gram	MCV	mean corpuscular volume
gr.	grain	MD	muscular dystrophy
GTT	glucose tolerance test	mEq/L	milliequivalents per liter
gtt.	drops	Mg	magnesium
GU	genitourinary	mg.	milligram
gyn	gynecology	MH	mental health, marital history
hb	hemoglobin	MI	myocardial infarction
HBP	high blood pressure	min.	minim, minute
hct.	hematocrit	ml.	milliliter
HCTZ	hydrochlorothiazide	mm.	millimeter
hgb	hemoglobin	MMT	manual muscle test
H & H	hemoglobin and hematocrit	MOM	milk of magnesia
HHA	home health aide	MS	mitral stenosis, multiple sclerosis
H_2O	water	Na	sodium
H_2O_2	hydrogen peroxide	NaCl	sodium chloride
H & P	history and physical	NAD	no acute distress
HPI	history of present illness	NAS	no added salt
hs	hour of sleep	NB	newborn
HSV	herpes simplex virus	neg.	negative
HT, HTN	hypertension	N-G	nasogastric
HVD	hypertensive vascular disease	NKA	no known allergies
Hx	history	NPO	nothing by mouth
hyp.	hypodermic	NSAID	nonsteroidal anti-inflammatory drug
ICU	intensive care unit	NSR	normal sinus rhythm
I & D	incision and drainage	NSS	normal saline solution
IM	intramuscular (injection)	NSVD	normal spontaneous vaginal delivery
I & O	intake and output	N & V	nausea and vomiting
IOP	intraocular pressure	NWB	non weight bearing
IPPB	intermittent positive pressure breathing	O_2	oxygen
ITP	idiopathic thrombocytopenic purpura	OA	osteoarthritis, occiput anterior
IU	international unit	OB	obstetrics
IUD	intrauterine device	OBS	organic brain syndrome
IV	intravenous	OD	right eye
IVP	intravenous pyelogram	od	daily
		OOB	out of bed
jt.	joint	OP	occiput posterior
		OS	left eye
K	potassium	OT	occupational therapy
kg.	kilogram	OTC	over the counter
KVO	keep vein open	OU	both eyes
		oz.	ounce
L	left		
L(x)	L followed by a number indicates a specific lumbar vertebra	P	pulse
		$\bar{p}$	after
l	liter	PA	pernicious anemia
lat.	lateral	P & A	percussion and auscultation
lb.	pound	PAC	premature atrial contractions
LBP	low back pain, low blood pressure	PAP	Papanicolaou (test)
LE	lupus erythematosus, lower extremity	para	number of pregnancies
LGA	large for gestational age	p.c.	after meals
LLE	left lower extremity	pct.	percent
LLL	left lower lobe	PDR	Physician's Desk Reference
LLQ	left lower quadrant	PE	physical examination
LMP	last menstrual period	P.E.	physical examination, pulmonary embolism
LOA	left occiput anterior		
LOM	limitation of motion	PERLA	pupils equal, react to light and accommodation
LOP	left occiput posterior		
LOT	left occiput transverse	PH	past history
LP	lumbar puncture	PI	present illness
LQ	lower quadrant	PID	pelvic inflammatory disease
LUE	left upper extremity	PKU	phenylketonuria
LUL	left upper lobe	PM	afternoon
LUQ	left upper quadrant	P.M.	perceptual motor

Table continued on following page

ABBREVIATIONS COMMONLY USED BY HOSPITALS Continued

PMH	past medical history	SGPT	serum glutamic-pyruvic transaminase
PMP	previous menstrual period	SH	social history, serum hepatitis
PND	paroxysmal noctural dyspnea	sib.	sibling
p.o.	by mouth	SID	sudden infant death syndrome
P.O.R.	problem oriented record	SIDS	sudden infant death syndrome
pp	post partum, postprandial	sig.	label
PPD	purified protein derivative (tuberculin)	SLE	systemic lupus erythematosus
pr	per rectum	SNF	skilled nursing facility
PRE	progressive resistive exercise	S.O.A.P.	subjective, objective, assessment, plan
prn	as needed	SOB	shortness of breath
PROM	passive range of motion	s/p	status post
pro time	prothrombin time	SPF	sun protection factor
PSS	physiologic saline solution	sp. gr.	specific gravity
pt.	patient, pint	ss	one half
PT	prothrombin time, physical therapy	SSE	soapsuds enema
PTA	prior to admission	S&Sx	signs and symptoms
PTT	partial thromboplastin time	stat	immediately
PVC	premature ventricular contraction	STS	serologic test for syphilis
PWB	partial weight bearing	sub. q.	subcutaneous
		SUID	sudden unexplained infant death
q	every	SVD	spontaneous vaginal delivery
qd	every day	SVT	supraventricular tachycardia
qh	every hour	Sx.	symptoms
q.n.s.	quantity not sufficient		
q.o.d.	every other day	T.	tablespoon
q.s.	quantity sufficient	T(x)	T followed by a number indicates a specific thoracic vertebra
qt.	quart	TB	tuberculosis
		tbsp	tablespoon
RA	rheumatoid arthritis	TIA	transient ischemic attack
RBC	red blood cell count	t.i.d.	three times a day
RDA	recommended dietary allowance	T.O.	telephone order
RDS	respiratory distress syndrome	TPR	temperature, pulse, respiration
Rh	Rhesus factor	tsp.	teaspoon
RHD	rheumatic heart disease	TUR	transurethral resection
RLE	right lower extremity		
RLL	right lower lobe	U	unit
RLQ	right lower quadrant	UA	urinalysis
RML	right middle lobe	UE	upper extremity
r/o	rule out	ung.	ointment
ROA	right occiput anterior	UQ	upper quadrant
ROM	range of motion	URI	upper respiratory infection
ROP	right occiput posterior	UTI	urinary tract infection
ROS	review of systems	VA	Veterans Administration
ROT	right occiput transverse	VD	veneral disease
RPRC	rapid plasma reagin card test (for syphilis)	V.O.	verbal order
		v.s.	vital signs
RR	respiratory rate		
rt.	right	WBAT	weight bearing as tolerated
RUE	right upper extremity	WBC	white blood cell count
RUL	right upper lobe	w.b.c.	white blood cell
RUQ	right upper quadrant	w/c	wheel chair
Rx	treatment, therapy, prescription	WDWN	well developed, well nourished
		wk.	week
s̄	without	WNL	within normal limits
sc.	subcutaneous	wo	without
SGA	small for gestational age	wt.	weight
SGOT	serum glutamic-oxaloacetic transaminase	x	times

From Miller BF, Keane CB: *Encyclopedia and Dictionary of Medicine, Nursing, and Allied Health*, 5th ed. Philadelphia: W.B. Saunders, 1992, pp. 1733–1735.

B-2
ACRONYMS FOR SELECTED HEALTH CARE ORGANIZATIONS, ASSOCIATIONS, AND AGENCIES

AAAA	American Academy of Anesthesiologist's Assistants
AAATP	Association for Anesthesiologist's Assistants Training Program
AAB	American Association of Bioanalysts
AABB	American Association of Blood Banks
AACAHPO	American Association of Certified Allied Health Personnel in Ophthalmology
AACC	American Association for Clinical Chemistry
AACCN	American Association of Critical Care Nurses
AACN	American Association of Colleges of Nursing
AADS	American Association of Dental Schools
AAFP	American Academy of Family Physicians
AAHA	American Academy of Health Administration
AAHC	Association of Academic Health Centers
AAHE	Association for the Advancement of Health Education
AAHP	American Association of Hospital Planners
AAHPER	American Association for Health, Physical Education, and Recreation
AAMA	American Association of Medical Assistants
AAMC	Association of American Medical Colleges
AAMI	Association for the Advancement of Medical Instrumentation
AAMT	American Association for Music Therapy
AAN	American Academy of Neurology
AANA	American Association of Nurse Anesthetists
AAO	American Association of Ophthalmology
AAO	American Association of Orthodontists
AAOHN	American Association of Occupational Health Nurses
AAP	American Academy of Pediatrics
AAPA	American Academy of Physicians Assistants
AAPMR	American Academy of Physical Medicine and Rehabilitation
AARC	American Association for Respiratory Care
AART	American Association for Rehabilitation Therapy
AATA	American Art Therapy Association
AATS	American Association for Thoracic Surgery
ABCP	American Board of Cardiovascular Perfusion
ABNF	Association of Black Nursing Faculty in Higher Education
ACC	American College of Cardiology
ACCP	American College of Chest Physicians
ACEP	American College of Emergency Physicians
ACHA	American College of Hospital Administrators
ACNM	American College of Nurse-Midwives
ACP	American College of Physicians
ACR	American College of Radiology
ACS	American College of Surgeons
ACTA	American Cardiovascular Technologists Association
ACTA	American Corrective Therapy Association
ADA	American Dental Association
ADA	American Dietetic Association
ADAA	American Dental Assistants Association
ADHA	American Dental Hygienists' Association
ADTA	American Dance Therapy Association
AES	American Electroencephalographic Society
AHA	American Hospital Association
AHPA	American Health Planning Association
AIBS	American Institute of Biological Sciences
AIHA	American Industrial Hygiene Association
AIUM	American Institute of Ultrasound in Medicine
AMA	American Medical Association
AMEA	American Medical Electroencephalographic Association
AMI	Association of Medical Illustrators
AmSECT	American Society of Extra-Corporeal Technology
AMT	American Medical Technologists
ANA	American Nurses Association
ANF	American Nurses Foundation
ANRC	American National Red Cross
AOA	American Optometric Association
AOA	American Osteopathic Association
AONE	American Organization of Nurse Executives
AORN	Association of Operating Room Nurses
AOTA	American Occupational Therapy Association
APA	American Podiatry Association

Table continued on following page

B-2
ACRONYMS FOR SELECTED HEALTH CARE ORGANIZATIONS, ASSOCIATIONS, AND AGENCIES Continued

APA	American Psychiatric Association
APA	American Psychological Association
APAP	Association of Physician Assistants Programs
APHA	American Public Health Association
APIC	Association of Practioners in Infection Control
APTA	American Physical Therapy Association
ARCA	American Rehabilitation Counseling Association
ARN	Association of Rehabilitation Nurses
ASA	American Society of Anesthesiologists
ASAHP	American Society of Allied Health Professionals
ASC	American Society of Cytotechnology
ASCP	American Society of Clinical Pathologists
ASE	American Society of Echocardiography
ASET	American Society of Electroencephalographic Technologists
ASHA	American Speech and Hearing Association
ASIA	American Spinal Injury Association
ASIM	American Society of Internal Medicine
ASM	American Society of Microbiology
ASMT	American Society for Medical Technology
ASNSA	American Society of Nursing Service Administrators
ASPAN	American Association of Post Anesthesia Nurses
ASPH	Association of Schools of Public Health
ASRT	American Society of Radiologic Technologists
AST	Association of Surgical Technologists
ASUTS	American Society of Ultrasound Technical Specialists
ATS	American Thoracic Society
AUPHA	Association of University Programs in Health Administration
AVA	American Vocational Association
AVMA	American Veterinary Medical Association
CAP	College of American Pathologists
CAHEA (AMA)	Committee on Allied Health Education and Accreditation
CDC	Centers for Disease Control
CGFNS	Commission on Graduates of Foreign Nursing Schools
CGNA	Canadian Gerontological Nursing Association
CME(AMA)	Council on Medical Education of the American Medical Association
CNA	Canadian Nurses Association
COEAMRA	Council on Education of the American Medical Record Association
DHHS	Department of Health and Human Services
ENA	Emergency Nurses Association
FDA	Food and Drug Administration
HCFA	Health Care Financing Administration
HRA	Health Resources Administration
HSCA	Health Sciences Communications Association
HSRA	Health Services and Resources Administration
IAET	International Association for Enterostomal Therapy
ISCV	International Society for Cardiovascular Surgery
JCAHO	Joint Commission on the Accreditation of Healthcare Organizations
JCAHPO	Joint Commission on Allied Health Personnel in Ophthalmology
MLA	Medical Library Association
NAACLS	National Accrediting Agency for Clinical Laboratory Science
NAACOG	Nurses Association of the American Association of Obstetrics and Gynecology
NACA	National Advisory Council on Aging—Canadian
NACT	National Alliance of Cardiovascular Technologists
NADONA/LTC	National Association of Directors of Nursing Administration in Long Term Care
NAEMT	National Association of Emergency Medical Technicians
NAHC	National Association of Home Care
NAHM	National Association for Mental Health
NAHSR	National Association of Human Services Technologists
NAMT	National Association for Music Therapy
NANDA	North American Nursing Diagnosis Association
NANPHR	National Association of Nurse Practitioners in Reproductive Health
NAPNES	National Association for Practical Nurse Education and Services
NARF	National Association of Rehabilitation Facilities
NASW	National Association of Social Workers
NATTS	National Association of Trade and Technical Schools
NCEHPHP	National Council on the Education of Health Professionals in Health Promotion

B-2
ACRONYMS FOR SELECTED HEALTH CARE ORGANIZATIONS, ASSOCIATIONS, AND AGENCIES Continued

NCRE	National Council on Rehabilitation Education
NEHA	National Environmental Health Education
NFLPN	National Federation of Licensed Practical Nurses
NHC	National Health Council
NIH	National Institutes of Health
NIOSH	National Institute of Occupational Safety and Health
NLN	National League for Nursing
NNBA	National Nurses in Business Association
NRCA	National Rehabilitation Counseling Association
NREMT	National Registry of Emergency Medical Technicians
NSCPT	National Society for Cardiopulmonary Technology
NSH	National Society for Histotechnology
NSNA	National Student Nurses Association
NTRS	National Therapeutic Recreation Society
OAA	Opticians Association of America
ONS	Oncology Nurses Association
SAAABB	Subcommittee on Accreditation of the American Association of Blood Banks
SDMS	Society of Diagnostic Medical Sonographers
SNIVT	Society of Non-Invasive Vascular Technology
SNM	Society of Nuclear Medicine
SNM-TS	Society for Nuclear Medicine—Technologists Section
SPHE	Society of Public Health Educators
STS	Society of Thoracic Surgeons
SVS	Society for Vascular Surgery
TAANA	American Association of Nurse Attorneys
USPHS	United States Public Health Services
VA	Veterans Administration
WHO	World Health Organization

From Miller BF, Keane CB: *Encyclopedia and Dictionary of Medicine, Nursing, and Allied Health,* 5th ed. Philadelphia: W.B. Saunders, 1992, pp. 1754–1756.

B-3
ALPHABET SOUP OF HEALTH CARE

There are a variety of health care providers and insurers that are referred to only by letter. When these terms are being discussed together, they are often referred to as the alphabet soup of health care.

BC/BS—Blue Cross, Blue Shield, a national insurance organization that makes payments for a wide variety of health care services for its subscribers. Frequently referred to as the "Blues."

CHAMPUS—the civilian health and medical program of the uniformed services, a program that is administered by the Department of Defense. CHAMPUS pays for health care services to active and retired members of the uniformed services and reimburses providers for the health care of the dependents of eligible personnel.

HMO—health maintenance organization, an organization that provides preventive health services as well as medical, hospital, and emergency care for members. There is a fee, paid in advance, to belong to a HMO.

IPA—Independent Practice Association, a type of health maintenance organization in which the organization contracts with physicians who see patients in their own offices, rather than at a specific location designated as an HMO. The physicians are reimbursed by the HMO.

Medicare, Part A—Title XVIII of Health Insurance for the Aged of the Social Security Act. Medicare, Part A reimburses the hospital for services provided to eligible patients.

Medicare, Part B—Title XVIII of Health Insurance for the Aged of the Social Security Act. Medicare, Part B reimburses physicians for service provided to eligible patients. This insurance is provided to eligible citizens only when a supplementry payment is made.

PPO—Preferred Provider Organization, an association of hospitals, physicians, and agencies that provides health care to a specific group of individuals at agreed-upon rates.

From Miller BF, Keane CB: *Encyclopedia and Dictionary of Medicine, Nursing, and Allied Health,* 5th ed. Philadelphia: W.B. Saunders, p. 1748.

B-4
COMBINING FORMS IN MEDICAL TERMINOLOGY

Combining Forms In Medical Terminology*

The following is a list of combining forms encountered frequently in the vocabulary of medicine. A dash or dashes are appended to indicate whether the form usually precedes (as *ante-*) or follows (as *-agra*) the other elements of the compound or usually appears between the other elements (as *-em-*). Following each combining form, the first item of information is the Greek or Latin word, or both a Greek and a Latin word, from which it is derived. Greek words have been transliterated into Roman characters. Latin words are identified by [L.], Greek words by [Gr.]. Information necessary to an understanding of the form appears next in parentheses. Then the meaning or meanings of the words are given, followed where appropriate by reference to a synonymous combining form. Finally, an example is given to illustrate the use of the combining form in a compound English derivative.

a-	*a-* [L.] (*n* is added before words beginning with a vowel) negative prefix. Cf. in-³. *a*metria	-agogue	*agōgos* [Gr.] leading, inducing. galact*agogue*
ab-	*ab* [L.] away from. Cf. apo-. *ab*ducent	-agra	*agra* [Gr.] catching, seizure. po*dagra*
abdomin-	*abdomen, abdominis* [L.] abdomen. *abdomin*oscopy	alb-	*albus* [L.] white. Cf. leuk-. *alb*ocinereous
ac-	See ad-. *ac*cretion	alg-	*algos* [Gr.] pain. neur*alg*ia
acet-	*acetum* [L.] vinegar. *acet*ometer	all-	*allos* [Gr.] other, different. *al*lergy
acid-	*acidus* [L.] sour. *acid*uric	alve-	*alveus* [L.] trough, channel, cavity. *alve*olar
acou-	*akouō* [Gr.] hear. *acou*ethesia. (Also spelled acu-)	amph-	See amphi-. *amph*eclexis
acr-	*akron* [Gr.] extremity, peak. *acr*omegaly	amphi-	*amphi* [Gr.] (*i* is dropped before words beginning with a vowel) both, doubly. *amphi*celous
act-	*ago, actus* [L.] do, drive, act. re*act*ion	amyl-	*amylon* [Gr.] starch. *amyl*osynthesis
actin-	*aktis, aktinos* [Gr.] ray, radius. Cf. radi-. *actin*ogenesis	an-¹	See ana-. *an*agogic
acu-	See acou-. oste*oacu*sis	an-²	See a-. *an*omalous
ad-	*ad* [L.] (*d* changes to *c, f, g, p, s,* or *t* before words beginning with those consonants) to. *ad*renal	ana-	*ana* [Gr.] (final *a* is dropped before words beginning with a vowel) up, positive. *ana*phoresis
aden-	*adēn* [Gr.] gland. Cf. gland-. *aden*oma	ancyl-	See ankyl-. *ancyl*ostomiasis
adip-	*adeps, adipis* [L.] fat. Cf. lip- and stear-. *adip*ocellular	andr-	*anēr, andros* [Gr.] man. gyn*andr*oid
aer-	*aēr* [Gr.] air. an*aer*obiosis	angi-	*angeion* [Gr.] vessel. Cf. vas-. *angi*emphraxis
aesthe-	See esthe-. *aesthe*sioneurosis	ankyl-	*ankylos* [Gr.] crooked, looped. *ankylo*dactylia. (Also spelled ancyl-)
af-	See ad-. *af*ferent		
ag-	See ad-. *ag*glutinant		

*Compiled by Lloyd W. Daly, A.M., Ph.D., Litt. D., Allen Memorial Professor of Greek Emeritus, University of Pennsylvania.

Table continued on following page

B-4

COMBINING FORMS IN MEDICAL TERMINOLOGY Continued

ant-	See anti-. *ant*ophthalmic	cac-	*kakos* [Gr.] bad, abnormal. Cf. mal*cac*odontia, arthro*cac*e. (See also dys-)
ante-	*ante* [L.] before. *ante*flexion		
anti-	*anti* [Gr.] (*i* is dropped before words beginning with a vowel) against, counter. Cf. contra*anti*pyogenic	calc-¹	*calx, calcis* [L.] stone (cf. lith-), limestone, lime. *calc*ipexy
		calc-²	*calx, calcis* [L.] heel. *calc*aneotibial
antr-	*antron* [Gr.] cavern. *antro*dynia	calor-	*calor* [L.] heat. Cf. therm-. *cal*orimeter
ap-¹	See apo-. *ap*heter	cancr-	*cancer, cancri* [L.] crab, cancer. Cf. carcin-. *cancr*ology. (Also spelled chancr-)
ap-²	See ad-. *ap*pend		
-aph-	*haptō, haph-* [Gr.] touch. dys*aph*ia. (See also hapt-)	capit-	*caput, capitis* [L.] head. Cf. cephal-. de*capit*ator
apo-	*apo* [Gr.] (*o* is dropped before words beginning with a vowel) away from, detached. Cf. ab-. *apo*physis	caps-	*capsa* [L.] (from *capio*; see cept-) container. en*caps*ulation
		carbo(n)-	*carbo, carbonis* [L.] coal, charcoal. *carbo*hydrate, *carbon*uria
arachn-	*arachnē* [Gr.] spider. *arachno*dactyly		
arch-	*archē* [Gr.] beginning, origin. *arch*enteron	carcin-	*karkinos* [Gr.] crab, cancer. Cf. cancr-. *carcin*oma
arter(i)-	*arteria* [Gr.] windpipe, artery. *arterio*sclerosis, peri*arter*itis	cardi-	*kardia* [Gr.] heart. lipo*cardi*ac
		cary-	See kary-. *cary*okinesis
arthr-	*arthron* [Gr.] joint. Cf. articul-. syn*arthr*osis	cat-	See cata-. *cat*hode
articul-	*articulus* [L.] joint. Cf. arthr-. dis*articul*ation	cata-	*kata* [Gr.] (final *a* is dropped before words beginning with a vowel) down, negative. *cat*abatic
as-	See ad-. *as*similation		
at-	See ad-. *at*trition	caud-	*cauda* [L.] tail. *caud*ad
aur-	*auris* [L.] ear. Cf. ot-. *aur*inasal	cav-	*cavus* [L.] hollow. Cf. coel-. con*cav*e
aux-	*auxō* [Gr.] increase. enter*aux*e		
ax-	*axōn* [Gr.] or *axis* [L.] axis. *ax*ofugal	cec-	*caecus* [L.] blind. Cf. typhl-. *cec*opexy
		cel-¹	See coel-. amphi*cel*ous
axon-	*axōn* [Gr.] axis. *axon*ometer	cel-²	See -cele. *cel*ectome
ba-	*bainō, ba-* [Gr.] go, walk, stand. hypno*ba*tia	-cele	*kēlē* [Gr.] tumor, hernia. gastro*cele*
bacill-	*bacillus* [L.] small staff, rod. Cf. bacter-. actino*bacill*osis	cell-	*cella* [L.] room, cell. Cf. cyt-. *cell*iferous
bacter-	*bactērion* [Gr.] small staff, rod. Cf. bacill-. *bacter*iophage	cen-	*koinos* [Gr.] common. *cen*esthesia
ball-	*ballō, bol-* [Gr.] throw. *ball*istics. (See also bol-)	cent-	*centum* [L.] hundred. Cf. hect-. Indicates fraction in metric system. [This exemplifies the custom in the metric system of identifying fractions of units by stems from the Latin, as centimeter, decimeter, millimeter, and multiples of units by the similar stems from the Greek, as hectometer, decameter, and kilometer.] *cent*imeter, *cent*ipede
bar-	*baros* [Gr.] weight. pedo*bar*ometer		
bi-¹	*bios* [Gr.] life. Cf. vit-. aero*bi*c		
bi-²	*bi-* [L.] two (see also di-¹). *bi*lobate		
bil-	*bilis* [L.] bile. Cf. chol-. *bil*iary		
blast-	*blastos* [Gr.] bud, child, a growing thing in its early stages. Cf. germ-. *blast*oma, zygoto*blast*		
blep-	*blepō* [Gr.] look, see. hemia*blep*sia		
		cente-	*kenteō* [Gr.] to puncture. Cf. punct-. entero*cente*sis
blephar-	*blepharon* [Gr.] (from *blepō*; see blep-) eyelid. Cf. cili-. *blephar*oncus	centr-	*kentron* [Gr.] or *centrum* [L.] point, center. neuro*centr*al
		cephal-	*kephalē* [Gr.] head. Cf. capit-. en*cephal*itis
bol-	See ball-. em*bol*ism		
brachi-	*brachiōn* [Gr.] arm. *brachio*cephalic	cept-	*capio, -cipientis, -ceptus* [L.] take, receive. re*cept*or
brachy-	*brachys* [Gr.] short. *brachy*cephalic	cer-	*kēros* [Gr.] or *cera* [L.] wax. *cer*oplasty, *cer*omel
brady-	*bradys* [Gr.] slow. *brady*cardia	cerat-	See kerat-. a*cerat*osis
brom-	*brōmos* [Gr.] stench. podo*brom*idrosis	cerebr-	*cerebrum* [L.] brain. *cerebro*spinal
bronch-	*bronchos* [Gr.] windpipe. *bron*choscopy		
bry-	*bryō* [Gr.] be full of life. em*bry*onic		
bucc-	*bucca* [L.] cheek. disto*bucc*al		

COMBINING FORMS IN MEDICAL TERMINOLOGY Continued

cervic-	*cervix, cervicis* [L.] neck. Cf. trachel-. *cervic*itis	creat-	*kreas, kreato-* [Gr.] meat, flesh. *creat*orrhea
chancr-	See cancr-. *chancr*iform	-crescent	*cresco, crescentis, cretus* [L.] grow. ex*crescent*
cheil-	*cheilos* [Gr.] lip. Cf. labi-. *chei*loschisis	cret-¹	*cerno, cretus* [L.] distinguish, separate off. Cf. crin-. dis*crete*
cheir-	*cheir* [Gr.] hand. Cf. man-. mac*rocheir*ia. (Also spelled chir-)	cret-²	See -crescent. ac*cret*ion
chir-	See cheir-. *chir*omegaly	crin-	*krinō* [Gr.] distinguish, separate off. Cf. cret-¹. endo*crin*ology
chlor-	*chlōros* [Gr.] green. a*chlor*opsia		
chol-	*cholē* [Gr.] bile. Cf. bil-. hepato*chol*angeitis	crur-	*crus, cruris* [L.] shin, leg. brachio*crur*al
chondr-	*chondros* [Gr.] cartilage. *chondr*omalacia	cry-	*kryos* [Gr.] cold. *cry*esthesia
chord-	*chordē* [Gr.] string, cord. peri*chord*al	crypt-	*kryptō* [Gr.] hide, conceal. *crypt*orchism
chori-	*chorion* [Gr.] protective fetal membrane. endo*chori*on	cult-	*colo, cultus* [L.] tend, cultivate. *cult*ure
chro-	*chrōs* [Gr.] color. poly*chro*matic	cune-	*cuneus* [L.] wedge. Cf. sphen-. *cune*iform
chron-	*chronos* [Gr.] time. syn*chron*ous	cut-	*cutis* [L.] skin. Cf. derm(at)-. sub*cut*aneous
chy-	*cheō, chy-* [Gr.] pour. ec*chy*mosis	cyan-	*kyanos* [Gr.] blue. antho*cyan*in
-cid(e)	*caedo, -cisus* [L.] cut, kill. infanti*cide*, germi*cid*al	cycl-	*kyklos* [Gr.] circle, cycle. *cyclo*phoria
cili-	*cilium* [L.] eyelid. Cf. blephar-. super*cili*ary	cyst-	*kystis* [Gr.] bladder. Cf. vesic-. nephro*cyst*itis
cine-	See kine-. auto*cine*sis	cyt-	*kytos* [Gr.] cell. Cf. cell-. plasmo*cyt*oma
-cipient	See cept-. in*cipient*	dacry-	*dakry* [Gr.] tear. *dacry*ocyst
circum-	*circum* [L.] around. Cf. peri-. *circum*ferential	dactyl-	*daktylos* [Gr.] finger, toe. Cf. digit-. hexa*dactyl*ism
-cis-	*caedo, -cisus* [L.] cut, kill. ex*cis*ion	de-	*de* [L.] down from. *de*composition
clas-	*klaō* [Gr.] break. cranio*clas*t	dec-¹	*deka* [Gr.] ten. Indicates multiple in metric system. Cf. dec-². *dec*agram
clin-	*klinō* [Gr.] bend, incline, make lie down. *clin*ometer	dec-²	*decem* [L.] ten. Indicates fraction in metric system. Cf. dec-¹. *dec*ipara, *dec*imeter
clus-	*claudo, -clusus* [L.] shut. Maloc*clus*ion		
co-	See con-. *co*hesion	dendr-	*dendron* [Gr.] tree. neuro*dendr*ite
cocc-	*kokkos* [Gr.] seed, pill. gono*cocc*us	dent-	*dens, dentis* [L.] tooth. Cf. odont-. inter*dent*al
coel-	*koilos* [Gr.] hollow. Cf. cav-. *coel*enteron. (Also spelled cel-)	derm(at)-	*derma, dermatos* [Gr.] skin. Cf. cut-. endo*derm*, *dermat*itis
col-¹	See colon-. *col*ic	desm-	*desmos* [Gr.] band, ligament. syn*desm*opexy
col-²	See con-. *col*lapse	dextr-	*dexter, dextr-* [L.] right-hand. ambi*dextr*ous
colon-	*kolon* [Gr.] lower intestine. *colon*ic	di-¹	*di-* [Gr.] two. *di*morphic. (See also bi-²)
colp-	*kolpos* [Gr.] hollow, vagina. Cf. sin-. endo*colp*itis	di-²	See dia-. *di*uresis
com-	See con-. *com*masculation	di-³	See dis-. *di*vergent
con-	*con-* [L.] (becomes co- before vowels or *h*; col- before *l*; com- before *b, m,* or *p*; cor- before *r*) with, together. Cf. syn-. *con*traction	dia-	*dia* [Gr.] (*a* is dropped before words beginning with a vowel) through, apart. Cf. per-. *dia*gnosis
		didym-	*didymos* [Gr.] twin. Cf. gemin-. epi*didym*al
contra-	*contra* [L.] against, counter. Cf. anti-. *contra*indication	digit-	*digitus* [L.] finger, toe. Cf. dactyl-. *digit*igrade
copr-	*kopros* [Gr.] dung. Cf. sterco-. *copr*oma	diplo-	*diploos* [Gr.] double. *diplo*myelia
cor-₁	*korē* [Gr.] doll, little image, pupil. iso*cor*ia	dis-	*dis-* [L.] (*s* may be dropped before a word beginning with a consonant) apart, away from. *dis*location
cor-²	See con-. *cor*rugator		
corpor-	*corpus, corporis* [L.] body. Cf. somat-. intra*corpor*al		
cortic-	*cortex, corticis* [L.] bark, rind. *cortic*osterone		
cost-	*costa* [L.] rib. Cf. pleur-. inter*cost*al		
crani-	*kranion* [Gr.] or *cranium* [L.] skull. peri*crani*um		

Table continued on following page

COMBINING FORMS IN MEDICAL TERMINOLOGY Continued

disc-	*diskos* [Gr.] or *discus* [L.] disk. *disc*oplacenta	-fect-	See -facient. de*fect*ive
dors-	*dorsum* [L.] back. ventro*dors*al	-ferent	*fero, ferentis, latus* [L.] bear, carry. Cf. phor-. ef*ferent*
drom-	*dromos* [Gr.] course. hemo*dro*mometer	ferr-	*ferrum* [L.] iron. *ferr*oprotein
-ducent	See duct-. ad*ducent*	fibr-	*fibra* [L.] fiber. Cf. in-¹. chondro*fibr*oma
-duct	*duco, ducentis, ductus* [L.] lead, conduct. ovi*duct*	fil-	*filum* [L.] thread. *fil*iform
dur-	*durus* [L.] hard. Cf. scler-. in*dur*ation	fiss-	*findo, fissus* [L.] split. Cf. schis-. *fiss*ion
dynam(i)-	*dynamis* [Gr.] power. *dynam*oneure, neuro*dynam*ic	flagell-	*flagellum* [L.] whip. *flagell*ation
dys-	*dys-* [Gr.] bad, improper. Cf. mal-. *dys*trophic. (See also cac-)	flav-	*flavus* [L.] yellow. Cf. xanth-. ribo*flav*in
e-	*e* [L.] out from. Cf. ec- and ex-. *e*mission	-flect-	*flecto, flexus* [L.] bend, divert. de*flect*ion
ec-	*ek* [Gr.] out of. Cf. e- *ec*centric	-flex-	See -flect-. re*flex*ometer
-ech-	*echō* [Gr.] have, hold, be. syn*ech*otomy	flu-	*fluo, fluxus* [L.] flow. Cf. rhe-. *flu*id
ect-	*ektos* [Gr.] outside. Cf. extra-. *ect*oplasm	flux-	See flu-. af*flux*ion
ede-	*oideō* [Gr.] swell. *ede*matous	for-	*foris* [L.] door, opening. per*fo*rated
ef-	See ex-. *ef*florescent	-form	*forma* [L.] shape. Cf. oid. ossi*form*
-elc-	*helkos* [Gr.] sore, ulcer. enter*elc*osis. (See also helc-)	fract-	*frango, fractus* [L.] break. re*fract*ive
electr-	*ēlectron* [Gr.] amber. *electr*otherapy	front-	*frons, frontis* [L.] forehead, front. naso*front*al
em-	See en-. *em*bolism, *em*pathy, *em*physis	-fug(e)	*fugio* [L.] flee, avoid. vermi*fuge*, centri*fug*al
-em-	*haima* [Gr.] blood. an*em*ia. (See also hem(at)-)	funct-	*fungor, functus* [L.] perform, serve, function. mal*funct*ion
en-	*en* [Gr.] (*n* changes to *m* before *b, p* or *ph*) in, on. Cf. in-². *en*celitis	fund-	*fundo, fusus* [L.] pour. in*fund*ibulum
end-	*endon* [Gr.] inside. Cf. intra-. *end*angium	fus-	See fund-. dif*fus*ible
enter-	*enteron* [Gr.] intestine. dys*enter*y	galact-	*gala, galactos* [Gr.] milk. Cf. lact-. dys*galact*ia
ep-	See epi-. *ep*axial	gam-	*gamos* [Gr.] marriage, reproductive union. a*gam*ont
epi-	*epi* [Gr.] (*i* is dropped before words beginning with a vowel) upon, after, in addition. *epi*glottis	gangli-	*ganglion* [Gr.] swelling, plexus. neuro*gangli*itis
erg-	*ergon* [Gr.] work, deed. en*erg*y	gastr-	*gastēr, gastros* [Gr.] stomach. cholangio*gastr*ostomy
erythr-	*erythros* [Gr.] red. Cf. rub(r)-. *erythr*ochromia	gelat-	*gelo, gelatus* [L.] freeze, congeal. *gelat*in
eso-	*esō* [Gr.] inside. Cf. intra-. *eso*phylactic	gemin-	*geminus* [L.] twin, double. Cf. didym-. quadri*gemin*al
esthe-	*aisthanomai, aisthē-* [Gr.] perceive, feel. Cf. sens-. an*esthe*sia	gen-	*gignomai, gen-, gon-* [Gr.] become, be produced, originate, or *gennaō* [Gr.] produce, originate. cyto*gen*ic
eu-	*eu* [Gr.] good, normal. *eu*pepsia	germ-	*germen, germinis* [L.] bud, a growing thing in its early stages. Cf. blast-. *germ*inal, ovi*germ*
ex-	*ex* [Gr.] or *ex* [L.] out of. Cf. e-. *ex*cretion	gest-	*gero, gerentis, gestus* [L.] bear, carry. con*gest*ion
exo-	*exō* [Gr.] outside. Cf. extra-. *exo*pathic	gland-	*glans, glandis* [L.] acorn. Cf. aden-. intra*gland*ular
extra-	*extra* [L.] outside of, beyond. Cf. ect- and exo-. *extra*cellular	-glia	*glia* [Gr.] glue. neuro*glia*
faci-	*facies* [L.] face. Cf. prosop-. brachio*faci*olingual	gloss-	*glōssa* [Gr.] tongue. Cf. lingu-. tricho*gloss*ia
-facient	*facio, facientis, factus, -fectus* [L.] make. Cf. poie-. cale*facient*	glott-	*glōtta* [Gr.] tongue, language. *glott*ic
-fact-	See facient-. arte*fact*	gluc-	See glyc(y)-. *gluc*ophenetidin
fasci-	*fascia* [L.] band. *fasci*orrhaphy	glutin-	*gluten, glutinis* [L.] glue. ag*glutin*ation
febr-	*febris* [L.] fever. Cf. pyr-. *febr*icide	glyc(y)-	*glykys* [Gr.] sweet. *glyc*emia, *glycy*rrhizin. (Also spelled gluc-)

B-4
COMBINING FORMS IN MEDICAL TERMINOLOGY Continued

gnath-	*gnathos* [Gr.] jaw. ortho*gnath*ous
gno-	*gignōsiō, gnō-* [Gr.] know, discern. dia*gno*sis
gon-	See gen-. anphi*gon*y
grad-	*gradior* [L.] walk, take steps. retro*grad*e
-gram	*gramma* [Gr.] letter, drawing. cardio*gram*
gran-	*granum* [L.] grain, particle. lipo*gran*uloma
graph-	*graphō* [Gr.] scratch, write, record. histo*graph*y
grav-	*gravis* [L.] heavy. multi*grav*ida
gyn(ec)-	*gynē, gynaikos* [Gr.] woman, wife. andro*gyn*y, *gyn*ecologic
gyr-	*gyros* [Gr.] ring, circle. *gyr*ospasm
haem(at)-	See hem(at)-. *haem*orrhagia, *haemat*oxylon
hapt-	*haptō* [Gr.] touch. *hapt*ometer
hect-	*hekt-* [Gr.] hundred. Cf. cent-. Indicates multiple in metric system. *hect*ometer
helc-	*helkos* [Gr.] sore, ulcer. *helc*osis
hem(at)-	*haima, haimatos* [Gr.] blood. Cf. sanguin-. *hem*angioma, *hemat*ocyturia. (See also -em-)
hemi-	*hēmi-* [Gr.] half. Cf. semi-. *hemi*ageusia
hen-	*heis, henos* [Gr.] one. Cf. un-. *hen*ogenesis
hepat-	*hēpar, hēpatos* [Gr.] liver. gastro*hepat*ic
hept(a)-	*hepta* [Gr.] seven. Cf. sept-². *hept*atomic, *hept*avalent
hered-	*heres, heredis* [L.] heir. *hered*oimmunity
hex-¹	*hex* [Gr.] six. Cf. sex-. *hex*yl-. An *a* is added in some combinations
hex-²	*echō, hex-* [Gr.] (added to *s* becomes *hex*-) have, hold, be. cache*x*ia
hexa-	See hex-¹. *hexa*chromic
hidr-	*hidros* [Gr.] sweat. hyper*hidr*osis
hist-	*histos* [Gr.] web, tissue. *hist*odialysis
hod-	*hodos* [Gr.] road, path. *hod*oneuromere. (See also od- and -ode¹)
hom-	*homos* [Gr.] common, same. *hom*omorphic
horm-	*ormē* [Gr.] impetus, impulse. *horm*one
hydat-	*hydōr, hydatos* [Gr.] water. *hydat*ism
hydr-	*hydōr, hydr-* [Gr.] water. Cf. lymph-. anclor*hydr*ia
hyp-	See hypo-. *hyp*axial
hyper-	*hyper* [Gr.] above, beyond, extreme. Cf. super-. *hyper*trophy
hypn-	*hypnos* [Gr.] sleep. *hypn*otic
hypo-	*hypo* [Gr.] (*o* is dropped before words beginning with a vowel) under, below. Cf. sub-. *hypo*metabolism
hyster-	*hystera* [Gr.] womb. colpo*hyster*opexy
iatr-	*iatros* [Gr.] physician. ped*iatr*ics
idi-	*idios* [Gr.] peculiar, separate, distinct. *idi*osyncrasy
il-	See in-²,³. *il*linition (in, on), *il*legible (negative prefix)
ile-	See ili- [ile- is commonly used to refer to the portion of the intestines known as the ileum]. *ile*ostomy
ili-	*ilium (ileum)* [L.] lower abdomen, intestines [ili- is commonly used to refer to the flaring part of the hip bone known as the ilium]. *ili*osacral
im-	See in-²,³. *im*mersion (in, on), *im*perforation (negative prefix)
in-¹	*is, inos* [Gr.] fiber. Cf. fibr-. *in*osteatoma
in-²	*in* [L.] (*n* changes to *l, m,* or *r* before words beginning with those consonants) in, on. Cf. en-. *in*sertion
in-³	*in-* [L.] (*n* changes to *l, m,* or *r* before words beginning with those consonants) negative prefix. Cf. a-. *in*valid
infra-	*infra* [L.] beneath. *infra*orbital
insul-	*insula* [L.] island. *insul*in
inter-	*inter* [L.] among, between. *inter*carpal
intra-	*intra* [L.] inside. Cf. end- and eso-. *intra*venous
ir-	See in-²,³. *ir*radiation (in, on), *ir*reducible (negative prefix)
irid-	*iris, iridos* [Gr.] rainbow, colored circle. kerato*irid*ocyclitis
is-	*isos* [Gr.] equal. *is*otope
ischi-	*ischion* [Gr.] hip, haunch. *ischi*opubic
jact-	*iacio, iactus* [L.] throw. *jact*itation
-ject	*iacio, -iectus* [L.] throw. in*ject*ion
jejun-	*ieiunus* [L.] hungry, not partaking of food. gastro*jejun*ostomy
jug-	*iugum* [L.] yoke. con*jug*ation
junct-	*iungo, iunctus* [L.] yoke, join. con*junct*iva
kary-	*karyon* [Gr.] nut, kernel, nucleus. Cf. nucle-. mega*kary*ocyte. (Also spelled cary-)
kerat-	*keras, keratos* [Gr.] horn. *kerat*olysis. (Also spelled cerat-)
kil-	*chilioi* [Gr.] one thousand. Cf. mill-. Indicates multiple in metric system. *kil*ogram
kine-	*kineō* [Gr.] move. *kine*matograph. (Also spelled cine-)
labi-	*labium* [L.] lip. Cf. cheil-. gingivo*labi*al

Table continued on following page

COMBINING FORMS IN MEDICAL TERMINOLOGY Continued

lact-	*lac, lactis* [L.] milk. Cf. galact-. gluco*lact*one	mening-	*mēninx, mēningos* [Gr.] membrane. encephalo*mening*itis
lal-	*laleō* [Gr.] talk, babble. glosso*lal*ia	ment-	*mens, mentis* [L.] mind. Cf. phren-, psych- and thym-. de*ment*ia
lapar-	*lapara* [Gr.] flank. *lapar*otomy	mer-	*meros* [Gr.] part. poly*mer*ic
laryng-	*larynx, laryngos* [Gr.] windpipe. *laryng*endoscope	mes-	*mesos* [Gr.] middle. Cf. medi-. *mes*oderm
lat-	*fero, latus* [L.] bear, carry. See -ferent. trans*lat*ion	met-	See meta-. *met*allergy
later-	*latus, lateris* [L.] side. ventro*later*al	meta-	*meta* [Gr.] (*a* is dropped before words beginning with a vowel) after, beyond, accompanying. *meta*carpal
lent-	*lens, lentis* [L.] lentil. Cf. phac-. *lent*iconus	metr-¹	*metron* [Gr.] measure. stereo*metr*y
lep-	*lambanō, lēp-* [Gr.] take, seize. cata*lep*tic	metr-²	*metra* [Gr.] womb. endo*metr*itis
leuc-	See leuk-. *leuc*inuria	micr-	*mikros* [Gr.] small. photo*micr*ograph
leuk-	*leukos* [Gr.] white. Cf. alb-. *leuk*orrhea. (Also spelled leuc-)	mill-	*mille* [L.] one thousand. Cf. kil-. Indicates fraction in metric system. *mill*igram, *mill*ipede
lien-	*lien* [L.] spleen. Cf. splen-. *lien*ocele	miss-	See -mittent. intro*miss*ion
lig-	*ligo* [L.] tie, bind. *lig*ate	-mittent	*mitto, mittentis, missus* [L.] send. inter*mittent*
lingu-	*lingua* [L.] tongue. Cf. gloss-. sub*lingu*al	mne-	*mimnērcō, mnē-* [Gr.] remember. pseud*omne*sia
lip-	*lipos* [Gr.] fat. Cf. adip-. gly-co*lip*in	mon-	*monos* [Gr.] only, sole. *mon*oplegia
lith-	*lithos* [Gr.] stone. Cf. calc-¹. nephro*lith*otomy	morph-	*morphē* [Gr.] form, shape. poly*morph*onuclear
loc-	*locus* [L.] place. Cf. top-. *lo*comotion	mot-	*moveo, motus* [L.] move. vaso*mot*or
log-	*legō, log-* [Gr.] speak, give an account. *log*orrhea, embryo*log*y	my-	*mys, myos* [Gr.] muscle. ino-leio*my*oma
lumb-	*lumbus* [L.] loin. dorso*lumb*ar	-myces	*mykēs, mykētos* [Gr.] fungus. myelo*myces*
lute-	*luteus* [L.] yellow. Cf. xanth-. *lute*oma	myc(et)-	See -myces. asco*mycet*es, strepto*myc*in
ly-	*lyō* [Gr.] loose, dissolve. Cf. solut-. kerato*ly*sis	myel-	*myelos* [Gr.] marrow. polio*myel*itis
lymph-	*lympha* [Gr.] water. Cf. hydr-. *lymph*adenosis	myx-	*myxa* [Gr.] mucus. *myx*edema
macr-	*makros* [Gr.] long, large. *macr*omyeloblast	narc-	*narkē* [Gr.] numbness. topo*narc*osis
mal-	*malus* [L.] bad, abnormal. Cf. cac- and dys-. *mal*function	nas-	*nasus* [L.] nose. Cf. rhin-. palato*nas*al
malac-	*malakos* [Gr.] soft. osteo*malac*ia	ne-	*neos* [Gr.] new, young. *ne*ocyte
mamm-	*mamma* [L.] breast. Cf. mast-. sub*mamm*ary	necr-	*nekros* [Gr.] corpse. *necr*ocytosis
man-	*manus* [L.] hand. Cf. cheir-. *man*iphalanx	nephr-	*nephros* [Gr.] kidney. Cf. ren-. para*nephr*ic
mani-	*mania* [Gr.] mental aberration. *mani*graphy, klepto*mani*a	neur-	*neuron* [Gr.] nerve. esthesio*neur*e
mast-	*mastos* [Gr.] breast. Cf. mamm-. hyper*mast*ia	nod-	*nodus* [L] knot. *nod*osity
medi-	*medius* [L.] middle. Cf. mes-. *medi*frontal	nom-	*nomos* [Gr.] (from *nemō* deal out, distribute) law, custom. taxo*nom*y
mega-	*megas* [Gr.] great, large. Also indicates multiple (1,000,000) in metric system. *mega*colon, *mega*dyne. (See also megal-)	non-	*nona* [L.] nine. *non*acosane
		nos-	*nosos* [Gr.] disease. *nos*ology
megal-	*megas, megalou* [Gr.] great, large. acro*megal*y	nucle-	*nucleus* [L.] (from *nux, nucis* nut) kernel. Cf. kary-. *nucle*ide
mel-	*melos* [Gr.] limb, member. sym*mel*ia	nutri-	*nutrio* [L.] nourish. mal*nutri*tion
melan-	*melas, melanos* [Gr.] black. hippo*melan*in	ob-	*ob* [L.] (*b* changes to *c* before words beginning with that
men-	*mēn* [Gr.] month. dys*men*orrhea		

B-4
COMBINING FORMS IN MEDICAL TERMINOLOGY *Continued*

	consonant) against, toward, etc. ob*tuse*	pell-	*pellis* [L.] skin, hide. *pell*agra
oc-	See ob-. oc*clude*	-pellent	*pello, pellentis, pulsus* [L.] drive. re*pellent*
ocul-	*oculus* [L.] eye. Cf. ophthalm-. *ocul*omotor	pen-	*penomai* [Gr.] need, lack. erythrocyto*pen*ia
-od-	See -ode¹. peri*od*ic	pend-	*pendeo* [L.] hang down. ap*pend*ix
-ode¹	*hodos* [Gr.] road, path. cath*ode*. (See also hod-)	pent(a)-	*pente* [Gr.] five. Cf. quinque-. *pent*ose, *penta*ploid
-ode²	See -oid. nemat*ode*	peps-	*peptō, peps-* [Gr.] digest. brady*peps*ia
odont-	*odous, odontos* [Gr.] tooth. Cf. dent-. orth*odont*ia	pept-	*peptō* [Gr.] digest. dys*pept*ic
-odyn-	*odynē* [Gr.] pain, distress. gastr*odyn*ia	per-	*per* [L.] through. Cf. dia-. *per*nasal
-oid	*eidos* [Gr.] form. Cf. -form. hy*oid*	peri-	*peri* [Gr.] around. Cf. circum-. *peri*phery
-ol	See ole-. cholester*ol*	pet-	*peto* [L.] seek, tend toward. centri*pet*al
ole-	*oleum* [L.] oil. *ole*oresin	pex-	*pēgnumi, pēg-* [Gr.] (added to s becomes *pēx*) fix, make fast. hepato*pex*y
olig-	*oligos* [Gr.] few, small. *olig*ospermia		
omphal-	*omphalos* [Gr.] navel. peri*omphal*ic	pha-	*phēmi, pha-* [Gr.] say, speak. dys*pha*sia
onc-	*onkos* [Gr.] bulk, mass. hemat*onc*ometry	phac-	*phakos* [Gr.] lentil, lens. Cf. lent-. *phac*osclerosis. (Also spelled phak-)
onych-	*onyx, onychos* [Gr.] claw, nail. an*onych*ia	phag-	*phagein* [Gr.] eat. lipo*phag*ic
oo-	*ōon* [Gr.] egg. Cf. ov-. peri*oo*thecitis	phak-	See phac-. *phak*itis
op-	*horaō, op-* [Gr.] see. erythr*op*sia	phan-	See phen-. dia*phan*oscopy
ophthalm-	*ophthalmos* [Gr.] eye. Cf. ocul-. ex*ophthalm*ic	pharmac-	*pharmakon* [Gr.] drug. *pharmac*ognosy
or-	*os, oris* [L.] mouth. Cf. stom(at)-. intra*or*al	pharyng-	*pharynx, pharyng-* [Gr.] throat, glosso*pharyng*eal
orb-	*orbis* [L.] circle. sub*orb*ital	phen-	*phainō, phan-* [Gr.] show, be seen. phos*phen*e
orchi-	*orchis* [Gr.] testicle. Cf. test-. *orchi*opathy	pher-	*pherō, phor-* [Gr.] bear, support. peri*pher*y
organ-	*organon* [Gr.] implement, instrument. *organ*oleptic	phil-	*phileō* [Gr.] like, have affinity for. eosino*phil*ia
orth-	*orthos* [Gr.] straight, right, normal. *orth*opedics	phleb-	*phleps, phlebos* [Gr.] vein. peri*phleb*itis
oss-	*os, ossis* [L.] bone. Cf. ost(e)-. *oss*iphone	phleg-	*phlogō, phlog-* [Gr.] burn, inflame. adeno*phleg*mon
ost(e)-	*osteon* [Gr.] bone. Cf. oss-. en*ost*osis, *oste*anaphysis	phlog-	See phleg-. anti*phlog*istic
ot-	*ous, ōtos* [Gr.] ear. Cf. aur-. par*ot*id	phob-	*phobos* [Gr.] fear, dread. claustro*phob*ia
ov-	*ovum* [L.] egg. Cf. oo-. syn*ov*ia	phon-	*phōne* [Gr.] sound. echo*phon*y
oxy-	*oxys* [Gr.] sharp. *oxy*cephalic	phor-	See pher-. Cf. -ferent. exo*phor*ia
pachy(n)-	*pachynō* [Gr.] thicken. *pachy*derma, myo*pachyn*sis	phos-	See phot-. *phos*phorus
pag-	*pēgnymi, pag-* [Gr.] fix, make fast. thoraco*pag*us	phot-	*phōs, phōtos* [Gr.] light. *phot*erythrous
par-¹	*pario* [L.] bear, give birth to. primi*par*ous	phrag-	*phrassō, phrag-* [Gr.] fence, wall off, stop up. Cf. sept-¹. dia*phrag*m
par-²	See para-. *par*epigastric		
para-	*para* [Gr.] (final *a* is dropped before words beginning with a vowel) beside, beyond. *para*mastoid	phrax-	*phrassō, phrag-* [Gr.] (added to s becomes *phrax-*) fence, wall off, stop up. em*phrax*is
		phren-	*phrēn* [Gr.] mind, midriff. Cf. ment-. meta*phren*ia, meta*phren*on
part-	*pario, partus* [L.] bear, give birth to. *part*urition		
path-	*pathos* [Gr.] that which one undergoes, sickness. psycho*path*ic	phthi-	*phthinō* [Gr.] decay, waste away. *phthi*sis
		phy-	*phyō* [Gr.] beget, bring forth, produce, be by nature. noso*phy*te
pec-	*pēgnymi, pēg-* [Gr.] (*pēk-* before *t*) fix, make fast. sym*pec*tothiene. (See also pex-)		
		phyl-	*phylon* [Gr.] tribe, kind. *phyl*ogeny
ped-	*pais, paidos* [Gr.] child. orth*oped*ic		

Table continued on following page

B-4
COMBINING FORMS IN MEDICAL TERMINOLOGY Continued

-phyll	*phyllon* [Gr.] leaf. xantho*phyll*		adult. ischio*pub*ic. (See also *puber*-)
phylac-	*phylax* [Gr.] guard. pro*phylac*tic	puber-	*puber* [L.] adult. *puber*ty
phys(a)-	*physaō* [Gr.] blow, inflate. *phys*ocele, *phys*alis	pulmo(n)-	*pulmo, pulmonis* [L.] lung. Cf. pneumo(n)-. *pulmo*lith, cardio*pulmon*ary
physe-	*physō, physē-* [Gr.] blow, inflate. em*physe*ma	puls-	*pello, pellentis, pulsus* [L.] drive. pro*puls*ion
pil-	*pilus* [L.] hair. e*pil*ation	punct-	*pungo, punctus* [L.] prick, pierce. Cf. cente-. *puncti*form
pituit-	*pituita* [L.] phlegm, rheum. *pituit*ous	pur-	*pus, puris* [L.] pus. Cf. py-. sup*pur*ation
placent-	*placenta* [L.] (from *plakous* [Gr.]) cake. extra*placent*al	py-	*pyon* [Gr.] pus. Cf. pur-. ne*phropy*osis
plas-	*plassō* [Gr.] mold, shape. cine*plas*ty	pyel-	*pyelos* [Gr.] trough, basin, pelvis. nephro*pyel*itis
platy-	*platys* [Gr.] broad, flat. *platy*rrhine	pyl-	*pylē* [Gr.] door, orifice. *pyle*phlebitis
pleg-	*plēssō* [Gr.] strike. di*pleg*ia	pyr-	*pyr* [Gr.] fire. Cf. febr-. galacto*pyr*a
plet-	*pleo, -pletus* [L.] fill. de*plet*ion	quadr-	*quadr-* [L.] four. Cf. tetra-. *quadr*igeminal
pleur-	*pleura* [Gr.] rib, side. Cf. cost-. peri*pleur*al	quinque-	*quinque* [L.] five. Cf. pent(a)-. *quinque*cuspid
plex-	*plēssō, plēg-* (added to s becomes *plēx-*) strike. apo*plex*y	rachi-	*rachis* [Gr.] spine. Cf. spin-. encephalo*rachi*dian
plic-	*plico* [L.] fold. com*plic*ation	radi-	*radius* [L.] ray. Cf. actin-. ir*radi*ation
pne-	*pneuma, pneumatos* [Gr.] breathing. traumato*pne*a	re-	*re-* [L.] back, again. *re*traction
pneum(at)-	*pneuma, pneumatos* [Gr.] breath, air. *pneum*odynamics, *pneumat*othorax	ren-	*renes* [L.] kidneys. Cf. nephr-. ad*ren*al
pneumo(n)-	*pneumōn* [Gr.] lung. Cf. pulmo(n)-. *pneumo*centesis, *pneumon*otomy	ret-	*rete* [L.] net. *ret*othelium
		retro-	*retro* [L.] backwards. *retro*deviation
pod-	*pous, podos* [Gr.] foot. *pod*iatry	rhag-	*rhēgnymi, rhag-* [Gr.] break, burst. hemor*rhag*ic
poie-	*poieō* [Gr.] make, produce. Cf. -facient. sarco*poie*tic	rhaph-	*rhaphē* [Gr.] suture. gastror*rhaph*y
pol-	*polos* [Gr.] axis of a sphere. peri*pol*ar	rhe-	*rhaphē* [Gr.] flow. Cf. flu-. diar*rhe*al
poly-	*polys* [Gr.] much, many. *poly*spermia	rhex-	*rhēgnymi, rhēg-* [Gr.] (added to s becomes *rhēx*) break, burst. metror*rhex*is
pont-	*pons, pontis* [L.] bridge. *pont*ocerebellar	rhin-	*rhis, rhinos* [Gr.] nose. Cf. nas-. basi*rhin*al
por-¹	*poros* [Gr.] passage. myelo*por*e	rot-	*rota* [L.] wheel. *rot*ator
por-²	*pōros* [Gr.] callus. *por*ocele	rub(r)-	*ruber, rubri* [L.] red. Cf. erythr-. bili*rub*in, *rub*rospinal
posit-	*pono, positus* [L.] put, place. re*posit*or	salping-	*salpinx, salpingos* [Gr.] tube, trumpet. *salping*itis
post-	*post* [L.] after, behind in time or place. *post*natal, *post*oral	sanguin-	*sanguis, sanguinis* [L.] blood. Cf. hem(at)-. *sanguin*eous
pre-	*prae* [L.] before in time or place. *pre*natal, *pre*vesical	sarc-	*sarx, sarkos* [Gr.] flesh. *sarc*oma
press-	*premo, pressus* [L.] press. *press*oreceptive	schis-	*schizō, schid-* [Gr.] (before t or added to s becomes *schis-*) split. Cf. fiss-. *schis*torachis, rachi*schis*is
pro-	*pro* [Gr.] or *pro* [L.] before in time or place. *pro*gamous, *pro*cheilon, *pro*lapse	scler-	*sklēros* [Gr.] hard. Cf. dur-. *scler*osis
proct-	*prōktos* [Gr.] anus. entero*proct*ia	scop-	*skopeō* [Gr.] look at, observe. endo*scop*e
prosop-	*prosōpon* [Gr.] face. Cf. faci-. di*prosop*us	sect-	*seco, sectus* [L.] cut. Cf. tom-. *sect*ile
pseud-	*pseudēs* [Gr.] false. *pseud*oparaplegia	semi-	*semi* [L.] half. Cf. hemi-. *semi*flexion
psych-	*psychē* [Gr.] soul, mind. Cf. ment-. *psych*osomatic	sens-	*sentio, sensus* [L.] perceive, feel. Cf. esthe-. *sens*ory
pto-	*piptō, ptō-* [Gr.] fall. nephro*pto*sis		
pub-	*pubes* and *puber, puberis* [L.]		

COMBINING FORMS IN MEDICAL TERMINOLOGY Continued

sep-	*sepō* [Gr.] rot, decay. *sep*sis		orifice. Cf. or-. ana*stom*osis, *stomat*ogastric
sept-[1]	*saepio, saeptio* [L.] fence, wall off, stop up. Cf. phrag-. naso*sept*al	strep(h)-	*strephō, strep-* (before *t*) [Gr.] twist. Cf. tors-. *streph*osymbolia, *strep*tomycin. (See also stroph-)
sept-[2]	*septem* [L.] seven. Cf. hept(a)-. *sept*an	strict-	*stringo, stringentis, strictus* [L.] draw tight, compress, cause pain. con*strict*ion
ser-	*serum* [L.] whey, watery substance. *ser*osynovitis	-stringent	See strict-. a*stringent*
sex-	*sex* [L.] six. Cf. hex-[1]. *sex*digitate	stroph-	*strephō, stroph-* [Gr.] twist. ana*stroph*ic. (See also strep(h)-)
sial-	*sialon* [Gr.] saliva. poly*sial*ia	struct-	*struo, structus* [L.] pile up (against). ob*struct*ion
sin-	*sinus* [L.] hollow, fold. Cf. colp-. *sin*obronchitis	sub-	*sub* [L.] (*b* changes to *f* or *p* before words beginning with those consonants) under, below. Cf. hypo-. *sub*lumbar
sit-	*sitos* [Gr.] food. para*sit*ic		
solut-	*solvo, solventis, solutus* [L.] loose, dissolve, set free. Cf. ly-. dis*solut*ion		
-solvent	See solut-. dis*solvent*	suf-	See sub-. *suf*fusion
somat-	*sōma, somatos* [Gr.] body. Cf. corpor-. psycho*somat*ic	sup-	See sub-. *sup*pository
		super-	*super* [L.] above, beyond, extreme. Cf. hyper-. *super*motility
-some	See somat-. dictyo*some*		
spas-	*spaō, spas-* [Gr.] draw, pull. *spas*m, *spas*tic	sy-	See syn-. *sy*stole
spectr-	*spectrum* [L.] appearance, what is seen. micro*spectr*oscope	syl-	See syn-. *syl*lepsiology
		sym-	See syn-. *sym*biosis, *sym*metry, *sym*pathetic, *sym*physis
sperm(at)-	*sperma, spermatos* [Gr.] seed. *sperm*acrasia, *spermat*ozoon		
		syn-	*syn* [Gr.] (*n* disappears before *s*, changes to *l* before *l*, and changes to *m* before *b, m, p,* and *ph*) with, together. Cf. con-. myo*syn*izesis
spers-	*spargo, -spersus* [L.] scatter. di*spers*ion		
sphen-	*sphēn* [Gr.] wedge. Cf. cune-. *sphen*oid		
spher-	*sphaira* [Gr.] ball. hemi*spher*e	ta-	See ton-. *ect*asis
		tac-	*tassō, tag-* [Gr.] (*tak-* before *t*) order, arrange. a*tac*tic
sphygm-	*sphygmos* [Gr.] pulsation. *sphygm*omanometer	tact-	*tango, tactus* [L.] touch. con*tact*
spin-	*spina* [L.] spine. Cf. rachi-. cerebro*spin*al	tax-	*tassō, tag-* [Gr.] (added to *s* becomes *tax-*) order, arrange. a*tax*ia
spirat-	*spiro, spiratus* [L.] breathe. in*spirat*ory		
splanchn-	*splanchna* [Gr.] entrails, viscera. neuro*splanchn*ic	tect-	See teg-. pro*tect*ive
		teg-	*tego, tectus* [L.] cover. in*teg*ument
splen-	*splēn* [Gr.] spleen. Cf. lien-. *splen*omegaly	tel-	*telos* [Gr.] end. *tel*osynapsis
spor-	*sporos* [Gr.] seed. *spor*ophyte, zygo*spor*e	tele-	*tēle* [Gr.] at a distance. *tele*ceptor
squam-	*squama* [L.] scale. de*squam*ation	tempor-	*tempus, temporis* [L.] time, timely or fatal spot, temple. *tempor*omalar
sta-	*histēmi, sta-* [Gr.] make stand, stop. genesi*sta*sis	ten(ont)-	*tenōn, tenontos* [Gr.] (from *teinō* stretch) tight stretched band. *ten*odynia, *ten*onitis, *tenont*agra
stal-	*stellō, stal-* [Gr.] send. peri*stal*sis. (See also stol-)		
staphyl-	*staphylē* [Gr.] bunch of grapes, uvula. *staphyl*ococcus, *staphyl*ectomy		
		tens-	*tendo, tensus* [L.] stretch. Cf. ton-. ex*tens*or
stear-	*stear, steatos* [Gr.] fat. Cf. adip-. *stear*odermia	test-	*testis* [L.] testicle. Cf. orchi-. *test*itis
steat-	See stear-. *steat*opygous	tetra-	*tetra-* [Gr.] four. Cf. quadr-. *tetra*genous
sten-	*stenos* [Gr.] narrow, compressed. *sten*ocardia		
ster-	*stereos* [Gr.] solid. chole*ster*ol	the-	*tithēmi, thē-* [Gr.] put, place. syn*the*sis
sterc-	*stercus* [L.] dung. Cf. copr-. *sterc*oporphyrin	thec-	*thēkē* [Gr.] repository, case. *thec*ostegnosis
sthen-	*sthenos* [Gr.] strength. a*sthen*ia	thel-	*thēlē* [Gr.] teat, nipple. *thel*erethism
stol-	*stellō, stol-* [Gr.] send. dia*stol*e		
stom(at)-	*stoma, stomatos* [Gr.] mouth,		

Table continued on following page

B-4
COMBINING FORMS IN MEDICAL TERMINOLOGY Continued

therap-	*therapeia* [Gr.] treatment. hydro*therapy*	**trip-**	*tribō* [Gr.] rub. en*trip*sis
therm-	*thermē* [Gr.] heat. Cf. calor-. dia*thermy*	**trop-**	*trepō, trop-* [Gr.] turn, react. sito*tropism*
thi-	*theion* [Gr.] sulfur. *thio*genic	**troph-**	*trepō, troph-* [Gr.] nurture. a*trophy*
thorac-	*thōrax, thōrakos* [Gr.] chest. *thoraco*plasty	**tuber-**	*tuber* [L.] swelling, node. *tuber*cle
thromb-	*thrombos* [Gr.] lump, clot. *thromb*openia	**typ-**	*typos* [Gr.] (from *typto* strike) type. a*typ*ical
thym-	*thymos* [Gr.] spirit. Cf. ment-. dys*thym*ia	**typh-**	*typhos* [Gr.] fog, stupor. adeno*typh*us
thyr-	*thyreos* [Gr.] shield (shaped like a door *thyra*). *thyr*oid	**typhl-**	*typhlos* [Gr.] blind. Cf. cec-. *typhl*ectasis
tme-	*temnō, tmē-* [Gr.] cut. axon*otmesis*	**un-**	*unus* [L.] one. Cf. hen-. *un*ioval
toc-	*tokos* [Gr.] childbirth. dys*toc*ia	**ur-**	*ouron* [Gr.] urine. poly*ur*ia
tom-	*temnō, tom-* [Gr.] cut. Cf. sect-. appendec*tomy*	**vacc-**	*vacca* [L.] cow. *vacc*ine
ton-	*teino, ton-* [Gr.] stretch, put under tension. Cf. tens-. peri*ton*eum	**vagin-**	*vagina* [L.] sheath. in*vagin*ated
top-	*topos* [Gr.] place. Cf. loc-. *top*esthesia	**vas-**	*vas* [L.] vessel. Cf. angi-. *vas*cular
tors-	*torqueo, torsus* [L.] twist. Cf. strep-. ec*tors*ion	**vers-**	See vert-. in*vers*ion
tox-	*toxicon* [Gr.] (from *toxon* bow) arrow poison, poison. *tox*emia	**vert-**	*verto, versus* [L.] turn. di*vert*iculum
trache-	*tracheia* [Gr.] windpipe. *trache*otomy	**vesic-**	*vesica* [L.] bladder. Cf. cyst-. *vesic*ovaginal
trachel-	*trachēlos* [Gr.] neck. Cf. cervic-. *trachel*opexy	**vit-**	*vita* [L.] life. Cf. bi-¹. de*vit*alize
tract-	*traho, tractus* [L.] draw, drag. pro*tract*ion	**vuls-**	*vello, vulsus* [L.] pull, twitch. con*vuls*ion
traumat-	*trauma, traumatos* [Gr.] wound. *traumat*ic	**xanth-**	*xanthos* [Gr.] yellow, blond. Cf. flav- and lute-. *xantho*phyll
tri-	*treis, tria* [Gr.] or *tri-* [L.] three. *tri*gonid	**-yl-**	*hyte* [Gr.] substance. cacod*yl*
trich-	*thrix, trichos* [Gr.] hair. *tri*choid	**zo-**	*zoē* [Gr.] life, *zōon* [Gr.] animal. micro*zo*aria
		zyg-	*zygon* [Gr.] yoke, union. *zyg*odactyly
		zym-	*zymē* [Gr.] ferment. en*zyme*

From Miller BF, Keane CB: *Encyclopedia and Dictionary of Medicine, Nursing, and Allied Health,* 5th ed. Philadelphia: W.B. Saunders, 1992, pp. xxi–xxx.

B-5
MEDICARE PHYSICIAN PAYMENT REFORM (PPR)

PHYSICIAN FEE SCHEDULE — WHAT AND WHY

Congress Enacted Three Part Physician Payment Reform in 1989.

Three major elements include:

- Establishes physician fee schedule, effective January 1, 1992.
- Sets goals for rate of increase in Medicare physician expenditures.
- Establishes financial protection for beneficiaries.

Health Care Financing Administration, November 1991.

HOW TO OBTAIN COPIES OF FINAL FEE SCHEDULE

Contact GOVERNMENT PRINTING OFFICE

Write:
Superintendent of Documents
Government Printing Office
Washington, D.C. 20402

Paper or Microfiche

Call: (202) 783-3238

Ask for:
Stock # 069-001-000-37-8

Diskette (3.5)

Call: (202) 783-3238

Ask for:
Stock # 069-001-000-38-6

SUMMARY OF FINAL RULE CHANGES

Major changes in Final Rules (compared to Proposed Rules as published in June 1991 Federal Register) include:

	Final Rule	Proposed Rule
Conversion Factor (Incl. 1.9% adj. — CY 1992)	$31.001	$26.873
Global Surgery (Pre-Op)	1 Day	30 Days
Post-Op	0 Days	30 Days
Endoscopy		
Minor Surgery	0 or 10 Days	30 Days
Anesthesia "Time"	Continued Separate Payments	Elimination of Separate Payments
Drugs	Payments at Lower of Est. Cost or National Wholesale Price	Payments at 85% of Average Wholesale Price

Health Care Financing Administration, November 1991.

Table continued on following page

B-5
MEDICARE PHYSICIAN PAYMENT REFORM (PPR) Continued

MEDICARE FEE SCHEDULE COMPONENTS

- Relative Value Units (RVUs)
- Geographic Practice Cost Index (GPCI)
- Conversion Factor (CF)

Health Care Financing Administration, November 1991.

FEE SCHEDULE COMPUTATION

Fee Schedule Amount =

- Total RVUs × CF
- (W + PE + MP) × CF
- [(RVUw × GPCIw) + (RVUpe × GPCIpe) + (RVUmp × GPCImp)] × $31.001

Variables:

- RVUs = Relative Value Units
- W = Work
- PE = Practice Expense (i.e., Overhead)
- MP = Malpractice Expense
- CF = Conversion Factor
- GPCI = Geographic Price Cost Index ("gypsy")

Health Care Financing Administration, November 1991.

FEE SCHEDULE COMPUTATION

(RVUw) × (GPCIw)
+(RVUpe) × (GPCIpe)
+(RVUmp) × (GPCImp)
TOTAL × CF = PAYMENT

Substituting figures for procedure code 99213 in locality 01 of Maryland (Baltimore and surrounding counties):

.58 × 1.027 = .596
+.39 × 1.040 = .406
+.03 × .927 = .028
Total = 1.023 × 31.001 = $31.90

Health Care Financing Administration, January 1992.

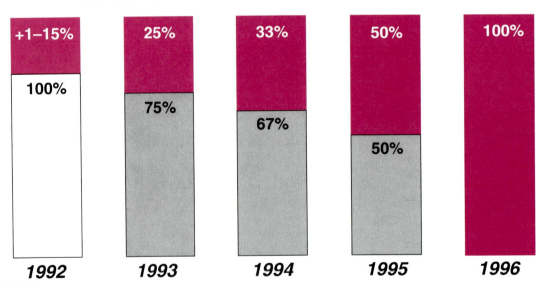

TRANSITION FEE COMPONENTS 1992–1996

- % of current fee schedule amount
- % of previous year's transition payment amount
- Adjusted Historical Payment Base (AHPB)

Health Care Financing Administration
November 1991

B-5

MEDICARE PHYSICIAN PAYMENT REFORM (PPR) Continued

1992 PAYMENT — MARYLAND

Locality: 01

HCPCS	AHPB	Fee Schedule	Transition
99213	$31.60	$31.90	N/A
99254	$108.31	$117.66	N/A
52601	$1,022.13	$824.59	$898.44

Health Care Financing Administration, December 1991.

1992 PAYMENT — D.C.

HCPCS	AHPB	Fee Schedule	Transition
99213	$34.79	$34.04	N/A
99254	$109.46	$125.09	N/A
52601	$1,052.21	$887.02	$919.16

Health Care Financing Administration, December 1991.

NEW EVALUATION AND MANAGEMENT CODES

Category/Subcategory	CPT Codes	No. of Levels
Office or Other Outpatient		
• New Patient	99201–99205	5
• Established Patient	99211–99215	5
Hospital Inpatient Services		
• Initial Hospital Care	99221–99223	3
• Subsequent Hospital Care	99231–99233	3
• Hospital Discharge Services	99238	1
Consultations		
• Office	99241–99245	5
• Initial Inpatient	99251–99255	5
• Follow-up Inpatient	99261–99263	3
• Confirmatory	99271–99275	5
Emergency Department Services	99281–99285	5
Critical Care Services	99291–99292	2
Nursing Facility Services		
• Comprehensive Assessments	99301–99303	3
• Subsequent Care	99311–99313	3
Domiciliary/Custodial Care		
• New Patient	99321–99323	3
• Established Patient	99331–99333	3
Home Services		
• New Patient	99341–99343	3
• Established Patient	99351–99353	3

Health Care Financing Administration, November 1991; January 1992.

Table continued on following page

B-5

MEDICARE PHYSICIAN PAYMENT REFORM (PPR) Continued

EVALUATION AND MANAGEMENT SERVICE DESCRIPTORS

Descriptor	Component Levels	Definitions
Key Descriptors*		
• History	Four types of history recognized	Problem Focused Expanded Problem Focused Detailed Comprehensive
• Examination	Four types of examination recognized	Problem Focused Expanded Problem Focused Detailed Comprehensive
• Medical Decision Making	Four types of medical decision making	Straightforward Low Complexity Moderate Complexity High Complexity

* Must meet all or two of three key components for particular levels of E&M services.

Contributory Descriptors

• Counseling		Not required to be performed in every patient encounter
• Coordination of Care		
• Nature of Presenting Problem	Five types of presenting problems recognized	Minimal Self-limited or Minor Low Severity Moderate Severity High Severity
• Time*	Office and Outpt. Visits Hospital and Nursing Facility Care	Face-to-Face Time Unit/Floor Time

* The key descriptor when counseling and/or coordination of care dominates (more than 50%).

Health Care Financing Administration, November 1991.

MAJOR SURGICAL GLOBAL PACKAGE

Service	PPR Policy
• Initial Consult	Separate payment
• Pre-Operative Visits	Includes 1 day pre-operative period
• Intraoperative Services	Includes usual and necessary intraoperative services
• Complications	Includes additional medical and surgical services except additional trips to operating room (reduced payment)
• Post-Operative Visits	Includes 90-day post-operative period

Health Care Financing Administration, January 1992.

GLOBAL PACKAGE MINOR SURGERY AND NON-INCISIONAL PROCEDURES

Service	PPR Policy
• Visits (same day)	No separate payment *unless separate* service provided
• Post-Op Visits	Minor Surgery: 0 or 10 days Endoscopy (Non-incisional): None

Health Care Financing Administration, January 1992.

B-5

MEDICARE PHYSICIAN PAYMENT REFORM (PPR) *Continued*

NEW SURGICAL MODIFIER CODES

Description	Modifier	Payment
Postoperative E&M service unrelated to surgery	−24	Based on E&M code
Unrelated E&M service same day as surgery	−25	Based on E&M code
Return to O.R. for related procedure during postoperative period	−78	Based on 50% intraoperative payment for surgery or intraoperative for code for reoperation due to complications

Health Care Financing Administration, January 1992.

SURGICAL MODIFIER CODES

Description	Modifier	Payment
Postoperative Unrelated Surgical Procedure	−79	Global Surgical Fee
Bilateral Surgery	−50	150% of Global Surgical Fee
Multiple Surgery	−51	100%—1st Surgery 50%—2nd Surgery 25%—3rd through 5th Surgery
Surgical Care Only	−54	Pre-operative and intra-operative component of surgical fee (includes post-operative inpatient visits)
Post-operative Care Only	−55	Post-operative component of fee
Co-Surgeon	−62	Total Payment limited to 125% of Global Surgical Fee (National Codes Only)
Team Surgeon	−66	By Report (National Codes Only)
Assistant-at-Surgery	−80 or −82	16% of Global Surgical Fee (National Codes Only)

Health Care Financing Administration, December 1991.

BALANCE BILLING LIMITS

Limiting charge (L.C.) percentages:

- CY 1991—125% All Other Services
    —140% Evaluation & Management
- CY 1992—120% All Services (Net 114%)
    (Net = 95% of F.S. times 120%)
- CY 1993—115% All Services (Net 109.25%)
    (Net = 95% of F.S. times 115%)

Health Care Financing Administration, January 1992.

NEW PHYSICIAN PAYMENT

- No longer an exclusion for joining a "group practice."
- Effective January 1, 1992, retroactively identifies those already in practice (less than 5 years).
- Expands reduction from 2 to 4 years, as follows:
    80%—1st Year
    85%—2nd Year
    90%—3rd Year
    95%—4th Year
    100%—5th Year
- Exceptions:
    Primary Care Services
        99201–99215 (Office Visit)
        99281–99285 (Emer. Room)
        99301–99313 (Nursing Facility)
        99321–99333 (Dom. Facility)
        99341–99353 (Home Services)
        92002 and 92004 (Eye Care)
    Rural Health Professional Shortage Areas
- Non-participating (new physicians)—"Limiting Charge"
    Determined after all adjustments (i.e., 5% reduced payment due to non-participation status and the standard % reduction for "new physicians").
    Multiple "Limiting Charge" schedules may be necessary for group practices.

Health Care Financing Administration, November 1991.

B-6

MEDICARE PPR PROCEDURE CODES SUBJECT TO THE OUTPATIENT LIMIT

HCPCS*	Description	HCPCS*	Description
10040	Acne surgery	21030	Removal of face bone lesion
10060	Drainage of skin abscess	21040	Removal of jaw bone lesion
10061	Drainage of skin abscess	23066	Biopsy shoulder tissues
10080	Drainage of pilonidal cyst	24650	Treat radius fracture
10120	Remove foreign body	25500	Treat fracture of radius
10121	Remove foreign body	25600	Treat fracture radius/ulna
10140	Drainage of hematoma	26010	Drainage of finger abscess
10141	Drainage of hematoma	26600	Treat metacarpal fracture
10160	Puncture drainage of lesion	26605	Treat metacarpal fracture
11000	Surgical cleansing of skin	26720	Treat finger fracture, each
11001	Additional cleansing of skin	27520	Treat kneecap fracture
11040	Surgical cleansing, abrasion	27780	Treatment of fibula fracture
11041	Surgical cleansing of skin	27786	Treatment of ankle fracture
11042	Cleansing of skin/tissue	28001	Drainage of bursa of foot
11050	Trim skin lesion	28010	Incision of toe tendon
11051	Trim 2 to 4 skin lesions	28090	Removal of foot lesion
11052	Trim over 4 skin lesions	28108	Removal of toe lesion
11100	Biopsy of lesion	28124	Partial removal of toe
11101	Biopsy, each additional lesion	28126	Partial removal of toe
11200	Removal of skin tags	28153	Partial removal of toe
11201	Removal of added skin tags	28160	Partial removal of toe
11400	Removal of skin lesion	28190	Removal of foot foreign body
11401	Removal of skin lesion	28230	Incision of foot tendon(s)
11402	Removal of skin lesion	28232	Incision of toe tendon
11403	Removal of skin lesion	28234	Incision of foot tendon
11404	Removal of skin lesion	28270	Release of foot contracture
11420	Removal of skin lesion	28272	Release of toe joint, each
11421	Removal of skin lesion	28285	Revision of hammertoe
11422	Removal of skin lesion	28298	Correction of bunion
11423	Removal of skin lesion	28308	Incision of metatarsal
11424	Removal of skin lesion	28400	Treatment of heel fracture
11440	Removal of skin lesion	28470	Treat metatarsal fracture
11441	Removal of skin lesion	28475	Treat metatarsal fracture
11442	Removal of skin lesion	28490	Treat big toe fracture
11443	Removal of skin lesion	28510	Treatment of toe fracture
11444	Removal of skin lesion	28515	Treatment of toe fracture
11446	Removal of skin lesion	29065	Application of long arm cast
11600	Removal of skin lesion	29075	Application of forearm cast
11601	Removal of skin lesion	29085	Apply hand/wrist cast
11602	Removal of skin lesion	29105	Apply long arm splint
11603	Removal of skin lesion	29125	Apply forearm splint
11604	Removal of skin lesion	29126	Apply forearm splint
11620	Removal of skin lesion	29130	Application of finger splint
11621	Removal of skin lesion	29200	Strapping of chest
11622	Removal of skin lesion	29260	Strapping of elbow or wrist
11623	Removal of skin lesion	29345	Application of long leg cast
11624	Removal of skin lesion	29355	Application of long leg cast
17306	3rd stage chemosurgery	29365	Application of long leg cast
17307	Followup skin lesion therapy	29405	Apply short leg cast
17310	Extensive skin chemosurgery	29425	Apply short leg cast
17340	Cryotherapy of skin	29435	Apply short leg cast
17360	Skin peel therapy	29440	Addition of walker to cast
19000	Drainage of breast lesion	29515	Application lower leg splint
19100	Biopsy of breast	29520	Strapping of hip
20000	Incision of abscess	29530	Strapping of knee
20500	Injection of sinus tract	29540	Strapping of ankle
20520	Removal of foreign body	29550	Strapping of toes
20550	Injection treatment	29580	Application of paste boot
20600	Drainage joint/bursa/cyst	29700	Removal/revision of cast
20605	Drainage joint/bursa/cyst	29705	Removal/revision of cast
20610	Inject/drain joint/bursa	30100	Intranasal biopsy
20615	Treatment of bone cyst	30110	Removal of nose polyp(s)
20670	Removal of support implant	30200	Injection treatment of nose

B-6
MEDICARE PPR PROCEDURE CODES SUBJECT TO THE OUTPATIENT LIMIT Continued

HCPCS*	Description	HCPCS*	Description
30210	Nasal sinus therapy	92225	Extended ophthalmoscopy, new
30901	Control of nosebleed	92226	Extended ophthalmoscopy
31000	Irrigation maxillary sinus	92230	Ophthalmoscopy/angioscopy
31250	Nasal endoscopy, diagnostic	92235	Ophthalmoscopy/angiography
31505	Diagnostic laryngoscopy	92270	Electro-oculography
31525	Diagnostic laryngoscopy	92275	Electroretinography
31575	Fiberscopic laryngoscopy	92280	Special eye evaluation
36400	Establish access to vein	92283	Color vision examination
36425	Establish access to vein	92284	Dark adaptation eye exam
36470	Injection therapy of vein	92286	Internal eye photography
36471	Injection therapy of veins	92311	Special contact lens fitting
36500	Insertion of catheter, vein	92312	Special contact lens fitting
38505	Needle biopsy, lymph node(s)	92352	Special spectacles fitting
40490	Biopsy of lip	92353	Special spectacles fitting
40808	Biopsy of mouth lesion	92504	Ear microscopy examination
56600	Biopsy of vulva	92506	Speech & hearing evaluation
57100	Biopsy of vagina	92507	Speech/hearing therapy
57150	Treat vagina infection	92511	Nasopharyngoscopy
57160	Insertion of pessary	92516	Facial nerve function test
57452	Examination of vagina	93797	Cardiac rehab
57454	Vagina examination & biopsy	93798	Cardiac rehab/monitor
57500	Biopsy of cervix	95831	Limb muscle testing, manual
57505	Endocervical curettage	95832	Hand muscle testing, manual
57510	Cauterization of cervix	95833	Body muscle testing, manual
57511	Cryocautery of cervix	95834	Body muscle testing, manual
58100	Biopsy of uterus lining	95851	Range of motion measurements
58102	Curettage of uterus lining	95852	Range of motion measurements
59420	Care before delivery	95857	Tensilon test
60100	Biopsy of thyroid	96440	Chemotherapy, intracavitary
61070	Brain canal shunt procedure	99201	Office and other outpatient, new patient, Level 1
64400	Injection for nerve block	99202	Office and other outpatient, new patient, Level 2
64405	Injection for nerve block	99203	Office and other outpatient, new patient, Level 3
64413	Injection for nerve block	99204	Office and other outpatient, new patient, Level 4
64415	Injection for nerve block	99205	Office and other outpatient, new patient, Level 5
64418	Injection for nerve block	99211	Office and other outpatient, established patient, Level 1
64420	Injection for nerve block		
64425	Injection for nerve block	99212	Office and other outpatient, established patient, Level 1
64440	Injection for nerve block		
64441	Injection for nerve block	99213	Office and other outpatient, established patient, Level 1
64445	Injection for nerve block		
64450	Injection for nerve block	99214	Office and other outpatient, established patient, Level 1
64505	Injection for nerve block		
64550	Apply neurostimulator	99215	Office and other outpatient, established patient, Level 1
64565	Implant neuroelectrodes		
64640	Injection treatment of nerve	A2000	Manipulation of spine by chiropractor
65205	Remove foreign body from eye	H5300	Occupational therapy
65210	Remove foreign body from eye	M0005	Office visits with two or more modalities to the same area
65220	Remove foreign body from eye		
65222	Remove foreign body from eye	M0006	Office visits with one of the above mentioned treatment
65430	Corneal smear		
65435	Curette/treat cornea	M0007	Office visit including combination of any modality(s) and
66761	Revision of iris		
66762	Revision of iris	M0008	Office visit including combination of any modality(s) and
67031	Laser surgery, eye strands		
67105	Repair, detached retina	M0101	Cutting or removal of corns, calluses and/or trimming of nails, application
67141	Treatment of retina		
67145	Treatment of retina	M0702	Brief, osteopathic manipulative therapy performed in office, or
67208	Treatment of retinal lesion		
67210	Treatment of retinal lesion		
67228	Treatment of retinal lesion		
67505	Inject/treat eye socket		
67515	Inject/treat eye socket		

* All CPT codes and descriptors, copyright 1991 AMA.
From the Federal Register, Vol. 56, No. 227, November 25, 1991, Rules and Regulations.

B-7

MEDICARE PPR FACILITY-BASED PROCEDURES FOR WHICH ADDITIONAL AMOUNT FOR SUPPLIES MAY BE PAYABLE IF PERFORMED IN A PHYSICIAN'S OFFICE

HCPCS*	Description
19101	Biopsy of breast
19120	Removal of breast lesion
20200	Muscle biopsy
20205	Deep muscle biopsy
20220	Bone biopsy, trocar/needle
20225	Bone biopsy, trocar/needle
20240	Bone biopsy, excisional
25111	Remove wrist tendon lesion
28290	Correction of bunion
28292	Correction of bunion
28293	Correction of bunion
28294	Correction of bunion
28296	Correction of bunion
28297	Correction of bunion
28298	Correction of bunion
28299	Correction of bunion
32000	Drainage of chest
37609	Temporal artery procedure
38500	Biopsy/removal, lymph node(s)
43200	Esophagus endoscopy
43202	Esophagus endoscopy, biopsy
43220	Esophagus endoscopy, dilation
43226	Esophagus endoscopy, dilation
43234	Upper GI endoscopy, exam
43235	Upper GI endoscopy, diagnosis
43239	Upper GI endoscopy, biopsy
43245	Operative upper GI endoscopy
43247	Operative upper GI endoscopy
43251	Operative upper GI endoscopy
45378	Diagnostic colonoscopy
45379	Colonoscopy
45380	Colonoscopy and biopsy
45382	Colonoscopy, control bleeding
45383	Colonoscopy, lesion removal
45385	Colonoscopy, lesion removal
49080	Puncture, peritoneal cavity
57520	Biopsy of cervix
58120	Dilation and curettage
62270	Spinal fluid tap, diagnostic
85095	Bone marrow aspiration
85102	Bone marrow biopsy
96440	Chemotherapy, intracavitary
96445	Chemotherapy, intracavitary
96450	Chemotherapy, into CNS

* All CPT codes and descriptors, copyright 1991, AMA.
From the Federal Register, Vol, 56, No. 227, November 25, 1991, Rules and Regulations.

B-8
MEDICARE PPR EVALUATION AND MANAGEMENT CODES
Office or Other Outpatient Services
New Patient

Service Category Code	Key Components		Contributory Components		Secondary
	History/ Examination	Medical Decision Making	Nature of Presenting Problem	Counseling Coordination Of Care	Time
99201	Problem focused	Straightforward	Self/limited or minor	Definition for all codes: Counseling and/or coordination of care with other providers or agencies consistent with the nature of the problem(s) and the patient's and/ or family's needs.	10 minutes
99202	Expanded problem focused	Straightforward	Low to moderate severity		20 minutes
99203	Detailed	Low complexity	Moderate severity		30 minutes
99204	Comprehensive	Moderate complexity	Moderate to high severity		45 minutes
99205	Comprehensive	High complexity	Moderate to high severity		60 minutes

Office or Other Outpatient Services
Established Patient

Service Category Code	Key Components		Contributory Components		Secondary
	History/ Examination	Medical Decision Making	Nature of Presenting Problem	Counseling Coordination Of Care	Time
99211	Usually a follow-up and/or periodic reevaluation (see definition)		Minimal	Definition for all codes: Counseling and/or coordination of care with other providers or agencies consistent with the nature of the problem(s) and the patient's and/ or family's needs.	5 minutes
99212	Problem focused	Straightforward	Self/limited or minor		10 minutes
99213	Expanded problem focused	Low complexity	Low to moderate severity		15 minutes
99214	Detailed	Moderate complexity	Moderate to high severity		25 minutes
99215	Comprehensive	High complexity	Moderate to high complexity		40 minutes

New or Established Patient
Initial Hospital Care

Service Category Code	Key Components		Contributory Components		Secondary Time Bedside/ Unit
	History/ Examination	Medical Decision Making	Nature of Presenting Problem	Counseling Coordination Of Care	
99221	Comprehensive	Straightforward or low complexity	Low severity	Definition for all codes: Counseling and/or coordination of care with other providers or agencies consistent with the nature of the problem(s) and the patient's and/or family's needs.	30 minutes
99222	Comprehensive	Moderate severity	Moderate severity		50 minutes
99223	Comprehensive	High complexity	High severity		70 minutes

Table continued on following page

B-8

MEDICARE PPR EVALUATION AND MANAGEMENT CODES *Continued*
Subsequent Hospital Care

Service Category	Key Components		Contributory Components		Secondary
Code	History/ Examination	Medical Decision Making	Nature of Presenting Problem (Definition change)	Counseling Coordination Of Care	Time Bedside/ Unit
99231	Problem focused	Straightforward or low complexity	Stable, recovering or improving	Definition for all codes: Counseling and/or coordination of care with other providers or agencies consistent with the nature of the problem(s) and the patient's and/ or family's needs.	15 minutes
99232	Expanded problem focused	Moderate complexity	Inadequate response to therapy or minor complication		25 minutes
99233	Detailed	High complexity	Unstable new problem or serious complication		35 minutes
99238	Discharge day management				

Office or Other Outpatient Consultation
New or Established Patient

Service Category	Key Components		Contributory Components		Secondary
Code	History/ Examination	Medical Decision Making	Nature of Presenting Problem	Counseling Coordination Of Care	Time
99241	Problem focused	Straightforward	Self/limited or minor	Definition for all codes: Counseling and/or coordination of care with other providers or agencies consistent with the nature of the problem(s) and the patient's and/ or family's needs.	15 minutes
99242	Expanded problem focused	Straightforward	Low severity		30 minutes
99243	Detailed	Low complexity	Moderate severity		40 minutes
99244	Comprehensive	Moderate complexity	Moderate to high complexity		60 minutes
99245	Comprehensive	High complexity	Moderate to high severity		80 minutes

Initial Inpatient Consultation
New or Established Patient

Service Category	Key Components		Contributory Components		Secondary
Code	History/ Examination	Medical Decision Making	Nature of Presenting Problem	Counseling Coordination Of Care	Time Bedside/ Unit
99251	Problem focused	Straightforward	Self/limited or minor	Definition for all codes: Counseling and/or coordination of care with other providers or agencies consistent with the nature of the problem(s) and the patient's and/ or family's needs.	20 minutes
99252	Expanded problem focused	Straightforward	Low severity		40 minutes
99253	Detailed	Low complexity	Moderate severity		55 minutes
99254	Comprehensive	Moderate complexity	Moderate to high severity		80 minutes
99255	Comprehensive	High complexity	Moderate to high severity		110 minutes

B-8
MEDICARE PPR EVALUATION AND MANAGEMENT CODES Continued
Follow-up Inpatient Consultations
Established Patient

Service Category	Key Components		Contributory Components		Secondary
Code	History/ Examination	Medical Decision Making	Nature of Presenting Problem	Counseling Coordination Of Care	Time Bedside/ Unit
99261	Problem focused	Straightforward or low complexity	Stable, recovering or improving	Definition for all codes: Counseling and/or coordination of care with other providers or agencies consistent with the nature of the problem(s) and the patient's and/ or family's needs.	10 minutes
99262	Expanded problem focused	Moderate complexity	Inadequate therapy response or minor complication		20 minutes
99263	Detailed	High complexity	Unstable or significant complication or new problem		30 minutes

Confirmatory Consultations
New or Established Patient

Service Category	Key Components		Contributory Components		Secondary
Code	History/ Examination	Medical Decision Making	Nature of Presenting Problem	Counseling Coordination Of Care	Time
99271	Problem focused	Straightforward	Self/limited or minor	Definition for all codes: Counseling and/or coordination of care with other providers or agencies consistent with the nature of the problem(s) and the patient's and/ or family's needs.	None
99272	Expanded problem focused	Straightforward	Low severity		None
99273	Detailed	Low complexity	Moderate severity		None
99274	Comprehensive	Moderate complexity	Moderate to high severity		None
99275	Comprehensive	High complexity	Moderate to high complexity		None

Emergency Department Services
New or Established Patient

Service Category	Key Components		Contributory Components		Secondary
Code	History/ Examination	Medical Decision Making	Nature of Presenting Problem	Counseling Coordination Of Care	Time
99281	Problem focused	Straightforward	Self/limited or minor	Definition for all codes: Counseling and/or coordination of care with other providers or agencies consistent with the nature of the problem(s) and the patient's and/ or family's needs.	None
99282	Expanded problem focused	Low complexity	Low to moderate severity		None
99283	Expanded problem focused	Low to moderate complexity	Moderate severity		None
99284	Detailed	Moderate complexity	High severity		None
99285	Comprehensive	High complexity	High severity		None

B-8

MEDICARE PPR EVALUATION AND MANAGEMENT CODES *Continued*
Comprehensive Nursing Facility Assessments
New or Established Patient

Service Category	Key Components			Contributory Components		Secondary
Code	History	Examination	Medical Decision Making	Nature of Presenting Problem	Counseling Coordination Of Care	Time Bedside/ Unit
99301	Detailed	Comprehensive	Straightforward or low complexity	Stable, recovering or improving	Definition for all codes: Counseling and/or coordination of care with other providers or agencies consistent with the nature of the problem(s) and the patient's and/or family's needs.	30 minutes
99302	Detailed	Comprehensive	Moderate to high complexity	Complication, new problem or major status change		40 minutes
99303	Comprehensive	Comprehensive	Moderate to high complexity	None given in AMA/HCFA literature		50 minutes

Subsequent NF Care
New or Established Patient

Service Category	Key Components		Contributory Components		Secondary
Code	History/ Examination	Medical Decision Making	Nature of Presenting Problem	Counseling Coordination Of Care	Time Bedside/ Unit
99311	Problem focused	Straightforward or low complexity	Stable, recovering or improving	Definition for all codes: Counseling and/or coordination of care with other providers or agencies consistent with the nature of the problem(s) and the patient's and/or family's needs.	15 minutes
99312	Expanded problem focused	Moderate complexity	Inadequate response to therapy or minor complication		25 minutes
99313	Detailed	Moderate to high complexity	Significant complication or new problem		35 minutes

Domiciliary, Rest Home or Custodial Care
New Patient

Service Category	Key Components		Contributory Components		Secondary
Code	History/ Examination	Medical Decision Making	Nature of Presenting Problem	Counseling Coordination Of Care	Time
99321	Problem focused	Straightforward or low complexity	Low severity	Definition for all codes: Counseling and/or coordination of care with other providers or agencies consistent with the nature of the problem(s) and the patient's and/or family's needs.	None
99322	Expanded problem focused	Moderate complexity	Moderate severity		None
99323	Detailed	High complexity	High severity		None

B-8
MEDICARE PPR EVALUATION AND MANAGEMENT CODES Continued
Domiciliary, Rest Home or Custodial Care
Established Patient

Service Category	Key Components		Contributory Components		Secondary
Code	History/ Examination	Medical Decision Making	Nature of Presenting Problem	Counseling Coordination Of Care	Time
99331	Problem focused	Straightforward or low complexity	Stable, recovering or improving	Definition for all codes: Counseling and/or coordination of care with other providers or agencies consistent with the nature of the problem(s) and the patient's and/ or family's needs.	None
99332	Expanded problem focused	Moderate complexity	Inadequate therapy response or minor complication		None
99333	Detailed	High complexity	Complication or new problem		None

Home Services
New Patient

Service Category	Key Components		Contributory Components		Secondary
Code	History/ Examination	Medical Decision Making	Nature of Presenting Problem	Counseling Coordination Of Care	Time
99341	Problem focused	Straightforward or low complexity	Low severity	Definition for all codes: Counseling and/or coordination of care with other providers or agencies consistent with the nature of the problem(s) and the patient's and/ or family's needs.	None
99342	Expanded problem focused	Moderate complexity	Moderate severity		None
99343	Detailed	High complexity	High severity		None

Home Services
Established Patient

Service Category	Key Components		Contributory Components		Secondary
Code	History/ Examination	Medical Decision Making	Nature of Presenting Problem	Counseling Coordination Of Care	Time
99351	Problem focused	Straightforward or low complexity	Stable recovering or improving	Definition for all codes: Counseling and/or coordination of care with other providers or agencies consistent with the nature of the problem(s) and the patient's and/ or family's needs.	None
99352	Expanded problem focused	Moderate complexity	Inadequate therapy response or minor complication		None
99353	Detailed	High complexity	Complication or new problem		None

Courtesy of The Travelers Insurance Company.

B-9

PROFESSIONAL DESIGNATIONS FOR HEALTH CARE PROVIDERS

Degrees, certifications, memberships and other initials that precede or follow the names of health care providers often provide helpful information regarding their area of expertise and level of practice. The following list identifies commonly used designations in English speaking countries, particularly the United States and Canada.

ANP	Adult Nurse Practitioner
ARNP	Advanced Registered Nurse Practitioner
BA	Bachelor of Arts
BB(ASCP)	Technologist in Blood Banking certified by The American Society of Clinical Pathologists
BDentSci	Bachelor of Dental Science
BDS	Bachelor of Dental Surgery
BDSc	Bachelor of Dental Science
BHS	Bachelor of Health Science
BHyg	Bachelor of Hygiene
BM	Bachelor of Medicine
BMed	Bachelor of Medicine
BMedBiol	Bachelor of Medical Biology
BMedSci	Bachelor of Medical Science
BMic	Bachelor of Microbiology
BMS	Bachelor of Medical Science
BMT	Bachelor of Medical Technology
BO	Bachelor of Osteopathy
BP	Bachelor of Pharmacy
BPH	Bachelor of Public Health
BPharm	Bachelor of Pharmacy
BPHEng	Bachelor of Public Health Engineering
BPHN	Bachelor of Public Health Nursing
BPsTh	Bachelor of Psychotherapy
BS	Bachelor of Science
BSM	Bachelor of Science in Medicine
BSN	Bachelor of Science in Nursing
BSPh	Bachelor of Science in Pharmacy
BSS	Bachelor of Sanitary Science
BVMS	Bachelor of Veterinary Medicine and Science
BVSc	Bachelor of Veterinary Science
C(ASCP)	Technologist in Chemistry certified by the American Society of Clinical Pathologists
CB	Bachelor of Surgery
CCRN	Critical Care Registered Nurse
CDA	Certified Dental Assistant
CEN	Certificate for Emergency Nursing
CEO	Chief Executive Officer
ChB	Bachelor of Surgery
ChD	Doctor of Surgery
ChM	Master of Surgery
CIH	Certificate in Industrial Health
CLA	Certified Laboratory Assistant
CLS	Clinical Laboratory Scientist
CLS(NCA)	Clinical Laboratory Scientist certified by the National Certification Agency for Medical Laboratory Personnel
CLT	Certified Laboratory Technician; Clinical Laboratory Technician
CLT(NCA)	Laboratory Technician certified by the National Certification Agency for Medical Laboratory Personnel
CM	Master of Surgery
CMA	Certified Medical Assistant
CMO	Chief Medical Officer
CNM	Certified Nurse Midwife
CNMT	Certified Nuclear Medicine Technologist
CNP	Community Nurse Practitioner
CNS	Clinical Nurse Specialist
CORN	Certified Operating Room Nurse
COTA	Certified Occupational Therapy Assistant
CPAN	Certified Post Anesthesia Nurse
CPH	Certificate in Public Health
CRNA	Certified Registered Nurse Anesthetist
CRRN	Certified Registered Rehabilitation Nurse
CRTT	Certified Respiratory Therapy Technician

B-9
PROFESSIONAL DESIGNATIONS FOR HEALTH CARE PROVIDERS Continued

CT(ASCP)	Cytotechnologist certified by the American Society of Clinical Pathologists
CURN	Certified Urological Registered Nurse
CVO	Chief Veterinary Officer
DA	Dental Assistant; Diploma in Anesthetics
DC	Doctor of Chiropractic
DCH	Diploma in Child Health
DCh	Doctor of Surgery
DChO	Doctor of Ophthalmic Surgery
DCM	Doctor of Comparative Medicine
DCOG	Diploma of the College of Obstetricians and Gynaecologists
DCP	Diploma in Clinical Pathology; Diploma in Clinical Psychology
DDH	Diploma in Dental Health
DDM	Doctor of Dental Medicine; Diploma in Dermatologic Medicine
DDO	Diploma in Dental Orthopaedics
DDR	Diploma in Diagnostic Radiology
DDS	Doctor of Dental Surgery
DDSc	Doctor of Dental Science
DFHom	Diploma of the Faculty of Homeopathy
DHg	Doctor of Hygiene
DHy	Doctor of Hygiene
DHyg	Doctor of Hygiene
Dip	Diplomate
DipBact	Diploma in Bacteriology
DipChem	Diploma in Chemistry
DipClinPath	Diploma in Clinical Pathology
DipMicrobiol	Diploma in Microbiology
DipSocMed	Diploma in Social Medicine
DLM(ASCP)	Diplomate in Laboratory Management
DMD	Doctor of Dental Medicine
DMT	Doctor of Medical Technology
DMV	Doctor of Veterinary Medicine
DN	Doctor of Nursing
DNE	Doctor of Nursing Education
DNS	Doctor of Nursing Science
DNSc	Doctor of Nursing Science
DO	Doctor of Osteopathy; Doctor of Optometry; Doctor of Ophthalmology
DON	Director of Nursing
DOS	Doctor of Ocular Science; Doctor of Optical Science
DP	Doctor of Pharmacy; Doctor of Podiatry
DPH	Doctor of Public Hygiene; Doctor of Public Health
DPhC	Doctor of Pharmaceutical Chemistry
DPHN	Doctor of Public Health Nursing
DPhys	Diploma in Physiotherapy
DPM	Doctor of Podiatric Medicine; Doctor of Physical Medicine; Doctor of Preventive Medicine; Doctor of Psychiatric Medicine
Dr	Doctor
DrHyg	Doctor of Hygiene
DrMed	Doctor of Medicine
DrPH	Doctor of Public Health; Doctor of Public Hygiene
DSc	Doctor of Science
DSE	Doctor of Sanitary Engineering
DSIM	Doctor of Science in Industrial Medicine
DSSc	Diploma in Sanitary Science
DVM	Doctor of Veterinary Medicine
DVMS	Doctor of Veterinary Medicine and Surgery
DVR	Doctor of Veterinary Radiology
DVS	Doctor of Veterinary Science; Doctor of Veterinary Medicine
DVSc	Doctor of Veterinary Science
Ed.D.	Doctor of Education
ET	Enterostomal Therapist
FAAN	Fellow of the American Academy of Nurses
FACA	Fellow of the American College of Anesthetists; Fellow of the American College of Angiology; Fellow of the American College of Apothecaries
FACAI	Fellow of the American College of Allergists
FACC	Fellow of the American College of Cardiologists
FACCP	Fellow of the American College of Chest Physicians
FACD	Fellow of the American College of Dentists
FACFP	Fellow of the American College of Family Physicians

Table continued on following page

B-9
PROFESSIONAL DESIGNATIONS FOR HEALTH CARE PROVIDERS Continued

FACG	Fellow of the American College of Gastroenterology
FACHA	Fellow of the American College of Health Administrators
FACOG	Fellow of the American College of Obstetricians and Gynecologists
FACP	Fellow of the American College of Physicians
FACPM	Fellow of the American College of Preventive Medicine
FACS	Fellow of the American College of Surgeons
FACSM	Fellow of the American College of Sports Medicine
FAMA	Fellow of the American Medicine Association
FAOTA	Fellow of the American Occupational Therapy Association
FAPA	Fellow of the American Psychiatric Association
FAPHA	Fellow of the American Public Health Association
FBPsS	Fellow of the British Psychological Association
FCAP	Fellow of the College of American Pathologists
FCMS	Fellow of the College of Medicine and Surgery
FCO	Fellow of the College of Osteopathy
FCPS	Fellow of the College of Physicians and Surgeons
FCSP	Fellow of the Chartered Society of Physiotherapy
FCST	Fellow of the College of Speech Therapists
FDS	Fellow in Dental Surgery
FDSRCSEng	Fellow in Dental Surgery of the Royal College of Surgeons of England
FFA	Fellow of the Faculty of Anesthetists
FFCM	Fellow of the Faculty of Community Medicine
FFD	Fellow in the Faculty of Dentistry
FFOM	Fellow of the Faculty of Occupational Medicine
FFR	Fellow of the Faculty of Radiologists
FIB	Fellow in the Institute of Biology
FICD	Fellow of the Institute of Canadian Dentists; Fellow of the International College of Dentists
FIMLT	Fellow of the Institute of Medical Laboratory Technology
FNP	Family Nurse Practitioner
FPS	Fellow of the Pathological Society
FRCD	Fellow of the Royal College of Dentists
FRCGP	Fellow of the Royal College of General Practitioners
FRCOG	Fellow of the Royal College of Obstetricians and Gynaecologists
FRCP	Fellow of the Royal College of Physicians
FRCPath	Fellow of the Royal College of Pathologists
FRCP(C)	Fellow of the Royal College of Physicians of Canada
FRCS	Fellow of the Royal College of Surgeons
FRCS(C)	Fellow of the Royal College of Surgeons of Canada
GNP	Gerontological Nurse Practitioner
H(ASCP)	Technologist in Hematology certified by the American Society of Clinical Pathologists
HT(ASCP)	Histologic Technician certified by the American Society of Clinical Pathologists
HTL(ASCP)	Histotechnologist certified by the American Society of Clinical Pathologists
I(ASCP)	Technologist in Immunology certified by the American Society of Clinical Pathologists
LMCC	Licentiate of the Medical Council of Canada
LMRCP	Licentiate in Midwifery of the Royal College of Physicians
LPN	Licensed Practical Nurse
LVN	Licensed Vocational Nurse
MA	Master of Arts
M(ASCP)	Technologist in Microbiology certified by the American Society of Clinical Pathologists
MB	Bachelor of Medicine
MC	Mastery of Surgery
MCPS	Member of the College of Physicians and Surgeons
MD	Doctor of Medicine
MDentSc	Master of Dental Science
MDS	Master of Dental Surgery
MLT	Medical Laboratory Technician
MLT(ASCP)	Medical Laboratory Technician certified by the American Society of Clinical Pathologists
MMS	Master of Medical Science
MMSA	Master of Midwifery
MPH	Master of Public Health
MPharm	Master of Pharmacy
MRad	Master of Radiology
MRL	Medical Records Librarian
MS	Master of Science; Master of Surgery
MSB	Master of Science in Bacteriology

B-9
PROFESSIONAL DESIGNATIONS FOR HEALTH CARE PROVIDERS Continued

MSc	Master of Science
MScD	Master of Dental Science
MScN	Master of Science in Nursing
MSN	Master of Science in Nursing
MSPH	Master of Science in Public Health
MSPhar	Master of Science in Pharmacy
MSSc	Master of Sanitary Science
MSW	Master of Social Work; Medical Social Worker
MT	Medical Technologist
MT(ASCP)	Medical Technologist certified by the American Society of Clinical Pathologists
MVD	Doctor of Veterinary Medicine
ND	Doctor of Nursing
NM(ASCP)	Technologist in Nuclear Medicine certified by the American Society of Clinical Pathologists
NP	Nurse Practitioner
OD	Doctor of Optometry
ONC	Orthopedic Nursing Certificate
OT	Occupational Therapist
OTL	Occupational Therapist, Licensed
OTR	Occupational Therapist, Registered
OTReg	Occupational Therapist, Registered
PA	Physician's Assistant
PBT(ASCP)	Phlebotomy Technician certified by the American Society of Clinical Pathologists
PCP	Primary Care Physician
PD	Doctor of Pharmacy
Ph.D.	Doctor of Philosophy; Doctor of Pharmacy
PNP	Pediatric Nurse Practitioner
PT	Physical Therapist
RDA	Registered Dental Assistant
Reg	Registered
RMA	Registered Medical Assistant
RN	Registered Nurse
RNA	Registered Nurse Anesthetist
RN,C.	Registered Nurse Certified (used to identify nurses certified by the American Nurses Credentialing Center; areas of practice are medical-surgical nurse, gerontological nurse, psychiatric and mental health nurse, pediatric nurse, perinatal nurse, community health nurse, school nurse, general nursing practice, college health nurse, gerontologic nurse practitioner, pediatric nurse practitioner, adult nurse practitioner, family nurse practitioner, and school nurse practitioner)
RN,C.N.A.	Registered Nurse, Certified in Nursing Administration
RN, CNNA	Registered Nurse, Certified in Nursing Administration, Advanced
RN,C.S.	Registered Nurse, Certified Specialist (used to identify nurses certified by the American Nurses Credentialing Center; this certification recognizes clinical specialists in the following areas: gerontological nursing, medical surgical nursing, adult psychiatric and mental health nursing, child and adolescent psychiatric and mental health nursing, and community health nursing)
RPh	Registered Pharmacist
RPT	Registered Physical Therapist
RRA	Registered Record Administrator
RRL	Registered Record Librarian
RRT	Registered Respiratory Therapist
RT	Radiologic Technologist; Respiratory Therapist
RT(N)	Nuclear Medicine Technologist
RT(R)	Technologist in Diagnostic Radiology
RTR	Registered Recreational Therapist
RT(T)	Radiation Therapy Technologist
SBB(ASCP)	Specialist in Blood Banking certified by the American Society of Clinical Pathologists
ScD	Doctor of Science
SCT(ASCP)	Specialist in Cytotechnology certified by the American Society of Clinical Pathologists
SNP	School Nurse Practitioner
SW	Social Worker

From Miller BF, Keane CB: *Encyclopedia and Dictionary of Medicine, Nursing, and Allied Health*, 5th ed. Philadelphia: W.B. Saunders, 1992, pp. 1757–1760.

B-10

SPECIALIZED TERMS USED IN MEDICAL RECORDS

The American Health Information Management Association has identified a group of terms used to compile statistical health care data, and has defined them in an attempt at standardization. Some of the terms are presented here in an appendix to highlight the importance of using standardized terms for research initiatives and the reporting of statistical data. The definitions are the exact ones used by the American Health Information Management Association. Some of the terms are defined in other ways in the entries section of this dictionary, but terms often have multiple meanings. *The Glossary of Health Care Terms* is a complete list of terms and definitions used in medical records; it is available from the American Health Information Management Association, 919 N. Michigan Ave., Suite 1400, Chicago, Illinois 60611.

Diagnosis—A word or phrase used by a physician to identify a disease from which an individual patient suffers or a condition for which a patient needs, seeks, or receives medical care.

Principal Diagnosis—The diagnosis of the condition established after study, chiefly responsible for occasioning the admission of the patient to the hospital for care.

Other Diagnosis—A diagnosis, other than the principal diagnosis, that describes a condition for which a patient receives treatment or which the physician considers of sufficient significance to warrant inclusion for investigative medical studies.

Complication—An additional diagnosis that describes a condition arising after the beginning of hospital observation and treatment and modifying the course of the patient's illness or the medical care required.

Most Significant Diagnosis—The one diagnosis, often but not necessarily the principal diagnosis, that describes the most important or significant condition of a patient in terms of its implications for his health, his medical care, and the use of the hospital.

Discharge Diagnosis—Any one of the diagnoses recorded after all data is accumulated in the course of a patient's hospitalization or other circumscribed episode of medical care have been studied.

Discharge Diagnoses (List of Discharge Diagnoses)—The complete set or list of discharge diagnoses applicable to a single patient experience such as inpatient hospitalization.

Facility—Those objects, including plant, equipment, or supplies, necessary for implementation of services by personnel.

Hospital—Health care institution with an organized and professional staff and with inpatient beds available around the clock, whose primary function is to provide inpatient medical, nursing, and other health related services to patients for both surgical and nonsurgical conditions, and that usually provides some outpatient services, particularly emergency care; for licensure purposes, each state has its own definition of hospital.

Hospital Patient—An individual receiving, in person, hospital based or coordinated medical services for which the hospital is responsible.

Hospital Inpatient—A hospital patient who is provided with room, board, and continuous general nursing service in an area of the hospital where patients generally stay at least overnight.

Hospital Newborn Inpatient—A hospital patient who was born in the hospital at the beginning of his current inpatient hospitalization.

Hospital Boarder—An individual who receives lodging in the hospital but is not a hospital inpatient.

Hospital Inpatient Beds—Accommodations with supporting services (such as food, laundry, housekeeping) for hospital inpatients, excluding those for the newborn nursery.

Hospital Newborn Bassinets—Accommodations with supporting services (such as food, laundry, housekeeping) for hospital newborn inpatients. These include bassinets, incubators, and isolettes in the newborn nursery.

Medical Services—The activities related to medical care performed by physicians, nurses, and other professional and technical personnel under the direction of a physician.

Operating room—An area of a hospital equipped and staffed to provide facilities and personnel services for the performance of surgical procedures.

Delivery room—A special operating room for obstetric delivery and infant resuscitation.

Unit—An organizational entity of a hospital. Hospitals are organized both physically and functionally into units.

Medical Staff Unit—One of the departments, divisions, or specialties into which the organized medical staff of a hospital is divided in order to fulfill medical staff responsibility.

Medical Care Unit—An assemblage of inpatient beds (or newborn bassinets) and related facilities and assigned personnel in which medical services are provided to a defined and limited class of patients according to their particular medical care needs.

Special Care Unit—A medical care unit in which there is appropriate equipment and a concentration of physicians, nurses, and others who have special skills and experience to provide optimal medical care for critically ill patients, or continuous care of patients in special diagnostic categories.

Adjunct Diagnostic or Therapeutic Unit (Ancillary Unit)—An organized unit of a hospital, other than the operating room, delivery room, or medical care unit, with facilities and personnel to aid physicians in the diagnosis and treatment of patients through the performance of diagnostic or therapeutic procedures.

From Miller BF, Keane CB: *Encyclopedia and Dictionary of Medicine, Nursing, and Allied Health,* 5th ed. Philadelphia: W.B. Saunders, 1992, p. 1736.

B-11
SYMBOLS COMMONLY USED IN CLINICAL PRACTICE

$\bar{a}$	before
$\bar{p}$	after
$\bar{c}$	with
$\bar{s}$	without
=	equal
≠	unequal
>	greater than
<	less than
↑	increase
↗	increasing
↓	decrease
↘	decreasing
−	negative, minus, deficiency, alkaline reaction
±	very slight trace or reaction, indefinite
+	slight trace or reaction, positive, plus, excess, acid reaction
+ +	trace or notable reaction
+ + +	moderate amount or reaction
+ + + +	large amount or pronounced reaction
#	number, pound, has been given or done
→	yields, leads to
←	resulting from or secondary to
$\xrightarrow{\text{(catalyst)}}$	accelerant, increases velocity of a chemical reaction or process
♂ ○ ○ or □	male
♀ or ○	female
ʒ	dram
℥	ounce
1°, 2°	primary, secondary

From Miller BF, Keane CB: *Encyclopedia and Dictionary of Medicine, Nursing, and Allied Health,* 5th ed. Philadelphia: W.B. Saunders, 1992, p. 1671.

Appendix B: ADMINISTRATIVE INFORMATION

B-12
WORDS AND PHRASES COMMONLY MISINTERPRETED

Health care professionals who have difficulty with the English language may face particular challenges with terms commonly used in a health care setting. The unique application of words may cause confusion. The words and phrases listed below have been identified as frequently causing problems for health care providers.

Word or Phrase	Definition/Example	Word or Phrase	Definition/Example
Adequate	*Definition* enough; sufficient. *Example* A well balanced diet should contain ADEQUATE amounts of protein and vitamins. *Alternate Wording* A well balanced diet should contain sufficient amounts of protein and vitamins.		*Example* A patient receiving continuous tube feedings should have the head of the bed elevated AT LEAST 30 degrees. *Alternate Wording* A patient receiving continuous tube feedings should have the head of the bed elevated at a minimum of 30 degrees.
Aggravate	*Definition* to make worse. *Example* Heat AGGRAVATES an itch. *Alternate Wording* Heat makes an itch worse.	Avoid	*Definition* to abstain from a substance or activity; to keep at a distance. *Example* A patient with cardiac disease should AVOID salty foods. *Alternate Wording* A patient with cardiac disease should not eat any salty foods.
Allay anxiety	*Definition* to decrease worry, tension, or apprehension. *Example* Telling a patient what to expect during a procedure helps to ALLAY ANXIETY. *Alternate Wording* Telling a patient what to expect during a procedure helps to decrease the patient's tension or apprehension.	Competitive	*Definition* striving for the same thing or goal as another. A person who is competitive feels a need to succeed or to be beter than others. (There does not always need to be a formal competition for a person who is competitive to want to be the best.)
Anticipate	*Definition* to expect an event or symptoms; to foresee a patient problem *Example* The nurse ANTICIPATES the need for pain medication in the postoperative patient. *Alternate Wording* The nurse expects to administer pain medication to the post-operative patient.		*Example* COMPETITIVE sports may be too stressful for a patient with cardiac disease. *Alternate Wording* Sports in which participants play to win may be too stressful for the patient with cardiac disease.
Assume responsibility	*Definition* to take on as one's duty. *Example* The nurses ASSUMED RESPONSIBILITY for the patient's discharge plan. *Alternate Wording* The nurse accepted as a duty the obligation to complete the patient's discharge plan.	Compromise	*Definitions* (1) to adjust or settle a difference between parties by mutual concessions; (2) to endanger or put in jeopardy. *Example (1)* The physical therapist and occupational therapist COMPROMISED on the patient's schedule. *Alternate Wording* The physical therapist and occupational therapist both modified the patient's schedule after they discussed the patient's needs.
At least	*Definition* at a minimum of, the smallest amount acceptable.		

B-12
WORDS AND PHRASES COMMONLY MISINTERPRETED Continued

Word or Phrase	Definition/Example	Word or Phrase	Definition/Example
	Example (2) Heart disease may COMPROMISE respiratory function.	Energy Requirements	*Definition* that which is needed to act, or work, or have strength.
	Alternate Wording In the presence of heart disease, respiratory function may be less than optimal or may even be endangered.		*Example* A balanced diet provides the body with its ENERGY REQUIREMENTS.
Confer	*Definitions* (1) to give; (2) to advise.		*Alternate Wording* A balanced diet provides the body with what it needs to have strength.
	Example (1) The Hepatitis B vaccine CONFERS immunity to that disease.	Enhance	*Definition* to make greater; to increase in value, attractiveness, or effectiveness.
	Alternate Wording The Hepatitis B vaccine gives immunity to that disease.		*Example* A clearly stated message ENHANCES communication.
	Example (2) The doctor and nurse CONFER about a patient's progress.		*Alternate Wording* A clearly stated message makes communication more effective.
	Alternate Wording The doctor and nurse advise each other about a patient's progress.	Exacerbate	*Definition* to irritate; to annoy; to make more intense; to make worse.
Deny	*Definition* to state that something is not true or does not exist.		*Example* Spicy foods EXACERBATE the pain of a duodenal ulcer.
	Example The patient DENIES a history of heart disease in his family.		*Alternate Wording* Spicy foods make the pain of a duodenal ulcer worse.
	Alternate Wording The patient states that there is no heart disease in his family.	Except	*Definition* excluding or omitting.
Determine	*Definition* to find out exactly.		*Example* (this is a common wording for multiple choice test questions) All of the following foods contain protein EXCEPT (1) meat (2) fish (3) celery (4) eggs. (The correct answer is (3) celery because that does not contain protein.)
	Example The dietician should DETERMINE the patient's food preferences.		
	Alternate Wording The dietician should find out what food the patient prefers.		*Alternate Wording* All of the following foods contain protein if you exclude (1) meat (2) fish (3) celery (4) eggs.
Differentiate	*Definition* to distinguish; to discriminate; to mark or show the difference in.	Excessively	*Definition* Much more than normal or desirable; a great deal.
	Example DIFFERENTIATE the symptoms of angina pectoris and a myocardial infarction.		*Example* The patient bled EXCESSIVELY.
	Alternate Wording Show how the symptoms of angina pectoris and a myocardial infarction differ from each other.		*Alternate Wording* The patient bled a great deal.
		Expectorate	*Definition* to cough up and spit.

Table continued on following page

B-12
WORDS AND PHRASES COMMONLY MISINTERPRETED *Continued*

Word or Phrase	Definition/Example	Word or Phrase	Definition/Example
	Example The patient EXPECTORATED thick mucus. *Alternate Wording* The patient coughed up and spit thick mucus.		*Example* (1) The patient's condition is GUARDED. *Alternate Wording* The patient's condition is precarious. *Example* (2) The patient GUARDED his wound during the physical examination. *Alternate Wording* The patient tensed the abdominal muscles to avoid pain during the physical examination.
Flaccid	*Definition* weak, ineffective, limp. *Example* Those who do not exercise have FLACCID muscles. *Alternate Wording* Those who do not exercise have weak, ineffective muscles.		
Flushed	*Definition* reddened; feeling warm or hot. *Example* The nurse checks the temperature of the patient who has a FLUSHED face. *Alternate Wording* The nurse checks the temperature of the patient whose face is reddened.	Herb	*Definition* a plant or plant part that is valued for its medicinal, savory, or aromatic qualities. *Example* Many people include HERBS in their diet to promote healing. *Alternate Wording* Many people include in their diet plant substances believed to have medicinal qualities.
Garter	*Definition* a narrow elastic strap that usually encircles the leg to hold up a stocking; sometimes a piece of elastic with a fastener that is attached to a girdle to hold up a stocking. *Example* Wearing tight GARTERS will interfere with circulation. *Alternate Wording* Wearing tight elastic straps around the legs to hold up the stockings will interfere with circulation.	Hoarseness	*Definition* harshness of sound or voice; an unpleasantly rough sound or voice. *Example* HOARSENESS may be an early sign of cancer of the larynx. *Alternate Wording* A rough sounding voice may be an early sign of cancer of the larynx.
Girdle	*Definition* corset; a close fitting, usually elastic undergarment that encircles a part of the body. *Example* Very tight GIRDLES will interfere with circulation. *Alternate Wording* Very tight undergarments or corsets will interfere with circulation.	Impinge	*Definition* to strike, clash, hit against, or interfere with something. *Example* The mumbling of words IMPINGES upon effective communication. *Alternate Wording* The mumbling of words interferes with effective communication.
Guarded	*Definition* (1) in a precarious state of health; (2) a term used when a patient has taken an action to protect from pain or discomfort.	Inept	*Definition* likely to fail; inadequate, out of place. *Example* The depressed man may feel INEPT as a father and provider.

B-12
WORDS AND PHRASES COMMONLY MISINTERPRETED Continued

Word or Phrase	Definition/Example	Word or Phrase	Definition/Example
Insulation	*Alternate Wording* The depressed man may feel inadequate as a father and provider. *Definition* material used to shield from the transfer of electricity, heat, or sound. *Example* A house must have proper INSULATION if it is to stay warm in the winter. *Alternate Wording* A house must be shielded from the loss of heat to stay warm in the winter.	Permit	*Alternate Wording* Patients on regular diets may use spices in large amounts. *Definition* to allow; to make possible. *Example* The doctor will PERMIT the patient with cardiac disease to ambulate when his condition remains stable. *Alternate Wording* The doctor will allow the patient with cardiac disease to ambulate when his condition remains stable.
Isolation	*Definition* the state of being separated or placed apart from other persons or things. *Example* The patient with chickenpox was placed in ISOLATION. *Alternate Wording* The patient with chickenpox was separated from other patients.	Predispose	*Definition* to make susceptible; to create a tendency toward. *Example* Smoking PREDISPOSES a person to lung cancer. *Alternate Wording* Smoking makes a person more likely to develop lung cancer.
Lead to	*Definition* to cause; to precede. *Example* Heavy smoking may LEAD TO lung cancer. *Alternate Wording* Heavy smoking may cause lung cancer.	Profusely	*Definition* pouring freely and abundantly; a great deal. *Example* The patient bled PROFUSELY. *Alternate Wording* The patient bled a great deal.
Least likely	*Definition* most probably not; in a series of choices, the one that is not likely to occur or be true. *Example* Among men over 40 years of age, those who exercise regularly and eat well balanced diets are LEAST LIKELY to develop heart disease. *Alternate Wording* Among men over 40 years of age, those who exercise regularly and eat well balanced diets will probably not develop heart disease.	Refrain	*Definition* to hold back; to avoid. *Example* A person with poor circulation must REFRAIN from smoking. *Alternate Wording* A person with poor circulation must avoid smoking.
		Sniffles	*Definition* an upper respiratory infection; breathing in through the nose so as to check or stop mucus from running out of the nose. *Example* The child has the SNIFFLES. *Alternate Wording* The child has an upper respiratory infection.
Liberally	*Definition* in a large amount; abundantly. *Example* Patients on regular diets may use spices LIBERALLY.	Sparingly	*Definition* infrequently; used very little. *Example* Patients on low cholesterol diets should eat eggs SPARINGLY.

Table continued on following page

B-12

WORDS AND PHRASES COMMONLY MISINTERPRETED *Continued*

Word or Phrase	Definition/Example	Word or Phrase	Definition/Example
	Alternate Wording Patients on low cholesterol diets should eat eggs infrequently.		*Alternate Wording* The nurse supports the incision with a pillow following surgery while the patient coughs and deep breathes.
Spasm	*Definition* an involuntary or abnormal contraction of a muscle or muscle fibers.	Support hose	*Definition* elastic stockings.
	Example Muscle SPASMS of the lower back can be very painful.		*Example* People with varicose veins are encouraged to wear SUPPORT HOSE.
	Alternate Wording Involuntary contractions of the muscles of the lower back can be very painful.		*Alternate Wording* People with varicose veins are encouraged to wear special elastic stockings.
Splint	*Definition* to support or brace; to protect against pain by limiting motion.		
	Example The nurse SPLINTS the incision of the patient following surgery while he coughs and deep breathes.		

From Miller BF, Keane CB: *Encyclopedia and Dictionary of Medicine, Nursing, and Allied Health*, 5th ed. Philadelphia: W.B. Saunders, 1992, pp. 1737–1741.

APPENDIX C
CLINICAL INFORMATION

C-1	Poisoning by Common Chemicals
C-2	Drugs for Treating Poisoning
C-3	Uses and Effects of Controlled Substances
C-4	Selected Skin Tests
C-5	Tables of Weights and Measures
C-6	Approximate Household Equivalents
C-7	Desirable Weights for Men and Women, According to Height and Frame, Ages 25 to 29
C-8	Ideal Weights for Boys and Girls, According to Height and Age
C-9	Recommended Daily Dietary Allowances (RDAs)
C-10	The Principal Micronutrients (Vitamins and Minerals)
C-11	Laboratory Values of Clinical Importance

C-1

POISONING BY COMMON CHEMICALS

Poison and sources	Assessment factors	Emergency treatment
Acids (corrosive) Hydrochloric Sulfuric Nitric Phosphoric (toilet bowl cleaners)	1. Burns about mouth and throat 2. Abdominal pain, nausea, vomiting 3. Circulatory collapse: ↓ BP, ↑ P, cold and clammy 4. Respiratory tract edema, asphyxia 5. Long-term effects: respiratory strictures, stenoses	1. *Do not use emetics or lavage.* 2. Give milk of magnesia, aluminum hydroxide gel, or dilute soap solution. 3. Have victim drink large quantities of water. 4. Give demulcents such as milk, egg whites, or olive oil. 5. Flood external skin burns with large amounts of water, followed by application of sodium bicarbonate paste. 6. Flush eye burns with water, possibly after use of topical anesthetic.
Alkali (caustic) "Lye": sodium hydroxide, potassium hydroxide, caustic soda, alkaline carbonates (drain cleaners, paint removers, Clinitest urine tablets, stove grease removers, solid household bleaches)	1. Burns about the mouth and throat; throat edematous, white, then turning brown 2. Burning pain in esophagus and stomach; mucoid, then bloody vomitus 3. Circulatory collapse indicated by cold clammy skin and by ↑ P, ↓ BP 4. Death may result rapidly from shock or asphyxia, or occur later from shock as a result of perforation of viscera or from more slowly developing respiratory tract infections	1. *Do not induce emesis or employ gastric lavage.* 2. Have patient drink large quantities of water or milk to dilute the alkali. 3. Give demulcents, including olive oil and egg white. 4. Wash external burns with large amounts of water or with dilute vinegar. 5. Give potent analgesics, IV fluids, and electrolytes, antibiotics, and corticosteroids, as appropriate.
Arsenic compounds Arsenic trioxide Arsenic pentoxide Sodium arsenite Sodium arsenate (weed killers, rat poison, insecticides, paints)	1. Burning, cramping abdominal pain; difficulty swallowing; severe, watery or bloody diarrhea 2. Signs of dehydration 3. Complaints of metallic taste; garliclike odor on breath 4. Death may result from cardiovascular collapse, or from fluid and electrolyte imbalances 5. Chronic effects: headache, dizziness, delirium, coma, convulsions	1. Use emetics, gastric lavage, and saline cathartics. 2. Give milk; give penicillamine orally. 3. Administer dimercaprol (BAL) intramuscularly. 4. Give IV fluids and electrolytes to correct dehydration and deficiencies and to counteract shock.

(continued)

C-1
POISONING BY COMMON CHEMICALS Continued

Poison and sources	Assessment factors	Emergency treatment
Aromatic hydrocarbons		
Benzene Toluene Xylene (solvents, paint removers, insecticide solutions, glue)	1. Inflammatory reaction at site of local skin contact 2. Nausea, vomiting, increased salivation; if swallowed, patient reports a burning sensation on swallowing 3. Acute inhalation exposure results in signs and symptoms of alcohol intoxication; continued inhalation results in coma, hyperactive reflexes, death 4. Chronic exposure: bone marrow suppression ($\downarrow$ WBC, $\downarrow$ RBC, $\downarrow$ platelets)	1. Wash skin and eyes thoroughly. 2. Use gastric lavage; instill mineral oil or saline cathartic into stomach. 3. Institute supportive measures to maintain respirations and fluid balance. 4. Do not give epinephrine, alcohol, or vegetable fats.
Bleaches (household)		
Liquid: sodium hypochlorite (Clorox)—releases hypochlorous acid in acidic gastric juice (*Caution:* combining liquid bleach with acidic toilet bowl cleaners may produce dangerous chlorine gas) Solid: sodium perborate	1. Vomiting; complaints of upper GI burning 2. Tearing, red eyes; irritation of nose and throat 3. Gastrointestinal signs and symptoms; shock; CNS effects leading to convulsions and coma	1. Give milk to dilute; antacids may also be given. 2. Wash areas exposed to local contact. 3. Supportive and protective measures.
Camphor		
(Liniment, camphorated oil, moth repellents)	1. Nausea, vomiting—vomitus smells like camphor 2. CNS signs: headache, dizziness, confusion, restlessness, delirium 3. Grand mal seizures, coma, respiratory failure, death	1. Use gastric lavage or induce vomiting if CNS excitement has not occurred. 2. Sedate with IV barbiturates.
Carbon monoxide—CO combines with hemoglobin to form carboxyhemoglobin, which cannot carry oxygen to tissues		
(Automobile exhaust; exhaust from heaters, stoves; fumes from burning of certain synthetic materials)	1. Headache in varying degrees, depending on dose 2. CNS effects: confusion, ataxia, loss of consciousness, coma 3. Skin: cherry-red color	1. Provide fresh air or pure oxygen, if possible (hyperbaric O_2 is very effective). 2. Provide respiratory support if needed.

(continued)

C-1

POISONING BY COMMON CHEMICALS *Continued*

Poison and sources	Assessment factors	Emergency treatment
Carbon tetrachloride (Dry cleaning stain remover, industrial degreasers, some home fire extinguishers)	1. Nausea, vomiting, abdominal pain 2. CNS effects: headache, confusion, dizziness, drowsiness, visual changes, coma, respiratory failure 3. Chronic effects: liver failure; anorexia, nausea, vomiting, jaundice; renal failure: oliguria, anuria, albuminuria, edema, weight gain	1. Provide fresh air if inhaled; use gastric lavage or induce vomiting if ingested; flush with soap and water if skin contact has occurred. 2. Provide oxygen to help protect liver from anoxia. 3. Provide support and prophylaxis for liver and kidney complications.
Cyanides (Exterminator's fumigants, salts used in metal polishes and in photography, electroplating, metallurgy)	1. Rapid respiratory failure and death 2. CNS signs and symptoms of hypoxia, if minute doses; headache, dizziness, respiratory difficulty, tremors to convulsions	1. Give artificial respiration; positive pressure oxygen. 2. Have patient inhale amyl nitrite (smelling salts) or give IV sodium nitrite, both of which form methemoglobin, which in turn will combine with cyanide. 3. Inject sodium thiosulfate to convert cyanide to thiocyanate, a safer substance. 4. Provide for whole blood transfusion, in extreme cases.
Fluorides Sodium fluoride Sodium fluorsilicate (insecticides, roach powders) (*Note:* fluoridated water supplies are *not* toxic)	1. Abdominal pain and cramps; nausea, vomiting, diarrhea 2. Dehydration; shock: weak, rapid pulse; pallor; weakness 3. Muscular effects: tremors, partial paralysis, spasms, convulsions 4. Death from shock or respiratory or cardiac failure	1. Give milk or fluid with calcium salts. 2. IV calcium salts may be used to treat muscle spasms. 3. Give parenteral fluids to counteract dehydration and to prevent shock.
Nicotine (Black Leaf 40, tobacco products)	1. Abdominal pain, nausea, vomiting, diarrhea 2. CNS effects: headache, dizziness, weakness, visual disturbances, confusion 3. Cardiovascular effects: ↑ BP, arrhythmias 4. In severe cases, shock, respiratory failure, convulsions, loss of reflexes, respiratory paralysis, death	1. Use gastric lavage with potassium permanganate 1:5000; give universal antidote in water. 2. Wash skin to prevent absorption. 3. Provide respiratory support and give diazepam if convulsions occur.

(continued)

C-1
POISONING BY COMMON CHEMICALS Continued

Poison and sources	Assessment factors	Emergency treatment
Petroleum distillates Kerosene Gasoline Other oils (fuels, furniture waxes, paint thinners, cleaning fluids)	1. Nausea, vomiting, complaints of GI burning; coughing and choking if inhaled 2. CNS effects: drowsiness, stupor, coma 3. Rapidly developing pulmonary edema: rales, dyspnea, cyanosis; fever, tachycardia; death occurs frequently	1. *Do not induce emesis.* 2. Use careful gastric lavage with water and sodium bicarbonate solution. 3. Use olive oil, mineral oil, or saline cathartic to prevent absorption. 4. Provide supportive treatment: give oxygen, steroids, antibiotics; do not use epinephrine.
Phenol (carbolic acid) (Disinfectants: if used appropriately, in small doses, should not be toxic to skin)	1. White burns of skin, mucous membranes 2. Upper GI burning, nausea, vomiting, diarrhea 3. Cardiovascular effects: weak pulse, arrhythmias, pale, cyanotic skin, shallow respirations, shock 4. CNS effects: excitement followed by depression 5. Death from respiratory failure; chronic kidney damage: oliguria, dark urine	1. Give olive oil or vegetable oils as a solvent; use gastric lavage, milk, eggs 2. Wash skin with water if there are contact burns. 3. Provide supportive measures and protection.
Turpentine (Varnish and paint solvent; disinfectants; cleansing solutions)	1. Upper GI and abdominal pain; nausea, vomiting, diarrhea 2. Choking, coughing if inhaled 3. CNS effects: excitement followed by depression 4. Kidney damage: albuminuria, hematuria, urine smells like violets	1. Lavage stomach with water or sodium bicarbonate solution. 2. Instill milk or mineral oil to allay GI irritation. 3. Force fluids to prevent kidney damage. 4. Provide supportive and protective measures.

Rodman M, et al: *Pharmacology and Drug Therapy in Nursing*, 3rd ed. Philadelphia: J.B. Lippincott, 1985, pp. 97–100.

C-2
DRUGS FOR TREATING POISONING

Acetic acid (diluted vinegar)—neutralizes alkali
Activated charcoal—adsorbs most chemicals
Ammonium acetate—neutralizes formaldehyde
Ammonium hydroxide—neutralizes formaldehyde
Apomorphine HCl—emetic
Calcium salts (chloride, gluconate, lactate)—neutralize fluorides and oxalic acid
Copper sulfate—neutralizes phosphorus
Ipecac syrup—emetic
Iodine tincture—neutralizes some metals and alkaloids
Magnesium oxide and hydroxide (milk of magnesia)—neutralize acids, including acid from bleach; also demulcent and cathartic
Magnesium sulfate (Epsom salt)—cathartic
Milk, diluted dairy or evaporated—demulcent, diluent, precipitant
Olive oil—demulcent, laxative
Petrolatum, liquid—demulcent, solvent
Potassium permanganate—oxidizes alkaloids
Sodium bicarbonate—neutralizes ferrous sulfate and other iron salts; externally only to neutralize acids
Sodium chloride (normal saline solution)—neutralizes silver nitrate
Sodium sulfate—cathartic
Sodium thiosulfate—neutralizes iodine
Starch solution—neutralizes iodine
Tannic acid—neutralizes metals, alkaloids, other organic substances
Universal antidote (activated charcoal, magnesium oxide, tannic acid)—neutralizes most poisons (theoretically; practically, activated charcoal alone is preferred)

Rodman M, et al: *Pharmacology and Drug Therapy in Nursing*, 3rd ed. Philadelphia: J.B. Lippincott, 1985, p. 102.

C-3
USES AND EFFECTS OF CONTROLLED SUBSTANCES

	Drugs	Schedule	Trade or Other Name	Medical Uses	Physical Dependence
Narcotics	Opium	I, III, V	Dover's Powder, paregoric, Parepectolin	Analgesic, antidiarrheal	High
	Morphine	II, III	Morphine, Pectoral Syrup	Analgesic, antitussive	High
	Codeine	II, III, V	Codeine, Empirin Compound with Codeine, Robitussin A-C	Analgesic, antitussive	Moderate
	Heroin	I	Diacetylmorphine, horse, smack	Under investigation	High
	Hydromorphone	II	Dilaudid	Analgesic	High
	Meperidine (penthidine)	II	Demerol	Analgesic	High
	Methadone	II	Dolophine, Methadone, Methadose	Analgesic, heroin substitute	High
	Other narcotics	I, II, III, IV, V	LAAM, Leritine, Levo-Dromoran, Percodan, Tussionex, Fentanyl, Darvon*, Talwin*, Lomotil	Analgesic, antidiarrheal, antitussive	High–low
Depressants	Chloral hydrate	IV	Noctec, Somnos	Hypnotic	Moderate
	Barbiturates	II, III, V	Amobarbital, phenobarbital, Butisol, Phenobarbital, Secobarbital, Tuinal	Anesthetic, anticonvulsant, sedative, hypnotic	High–moderate
	Glutethimide	III	Doriden	Sedative, hypnotic	High
	Methaqualone	II	Optimil, Parest, Quaalude, Somnafac, Sopor	Sedative, hypnotic	High
	Benzodiazepines	IV	Ativan, Azene, Clonopin, Dalmane, Diazepam, Librium, Serax, Tranxene, Valium, Verstran	Anti-anxiety, anticonvulsant, sedative, hypnotic	Low
	Other depressants	III, IV	Equanil, Miltown, Noludar, Placidyl, Valmid	Anti-anxiety, sedative, hypnotic	Moderate
Stimulants	Cocaine†	II	Coke, flake, snow	Local anesthetic	Possible
	Amphetamines	II, III	Biphetamine, Delcobese, Desoxyn, Dexedrine, Mediatric		Possible
	Phenmetrazine	II	Preludin		Possible
	Methylphenidate	II	Ritalin	Hyperkinesis, narcolepsy, weight control	Possible
	Other stimulants	III, IV	Adipex, Bacarate, Cylert, Didrex, Ionamin, Plegine, Pre-Sate, Sanorex, Tenuate, Tepanil, Voranil		Possible
Hallucinogens	LSD	I	Acid, microdot	None	None
	Mescaline and peyote	I	Mesc, buttons, cactus	None	None
	Amphetamine variants	I	2,5-DMA, PMA, STP, MDA, MMDA, TMA, DOM, DOB	None	Unknown
	Phencyclidine	II	PCP, angle dust, hog	Veterinary anesthetic	Degree unknown
	Phencyclidine analogs	I	PCE, PCPy, TCP	None	Degree unknown
	Other hallucinogens	I	Bufotenine, ibogaine, DMT, DET, psilocybin, psilocin	None	None

*Not designated a narcotic under the Controlled Substances Act.
†Designated a narcotic under the Controlled Substances Act.
Data from the Drug Enforcement Administration, United States Department of Justice.

C-3
USES AND EFFECTS OF CONTROLLED SUBSTANCES *Continued*

Psychological Dependence	Tolerance	Duration of Effects (In Hours)	Usual Method of Administration	Possible Effects	Effects of Overdose	Withdrawal Syndrome
High	Yes	3–6	Oral, smoked			
High	Yes	3–6	Oral, injected, smoked			
High	Yes	3–6	Oral, injected			
High	Yes	3–6	Injected, sniffed, smoked	Euphoria, drowsiness, respiratory depression, constricted pupils, nausea	Slow and shallow breathing, clammy skin, convulsions, coma, possible death	Watery eyes, runny nose, yawning, loss of appetite, irritability, tremors, panic, chills and sweating, cramps, nausea
High	Yes	3–6	Oral, injected			
High	Yes	3–6	Oral, injected			
High	Yes	12–24	Oral, injected			
High–low	Yes	Variable	Oral, injected			
Moderate	Possible	5–8	Oral			
High–moderate	Yes	1–16	Oral, injected			
High	Yes	4–8	Oral, injected	Slurred speech, disorientation, drunken behavior without odor of alcohol	Shallow respiration, cold and clammy skin, dilated pupils, weak and rapid pulse, coma, possible death	Anxiety, insomnia, tremors, delirium, convulsions, possible death
High	Yes	4–8	Oral, injected			
Low	Yes	4–8	Oral injected			
Moderate	Yes	4–8	Oral, injected			
High	Possible	1–2	Sniffed, injected	Increased alertness, excitation, euphoria, increased pulse rate and blood pressure, insomnia, loss of appetite	Agitation, increase in body temperature, hallucinations, convulsions, possible death	Apathy, long periods of sleep, irritability, depression, disorientation
High	Yes	2–4	Oral, injected			
High	Yes	2–4	Oral, injected			
High	Yes	2–4	Oral, injected			
High	Yes	2–4	Oral, injected			
Degree unknown	Yes	8–12	Oral			
Degree unknown	Yes	8–12	Oral, injected			
Degree unknown	Yes	Up to days	Oral, injected	Illusions and hallucinations, poor perception of time and distance	Longer more intense "trip" episodes, psychosis, possible death	Withdrawal syndrome not reported
High	Yes	Variable	Smoked, oral, injected			
Degree unknown	Yes	Variable	Smoked, oral, injected			
Degree unknown	Possible	Variable	Oral, injected, smoked, sniffed			

Table continued on following page

USES AND EFFECTS OF CONTROLLED SUBSTANCES *Continued*

Cannabis	Marijuana	I	Pot, Acapulco gold, grass, reefer, sinsemilla, Thai sticks	Under investigation	Degree unknown
	Tetrahydro-cannabinol	I	THC		Degree unknown
	Hashish	I	Hash	None	Degree unknown
	Hashish oil	I	Hash oil	None	Degree unknown

C-3

USES AND EFFECTS OF CONTROLLED SUBSTANCES Continued

Moderate	Yes	2–4	Smoked, oral			
Moderate	Yes	2–4	Smoked, oral	Euphoria, relaxed inhibitions, increased appetite, disoriented behavior	Fatigue, paranoia, possible psychosis	Insomnia, hyperactivity, and decreased appetite occasionally reported
Moderate	Yes	2–4	Smoked, oral			
Moderate	Yes	2–4	Smoked, oral			

From Miller BK, Keane CB: *Encyclopedia and Dictionary of Medicine, Nursing, and Allied Health*, 5th ed. Philadelphia: W.B. Saunders, 1992, pp. 450–453.

C-4

SELECTED SKIN TESTS

Disease	Test	Antigen	Time to Read	Positive Reaction
Diphtheria susceptibility	Schick	Diphtheria toxin	3–6 days	>10 mm
Echinococcosis	Casoni	Fluid from hydatid cyst	15–20 minutes	Immediate erythema and swelling
Lymphogranuloma venereum	Frei	Killed virus	48–72 hours	6 × 6 mm raised papule
Sarcoidosis	Kveim-Siltzback	Sarcoid tissue	6 weeks	Palpable nodule
Scarlet fever	Schultz-Charlton	Antitoxin	24 hours	Blanched area
Scarlet fever susceptibility	Dick	Erythrogenic toxin	24 hours	>10 mm
Systemic fungal infection	Histoplasmin, etc.	Killed fungi	48 hours	>5 mm
Toxoplasmosis	Toxoplasm	Antigen	24–48 hours	>10 mm
Trichinosis	*Trichinella*	Killed larvae	15–20 minutes	Blanched wheal surrounded by erythema
Tuberculosis	PPD	Tuberculin antigen	48–72 hours	>10 mm
Tularemia	Foshay	Killed bacteria	48 hours	Erythema and induration

From Pagana KD, Pagana TJ: *Pocket Nurse Guide to Laboratory and Diagnostic Tests.* St. Louis, C.V. Mosby, 1986, p. 431.

C-5
TABLES OF WEIGHTS AND MEASURES

MEASURES OF MASS

AVOIRDUPOIS WEIGHT

Grains	Drams	Ounces	Pounds	Metric Equivalents, Grams
1	0.0366	0.0023	0.00014	0.0647989
27.34	1	0.0625	0.0039	1.772
437.5	16	1	0.0625	28.350
7000	256	16	1	453.5924277

APOTHECARIES' WEIGHT

Grains	Scruples (Ə)	Drams (ʒ)	Ounces (ʒ)	Pounds (lb.)	Metric Equivalents, Grams
1	0.05	0.0167	0.0021	0.00017	0.0647989
20	1	0.333	0.042	0.0035	1.296
60	3	1	0.125	0.0104	3.888
480	24	8	1	0.0833	31.103
5760	288	96	12	1	373.24177

TROY WEIGHT

Grains	Pennyweights	Ounces	Pounds	Metric Equivalents, Grams
1	0.042	0.002	0.00017	0.0647989
24	1	0.05	0.0042	1.555
480	20	1	0.083	31.103
5760	240	12	1	373.24177

METRIC WEIGHT

Microgram	Milligram	Centigram	Decigram	Gram	Dekagram	Hectogram	Kilogram	Equivalents Avoirdupois	Apothecaries'
1	—	—	—	—	—	—	—	0.000015 grains	
10^3	1	—	—	—	—	—	—	0.015432 grains	
10^4	10	1	—	—	—	—	—	0.154323 grains	
10^5	10^2	10	1	—	—	—	—	1.543235 grains	
10^6	10^3	10^2	10	1	—	—	—	15.432356 grains	
10^7	10^4	10^3	10^2	10	1	—	—	5.6438 dr.	7.7162 scr.
10^8	10^5	10^4	10^3	10^2	10	1	—	3.527 oz.	3.215 oz.
10^9	10^6	10^5	10^4	10^3	10^2	10	1	2.2046 lb.	2.6792 lb.
10^{12}	10^9	10^8	10^7	10^6	10^5	10^4	10^3	2204.6223 lb.	2679.2285 lb.

MEASURES OF CAPACITY

APOTHECARIES' (WINE) MEASURE

Minims	Fluid Drams	Fluid Ounces	Gills	Pints	Quarts	Gallons	Cubic Inches	Milliliters	Cubic Centimeters
1	0.0166	0.002	0.0005	0.00013	—	—	0.00376	0.06161	0.06161
60	1	0.125	0.0312	0.0078	0.0039	—	0.22558	3.6967	3.6967
480	8	1	0.25	0.0625	0.0312	0.0078	1.80468	29.5737	29.5737
1920	32	4	1	0.25	0.125	0.0312	7.21875	118.2948	118.2948
7680	128	16	4	1	0.5	0.125	28.875	473.179	473.179
15360	256	32	8	2	1	0.25	57.75	946.358	946.358
61440	1024	128	32	8	4	1	231	3785.434	3785.434

TABLES OF WEIGHTS AND MEASURES Continued

METRIC MEASURE

Microliter	Milliliter	Centiliter	Deciliter	Liter	Dekaliter	Hectoliter	Kiloliter	Myrialiter	Equivalents (Apothecaries' Fluid)	
1	—	—	—	—	—	—	—	—	0.01623108	minim
10^3	1	—	—	—	—	—	—	—	16.23	minims
10^4	10	1	—	—	—	—	—	—	2.7	fluid drams
10^5	10^2	10	1	—	—	—	—	—	3.38	fluid ounces
10^6	10^3	10^2	10	1	—	—	—	—	2.11	pints
10^7	10^4	10^3	10^2	10	1	—	—	—	2.64	gallons
10^8	10^5	10^4	10^3	10^2	10	1	—	—	26.418	gallons
10^9	10^6	10^5	10^4	10^3	10^2	10	1	—	264.18	gallons
10^{10}	10^7	10^6	10^5	10^4	10^3	10^2	10	1	2641.8	gallons

1 liter = 2.113363738 pints (Apothecaries').

MEASURES OF LENGTH

Micrometer	Millimeter	Centimeter	Decimeter	Meter	Dekameter	Hectometer	Kilometer	Myriameter	Megameter	Equivalents	
1	0.001	10^{-4}	—	—	—	—	—	—	—	0.000039	inch
10^3	1	10^{-1}	—	—	—	—	—	—	—	0.03937	inch
10^4	10	1	—	—	—	—	—	—	—	0.3937	inch
10^5	10^2	10	1	—	—	—	—	—	—	3.937	inches
10^6	10^3	10^2	10	1	—	—	—	—	—	39.37	inches
10^7	10^4	10^3	10^2	10	1	—	—	—	—	10.9361	yards
10^8	10^5	10^4	10^3	10^2	10	1	—	—	—	109.3612	yards
10^9	10^6	10^5	10^4	10^3	10^2	10	1	—	—	1093.6121	yards
10^{10}	10^7	10^6	10^5	10^4	10^3	10^2	10	1	—	6.2137	miles
10^{12}	10^9	10^8	10^7	10^6	10^5	10^4	10^3	10^2	1	621.37	miles

Table continued on following page

C-5

TABLES OF WEIGHTS AND MEASURES Continued

CONVERSION TABLES

AVOIRDUPOIS—METRIC WEIGHT

Ounces	Grams	
1/16	1.772	
1/8	3.544	
1/4	7.088	
1/2	14.175	
1	28.350	
2	56.699	
3	85.049	
4	113.398	
5	141.748	
6	170.097	
7	198.447	
8	226.796	
9	255.146	
10	283.495	
11	311.845	
12	340.194	
13	368.544	
14	396.893	
15	425.243	
16 (1 lb.)	453.59	

Pounds	Grams	
1 (16 oz.)	453.69	
2	907.18	
3	1360.78	(1.36 kg.)
4	1814.37	(1.81 kg.)
5	2267.96	(2.27 kg.)
6	2721.55	(2.72 kg.)
7	3175.15	(3.18 kg.)
8	3628.74	(3.63 kg.)
9	4082.33	(4.08 kg.)
10	4535.92	(4.54 kg.)

METRIC—AVOIRDUPOIS WEIGHT

Grams	Ounces
0.001 (1 mg.)	0.000035274
1	0.035274
1000 (kg.)	35.274 (2.2046 lb.)

APOTHECARIES'—METRIC LIQUID MEASURE

Minims	Milliliters
1	0.06
2	0.12
3	0.19
4	0.25
5	0.31
10	0.62
15	0.92
20	1.23
25	1.54
30	1.85
35	2.16
40	2.46
45	2.77
50	3.08
55	3.39
60 (1 fl. dr.)	3.70

Fluid Drams	Milliliters
1	3.70
2	7.39
3	11.09
4	14.79
5	18.48
6	22.18
7	25.88
8 (1 fl. oz.)	29.57

Fluid Ounces	Milliliters
1	29.57
2	59.15
3	88.72
4	118.29
5	147.87
6	177.44
7	207.01
8	236.58
9	266.16
10	295.73
11	325.30
12	354.88
13	384.45
14	414.02
15	443.59
16 (1 pt.)	473.18
32 (1 qt.)	946.36
128 (1 gal.)	3785.43

METRIC—APOTHECARIES' LIQUID MEASURE

Milliliters	Minims	Milliliters	Fluid Drams	Milliliters	Fluid Ounces
1	16.231	5	1.35	30	1.01
2	32.5	10	2.71	40	1.35
3	48.7	15	4.06	50	1.69
4	64.9	20	5.4	500	16.91
5	81.1	25	6.76	1000 (1 L.)	33.815
		30	7.1		

C-5
TABLES OF WEIGHTS AND MEASURES *Continued*

APOTHECARIES'—METRIC WEIGHT		METRIC—APOTHECARIES' WEIGHT	
Grains	*Grams*	*Milligrams*	*Grains*
1/150	0.0004	1	0.015432
1/120	0.0005	2	0.030864
1/100	0.0006	3	0.046296
1/80	0.0008	4	0.061728
1/64	0.001	5	0.077160
1/50	0.0013	6	0.092592
1/48	0.0014	7	0.108024
1/30	0.0022	8	0.123456
1/25	0.0026	9	0.138888
1/16	0.004	10	0.154320
1/12	0.005	15	0.231480
1/10	0.006	20	0.308640
1/9	0.007	25	0.385800
1/8	0.008	30	0.462960
1/7	0.009	35	0.540120
1/6	0.01	40	0.617280
1/5	0.013	45	0.694440
1/4	0.016	50	0.771600
1/3	0.02	100	1.543240
1/2	0.032		
1	0.065	*Grams*	
1 1/2	0.097 (0.1)	0.1	1.5432
2	0.125	0.2	3.0864
3	0.20	0.3	4.6296
4	0.25	0.4	6.1728
5	0.30	0.5	7.7160
6	0.40	0.6	9.2592
7	0.45	0.7	10.8024
8	0.50	0.8	12.3456
9	0.60	0.9	13.8888
10	0.65	1.0	15.4320
15	1.00	1.5	23.1480
20 (19)	1.30	2.0	30.8640
30	2.00	2.5	38.5800
Scruples		3.0	46.2960
1	1.296 (1.3)	3.5	54.0120
2	2.592 (2.6)	4.0	61.728
3 (1ℨ)	3.888 (3.9)	4.5	69.444
Drams		5.0	77.162
1	3.888	10.0	154.324
2	7.776		
3	11.664		*Equivalents*
4	15.552	10	2.572 drams
5	19.440	15	3.858 drams
6	23.328	20	5.144 drams
7	27.216	25	6.430 drams
8 (1 ℥)	31.103	30	7.716 drams
Ounces		40	1.286 oz.
1	31.103	45	1.447 oz.
2	62.207	50	1.607 oz.
3	93.310	100	3.215 oz.
4	124.414	200	6.430 oz.
5	155.517	300	9.644 oz.
6	186.621	400	12.859 oz.
7	217.724	500	1.34 lb.
8	248.828	600	1.61 lb.
9	279.931	700	1.88 lb.
10	311.035	800	2.14 lb.
11	342.138	900	2.41 lb.
12 (1 lb.)	373.242	1000	2.68 lb.

Table continued on following page

TABLES OF WEIGHTS AND MEASURES Continued

METRIC DOSES WITH APPROXIMATE APOTHECARY EQUIVALENTS*

These *approximate* dose equivalents represent the quantities usually prescribed, under identical conditions, by physicians trained, respectively, in the metric or in the apothecary system of weights and measures. In labeling dosage forms in both the metric and the apothecary systems, if one is the approximate equivalent of the other, the approximate figure shall be enclosed in parentheses.

When prepared dosage forms such as tablets, capsules, pills, etc., are prescribed in the metric system, the pharmacist may dispense the corresponding *approximate* equivalent in the apothecary system, and vice versa, as indicated in the following table.

Caution—For the conversion of specific quantities in a prescription which requires compounding, or in converting a pharmaceutical formula from one system of weights or measures to the other, *exact* equivalents must be used.

Liquid Measure Metric	Approx. Apothecary Equivalents	Liquid Measure Metric	Approx. Apothecary Equivalents
1000 ml.	1 quart	3 ml.	45 minims
750 ml.	1 1/2 pints	2 ml.	30 minims
500 ml.	1 pint	1 ml.	15 minims
250 ml.	8 fluid ounces	0.75 ml.	12 minims
200 ml.	7 fluid ounces	0.6 ml.	10 minims
100 ml.	3 1/2 fluid ounces	0.5 ml.	8 minims
50 ml.	1 3/4 fluid ounces	0.3 ml.	5 minims
30 ml.	1 fluid ounce	0.25 ml.	4 minims
15 ml.	4 fluid drams	0.2 ml.	3 minims
10 ml.	2 1/2 fluid drams	0.1 ml.	1 1/2 minims
8 ml.	2 fluid drams	0.06 ml.	1 minim
5 ml.	1 1/4 fluid drams	0.05 ml.	3/4 minim
4 ml.	1 fluid dram	0.03 ml.	1/2 minim

Weight Metric	Approx. Apothecary Equivalents	Weight Metric	Approx. Apothecary Equivalents
30 gm.	1 ounce	30 mg.	1/2 grain
15 gm.	4 drams	25 mg.	3/8 grain
10 gm.	2 1/2 drams	20 mg.	1/3 grain
7.5 gm.	2 drams	15 mg.	1/4 grain
6 gm.	90 grains	12 mg.	1/5 grain
5 gm.	75 grains	10 mg.	1/6 grain
4 gm.	60 grains (1 dram)	8 mg.	1/8 grain
3 gm.	45 grains	6 mg.	1/10 grain
2 gm.	30 grains (1/2 dram)	5 mg.	1/12 grain
1.5 gm.	22 grains	4 mg.	1/15 grain
1 gm.	15 grains	3 mg.	1/20 grain
0.75 gm.	12 grains	2 mg.	1/30 grain
0.6 gm.	10 grains	1.5 mg.	1/40 grain
0.5 gm.	7 1/2 grains	1.2 mg.	1/50 grain
0.4 gm.	6 grains	1 mg.	1/60 grain
0.3 gm.	5 grains	0.8 mg.	1/80 grain
0.25 gm.	4 grains	0.6 mg.	1/100 grain
0.2 gm.	3 grains	0.5 mg.	1/120 grain
0.15 gm.	2 1/2 grains	0.4 mg.	1/150 grain
0.12 gm.	2 grains	0.3 mg.	1/200 grain
0.1 gm.	1 1/2 grains	0.25 mg.	1/250 grain
75 mg.	1 1/4 grains	0.2 mg.	1/300 grain
60 mg.	1 grain	0.15 mg.	1/400 grain
50 mg.	3/4 grain	0.12 mg.	1/500 grain
40 mg.	2/3 grain	0.1 mg.	1/600 grain

Note: A milliliter (ml.) is the approximate equivalent of a cubic centimeter (cc.).

*Adopted by the latest Pharmacopeia, National Formulary, and New and Nonofficial Remedies, and approved by the Federal Food and Drug Administration.

From Miller BF, Keane CB: *Encyclopedia and Dictionary of Medicine, Nursing, and Allied Health,* 5th ed. Philadelphia: W.B. Saunders, 1992, pp. 1664–1668.

C-6
APPROXIMATE HOUSEHOLD EQUIVALENTS

			LIQUID	WEIGHT
		1 teaspoon	5 ml.	5 gm.
	1 tablespoon	= 3 teaspoons	15 ml.	15 gm.
1 cup	= 16 tablespoons		237 ml.	240 gm.
1 pint = 2 cups			473 ml.	480 gm.
1 quart = 2 pints = 4 cups			946 ml.	960 ml.

1	pound of butter	=	2 cups
8	average eggs	=	1 cup
4	cups sifted flour	=	1 pound
2	cups granulated sugar	=	1 pound
$2^{2}/_{3}$	cups confectioner's sugar	=	1 pound
$2^{2}/_{3}$	cups brown sugar	=	1 pound

From Miller BF, Keane CB: *Encyclopedia and Dictionary of Medicine, Nursing, and Allied Health,* 5th ed. Philadelphia: W.B. Saunders, 1992, p. 1669.

C-7
DESIRABLE WEIGHTS FOR MEN AND WOMEN, ACCORDING TO HEIGHT AND FRAME, AGES 25 TO 29

HEIGHT (IN 1-INCH HEELS)		WEIGHT (IN INDOOR CLOTHING)					
		SMALL FRAME		MEDIUM FRAME		LARGE FRAME	
	Cm	Lb	Kg	Lb	Kg	Lb	Kg
MEN							
5 ft 2 in	158	128–134	58–61	131–141	59–64	138–150	63–68
5 ft 3 in	160	130–136	59–62	133–143	60–65	140–153	64–69
5 ft 4 in	163	132–138	60–63	135–145	61–66	142–156	64–71
5 ft 5 in	165	134–140	61–64	137–148	62–67	144–160	65–73
5 ft 6 in	168	136–142	62–64	139–151	63–68	146–164	66–74
5 ft 7 in	170	138–145	63–66	142–154	64–70	149–168	68–76
5 ft 8 in	173	140–148	64–67	145–157	66–71	152–172	69–78
5 ft 9 in	176	142–151	64–68	148–160	67–73	155–176	70–80
5 ft 10 in	178	144–154	65–70	151–163	68–74	158–180	72–82
5 ft 11 in	180	146–157	66–71	154–166	70–75	161–184	73–83
6 ft	183	149–160	68–73	157–170	71–77	164–188	74–85
6 ft 1 in	185	152–164	69–74	160–174	73–79	168–192	76–87
6 ft 2 in	188	155–168	70–76	164–174	74–81	172–197	78–89
6 ft 3 in	191	158–172	72–78	167–182	76–83	176–202	80–92
6 ft 4 in	193	162–176	74–80	171–187	78–85	181–207	82–93
WOMEN							
4 ft 10 in	147	102–111	46–50	109–121	49–55	118–131	54–59
4 ft 11 in	150	103–113	47–51	111–123	50–56	120–134	54–61
5 ft	152	104–115	47–52	113–126	51–57	122–137	55–62
5 ft 1 in	155	106–118	48–54	115–129	52–59	125–140	57–64
5 ft 2 in	158	108–121	49–55	118–132	54–60	128–143	58–65
5 ft 3 in	160	111–124	50–56	121–135	55–61	131–147	59–66
5 ft 4 in	163	114–127	52–58	124–138	56–62	134–151	61–68
5 ft 5 in	165	117–130	53–59	127–141	58–64	137–155	62–70
5 ft 6 in	168	120–133	54–60	130–144	59–65	140–159	64–72
5 ft 7 in	170	123–136	56–62	133–147	60–66	143–163	65–74
5 ft 8 in	173	126–139	57–63	136–150	62–68	146–167	66–76
5 ft 9 in	175	129–142	58–64	139–153	63–69	149–170	68–77
5 ft 10 in	178	132–145	60–66	142–156	64–70	152–173	69–78
5 ft 11 in	180	135–148	61–67	145–159	66–72	155–176	70–80
6 ft	183	138–151	63–69	148–162	67–73	158–179	72–81

Courtesy of The Metropolitan Life Insurance Co.

C-8

IDEAL WEIGHTS FOR BOYS AND GIRLS, ACCORDING TO HEIGHT AND AGE

Height		Boys, Aged 14 to 19 Years — Weight										
		Age 14		15		16		17		18		19	
	Cm	Lb	Kg	Lb	Kg	Lb	Kg	Lb	Kg	Lb	Kg	Lb	Kg
4 ft 6 in	137	72	33										
4 ft 7 in	140	74	34										
4 ft 8 in	142	78	35	80	36								
4 ft 9 in	145	83	38	83	38								
4 ft 10 in	147	86	39	87	39								
4 ft 11 in	150	90	41	90	41	90	41						
5 ft	152	94	43	95	43	96	44						
5 ft 1 in	155	99	45	100	45	103	47	106	48				
5 ft 2 in	158	103	47	104	47	107	49	111	50	116	53		
5 ft 3 in	160	108	49	110	50	113	51	118	54	123	56	127	58
5 ft 4 in	163	113	51	115	52	117	53	121	55	126	57	130	59
5 ft 5 in	165	118	54	120	54	122	55	127	58	131	59	134	61
5 ft 6 in	168	122	55	125	57	128	58	132	60	136	62	139	63
5 ft 7 in	170	128	58	130	59	134	61	136	62	139	63	142	64
5 ft 8 in	173	134	61	134	61	137	62	141	64	143	65	147	67
5 ft 9 in	175	137	62	139	63	143	65	146	66	149	67	152	69
5 ft 10 in	178	143	65	144	65	145	66	148	67	151	68	155	70
5 ft 11 in	180	148	67	150	68	151	68	152	69	154	70	159	72
6 ft	183			153	69	155	70	156	71	158	72	163	74
6 ft 1 in	185			157	71	160	73	162	73	164	73	167	76
6 ft 2 in	188			160	73	164	74	168	76	170	77	171	78

Height		Girls, Aged 14 to 18 Years — Weight									
		Age 14		15		16		17		18	
	Cm	Lb	Kg	Lb	Kg	Lb	Kg	Lb	Kg	Lb	Kg
4 ft 7 in	140	78	35								
4 ft 8 in	142	83	38								
4 ft 9 in	145	88	40	92	42						
4 ft 10 in	147	93	42	96	44	101	46				
4 ft 11 in	150	96	44	100	45	103	47	104	47		
5 ft	152	101	46	105	48	108	49	109	49	111	50
5 ft 1 in	155	105	48	108	49	112	51	113	51	116	53
5 ft 2 in	158	109	49	113	51	115	52	117	53	118	54
5 ft 3 in	160	112	51	116	53	117	53	119	54	120	55
5 ft 4 in	163	117	53	119	54	120	54	122	55	123	56
5 ft 5 in	165	121	55	122	55	123	56	125	57	126	57
5 ft 6 in	168	124	56	124	56	125	57	128	58	130	59
5 ft 7 in	170	130	59	131	59	133	60	133	60	135	61
5 ft 8 in	173	133	60	135	61	136	62	138	63	138	63
5 ft 9 in	175	135	61	137	62	138	63	140	64	142	64
5 ft 10 in	178	136	62	138	63	140	64	142	64	144	65
5 ft 11 in	180	138	63	140	64	142	64	144	65	145	66

From Miller BF, Keane CB: *Encyclopedia and Dictionary of Medicine, Nursing, and Allied Health,* 5th ed. Philadelphia: W.B. Saunders, 1992, p. 1652.

C-9
FOOD AND NUTRITION BOARD, NATIONAL ACADEMY OF SCIENCES—NATIONAL RESEARCH COUNCIL RECOMMENDED DAILY DIETARY ALLOWANCES (RDA),[a] REVISED 1980

Designed for the maintenance of good nutrition of practically all healthy people in the U.S.A.

	Age (years)	Weight (kg)	Weight (lb)	Height (cm)	Height (in)	Protein (g)	Fat-Soluble Vitamins			Water-Soluble Vitamins							Minerals				
							Vita-min A (μg RE)[b]	Vita-min D (μg)[c]	Vita-min E (mg α-TE)[d]	Vita-min C (mg)	Thia-min (mg)	Ribo-fla-vin (mg)	Nia-cin (mg NE)[e]	Vita-min B-6 (mg)	Fola-cin[f] (μg)	Vita-min B-12 (μg)	Cal-cium (mg)	Phos-pho-rus (mg)	Mag-nes-ium (mg)	Iron (mg)	Zinc (mg)	Io-dine (μg)
Infants	0.0–0.5	6	13	60	24	kg×2.2	420	10	3	35	0.3	0.4	6	0.3	30	0.5[g]	360	240	50	10	3	40
	0.5–1.0	9	20	71	28	kg×2.0	400	10	4	35	0.5	0.6	8	0.6	45	1.5	540	360	70	15	5	50
Children	1–3	13	29	90	35	23	400	10	5	45	0.7	0.8	9	0.9	100	2.0	800	800	150	15	10	70
	4–6	20	44	112	44	30	500	10	6	45	0.9	1.0	11	1.3	200	2.5	800	800	200	10	10	90
	7–10	28	62	132	52	34	700	10	7	45	1.2	1.4	16	1.6	300	3.0	800	800	250	10	10	120
Males	11–14	45	99	157	62	45	1000	10	8	50	1.4	1.6	18	1.8	400	3.0	1200	1200	350	18	15	150
	15–18	66	145	176	69	56	1000	10	10	60	1.4	1.7	18	2.0	400	3.0	1200	1200	400	18	15	150
	19–22	70	154	177	70	56	1000	7.5	10	60	1.5	1.7	19	2.2	400	3.0	800	800	350	10	15	150
	23–50	70	154	178	70	56	1000	5	10	60	1.4	1.6	18	2.2	400	3.0	800	800	350	10	15	150
	51+	70	154	178	70	56	1000	5	10	60	1.2	1.4	16	2.2	400	3.0	800	800	350	10	15	150
Females	11–14	46	101	157	62	46	800	10	8	50	1.1	1.3	15	1.8	400	3.0	1200	1200	300	18	15	150
	15–18	55	120	163	64	46	800	10	8	60	1.1	1.3	14	2.0	400	3.0	1200	1200	300	18	15	150
	19–22	55	120	163	64	44	800	7.5	8	60	1.0	1.3	14	2.0	400	3.0	800	800	300	18	15	150
	23–50	55	120	163	64	44	800	5	8	60	1.0	1.2	13	2.0	400	3.0	800	800	300	18	15	150
	51+	55	120	163	64	44	800	5	8	60	1.0	1.2	13	2.0	400	3.0	800	800	300	10	15	150
Pregnant						+30	+200	+5	+2	+20	+0.4	+0.3	+2	+0.6	+400	+1.0	+400	+400	+150	h	+5	+25
Lactating						+20	+400	+5	+3	+40	+0.5	+0.5	+5	+0.5	+100	+1.0	+400	+400	+150	h	+10	+50

[a]The allowances are intended to provide for individual variations among most normal persons as they live in the United States under usual environmental stresses. Diets should be based on a variety of common foods in order to provide other nutrients for which human requirements have been less well defined.

[b]Retinol equivalents. 1 retinol equivalent = 1 μg retinol or 6 μg carotene.

[c]As cholecalciferol. 10 μg cholecalciferol = 400 IU of vitamin D.

[d]α-tocopherol equivalents. 1 mg d-α-tocopherol = 1 α-TE.

[e]1 NE (niacin equivalent) is equal to 1 mg of niacin or 60 mg of dietary tryptophan.

[f]The folacin allowances refer to dietary sources as determined by *Lactobacillus casei* assay after treatment with enzymes (conjugases) to make polyglutamyl forms of the vitamin available to the test organism.

[g]The recommended dietary allowance for vitamin B-12 in infants is based on average concentration of the vitamin in human milk. The allowances after weaning are based on energy intake (as recommended by the American Academy of Pediatrics) and consideration of other factors, such as intestinal absorption.

[h]The increased requirement during pregnancy cannot be met by the iron content of habitual American diets nor by the existing iron stores of many women; therefore the use of 30–60 mg of supplemental iron is recommended. Iron needs during lactation are not substantially different from those of nonpregnant women, but continued supplementation of the mother for 2–3 months after parturition is advisable in order to replenish stores depleted by pregnancy.

From Miller BF, Keane CB: *Encyclopedia and Dictionary of Medicine, Nursing, and Allied Health*, 5th ed. Philadelphia: W.B. Saunders, 1992, p. 1653.

C-10

THE PRINCIPAL MICRONUTRIENTS (VITAMINS AND MINERALS)

Micronutrient	Principal Sources	Functions	Effects of Deficiency and Toxicity	Usual Therapeutic Dosage
Vitamin A	Fish liver oils, liver, egg yolk, butter, cream, vitamin A-fortified margarine, green leafy or yellow vegetables	Photoreceptor mechanism of retina; integrity of epithelia; lysosome stability; glycoprotein synthesis	*Deficiency:* Night blindness, perifollicular hyperkeratosis; xerophthalmia, keratomalacia *Toxicity:* Headache; peeling of skin; hepatosplenomegaly; bone thickening	10,000–20,000 µg (30,000–60,000 IU/day)
Vitamin D	Fortified milk is main dietary source; fish liver oils, butter, egg yolk, liver, ultraviolet irradiation	Calcium and phosphorus absorption; resorption, mineralization, & collagen maturation of bone; tubular reabsorption of phosphorus (?)	*Deficiency:* Rickets (tetany sometimes associated); osteomalacia *Toxicity:* Anorexia; renal failure; metastatic calcification	*Primary Deficiency:* 10–40 µg (1400–1600 IU)/day *Metabolic Deficiency:* 1–2 µg/day 1,25-$(OH)_2D_3$ or 1α-$(OH)D_3$
Vitamin E group	Vegetable oil, wheat germ, leafy vegetables, egg yolk, margarine, legumes	Intracellular antioxidant; stability of biologic membranes	*Deficiency:* RBC hemolysis; creatinuria; ceroid deposition in muscle	30–100 mg/day
Vitamin K (activity) Vitamin K_1 (phytonadione) Vitamin K_2 (menaquinone)	Leafy vegetables, pork, liver, vegetable oils, intestinal flora after newborn period	Prothrombin formation; normal blood coagulation	*Deficiency:* Hemorrhage from deficient prothrombin *Toxicity:* Kernicterus	In situations conducive to neonatal hemorrhage, 2–5 mg during labor or daily for 1 wk prior; or 1–2 mg to newborn
Essential fatty acids (linoleic, linolenic, arachidonic acids)	Vegetable seed oils (corn, sunflower, safflower); margarines blended with vegetable oils	Synthesis of prostaglandins, membrane structure	Growth cessation, dermatosis	Up to 10 gm/day
Thiamine (vitamin B_1)	Dried yeast; whole grains; meat (especially pork, liver); enriched cereal products; nuts; legumes; potatoes	Carbohydrate metabolism; central & peripheral nerve cell function; myocardial function	Beriberi; infantile & adult (peripheral neuropathy, cardiac failure; Wernicke-Korsakoff syndrome)	30–100 mg/day
Riboflavin (vitamin B_2)	Milk, cheese, liver, meat, eggs, enriched cereal products	Many aspects of energy & protein metabolism; integrity of mucous membranes	Cheilosis; angular stomatitis; corneal vascularization; amblyopia; sebaceous dermatosis	10–30 mg/day
Niacin (nicotinic acid, niacinamide)	Dried yeast, liver, meat, fish, legumes, whole-grain enriched cereal products	Oxidation-reduction reactions; carbohydrate metabolism	Pellagra (dermatosis glossitis, GI & CNS dysfunction)	Niacinamide 100–1000 mg/day
Vitamin B_6 group (pyridoxine)	Dried yeast, liver, organ meats, whole-grain cereals, fish, legumes	Many aspects of nitrogen metabolism, e.g., transaminations, porphyrin & heme synthesis, tryptophan conversion to niacin. Linoleic acid metabolism	Convulsions in infancy; anemias; neuropathy; seborrhealike skin lesions Dependency states	25–100 mg/day
Folic acid	Fresh green leafy vegetables, fruit, organ meats, liver, dried yeast	Maturation of RBCs; synthesis of purines & pyrimidines	Pancytopenia; megaloblastosis (especially pregnancy, infancy, malabsorption)	1 mg/day
Vitamin B_{12} (cobalamins)	Liver; meats (especially beef, pork, organ meats); eggs; milk & milk products	Maturation of RBCs; neural function; DNA synthesis, related to folate coenzymes; methionine & acetate synthesis	Pernicious anemia; fish tapeworm & vegan anemias; some psychiatric syndromes; nutritional amblyopia Dependency states	In pernicious anemia 50 µg/day IM first 2 wk, 100 µg twice/wk next 2 mo, thereafter 100 µg/mo

THE PRINCIPAL MICRONUTRIENTS (VITAMINS AND MINERALS) Continued

Micronutrient	Principal Sources	Functions	Effects of Deficiency and Toxicity	Usual Therapeutic Dosage
Biotin	Liver, kidney, egg yolk, yeast, cauliflower, nuts, legumes	Carboxylation & decarboxylation of oxaloacetic acid; amino acid & fatty acid metabolism	Dermatitis, glossitis Dependency states	150–300 µg/day
Vitamin C (ascorbic acid)	Citrus fruits, tomatoes, potatoes, cabbage, green peppers	Essential to osteoid tissue; collagen formation; vascular function; tissue respiration & wound healing	Scurvy (hemorrhages, loose teeth, gingivitis)	100–1000 mg/day
Sodium	Wide distribution—beef, pork, sardines, cheese, green olives, corn bread, potato chips, sauerkraut	Acid-base balances; osmotic pressure; pH of blood; muscle contractility; nerve transmission; sodium pumps	*Deficiency:* Hyponatremia *Toxicity:* Hypernatremia; confusion, coma	
Potassium	Wide distribution—whole and skim milk, bananas, prunes, raisins	Muscle activity, nerve transmission; intracellular acid-base balance and water retention	*Deficiency:* Hypokalemia; paralysis, cardiac disturbances *Toxicity:* Hyperkalemia; paralysis, cardiac disturbances	
Calcium	Milk and milk products, meat, fish, eggs, cereal products, beans, fruits, vegetables	Bone and tooth formation; blood coagulation; neuromuscular irritability; muscle contractility; myocardial conduction	*Deficiency:* Hypocalcemia and tetany; neuromuscular hyperexcitability *Toxicity:* Hypercalcemia; GI atony; renal failure; psychosis	10–30 ml 10% calcium gluconate soln IV in 24 h
Phosphorus	Milk, cheese, meat, poultry, fish, cereals, nuts, legumes	Bone and tooth formation, acid-base balance, component of nucleic acids, energy production	*Deficiency:* Irritability; weakness; blood cell disorders; GI tract & renal dysfunction *Toxicity:* Hyperphosphatemia in renal failure	Potassium acid and dibasic phosphate parenteral 600 mg (18.8 mEq)/day
Magnesium	Green leaves, nuts, cereal grains, seafoods	Bone and tooth formation; nerve conduction; muscle contraction; enzyme activation	*Deficiency:* Hypomagnesemia; neuromuscular irritability *Toxicity:* Hypermagnesemia; hypotension, respiratory failure, cardiac disturbances	2–4 ml 50% magnesium sulfate soln/day IM
Iron	Wide distribution (except dairy products)—soybean flour, beef, kidney, liver, beans, clams, peaches Much unavailable (<20% absorbed)	Hemoglobin, myoglobin formation, enzymes	*Deficiency:* Anemia; dysphagia; koilonychia; enteropathy *Toxicity:* Hemochromatosis; cirrhosis; diabetes mellitus; skin pigmentation	Ferrous sulphate or gluconate 300 mg orally t.i.d.
Iodine	Seafoods, iodized salt, dairy products Water variable	Thyroxine (T_4) & triiodothyronine (T_3) formation and energy control mechanisms	*Deficiency:* Simple (colloid, endemic) goiter; cretinism; deaf-mutism *Toxicity:* Occasional myxedema	150 µg iodine/day as potassium iodide added to salt 1:10–40,000 ppm
Fluorine	Wide distribution—tea, coffee Fluoridation of water supplies sodium fluoride 1.0–2.0 ppm	Bone and tooth formation	*Deficiency:* Predisposition to dental caries; osteoporosis (?) *Toxicity:* Fluorosis, mottling, pitting of permanent teeth; exostoses of spine	Sodium fluoride 1.1–2.2 mg/day orally

Table continued on following page

THE PRINCIPAL MICRONUTRIENTS (VITAMINS AND MINERALS) Continued

Micronutrient	Principal Sources	Functions	Effects of Deficiency and Toxicity	Usual Therapeutic Dosage
Zinc	Wide distribution—vegetable sources Much unavailable	Component of enzymes and insulin; wound healing; growth	*Deficiency:* Growth retardation; hypogonadism; hypogeusia; in cirrhosis; acrodermatitis enteropathica	30–150 mg zinc sulfate/day orally
Copper	Wide distribution—organ meats, oysters, nuts, dried legumes, whole-grain cereals	Enzyme component	*Deficiency:* Anemia in malnourished children; Menkes' kinky hair syndrome *Toxicity:* Hepatolenticular degeneration; some biliary cirrhosis (?)	0.3 mg/kg/day copper sulfate, orally
Cobalt	Green leafy vegetables	Part of vitamin B_{12} molecule	*Deficiency:* Anemia in children (?) *Toxicity:* Beer-drinker's cardiomyopathy	20–30 mg/day cobaltous chloride, orally
Chromium	Wide distribution—brewer's yeast	Part of glucose tolerance factor (GTF)	*Deficiency:* Impaired glucose tolerance in malnourished children; some diabetics (?)	

From *The Merck Manual of Diagnosis and Therapy,* Edition 14, pages 871–875, edited by Robert Berkow. Copyright 1982 by Merck & Co., Inc. Used with permission.

C-11
LABORATORY VALUES OF CLINICAL IMPORTANCE*

method of
REX B. CONN, M.D.
Thomas Jefferson University
Philadelphia, Pennsylvania

Reference values for laboratory tests serve as indispensible benchmarks when evaluating laboratory data on an individual patient. However, reference values should not be considered equivalent to normal values, because in medicine it is a logical impossibility to define normality. There can be no sharp dividing line between normal and abnormal values, and there is a gradual transition during any pathologic process from what is clearly normal to a value that is clearly abnormal.

Reference values are derived from statistical studies on subjects believed to have no condition that might affect the measurement being evaluated. An important consideration is that the reference ranges derived by these statistical methods encompass only 95% of the reference population. Thus, a value slightly outside the range might be due to a chance distribution or to an underlying pathologic process.

A single reference range for all individuals may be inadequate for some measurements. Values obtained on presumably normal persons may vary because of age, sex, body build, race, environment, and state of gastrointestinal absorption. Another consideration is that values for some constituents found in a "normal" population may reflect a general disorder in the population rather than normality. Thus, reference values for serum cholesterol level now indicate the "desirable" range rather than that actually found in the reference population.

Tables of reference values must be revised and updated frequently to reflect the addition of new tests, the deletion of obsolete tests, and changes in techniques used in the clinical laboratory. As with many other aspects of medicine, widespread use of computers has both simplified and complicated application of reference ranges. Most laboratory computer systems permit use of as many as one or two dozen age- and sex-corrected ranges for each constituent, and the appropriate range is indicated on each patient's report. Serum alkaline phosphatase determination is an example of a test in which the values change dramatically with age and differ between sexes. The computer handles this well, but one can imagine how the following tables would appear if up to a dozen ranges were included for each test listed.

THE INTERNATIONAL SYSTEM OF UNITS FOR LABORATORY MEASUREMENTS (LE SYSTÈME INTERNATIONAL D'UNITÉS)

The United States is the only major industrialized country that has not adopted the International System of Units (abbreviated SI units) for expressing measurements in all areas of science and industry. The medical profession in the United States has been remarkably firm in its opposition to introduction of SI units, even though many American medical journals express laboratory data only in SI units. A much more significant change occurred some 35 years ago when the apothecaries' system was abandoned in favor of the metric system for expressing drug dosages, and it appears to be only a matter of time until the International System is adopted. Because of this, the following information on SI units is being reprinted from *Current Therapy 1991*.

The International System is a coherent approach to all types of measurement that uses seven dimensionally independent basic quantities: mass, length, time, thermodynamic temperature, electrical current, luminous intensity, and amount of substance. Each of these quantities is expressed in a clearly defined *base unit* (Table 1).

Two or more base units may be combined to provide *derived units* (Table 2) for expressing other measurements such as mass concentration (kilograms per cubic meter) and velocity (meters per second). Standardized prefixes (Table 3) for base and derived units are used to express fractions or multiples of the base units so that any measurement can be expressed in a value between 0.001 and 1000.

Medical Applications

The most profound change in laboratory reports will result from expressing concentration as amount per volume (moles per liter) rather than mass per volume (milligrams per 100 mil-

---

*From Rakel RE (ed): *Conn's Current Therapy 1992*. Philadelphia: W. B. Saunders.

TABLE 1. BASE UNITS

PROPERTY	BASE UNIT	SYMBOL
Length	meter	m
Mass	kilogram	kg
Amount of substance	mole	mol
Time	second	s
Thermodynamic temperature	kelvin	K
Electrical current	ampere	A
Luminous intensity	candela	cd

LABORATORY VALUES OF CLINICAL IMPORTANCE Continued

TABLE 2. DERIVED UNITS

DERIVED PROPERTY	DERIVED UNIT	SYMBOL
Area	square meter	m^2
Volume	cubic meter	m^3
	liter	L
Mass concentration	kilogram/cubic meter	kg/m^3
	gram/liter	g/L
Substance concentration	mole/cubic meter	mol/m^3
	mole/liter	mol/L
Temperature	degree Celsius	C = K − 273.15

liliters). The advantages of the former expression can be seen in the following:

Conventional Units

1.0 gram of hemoglobin
Combines with 1.37 ml of oxygen
Contains 3.4 mg of iron
Forms 34.9 mg of bilirubin

SI Units

1.0 mmol of hemoglobin
Combines with 4.0 mmol of oxygen
Contains 4.0 mmol of iron
Forms 4.0 mmol of bilirubin

Chemical relationships between lactic acid and pyruvic acid and the glucose from which both are derived, as well as the relationship between bilirubin and the binding capacity of albumin, are other examples of chemical relationships that will be clarified by using the new system.

There are a number of laboratory and other medical measurements for which the SI units appear to offer little advantage, and some that are disadvantageous because the change would require replacement or revision of instruments such as the sphygmomanometer. The cubic meter is the derived unit for volume; however it is inappropriately large for medical measure-

TABLE 3. STANDARD PREFIXES

PREFIX	MULTIPLICATION FACTOR	SYMBOL
atto	10^{-18}	a
femto	10^{-15}	f
pico	10^{-12}	p
nano	10^{-9}	n
micro	10^{-6}	μ
milli	10^{-3}	m
centi	10^{-2}	c
deci	10^{-1}	d
deca	10^{1}	da
hecto	10^{2}	h
kilo	10^{3}	k
mega	10^{6}	M
giga	10^{9}	G
tera	10^{12}	T

ments, and the liter has been retained. Thermodynamic temperature expressed in kelvins is not more informative for medical measurements. Since the Celsius degree is the same as the Kelvin degree, the Celsius scale is used. Celsius rather than centigrade is the preferred term.

Selection of units for expressing enzyme activity presents certain difficulties. Literally dozens of different units have been used in expressing enzyme activity, and interlaboratory comparison of enzyme results is impossible unless the assay system is precisely defined. In 1964, the International Union of Biochemistry attempted to remedy the situation by proposing the International Unit for enzymes. This unit was defined as the amount of enzyme that will catalyze the conversion of 1 μmol of substrate per minute under standard conditions. Difficulties remain, however, as enzyme activity is affected by temperature, pH, the type and amount of substrate, the presence of inhibitors, and other factors. Enzyme activity can be expressed in SI units, and the katal has been proposed to express activities of all catalysts, including enzymes. The katal is that amount of enzyme that catalyzes a reaction rate of 1 mol per second. Thus, adoption of the katal as the unit of enzyme activity would provide no more information than is obtained when results are expressed in International Units.

Hydrogen ion concentration in blood is customarily expressed as pH, but in SI units it would be expressed in nanomoles per liter. It appears unlikely that the very useful pH scale will be discarded.

Pressure measures, such as blood pressure and partial pressures of blood gases, would be expressed in SI units using the pascal, a unit that can be derived from the base units for mass, length, and time. This change probably will not be adopted in the early phases of the conversion to SI units. Similarly, a proposed change in expressing osmolality in terms of the depression of freezing point is inappropriate, because osmolality may be calculated from vapor pressure as well as freezing point measurement.

In the following tables, reference ranges for the most commonly used diagnostic tests are given in conventional units and in SI units. The conversion of weight per volume (conventional units) to amount per volume (SI units) is based on the molecular weight of the analyte. For heterogeneous analytes, for example, gamma globulins, weight per volume must be retained as the unit; however, volume is expressed as the liter rather than as the deciliter as in conventional units. Weight per volume is retained for albumin, to be consistent with the other serum proteins. Hemoglobin is expressed here in SI units as the tetramer; in some countries it is expressed as the monomer, in which case the numerical values in SI units are four times as great as those shown. Plasma drug concentrations for therapeutic monitoring are not given in SI units, since it is unlikely that pharmaceutical manufacturers will change to molar quantities for expressing drug dosages.

LABORATORY VALUES OF CLINICAL IMPORTANCE Continued

Reference Values in Hematology

		Conventional Units	SI Units
Acid hemolysis test (Ham)		No hemolysis	No hemolysis
Alkaline phosphatase, leukocyte		Total score 14–100	Total score 14–100
Cell counts			
Erythrocytes			
Males		4.6–6.2 million/mm^3	4.6–6.2 × 10^{12}/L
Females		4.2–5.4 million/mm^3	4.2–5.4 × 10^{12}/L
Children (varies with age)		4.5–5.1 million/mm^3	4.5–5.1 × 10^{12}/L
Leukocytes			
Total		4500–11,000 mm^3	4.5–11.0 × 10^9/L
Differential	*Percentage*	*Absolute*	*Absolute*
Myelocytes	0	0/mm^3	0/L
Band neutrophils	3–5	150–400/mm^3	150–400 × 10^6/L
Segmented neutrophils	54–62	3000–5800/mm^3	3000–5800 × 10^6/L
Lymphocytes	25–33	1500–3000/mm^3	1500–3000 × 10^6/L
Monocytes	3–7	300–500/mm^3	300–500 × 10^6/L
Eosinophils	1–3	50–250/mm^3	50–250 × 10^6/L
Basophils	0–0.75	15–50/mm^3	15–50 × 10^6/L
Platelets		150,000–350,000/mm^3	150–350 × 10^9/L
Reticulocytes		25,000–75,000/mm^3	25–75 × 10^9/L
		0.5–1.5% of erythrocytes	
Coagulation tests			
Bleeding time (template)		2.75–8.0 min	2.75–8.0 min
Coagulation time (glass tubes)		5–15 min	5–15 min
Factor VIII and other coagulation factors		50–150% of normal	0.5–1.5 of normal
Fibrin split products (Thrombo-Welco test)		<10 μg/mL	<10 mg/L
Fibrinogen		200–400 mg/dL	2.0–4.0 g/L
Partial thromboplastin time (PTT)		20–35 sec	20–35 s
Prothrombin time (PT)		12.0–14.0 sec	12.0–14.0 s
Coombs' test			
Direct		Negative	Negative
Indirect		Negative	Negative
Corpuscular values of erythrocytes			
Mean corpuscular hemoglobin (MCH)		26–34 pg	0.40–0.53 fmol
Mean corpuscular volume (MCV)		80–96 μm^3	80–96 fL
Mean corpuscular hemoglobin concentration (MCHC)		32–36%	0.32–0.36
Haptoglobin		26–185 mg/dL	260–1850 mg/L
Hematocrit			
Males		40–54 mL/dL	0.40–0.54 volume fraction
Females		37–47 mL/dL	0.37–0.47 volume fraction
Newborns		49–54 mL/dL	0.49–0.54 volume fraction
Children (varies with age)		35–49 mL/dL	0.35–0.49 volume fraction
Hemoglobin			
Males		14.0–18.0 gm/dL	2.17–2.79 mmol/L
Females		12.0–16.0 gm/dL	1.86–2.48 mmol/L
Newborns		16.5–19.5 gm/dL	2.56–3.02 mmol/L
Children (varies with age)		11.2–16.5 gm/dL	1.74–2.56 mmol/L
Hemoglobin, fetal		<1.0% of total	<0.01 of total
Hemoglobin A$_{1C}$		3–5% of total	0.03–0.05 of total
Hemoglobin A$_2$		1.5–3.0% of total	0.015–0.03 of total
Hemoglobin, plasma		0–5.0 mg/dL	0–0.8 μmol/L
Methemoglobin		30–130 mg/dL	4.7–20 μmol/L
Sedimentation rate (ESR)			
Wintrobe: Males		0–5 mm/hr	0–5 mm/h
Females		0–15 mm/hr	0–15 mm/h
Westergren: Males		0–15 mm/hr	0–15 mm/h
Females		0–20 mm/hr	0–20 mm/h

LABORATORY VALUES OF CLINICAL IMPORTANCE *Continued*

Reference Values for Blood, Plasma, and Serum
(For some procedures the reference values may vary depending on the method used)

	Conventional Units	SI Units
Acetoacetate plus acetone, serum		
Qualitative	Negative	Negative
Quantitative	0.3–2.0 mg/dL	3–20 mg/L
Acid phosphatase (thymolphthalein monophosphate substrate), serum	0.11–0.60 U/L	0.11–0.60 U/L
Adrenocorticotropin (ACTH), plasma		
6 a.m.	10–80 pg/mL	10–80 ng/L
6 p.m.	<50 pg/mL	<50 ng/L
Alanine aminotransferase (ALT, SGPT), serum	5–30 U/L	5–30 U/L
Albumin, serum	3.5–5.5 gm/dL	35–55 g/L
Aldolase, serum	1.5–12.0 U/L	1.5–12.0 U/L
Aldosterone, plasma		
Supine	3–10 ng/dL	0.08–0.30 nmol/L
Standing		
Males	6–22 ng/dL	0.17–0.61 nmol/L
Females	5–30 ng/dL	0.14–0.83 nmol/L
Alkaline phosphatase (ALP), serum	20–90 U/L (30° C)	20–90 U/L (30° C)
Ammonia nitrogen, plasma	15–49 µg/dL	11–35 µmol/L
Amylase, serum	25–125 U/L	25–125 U/L
Anion gap	8–16 mEq/L	8–16 mmol/L
Ascorbic acid, blood	0.4–1.5 mg/dL	23–85 µmol/L
Aspartate aminotransferase (AST, SGOT), serum	10–30 U/L	10–30 U/L
Base excess, blood	0 ± 2 mEq/L	0 ± 2 mmol/L
Bicarbonate		
Venous plasma	23–29 mEq/L	23–29 mmol/L
Arterial blood	18–23 mEq/L	18–23 mmol/L
Bile acids, serum	0.3–3.0 mg/dL	3–30 mg/L
Bilirubin, serum		
Conjugated	0.1–0.4 mg/dL	1.7–6.8 µmol/L
Unconjugated	0.2–0.7 mg/dL	3.4–12 µmol/L
Total	0.3–1.1 mg/dL	5.1–19 µmol/L
Calcium, serum	9.0–11.0 mg/dL	2.25–2.75 mmol/L
Calcium, ionized, serum	4.25–5.25 mg/dL	1.05–1.30 mmol/L
Carbon dioxide, total, serum or plasma	24–30 mEq/L	24–30 mmol/L
Carbon dioxide tension (P_{CO_2}), blood	35–45 mmHg	35–45 mmHg
β-Carotene, serum	40–200 µg/dL	0.74–3.72 µmol/L
Ceruloplasmin, serum	23–44 mg/dL	230–44 mg/L
Chloride, serum or plasma	96–106 mEq/L	96–106 mmol/L
Cholesterol, serum or EDTA plasma		
Desirable range	<200 mg/dL	<5.18 mmol/L
LDL cholesterol	60–180 mg/dL	600–1800 mg/L
HDL cholesterol	30–80 mg/dL	300–800 mg/L
Copper		
Males	70–140 µg/dL	11–22 µmol/L
Females	85–155 µg/dL	13–24 µmol/L
Cortisol, plasma		
8 A.M.	6–23 µg/dL	170–635 nmol/L
4 P.M.	3–15 µg/dL	82–413 nmol/L
10 P.M.	<50% of 8 A.M. value	<0.5 of 8 A.M. value
Creatine, serum	0.2–0.8 mg/dL	15–61 µmol/L
Creatine kinase (CK, CPK), serum		
Males	55–170 U/L	55–170 U/L
Females	30–135 U/L	30–135 U/L
Creatine kinase MB isozyme, serum	0.0–4.7 ng/mL	0.0–4.7 µg/L
Creatinine, serum	0.6–1.2 mg/dL	53–106 µmol/L
Ferritin, serum	20–200 ng/mL	20–200 µg/L
Fibrinogen, plasma	200–400 mg/dL	2.0–4.0 g/L
Folate, serum	1.8–9.0 ng/mL	4.1–20.4 nmol/L
Erythrocytes	150–450 ng/mL	340–1020 nmol/L
Follicle-stimulating hormone (FSH), plasma		
Males	4–25 mU/mL	4–25 U/L
Females	4–30 mU/mL	4–30 U/L
Postmenopausal	40–250 mU/mL	40–250 U/L
γ-Glutamyltransferase, serum		
Males	5–38 U/L	5–38 U/L
Females	5–29 U/L	5–29 U/L
Gastrin, serum	0–200 pg/mL	0–200 ng/L

LABORATORY VALUES OF CLINICAL IMPORTANCE Continued

Reference Values for Blood, Plasma, and Serum Continued
(For some procedures the reference values may vary depending on the method used)

	Conventional Units	SI Units
Glucose (fasting), plasma or serum	70–115 mg/dL	3.89–6.38 mmol/L
Growth hormone (hGH), plasma	0–10 ng/mL	0–10 µg/L
Haptoglobin, serum	26–185 mg/dL	260–1850 mg/L
Immunoglobulins, serum		
IgG	550–1900 mg/dL	5.5–19.0 g/L
IgA	60–333 mg/dL	0.60–3.3 g/L
IgM	45–145 mg/dL	0.45–1.5 g/L
IgD	0.5–3.0 mg/dL	5–30 mg/L
IgE	<500 ng/mL	<500 µg/L
Insulin (fasting), plasma	5–25 µU/mL	36–179 pmol/L
Iron, serum	75–175 µg/dL	13–31 µmol/L
Iron binding capacity, serum		
Total	250–410 µg/dL	45–73 µmol/L
Saturation	20–55%	0.20–0.55
Lactate		
Venous blood	4.5–19.8 mg/dL	0.50–2.2 mmol/L
Arterial blood	4.5–14.4 mg/dL	0.50–1.6 mmol/L
Lactate dehydrogenase (LD, LDH), serum	100–190 U/L	100–190 U/L
Lipase, serum	10–140 U/L	10–140 U/L
Lipids, total, serum	450–850 mg/dL	4.5–8.5 g/L
Luteinizing (LH), serum		
Males	6–18 IU/L	6–18 U/L
Females		
Premenopausal	5–22 IU/L	5–22 U/L
Mid-cycle	3 times baseline	3 times baseline
Postmenopausal	>30 IU/L	>30 U/L
Magnesium, serum	1.8–3.0 mg/dL	0.75–1.25 mmol/L
Osmolality	286–295 mOsm/kg water	285–295 mmol/kg water
Oxygen, blood		
Capacity (varies with hemoglobin)	16–24 vol %	7.14–10.7 mmol/L
Content, arterial	15–23 vol %	6.69–10.3 mmol/L
Saturation, arterial	94–100 %	0.94–1.00
Oxygen tension (P_{O_2}), blood	75–100 mmHg	75–100 mmHg
P_{50}	26–27 mmHg	26–27 mmHg
pH, arterial blood	7.35–7.45	7.35–7.45
Phenylalanine, serum	<3 mg/dL	<0.18 mmol/L
Phosphate, inorganic, serum	3.0–4.5 mg/dL	1.0–1.5 mmol/L
Potassium, serum or plasma	3.5–5.0 mEq/L	3.5–5.0 mmol/L
Prolactin		
Males	1–20 ng/mL	1–20 µg/L
Females	1–25 ng/mL	1–25 µg/L
Protein, serum		
Total	6.0–8.0 gm/dL	60–80 g/L
Albumin	3.5–5.5 gm/dL	35–55 g/L
Alpha$_1$ globulin	0.2–0.4 gm/dL	2–4 g/L
Alpha$_2$ globulin	0.5–0.9 gm/dL	5–9 g/L
Beta globulin	0.6–1.1 gm/dL	6–11 g/L
Gamma globulin	0.7–1.7 gm/dL	7–17 g/L
Pyruvate, blood	0.3–0.9 mg/dL	0.03–0.10 mmol/L
Sodium, serum or plasma	136–145 mEq/L	136–145 mmol/L
Testosterone, plasma		
Males	275–875 ng/dL	9.5–30 nmol/L
Females	23–75 ng/dL	0.8–2.6 nmol/L
Pregnant	38–190 ng/dL	1.3–6.6 nmol/L
Thyroid-stimulating hormone (TSH), serum	0–7 µU/mL	0–7 mU/L
Thyroxine, free (FT), serum	1.0–2.1 ng/dL	13–27 pmol/L
Thyroxine (T_4), serum	4.4–9.9 µg/dL	57–128 nmol/L
Triglycerides, serum	40–150 mg/dL	0.4–1.5 g/L
Triiodothyronine (T_3), serum	150–250 ng/dL	2.3–3.9 nmol/L
Triiodothyronine uptake, resin (T_3RU)	25–38% uptake	0.25–0.38 uptake
Urate, serum		
Males	2.5–8.0 mg/dL	0.15–0.48 mmol/L
Females	1.5–7.0 mg/dL	0.09–0.42 mmol/L

Table continued on following page

LABORATORY VALUES OF CLINICAL IMPORTANCE Continued

Reference Values for Blood, Plasma, and Serum Continued
(For some procedures the reference values may vary depending on the method used)

	Conventional Units	SI Units
Urea, serum or plasma	24–49 mg/dL	4.0–8.2 mmol/L
Urea nitrogen, serum or plasma	11–23 mg/dL	3.9–8.2 mmol/L
Viscosity, serum	1.4–1.8 times water	1.4–1.8 times water
Vitamin A, serum	20–80 µg/dL	0.70–2.80 µmol/L
Vitamin B_{12}, serum	180–900 pg/mL	133–664 pmol/L

Reference Values for Urine
(For some procedures the reference values may vary depending on the method used)

	Conventional Units	SI Units
Acetone and acetoacetate, qualitative	Negative	Negative
Albumin		
Qualitative	Negative	Negative
Quantitive	10–100 mg/24 hr	0.15–1.5 µmol/24 h
Aldosterone	3–20 µg/24 hr	8.3–55 nmol/24 h
δ-Aminolevulinic acid	1.3–7.0 mg/24 hr	10–53 µmol/24 h
Amylase	3–20 U/hr	3–20 U/h
Amylase/creatinine clearance ratio	1–4%	0.01–0.04
Bilirubin, qualitative	Negative	Negative
Calcium (usual diet)	<250 mg/24 hr	<6.3 mmol/24 h
Catecholamines		
Epinephrine	<10 µg/24 hr	<55 nmol/24 h
Norepinephrine	<100 µg/24 hr	<590 nmol/24 h
Total free catecholamines	4–126 µg/24 hr	24–745 nmol/24 h
Total metanephrines	0.1–1.6 mg/24 hr	0.5–8.1 µmol/24 h
Chloride (varies with intake)	110–250 mEq/24 hr	110–250 mmol/24 h
Copper	0–50 µg/24 hr	0–0.80 µmol/24 h
Cortisol, free	10–100 µg/24 hr	27.6–276 nmol/24 h
Creatinine	15–25 mg/kg body weight/24 hr	0.13–0.22 mmol/kg body weight/24 h
Creatinine clearance (corrected to 1.73 m² body surface area)		
Males	110–150 mL/min	110–150 ml/min
Females	105–132 mL/min	105–132 ml/min
Dehydroepiandrosterone		
Males	0.2–2.0 mg/24 hr	0.7–6.9 µmol/24 h
Females	0.2–1.8 mg/24 hr	0.7–6.2 µmol/24 h
Estrogens, total		
Males	4–25 µg/24 hr	14–90 nmol/24 h
Females	5–100 µg/24 hr	18–360 nmol/24 h
Glucose (as reducing substance)	<250 mg/24 hr	<250 mg/24 h
Hemoglobin and myoglobin, qualitative	Negative	Negative
17-Hydroxycorticosteroids		
Males	3–9 mg/24 hr	8.3–25 µmol/24 h
Females	2–8 mg/24 hr	5.5–22 µmol/24 h
5-Hydroxyindoleacetic acid		
Qualitative	Negative	Negative
Quantitative	<9 mg/24 hr	<47 µmol/24 h
17-Ketosteroids		
Males	6–18 mg/24 hr	21–62 µmol/24 h
Females	4–13 mg/24 hr	14–45 µmol/24 h
Magnesium	6.0–8.5 mEq/24 hr	3.0–4.2 mmol/24 h
Metanephrines (see Catecholamines)		
Osmolality	38–1400 mOsm/kg water	38–1400 mmol/kg water
pH	4.6–8.0	4.6–8.0
Phenylpyruvic acid, qualitative	Negative	Negative
Phosphate	0.9–1.3 grams/24 hr	29–42 mmol/24 h
Porphobilinogen		
Qualitative	Negative	Negative
Quantitative	<2.0 mg/24 hr	<9 µmol/24 h
Porphyrins		
Coproporphyrin	50–250 µg/24 hr	77–380 nmol/24 h
Uroporphyrin	10–30 µg/24 hr	12–36 nmol/24 h
Potassium	25–100 mEq/24 hr	25–100 mmol/24 h

LABORATORY VALUES OF CLINICAL IMPORTANCE Continued

Reference Values for Urine Continued
(For some procedures the reference values may vary depending on the method used)

	Conventional Units	SI Units
Pregnanediol		
Males	0.4–1.4 mg/24 hr	1.2–4.4 μmol/24 h
Females		
Proliferative phase	0.5–1.5 mg/24 hr	1.6–4.7 μmol/24 h
Luteal phase	2.0–7.0 mg/24 hr	6.2–22 μmol/24 h
Postmenopausal	0.2–1.0 mg/24 hr	0.6–3.1 μmol/24 h
Pregnanetriol	<2.5 mg/24 hr	<7.4 μmol/24 h
Protein		
Qualitative	Negative	Negative
Quantitative	10–150 mg/24 hr	10–150 mg/24 h
Sodium	130–260 mEq/24 hr	130–260 mmol/24 h
Specific gravity	1.003–1.030	1.003–1.030
Urate	200–500 mg/24 hr	1.2–3.0 mmol/24 h
Urobilinogen	<4.0 mg/24 hr	<6.8 μmol/24 h
Vanillylmandelic acid (VMA, 4-hydroxy-3-methoxymandelic acid)	1–8 mg/24 hr	5–40 μmol/24 h

Reference Values for Therapeutic Drug Monitoring

	Therapeutic Range	Toxic Levels	Proprietary Names
Antibiotics			
Amikacin, serum	25–30 μg/mL	Peak: >35 μg/mL Trough: >5–7 μg/mL	Amikin
Chloramphenicol, serum	10–20 μg/mL	>25 μg/mL	Chloromycetin
Gentamicin, serum	5–10 μg/mL	Peak: >12 μg/mL Trough: >2 μg/mL	Garamycin
Tobramycin, serum	5–10 μg/mL	Peak: >12 μg/mL Trough: >2 μg/mL	Nebcin
Anticonvulsants			
Carbamazepine, serum	5–12 μg/mL	>12 μg/mL	Tegretol
Ethosuximide, serum	40–100 μg/mL	>100 μg/mL	Zarontin
Phenobarbital, serum	10–30 μg/mL	Vary widely because of developed tolerance	
Phenytoin, serum	10–20 μg/mL	>20 μg/mL	Dilantin
Primidone, serum	5–12 μg/mL	>15 μg/mL	Mysoline
Valproic acid, serum	50–100 μg/mL	>100 μg/mL	Depakene
Analgesics			
Acetaminophen, serum	10–20 μg/mL	>250 μg/mL	Tylenol
Salicylate, serum	100–250 μg/mL	>300 μg/mL	Disalcid
Bronchodilator			
Theophylline (aminophylline), serum	10–20 μg/mL	>20 μg/mL	
Cardiovascular Drugs			
Digitoxin, serum (specimen must be obtained 12–24 hr after last dose)	15–25 ng/mL	>25 ng/ml	Crystodigin
Digoxin, serum (specimen must be obtained 12–24 hr after last dose)	0.8–2.0 ng/mL	>2.4 ng/mL	Lanoxin
Disopyramide, serum	2–5 μg/mL	>5 μg/mL	Norpace
Lidocaine, serum	1.5–5.0 μg/mL	>6–8 μg/mL	Xylocaine
Procainamide, serum (measured as procainamide + N-acetylprocainamide)	4–10 μg/mL	>16 μg/mL	Pronestyl
Propranolol, serum	50–100 ng/mL	Variable	Inderal
Quinidine, serum	2–5 μg/mL	>10 μg/mL	Cardioquin Quinaglute Quinidex Quinora
Psychopharmacologic Drugs			
Amitriptyline, serum (measured as amitriptyline + nortriptyline)	120–150 ng/mL	>500 ng/mL	Amitril Elavil Endep Limbitrol Triavil

Table continued on following page

LABORATORY VALUES OF CLINICAL IMPORTANCE Continued

Reference Values for Therapeutic Drug Monitoring Continued

	Therapeutic Range	Toxic Levels	Proprietary Names
Desipramine, serum (measured as desipramine + imipramine)	150–300 ng/mL	>500 ng/mL	Norpramin Pertofrane
Imipramine, serum (measured as imipramine + desipramine)	150–300 ng/mL	>500 ng/mL	Antipress Imavate Janimine Presamine Tofranil
Lithium, serum (obtain specimen 12 hr after last dose)	0.8–1.2 mEq/L	>2.0 mEq/L	Lithobid
Nortriptyline, serum	50–150 ng/mL	>500 ng/mL	Aventyl Pamelor

Reference Values in Toxicology

	Conventional Units	SI Units
Arsenic		
Blood	3.5–7.2 µg/dL	0.47–0.96 µmol/L
Urine	<100 µg/24 hr	<1.3 µmol/24 h
Bromides, serum	0	0
	Toxic: >17 mEq/L	Toxic: >17 mmol/L
Carboxyhemoglobin, blood	<5% saturation	<0.05 saturation
Symptoms occur	>20% saturation	>0.20 saturation
Ethanol, blood	<0.05 mg/dL (<0.005%)	<1.0 mmol/L
Marked intoxication	300–400 mg/dL (0.3–0.4%)	65–87 mmol/L
Alcoholic stupor	400–500 mg/dL (0.4–0.5%)	87–109 mmol/L
Coma	>500 mg/dL (0.5%)	>109 mmol/L
Lead		
Blood	0–40 µg/dL	0–2 µmol/L
Urine	<100 µg/24 hr	<0.48 µmol/24 h
Mercury, urine	<100 µg/24 hr	<50 nmol/24 h

Reference Values for Cerebrospinal Fluid

	Conventional Units	SI Units
Cells	<5/mm^3; all mononuclear	<5 × 10^6/L, all mononuclear
Electrophoresis	Predominantly albumin	Predominantly albumin
Glucose	50–75 mg/dL (20 mg/dL less than serum)	2.8–4.2 mmol/L (1.1 mmol less than serum)
IgG		
Children under 14	<8% of total protein	<0.08 of total protein
Adults	<14% of total protein	<0.14 of total protein
IgG index $\left(\dfrac{\text{CSF/serum IgG ratio}}{\text{CSF/serum albumin ratio}}\right)$	0.3–0.6	0.3–0.6
Oligoclonal banding on electrophoresis	Absent	Absent
Pressure	70–180 mm water	70–180 mm water
Protein, total	15–45 mg/dL	150–450 mg/L

Reference Values for Semen

	Conventional Units	SI Units
Volume	2–5 mL	2–5 mL
Liquefaction	Complete in 15 min	Complete in 15 min
Leukocytes	Occasional or absent	Occasional or absent
Count	60–150 million/mL	60–150 × 10^6/mL
Motility	>80% motile	>0.80 motile
Morphology	80–90% normal forms	0.80–0.90 normal forms
Fructose	>150 mg/dL	>8.33 mmol/L

C-11
LABORATORY VALUES OF CLINICAL IMPORTANCE Continued

	Reference Values for Feces	
	Conventional Units	**SI Units**
Bulk	100–200 gm/24 hr	100–200 g/24 h
Dry matter	23–32 gm/24 hr	23–32 g/24 h
Fat, total	<6.0 gm/24 hr	<6.0 g/24 h
Nitrogen, total	<2.0 gm/24 hr	<2.0 g/24 h
Water	Approximately 65%	Approximately 0.65

REFERENCES

1. Brown SS, Mitchell FL, and Young DS (eds): Chemical Diagnosis of Disease. Amsterdam, Elsevier/North-Holland Biomedical Press, 1979.
2. Conn RB (ed): Current Diagnosis. 8th ed. Philadelphia, WB Saunders Co, 1991.
3. Goodman AG, Gilman LS, Rall TW, and Murad F: Goodman and Gilman's The Pharmacological Basis of Therapeutics. 7th ed. New York, Macmillan Co, 1985.
4. Henry JB (ed): Clinical Diagnosis and Management by Laboratory Methods. 18th ed. Philadelphia, WB Saunders Co, 1991.
5. Lundberg GD, Iverson C, and Radulescu G: JAMA 255:2247, 1986.
6. Miale JB: Laboratory Medicine-Hematology. 6th ed. St. Louis, CV Mosby, 1982.
7. Physicians' Desk Reference. 45th ed. Oradell, NJ, Medical Economics Co, 1991.
8. Tietz NW: Clinical Guide to Laboratory Tests. 2nd ed. Philadelphia, WB Saunders Co, 1990.
9. Tietz NW: Textbook of Clinical Chemistry. Philadelphia, WB Saunders Co, 1986.
10. Williams WJ, Beutler E, Erslev AJ, and Lichtman MA: Hematology. 3rd ed. New York, McGraw-Hill Book Co, 1983.

Some of these values have been established by the Clinical Laboratories at Thomas Jefferson University Hospital, Philadelphia, PA, and have not been published elsewhere.

APPENDIX D
STANDARDS AND REGULATIONS

D–1	CDC Recommendations for Prevention of HIV Transmission in Health-Care Settings
D–2	CDC Update: Universal Precautions for Prevention of Transmission of Human Immunodeficiency Virus, Hepatitis B Virus, and Other Bloodborne Pathogens in Health-Care Settings
D–3	CLIA (Clinical Laboratory Improvement Amendments): 1988 Regulations and Requirements
D–4	DACUM (Developing a Curriculum): 1990 Guidelines
D–5	Diagnosis-Related Groups (DRGs)
D–6	OSHA Bloodborne Pathogens Final Standard: Summary of Key Provisions
D–7	OSHA Joint Advisory Notice of the Department of Labor and the Department of Health and Human Services for the Protection Against Occupational Exposure to Hepatitis B Virus (HBV) and Human Immunodeficiency Virus (HIV)
D–8	OSHA Guidelines to Developing a Facility Bloodborne Pathogens Exposure Control Plan
D–9	OSHA Hepatitis B Vaccination Protection
D–10	States with OSHA-Approved Plans

Recommendations for Prevention of HIV Transmission in Health-Care Settings

Introduction

Human immunodeficiency virus (HIV), the virus that causes acquired immunodeficiency syndrome (AIDS), is transmitted through sexual contact and exposure to infected blood or blood components and perinatally from mother to neonate. HIV has been isolated from blood, semen, vaginal secretions, saliva, tears, breast milk, cerebrospinal fluid, amniotic fluid, and urine and is likely to be isolated from other body fluids, secretions, and excretions. However, epidemiologic evidence has implicated only blood, semen, vaginal secretions, and possibly breast milk in transmission.

The increasing prevalence of HIV increases the risk that health-care workers will be exposed to blood from patients infected with HIV, especially when blood and body-fluid precautions are not followed for all patients. Thus, this document emphasizes the need for health-care workers to consider **all** patients as potentially infected with HIV and/or other blood-borne pathogens and to adhere rigorously to infection-control precautions for minimizing the risk of exposure to blood and body fluids of all patients.

The recommendations contained in this document consolidate and update CDC recommendations published earlier for preventing HIV transmission in health-care settings: precautions for clinical and laboratory staffs (*1*) and precautions for health-care workers and allied professionals (*2*); recommendations for preventing HIV transmission in the workplace (*3*) and during invasive procedures (*4*); recommendations for preventing possible transmission of HIV from tears (*5*); and recommendations for providing dialysis treatment for HIV-infected patients (*6*). These recommendations also update portions of the "Guideline for Isolation Precautions in Hospitals" (*7*) and reemphasize some of the recommendations contained in "Infection Control Practices for Dentistry" (*8*). The recommendations contained in this document have been developed for use in health-care settings and emphasize the need to treat blood and other body fluids from **all** patients as potentially infective. These same prudent precautions also should be taken in other settings in which persons may be exposed to blood or other body fluids.

Definition of Health-Care Workers

Health-care workers are defined as persons, including students and trainees, whose activities involve contact with patients or with blood or other body fluids from patients in a health-care setting.

D-1

CDC RECOMMENDATIONS FOR PREVENTION OF HIV TRANSMISSION IN HEALTH-CARE SETTINGS *Continued*

Health-Care Workers with AIDS

As of July 10, 1987, a total of 1,875 (5.8%) of 32,395 adults with AIDS, who had been reported to the CDC national surveillance system and for whom occupational information was available, reported being employed in a health-care or clinical laboratory setting. In comparison, 6.8 million persons—representing 5.6% of the U.S. labor force—were employed in health services. Of the health-care workers with AIDS, 95% have been reported to exhibit high-risk behavior; for the remaining 5%, the means of HIV acquisition was undetermined. Health-care workers with AIDS were significantly more likely than other workers to have an undetermined risk (5% versus 3%, respectively). For both health-care workers and non-health-care workers with AIDS, the proportion with an undetermined risk has not increased since 1982.

AIDS patients initially reported as not belonging to recognized risk groups are investigated by state and local health departments to determine whether possible risk factors exist. Of all health-care workers with AIDS reported to CDC who were initially characterized as not having an identified risk and for whom follow-up information was available, 66% have been reclassified because risk factors were identified or because the patient was found not to meet the surveillance case definition for AIDS. Of the 87 health-care workers currently categorized as having no identifiable risk, information is incomplete on 16 (18%) because of death or refusal to be interviewed; 38 (44%) are still being investigated. The remaining 33 (38%) health-care workers were interviewed or had other follow-up information available. The occupations of these 33 were as follows: five physicians (15%), three of whom were surgeons; one dentist (3%); three nurses (9%); nine nursing assistants (27%); seven housekeeping or maintenance workers (21%); three clinical laboratory technicians (9%); one therapist (3%); and four others who did not have contact with patients (12%). Although 15 of these 33 health-care workers reported parenteral and/or other non-needlestick exposure to blood or body fluids from patients in the 10 years preceding their diagnosis of AIDS, none of these exposures involved a patient with AIDS or known HIV infection.

Risk to Health-Care Workers of Acquiring HIV in Health-Care Settings

Health-care workers with documented percutaneous or mucous-membrane exposures to blood or body fluids of HIV-infected patients have been prospectively evaluated to determine the risk of infection after such exposures. As of June 30, 1987, 883 health-care workers have been tested for antibody to HIV in an ongoing surveillance project conducted by CDC (*9*). Of these, 708 (80%) had percutaneous exposures to blood, and 175 (20%) had a mucous membrane or an open wound contaminated by blood or body fluid. Of 396 health-care workers, each of whom had only a convalescent-phase serum sample obtained and tested ≥90 days post-exposure, one—for whom heterosexual transmission could not be ruled out—was seropositive for HIV antibody. For 425 additional health-care workers, both acute- and convalescent-phase serum samples were obtained and tested; none of 74 health-care workers with nonpercutaneous exposures seroconverted, and three (0.9%) of 351 with percutaneous exposures seroconverted. None of these three health-care workers had other documented risk factors for infection.

Two other prospective studies to assess the risk of nosocomial acquisition of HIV infection for health-care workers are ongoing in the United States. As of April 30, 1987, 332 health-care workers with a total of 453 needlestick or mucous-membrane exposures to the blood or other body fluids of HIV-infected patients were tested for HIV antibody at the National Institutes of Health (10). These exposed workers included 103 with needlestick injuries and 229 with mucous-membrane exposures; none had seroconverted. A similar study at the University of California of 129 health-care workers with documented needlestick injuries or mucous-membrane exposures to blood or other body fluids from patients with HIV infection has not identified any seroconversions (11). Results of a prospective study in the United Kingdom identified no evidence of transmission among 150 health-care workers with parenteral or mucous-membrane exposures to blood or other body fluids, secretions, or excretions from patients with HIV infection (12).

In addition to health-care workers enrolled in prospective studies, eight persons who provided care to infected patients and denied other risk factors have been reported to have acquired HIV infection. Three of these health-care workers had needlestick exposures to blood from infected patients (13-15). Two were persons who provided nursing care to infected persons; although neither sustained a needlestick, both had extensive contact with blood or other body fluids, and neither observed recommended barrier precautions (16,17). The other three were health-care workers with non-needlestick exposures to blood from infected patients (18). Although the exact route of transmission for these last three infections is not known, all three persons had direct contact of their skin with blood from infected patients, all had skin lesions that may have been contaminated by blood, and one also had a mucous-membrane exposure.

A total of 1,231 dentists and hygienists, many of whom practiced in areas with many AIDS cases, participated in a study to determine the prevalence of antibody to HIV; one dentist (0.1%) had HIV antibody. Although no exposure to a known HIV-infected person could be documented, epidemiologic investigation did not identify any other risk factor for infection. The infected dentist, who also had a history of sustaining needlestick injuries and trauma to his hands, did not routinely wear gloves when providing dental care (19).

Precautions To Prevent Transmission of HIV

Universal Precautions
Since medical history and examination cannot reliably identify all patients infected with HIV or other blood-borne pathogens, blood and body-fluid precautions should be consistently used for **all** patients. This approach, previously recommended by CDC (3,4), and referred to as "universal blood and body-fluid precautions" or "universal precautions," should be used in the care of **all** patients, especially including those in emergency-care settings in which the risk of blood exposure is increased and the infection status of the patient is usually unknown (20).

D-1
CDC RECOMMENDATIONS FOR PREVENTION OF HIV TRANSMISSION IN HEALTH-CARE SETTINGS *Continued*

1. All health-care workers should routinely use appropriate barrier precautions to prevent skin and mucous-membrane exposure when contact with blood or other body fluids of any patient is anticipated. Gloves should be worn for touching blood and body fluids, mucous membranes, or non-intact skin of all patients, for handling items or surfaces soiled with blood or body fluids, and for performing venipuncture and other vascular access procedures. Gloves should be changed after contact with each patient. Masks and protective eyewear or face shields should be worn during procedures that are likely to generate droplets of blood or other body fluids to prevent exposure of mucous membranes of the mouth, nose, and eyes. Gowns or aprons should be worn during procedures that are likely to generate splashes of blood or other body fluids.
2. Hands and other skin surfaces should be washed immediately and thoroughly if contaminated with blood or other body fluids. Hands should be washed immediately after gloves are removed.
3. All health-care workers should take precautions to prevent injuries caused by needles, scalpels, and other sharp instruments or devices during procedures; when cleaning used instruments; during disposal of used needles; and when handling sharp instruments after procedures. To prevent needlestick injuries, needles should not be recapped, purposely bent or broken by hand, removed from disposable syringes, or otherwise manipulated by hand. After they are used, disposable syringes and needles, scalpel blades, and other sharp items should be placed in puncture-resistant containers for disposal; the puncture-resistant containers should be located as close as practical to the use area. Large-bore reusable needles should be placed in a puncture-resistant container for transport to the reprocessing area.
4. Although saliva has not been implicated in HIV transmission, to minimize the need for emergency mouth-to-mouth resuscitation, mouthpieces, resuscitation bags, or other ventilation devices should be available for use in areas in which the need for resuscitation is predictable.
5. Health-care workers who have exudative lesions or weeping dermatitis should refrain from all direct patient care and from handling patient-care equipment until the condition resolves.
6. Pregnant health-care workers are not known to be at greater risk of contracting HIV infection than health-care workers who are not pregnant; however, if a health-care worker develops HIV infection during pregnancy, the infant is at risk of infection resulting from perinatal transmission. Because of this risk, pregnant health-care workers should be especially familiar with and strictly adhere to precautions to minimize the risk of HIV transmission.

Implementation of universal blood and body-fluid precautions for **all** patients eliminates the need for use of the isolation category of "Blood and Body Fluid Precautions" previously recommended by CDC (*7*) for patients known or suspected to be infected with blood-borne pathogens. Isolation precautions (e.g., enteric, "AFB" [*7*]) should be used as necessary if associated conditions, such as infectious diarrhea or tuberculosis, are diagnosed or suspected.

Precautions for Invasive Procedures

In this document, an invasive procedure is defined as surgical entry into tissues, cavities, or organs or repair of major traumatic injuries 1) in an operating or delivery room, emergency department, or outpatient setting, including both physicians' and dentists' offices; 2) cardiac catheterization and angiographic procedures; 3) a vaginal or cesarean delivery or other invasive obstetric procedure during which bleeding may occur; or 4) the manipulation, cutting, or removal of any oral or perioral tissues, including tooth structure, during which bleeding occurs or the potential for bleeding exists. The universal blood and body-fluid precautions listed above, combined with the precautions listed below, should be the minimum precautions for **all** such invasive procedures.

1. All health-care workers who participate in invasive procedures must routinely use appropriate barrier precautions to prevent skin and mucous-membrane contact with blood and other body fluids of all patients. Gloves and surgical masks must be worn for all invasive procedures. Protective eyewear or face shields should be worn for procedures that commonly result in the generation of droplets, splashing of blood or other body fluids, or the generation of bone chips. Gowns or aprons made of materials that provide an effective barrier should be worn during invasive procedures that are likely to result in the splashing of blood or other body fluids. All health-care workers who perform or assist in vaginal or cesarean deliveries should wear gloves and gowns when handling the placenta or the infant until blood and amniotic fluid have been removed from the infant's skin and should wear gloves during post-delivery care of the umbilical cord.

2. If a glove is torn or a needlestick or other injury occurs, the glove should be removed and a new glove used as promptly as patient safety permits; the needle or instrument involved in the incident should also be removed from the sterile field.

Precautions for Dentistry*

Blood, saliva, and gingival fluid from **all** dental patients should be considered infective. Special emphasis should be placed on the following precautions for preventing transmission of blood-borne pathogens in dental practice in both institutional and non-institutional settings.

1. In addition to wearing gloves for contact with oral mucous membranes of all patients, all dental workers should wear surgical masks and protective eyewear or chin-length plastic face shields during dental procedures in which splashing or spattering of blood, saliva, or gingival fluids is likely. Rubber dams, high-speed evacuation, and proper patient positioning, when appropriate, should be utilized to minimize generation of droplets and spatter.

2. Handpieces should be sterilized after use with each patient, since blood, saliva, or gingival fluid of patients may be aspirated into the handpiece or waterline. Handpieces that cannot be sterilized should at least be flushed, the outside surface cleaned and wiped with a suitable chemical germicide, and then rinsed. Handpieces should be flushed at the beginning of the day and after use with each patient. Manufacturers' recommendations should be followed for use and maintenance of waterlines and check valves and for flushing of handpieces. The same precautions should be used for ultrasonic scalers and air/water syringes.

*General infection-control precautions are more specifically addressed in previous recommendations for infection-control practices for dentistry (8).

D-1

CDC RECOMMENDATIONS FOR PREVENTION OF HIV TRANSMISSION IN HEALTH-CARE SETTINGS *Continued*

3. Blood and saliva should be thoroughly and carefully cleaned from material that has been used in the mouth (e.g., impression materials, bite registration), especially before polishing and grinding intra-oral devices. Contaminated materials, impressions, and intra-oral devices should also be cleaned and disinfected before being handled in the dental laboratory and before they are placed in the patient's mouth. Because of the increasing variety of dental materials used intra-orally, dental workers should consult with manufacturers as to the stability of specific materials when using disinfection procedures.
4. Dental equipment and surfaces that are difficult to disinfect (e.g., light handles or X-ray-unit heads) and that may become contaminated should be wrapped with impervious-backed paper, aluminum foil, or clear plastic wrap. The coverings should be removed and discarded, and clean coverings should be put in place after use with each patient.

Precautions for Autopsies or Morticians' Services

In addition to the universal blood and body-fluid precautions listed above, the following precautions should be used by persons performing postmortem procedures:

1. All persons performing or assisting in postmortem procedures should wear gloves, masks, protective eyewear, gowns, and waterproof aprons.
2. Instruments and surfaces contaminated during postmortem procedures should be decontaminated with an appropriate chemical germicide.

Precautions for Dialysis

Patients with end-stage renal disease who are undergoing maintenance dialysis and who have HIV infection can be dialyzed in hospital-based or free-standing dialysis units using conventional infection-control precautions (*21*). Universal blood and body-fluid precautions should be used when dialyzing **all** patients.

Strategies for disinfecting the dialysis fluid pathways of the hemodialysis machine are targeted to control bacterial contamination and generally consist of using 500-750 parts per million (ppm) of sodium hypochlorite (household bleach) for 30-40 minutes or 1.5%-2.0% formaldehyde overnight. In addition, several chemical germicides formulated to disinfect dialysis machines are commercially available. None of these protocols or procedures need to be changed for dialyzing patients infected with HIV.

Patients infected with HIV can be dialyzed by either hemodialysis or peritoneal dialysis and do not need to be isolated from other patients. The type of dialysis treatment (i.e., hemodialysis or peritoneal dialysis) should be based on the needs of the patient. The dialyzer may be discarded after each use. Alternatively, centers that reuse dialyzers—i.e., a specific single-use dialyzer is issued to a specific patient, removed, cleaned, disinfected, and reused several times on the same patient only—may include HIV-infected patients in the dialyzer-reuse program. An individual dialyzer must never be used on more than one patient.

Precautions for Laboratories[†]

Blood and other body fluids from **all** patients should be considered infective. To supplement the universal blood and body-fluid precautions listed above, the following precautions are recommended for health-care workers in clinical laboratories.

[†]Additional precautions for research and industrial laboratories are addressed elsewhere (*22,23*).

D-1
CDC RECOMMENDATIONS FOR PREVENTION OF HIV TRANSMISSION IN HEALTH-CARE SETTINGS *Continued*

1. All specimens of blood and body fluids should be put in a well-constructed container with a secure lid to prevent leaking during transport. Care should be taken when collecting each specimen to avoid contaminating the outside of the container and of the laboratory form accompanying the specimen.
2. All persons processing blood and body-fluid specimens (e.g., removing tops from vacuum tubes) should wear gloves. Masks and protective eyewear should be worn if mucous-membrane contact with blood or body fluids is anticipated. Gloves should be changed and hands washed after completion of specimen processing.
3. For routine procedures, such as histologic and pathologic studies or microbiologic culturing, a biological safety cabinet is not necessary. However, biological safety cabinets (Class I or II) should be used whenever procedures are conducted that have a high potential for generating droplets. These include activities such as blending, sonicating, and vigorous mixing.
4. Mechanical pipetting devices should be used for manipulating all liquids in the laboratory. Mouth pipetting must not be done.
5. Use of needles and syringes should be limited to situations in which there is no alternative, and the recommendations for preventing injuries with needles outlined under universal precautions should be followed.
6. Laboratory work surfaces should be decontaminated with an appropriate chemical germicide after a spill of blood or other body fluids and when work activities are completed.
7. Contaminated materials used in laboratory tests should be decontaminated before reprocessing or be placed in bags and disposed of in accordance with institutional policies for disposal of infective waste (*24*).
8. Scientific equipment that has been contaminated with blood or other body fluids should be decontaminated and cleaned before being repaired in the laboratory or transported to the manufacturer.
9. All persons should wash their hands after completing laboratory activities and should remove protective clothing before leaving the laboratory.

Implementation of universal blood and body-fluid precautions for **all** patients eliminates the need for warning labels on specimens since blood and other body fluids from all patients should be considered infective.

Environmental Considerations for HIV Transmission

No environmentally mediated mode of HIV transmission has been documented. Nevertheless, the precautions described below should be taken routinely in the care of **all** patients.

Sterilization and Disinfection

Standard sterilization and disinfection procedures for patient-care equipment currently recommended for use (*25,26*) in a variety of health-care settings—including hospitals, medical and dental clinics and offices, hemodialysis centers, emergency-care facilities, and long-term nursing-care facilities—are adequate to sterilize or disinfect instruments, devices, or other items contaminated with blood or other body fluids from persons infected with blood-borne pathogens including HIV (*21,23*).

D-1
CDC RECOMMENDATIONS FOR PREVENTION OF HIV TRANSMISSION IN HEALTH-CARE SETTINGS *Continued*

Instruments or devices that enter sterile tissue or the vascular system of any patient or through which blood flows should be sterilized before reuse. Devices or items that contact intact mucous membranes should be sterilized or receive high-level disinfection, a procedure that kills vegetative organisms and viruses but not necessarily large numbers of bacterial spores. Chemical germicides that are registered with the U.S. Environmental Protection Agency (EPA) as "sterilants" may be used either for sterilization or for high-level disinfection depending on contact time.

Contact lenses used in trial fittings should be disinfected after each fitting by using a hydrogen peroxide contact lens disinfecting system or, if compatible, with heat (78 C-80 C [172.4 F-176.0 F]) for 10 minutes.

Medical devices or instruments that require sterilization or disinfection should be thoroughly cleaned before being exposed to the germicide, and the manufacturer's instructions for the use of the germicide should be followed. Further, it is important that the manufacturer's specifications for compatibility of the medical device with chemical germicides be closely followed. Information on specific label claims of commercial germicides can be obtained by writing to the Disinfectants Branch, Office of Pesticides, Environmental Protection Agency, 401 M Street, SW, Washington, D.C. 20460.

Studies have shown that HIV is inactivated rapidly after being exposed to commonly used chemical germicides at concentrations that are much lower than used in practice (27-30). Embalming fluids are similar to the types of chemical germicides that have been tested and found to completely inactivate HIV. In addition to commercially available chemical germicides, a solution of sodium hypochlorite (household bleach) prepared daily is an inexpensive and effective germicide. Concentrations ranging from approximately 500 ppm (1:100 dilution of household bleach) sodium hypochlorite to 5,000 ppm (1:10 dilution of household bleach) are effective depending on the amount of organic material (e.g., blood, mucus) present on the surface to be cleaned and disinfected. Commercially available chemical germicides may be more compatible with certain medical devices that might be corroded by repeated exposure to sodium hypochlorite, especially to the 1:10 dilution.

Survival of HIV in the Environment

The most extensive study on the survival of HIV after drying involved greatly concentrated HIV samples, i.e., 10 million tissue-culture infectious doses per milliliter (31). This concentration is at least 100,000 times greater than that typically found in the blood or serum of patients with HIV infection. HIV was detectable by tissue-culture techniques 1-3 days after drying, but the rate of inactivation was rapid. Studies performed at CDC have also shown that drying HIV causes a rapid (within several hours) 1-2 log (90%-99%) reduction in HIV concentration. In tissue-culture fluid, cell-free HIV could be detected up to 15 days at room temperature, up to 11 days at 37 C (98.6 F), and up to 1 day if the HIV was cell-associated.

When considered in the context of environmental conditions in health-care facilities, these results do not require any changes in currently recommended sterilization, disinfection, or housekeeping strategies. When medical devices are contaminated with blood or other body fluids, existing recommendations include the cleaning of these instruments, followed by disinfection or sterilization, depending on the type of medical device. These protocols assume "worst-case" conditions of

D-1

CDC RECOMMENDATIONS FOR PREVENTION OF HIV TRANSMISSION IN HEALTH-CARE SETTINGS Continued

extreme virologic and microbiologic contamination, and whether viruses have been inactivated after drying plays no role in formulating these strategies. Consequently, no changes in published procedures for cleaning, disinfecting, or sterilizing need to be made.

Housekeeping

Environmental surfaces such as walls, floors, and other surfaces are not associated with transmission of infections to patients or health-care workers. Therefore, extraordinary attempts to disinfect or sterilize these environmental surfaces are not necessary. However, cleaning and removal of soil should be done routinely.

Cleaning schedules and methods vary according to the area of the hospital or institution, type of surface to be cleaned, and the amount and type of soil present. Horizontal surfaces (e.g., bedside tables and hard-surfaced flooring) in patient-care areas are usually cleaned on a regular basis, when soiling or spills occur, and when a patient is discharged. Cleaning of walls, blinds, and curtains is recommended only if they are visibly soiled. Disinfectant fogging is an unsatisfactory method of decontaminating air and surfaces and is not recommended.

Disinfectant-detergent formulations registered by EPA can be used for cleaning environmental surfaces, but the actual physical removal of microorganisms by scrubbing is probably at least as important as any antimicrobial effect of the cleaning agent used. Therefore, cost, safety, and acceptability by housekeepers can be the main criteria for selecting any such registered agent. The manufacturers' instructions for appropriate use should be followed.

Cleaning and Decontaminating Spills of Blood or Other Body Fluids

Chemical germicides that are approved for use as "hospital disinfectants" and are tuberculocidal when used at recommended dilutions can be used to decontaminate spills of blood and other body fluids. Strategies for decontaminating spills of blood and other body fluids in a patient-care setting are different than for spills of cultures or other materials in clinical, public health, or research laboratories. In patient-care areas, visible material should first be removed and then the area should be decontaminated. With large spills of cultured or concentrated infectious agents in the laboratory, the contaminated area should be flooded with a liquid germicide before cleaning, then decontaminated with fresh germicidal chemical. In both settings, gloves should be worn during the cleaning and decontaminating procedures.

Laundry

Although soiled linen has been identified as a source of large numbers of certain pathogenic microorganisms, the risk of actual disease transmission is negligible. Rather than rigid procedures and specifications, hygienic and common-sense storage and processing of clean and soiled linen are recommended (26). Soiled linen should be handled as little as possible and with minimum agitation to prevent gross microbial contamination of the air and of persons handling the linen. All soiled linen should be bagged at the location where it was used; it should not be sorted or rinsed in patient-care areas. Linen soiled with blood or body fluids should be placed and transported in bags that prevent leakage. If hot water is used, linen should be washed

D-1
CDC RECOMMENDATIONS FOR PREVENTION OF HIV TRANSMISSION IN HEALTH-CARE SETTINGS *Continued*

with detergent in water at least 71 C (160 F) for 25 minutes. If low-temperature(≤70 C [158 F]) laundry cycles are used, chemicals suitable for low-temperature washing at proper use concentration should be used.

Infective Waste

There is no epidemiologic evidence to suggest that most hospital waste is any more infective than residential waste. Moreover, there is no epidemiologic evidence that hospital waste has caused disease in the community as a result of improper disposal. Therefore, identifying wastes for which special precautions are indicated is largely a matter of judgment about the relative risk of disease transmission. The most practical approach to the management of infective waste is to identify those wastes with the potential for causing infection during handling and disposal and for which some special precautions appear prudent. Hospital wastes for which special precautions appear prudent include microbiology laboratory waste, pathology waste, and blood specimens or blood products. While any item that has had contact with blood, exudates, or secretions may be potentially infective, it is not usually considered practical or necessary to treat all such waste as infective (*23,26*). Infective waste, in general, should either be incinerated or should be autoclaved before disposal in a sanitary landfill. Bulk blood, suctioned fluids, excretions, and secretions may be carefully poured down a drain connected to a sanitary sewer. Sanitary sewers may also be used to dispose of other infectious wastes capable of being ground and flushed into the sewer.

Implementation of Recommended Precautions

Employers of health-care workers should ensure that policies exist for:
1. Initial orientation and continuing education and training of all health-care workers—including students and trainees—on the epidemiology, modes of transmission, and prevention of HIV and other blood-borne infections and the need for routine use of universal blood and body-fluid precautions for **all** patients.
2. Provision of equipment and supplies necessary to minimize the risk of infection with HIV and other blood-borne pathogens.
3. Monitoring adherence to recommended protective measures. When monitoring reveals a failure to follow recommended precautions, counseling, education, and/or re-training should be provided, and, if necessary, appropriate disciplinary action should be considered.

Professional associations and labor organizations, through continuing education efforts, should emphasize the need for health-care workers to follow recommended precautions.

CDC RECOMMENDATIONS FOR PREVENTION OF HIV TRANSMISSION IN HEALTH-CARE SETTINGS *Continued*

Serologic Testing for HIV Infection

Background

A person is identified as infected with HIV when a sequence of tests, starting with repeated enzyme immunoassays (EIA) and including a Western blot or similar, more specific assay, are repeatedly reactive. Persons infected with HIV usually develop antibody against the virus within 6-12 weeks after infection.

The sensitivity of the currently licensed EIA tests is at least 99% when they are performed under optimal laboratory conditions on serum specimens from persons infected for ≥12 weeks. Optimal laboratory conditions include the use of reliable reagents, provision of continuing education of personnel, quality control of procedures, and participation in performance-evaluation programs. Given this performance, the probability of a false-negative test is remote except during the first several weeks after infection, before detectable antibody is present. The proportion of infected persons with a false-negative test attributed to absence of antibody in the early stages of infection is dependent on both the incidence and prevalence of HIV infection in a population (Table 1).

The specificity of the currently licensed EIA tests is approximately 99% when repeatedly reactive tests are considered. Repeat testing of initially reactive specimens by EIA is required to reduce the likelihood of laboratory error. To increase further the specificity of serologic tests, laboratories must use a supplemental test, most often the Western blot, to validate repeatedly reactive EIA results. Under optimal laboratory conditions, the sensitivity of the Western blot test is comparable to or greater than that of a repeatedly reactive EIA, and the Western blot is highly specific when strict criteria are used to interpret the test results. The testing sequence of a repeatedly reactive EIA and a positive Western blot test is highly predictive of HIV infection, even in a population with a low prevalence of infection (Table 2). If the Western blot test result is indeterminant, the testing sequence is considered equivocal for HIV infection.

TABLE 1. Estimated annual number of patients infected with HIV not detected by HIV-antibody testing in a hypothetical hospital with 10,000 admissions/year*

Beginning prevalence of HIV infection	Annual incidence of HIV infection	Approximate number of HIV-infected patients	Approximate number of HIV-infected patients not detected
5.0%	1.0%	550	17-18
5.0%	0.5%	525	11-12
1.0%	0.2%	110	3-4
1.0%	0.1%	105	2-3
0.1%	0.02%	11	0-1
0.1%	0.01%	11	0-1

*The estimates are based on the following assumptions: 1) the sensitivity of the screening test is 99% (i.e., 99% of HIV-infected persons with antibody will be detected); 2) persons infected with HIV will not develop detectable antibody (seroconvert) until 6 weeks (1.5 months) after infection; 3) new infections occur at an equal rate throughout the year; 4) calculations of the number of HIV-infected persons in the patient population are based on the mid-year prevalence, which is the beginning prevalence plus half the annual incidence of infections.

D-1
CDC RECOMMENDATIONS FOR PREVENTION OF HIV TRANSMISSION IN HEALTH-CARE SETTINGS *Continued*

When this occurs, the Western blot test should be repeated on the same serum sample, and, if still indeterminant, the testing sequence should be repeated on a sample collected 3-6 months later. Use of other supplemental tests may aid in interpreting of results on samples that are persistently indeterminant by Western blot.

Testing of Patients

Previous CDC recommendations have emphasized the value of HIV serologic testing of patients for: 1) management of parenteral or mucous-membrane exposures of health-care workers, 2) patient diagnosis and management, and 3) counseling and serologic testing to prevent and control HIV transmission in the community. In addition, more recent recommendations have stated that hospitals, in conjunction with state and local health departments, should periodically determine the prevalence of HIV infection among patients from age groups at highest risk of infection (*32*).

Adherence to universal blood and body-fluid precautions recommended for the care of all patients will minimize the risk of transmission of HIV and other blood-borne pathogens from patients to health-care workers. The utility of routine HIV serologic testing of patients as an adjunct to universal precautions is unknown. Results of such testing may not be available in emergency or outpatient settings. In addition, some recently infected patients will not have detectable antibody to HIV (Table 1).

Personnel in some hospitals have advocated serologic testing of patients in settings in which exposure of health-care workers to large amounts of patients' blood may be anticipated. Specific patients for whom serologic testing has been advocated include those undergoing major operative procedures and those undergoing treatment in critical-care units, especially if they have conditions involving uncontrolled bleeding. Decisions regarding the need to establish testing programs for patients should be made by physicians or individual institutions. In addition, when deemed appropriate, testing of individual patients may be performed on agreement between the patient and the physician providing care.

In addition to the universal precautions recommended for all patients, certain additional precautions for the care of HIV-infected patients undergoing major surgical operations have been proposed by personnel in some hospitals. For example, surgical procedures on an HIV-infected patient might be altered so that hand-to-hand passing of sharp instruments would be eliminated; stapling instruments rather than

TABLE 2. Predictive value of positive HIV-antibody tests in hypothetical populations with different prevalences of infection

	Prevalence of infection	Predictive value of positive test[*]
Repeatedly reactive enzyme immunoassay (EIA)[†]	0.2%	28.41%
	2.0%	80.16%
	20.0%	98.02%
Repeatedly reactive EIA followed by positive Western blot (WB)[§]	0.2%	99.75%
	2.0%	99.97%
	20.0%	99.99%

[*]Proportion of persons with positive test results who are actually infected with HIV.
[†]Assumes EIA sensitivity of 99.0% and specificity of 99.5%.
[§]Assumes WB sensitivity of 99.0% and specificity of 99.9%.

D-1

CDC RECOMMENDATIONS FOR PREVENTION OF HIV TRANSMISSION IN HEALTH-CARE SETTINGS *Continued*

hand-suturing equipment might be used to perform tissue approximation; electrocautery devices rather than scalpels might be used as cutting instruments; and, even though uncomfortable, gowns that totally prevent seepage of blood onto the skin of members of the operative team might be worn. While such modifications might further minimize the risk of HIV infection for members of the operative team, some of these techniques could result in prolongation of operative time and could potentially have an adverse effect on the patient.

Testing programs, if developed, should include the following principles:

- Obtaining consent for testing.
- Informing patients of test results, and providing counseling for seropositive patients by properly trained persons.
- Assuring that confidentiality safeguards are in place to limit knowledge of test results to those directly involved in the care of infected patients or as required by law.
- Assuring that identification of infected patients will not result in denial of needed care or provision of suboptimal care.
- Evaluating prospectively 1) the efficacy of the program in reducing the incidence of parenteral, mucous-membrane, or significant cutaneous exposures of health-care workers to the blood or other body fluids of HIV-infected patients and 2) the effect of modified procedures on patients.

Testing of Health-Care Workers

Although transmission of HIV from infected health-care workers to patients has not been reported, transmission during invasive procedures remains a possibility. Transmission of hepatitis B virus (HBV)—a blood-borne agent with a considerably greater potential for nosocomial spread—from health-care workers to patients has been documented. Such transmission has occurred in situations (e.g., oral and gynecologic surgery) in which health-care workers, when tested, had very high concentrations of HBV in their blood (at least 100 million infectious virus particles per milliliter, a concentration much higher than occurs with HIV infection), and the health-care workers sustained a puncture wound while performing invasive procedures or had exudative or weeping lesions or microlacerations that allowed virus to contaminate instruments or open wounds of patients (*33,34*).

The hepatitis B experience indicates that only those health-care workers who perform certain types of invasive procedures have transmitted HBV to patients. Adherence to recommendations in this document will minimize the risk of transmission of HIV and other blood-borne pathogens from health-care workers to patients during invasive procedures. Since transmission of HIV from infected health-care workers performing invasive procedures to their patients has not been reported and would be expected to occur only very rarely, if at all, the utility of routine testing of such health-care workers to prevent transmission of HIV cannot be assessed. If consideration is given to developing a serologic testing program for health-care workers who perform invasive procedures, the frequency of testing, as well as the issues of consent, confidentiality, and consequences of test results—as previously outlined for testing programs for patients—must be addressed.

D-1
CDC RECOMMENDATIONS FOR PREVENTION OF HIV TRANSMISSION IN HEALTH-CARE SETTINGS *Continued*

Management of Infected Health-Care Workers

Health-care workers with impaired immune systems resulting from HIV infection or other causes are at increased risk of acquiring or experiencing serious complications of infectious disease. Of particular concern is the risk of severe infection following exposure to patients with infectious diseases that are easily transmitted if appropriate precautions are not taken (e.g., measles, varicella). Any health-care worker with an impaired immune system should be counseled about the potential risk associated with taking care of patients with any transmissible infection and should continue to follow existing recommendations for infection control to minimize risk of exposure to other infectious agents (*7,35*). Recommendations of the Immunization Practices Advisory Committee (ACIP) and institutional policies concerning requirements for vaccinating health-care workers with live-virus vaccines (e.g., measles, rubella) should also be considered.

The question of whether workers infected with HIV—especially those who perform invasive procedures—can adequately and safely be allowed to perform patient-care duties or whether their work assignments should be changed must be determined on an individual basis. These decisions should be made by the health-care worker's personal physician(s) in conjunction with the medical directors and personnel health service staff of the employing institution or hospital.

Management of Exposures

If a health-care worker has a parenteral (e.g., needlestick or cut) or mucous-membrane (e.g., splash to the eye or mouth) exposure to blood or other body fluids or has a cutaneous exposure involving large amounts of blood or prolonged contact with blood—especially when the exposed skin is chapped, abraded, or afflicted with dermatitis—the source patient should be informed of the incident and tested for serologic evidence of HIV infection after consent is obtained. Policies should be developed for testing source patients in situations in which consent cannot be obtained (e.g., an unconscious patient).

If the source patient has AIDS, is positive for HIV antibody, or refuses the test, the health-care worker should be counseled regarding the risk of infection and evaluated clinically and serologically for evidence of HIV infection as soon as possible after the exposure. The health-care worker should be advised to report and seek medical evaluation for any acute febrile illness that occurs within 12 weeks after the exposure. Such an illness—particularly one characterized by fever, rash, or lymphadenopathy—may be indicative of recent HIV infection. Seronegative health-care workers should be retested 6 weeks post-exposure and on a periodic basis thereafter (e.g., 12 weeks and 6 months after exposure) to determine whether transmission has occurred. During this follow-up period—especially the first 6-12 weeks after exposure, when most infected persons are expected to seroconvert—exposed health-care workers should follow U.S. Public Health Service (PHS) recommendations for preventing transmission of HIV (*36,37*).

No further follow-up of a health-care worker exposed to infection as described above is necessary if the source patient is seronegative unless the source patient is at high risk of HIV infection. In the latter case, a subsequent specimen (e.g., 12 weeks following exposure) may be obtained from the health-care worker for antibody

D-1
CDC RECOMMENDATIONS FOR PREVENTION OF HIV TRANSMISSION IN HEALTH-CARE SETTINGS Continued

testing. If the source patient cannot be identified, decisions regarding appropriate follow-up should be individualized. Serologic testing should be available to all health-care workers who are concerned that they may have been infected with HIV.

If a patient has a parenteral or mucous-membrane exposure to blood or other body fluid of a health-care worker, the patient should be informed of the incident, and the same procedure outlined above for management of exposures should be followed for both the source health-care worker and the exposed patient.

References
1. CDC. Acquired immunodeficiency syndrome (AIDS): Precautions for clinical and laboratory staffs. MMWR 1982;31:577-80.
2. CDC. Acquired immunodeficiency syndrome (AIDS): Precautions for health-care workers and allied professionals. MMWR 1983;32:450-1.
3. CDC. Recommendations for preventing transmission of infection with human T-lymphotropic virus type III/lymphadenopathy-associated virus in the workplace. MMWR 1985;34:681-6, 691-5.
4. CDC. Recommendations for preventing transmission of infection with human T-lymphotropic virus type III/lymphadenopathy-associated virus during invasive procedures. MMWR 1986;35:221-3.
5. CDC. Recommendations for preventing possible transmission of human T-lymphotropic virus type III/lymphadenopathy-associated virus from tears. MMWR 1985;34:533-4.
6. CDC. Recommendations for providing dialysis treatment to patients infected with human T-lymphotropic virus type III/lymphadenopathy-associated virus infection. MMWR 1986;35:376-8, 383.
7. Garner JS, Simmons BP. Guideline for isolation precautions in hospitals. Infect Control 1983;4 (suppl) :245-325.
8. CDC. Recommended infection control practices for dentistry. MMWR 1986;35:237-42.
9. McCray E, The Cooperative Needlestick Surveillance Group. Occupational risk of the acquired immunodeficiency syndrome among health care workers. N Engl J Med 1986;314:1127-32.
10. Henderson DK, Saah AJ, Zak BJ, et al. Risk of nosocomial infection with human T-cell lymphotropic virus type III/lymphadenopathy-associated virus in a large cohort of intensively exposed health care workers. Ann Intern Med 1986;104:644-7.
11. Gerberding JL, Bryant-LeBlanc CE, Nelson K, et al. Risk of transmitting the human immunodeficiency virus, cytomegalovirus, and hepatitis B virus to health care workers exposed to patients with AIDS and AIDS-related conditions. J Infect Dis 1987;156:1-8.
12. McEvoy M, Porter K, Mortimer P, Simmons N, Shanson D. Prospective study of clinical, laboratory, and ancillary staff with accidental exposures to blood or other body fluids from patients infected with HIV. Br Med J 1987;294:1595-7.
13. Anonymous. Needlestick transmission of HTLV-III from a patient infected in Africa. Lancet 1984;2:1376-7.
14. Oksenhendler E, Harzic M, Le Roux JM, Rabian C, Clauvel JP. HIV infection with seroconversion after a superficial needlestick injury to the finger. N Engl J Med 1986;315:582.
15. Neisson-Vernant C, Arfi S, Mathez D, Leibowitch J, Monplaisir N. Needlestick HIV seroconversion in a nurse. Lancet 1986;2:814.
16. Grint P, McEvoy M. Two associated cases of the acquired immune deficiency syndrome (AIDS). PHLS Commun Dis Rep 1985;42:4.
17. CDC. Apparent transmission of human T-lymphotropic virus type III/lymphadenopathy-associated virus from a child to a mother providing health care. MMWR 1986;35:76-9.
18. CDC. Update: Human immunodeficiency virus infections in health-care workers exposed to blood of infected patients. MMWR 1987;36:285-9.
19. Kline RS, Phelan J, Friedland GH, et al. Low occupational risk for HIV infection for dental professionals [Abstract]. In: Abstracts from the III International Conference on AIDS, 1-5 June 1985. Washington, DC: 155.
20. Baker JL, Kelen GD, Sivertson KT, Quinn TC. Unsuspected human immunodeficiency virus in critically ill emergency patients. JAMA 1987;257:2609-11.
21. Favero MS. Dialysis-associated diseases and their control. In: Bennett JV, Brachman PS, eds. Hospital infections. Boston: Little, Brown and Company, 1985:267-84.

D-1

CDC RECOMMENDATIONS FOR PREVENTION OF HIV TRANSMISSION IN HEALTH-CARE SETTINGS Continued

22. Richardson JH, Barkley WE, eds. Biosafety in microbiological and biomedical laboratories, 1984. Washington, DC: US Department of Health and Human Services, Public Health Service. HHS publication no. (CDC) 84-8395.
23. CDC. Human T-lymphotropic virus type III/lymphadenopathy-associated virus: Agent summary statement. MMWR 1986;35:540-2, 547-9.
24. Environmental Protection Agency. EPA guide for infectious waste management. Washington, DC: U.S. Environmental Protection Agency, May 1986 (Publication no. EPA/530-SW-86-014).
25. Favero MS. Sterilization, disinfection, and antisepsis in the hospital. In: Manual of clinical microbiology. 4th ed. Washington, DC: American Society for Microbiology, 1985;129-37.
26. Garner JS, Favero MS. Guideline for handwashing and hospital environmental control, 1985. Atlanta: Public Health Service, Centers for Disease Control, 1985. HHS publication no. 99-1117.
27. Spire B, Montagnier L, Barré-Sinoussi F, Chermann JC. Inactivation of lymphadenopathy associated virus by chemical disinfectants. Lancet 1984;2:899-901.
28. Martin LS, McDougal JS, Loskoski SL. Disinfection and inactivation of the human T lymphotropic virus type III/lymphadenopathy-associated virus. J Infect Dis 1985; 152:400-3.
29. McDougal JS, Martin LS, Cort SP, et al. Thermal inactivation of the acquired immunodeficiency syndrome virus-III/lymphadenopathy-associated virus, with special reference to antihemophilic factor. J Clin Invest 1985;76:875-7.
30. Spire B, Barré-Sinoussi F, Dormont D, Montagnier L, Chermann JC. Inactivation of lymphadenopathy-associated virus by heat, gamma rays, and ultraviolet light. Lancet 1985;1:188-9.
31. Resnik L, Veren K, Salahuddin SZ, Tondreau S, Markham PD. Stability and inactivation of HTLV-III/LAV under clinical and laboratory environments. JAMA 1986;255:1887-91.
32. CDC. Public Health Service (PHS) guidelines for counseling and antibody testing to prevent HIV infection and AIDS. MMWR 1987;3:509-15..
33. Kane MA, Lettau LA. Transmission of HBV from dental personnel to patients. J Am Dent Assoc 1985;110:634-6.
34. Lettau LA, Smith JD, Williams D, et. al. Transmission of hepatitis B with resultant restriction of surgical practice. JAMA 1986;255:934-7.
35. Williams WW. Guideline for infection control in hospital personnel. Infect Control 1983;4 (suppl) :326-49.
36. CDC. Prevention of acquired immune deficiency syndrome (AIDS): Report of inter-agency recommendations. MMWR 1983;32:101-3.
37. CDC. Provisional Public Health Service inter-agency recommendations for screening donated blood and plasma for antibody to the virus causing acquired immunodeficiency syndrome. MMWR 1985;34:1-5.

From Morbidity and Mortality Weekly Report, Supplement, August 21, 1987, Vol. 36, No. 2S. U.S. Department of Health and Human Services, Public Health Service, Centers for Disease Control, Atlanta, Georgia.

D-2
CDC UPDATE: UNIVERSAL PRECAUTIONS FOR PREVENTION OF TRANSMISSION OF HUMAN IMMUNODEFICIENCY VIRUS, HEPATITIS B VIRUS, AND OTHER BLOODBORNE PATHOGENS IN HEALTH-CARE SETTINGS

Update: Universal Precautions for Prevention of Transmission of Human Immunodeficiency Virus, Hepatitis B Virus, and Other Bloodborne Pathogens in Health-Care Settings

Introduction

The purpose of this report is to clarify and supplement the CDC publication entitled "Recommendations for Prevention of HIV Transmission in Health-Care Settings" (1).*

In 1983, CDC published a document entitled "Guideline for Isolation Precautions in Hospitals" (2) that contained a section entitled "Blood and Body Fluid Precautions." The recommendations in this section called for blood and body fluid precautions when a patient was known or suspected to be infected with bloodborne pathogens. In August 1987, CDC published a document entitled "Recommendations for Prevention of HIV Transmission in Health-Care Settings" (1). In contrast to the 1983 document, the 1987 document recommended that blood and body fluid precautions be consistently used for all patients regardless of their bloodborne infection status. This extension of blood and body fluid precautions to **all** patients is referred to as "Universal Blood and Body Fluid Precautions" or "Universal Precautions." Under universal precautions, blood and certain body fluids of all patients are considered potentially infectious for human immunodeficiency virus (HIV), hepatitis B virus (HBV), and other bloodborne pathogens.

---

*The August 1987 publication should be consulted for general information and specific recommendations not addressed in this update.

Copies of this report and of the *MMWR* supplement entitled *Recommendations for Prevention of HIV Transmission in Health-Care Settings* published in August 1987 are available through the National AIDS Information Clearinghouse, P.O. Box 6003, Rockville, MD 20850.

D-2

CDC UPDATE: UNIVERSAL PRECAUTIONS FOR PREVENTION OF TRANSMISSION OF HUMAN IMMUNODEFICIENCY VIRUS, HEPATITIS B VIRUS, AND OTHER BLOODBORNE PATHOGENS IN HEALTH-CARE SETTINGS *Continued*

Universal precautions are intended to prevent parenteral, mucous membrane, and nonintact skin exposures of health-care workers to bloodborne pathogens. In addition, immunization with HBV vaccine is recommended as an important adjunct to universal precautions for health-care workers who have exposures to blood (*3,4*).

Since the recommendations for universal precautions were published in August 1987, CDC and the Food and Drug Administration (FDA) have received requests for clarification of the following issues: 1) body fluids to which universal precautions apply, 2) use of protective barriers, 3) use of gloves for phlebotomy, 4) selection of gloves for use while observing universal precautions, and 5) need for making changes in waste management programs as a result of adopting universal precautions.

Body Fluids to Which Universal Precautions Apply

Universal precautions apply to blood and to other body fluids containing visible blood. Occupational transmission of HIV and HBV to health-care workers by blood is documented (*4,5*). **Blood is the single most important source of HIV, HBV, and other bloodborne pathogens in the occupational setting. Infection control efforts for HIV, HBV, and other bloodborne pathogens must focus on preventing exposures to blood as well as on delivery of HBV immunization.**

Universal precautions also apply to semen and vaginal secretions. Although both of these fluids have been implicated in the sexual transmission of HIV and HBV, they have not been implicated in occupational transmission from patient to health-care worker. This observation is not unexpected, since exposure to semen in the usual health-care setting is limited, and the routine practice of wearing gloves for performing vaginal examinations protects health-care workers from exposure to potentially infectious vaginal secretions.

Universal precautions also apply to tissues and to the following fluids: cerebrospinal fluid (CSF), synovial fluid, pleural fluid, peritoneal fluid, pericardial fluid, and amniotic fluid. The risk of transmission of HIV and HBV from these fluids is unknown; epidemiologic studies in the health-care and community setting are currently inadequate to assess the potential risk to health-care workers from occupational exposures to them. However, HIV has been isolated from CSF, synovial, and amniotic fluid (*6–8*), and HBsAg has been detected in synovial fluid, amniotic fluid, and peritoneal fluid (*9–11*). One case of HIV transmission was reported after a percutaneous exposure to bloody pleural fluid obtained by needle aspiration (*12*). Whereas aseptic procedures used to obtain these fluids for diagnostic or therapeutic purposes protect health-care workers from skin exposures, they cannot prevent penetrating injuries due to contaminated needles or other sharp instruments.

Body Fluids to Which Universal Precautions Do Not Apply

Universal precautions do not apply to feces, nasal secretions, sputum, sweat, tears, urine, and vomitus unless they contain visible blood. The risk of transmission of HIV and HBV from these fluids and materials is extremely low or nonexistent. HIV has been isolated and HBsAg has been demonstrated in some of these fluids; however, epidemiologic studies in the health-care and community setting have not implicated these fluids or materials in the transmission of HIV and HBV infections (*13,14*). Some of the above fluids and excretions represent a potential source for nosocomial and community-acquired infections with other pathogens, and recommendations for preventing the transmission of nonbloodborne pathogens have been published (*2*).

CDC UPDATE: UNIVERSAL PRECAUTIONS FOR PREVENTION OF TRANSMISSION OF HUMAN IMMUNODEFICIENCY VIRUS, HEPATITIS B VIRUS, AND OTHER BLOODBORNE PATHOGENS IN HEALTH-CARE SETTINGS Continued

Precautions for Other Body Fluids in Special Settings

Human breast milk has been implicated in perinatal transmission of HIV, and HBsAg has been found in the milk of mothers infected with HBV (10,13). However, occupational exposure to human breast milk has not been implicated in the transmission of HIV nor HBV infection to health-care workers. Moreover, the health-care worker will not have the same type of intensive exposure to breast milk as the nursing neonate. Whereas universal precautions do not apply to human breast milk, gloves may be worn by health-care workers in situations where exposures to breast milk might be frequent, for example, in breast milk banking.

Saliva of some persons infected with HBV has been shown to contain HBV-DNA at concentrations 1/1,000 to 1/10,000 of that found in the infected person's serum (15). HBsAg-positive saliva has been shown to be infectious when injected into experimental animals and in human bite exposures (16–18). However, HBsAg-positive saliva has not been shown to be infectious when applied to oral mucous membranes in experimental primate studies (18) or through contamination of musical instruments or cardiopulmonary resuscitation dummies used by HBV carriers (19,20). Epidemiologic studies of nonsexual household contacts of HIV-infected patients, including several small series in which HIV transmission failed to occur after bites or after percutaneous inoculation or contamination of cuts and open wounds with saliva from HIV-infected patients, suggest that the potential for salivary transmission of HIV is remote (5,13,14,21,22). One case report from Germany has suggested the possibility of transmission of HIV in a household setting from an infected child to a sibling through a human bite (23). The bite did not break the skin or result in bleeding. Since the date of seroconversion to HIV was not known for either child in this case, evidence for the role of saliva in the transmission of virus is unclear (23). Another case report suggested the possibility of transmission of HIV from husband to wife by contact with saliva during kissing (24). However, follow-up studies did not confirm HIV infection in the wife (21).

Universal precautions do not apply to saliva. General infection control practices already in existence — including the use of gloves for digital examination of mucous membranes and endotracheal suctioning, and handwashing after exposure to saliva — should further minimize the minute risk, if any, for salivary transmission of HIV and HBV (1,25). Gloves need not be worn when feeding patients and when wiping saliva from skin.

Special precautions, however, are recommended for dentistry (1). Occupationally acquired infection with HBV in dental workers has been documented (4), and two possible cases of occupationally acquired HIV infection involving dentists have been reported (5,26). During dental procedures, contamination of saliva with blood is predictable, trauma to health-care workers' hands is common, and blood spattering may occur. Infection control precautions for dentistry minimize the potential for nonintact skin and mucous membrane contact of dental health-care workers to blood-contaminated saliva of patients. In addition, the use of gloves for oral examinations and treatment in the dental setting may also protect the patient's oral mucous membranes from exposures to blood, which may occur from breaks in the skin of dental workers' hands.

Use of Protective Barriers

Protective barriers reduce the risk of exposure of the health-care worker's skin or mucous membranes to potentially infective materials. For universal precautions,

D-2
CDC UPDATE: UNIVERSAL PRECAUTIONS FOR PREVENTION OF TRANSMISSION OF HUMAN IMMUNODEFICIENCY VIRUS, HEPATITIS B VIRUS, AND OTHER BLOODBORNE PATHOGENS IN HEALTH-CARE SETTINGS *Continued*

protective barriers reduce the risk of exposure to blood, body fluids containing visible blood, and other fluids to which universal precautions apply. Examples of protective barriers include gloves, gowns, masks, and protective eyewear. Gloves should reduce the incidence of contamination of hands, but they cannot prevent penetrating injuries due to needles or other sharp instruments. Masks and protective eyewear or face shields should reduce the incidence of contamination of mucous membranes of the mouth, nose, and eyes.

Universal precautions are intended to supplement rather than replace recommendations for routine infection control, such as handwashing and using gloves to prevent gross microbial contamination of hands (*27*). Because specifying the types of barriers needed for every possible clinical situation is impractical, some judgment must be exercised.

The risk of nosocomial transmission of HIV, HBV, and other bloodborne pathogens can be minimized if health-care workers use the following general guidelines:[†]

1. Take care to prevent injuries when using needles, scalpels, and other sharp instruments or devices; when handling sharp instruments after procedures; when cleaning used instruments; and when disposing of used needles. Do not recap used needles by hand; do not remove used needles from disposable syringes by hand; and do not bend, break, or otherwise manipulate used needles by hand. Place used disposable syringes and needles, scalpel blades, and other sharp items in puncture-resistant containers for disposal. Locate the puncture-resistant containers as close to the use area as is practical.
2. Use protective barriers to prevent exposure to blood, body fluids containing visible blood, and other fluids to which universal precautions apply. The type of protective barrier(s) should be appropriate for the procedure being performed and the type of exposure anticipated.
3. Immediately and thoroughly wash hands and other skin surfaces that are contaminated with blood, body fluids containing visible blood, or other body fluids to which universal precautions apply.

Glove Use for Phlebotomy

Gloves should reduce the incidence of blood contamination of hands during phlebotomy (drawing blood samples), but they cannot prevent penetrating injuries caused by needles or other sharp instruments. The likelihood of hand contamination with blood containing HIV, HBV, or other bloodborne pathogens during phlebotomy depends on several factors: 1) the skill and technique of the health-care worker, 2) the frequency with which the health-care worker performs the procedure (other factors being equal, the cumulative risk of blood exposure is higher for a health-care worker who performs more procedures), 3) whether the procedure occurs in a routine or emergency situation (where blood contact may be more likely), and 4) the prevalence of infection with bloodborne pathogens in the patient population. The likelihood of infection after skin exposure to blood containing HIV or HBV will depend on the concentration of virus (viral concentration is much higher for hepatitis B than for HIV), the duration of contact, the presence of skin lesions on the hands of the health-care worker, and — for HBV — the immune status of the health-care worker. Although not accurately quantified, the risk of HIV infection following intact skin contact with infective blood is certainly much less than the 0.5% risk following percutaneous

---
[†]The August 1987 publication should be consulted for general information and specific recommendations not addressed in this update.

D-2

CDC UPDATE: UNIVERSAL PRECAUTIONS FOR PREVENTION OF TRANSMISSION OF HUMAN IMMUNODEFICIENCY VIRUS, HEPATITIS B VIRUS, AND OTHER BLOODBORNE PATHOGENS IN HEALTH-CARE SETTINGS Continued

needlestick exposures (5). In universal precautions, *all* blood is assumed to be potentially infective for bloodborne pathogens, but in certain settings (e.g., volunteer blood-donation centers) the prevalence of infection with some bloodborne pathogens (e.g., HIV, HBV) is known to be very low. Some institutions have relaxed recommendations for using gloves for phlebotomy procedures by skilled phlebotomists in settings where the prevalence of bloodborne pathogens is known to be very low.

Institutions that judge that routine gloving for *all* phlebotomies is not necessary should periodically reevaluate their policy. Gloves should always be available to health-care workers who wish to use them for phlebotomy. In addition, the following general guidelines apply:

1. Use gloves for performing phlebotomy when the health-care worker has cuts, scratches, or other breaks in his/her skin.
2. Use gloves in situations where the health-care worker judges that hand contamination with blood may occur, for example, when performing phlebotomy on an uncooperative patient.
3. Use gloves for performing finger and/or heel sticks on infants and children.
4. Use gloves when persons are receiving training in phlebotomy.

Selection of Gloves

The Center for Devices and Radiological Health, FDA, has responsibility for regulating the medical glove industry. Medical gloves include those marketed as sterile surgical or nonsterile examination gloves made of vinyl or latex. General purpose utility ("rubber") gloves are also used in the health-care setting, but they are not regulated by FDA since they are not promoted for medical use. There are no reported differences in barrier effectiveness between intact latex and intact vinyl used to manufacture gloves. Thus, the type of gloves selected should be appropriate for the task being performed.

The following general guidelines are recommended:

1. Use sterile gloves for procedures involving contact with normally sterile areas of the body.
2. Use examination gloves for procedures involving contact with mucous membranes, unless otherwise indicated, and for other patient care or diagnostic procedures that do not require the use of sterile gloves.
3. Change gloves between patient contacts.
4. Do not wash or disinfect surgical or examination gloves for reuse. Washing with surfactants may cause "wicking," i.e., the enhanced penetration of liquids through undetected holes in the glove. Disinfecting agents may cause deterioration.
5. Use general-purpose utility gloves (e.g., rubber household gloves) for housekeeping chores involving potential blood contact and for instrument cleaning and decontamination procedures. Utility gloves may be decontaminated and reused but should be discarded if they are peeling, cracked, or discolored, or if they have punctures, tears, or other evidence of deterioration.

Waste Management

Universal precautions are not intended to change waste management programs previously recommended by CDC for health-care settings (1). Policies for defining, collecting, storing, decontaminating, and disposing of infective waste are generally determined by institutions in accordance with state and local regulations. Information

D-2

CDC UPDATE: UNIVERSAL PRECAUTIONS FOR PREVENTION OF TRANSMISSION OF HUMAN IMMUNODEFICIENCY VIRUS, HEPATITIS B VIRUS, AND OTHER BLOODBORNE PATHOGENS IN HEALTH-CARE SETTINGS Continued

regarding waste management regulations in health-care settings may be obtained from state or local health departments or agencies responsible for waste management.

Reported by: Center for Devices and Radiological Health, Food and Drug Administration. Hospital Infections Program, AIDS Program, and Hepatitis Br, Div of Viral Diseases, Center for Infectious Diseases, National Institute for Occupational Safety and Health, CDC.

Editorial Note: Implementation of universal precautions does not eliminate the need for other category- or disease-specific isolation precautions, such as enteric precautions for infectious diarrhea or isolation for pulmonary tuberculosis (*1,2*). In addition to universal precautions, detailed precautions have been developed for the following procedures and/or settings in which prolonged or intensive exposures to blood occur: invasive procedures, dentistry, autopsies or morticians' services, dialysis, and the clinical laboratory. These detailed precautions are found in the August 21, 1987, "Recommendations for Prevention of HIV Transmission in Health-Care Settings" (*1*). In addition, specific precautions have been developed for research laboratories (*28*).

References
1. Centers for Disease Control. Recommendations for prevention of HIV transmission in health-care settings. MMWR 1987;36(suppl no. 2S).
2. Garner JS, Simmons BP. Guideline for isolation precautions in hospitals. Infect Control 1983:4;245–325.
3. Immunization Practices Advisory Committee. Recommendations for protection against viral hepatitis. MMWR 1985:34:313-24,329–35.
4. Department of Labor, Department of Health and Human Services. Joint advisory notice: protection against occupational exposure to hepatitis B virus (HBV) and human immunodeficiency virus (HIV). Washington, DC:US Department of Labor, US Department of Health and Human Services, 1987.
5. Centers for Disease Control. Update: Acquired immunodeficiency syndrome and human immunodeficiency virus infection among health-care workers. MMWR 1988;37:229–34,239.
6. Hollander H, Levy JA. Neurologic abnormalities and recovery of human immunodeficiency virus from cerebrospinal fluid. Ann Intern Med 1987;106:692–5.
7. Wirthrington RH, Cornes P, Harris JRW, et al. Isolation of human immunodeficiency virus from synovial fluid of a patient with reactive arthritis. Br Med J 1987;294:484.
8. Mundy DC, Schinazi RF, Gerber AR, Nahmias AJ, Randall HW. Human immunodeficiency virus isolated from amniotic fluid. Lancet 1987;2:459–60.
9. Onion DK, Crumpacker CS, Gilliland BC. Arthritis of hepatitis associated with Australia antigen. Ann Intern Med 1971;75:29–33.
10. Lee AKY, Ip HMH, Wong VCW. Mechanisms of maternal-fetal transmission of hepatitis B virus. J Infect Dis 1978;138:668–71.
11. Bond WW, Petersen NJ, Gravelle CR, Favero MS. Hepatitis B virus in peritoneal dialysis fluid: A potential hazard. Dialysis and Transplantation 1982;11:592–600.
12. Oskenhendler E, Harzic M, Le Roux J-M, Rabian C, Clauvel JP. HIV infection with seroconversion after a superficial needlestick injury to the finger [Letter]. N Engl J Med 1986;315:582.
13. Lifson AR. Do alternate modes for transmission of human immunodeficiency virus exist? A review. JAMA 1988;259:1353–6.
14. Friedland GH, Saltzman BR, Rogers MF, et al. Lack of transmission of HTLV-III/LAV infection to household contacts of patients with AIDS or AIDS-related complex with oral candidiasis. N Engl J Med 1986;314:344–9.
15. Jenison SA, Lemon SM, Baker LN, Newbold JE. Quantitative analysis of hepatitis B virus DNA in saliva and semen of chronically infected homosexual men. J Infect Dis 1987;156:299–306.
16. Cancio-Bello TP, de Medina M, Shorey J, Valledor MD, Schiff ER. An institutional outbreak of hepatitis B related to a human biting carrier. J Infect Dis 1982;146:652–6.
17. MacQuarrie MB, Forghani B, Wolochow DA. Hepatitis B transmitted by a human bite. JAMA 1974;230:723–4.

D-2

CDC UPDATE: UNIVERSAL PRECAUTIONS FOR PREVENTION OF TRANSMISSION OF HUMAN IMMUNODEFICIENCY VIRUS, HEPATITIS B VIRUS, AND OTHER BLOODBORNE PATHOGENS IN HEALTH-CARE SETTINGS Continued

18. Scott RM, Snitbhan R, Bancroft WH, Alter HJ, Tingpalapong M. Experimental transmission of hepatitis B virus by semen and saliva. J Infect Dis 1980;142:67–71.
19. Glaser JB, Nadler JP. Hepatitis B virus in a cardiopulmonary resuscitation training course: Risk of transmission from a surface antigen-positive participant. Arch Intern Med 1985;145:1653–5.
20. Osterholm MT, Bravo ER, Crosson JT, et al. Lack of transmission of viral hepatitis type B after oral exposure to HBsAg-positive saliva. Br Med J 1979;2:1263–4.
21. Curran JW, Jaffe HW, Hardy AM, et al. Epidemiology of HIV infection and AIDS in the United States. Science 1988;239:610–6.
22. Jason JM, McDougal JS, Dixon G, et al. HTLV-III/LAV antibody and immune status of household contacts and sexual partners of persons with hemophilia. JAMA 1986;255:212–5.
23. Wahn V, Kramer HH, Voit T, Brüster HT, Scrampical B, Scheid A. Horizontal transmission of HIV infection between two siblings [Letter]. Lancet 1986;2:694.
24. Salahuddin SZ, Groopman JE, Markham PD, et al. HTLV-III in symptom-free seronegative persons. Lancet 1984;2:1418–20.
25. Simmons BP, Wong ES. Guideline for prevention of nosocomial pneumonia. Atlanta: US Department of Health and Human Services, Public Health Service, Centers for Disease Control, 1982.
26. Klein RS, Phelan JA, Freeman K, et al. Low occupational risk of human immunodeficiency virus infection among dental professionals. N Engl J Med 1988;318:86–90.
27. Garner JS, Favero MS. Guideline for handwashing and hospital environmental control, 1985. Atlanta: US Department of Health and Human Services, Public Health Service, Centers for Disease Control, 1985; HHS publication no. 99-1117.
28. Centers for Disease Control. 1988 Agent summary statement for human immunodeficiency virus and report on laboratory-acquired infection with human immunodeficiency virus. MMWR 1988;37(suppl no. S4:1S-22S).

From Morbidity and Mortality Weekly Report, June 24, 1988, Vol. 37, No. 24, pp. 377–382, 387–388. U.S. Department of Health and Human Services, Public Health Service, Centers for Disease Control, Atlanta, Georgia.

D-3
CLIA (CLINICAL LABORATORY IMPROVEMENT AMENDMENTS): 1988 REGULATIONS AND REQUIREMENTS

SPECIAL ISSUE: CLIA '88 FINAL RULE RELEASED

From the Chairman of the Board...

The Final Rules are here at last! It was four years ago that Congress began its debate about regulating all laboratory test sites. Prompted by articles in the Wall Street Journal and the Washington Post, and television reports of deaths resulting from mis-diagnosed Pap smears, Congress passed the landmark Clinical Laboratories Improvement Amendments of 1988 (CLIA '88). Intended to regulate all human testing, CLIA affects over 200,000 testing sites, more than half of which are office laboratories.

Two years after the law was passed, the Health Care Financing Administration (HCFA) published a proposed rule that was so unreasonable it provoked a record 60,000 written comments, most from physicians telling HCFA the adverse impact the regulations would have on their ability to care for their patients. Stunned, HCFA turned to the Centers for Disease Control (CDC) for technical assistance in developing new regulations. In addition to reading your letters, the CDC convened panels of laboratory experts (including COLA Board member Paul Fischer, MD, COLA CEO J. Stephen Kroger, MD, and myself) to advise them about the revised quality standards. The result of this effort was released by HCFA on February 20, 1992...a summary follows.

You will find that the moderate complexity requirements look very much like COLA's current standards. You will have to meet new personnel standards (see page 4) and new PT grading criteria, which are very similar to COLA's current criteria. While nobody likes to be regulated, I think you will agree with me that CDC and HCFA have responded to your comments and concerns with a surprising sensitivity to practicing physician's needs.

Darroll J. Loschen, MD
Chairman of the Board

CLIA regulations finalized

The following summary is derived from the CLIA '88 Final Rule, which was published in the Federal Register on February 28, 1992. We have identified the key issues of this now mandatory regulation, and offered some suggestions for compliance. The Clinical Laboratory Improvement Amendments of 1988 take effect September 1 of this year; inspections are also expected to begin at that time. Enrollment in proficiency testing is required in 1993, with participation required in 1994. Sanctions will not be imposed until 1995. We have not included information here regarding Cytology since most office laboratories do not read Pap smears.

To whom does CLIA '88 apply?

CLIA '88 applies to anyone who performs testing of human specimens for the diagnosis, prevention or treatment of disease or health problems. This includes everyone from physicians performing the most basic tests to those who operate physician office laboratories (POLs). The only exceptions are facilities that perform testing for forensic purposes, research labs that do not report patient results, and facilities certified by the National Institute on Drug Abuse to perform only urine drug testing.

States can seek exemption from the federal standards if they have regulations that are equivalent to CLIA. If the federal government grants the exemption, laboratories in these states will be subject to state standards and fees, instead of federal standards and fees. You may wish to call your state health department to find out what they plan to do.

Certificates

If you perform only waived tests, you are eligible for a waiver certificate. Otherwise, you must initially apply for a registration certificate, which is valid for up to 2 years, followed by a certificate or certificate of accreditation.

TIMETABLE FOR CLIA IMPLEMENTATION

Release of Final Rule	February 28, 1992
Registration Certificate Mailings Begin	April-May, 1992
HHS or Accreditation Certificate Mailings	July-Sept. 1992
Complete Moderate Complexity Analyte List Available	July-Sept. 1992
Effective Date of Registration	September 1, 1992
Enroll in Proficiency Testing	1993
Participate in Proficiency Testing	January 1, 1994
Sanctions Begin for Proficiency Testing	January 1, 1995
Limited QC for Moderate Complexity Labs	Until Sept. 1, 1994

CLIA (CLINICAL LABORATORY IMPROVEMENT AMENDMENTS): 1988 REGULATIONS AND REQUIREMENTS
Continued

How do I apply for a certificate? Is COLA approved for CLIA?

HCFA has already sent a questionnaire to over 600,000 laboratories requesting information about testing instruments, methods, menus and number of tests performed, and lab personnel training and experience. From this questionnaire, HCFA expects to identify all labs that must be certified under CLIA. (If you did not receive this questionnaire or did not return it, you should contact HCFA.) Next, they will send you an application for a registration certificate...and a bill for the registration fee. Complete this and pay the correct fee. You are now registered under CLIA, you are in compliance with the law, and you will continue to be paid for your Medicare and Medicaid work.

In the next several months, HCFA will approve accrediting organizations such as COLA, the College of American Pathologists, and the Joint Commission. Sometime in the latter part of the year, you will receive another form and a bill from HCFA, this time for your HHS certificate or your certificate of accreditation. Since COLA expects to have HCFA approval by this time, you will want to apply for the Certificate of Accreditation and pay the correct fee to HCFA. (See page 5 for fee schedule.)

How is HCFA classifying laboratories?

The nature of the standards you must follow depends upon the complexity of tests which you perform. HCFA has designated three categories of testing: waived, moderate complexity and high complexity.

Waived tests are simple, stable and require a minimal degree of judgement and interpretation. This category includes tests cleared by the FDA for home use. (See sidebar for listing.)

HCFA has specified criteria for determining moderate or high complexity tests, such as necessary knowledge and training, stability or liability of materials, and degree of troubleshooting and maintenance required to perform tests. Moderate complexity tests include approximately 75% of the 10,000 tests and analytes in the following disciplines: Bacteriology, Mycobacteriology, Mycology, Parasitology, Virology, Immunology, Chemistry, Hematology and Immunohematology. In the next several months, HCFA will publish several lists of all the moderate complexity analytes and test methods. The best way of finding out whether your particular instrument or kit is in the moderate complexity category is by calling the manufacturer and asking. You can also obtain copies of the Federal Register when a list is published. High complexity tests include the more complex tests in the previously mentioned disciplines and Clinical Cytogenetics, Histopathology, Histocompatibility and Cytology.

Proficiency Testing

Moderate and high-complexity labs are required to enroll in proficiency testing (PT) in 1993. COLA has always required PT and will continue to do so, because it is an important part of good laboratory practice, and it will give you a better chance of success in the future when PT failures can stop your Medicare lab payments and force you to cease testing a failed analyte or discipline.

Under CLIA you are required to participate in three testing events per year, with five challenges per analyte, in contrast to current standards of four test events with two challenges. You must pass two consecutive or two out of three consecutive testing events. You must receive an 80% pass rate in Microbiology, Diagnostic Immunology, Chemistry, Hematology, Immunohematology and all their subspecialties; and a 100% pass rate in ABO/Rh and compatibility testing.

Additional requirements pertain to testing PT specimens in the same way as patient specimens and prohibit inter-lab communications of PT results prior to the PT program end date.

HCFA will impose the following sanctions for PT:

1) Failure to enroll--denial or revocation of certificate.
2) Nonparticipation in PT event--score of zero.
3) Failure to return results to PT program--score of zero.
4) Failure to meet required success rates--During the first year, you will be given a chance to correct deficiencies; however, beginning September 1, 1995, your certification will be suspended for the failed analyte, specialty, or subspecialty for at least 6 months and until you pass two consecutive PT challenges(s), and Medicare/Medicaid

---

TEST CATEGORIES

WAIVER TESTS
1. Dipstick or Tablet Reagent Urinalysis for: Bilirubin, Glucose, Hemoglobin, Ketone, Leukocytes, Nitrite, pH, Protein, Specific gravity, Urobilinogen.
2. Fecal occult blood
3. Ovulation tests--visual color tests for human luteinizing hormone
4. Urine pregnancy tests--visual color comparison tests
5. Erythrocyte sedimentation rate--nonautomated
6. Hemoglobin--copper sulfate--nonautomated
7. Spun micro-hematocrit
8. Blood glucose testing (using monitoring devices FDA cleared for home use)

MODERATE COMPLEXITY
Approximately 7500 tests and analytes (see Federal Register).

HIGH COMPLEXITY
Most complex tests and analytes, specifically Clinical Cytogenetics, Histopathology, Histocompatibility and Cytology.

Tests not on HCFA lists must be considered high complexity until they can be categorized.

D-3
CLIA (CLINICAL LABORATORY IMPROVEMENT AMENDMENTS): 1988 REGULATIONS AND REQUIREMENTS
Continued

payments will be terminated for the failed analyte, specialty, or subspecialty.
4) Sending of samples to or comparing of results with another lab--Your certification will be revoked for at least 1 year.

Quality Assurance
Physicians are familiar with quality assurance programs used in hospitals to monitor patient care. Similarly, CLIA requires every laboratory to have a QA program to monitor the activities of the laboratory. The CLIA requirements include written policies and procedures for patient preparation; specimen collection; labeling, preservation and transportation of specimens; corrective actions; using different testing methods; inconsistent results; personnel problems and corrective actions; and complaints and subsequent investigations.

Quality Control
Quality control procedures now vary depending on whether you use instruments and kits approved by the FDA, whether you have modified them, and whether you have developed your own tests in-house. For the next 2 years, if you do only moderate complexity testing and you have FDA-approved instruments and kits you must meet the following QC requirements:
1) follow manufacturer's instructions for operation and maintenance,
2) have a procedure manual,
3) perform and document calibration procedures every 6 months,
4) perform and document control procedures using at least 2 levels of control materials each day of testing,
5) perform and document applicable specialty and subspecialty control procedures,
6) perform and document remedial actions taken when problems or errors are identified.

If you do high complexity testing or you have modified your moderate complexity test instrument of kit, you must perform the following quality control procedures:
1) Establish an appropriate environment for testing and follow written safety policies and procedures.
2) Compile a procedure manual, follow test manufacturer instructions, and establish, perform, and document the following: calibration every 6 months, appropriate specialty and subspecialty quality control procedures, and necessary remedial actions.
3) Meet FDA requirements and lab-established performance requirements for equipment, instruments, reagents and materials.
4) Label reagents, solutions, culture media, controls and calibration materials to indicate identity and concentration, storage requirements, and preparation and expiration date.
5) Laboratory may not use expired reagents, solutions, media or kits, or interchange different lot numbers of reagents, solutions, or media.
6) Verify modified or in-house test methods using acceptable scientific protocols, and establish acceptable ranges, variables, interfering substances, specificity and sensitivity.
7) Establish and follow appropriate instrument and test system maintenance, calibration and recalibration.
8) Adhere to manufacturer instructions for control procedures. If you are using an in-house procedure, you must evaluate instrument and reagent stability and operator variance to determine necessary controls.
9) Each day of use, you must perform the following: for qualitative tests, a positive and negative control must be run; for quantitative tests, at least two samples of different concentrations must be run; the detection phase of direct antigen systems must be evaluated; and staining materials must be checked for intended reactivity.
10) Check culture media for reactivity, sterility, ability to support growth, inhibition and biochemical response.
11) Establish remedial actions for test systems that do not meet performance specifications for control results outside acceptable limits, for the inability to perform testing within acceptable limits, and for errors in reported results.

In general, the FDA-approved package insert or instrument manual will determine the frequency of quality control. However, you will need to determine appropriate procedures and values for your individual lab, such as panic values reportable range. Since these QC requirements are part of operating a quality lab, you already have most in place; the biggest challenge will be continuous documentation.

continued on page 5

COLA UPDATE
Editor: Paul Fischer, MD, Chairman, COLA Education Committee
Publisher: Theresa D. Henige

COLA is sponsored by the American Academy of Family Physicians (AAFP), the American Medical Association (AMA), the American Society of Internal Medicine (ASIM), and the College of American Pathologists (CAP).

COLA Board of Directors: Chairman Darroll J. Loschen, MD (AAFP); Secretary Frank B. Walker, MD (AMA); Treasurer Perry A. Lambird, MD (CAP); Paul Fischer, MD (AAFP); E. Rodney Hornbake III, MD (ASIM); James R. Weber, MD (AAFP); William E. Jacott, MD (AMA); A. Samuel Koenig III, MD (CAP); John H. Rippey, MD (CAP); M. Boyd Shook, MD (ASIM); Kathleen M. Weaver, MD (ASIM).

Copyright 1992. COLA Update is published three times per year by the Commission on Office Laboratory Accreditation (COLA), 8701 Georgia Avenue, Suite 610, Silver Spring, MD, 20910. Telephone (301) 588-5882. This publication may be obtained through enrollment in the COLA accreditation program or by subscription. Individual subscriptions are available at $45 per year. Corporate subscriptions are available for $150 per year. For further information contact the COLA office. ALL RIGHTS RESERVED. Reproduction in whole or in part without written permission is prohibited. COLA Update is a trade mark of the Commission on Office Laboratory Accreditation.

D-3

CLIA (CLINICAL LABORATORY IMPROVEMENT AMENDMENTS): 1988 REGULATIONS AND REQUIREMENTS
Continued

PERSONNEL REQUIREMENTS

MODERATE COMPLEXITY LABS

DIRECTOR
1. Laboratory director licence if required by State AND
2. Licensed MD, DO AND
   Certified in anatomic or clinical pathology OR
   Lab training or experience consisting of:
   1 year directing or supervising non-waived lab OR
   20 CME credits in lab practice about director responsibilities [effective in Feb 93] OR
   Training equivalent to 20 CME credits during medical residency
3. Doctoral degree in laboratory science AND
   Board certified OR
   1 year experience directing or supervising non-waived lab
4. Master's degree in lab science AND
   1 year lab training or experience AND
   1 year of supervisory experience
5. Bachelor's degree in lab science AND
   2 years lab training or experience AND
   2 years of supervisory experience

TECHNICAL CONSULTANT
1. License, if required by State AND
2. Licensed MD, DO AND
   Certified in anatomic or clinical pathology OR
   Lab training or experience consisting of:
   1 year laboratory training or experience in designated specialty/subspecialty in areas of service
3. Doctoral or Master's degree in laboratory science AND
   1 year laboratory training or experience in designated specialty/subspecialty in areas of service
4. Bachelor's degree in lab science AND
   2 years laboratory training or experience in designated specialty/subspecialty in areas of service

NOTE: "Training or experience" can be acquired concurrently in specialties and subspecialties

CLINICAL CONSULTANT
1. Licensed MD or DO OR
2. Qualified laboratory director (see Director's column)

TESTING PERSONNEL
1. Licensed by State, if required
2. Licensed MD or DO
3. Doctorate, masters, Bachelor, or Associate degree in laboratory science
4. High School graduate or equivalent AND
   50 week military training as Medical Lab Specialist OR
   Documentation of training appropriate to testing performed, TO INCLUDE:
   Specimen collection, labeling, preparation, etc...
   implement laboratory procedures
   perform tests assigned
   conduct preventive maintenance, troubleshooting, calibration
   knowledge of reagent stability and storage
   implement quality control procedures
   knowledge of factors influencing test results
   validate patient test results with QC before reporting

HIGH COMPLEXITY LABS

DIRECTOR
1. Laboratory director license if required by state AND
2. Licensed MD, DO AND
   Certified in anatomic or clinical pathology OR
   1 year of laboratory training during medical residency OR
   2 years of experience directing or supervising high complexity lab
3. Doctoral degree in laboratory science AND
   Board certified OR [until Feb '94]
   2 years laboratory training/experience AND
   2 years experience directing or supervising high complexity lab

TECHNICAL SUPERVISOR
Specific qualifications are required for each specialty or subspecialty.
FOR ALL SPECIALTIES/SUBSPECIALTIES EXCEPT FOR HISTOCOMPATIBILITY AND CYTOGENETICS:
1. Licensed MD or DO AND
   Certified in anatomic AND clinical pathology
FOR SUBSPECIALTIES OF BACTERIOLOGY, MYCOBACTERIOLOGY, MYCOLOGY, VIROLOGY, PARASITOLOGY:
1. Licensed MD, DO AND
   Certified in clinical pathology OR
   1 year training or experience in high complexity microbiology with a minimum of 6 months in the appropriate subspecialty
2. Doctoral degree in laboratory science AND
   1 year training or experience in high complexity microbiology with a minimum of 6 months in the appropriate subspecialty
3. Master's degree in laboratory science AND
   2 years training or experience in high complexity microbiology with a minimum of 6 months in the appropriate subspecialty
4. Bachelor's degree in laboratory science AND
   4 years training or experience in high complexity microbiology with a minimum of 6 months in the appropriate subspecialty
FOR DIAGNOSTIC IMMUNOLOGY, CHEMISTRY, HEMATOLOGY, RADIOBIOASSAY:
Same educational/experiential requirements EXCEPT no 6 month subspecialty requirement.
FOR PATHOLOGY AND ITS SUBSPECIALTIES, CYTOLOGY, HISTOPATHOLOGY, CYTOGENETICS, IMMUNOHEMATOLOGY:
There are specific requirements for each specialty or subspecialty See Regulation.

CLINICAL CONSULTANT
1. Licensed MD or DO OR
2. Qualified laboratory director

GENERAL SUPERVISOR
1. Licensed by State, if required
2. Qualified Director OR
3. Qualified Technical Supervisor OR
4. MD, DO, Doctorate, master's, or bachelor's degree in lab science AND
   1 year lab training/experience in high complexity testing OR
4. Associate's degree AND
   2 years lab training or experience
FOR BLOOD GASES:
If not qualified above,
5. Bachelor's or Associate's degree in respiratory therapy AND 1 or 2 years of training or *experience*
FOR CYTOLOGY, SEE REGULATION

TESTING PERSONNEL
1. Licensed MD or DO
2. Doctor, Master, Bachelor, or Associate degree in laboratory science
3. Previously qualified as technologist
4. [Until Feb '97]: Same as moderate complexity
FOR BLOOD GASES:
4. Bachelor or associate degree in respiratory therapy.

D-3

CLIA (CLINICAL LABORATORY IMPROVEMENT AMENDMENTS): 1988 REGULATIONS AND REQUIREMENTS
Continued

Personnel

The personnel requirements are listed in a sidebar on page 4. Overall, keep in mind that the standards become more stringent as the complexity of testing increases. Waived labs require only a laboratory director, while moderate and high complexity labs require all of the following. (Keep in mind that one person may serve in all required functions, if qualified; it is not necessary to have one person for each function.)

The laboratory director is responsible for the overall operation of the lab and the competency of all laboratory personnel. In addition to providing an appropriate working environment, the director must see that all tests are performed according to applicable requirements, that QC and QA programs are established, and that the lab is enrolled in PT.

Most physician directors already possess the necessary qualifications (see chart). If you have operated a laboratory doing moderate complexity testing for 1 year, you meet both the director and technical consultant requirements. If you do high complexity testing in your medical specialty, such as hematology or rheumatology, and you have had training in residency to do so, you qualify to direct a high complexity laboratory in that specialty. If you were qualified under your state law to operate a laboratory before publication of CLIA, you remain qualified, regardless of the new requirements.

The clinical consultant is responsible for determining appropriateness of testing ordered and test result interpretation where the director is not a physician.

The technical consultant is responsible for technical and scientific oversight. It is not necessary to be on-site, but you must be accessible. Specific responsibilities include selection and verification of testing, establishment of acceptable levels of analytical performance, identifying training needs and evaluating competency of testing personnel. The laboratory director may also perform this function, if qualified in the appropriate specialties.

The testing personnel are mainly responsible for specimen processing, test performance and reporting test results. The minimum requirements include a high school diploma and appropriate training.

In addition to the previously listed personnel, high-complexity laboratories must also employ one or more persons who can function as a technical supervisor and a general supervisor. Responsibilities of a general supervisor include on-site direct supervision of and accessibility to testing personnel.

Inspections

Beginning September 1, 1992, waiver labs will receive random unannounced inspections; moderate and high complexity labs will receive unannounced inspections every 2 years. COLA will soon begin inspection of all laboratories every 2 years. Inspectors must be allowed access to all areas and all records.

continued on page 6

FEES

Schedule of Labs	No. Tests Performed Annually	No. Specialties	Registration Fee (1)	Waiver Certificate (1)	Accreditation Certificate (1)	HHS User Fee (2)	Complaint Investigation (2)	Sanction/ Hearing (2)	Revised Certificate (1)	Accreditation Validation Survey (2)
A-Low Vol.	<2K	*	$100	$100	$100	$300	*	*	$50	*
A	5K-10K	<=3	$100	$100	$100	$840	$52	$280	$50	$42
B	<10K	>=4	$100	$100	$100	$1120	$595	$315	$50	$56
C	10K-25K	<=3	$100	$100	$100	$1400	$665	$350	$50	$70
D	10K-25K	>=4	$350	$100	$100	$1645	$735	$385	$50	$82
E	25K-50K	*	$350	$100	$100	$1890	$840	$420	$50	$95
F	50K-75K	*	$350	$100	$100	$2135	$910	$455	$50	$107
G	75K-100K	*	$350	$100	$100	$2380	$980	$490	$50	$119
H	100K-500K	*	$600	$100	$100	$2625	$1050	$525	$50	$131
I	500K-1M	*	$600	$100	$100	$2870	$1120	$560	$50	$144
J	>1M	*	$600	$100	$100	**	**	**	**	**

*Not defined.
**Based on complex formula--see Federal Register.
1 Fixed fees.
2 Estimated fee; this will vary from state to state.

D-3
CLIA (CLINICAL LABORATORY IMPROVEMENT AMENDMENTS): 1988 REGULATIONS AND REQUIREMENTS
Continued

Unannounced inspections will also take place when HCFA has substantive reason to believe testing is presenting imminent and serious risk to human health or to evaluate public complaints.

Fees

The CLIA statute requires that the costs for the administration and enforcement of CLIA regulations be completely covered by user fees. You will be charged a fee for registration, for issuance of a certificate, for inspections, and for any complaint investigations or sanctions. In general, fees are determined by annual testing volume and number of specialties (see table on page 5 with schedules A through J). Fixed fees include $100 for a waiver certificate, $100 for an accreditation certificate, and $50 for a revised certificate. Since HCFA must negotiate the cost of inspections (compliance fees) with each state, compliance fees, complaint inspection fees, and revisit fees will vary from one state to another. HCFA has computed average fees, which are presented here. Be aware, however, that the fees in your state may be higher than these. We will have no information on state-specific fees until HCFA completes its negotiations.

A COLA laboratory must pay the appropriate registration certificate fee (every laboratory must pay this one-time fee), an accreditation certificate fee ($100) and an additional accreditation validation survey fee of ($42-$156). These federal fees are in addition to COLA fees.

Sanctions

HCFA may impose sanctions against laboratories for failure to comply with the regulations. In cases posing immediate harm to patients or personnel, sanctions will be imposed prior to a hearing; in all other cases, sanctions will not be imposed until a hearing is conducted. These sanctions may include suspension of testing certain analytes or specialties, suspension of Medicare/Medicaid payments, civil money penalties, or suspension, limitation or revocation of certification.

HCFA has stated it will allow previously unregulated laboratories (such as POLs) opportunity to correct deficiencies found during the first inspection unless they pose an immediate threat. Likewise, PT sanctions will not be imposed during the first year, unless the unsuccessful participation somehow poses an immediate threat. However, previously regulated laboratories will be subject to sanctions when the regulation becomes effective 6 months from now.

COLA

The CLIA '88 Final Rule is very complex and expected to cause great confusion. However, laboratories who have already gone through the COLA accreditation process will find they are in an excellent position to move into the post-CLIA era. First, the experience completing the COLA application process will render transition into CLIA regulation much less onerous. Secondly, COLA will continue to serve as a conduit for information flow from HCFA's regulatory program to COLA laboratories, thus assuring timely information. Finally, as soon as possible, COLA will be applying for deeming authority from HCFA, making COLA accreditation an attractive alternative to federal certification.

We will continue to keep you up-to-date on CLIA '88. And, as always, our technical staff is available by phone to clear up any confusions you may face.

Copies of the CLIA '88 Final Rule may be obtained by writing: Superintendent of Documents, US Government Printing Office. Washington, DC 20402-9325, ph. (202) 783-3238 Ask for the Federal Register dated February 28, 1992, stock no. 069-001-00042-4. Enclose a check or money order for $3.50 for each copy ordered.

The Commission on Office Laboratory Accreditation (COLA) is a voluntary education and accreditation organization for physician office laboratories, with a program that addresses all facets of office laboratory quality assurance. COLA was founded by the American Academy of Family Physicians, American Society of Internal Medicine, American Medical Association, and College of American Clinical Endocrinologists and the American Academy of Neurology. COLA is located at: 8701 Georgia Avenue, Suite 610, Silver Spring, MD 20910, Phone: (301)588-5882, Fax: (301)588-7681.
Reprinted with permission.

D-4
DACUM (DEVELOPING A CURRICULUM): 1990 GUIDELINES

by Mary Lee Seibert, EdD, CMA, and
Patricia A. Amos, MS

In keeping with its responsibilities to the public and the members of the profession, the AAMA has recently updated its analysis of the occupation of medical assisting. The competencies needed to practice were described in 1979 and then updated in 1984. The most recent update occurred in January 1990.

The method used for all three analyses was the DACUM process, which derives its name from the words, Developing A Curriculum. The result is a chart which lists skills performed by medical assistants in their employment settings.

The DACUM chart has been an invaluable tool for defining to various publics the scope and substance of what medical assistants are and can do. Among its many uses have been continuing education program planning; curriculum content development for post-secondary medical assisting programs; and a means of self-assessment for practitioners.

An analysis of an occupation such as medical assisting must be updated frequently to remain current in the light of rapidly-changing forces in healthcare delivery and medical science. In the case of medical assisting, updating the DACUM was also necessary to identify changes in the roles and functions of medical assistants as perceived by practitioners in the field.

THE DACUM PROCESS

The 1990 DACUM process was conducted by AAMA January 27-29, 1990 in Birmingham, Alabama. Nine practicing medical assistants from a variety of backgrounds and geographic areas participated in the process. They represented urban and rural settings, group and individual physician practices, and clinical and administrative job focuses. The group was carefully selected to represent a balance of job responsibilities and years of experience. All are Certified Medical Assistants (CMAs), and all but one are graduates of CAHEA/AAMA accredited programs for medical assisting.

The technique used to conduct the analysis of medical assisting involved brainstorming and consensus. After a brief orientation to the process, participants began their work by listing, from their individual experiences, the categories into which they believed their work could be classified.

Once all the categories (general areas of competence) were named to the satisfaction of all participants, the group listed all the skill areas they believed should be included in the medical assistant's role. Both entry-level skills (those the medical assistant should be able to perform after completing a CAHEA-accredited program and starting a first job) and advanced skills (those beyond entry level) were identified. After nearly 12 hours, the initial set of skills for each category was identified.

The group then worked to achieve consensus on each individual skill. Was a skill worded so that it represented exactly the function of the medical assistant? Was it mutually exclusive of other skills listed or was it repetitive? Was it in the right category? Did everyone in the group understand the statement of a skill and agree with it?

Throughout the process, participants had to exercise impeccable communication and interpersonal skills. The result of this lengthy group process is the accompanying DACUM chart.

On the 1990 DACUM chart, the general areas of competence are listed in bold type in the left column. The skill statements within the general areas of competence are arranged from left to right in the order they would be taught to a new person on the job. The skill statements should be read, "The medical assistant should be able to (fill in with the words of each statement)."

With the exception of the advanced skills (asterisked), participants in the DACUM process believe that all skills should be taught in medical assisting education programs. It should be noted that the degree to which an entry-level medical assistant should be able to function in any of the skill areas on the chart may vary. Educators and evaluators must use their own judgment as to how much can be feasibly taught to a medical assisting student in each skill area.

In the 1990 session, eight general areas of competence were identified. Of the 79 individual skills, 14 were considered to be advanced and 65 were classified as entry level. This compares to 10 general areas of competence in 1979 and 7 in 1984, 13 advanced skills in 1979 and 15 in 1984, and 97 entry-level skills in 1979 and 63 in 1984.

As expected, many of the skills remained the same over the years and most likely, will continue to do so. The differences in the numbers of general areas of competence and individual skills often reflect variations in the way they are stated. The new chart should be examined, however, to discover new areas of emphasis indicating changes in medical assistant practice. One example, the general area of competence "Apply Legal Concepts To Practice" on the 1990 chart, indicates the expectations and use for these skills medical assistants will have in the future. Reasons for other apparent differences should be determined.

Mary Lee Seibert, EdD, CMA, and Patricia Amos, MS, served as consultants for the 1990 DACUM analysis. Dr. Seibert and Winifred Mauser were consultants for the 1979 and 1984 analyses. The 1990 CMA participants and consultants acknowledge with gratitude the work done by the previous DACUM participants, which provided a solid foundation for this updated chart.

Seibert, an honorary member of the AAMA, is dean of the College of Allied Health Professions, Temple University, Philadelphia, Pennsylvania.

Amos, Professor Emerita of the University of Alabama at Birmingham (UAB), is a former Assistant Dean of the School of Health Related Professions, UAB.

Appendix D: STANDARDS AND REGULATIONS

D-4

DACUM (DEVELOPING A CURRICULUM): 1990 GUIDELINES *Continued*

1.0	DISPLAY PROFES-SIONALISM	1.1 Project a Positive Attitude	1.2 Perform Within Ethical Boundaries	1.3 Practice Within the Scope of Education, Training and Personal Capabilities	1.4 Maintain Confidentiality	1.5 Work as a Team Member	1.6 Conduct Oneself in a Courteous and Diplomatic Manner	1.7 Adapt to Change
2.0	COMMUNICATE	2.1 Listen and Observe	2.2 Treat All Patients With Empathy and Impartiality	2.3 Adapt Communication to Individuals' Abilities to Understand	2.4 Recognize and Respond to Verbal and Non-verbal Communication	2.5 Serve as Liaison Between Physician and Others	2.6 Evaluate Understanding of Communication	2.7 Receive, Organize, Prioritize and Transmit Information
3.0	PERFORM ADMINISTRATIVE DUTIES	3.1 Perform Basic Secretarial Skills	3.2 Schedule and Monitor Appointments	3.3 Prepare and Maintain Medical Records	3.4 Apply Computer Concepts for Office Procedures	3.5 Perform Medical Transcription	3.6 Locate Resources and Information for Patients and Employers	3.7 Manage Physician's Professional Schedule and Travel
4.0	PERFORM CLINICAL DUTIES	4.1 Apply Principles of Aseptic Technique and Infection Control	4.2 Take Vital Signs	4.3 Recognize Emergencies	4.4 Perform First Aid and CPR	4.5 Prepare and Maintain Examination and Treatment Area	4.6 Interview and Take Patient History	4.7 Prepare Patients for Procedures
5.0	APPLY LEGAL CONCEPTS TO PRACTICE	5.1 Document Accurately	5.2 Determine Needs for Documentation and Reporting	5.3 Use Appropriate Guidelines When Releasing Records or Information	5.4 Follow Established Policy in Initiating or Terminating Medical Treatment	5.5 Dispose of Controlled Substances in Compliance With Government Regulations	5.6 Maintain Licenses and Accreditation	5.7 Monitor Legislation Related to Current Healthcare Issues and Practice
6.0	MANAGE THE OFFICE	6.1 Maintain the Physical Plant	6.2 Operate and Maintain Facilities and Equipment Safely	6.3 Inventory Equipment and Supplies	6.4 Evaluate and Recommend Equipment and Supplies for a Practice	6.5 Maintain Liability Coverage	6.6 Exercise Efficient Time Management	Supervise* Personnel
7.0	PROVIDE INSTRUCTION	7.1 Orient Patients to Office Policies and Procedures	7.2 Instruct Patients With Special Needs	7.3 Teach Patients Methods of Health Promotion and Disease Prevention	7.4 Orient and Train Personnel	Provide* Health Information for Public Use	Supervise* Student Practicums	Conduct* Continuing Education Activities
8.0	MANAGE PRACTICE FINANCES	8.1 Use Manual Bookkeeping Systems	8.2 Implement Current Procedural Terminology and ICD-9 Coding	8.3 Analyze and Use Current Third-Party Guidelines for Reimbursement	8.4 Manage Accounts Receivable	8.5 Manage Accounts Payable	8.6 Maintain Records for Accounting and Banking Purposes	8.7 Process Employee Payroll

D-4
DACUM (DEVELOPING A CURRICULUM): 1990 GUIDELINES Continued

| 1.8 Show Initiative and Responsibility | 1.9 Promote the Profession | Enhance* Skills Through Continuing Education | | | | | |

| 2.8 Use Proper Telephone Technique | 2.9 Interview Effectively | 2.10 Use Medical Terminology Appropriately | 2.11 Compose Written Communication Using Correct Grammar, Spelling and Format | Develop* and Conduct Public Relations Activities to Market Professional Services | | | |

| 4.8 Assist Physician With Examinations and Treatments | 4.9 Use Quality Control | 4.10 Collect and Process Specimens | 4.11 Perform Selected Tests That Assist With Diagnosis and Treatment | 4.12 Screen and Follow-up Patient Test Results | 4.13 Prepare and Administer Medications as Directed by Physician | 4.14 Maintain Medication Records | Respond* to Medical Emergencies |

| Develop* and Maintain Policy and Procedure Manuals | Establish* Risk Management Protocol for the Practice | | | | | | |

| Develop* Job Descriptions | Interview* and Recommend New Personnel | Negotiate* Leases and Prices for Equipment and Supply Contracts | | | | | |

Develop* Educational Materials

Manage* Personnel Benefits and Records

---

* Denotes advanced-level skills.
The medical assistant should be able to perform all other skills after completing a CAHEA-accredited program and starting a first job.

Developed by:

The American Association of Medical Assistants, Inc.

20 North Wacker Drive,
Suite 1575,
Chicago, Illinois 60606
312-899-1500
Toll-free
800-228-2262

Consultants:

Mary Lee Seibert, EdD, CMA, and Patricia A. Amos, MS

Reprinted from THE PROFESSIONAL MEDICAL ASSISTANT, May/June 1990. Copyright, The American Association of Medical Assistants, Inc., 1990.

D-5

DIAGNOSIS-RELATED GROUPS (DRGs)

DRG	Type of Case*	Title	DRG	Type of Case*	Title
\multicolumn{3}{l}{**Major Diagnostic Category 1—Diseases and Disorders of the Nervous System**}	30	M	Traumatic stupor and coma, coma <1 hour, age 0–17
1	S	Craniotomy, age >17 except for trauma	31	M	Concussion, age >69 and/or C.C.
2	S	Craniotomy for trauma, age >17	32	M	Concussion, age 18–69 without C.C.
3	S	Craniotomy, age <18	33	M	Concussion age 0–17
4	S	Spinal procedures	34	M	Other disorders of nervous system, age >69 and/or C.C.
5	S	Extracranial vascular procedures	35	M	Other disorders of nervous system, age <70 without C.C.
6	S	Carpal tunnel release			
7	S	Peripheral and cranial nerve and other nervous system procedures, age >69 and/or C.C.	\multicolumn{3}{l}{**Major Diagnostic Category 2—Diseases and Disorders of the Eye**}
8	S	Peripheral and cranial nerve and other nervous system procedures, age <70 without C.C.	36	S	Retinal procedures
			37	S	Orbital procedures
			38	S	Primary iris procedures
			39	S	Lens procedures with or without vitrectomy
9	M	Spinal disorders and injuries	40	S	Extraocular procedures except orbit, age >17
10	M	Nervous system neoplasms, age >69 and/or C.C.	41	S	Extraocular procedures except orbit, age 0–17
11	M	Nervous system neoplasms, age <70 without C.C.	42	S	Intraocular procedures except retina, iris, and lens
12	M	Degenerative nervous system disorders	43	M	Hyphema
13	M	Multiple sclerosis and cerebellar ataxia	44	M	Acute major eye infections
14	M	Specific cerebrovascular disorders except TIA	45	M	Neurological eye disorders
			46	M	Other disorders of the eye, age >17 with C.C.
15	M	Transient ischemic attack and precerebral occlusions	47	M	Other disorders of the eye, age >17 without C.C.
16	M	Nonspecific cerebrovascular disorders with C.C.	48	M	Other disorders of the eye, age 0–17
17	M	Nonspecific cerebrovascular disorders without C.C.			
18	M	Cranial and peripheral nerve disorders, age >69 and/or C.C.	\multicolumn{3}{l}{**Major Diagnostic Category 3—Diseases and Disorders of the Ear, Nose, and Throat**}
19	M	Cranial and peripheral nerve disorders, age <70 without C.C.	49	S	Major head and neck procedures
			50	S	Sialoadenectomy
20	M	Nervous system infection except viral meningitis	51	S	Salivary gland procedures except sialoadenectomy
21	M	Viral meningitis	52	S	Cleft lip and palate repair
22	M	Hypertensive encephalopathy	53	S	Sinus and mastoid procedures, age >17
23	M	Nontraumatic stupor and coma	54	S	Sinus and mastoid procedures, age 0–17
24	M	Seizure and headache, age >69 and/or C.C.	55	S	Miscellaneous ear, nose, and throat procedures
25	M	Seizure and headache, age 18–69 without C.C.	56	S	Rhinoplasty
26	M	Seizure and headache, age 0–17	57	S	Tonsil and adenoid procedures except tonsillectomy and/or adenoidectomy only, age >17
27	M	Traumatic stupor and coma, coma >1 hour	58	S	Tonsil and adenoid procedures except tonsillectomy and/or adenoidectomy only, age 0–17
28	M	Traumatic stupor and coma, coma <1 hour, age >69 and/or C.C.	59	S	Tonsillectomy and/or adenoidectomy only, age >17
29	M	Traumatic stupor and coma, coma <1 hour, age 18–69 without C.C.	60	S	Tonsillectomy and/or adenoidectomy only, age 0–17

*M, medical case; S, surgical case; C.C., Comorbidity or Complication
Data from the *Federal Register*, Vol. 50, No. 170, September 3, 1985.

D-5

DIAGNOSIS-RELATED GROUPS (DRGs) Continued

DRG	Type of Case*	Title	DRG	Type of Case*	Title
61	S	Myringotomy with tube insertion, age >17	94	M	Pneumothorax, age >69 and/or C.C.
62	S	Myringotomy with tube insertion, age 0–17	95	M	Pneumothorax, age <70 without C.C.
63	S	Other ear, nose, and throat O.R. procedures	96	M	Bronchitis and asthma, age >69 and/or C.C.
64	M	Ear, nose, and throat malignancy	97	M	Bronchitis and asthma, age 18–69 without C.C.
65	M	Dysequilibrium	98	M	Bronchitis and asthma, age 0–17
66	M	Epistaxis			
67	M	Epiglottitis	99	M	Respiratory signs and symptoms, age >69 and/or C.C.
68	M	Otitis media and URI, age >69 and/or C.C.			
69	M	Otitis media and URI, age 18–69 without C.C.	100	M	Respiratory signs and symptoms, age <70 without C.C.
70	M	Otitis media and URI, age 0–17	101	M	Other respiratory system diagnoses, age >69 and/or C.C.
71	M	Laryngotracheitis			
72	M	Nasal trauma and deformity			
73	M	Other ear, nose, and throat diagnoses, age >17	102	M	Other respiratory system diagnoses, age <70 without C.C.
74	M	Other ear, nose, and throat diagnoses, age 0–17			

Major Diagnostic Category 4—Diseases and Disorders of the Respiratory System

Major Diagnostic Category 5—Diseases and Disorders of the Circulatory System

DRG	Type of Case*	Title	DRG	Type of Case*	Title
75	S	Major chest procedures			
76	S	Other respiratory system O.R. procedures with C.C.	103	S	Heart transplant
			104	S	Cardiac valve procedure with pump and with cardiac catheterization
77	S	Other respiratory system O.R. procedures without C.C.			
78	M	Pulmonary embolism	105	S	Cardiac valve procedure with pump and without cardiac catheterization
79	M	Respiratory infections and inflammations, age >69 and/or C.C.			
			106	S	Coronary bypass with cardiac catheterization
80	M	Respiratory infections and inflammations, age 18–69 without C.C.	107	S	Coronary bypass without cardiac catheterization
81	M	Respiratory infections and inflammations, age 0–17	108	S	Other cardiovascular or thoracic procedures with pump
82	M	Respiratory neoplasms			
83	M	Major chest trauma, age >69 and/or C.C.	109	S	Cardiothoracic procedures without pump
84	M	Major chest trauma, age <70 without C.C.	110	S	Major reconstructive vascular procedure without pump, age >69 and/or C.C.
85	M	Pleural effusion, age >69 and/or C.C.			
86	M	Pleural effusion, age <70 without C.C.	111	S	Major reconstructive vascular procedure without pump, age <70 without C.C.
87	M	Pulmonary edema and respiratory failure	112	S	Vascular procedures except major reconstruction without pump
88	M	Chronic obstructive pulmonary disease			
89	M	Simple pneumonia and pleurisy, age >69 and/or C.C.	113	S	Amputation for circulatory system disorders except upper limb and toe
90	M	Simple pneumonia and pleurisy, age 18–69 without C.C.	114	S	Upper limb and toe amputation for circulatory system disorders
91	M	Simple pneumonia and pleurisy, age 0–17	115	S	Permanent cardiac pacemaker implant with AMI, heart failure, or shock
92	M	Interstitial lung disease, age >69 and/or C.C.			
93	M	Interstitial lung disease, age <70 without C.C.	116	S	Permanent cardiac pacemaker implant without AMI, heart failure, or shock

Table continued on following page

D-5

DIAGNOSIS-RELATED GROUPS (DRGs) Continued

DRG	TYPE OF CASE*	TITLE	DRG	TYPE OF CASE*	TITLE
117	S	Cardiac pacemaker replacement and revision except pulse generation replacement only			**Major Diagnostic Category 6—Diseases and Disorders of the Digestive System**
118	S	Cardiac pacemaker pulse generation replacement only	146	S	Rectal resection, age >69 and/or C.C.
119	S	Vein ligation and stripping	147	S	Rectal resection, age <70 without C.C.
120	S	Other circulatory system O.R. procedures	148	S	Major small and large bowel procedures, age >69 and/or C.C.
121	M	Circulatory disorders with AMI and cardiovascular complications discharged alive	149	S	Major small and large bowel procedures, age <70 without C.C.
122	M	Circulatory disorders with AMI without cardiovascular complications discharged alive	150	S	Peritoneal adhesiolysis, age >69 and/or C.C.
			151	S	Peritoneal adhesiolysis, age <70 without C.C.
123	M	Circulatory disorders with AMI, expired	152	S	Minor small and large bowel procedures, age >69 and/or C.C.
124	M	Circulatory disorders except AMI, with cardiac catheterization and complex diagnosis	153	S	Minor small and large bowel procedures, age <70 without C.C.
125	M	Circulatory disorders except AMI, with cardiac catheterization without complex diagnosis	154	S	Stomach, esophageal, and duodenal procedures, age >69 and/or C.C.
			155	S	Stomach, esophageal, and duodenal procedures, age 18–69 without C.C.
126	M	Acute and subacute endocarditis			
127	M	Heart failure and shock	156	S	Stomach, esophageal, and duodenal procedures, age 0–17
128	M	Deep vein thrombophlebitis			
129	M	Cardiac arrest, unexplained			
130	M	Peripheral vascular disorders, age >69 and/or C.C.	157	S	Anal and stomal procedures, age >69 and/or C.C.
131	M	Peripheral vascular disorders, age <70 without C.C.	158	S	Anal and stomal procedures, age <70 without C.C.
132	M	Atherosclerosis, age >69 and/or C.C.	159	S	Hernia procedures except inguinal and femoral, age >69 and/or C.C.
133	M	Atherosclerosis, age <70 without C.C.	160	S	Hernia procedures except inguinal and femoral, age 18–69 without C.C.
134	M	Hypertension			
135	M	Cardiac congenital and valvular disorders, age >69 and/or C.C.	161	S	Inguinal and femoral hernia procedures, age >69 and/or C.C.
136	M	Cardiac congenital and valvular disorders, age 18–69 without C.C.	162	S	Inguinal and femoral hernia procedures, age 18–69 without C.C.
137	M	Cardiac congenital and valvular disorders, age 0–17	163	S	Hernia procedures, age 0–17
138	M	Cardiac arrhythmia and conduction disorders, age >69 and/or C.C.	164	S	Appendectomy with complicated principal diagnosis, age >69 and/or C.C.
139	M	Cardiac arrhythmia and conduction disorders, age <70 without C.C.	165	S	Appendectomy with complicated principal diagnosis, age <70 without C.C.
140	M	Angina pectoris			
141	M	Syncope and collapse, age >69 and/or C.C.	166	S	Appendectomy without complicated principal diagnosis, age >69 and/or C.C.
142	M	Syncope and collapse, age <70 without C.C.			
143	M	Chest pain			
144	M	Other circulatory system diagnoses with C.C.	167	S	Appendectomy without complicated principal diagnosis, age <70 without C.C.
145	M	Other circulatory system diagnoses without C.C.			

D-5

DIAGNOSIS-RELATED GROUPS (DRGs) Continued

DRG	Type of Case*	Title	DRG	Type of Case*	Title
168	S	Mouth procedures, age >69 and/or C.C.	194	S	Biliary tract procedures except total cholecystectomy, age <70 without C.C.
169	S	Mouth procedures, age <70 without C.C.	195	S	Total cholecystectomy with common duct exploration, age >69 and/or C.C.
170	S	Other digestive system O.R. procedures, age >69 and/or C.C.	196	S	Total cholecystectomy with common duct exploration, age <70 without C.C.
171	S	Other digestive system O.R. procedures, age <70 without C.C.	197	S	Total cholecystectomy without common duct exploration, age >69 and/or C.C.
172	M	Digestive malignancy, age >69 and/or C.C.	198	S	Total cholecystectomy without common duct exploration, <70 without C.C.
173	M	Digestive malignancy, age <70 without C.C.	199	S	Hepatobiliary diagnostic procedure for malignancy
174	M	G.I. hemorrhage, age >69 and/or C.C.	200	S	Hepatobiliary diagnostic procedure for nonmalignancy
175	M	G.I. hemorrhage, age <70 without C.C.	201	S	Other hepatobiliary or pancreas O.R. procedures
176	M	Complicated peptic ulcer	202	M	Cirrhosis and alcoholic hepatitis
177	M	Uncomplicated peptic ulcer, age >69 and/or C.C.	203	M	Malignancy of hepatobiliary system or pancreas
178	M	Uncomplicated peptic ulcer, age <70 without C.C.	204	M	Disorders of pancreas except malignancy
179	M	Inflammatory bowel disease	205	M	Disorders of liver except malignancy, cirrhosis, alcoholic hepatitis, age >69 and or C.C.
180	M	G.I. obstruction, age >69 and/or C.C.			
181	M	G.I. obstruction, age <70 without C.C.	206	M	Disorders of liver except malignancy, cirrhosis, alcoholic hepatitis, age <70 without C.C.
182	M	Esophagitis, gastroenteritis, and miscellaneous digestive disorders age >69 and/or C.C.	207	M	Disorders of the biliary tract, age >69 and/or C.C.
183	M	Esophagitis, gastroenteritis, and miscellaneous digestive disorders, age 18–69 without C.C.	208	M	Disorders of the biliary tract, age <70 without C.C.
184	M	Esophagitis, gastroenteritis, and miscellaneous digestive disorders, age 0–17			
185	M	Dental and oral disorders except extractions and restorations, age >17			
186	M	Dental and oral disorders except extractions and restorations, age 0–17			**Major Diagnostic Category 8—Diseases and Disorders of the Musculoskeletal System and Connective Tissue**
187	M	Dental extractions and restorations	209	S	Major joint and limb reattachment procedure
188	M	Other digestive system diagnoses, age >69 and/or C.C.	210	S	Hip and femur procedures except major joint, age >69 and/or C.C.
189	M	Other digestive system diagnoses, age 18–69 without C.C.	211	S	Hip and femur procedures except major joint, age 18–69 without C.C.
190	M	Other digestive system diagnoses, age 0–17	212	S	Hip and femur procedures except major joint, age 0–17
		**Major Diagnostic Category 7—Diseases of the Hepatobiliary System and Pancreas**	213	S	Amputations for musculoskeletal system and connective tissue disorders
191	S	Major pancreas, liver, and shunt procedures	214	S	Back and neck procedures, age >69 and/or C.C.
192	S	Minor pancreas, liver, and shunt procedures	215	S	Back and neck procedures, age <70 without C.C.
193	S	Biliary tract procedures except total cholecystectomy, age >69 and/or C.C.	216	S	Biopsies of musculoskeletal system and connective tissue

Table continued on following page

DIAGNOSIS-RELATED GROUPS (DRGs) Continued

DRG	Type of Case*	Title	DRG	Type of Case*	Title
217	S	Wound débridement and skin graft except hand, for musculoskeletal and connective tissue disorders	245	M	Bone diseases and specific arthropathies, age <70 without C.C.
218	S	Lower extremity and humerus procedures except hip, foot, femur, age >69 and/or C.C.	246	M	Nonspecific arthropathies
			247	M	Signs and symptoms of musculoskeletal system and connective tissue
219	S	Lower extremity and humerus procedures except hip, foot, femur, age 18–69 without C.C.	248	M	Tendonitis, myositis, and bursitis
			249	M	Aftercare, musculoskeletal system and connective tissue
220	S	Lower extremity and humerus procedures except hip, foot, femur, age 0–17	250	M	Fractures, sprains, strains, and dislocations of forearm, hand, foot, age >69 and/or C.C.
221	S	Knee procedures, age >69 and/or C.C.	251	M	Fractures, sprains, strains, and dislocations of forearm, hand, foot, age 18–69 without C.C.
222	S	Knee procedures, age <70 without C.C.			
223	S	Upper extremity procedures except humerus and hand, age >69 and/or C.C.	252	M	Fractures, sprains, strains, and dislocations of forearm, hand, foot, age 0–17
224	S	Upper extremity procedures except humerus and hand, age <70 without C.C.	253	M	Fractures, sprains, strains, and dislocations of upper arm and lower leg except foot, age >69 and/or C.C.
225	S	Foot procedures			
226	S	Soft tissue procedures, age >69 and/or C.C.	254	M	Fractures, sprains, strains, and dislocations of upper arm and lower leg except foot, age 18–69 without C.C.
227	S	Soft tissue procedures, age <70 without C.C.			
228	S	Ganglion (hand) procedures	255	M	Fractures, sprains, strains, and dislocations of upper arm and lower leg except foot, age 0–17
229	S	Hand procedures except ganglion			
230	S	Local excision and removal of internal fixation devices of hip and femur	256	M	Other diagnoses of musculoskeletal system and connective tissue
231	S	Local excision and removal of internal fixation devices except hip and femur			
232	S	Arthroscopy			**Major Diagnostic Category 9—Diseases and Disorders of the Skin, Subcutaneous Tissue, and Breast**
233	S	Other musculoskeletal system and connective tissue O.R. procedures, age >69 and or C.C.	257	S	Total mastectomy for malignancy, age >69 and/or C.C.
234	S	Other musculoskeletal system and connective tissue O.R. procedures, age <70 without C.C.	258	S	Total mastectomy for malignancy, age <70 without C.C.
235	M	Fractures of femur	259	S	Subtotal mastectomy for malignancy, age >69 and/or C.C.
236	M	Fractures of hip and pelvis			
237	M	Sprains, strains, and dislocations of hip, pelvis, and thigh	260	S	Subtotal mastectomy for malignancy, age <70 without C.C.
238	M	Osteomyelitis			
239	M	Pathological fractures and musculoskeletal and connective tissue malignancy	261	S	Breast procedure for nonmalignancy except biopsy and local excision
240	M	Connective tissue disorders, age >69 and/or C.C.	262	S	Breast biopsy and local excision for nonmalignancy
241	M	Connective tissue disorders, age <70 without C.C.	263	S	Skin grafts and/or débridement, ulcer or cellulitis, age >69 and/or C.C.
242	M	Septic arthritis			
243	M	Medical back problems	264	S	Skin grafts and/or débridement, ulcer or cellulitis, age <70 without C.C.
244	M	Bone diseases and specific arthropathies, age >69 and/or C.C.			

DIAGNOSIS-RELATED GROUPS (DRGs) Continued

DRG	Type of Case*	Title	DRG	Type of Case*	Title
265	S	Skin graft and/or débridement, except skin ulcer or cellulitis with C.C.	292	S	Other endocrine, nutritional, and metabolic O.R. procedures, age >69 and/or C.C.
266	S	Skin graft and/or débridement, except skin ulcer or cellulitis without C.C.	293	S	Other endocrine, nutritional, and metabolic O.R. procedures, age <70 without C.C.
267	S	Perianal and pilonidal procedures	294	M	Diabetes, age ≥36
268	S	Skin, subcutaneous tissue, and breast plastic procedures	295	M	Diabetes, age 0–35
269	S	Other skin, subcutaneous tissue, and breast O.R. procedures, age >69 and/or C.C.	296	M	Nutritional and miscellaneous metabolic disorders, age >69 and/or C.C.
270	S	Other skin, subcutaneous tissue, and breast O.R. procedures, age <70 without C.C.	297	M	Nutritional and miscellaneous metabolic disorders, age 18–69 without C.C.
271	M	Skin ulcers	298	M	Nutritional and miscellaneous metabolic disorders, age 0–17
272	M	Major skin disorders, age >69 and/or C.C.	299	M	Inborn errors of metabolism
273	M	Major skin disorders, age <70 without C.C.	300	M	Endocrine disorders, age >69 and/or C.C.
274	M	Malignant breast disorders, age >69 and/or C.C.	301	M	Endocrine disorders, age <70 without C.C.
275	M	Malignant breast disorders, age <70 without C.C.			
276	M	Nonmalignant breast disorders			**Major Diagnostic Category 11—Diseases and Disorders of the Kidney and Urinary Tract**
277	M	Cellulitis, age >69 and/or C.C.	302	S	Kidney transplant
278	M	Cellulitis, age 18–69 without C.C.	303	S	Kidney, ureter, and major bladder procedure for neoplasm
279	M	Cellulitis, age 0–17	304	S	Kidney, ureter, and major bladder procedure for nonneoplasm, age >69 and/or C.C.
280	M	Trauma to the skin, subcutaneous tissue, and breast, age >69 and/or C.C.	305	S	Kidney, ureter, and major bladder procedure for nonneoplasm, age <70 without C.C.
281	M	Trauma to the skin, subcutaneous tissue, and breast, age 18–69 without C.C.	306	S	Prostatectomy, age >69 and/or C.C.
282	M	Trauma to the skin, subcutaneous tissue, and breast, age 0–17	307	S	Prostatectomy, age <70 without C.C.
283	M	Minor skin disorders, age >69 and/or C.C.	308	S	Minor bladder procedures, age >69 and/or C.C.
284	M	Minor skin disorders, age <70 without C.C.	309	S	Minor bladder procedures, age <70 without C.C.
			310	S	Transurethral procedures, age >69 and/or C.C.
		Major Diagnostic Category 10—Endocrine, Nutritional, and Metabolic Diseases and Disorders	311	S	Transurethral procedures, age <70 without C.C.
285	S	Amputation of lower limb for endocrine, nutritional, and metabolic disorders	312	S	Urethral procedures, age >69 and/or C.C.
286	S	Adrenal and pituitary procedures	313	S	Urethral procedures, age 18–69 without C.C.
287	S	Skin grafts and wound débridement for endocrine, nutritional, and metabolic disorders	314	S	Urethral procedures, age 0–17
			315	S	Other kidney and urinary tract O.R. procedures
288	S	O.R. procedures for obesity	316	M	Renal failure
289	S	Parathyroid procedures	317	M	Admit for renal dialysis
290	S	Thyroid procedures	318	M	Kidney and urinary tract neoplasms, age >69 and/or C.C.
291	S	Thyroglossal procedures			

Table continued on following page

D-5

DIAGNOSIS-RELATED GROUPS (DRGs) *Continued*

DRG	Type of Case*	Title
319	M	Kidney and urinary tract neoplasms, age <70 without C.C.
320	M	Kidney and urinary tract infections, age >69 and/or C.C.
321	M	Kidney and urinary tract infections, age 18–69 without C.C.
322	M	Kidney and urinary tract infections, age 0–17
323	M	Urinary stones, age >69 and/or C.C.
324	M	Urinary stones, age <70 without C.C.
325	M	Kidney and urinary tract signs and symptoms, age >69 and/or C.C.
326	M	Kidney and urinary tract signs and symptoms, age 18–69 without C.C.
327	M	Kidney and urinary tract signs and symptoms, age 0–17
328	M	Urethral stricture, age >69 and/or C.C.
329	M	Urethral stricture, age 18–69 without C.C.
330	M	Urethral stricture, age 0–17
331	M	Other kidney and urinary tract diagnoses, age >69 and/or C.C.
332	M	Other kidney and urinary tract diagnoses, age 18–69 without C.C.
333	M	Other kidney and urinary tract diagnoses, age 0–17
Major Diagnostic Category 12—Diseases and Disorders of the Male Reproductive System		
334	S	Major male pelvic procedures with C.C.
335	S	Major male pelvic procedures without C.C.
336	S	Transurethral prostatectomy, age >69 and/or C.C.
337	S	Transurethral prostatectomy, age <70 without C.C.
338	S	Testes procedures, for malignancy
339	S	Testes procedures, nonmalignant, age >17
340	S	Testes procedures, nonmalignant, age 0–17
341	S	Penis procedures
342	S	Circumcision, age >17
343	S	Circumcision, age 0–17
344	S	Other male reproductive system O.R. procedures for malignancy
345	S	Other male reproductive system O.R. procedures except for malignancy
346	M	Malignancy, male reproductive system, age >69 and/or C.C.
347	M	Malignancy, male reproductive system, age <70 without C.C.
348	M	Benign prostatic hypertrophy, age >69 and/or C.C.
349	M	Benign prostatic hypertrophy, age <70 without C.C.
350	M	Inflammation of the male reproductive system
351	M	Sterilization, male
352	M	Other male reproductive system diagnoses
Major Diagnostic Category 13—Diseases and Disorders of the Female Reproductive System		
353	S	Pelvic evisceration, radical hysterectomy, and vulvectomy
354	S	Nonradical hysterectomy, age >69 and/or C.C.
355	S	Nonradical hysterectomy, age <70 without C.C.
356	S	Female reproductive system reconstructive procedures
357	S	Uterus and adnexa procedures for malignancy
358	S	Uterus and adnexa procedures for nonmalignancy except tubal interruption
359	S	Incisional tubal interruption for nonmalignancy
360	S	Vagina, cervix, and vulva procedures
361	S	Laparoscopy and endoscopy (female) except tubal interruption
362	S	Laparoscopic tubal interruption
363	S	D & C, conization, and radioimplant, for malignancy
364	S	D & C, conization except for malignancy
365	S	Other female reproductive system O.R. procedures
366	M	Malignancy, female reproductive system, age >69 and/or C.C.
367	M	Malignancy, female reproductive system, age <70 without C.C.
368	M	Infections, female reproductive system
369	M	Menstrual and other female reproductive system disorders
Major Diagnostic Category 14—Pregnancy, Childbirth, and the Puerperium		
370	S	Cesarean section with C.C.
371	S	Cesarean section without C.C.
372	M	Vaginal delivery with complicating diagnoses

DIAGNOSIS-RELATED GROUPS (DRGs) Continued

DRG	TYPE OF CASE*	TITLE	DRG	TYPE OF CASE*	TITLE
373	M	Vaginal delivery without complicating diagnoses	401	S	Lymphoma or leukemia with other O.R. procedure, age >69 and/or C.C.
374	S	Vaginal delivery with sterilization and/or D & C	402	S	Lymphoma or leukemia with other O.R. procedure, age <70 without C.C.
375	S	Vaginal delivery with O.R. procedure except sterilization and/or D & C	403	M	Lymphoma or leukemia, age >69 and/or C.C.
376	M	Postpartum and postabortion diagnoses without O.R. procedure	404	M	Lymphoma or leukemia, age 18–69 without C.C.
377	S	Postpartum and postabortion diagnoses with O.R. procedure	405	M	Lymphoma or leukemia, age 0–17
378	M	Ectopic pregnancy	406	S	Myeloproliferative disorder or poorly differentiated neoplasm without major O.R. procedure and C.C.
379	M	Threatened abortion			
380	M	Abortion without D & C			
381	M	Abortion with D & C, aspiration curettage, or hysterotomy	407	S	Myeloproliferative disorder or poorly differentiated neoplasm with major O.R. procedure without C.C.
382	M	False labor			
383	M	Other antepartum diagnoses with medical complications	408	S	Myeloproliferative disorder or poorly differentiated neoplasm with other O.R. procedure
384	M	Other antepartum diagnoses without medical complications			
			409	M	Radiotherapy
			410	M	Chemotherapy
			411	M	History of malignancy without endoscopy

Major Diagnostic Category 15—Newborns and Other Neonates with Condition Originating in Perinatal Period

DRG	TYPE OF CASE*	TITLE	DRG	TYPE OF CASE*	TITLE
385		Neonates, died or transferred	412	M	History of malignancy with endoscopy
386		Extreme immaturity or respiratory distress syndrome, neonate	413	M	Other diagnoses of myeloproliferative disorder or poorly differentiated neoplasm, age >69 and/or C.C.
387		Prematurity with major problems			
388		Prematurity without major problems	414	M	Other diagnoses of myeloproliferative disorder or poorly differentiated neoplasm, age <70 without C.C.
389		Full-term neonate with major problems			
390		Neonates with other significant problems			
391		Normal newborns			

Major Diagnostic Category 16—Diseases and Disorders of Blood and Blood-Forming Organs

Major Diagnostic Category 18—Infectious and Parasitic Diseases

DRG	TYPE OF CASE*	TITLE	DRG	TYPE OF CASE*	TITLE
392	S	Splenectomy, age >17	415	S	O.R. procedure for infectious and parasitic diseases
393	S	Splenectomy, age 0–17	416	M	Septicemia, age >17
394	S	Other O.R. procedures of the blood and blood-forming organs	417	M	Septicemia, age 0–17
			418	M	Postoperative and posttraumatic infections
395	M	Red blood cell disorders, age >17	419	M	Fever of unknown origin, age >69 and/or C.C.
396	M	Red blood cell disorders, age 0–17	420	M	Fever of unknown origin, age 18–69 without C.C.
397	M	Coagulation disorders	421	M	Viral illness, age >17
398	M	Reticuloendothelial and immunity disorders, age >69 and/or C.C.	422	M	Viral illness and fever of unknown origin, age 0–17
399	M	Reticuloendothelial and immunity disorders, age <70 without C.C.	423	M	Other infectious and parasitic diseases

Major Diagnostic Category 17—Myeloproliferative Disorders

Major Diagnostic Category 19—Mental Diseases and Disorders

DRG	TYPE OF CASE*	TITLE	DRG	TYPE OF CASE*	TITLE
400	S	Lymphoma or leukemia with major O.R. procedure	424	S	O.R. procedures with principal diagnosis of mental illness

Table continued on following page

DIAGNOSIS-RELATED GROUPS (DRGs) Continued

DRG	TYPE OF CASE*	TITLE	DRG	TYPE OF CASE*	TITLE
425	M	Acute adjustment reaction and disturbances of psychosocial dysfunction	451	M	Poisoning and toxic effects of drugs, age 0–17
426	M	Depressive neuroses	452	M	Complications of treatment, age >69 and/or C.C.
427	M	Neuroses except depressive	453	M	Complications of treatment, age <70 without C.C.
428	M	Disorders of personality and impulse control	454	M	Other diagnoses of injuries, poisonings, and toxic effects, age >69 and/or C.C.
429	M	Organic disturbances and mental retardation			
430	M	Psychoses	455	M	Other diagnoses of injuries, poisonings, and toxic effects, age <70 without C.C.
431	M	Childhood mental disorders			
432	M	Other diagnoses of mental disorders			

Major Diagnostic Category 20—Substance Use and Substance-Induced Organic Mental Disorders

Major Diagnostic Category 22—Burns

DRG	TYPE OF CASE*	TITLE
433		Substance use and induced organic mental disorders, left against medical advice
434		Substance abuse, intoxicant-induced mental syndromes except dependency and/or other symptomatic treatment
435		Substance dependence, detoxification and/or other symptomatic treatment
436		Substance dependence with rehabilitation therapy
437		Substance dependence, combined rehabilitation and detoxification therapy
438		No longer valid

DRG	TYPE OF CASE*	TITLE
456		Burns, transferred to another acute care facility
457		Extensive burns
458	S	Nonextensive burns with skin grafts
459	S	Nonextensive burns with wound débridement and other O.R. procedure
460	M	Nonextensive burns without O.R. procedure

Major Diagnostic Category 23—Factors Influencing Health Status and Other Contacts with Health Services

DRG	TYPE OF CASE*	TITLE
461	S	O.R. procedure with diagnoses of other contact with health services
462	M	Rehabilitation
463	M	Signs and symptoms with C.C.
464	M	Signs and symptoms without C.C.
465	M	Aftercare with history of malignancy as secondary diagnosis
466	M	Aftercare without history of malignancy as secondary diagnosis
467	M	Other factors influencing health status

Major Diagnostic Category 21—Injuries, Poisonings, and Toxic Effects of Drugs

DRG	TYPE OF CASE*	TITLE
439	S	Skin grafts for injuries
440	S	Wound débridements for injuries
441	S	Hand procedures for injuries
442	S	Other O.R. procedures for injuries, age >69 and/or C.C.
443	S	Other O.R. procedures for injuries, age <70 without C.C.
444	M	Multiple trauma, age >69 and/or C.C.
445	M	Multiple trauma, age 18–69 without C.C.
446	M	Multiple trauma, age 0–17
447	M	Allergic reactions, age >17
448	M	Allergic reactions, age 0–17
449	M	Poisoning and toxic effects of drugs, age >69 and/or C.C.
450	M	Poisoning and toxic effects of drugs, age 18–69 without C.C.

DRGs Not Belonging to a Major Diagnostic Category

DRG	TYPE OF CASE*	TITLE
468		Unrelated O.R. procedure
469		Primary diagnosis invalid as discharge diagnosis
470		Ungroupable

Addition to Major Diagnostic Category 8

DRG	TYPE OF CASE*	TITLE
471	S	Bilateral or multiple major joint procedures of the lower extremity

From Miller BF, Keane CB: *Encyclopedia and Dictionary of Medicine, Nursing, and Allied Health*, 5th ed. Philadelphia: W.B. Saunders, 1992, pp. 1642–1650.

D-6

OSHA BLOODBORNE PATHOGENS FINAL STANDARD: SUMMARY OF KEY PROVISIONS

Purpose

Limits occupational exposure to blood and other potentially infectious materials, since any exposure could result in transmission of bloodborne pathogens, which could lead to disease or death.

Scope

Covers *all employees who* could be "reasonably anticipated," as the result of performing their job duties, to *face contact with blood* and other potentially infectious materials. OSHA has not attempted to list all occupations where exposures could occur. "Good Samaritan" acts such as assisting a coworker with a nosebleed would not be considered occupational exposure.

Infectious materials include semen, vaginal secretions, cerebrospinal fluid, synovial fluid, pleural fluid, pericardial fluid, peritoneal fluid, amniotic fluid, saliva in dental procedures, any body fluid visibly contaminated with blood, and all body fluids in situations where it is difficult or impossible to differentiate between body fluids. They also include any unfixed tissue or organ other than intact skin from a human (living or dead) and human immunodeficiency virus (HIV)–containing cell or tissue cultures, organ cultures and HIV or hepatitis B (HBV)–containing culture medium or other solutions as well as blood, organs or other tissues from experimental animals infected with HIV or HBV.

Exposure Control Plan

Requires employers to *identify, in writing,* tasks and procedures as well as job classifications *where occupational exposure to blood occurs*—without regard to personal protective clothing and equipment. It must also set forth the *schedule for implementing other provisions* of the standard and specify the procedure for evaluating circumstances surrounding exposure incidents. The plan must be accessible to employees and available to OSHA. Employers must review and update it at least annually—more often if necessary to accommodate workplace changes.

Methods of Compliance

Mandates *universal precautions* (treating body fluids/materials as if infectious) *emphasizing engineering and work practice controls*. The standard stresses handwashing and requires employers to provide facilities and ensure that employees use them following exposure to blood. It sets forth procedures to minimize needlesticks, minimize splashing and spraying of blood, ensure appropriate packaging of specimens and regulated wastes and decontaminate equipment or label it as contaminated before shipping to servicing facilities.

Employers must provide, at no cost, and require employees to use appropriate *personal protective equipment* such as gloves, gowns, masks, mouthpieces and resuscitation bags and must clean, repair, and replace these when necessary. Gloves are required for phlebotomy except in volunteer blood donation centers, where gloves must be made available to employees who want them.

The standard requires a *written schedule for cleaning,* identifying the method of decontamination to be used, in addition to cleaning following contact with blood or other potentially infectious materials. It specifies methods for disposing of contaminated sharps and sets forth standards for containers for these items and other regulated waste. Further, the standard includes provisions for handling contaminated laundry to minimize exposures.

HIV and HBV Research Laboratories and Production Facilities

Calls for these facilities to follow *standard microbiological practices* and specifies additional practices intended to minimize exposures of employees working with concentrated viruses and reduce the risk of accidental exposure for other employees at the facility. These facilities must include required containment equipment and an autoclave for decontamination of regulated waste and must be constructed to limit risks and enable easy clean-up. *Additional training and experience requirements* apply to workers in these facilities.

Hepatitis B Vaccination

Requires vaccinations to be made *available to all employees who have occupational exposure to blood* within 10 working days of assignment, at no cost, at a reasonable time and place, under the supervision of licensed physician/licensed health care professional and according to the latest recommendations of the U.S. Public Health Service (USPHS). *Prescreening may not be required* as a condition of receiving the vaccine. Employees must sign a *declination form* if they choose not to be vaccinated, but may later opt to receive the vaccine at no cost to the employee. Should booster doses later be recommended by the USPHS, employees must be offered them.

Post-Exposure Evaluation and Follow-up

Specifies procedures to be made *available to all employees who have had an exposure incident* plus any laboratory tests must be conducted by an accredited laboratory at no cost to the employee. Follow-up must include a *confidential medical evaluation* documenting the circumstances of exposure, identifying and testing the source individual if feasible, testing the exposed employee's blood if he/she consents, post-exposure prophylaxis, counseling, and evaluation of reported illness. Health care professionals must be provided specified information to facilitate the evaluation and their written opinion on the need for hepatitis B vaccination following the exposure. Information such as the employee's ability to receive the hepatitis B vaccine must be supplied to the employer. All diagnoses must remain confidential.

Hazard Communication

Requires *warning labels* including the *orange or orange-red biohazard symbol* affixed to containers of regulated waste, refrigerators and freezers, and other containers that are used to store or transport blood or other potentially infectious materials. *Red bags* or containers *may be used* instead of labeling. When a facility uses universal precautions in its handling of all specimens, labeling is not required within the facility. Likewise, when all laundry is handled with universal precautions, the laundry need not be labeled. Blood that has been tested and found free of HIV and HBV and released for clinical use, and regulated waste that has been decontaminated, need not be labeled. *Signs* must be used to *identify restricted areas* in HIV and HBV research laboratories and production facilities.

Information and Training

Mandates *training within 90 days* of effective date, *initially* upon assignment and *annually*—employees who have received appropriate training within the past year need only receive additional training in items not previously covered. Training must include making accessible a copy of the regulatory text of the standard and explanation of its contents, general discussion on bloodborne diseases and their transmission, exposure control

D-6
OSHA BLOODBORNE PATHOGENS FINAL STANDARD: SUMMARY OF KEY PROVISIONS Continued

plan, engineering and work practice controls, personal protective equipment, hepatitis B vaccine, response to emergencies involving blood, how to handle exposure incidents, the postgram, and signs/labels/color-coding. There must be *opportunity for questions and answers,* and the *trainer must be knowledgeable* in the subject matter. *Laboratory and production facility workers* must receive *additional specialized initial training.*

Record-Keeping

Calls for medical records to be kept for each employee with occupational exposure for the *duration of employment plus 30 years,* must be *confidential* and must include name and social security number; hepatitis B vaccination status (including dates); results of any examinations, medical testing, and follow-up procedures; a copy of the health care professional written opinion; and a copy of information provided to the healthcare professional. Training records must be maintained for 3 years and must include dates, contents of the training program or a summary, trainer's name and qualifications, and names and job titles of all persons attending the sessions. Medical records must be made *available to the subject employee,* anyone with written consent of the employee, OSHA and NIOSH—they are not available to the employer. Disposal of records must be in accord with OSHA's standard covering access to records.

Dates

Sets *effective date 90 days after publication in* the Federal Register. *Exposure control plan* must be completed within *60 days* of the effective data. *Information and training requirements* take effect *90 days* following the effective date. And the following *other provisions* take effect *120 days* after the effective date: engineering and work practice controls, personal protective equipment, housekeeping, special provisions covering HIV and HBV research laboratories and production facilities, hepatitis B vaccination and post-exposure evaluation and follow-up and labels and signs.

Produced by Occupational Safety and Health Administration, December, 1991, adapted by Epidemiology and Disease Control Program 2/92.

D-7

OSHA JOINT ADVISORY NOTICE OF THE DEPARTMENT OF LABOR AND THE DEPARTMENT OF HEALTH AND HUMAN SERVICES FOR THE PROTECTION AGAINST OCCUPATIONAL EXPOSURE TO HEPATITIS B VIRUS (HBV) AND HUMAN IMMUNODEFICIENCY VIRUS (HIV)

I. Background:

Hepatitis B (previously called serum hepatitis) is the major infectious occupational health hazard in the health-care industry, and a model for the transmission of blood-borne pathogens. In 1985 the Centers for Disease Control (CDC) estimated [1] that there were over 200,000 cases of hepatitis B virus (HBV) infection in the U.S. each year, leading to 10,000 hospitalizations, 250 deaths due to fulminant hepatitis, 4,000 deaths due to hepatitis-related cirrhosis, and 800 deaths due to hepatitis-related primary liver cancer. More recently [2] the CDC estimated the total number of HBV infections to be 300,000 per year with corresponding increases in numbers of hepatitis-related hospitalizations and deaths. The incidence of reported clinical hepatitis B has been increasing in the United States, from 6.9/100,000 in 1978 to 9.2/100,000 in 1981 and 11.5/100,000 in 1985 [2]. The Hepatitis Branch, CDC, has estimated [unpublished] that 500-600 health-care workers whose job entails exposure to blood are hospitalized annually, with over 200 deaths (12-15 due to fulminant hepatitis, 170-200 from cirrhosis, and 40-50 from liver cancer). Studies indicate that 10% to 40% of health-care or dental workers may show serologic evidence of past or present HBV infection [3]. Health-care costs for hepatitis B and non-A, non-B hepatitis in health-care workers were estimated to be $10 - $12 million annually [4]. A safe, immunogenic, and effective vaccine to prevent hepatitis B has been available since 1982 and is recommended by the CDC for health-care workers exposed to blood and body fluids [1,2,5-7]. According to unpublished CDC estimates, approximately 30-40% of health-care workers in high-risk settings have been vaccinated to date.

According to the most recent data available from the CDC [8], acquired immunodeficiency syndrome (AIDS) was the 13th leading cause of years of potential life lost (82,882 years) in 1984, increasing to 11th place in 1985 (152,595 years). As of August 10, 1987, a cumulative total of 40,051 AIDS cases (of which 558 were pediatric) had been reported to the CDC, with 23,165 (57.8%) of these known to have died [9]. Although occupational HIV infection has been documented [10], no AIDS case or AIDS-related death is believed to be occupationally related. Spending within the Public Health Service related to AIDS has also accelerated rapidly, from $5.6 million in 1982 to $494 million in 1987, with $791 million requested for 1988. Estimates of average lifetime costs for the care of an AIDS patient have varied considerably, but recent evidence suggests the amount is probably in the range of $50,000 to $75,000.

Infection with either HBV [1,2] or human immunodeficiency virus (HIV, previously called human T-lymphotrophic virus type III/lymphadenopathy-associated virus (HTLV III/LAV) or AIDS-associated retrovirus (ARV)) [11,12]

D-7

OSHA JOINT ADVISORY NOTICE OF THE DEPARTMENT OF LABOR AND THE DEPARTMENT OF HEALTH AND HUMAN SERVICES FOR THE PROTECTION AGAINST OCCUPATIONAL EXPOSURE TO HEPATITIS B VIRUS (HBV) AND HUMAN IMMUNODEFICIENCY VIRUS (HIV) Continued

can lead to a number of life-threatening conditions, including cancer. Therefore, exposure to HBV and HIV should be reduced to the maximum extent feasible by engineering controls, work practices, and protective equipment. (Engineering controls are those methods that prevent or limit the potential for exposure at or as near as possible to the point of origin, for example by eliminating a hazard by substitution or by isolating the hazard from the work environment.)

II. Modes Of Transmission:

In the U.S., the major mode of HBV transmission is sexual, both homosexual and heterosexual. Also important is parenteral (entry into the body by a route other than the gastrointestinal tract) transmission by shared needles among intravenous drug abusers and to a lesser extent in needlestick injuries or other exposures of health-care workers to blood. HBV is not transmitted by casual contact, fecal-oral or airborne routes, or by contaminated food or drinking water [1,2,13]. Workers are at risk of HBV infection to the extent they are exposed to blood and other body fluids; employment without that exposure, even in a hospital, carries no greater risk than that for the general population [1]. Thus, the high incidence of HBV infection in some clinical settings is particularly unfortunate because the modes of transmission are well known and readily interrupted by attention to work practices and protective equipment, and because transmission can be prevented by vaccination of those without serologic evidence of previous infection.

Identified risk factors for HIV transmission are essentially identical to those for HBV. Homosexual/bisexual males and male intravenous drug abusers account for 85.4% of all AIDS cases, female intravenous drug abusers for 3.4%, and heterosexual contact for 3.8% [9]. Blood transfusion and treatment of hemophilia/coagulation disorders account for 3.0% of cases, and 1.4% are pediatric cases. In only 3.0% of all AIDS cases has a risk factor not been identified [9]. Like HBV, there is no evidence that HIV is transmitted by casual contact, fecal-oral or airborne routes, or by contaminated food or drinking water [12-14], and barriers to HBV are effective against HIV. Workers are at risk of HIV infection to the extent they are directly exposed to blood and body fluids. Even in groups that presumably have high potential exposure to HIV-contaminated fluids and tissues, e.g., health-care workers specializing in treatment of AIDS patients and the parents, spouse, children, or other persons living with AIDS patients, transmission is recognized as occurring only between sexual partners or as a consequence of mucous membrane or parenteral (including open wound) exposure to blood or other body fluids [10,11,13-16].

Despite the similarities in the modes of transmission, the risk of HBV infection in health-care settings far exceeds that for HIV infection [13,14]. For example, it has been estimated [14,17,18] that the risk of acquiring HBV infection following puncture with a needle contaminated by an HBV carrier ranges from 6% to 30%—far in excess of the risk of HIV infection under similar circumstances, which the CDC and others estimated to be a less than 1% [10,13,16].

Health-care workers with documented percutaneous or mucous-membrane exposures to blood or body fluids of HIV-infected patients have

D-7

OSHA JOINT ADVISORY NOTICE OF THE DEPARTMENT OF LABOR AND THE DEPARTMENT OF HEALTH AND HUMAN SERVICES FOR THE PROTECTION AGAINST OCCUPATIONAL EXPOSURE TO HEPATITIS B VIRUS (HBV) AND HUMAN IMMUNODEFICIENCY VIRUS (HIV) Continued

been prospectively evaluated to determine the risk of infection after such exposures. As of June 30, 1987, 883 health-care workers have been tested for antibody to HIV in an ongoing surveillance project conducted by CDC [19]. Of these, 708 (80%) had percutaneous exposures to blood, and 175 (20%) had a mucous membrane or an open wound contaminated by blood or body fluid. Of 396 health-care workers, each of whom had only a convalescent-phase serum sample obtained and tested 90 days or more post-exposure, one—for whom heterosexual transmission could not be ruled out—was seropositive for HIV antibody. For 425 additional health-care workers, both acute- and convalescent-phase serum samples were obtained and tested; none of 74 health-care workers with nonpercutaneous exposures seroconverted, and three (0.9%) of 351 with percutaneous exposures seroconverted. None of these three health-care workers had other documented risk factors for infection.

Two other prospective studies to assess the risk of nosocomial acquisition of HIV infection for health-care workers are ongoing in the United States. As of April 30, 1987, 332 health-care workers with a total to 453 needlestick or mucous-membrane exposures to the blood or other body fluids of HIV-infected patients were tested for HIV antibody at the National Institutes of Health [20]. These exposed workers included 103 with needlestick injuries and 229 with mucous-membrane exposures; none had seroconverted. A similar study at the University of California of 129 health-care workers with documented needlestick injuries or mucous-membrane exposures to blood or other body fluids from patients with HIV infection has not identified any seroconversions [21]. Results of a prospective study in the United Kingdom identified no evidence of transmission among 150 health-care workers with parenteral or mucous-membrane exposure to blood or other body fluids, secretions, or excretions from patients with HIV infection [22].

Following needlestick injuries, one health-care worker contracted HBV but not HIV, and in another instance a health-care worker contracted cryptococcus but not HIV from patients infected with both [14]. This risk of infection by HIV and other blood-borne pathogens for which immunization is not available extends to all health-care workers exposed to blood, even those who have been immunized against HBV infection. Effective protection against blood-borne disease requires universal observation of common barrier precautions by all workers with potential exposure to blood, body fluids, and tissues [10,13].

HIV has been isolated from blood, semen, saliva, tears, urine, vaginal secretions, cerebrospinal fluid, breast milk, and amniotic fluid [10,23], but only blood and blood products, semen, vaginal secretions, and possibly breast milk (this needs to be confirmed) have been directly linked to transmission of HIV [10,13]. Contact with fluids such as saliva and tears has not been shown to result in infection [13-15]. Although other fluids have not been shown to transmit infection, all body fluids and tissues should be regarded as potentially contaminated by HBV or HIV, and treated as if they were infectious. Both HBV and HIV appear to be incapable of penetrating intact skin, but infection may result from infectious fluids coming into contact with mucous membranes or open wounds (including inapparent lesions) on the skin [14,16]. If a procedure involves the potential for skin contact with

D-7

OSHA JOINT ADVISORY NOTICE OF THE DEPARTMENT OF LABOR AND THE DEPARTMENT OF HEALTH AND HUMAN SERVICES FOR THE PROTECTION AGAINST OCCUPATIONAL EXPOSURE TO HEPATITIS B VIRUS (HBV) AND HUMAN IMMUNODEFICIENCY VIRUS (HIV) *Continued*

blood or mucous membranes, then appropriate barriers to skin contact should be worn, e.g., gloves. Investigations of HBV risks associated with dental and other procedures that might produce particulates in air, e.g., centrifuging and dialysis, indicated that the particulates generated were relatively large droplets (spatter), and not true aerosols of suspended particulates that would represent a risk of inhalation exposure [24-26]. Thus, if there is the potential for splashes or spatter of blood or fluids, face shields or protective eyewear and surgical masks should be worn. Detailed protective measures for health-care workers have been addressed by the CDC [10,13,23,27-33]. These can serve as general guides for the specific groups covered, and for the development of comparable procedures in other working environments.

HIV infection is known to have been transmitted by organ transplants [34] and blood transfusions [35] received from persons who were HIV seronegative at the time of donation. Falsely negative serology can be due to improperly performed tests or other laboratory error, or testing in that "window" of time during which a recently infected person is infective but has not yet converted from seronegative to seropositive. (Detectable levels of antibodies usually develop within 6 to 12 weeks of infection [36]. A recent report [37] suggesting that this "window" may extend to 14 months is not consistent with other data, and therefore requires confirmation.) If all body fluids and tissues are treated as infectious, no additional level of worker protection will be gained by identifying seropositive patients or workers. Conversely, if worker protection and work practices were upgraded only following the return of positive HBV or HIV serology, then workers would be inadequately protected during the time required for testing. By producing a false sense of safety with "silent" HBV- or HIV-positive patients, a seronegative test may significantly reduce the level of routine vigilance and result in virus exposure. Furthermore, developing, implementing, and administering a program of routine testing would shift resources and energy away from efforts to assure compliance with infection control procedures. Therefore, routine screening of workers or patients for HIV antibodies will not substantially increase the level of protection for workers above that achieved by adherence to strict infection control procedures.

On the other hand, workers who have had parenteral exposure to fluids or tissues may wish to know whether their own antibody status converts from negative to positive. Such a monitoring program can lead to prophylactic interventions in the case of HBV infection, and CDC has published guidelines on pre- and post-exposure prophylaxis of viral hepatitis [1,2]. Future developments may also allow effective intervention in the case of HIV infection. For the present, post-exposure monitoring for HIV at least can release the affected worker from unnecessary emotional stress if infection did not occur, or allow the affected worker to protect sexual partners in the event infection is detected [10,36].

III. Summary:

The cumulative epidemiologic data indicate that transmission of HBV and HIV requires direct, intimate contact with or parenteral inoculation of blood and blood products, semen, or tissues [10,11,13,14,16,23]. The mere pres-

D-7

OSHA JOINT ADVISORY NOTICE OF THE DEPARTMENT OF LABOR AND THE DEPARTMENT OF HEALTH AND HUMAN SERVICES FOR THE PROTECTION AGAINST OCCUPATIONAL EXPOSURE TO HEPATITIS B VIRUS (HBV) AND HUMAN IMMUNODEFICIENCY VIRUS (HIV) *Continued*

ence of, or casual contact with, an infected person cannot be construed as "exposure" to HBV or HIV. Although the theoretical possibility of rare or low-risk alternative modes of transmission cannot be totally excluded, the only documented occupational risks of HBV and HIV infection are associated with parenteral (including open wound) and mucous membrane exposure to blood and tissues [2,10,13,14,16]. Workers occupationally exposed to blood, body fluids, or tissues can be protected from the recognized risks of HBV and HIV infection by imposing barriers in the form of engineering controls, work practices, and protective equipment that are readily available, commonly used, and minimally intrusive.

IV. Recommendations:

General

"Exposure" (or "potential exposure") to HBV and HIV should be defined in terms of actual (or potential) skin, mucous membrane, or parenteral contact with blood, body fluids, and tissues. "Tissues" and "fluids" or "body fluids" should be understood to designate not only those materials from humans, but also potentially infectious fluids and tissues associated with laboratory investigations of HBV or HIV, e.g., organs and excreta from experimental animals, embryonated eggs, tissue or cell cultures and culture media, etc.

As the first step in determining what actions are required to protect worker health, every employer should evaluate all working conditions and the specific tasks that workers are expected to encounter as a consequence of employment. That evaluation should lead to the classification of work-related tasks to one of three categories of potential exposure (Table 1). These categories represent those tasks that require protective equipment to be worn during the task (Category I); tasks that do not require any protective equipment (Category III); and an intermediate grouping of tasks (Category II) that also do not require protective equipment, but that inherently include the predictable job-related requirement to perform Category I tasks unexpectedly or on short notice, so that these persons should have immediate access to some minimal set of protective devices. For example, law enforcement personnel or firefighters may be called upon to perform or assist in first aid or to be potentially exposed in some other way. This exposure classification applies to tasks rather than to individuals, who in the course of their daily activities may move from one exposure category to another as they perform various tasks.

For individual Category I and II tasks, engineering controls, work practices, and protective equipment should be selected after careful consideration, for each specific situation, of the overall risk associated with the task. Factors that should be included in that evaluation of risk include:

1. Type of body fluid with which there will or may be contact (e.g., blood is of greater concern than urine),
2. Volume of blood or body fluid likely to be encountered (e.g., hip replacement surgery can be very bloody while corneal transplantation is almost bloodless),

D-7

OSHA JOINT ADVISORY NOTICE OF THE DEPARTMENT OF LABOR AND THE DEPARTMENT OF HEALTH AND HUMAN SERVICES FOR THE PROTECTION AGAINST OCCUPATIONAL EXPOSURE TO HEPATITIS B VIRUS (HBV) AND HUMAN IMMUNODEFICIENCY VIRUS (HIV) Continued

3. Probability of an exposure taking place (e.g., drawing blood will more likely lead to exposure to blood than will performing a physical examination),
4. Probable route of exposure (e.g., needlestick injuries are of greater concern than contact with soiled linens), and
5. Virus concentration in the fluid or tissue. The number of viruses per milliliter of fluid in research laboratory cultures may be orders of magnitude higher than in blood. Similarly, viruses have been less frequently found in fluids such as sweat, tears, urine, and saliva.

Engineering controls, work practices, and protective equipment appropriate to the task being performed are critical to minimize HBV and HIV exposure and to prevent infection. Adequate protection can be assured only if the appropriate controls and equipment are provided and all workers know the applicable work practices and how to properly use the required controls or protective equipment. Therefore, employers should establish a detailed work practices program that includes standard operating procedures (SOPs) for all tasks or work areas having the potential for exposure to fluids or tissues, and a worker education program to assure familiarity with work practices and the ability to use properly the controls and equipment provided.

It is essential for both the patient and the health-care worker to be fully aware of the reasons for the preventive measures used. The health-care worker may incorrectly interpret the work practices and protective equipment as signifying that a task is unsafe. The patient may incorrectly interpret the work practices or protective garb as evidence that the health-care

TABLE 1. EXPOSURE CATEGORIES

CATEGORY I. Tasks That Involve Exposure To Blood, Body Fluids, Or Tissues.

All procedures or other job-related tasks that involve an inherent potential for mucous membrane or skin contact with blood, body fluids, or tissues, or a potential for spills or splashes of them, are Category I tasks. Use of appropriate protective measures should be required for every employee engaged in Category I tasks.

CATEGORY II. Tasks That Involve No Exposure To Blood, Body Fluids, Or Tissues, But Employment May Require Performing Unplanned Category I Tasks.

The normal work routine involves no exposure to blood, body fluids, or tissues, but exposure or potential exposure may be required as a condition of employment. Appropriate protective measures should be readily available to every employee engaged in Category II tasks.

CATEGORY III. Tasks That Involve No Exposure To Blood, Body Fluids, Or Tissues, And Category I Tasks Are Not A Condition Of Employment.

The normal work routine involves no exposure to blood, body fluids, or tissues (although situations can be imagined or hypothesized under which anyone, anywhere, might encounter potential exposure to body fluids). Persons who perform these duties are not called upon as part of their employment to perform or assist in emergency medical care or first aid or to be potentially exposed in some other way. Tasks that involve handling of implements or utensils, use of public or shared bathroom facilities or telephones, and personal contacts such as handshaking are Category III tasks.

D-7
OSHA JOINT ADVISORY NOTICE OF THE DEPARTMENT OF LABOR AND THE DEPARTMENT OF HEALTH AND HUMAN SERVICES FOR THE PROTECTION AGAINST OCCUPATIONAL EXPOSURE TO HEPATITIS B VIRUS (HBV) AND HUMAN IMMUNODEFICIENCY VIRUS (HIV) *Continued*

provider knows or believes the patient is infected with HBV or HIV. Therefore, worker education programs should strive to allow workers (and to the extent feasible, the clients or patients) to recognize the routine use of appropriate work practices and protective equipment as prudent steps that protect the health of all.

If the employer determines that Category I and II tasks do not exist in the workplace, then no specific personal hygiene or protective measures are required. However, these employers should ensure that workers are aware of the risk factors associated with transmission of HBV and HIV so that they can recognize situations which pose increased potential for exposure to HBV or HIV (Category I tasks) and know how to avoid or minimize personal risk. A comparable level of education is necessary for all citizens. Educational materials such as the Surgeon General's Report can provide much of the needed information [12,38].

If the employer determines that work-related Category I or II tasks exist, then the following procedures should be implemented.

Administrative

The employer should establish formal procedures to ensure that Category I and II tasks are properly identified, SOPs are developed, and employees who must perform these tasks are adequately trained and protected. If responsibility for implementation of these responsibilities is delegated to a committee, it should include both management and worker representatives. Administrative activities to enhance worker protection include:

1. Evaluating the workplace to:
    a. Establish category of risk classifications for all routine and reasonably anticipated job-related tasks.
    b. Identify all workers whose employment requires performance of Category I or II tasks.
    c. Determine for identified Category I or II tasks those body fluids to which workers most probably will be exposed and the potential extent and route of exposure.
2. Developing, or supervising the development of, Standard Operating Procedures (SOPs) for each Category I and II task. These SOPs should include mandatory work practices and protective equipment for each Category I and II task.
3. Monitoring the effectiveness of work practices and protective equipment. This includes:
    a. Surveillance of the workplace to ensure that required work practices are observed and that protective clothing and equipment are provided and properly used.
    b. Investigation of known or suspected parenteral exposures to body fluids or tissues to establish the conditions surrounding the exposure and to improve training, work practices, or protective equipment to prevent a recurrence.

OSHA JOINT ADVISORY NOTICE OF THE DEPARTMENT OF LABOR AND THE DEPARTMENT OF HEALTH AND HUMAN SERVICES FOR THE PROTECTION AGAINST OCCUPATIONAL EXPOSURE TO HEPATITIS B VIRUS (HBV) AND HUMAN IMMUNODEFICIENCY VIRUS (HIV) *Continued*

Training and Education

The employer should establish an initial and periodic training program for all employees who perform Category I and II tasks. No worker should engage in any Category I or II task before receiving training pertaining to the SOPs, work practices, and protective equipment required for that task. The training program should ensure that all workers:

1. Understand the modes of transmission of HBV and HIV.
2. Can recognize and differentiate Category I and II tasks.
3. Know the types of protective clothing and equipment generally appropriate for Category I and II tasks, and understand the basis for selection of clothing and equipment.
4. Are familiar with appropriate actions to take and persons to contact if unplanned Category I tasks are encountered.
5. Are familiar with and understand all the requirements for work practices and protective equipment specified in SOPs covering the tasks they perform.
6. Know where protective clothing and equipment is kept, how to use it properly, and how to remove, handle, decontaminate, and dispose of contaminated clothing or equipment.
7. Know and understand the limitations of protective clothing and equipment. For example, ordinary gloves offer no protection against needlestick injuries. Employers and workers should be on guard against a sense of security not warranted by the protective equipment being used.
8. Know the corrective actions to take in the event of spills or personal exposure to fluids or tissues, the appropriate reporting procedures, and the medical monitoring recommended in cases of suspected parenteral exposure.

Engineering Controls

Whenever possible, engineering controls should be used as the primary method to reduce worker exposure to harmful substances. The preferred approach in engineering controls is to use, to the fullest extent feasible, intrinsically safe substances, procedures, or devices. Substitution of a hazardous procedure or device with one that is less risky or harmful is an example of this approach, e.g., a laser scalpel reduces the risk of cuts and scrapes by eliminating the necessity to handle the conventional scalpel blade.

Isolation or containment of the hazard is an alternative engineering control technique. Disposable, puncture-resistant containers for used needles, blades, etc., isolate cut and needlestick injury hazards from the worker. Glove boxes, ventilated cabinets, or other enclosures for tissue homogenizers, sonicators, vortex mixers, etc. serve not only to isolate the hazard, but also to contain spills or splashes and prevent spatter and mist from reaching the worker.

After the potential for exposure has been minimized by engineering controls, further reductions can be achieved by work practices and, finally, personal protective equipment.

D-7
OSHA JOINT ADVISORY NOTICE OF THE DEPARTMENT OF LABOR AND THE DEPARTMENT OF HEALTH AND HUMAN SERVICES FOR THE PROTECTION AGAINST OCCUPATIONAL EXPOSURE TO HEPATITIS B VIRUS (HBV) AND HUMAN IMMUNODEFICIENCY VIRUS (HIV) *Continued*

Work Practices

For all identified Category I and II tasks, the employer should have written, detailed Standard Operating Procedures (SOPs). All employees who perform Category I or II tasks should have ready access to the SOPs pertaining to those tasks.

1. Work practices should be developed on the assumption that all body fluids and tissues are infectious. General procedures to protect healthcare workers against HBV or HIV transmission have been published elsewhere [1, 2, 23,28-33]. Each employer with Category I and II tasks in the workplace should incorporate those general recommendations, as appropriate, or equivalent procedures into work practices and SOPs. The importance of handwashing should be emphasized.

2. Work practices should include provision for safe collection of fluids and tissues and for disposal in accordance with applicable local, state, and federal regulations. Provision must be made for safe removal, handling, and disposal or decontamination of protective clothing and equipment, soiled linens, etc.

3. Work practices and SOPs should provide guidance on procedures to follow in the event of spills or personal exposure to fluids or tissues. These procedures should include instructions for personal and area decontamination as well as appropriate management or supervisory personnel to whom the incident should be reported.

4. Work practices should provide specific and detailed procedures to be observed with sharp objects, e.g., needles, scalpel blades. Puncture-resistant receptacles must be readily accessible for depositing these materials after use. These receptacles must be clearly marked and specific work practices provided to protect personnel responsible for disposing of them or processing their contents for reuse.

Personal Protective Equipment

Based upon the fluid or tissue to which there is potential exposure, the likelihood of exposure occurring, the potential volume of material, the probable route of exposure, and overall working conditions and job requirements, the employer should provide and maintain personal protective equipment appropriate to the specific requirements of each task.

For workers performing Category I tasks, a required minimum array of protective clothing or equipment should be specified by pertinent SOPs. All Category I tasks do not involve the same type or degree of risk, and therefore all do not require the same kind or extent of protection. Specific combinations of clothing and equipment must be tailored to specific tasks. Minimum levels of protection for Category I tasks in most cases would include use of appropriate gloves. If there is the potential for splashes, protective eyewear or face shields should be worn. Paramedics responding to an auto accident might protect against cuts on metal and glass by wearing gloves or gauntlets that are both puncture-resistant and impervious to blood. If the conditions of exposure include the potential for clothing becoming soaked with blood, protective outer garments such as impervious coveralls should be worn.

For workers performing Category II tasks, there should be ready access to appropriate protective equipment, e.g., gloves, protective eyewear, or surgi-

OSHA JOINT ADVISORY NOTICE OF THE DEPARTMENT OF LABOR AND THE DEPARTMENT OF HEALTH AND HUMAN SERVICES FOR THE PROTECTION AGAINST OCCUPATIONAL EXPOSURE TO HEPATITIS B VIRUS (HBV) AND HUMAN IMMUNODEFICIENCY VIRUS (HIV) Continued

cal masks, specified in pertinent SOPs. Workers performing Category II tasks need not be wearing protective equipment, but they should be prepared to put on appropriate protective garb on short notice.

Medical

In addition to any health-care or surveillance required by other rules, regulations, or labor-management agreement, the employer should make available at no cost to the worker:

1. Voluntary HBV immunization for all workers whose employment requires them to perform Category I tasks and who test negative for HBV antibodies. Detailed recommendations for protecting health-care workers from viral hepatitis have been published by the CDC [1]. These recommendations include procedures for both pre- and post-exposure prophylaxis, and should be the basis for the routine approach by management to the prevention of occupational hepatitis B.

2. Monitoring, at the request of the worker, for HBV and HIV antibodies following known or suspected parenteral exposure to blood, body fluids, or tissues. This monitoring program must include appropriate provisions to protect the confidentiality of test results for all workers who may elect to participate.

3. Medical counseling for all workers found, as a result of the monitoring described above, to be seropositive for HBV or HIV. Counseling guidelines have been published by the Public Health Service [1, 2, 36].

Recordkeeping

If any employee is required to perform Category I or II tasks, the employer should maintain records documenting:

1. The administrative procedures used to classify job tasks. Records should describe the factors considered and outline the rationale for classification.

2. Copies of all SOPs for Category I and II tasks, and documentation of the administrative review and approval process through which each SOP passed.

3. Training records, indicating the dates of training sessions, the content of those training sessions along with the names of all persons conducting the training, and the names of all those receiving training.

4. The conditions observed in routine surveillance of the workplace for compliance with work practices and use of protective clothing or equipment. If noncompliance is noted, the conditions should be documented along with corrective actions taken.

5. The conditions associated with each incident of mucous membrane or parenteral exposure to body fluids or tissue, an evaluation of those conditions, and a description of any corrective measures taken to prevent a recurrence or other similar exposure.

D-7
OSHA JOINT ADVISORY NOTICE OF THE DEPARTMENT OF LABOR AND THE DEPARTMENT OF HEALTH AND HUMAN SERVICES FOR THE PROTECTION AGAINST OCCUPATIONAL EXPOSURE TO HEPATITIS B VIRUS (HBV) AND HUMAN IMMUNODEFICIENCY VIRUS (HIV) *Continued*

References

1. Centers for Disease Control: Recommendations for protection against viral hepatitis. Morbidity and Mortality Weekly Report 34:313-24, 329-35, 7 June 1985.
2. Centers for Disease Control: Update on hepatitis B prevention. Morbidity and Mortality Weekly Report 36:353-60, 19 June 1987.
3. Palmer D. L., Barash, M., King, R., and Neil, F.: Hepatitis among hospital employees. Western J Med 138:519-523, 1983.
4. Grady, G. F. and Kane, M. A.: Hepatitis B infections account for multi-million dollar loss. Hosp Infect Contr 8:60-62, 1981.
5. Centers for Disease Control: Hepatitis B virus vaccine safety—Report of an inter-agency group. Morbidity and Mortality Weekly Report 31:465-67, 3 September 1982.
6. Centers for Disease Control: The safety of hepatitis B virus vaccine. Morbidity and Mortality Weekly Report 32:134-36, 18 March 1983.
7. Centers for Disease Control: Hepatitis B vaccine—Evidence confirming lack of AIDS transmission. Morbidity and Mortality Weekly Report 33:685-87, 14 December 1984.
8. Centers for Disease Control: Changes in premature mortality—United States, 1984-1985. Morbidity and Mortality Weekly Report 36:55-57, 6 February 1987.
9. Centers for Disease Control: Update—Acquired immunodeficiency syndrome—United States. Morbidity and Mortality Weekly Report Supplement, 36:522-526, 14 August 1987.
10. Centers for Disease Control: Recommendations for prevention of HIV transmission in health-care settings. Morbidity and Mortality Weekly Report Supplement, 36(2S):1S-16S, 21 August 1987.
11. Centers for Disease Control: Update—Acquired immunodeficiency syndrome—United States. Morbidity and Mortality Weekly Report 35:757-66, 12 December 1986.
12. Koop, C. E.: Surgeon General's Report on Acquired Immune Deficiency Syndrome, US DHHS, October, 1986, 36 pp.
13. Centers for Disease Control: Recommendations for preventing transmission of infection with human T-lymphotrophic virus type III/lymphadenopathy-associated virus in the workplace. Morbidity and Mortality Weekly Report 34:681-86, 691-95, 15 November 1985.
14. Vlahov, D., Polk, B. F.: Transmission of human immunodeficiency virus within the health care setting. Occup Med State of the Art Reviews 2:429-450, 1987.
15. Gestal, J. J.: Occupational hazards in hospitals—Risk of infection. Br J Ind Med 44:435-442, 1987.
16. Centers for Disease Control: Update—Human immunodeficiency virus infections in health-care workers exposed to blood of infected patients. Morbidity and Mortality Weekly Report 36:285-89, 22 May 1987.
17. Grady, G. F., Lee, V. A., Prince, A. m., et al.: Hepatitis B immune globulin for accidental exposures among medical personnel—Final report of a multicenter controlled trial. J Infect Dis 138:625-638, 1978.
18. Seeff, L. B., Wright, E. C., Zimmerman, H. J., et al.: Type B hepatitis after needlestick exposure—Prevention with hepatitis B immune globulin. Ann Intern Med 88:285-293, 1978.
19. McCray, E.: The cooperative needlestick surveillance group. Occupational risk of the acquired immunodeficiency syndrome among health care workers. N Engl J Med 314:1127-1132, 1986.
20. Henderson, D. K., Saah, A. J., Zak, B. J., et al.: Risk of nosocomial infection with human T-cell lymphotropic virus type III/lymphadenopathy-associated virus in a large cohort of intensively exposed health care workers. Ann Intern Med 104:644-647, 1986.
21. Gerberding J. L., Bryant-LeBlanc, C. E., Nelson, K., et al: Risk of transmitting the human immunodeficiency virus, cytomegalovirus, and hepatitis B virus to health care workers exposed to patients with AIDS and AIDS-related conditions. J Infect Dis 156:1-8, 1987.

D-7

OSHA JOINT ADVISORY NOTICE OF THE DEPARTMENT OF LABOR AND THE DEPARTMENT OF HEALTH AND HUMAN SERVICES FOR THE PROTECTION AGAINST OCCUPATIONAL EXPOSURE TO HEPATITIS B VIRUS (HBV) AND HUMAN IMMUNODEFICIENCY VIRUS (HIV) *Continued*

22. McEvoy, M., Porter, K., Mortimer, P., Simmons, N., Shanson, D.: Prospective study of clinical, laboratory, and ancillary staff with accidental exposures to blood or other body fluids from patients infected with HIV. Br Med J 294:1595-1597, 1987.
23. Centers for Disease Control: Human T-lymphotrophic virus, type III/lymphadenopathy-associated virus—Agent summary statement. Morbidity and Mortality Weekly Report 35:540-42, 547-49, 29 August 1986.
24. Petersen, N. J., Bond, W. W., Favero, M. S.: Air sampling for hepatitis B surface antigen in a dental operatory. J Am Dental Assoc 99:465-467, 1979.
25. Scarlett, M.: Infection control practices in dentistry, in Proceedings of the National Conference on Infection Control in Dentistry, Chicago, May 13-14, 1986, pp 41-51.
26. Bond, W. W.: Modes of transmission of infectious diseases, in Proceedings of the National Conference on Infection Control in Dentistry, Chicago, May 13-14, 1986, pp 29-35.
27. Centers for Disease Control: Recommendations for preventing transmission of infection with human T-lymphotrophic virus type III/lymphadenopathy- associated virus during invasive procedures. Morbidity and Mortality Weekly Report 35:221-23, 11 April 1986.
28. Centers for Disease Control: Acquired immune deficiency syndrome (AIDS)—Precautions for clinical and laboratory staffs. Morbidity and Mortality Weekly Report 31:577-80, 5 November 1982.
29. Centers for Disease Control: Acquired immunodeficiency syndrome (AIDS)—Precautions for health-care workers and allied professionals. Morbidity and Mortality Weekly Report 32:450-452, 2 September 1983.
30. Centers for Disease Control: Recommendations for preventing possible transmission of human T-lymphotrophic virus type III/lymphadenopathy- associated virus from tears. Morbidity and Mortality Weekly Report 34:533-34, 30 August 1985.
31. Centers for Disease Control: Recommended infection-control practices for dentistry. Morbidity and Mortality Weekly Report 35:237-42, 18 April 1986.
32. Centers for Disease Control: Recommendations for providing dialysis treatment to patients infected with human T-lymphotrophic virus, type III/lymphadenopathy- associated virus. Morbidity and Mortality Weekly Report 35:376-78, 383, 13 June 1986.
33. Williams, W. W.: Guidelines for infection control in hospital personnel. Infect Control 4:326-349, 1983.
34. Centers for Disease Control: Human immunodeficiency virus infections transmitted from an organ donor screened for HIV antibody—North Carolina. Morbidity and Mortality Weekly Report 36:306-8, 29 May 1987.
35. Centers for Disease Control: Transfusion-associated human T-lymphotrophic virus type III/lymphadenopathy-associated virus infection from a seronegative donor - Colorado. Morbidity and Mortality Weekly Report 35:389-91, 20 June 1986.
36. Centers for Disease Control: Public Health Service guidelines for counseling and antibody testing to prevent HIV infection and AIDS. Morbidity and Mortality Weekly Report, 36:509-515, 14 August 1987.
37. Ranki, A., Valle, S.-L., Krohn, M., Antonen, J., Allain, J.-P., Leuther, M., Franchini, G., and Krohn, K.: Long latency precedes overt seroconversion in sexually transmitted human-immunodeficiency-virus infection. Lancet 2(8559):589-593, 1987.
38. Centers for Disease Control: Facts About AIDS. US DHHS, Spring 1987, 9 pp.

D-7

OSHA JOINT ADVISORY NOTICE OF THE DEPARTMENT OF LABOR AND THE DEPARTMENT OF HEALTH AND HUMAN SERVICES FOR THE PROTECTION AGAINST OCCUPATIONAL EXPOSURE TO HEPATITIS B VIRUS (HBV) AND HUMAN IMMUNODEFICIENCY VIRUS (HIV) Continued

References Not Cited

Centers for Disease Control: Update on acquired immune deficiency syndrome (AIDS) United States. Morbidity and Mortality Weekly Report 31:507-14, 24 September 1982.

Centers for Disease Control: Prevention of acquired immune deficiency syndrome (AIDS)—Report of interagency recommendations. Morbidity and Mortality Weekly Report 32:101-4, 4 March 1983.

Centers for Disease Control: Acquired immunodeficiency syndrome (AIDS) update—United States. Morbidity and Mortality Weekly Report 32:309-11, 24 June 1983.

Centers for Disease Control: An evaluation of the acquired immunodeficiency syndrome (AIDS) reported in health-care personnel—United States. Morbidity and Mortality Weekly Report 32:358-60, 15 July 1983.

Centers for Disease Control: Update—Acquired immunodeficiency syndrome (AIDS)—United States. Morbidity and Mortality Weekly Report 32:389-91, 5 August 1983.

Centers for Disease Control: Update—Acquired immunodeficiency syndrome (AIDS)—United States. Morbidity and Mortality Weekly Report 32:465-67, 9 September 1983.

Centers for Disease Control: Update—Acquired immunodeficiency syndrome (AIDS)—United States. Morbidity and Mortality Weekly Report 32:688-91, 6 January 1984.

Centers for Disease Control: Prospective evaluation of health-care workers exposed via parenteral or mucous-membrane routes to blood and body fluids of patients with acquired immunodeficiency syndrome. Morbidity and Mortality Weekly Report 33:181-82, 6 April 1984.

Centers for Disease Control: Update—Acquired immunodeficiency syndrome (AIDS)—United States. Morbidity and Mortality Weekly Report 33:337-39, 22 June 1984.

Centers for Disease Control: Update—Acquired immunodeficiency syndrome (AIDS)—United States. Morbidity and Mortality Weekly Report 33:661-64, 30 November 1984.

Centers for Disease Control: Update—Prospective evaluation of health-care workers exposed via the parenteral or mucous-membrane route to blood and body fluids of patients with AIDS—United States. Morbidity and Mortality Weekly Report 34:101-3, 22 February 1985.

Centers for Disease Control: Update—Acquired immunodeficiency syndrome (AIDS)—United States. Morbidity and Mortality Weekly Report 34:245-48, 10 May 1985.

Centers for Disease Control: Education and foster care of children infected with human T-lymphotrophic virus type III/lymphadenopathy- associated virus. Morbidity and Mortality Weekly Report 34:517-21, 30 August 1985.

Centers for Disease Control: Update—Evaluation of human T-lymphotrophic virus type III/lymphadenopathy-associated virus infection in health-care personnel—United States. Morbidity and Mortality Weekly Report 34:575-78, 27 September 1985.

Centers for Disease Control: Update—Acquired immunodeficiency syndrome (AIDS)—United States. Morbidity and Mortality Weekly Report 35:17-21, 17 January 1986.

Centers for Disease Control: Apparent transmission of human T-lymphotrophic virus type III/lymphadenopathy-associated virus from a child to a mother providing health care. Morbidity and Mortality Weekly Report 35:76-79, 7 February 1986.

Centers for Disease Control: Safety of therapeutic immune globulin preparations with respect to transmission of human T-lymphotrophic virus type III/lymphadenopathy-associated virus infection. Morbidity and Mortality Weekly Report 35:231-33, 11 April 1986.

OSHA JOINT ADVISORY NOTICE OF THE DEPARTMENT OF LABOR AND THE DEPARTMENT OF HEALTH AND HUMAN SERVICES FOR THE PROTECTION AGAINST OCCUPATIONAL EXPOSURE TO HEPATITIS B VIRUS (HBV) AND HUMAN IMMUNODEFICIENCY VIRUS (HIV) *Continued*

Centers for Disease Control: Acquired immunodeficiency syndrome (AIDS) in Western Palm Beach County, Florida. Morbidity and Mortality Weekly Report 35:609-12, 3 October 1986.

Centers for Disease Control: Availability of informational material on AIDS. Morbidity and Mortality Weekly Report 35:819-20, 9 January 1987.

Centers for Disease Control: Survey of non-U.S. hemophilia treatment centers for HIV seroconversions following therapy with heat-treated factor concentrates. Morbidity and Mortality Weekly Report 36:121-24, 13 March 1987.

Centers for Disease Control: Tuberculosis and AIDS—Connecticut. Morbidity and Mortality Weekly Report 36:133-35, 13 March 1987.

Centers for Disease Control: Human immunodeficiency virus infection in transfusion recipients and their family members. Morbidity and Mortality Weekly Report 36:137-40, 20 March 1987.

Centers for Disease Control: Antibody to human immunodeficiency virus in female prostitutes. Morbidity and Mortality Weekly Report 36:157-61, 27 March 1987.

Centers for Disease Control: Self-reported changes in sexual behaviors among homosexual and bisexual men from the San Francisco City Clinic cohort. Morbidity and Mortality Weekly Report 36:187-89, 3 April 1987.

Centers for Disease Control: Classification system for human immunodeficiency virus (HIV) infection in children under 13 years of age. Morbidity and Mortality Weekly Report 36:225-30, 235-36, 24 April 1987.

Centers for Disease Control: Tuberculosis provisional data—United States, 1986. Morbidity and Mortality Weekly Report 36:254-55, 1 May 1987.

Centers for Disease Control: Trends in human immunodeficiency virus infection among civilian applicants for military service—United States, October 1985 - December 1986. Morbidity and Mortality Weekly Report 36:273-76, 15 May 1987.

For further information call: National OSHA Information Office, (202) 523-8148.

From the Department of Labor/Department of Health and Human Services: Joint Advisory Notice—Protection Against Occupational Exposure to Hepatitis B Virus (HBV) and Human Deficiency Virus (HIV), October 19, 1987.

D-8
OSHA GUIDELINES TO DEVELOPING A FACILITY BLOODBORNE PATHOGENS EXPOSURE CONTROL PLAN

Note: This sample plan is provided only as a guide to assist in complying with 29 CFR 1910.1030, OSHA's Bloodborne Pathogens standard. It is not intended to supersede the requirements detailed in the standard. Employers should review the standard for particular requirements which are applicable to their specific situation. It should be noted that this sample program does not include provisions for HIV/HBV laboratories and research facilities which are addressed in section (e) of the standard. Employers operating these laboratories need to include provisions as required by the standard. Employers will need to add information relevant to their particular facility in order to develop an effective, comprehensive exposure control plan. Employers should note that the exposure control plan is expected to be reviewed at least on an annual basis and updated when necessary.

(revision 1)

BLOODBORNE PATHOGENS EXPOSURE CONTROL PLAN

Facility Name: _____

Date of Preparation: _____

In accordance with the OSHA Bloodborne Pathogens standard, 29 CFR 1910.1030, the following exposure control plan has been developed:

1. Exposure Determination

OSHA requires employers to perform an exposure determination concerning which employees may incur occupational exposure to blood or other potentially infectious materials. The exposure determination is made without regard to the use of personal protective equipment (i.e., employees are considered to be exposed even if they wear personal protective equipment). This exposure determinization is required to list all job classifications in which all employees may be expected to incur such occupational exposure, regardless of frequency. At this facility the following job classifications are in this category:

In addition, if the employer has job classifications in which some employees may have occupational exposure, then a listing of those classifications is required. Since not all the employees in these categories would be expected to incur exposure to blood or other potentially infectious materials, tasks or procedures that would cause these employees to have occupational exposure are also required to be listed in order to clearly understand which employees in these categories are considered to have occupational exposure. The job classifications and associated tasks/procedures for these categories are as follows:

Job Classification	Tasks/Procedures

2. Implementation Schedule and Methodology

OSHA also requires that this plan also include a schedule and method of implementation for the various requirements of the standard. The following complies with this requirement:

Compliance Methods

Universal precautions will be observed at this facility in order to prevent contact with blood or other potentially infectious materials. All blood or other potentially infectious materials will be considered infectious regardless of the perceived status of the source individual.

Engineering and work practice controls will be utilized to eliminate or minimize exposure to employees at this facility. Where occupational exposure remains after institution of these controls, personal protective equipment shall also be utilized. At this facility the following engineering controls will be utilized: *(List controls, such as sharps containers, etc.)*

D-8

OSHA GUIDELINES TO DEVELOPING A FACILITY BLOODBORNE PATHOGENS EXPOSURE CONTROL PLAN
Continued

The above controls will be examined and maintained on a regular schedule. The schedule for reviewing the effectiveness of the controls is as follows: *(List schedule such as daily, once/week, etc. as well as list who has the responsibility to review the effectiveness of the individual controls, such as the supervisor for each department, etc.)*

Handwashing facilities are also available to the employees who incur exposure to blood or other potentially infectious materials. OSHA requires that these facilities be readily accessible after incurring exposure. At this facility handwashing facilities are located: *(List locations, such as patient rooms, procedure area, etc. If handwashing facilities are not feasible, the employer is required to provide either an antiseptic cleanser in conjunction with a clean cloth/paper towels or antiseptic towelettes. If these alternatives are used, then the hands are to be washed with soap and running water as soon as feasible. Employers who must provide alternatives to readily accessible handwashing facilities should list the location, tasks, and responsibilities to ensure maintenance and accessibility of these alternatives.)*

After removal of personal protective gloves, employees shall wash hands and any other potentially contaminated skin area immediately or as soon as feasible with soap and water.

If employees incur exposure to their skin or mucous membranes, then those areas shall be washed or flushed with water as appropriate as soon as feasible following contact.

Needles

Contaminated needles and other contaminated sharps will not be bent, recapped, removed, sheared or purposely broken. OSHA allows an exception to this if the procedure would require that the contaminated needle be recapped or removed and no alternative is feasible and the action is required by the medical procedure. If such action is required, then the recapping or removal of the needle must be done by the use of a mechanical device or a one-handed technique. At this facility recapping or removal is only permitted for the following procedures: *(List the procedures and also list the mechanical device to be used or alternately if a one-handed technique will be used.)*

Containers for Reusable Sharps

Contaminated sharps that are reusable are to be placed immediately, or as soon as possible, after use into appropriate sharps containers. At this facility the sharps containers are puncture resistant, labeled with a biohazard label, and are leak proof. *(Employers should list here where sharps containers are located as well as who has responsibility for removing sharps from containers and how often the containers will be checked to remove the sharps.)*

Work Area Restrictions

In work areas where there is a reasonable likelihood of exposure to blood or other potentially infectious materials, employees are not to eat, drink, apply cosmetics or lip balm, smoke, or handle contact lenses. Food and beverages are not to be kept in refrigerators, freezers, shelves, cabinets, or on counter tops or bench tops where blood or other potentially infectious materials are present.

Mouth pipetting/suctioning of blood or potentially infectious materials is prohibited.

All procedures will be conducted in a manner which will minimize splashing, spraying, splattering, and generation of droplets of blood or other potentially infectious materials. Methods which will be employed at this facility to accomplish this goal are: *(List methods, such as covers on centrifuges, usage of dental dams if appropriate, etc.).*

D-8

OSHA GUIDELINES TO DEVELOPING A FACILITY BLOODBORNE PATHOGENS EXPOSURE CONTROL PLAN
Continued

Specimens

Specimens of blood or other potentially infectious materials will be placed in a container which prevents leakage during the collection, handling, processing, storage, and transport of the specimens.

The container used for this purpose will be labeled or color coded in accordance with the requirements of the OSHA standard. *(Employers should note that the standard provides for an exemption for specimens from the labeling/color coding requirement of the standard provided that the facility utilizes universal precautions in the handling of all specimens and the containers are recognizable as containing specimens. This exemption applies only while the specimens remain in the facility. If the employer chooses to use this exemption then it should be stated here. _____)*

Any specimens which could puncture a primary container will be placed within a secondary container which is puncture resistant. *(The employer should list here how this will be carried out, e.g., which specimens, if any, could puncture a primary container, which containers can be used as secondary containers and where the secondary containers are located at the facility.)*

If outside contamination of the primary container occurs, the primary container shall be placed within a secondary container which prevents leakage during the handling, processing, storage, transport, or shipping of the specimen.

Contaminated Equipment

Equipment which has become contaminated with blood or other potentially infectious materials shall be examined prior to servicing or shipping and shall be decontaminated as necessary unless the decontamination of the equipment is not feasible. *(Employers should list here any equipment which it is felt can not be decontaminated prior to servicing or shipping. _____)*

Personal Protective Equipment

All personal protective equipment used at this facility will be provided without cost to employees. Personal protective equipment will be chosen based on the anticipated exposure to blood or other potentially infectious materials. The protective equipment will be considered appropriate only if it does not permit blood or other potentially infectious materials to pass through or reach the employees clothing, skin, eyes, mouth, or other mucous membranes under normal conditions of use and for the duration of time which the protective equipment will be used. Protective clothing will be provided to employees in the following manner: *(List how the clothing will be provided to employees, e.g., who has responsibility for distribution, etc., and also list which procedures would require the protective clothing and the type of protection required. This could also be listed as an appendix to this program.)*

(The employer could use a checklist as follows:)

Personal Protective Equipment	Task
Gloves	
Lab Coat	
Face Shield	
Clinic Jacket	
Protective Eyewear (with solid side shield)	
Surgical Gown	
Shoe Covers	

D-8

OSHA GUIDELINES TO DEVELOPING A FACILITY BLOODBORNE PATHOGENS EXPOSURE CONTROL PLAN
Continued

Utility Gloves

Examination Gloves

Other PPE (list)

All personal protective equipment will be cleaned, laundered, and disposed of by the employer at no cost to employees. All repairs and replacements will be made by the employer at no cost to employees.

All garments which are penetrated by blood shall be removed immediately or as soon as feasible. All personal protective equipment will be removed prior to leaving the work area. The following protocol has been developed to facilitate leaving the equipment at the work area: *(List where employees are expected to place the personal protective equipment upon leaving the work area, and other protocols, etc.)* _____

Gloves shall be worn where it is reasonably anticipated that employees will have hand contact with blood, other potentially infectious materials, non-intact skin, and mucous membranes. Gloves will be available from: *(State location and/or person who will be responsible for distribution of gloves.)* _____ Gloves will be used for the following procedures: _____

Disposable gloves used at this facility are not to be washed or decontaminated for re-use and are to be replaced as soon as practical when they become contaminated or as soon as feasible if they are torn, punctured, or when their ability to function as a barrier is compromised. Utility gloves may be decontaminated for re-use provided that the integrity of the glove is not compromised. Utility gloves will be discarded if they are cracked, peeling, torn, punctured, or exhibit other signs of deterioration or when their ability to function as a barrier is compromised.

Masks in combination with eye protection devices, such as goggles or glasses with solid side shield, or chin length face shields, are required to be worn whenever splashes, spray, splatter, or droplets of blood or other potentially infectious materials may be generated and eye, nose, or mouth contamination can reasonably be anticipated. Situations at this facility which would require such protection are as follows:

The OSHA standard also requires appropriate protective clothing to be used, such as lab coats, gowns, aprons, clinic jackets, or similar outer garments. The following situations require that such protective clothing be utilized:

This facility will be cleaned and decontaminated according to the following schedule: *(List area and schedule)*

Decontamination will be accomplished by utilizing the following materials: *(List the materials which will be utilized, such as bleach solutions or EPA registered germicides.)*

D-8

OSHA GUIDELINES TO DEVELOPING A FACILITY BLOODBORNE PATHOGENS EXPOSURE CONTROL PLAN
Continued

All contaminated work surfaces will be decontaminated after completion of procedures and immediately or as soon as feasible after any spill of blood or other potentially infectious materials, as well as the end of the work shift if the surface may have become contaminated since the last cleaning. *(Employers should add in any information concerning the usage of protective coverings, such as plastic wrap which they may be using to assist in keeping surfaces free of contamination.)*

All bins, pails, cans, and similar receptacles shall be inspected and decontaminated on a regularly scheduled basis. *(List frequency and by whom _____ .)*

Any broken glassware which may be contaminated will not be picked up directly with the hands. The following procedures will be used:

Regulated Waste Disposal

All contaminated sharps shall be discarded as soon as feasible in sharps containers which are located in the facility. Sharps containers are located in: *(Specify locations of sharps containers.)*

Regulated waste other than sharps shall be placed in appropriate containers. Such containers are located in: *(Specify locations of containers.)*

Laundry Procedures

Laundry contaminated with blood or other potentially infectious materials will be handled as little as possible. Such laundry will be placed in appropriately marked bags at the location where it was used. Such laundry will not be sorted or rinsed in the area of use.

All employees who handle contaminated laundry will utilize personal protective equipment to prevent contact with blood or other potentially infectious materials.

Laundry at this facility will be cleaned at _____. *(Employers should note here if the laundry is being sent off site. If the laundry is being sent off site, then the laundry service accepting the laundry is to be notified, in accordance with section (d) of the standard.)*

Hepatitis B Vaccine

All employees who have been identified as having exposure to blood or other potentially infectious materials will be offered the Hepatitis B vaccine, at no cost to the employee. The vaccine will be offered within 10 working days of their initial assignment to work involving the potential for occupational exposure to blood or other potentially infectious materials unless the employee has previously had the vaccine or who wishes to submit to antibody testing which shows the employee to have sufficient immunity.

Employees who decline the Hepatitis B vaccine will sign a waiver which uses the wording in Appendix A of the OSHA standard.

Employees who initially decline the vaccine but who later wish to have it may then have the vaccine provided at no cost. *(Employers should list here who has responsibility for assuring that the vaccine is offered, the waivers are signed, etc. Also the employer should list who will administer the vaccine.)*

D-8

OSHA GUIDELINES TO DEVELOPING A FACILITY BLOODBORNE PATHOGENS EXPOSURE CONTROL PLAN
Continued

Post-Exposure Evaluation and Follow-Up

When the employee incurs an exposure incident, it should be reported to: *(List who has responsibility to maintain records of exposure incidents.)* _____

All employees who incur an exposure incident will be offered post-exposure evaluation and follow-up in accordance with the OSHA standard.

This follow-up will include the following:

- Documentation of the route of exposure and the circumstances related to the incident.
- If possible, the identification of the source individual and, if possible, the status of the source individual. The blood of the source individual will be tested (after consent is obtained) for HIV/HBV infectivity.
- Results of testing of the source individual will be made available to the exposed employee with the exposed employee informed about the applicable laws and regulations concerning disclosure of the identity and infectivity of the source individual. *(Employers made need to modify this provision in accordance with applicable local laws on this subject. Modifications should be listed here: _____.)*
  _____
- The employee will be offered the option of having their blood collected for testing of the employees HIV/HBV serological status. The blood sample will be preserved for at least 90 days to allow the employee to decide if the blood should be tested for HIV serological status. However, if the employee decides prior to that time that testing will be conducted, then the appropriate action can be taken and the blood sample discarded.
- The employee will be offered post exposure prophylaxis in accordance with the current recommendations of the U.S. Public Health Service. These recommendations are currently as follows: *(These recommendations may be listed as an appendix to the plan.)*

- The employee will be given appropriate counseling concerning precautions to take during the period after the exposure incident. The employee will also be given information on what potential illnesses to be alert for and to report any related experiences to appropriate personnel.
- The following person(s) has been designated to assure that the policy outlined here is effectively carried out as well as to maintain records related to this policy: _____.

Interaction with Health Care Professionals

A written opinion shall be obtained from the health care professional who evaluates employees of this facility. Written opinions will be obtained in the following instances:

1. When the employee is sent to obtain the Hepatitis B vaccine.
2. Whenever the employee is sent to a health care professional following an exposure incident.

Health care professionals shall be instructed to limit their opinions to:

1. Whether the Hepatitis B vaccine is indicated and if the employee has received the vaccine, or for evaluation following an incident,
2. That the employee has been informed of the results of the evaluation, and
3. That the employee has been told about any medical conditions resulting from exposure to blood or other potentially infectious materials. *(Note that the written opinion to the employer is not to reference any personal medical information.)*

Training

Training for all employees will be conducted prior to initial assignment to tasks where occupational exposure may occur. Training will be conducted in the following manner:

D-8

OSHA GUIDELINES TO DEVELOPING A FACILITY BLOODBORNE PATHOGENS EXPOSURE CONTROL PLAN
Continued

Training for employees will include the following an explanation of:

1. The OSHA standard for Bloodborne Pathogens.
2. Epidemiology and symptomatology of bloodborne diseases.
3. Modes of transmission of bloodborne pathogens.
4. This Exposure Control Plan, (i.e., points of the plan, lines of responsibility, how the plan will be implemented, etc.).
5. Procedures which might cause exposure to blood or other potentially infectious materials at this facility.
6. Control methods which will be used at the facility to control exposure to blood or other potentially infectious materials.
7. Personal protective equipment available at this facility and who should be contacted concerning.
8. Post-Exposure evaluation and follow-up.
9. Signs and labels used at the facility.
10. Hepatitis B vaccine program at the facility.

(Employers should list here if training will be conducted using videotapes, written material, etc. Also the employer should indicate who is responsible for conducting the training.)

All employees will receive annual refresher training. *(Note that this training is to be conducted within one year of the employee's previous training.)*

The outline for the training material is located: *(List where the training materials are located.)*

Recordkeeping

All records required by the OSHA standard will be maintained by: *(Insert name or department responsible for maintaining records.)*

Dates

All provisions required by the standard will be implemented by: *(Insert date for implementation of the provisions of the standard.)*

From Occupational Safety and Health Administration, Department of Labor, Regional Office, Region 3, Philadelphia, 1992.

D-9

OSHA HEPATITIS B VACCINATION PROTECTION

WHAT IS HBV?

Hepatitis B virus (HBV) is a potentially life-threatening bloodborne pathogen. Centers for Disease Control estimates there are approximately 280,000 HBV infections each year in the U.S.

Approximately 8,700 health care workers each year contact hepatitis B, and about 200 will die as a result. In addition, some who contact HBV will become carriers, passing the disease on to others. Carriers also face a significantly higher risk for other liver ailments which can be fatal, including cirrhosis of the liver and primary liver cancer.

HBV infection is transmitted through exposure to blood and other infectious body fluids and tissues. Anyone with occupational exposure to blood is at risk of contracting the infection.

Employers must provide engineering controls; workers must use work practices and protective clothing and equipment to prevent exposure to potential infectious materials. However, the best defense against hepatitis B is vaccination.

WHO NEEDS VACCINATION?

The new OSHA standard covering bloodborne pathogens requires employers to offer the three-injection vaccination series free to all employees who are exposed to blood or other potentially infectious materials as part of their job duties. This includes health care workers, emergency responders, morticians, first-aid personnel, law enforcement officers, correctional facilities staff, launderers, as well as others.

The vaccination must be offered within 10 days of initial assignment to a job where exposure to blood or other potentially infectious materials can be "reasonably anticipated." The requirements for vaccinations of those already on the job take effect July 6, 1992.

WHAT DOES VACCINATION INVOLVE?

The hepatitis B vaccination is a noninfectious, yeast-based vaccine given in three injections in the arm. It is prepared from recombinant yeast cultures, rather than human blood or plasma. Thus, there is no risk of contamination from other bloodborne pathogens nor is there any chance of developing HBV from the vaccine.

The second injection should be given one month after the first and the third injection six months after the initial dose.

More than 90 percent of those vaccinated will develop immunity to the hepatitis B virus. To ensure immunity, it is important for individuals to receive all three injections. At this point it is unclear how long the immunity lasts, so booster shots may be required at some point in the future.

The vaccine causes no harm to those who are already immune or to those who may be HBV carriers. Although employees may opt to have their blood tested for antibodies to determine need for the vaccine, employers may not make such screening a condition of receiving vaccination nor are employers required to provide prescreening.

Each employee should receive counseling from a health care professional when vaccination is offered. This discussion will help an employee determine whether inoculation is necessary.

WHAT IF I DECLINE VACCINATION?

Workers who decide to decline vaccination must complete a declination form. Employers must keep these forms on file so that they know the vaccination status of everyone who is exposed to blood. At any time after a worker initially declines to receive the vaccine, he or she may opt to take it.

WHAT IF I AM EXPOSED BUT HAVE NOT YET BEEN VACCINATED?

If a worker experiences an exposure incident, such as a needlestick or a blood spash in the eye, he or she must receive confidential medical evaluation from a licensed health care professional with appropriate follow-up. To the extent possible by law, the employer is to determine the source individual for HBV as well as human immunodeficiency virus (HIV) infectivity. The worker's blood will also be screened if he or she agrees.

The health care professional is to follow the guidelines of the U.S. Public Health Service in providing treatment. This would include hepatitis B vaccination. The health care professional must give a written opinion on whether or not vaccination is recommended and whether the employee received it. Only this information is reported to the employer. Employee medical records must remain confidential. HIV or HBV status must NOT be reported to the employer.

This is one of a series of fact sheets which discuss various requirements of the Occupational Safety and Health Administration's standard covering exposure to blood borne pathogens. Single copies of fact sheets are available from OSHA Publications, Room N3101, 200 Constitution Ave, N.W., Washington, D.C. 20210 and from OSHA regional offices.

U.S. Department of Labor, Occupational Safety and Health Administration

D-10

STATES WITH OSHA-APPROVED PLANS

Alaska Department of Labor
P.O. Box 21149
Juneau, ALASKA 99802-1149
(907) 465-2700

Industrial Commission of Arizona
800 W. Washington
Phoenix, ARIZONA 85007
(602) 255-5795

California Department of Industrial
  Relations
395 Oyster Point Boulevard
3rd Floor, Wing C
S. San Francisco, CALIFORNIA
  94080
(415) 737-2960

Connecticut Department of Labor
200 Folly Brook Boulevard
Wethersfield, CONNECTICUT
  06109
(203) 566-5123

Hawaii Department of Labor and
  Industrial Relations
830 Punchbowl Street
Honolulu, HAWAII 96813
(808) 548-3150

Indiana Department of Labor
1013 State Office Building
100 North Senate Avenue
Indianapolis, INDIANA 46204-2287
(317) 232-2665

Iowa Division of Labor Services
1000 E. Grand Avenue
Des Moines, IOWA 50319
(515) 281-3447

Kentucky Labor Cabinet
U.S. Highway 127 South
Frankfort, KENTUCKY 40601
(502) 564-3070

Maryland Division of Labor and
  Industry
Department of Licensing and
  Regulation
501 St. Paul Place, 15th Floor
Baltimore, MARYLAND 21202-
  2272
(301) 333-4176

Michigan Department of Labor
309 N. Washington
P.O. Box 30015
Lansing, MICHIGAN 48909
(517) 373-9600

Michigan Department of Public
  Health
3423 North Logan Street
Box 30195
Lansing, MICHIGAN 48909
(517) 335-8022

Minnesota Department of Labor
  and Industry
443 Lafayette Road
St. Paul, MINNESOTA 55155
(612) 296-2342

Nevada Department of Industrial
  Relations
Division of Occupational Safety and
  Health
Capitol Complex
1370 S. Curry Street
Carson City, NEVADA 89710
(702) 885-5240

New Mexico Environmental
  Improvement Division
Health and Environment
  Department
1190 St. Francis Drive N2200
Santa Fe, NEW MEXICO 87503-
  0968
(505) 827-2850

New York Department of Labor
One Main Street
Brooklyn, NEW YORK 11201
(518) 457-3518

North Carolina Department of
  Labor
4 West Edenton Street
Raleigh, NORTH CAROLINA 27603
(919) 733-7166

Oregon Occupational Safety and
  Health Division
Oregon Department of Insurance
  and Finance
21 Labor and Industries Building
Salem, OREGON 97310
(503) 378-3304

Puerto Rico Department of Labor
  and Human Resources
Prudencio Rivera Martinez Building
505 Munoz Rivera Avenue
Hato Rey, PUERTO RICO 00918
(809) 754-2119-22

South Carolina Department of
  Labor
3600 Forest Drive
P.O. Box 11329
Columbia, SOUTH CAROLINA
  29211-1329
(803) 734-9594

Tennessee Department of Labor
501 Union Building
Suite "A"—2nd Floor
Nashville, TENNESSEE 37219
(615) 741-2582

Utah Occupational Safety and
  Health
160 East 300 South
P.O. Box 5800
Salt Lake City, UTAH 84110-5800
(801) 530-6900

D-10

STATES WITH OSHA-APPROVED PLANS *Continued*

Vermont Department of Labor and Industry
120 State Street
Montpelier, VERMONT 05602
(802) 828-2765

Virgin Islands Department of Labor
Box 890
Christiansted
St. Croix, VIRGIN ISLANDS 00820
(809) 773-1994

Virginia Department of Labor and Industry
P.O. Box 12064
Richmond, VIRGINIA 23241-0064
(804) 786-2376

Washington Department of Labor and Industries
General Administration Building
Room 334—AX-31
Olympia, WASHINGTON 98504-0631
(206) 753-6307

Wyoming Occupational Health and Safety
Herchier Building, 2nd Floor East
Cheyenne, WYOMING 82002
(309) 777-7786 or 777-7787

SUBJECT INDEX

Note: Page numbers in *italics* refer to illustrations; page numbers followed by t refer to tables.

AAMA. See *American Association of Medical Assistants*.
Abbreviation, for reasons for office visit, 10t
   in blood chemistry tests, 598t–600t
   in hospital terminology, 696–698
   in mailing address, 39
      for Canadian provinces, 35, 35t
      for individual states, 35, 35t
   in medication orders, 336, 337t–339t
Abdomen, examination of, position for, *320*
   ultrasonography in, 418, *421*, 422
   injury to, child abuse and, 438
   radiography of, 478
Aberration, 515, *515*
Abortion, definition of, 466
   ethics of, 272
   legislation and, 272
   missed, 470
   patient's rights and, 271
   septic, 470
   spontaneous, 469–470
Abortus, 467t
   definition of, 466
Abruptio placentae, 471
Abscess, breast, 452, *453*
Abstract, research, 42
Abuse. See specific type, e.g., *Drug abuse*.
Accident, cerebrovascular, 671
   claim form for, 175, *176*
   in medical office, report form for, *73*
   prevention of, 249
Accountant, selection of, 258, 259
Accounting. See also *Bookkeeping*.
   accrual, 124
   balance sheet in, *141*, 142
   budget in, 144–145, *146*
   cash basis, 124
      revenue in, 127
   chart of accounts in, 124, *125*, 131
   check writing and, 141
   checking *v* savings account in, 141
   cost analysis in, 123, 144, *145*
   expenditures in, 143
      benefits package and, 136, 138, *138*. See also *Benefits package*.
      chart of accounts and, 124, *125*, 131
      insurance premiums and, 138–140, *139*
      payroll and. See *Payroll*.
      physical plant and, 131
      supplies and, *140*, 140–141

Accounting *(Continued)*
   income statement in, *142*, 143
   methods of, 123–124
   net profit and loss in, 143–144
   practice goals and, 124, *124*
   profit and loss analysis in, *143*, 143–144
   revenue in, 123, 124, *125–128*, 131, 143
      accounts receivable control and, *127*, 127
      aged accounts receivable and, 127, *128*, 129
      computer mistakes and, 129
      credit and collections and, 129, 131
      day sheet and, 124, 126, *126*
      definition of, 123
      outside medical services and, 129
      sources of, 126–127
      taxes and. See *Tax(es)*.
   terminology in, 123
Accounts payable, definition of, 123
Accounts receivable, definition of, 123
   monthly analysis of, *122*, 122
Accounts receivable aging record, *121*, 122
Accounts receivable control, *127*, 127
Accrual, accounting, 124. See also *Accounting*.
Accucheck II glucose meter, 602–605, *603–605*
   calibration of, *604*, 604–605, *605*
Acids, poisoning by, 738t
Acquired immune deficiency syndrome. See also *Human immunodeficiency virus*.
   blood and body fluid precautions for. See *Centers for Disease Control, universal precautions for blood and body fluid from*.
   financial considerations in, 811
   information and resources for, 678
   manifestation in female, 447t
   pediatric, 429
Acronyms, for selected health care organizations, 699–702
Acyclovir, 447t
ADA. See *Americans with Disabilities Act of 1990*.
Address for Success brochure, 40
Administrator. See also *Personnel*.
   overtime exemption and, 236–237
Advertising, in personnel recruitment, 227
Affirmative action policy, 251–252
Agar, group A beta-hemolytic streptococcus and, 631
   in urine testing, 635t
Age, medication dosage and, 346
Aged accounts receivable, 127, *128*, 129
Agglutination inhibition test, 646
AHA. See *American Hospital Association*.
AIDS. See *Acquired immune deficiency syndrome; Human immunodeficiency virus*.
Airway, obstruction of, 667–668, *668–669*
Alcohol abuse, 250–251. See also *Drug abuse*.

835

Alcohol abuse *(Continued)*
  ICD-9-CM coding for, 197
  medical record release and, 33
Alcoholism Prevention, Treatment, and Rehabilitation Act (42 U.S.C. Section 290dd-3), 33
Aldosterone, in urinalysis, 561t
Aliquot, definition of, 525
Alkali poisoning, 738t
Alkaline phosphate, in blood chemistry test, 598t
Allergy, pediatric, 429
  to medication, 365
Alpha-fetoprotein, 472
Alphabetic coding, for medical record, 20
Ambulatory Health Care Standards Manual, 67
Amebic dysentry, pediatric, 436
Amenorrhea, definition of, 441
American Association of Medical Assistants, 258
  certification department of, 279
  code of ethics from, 267–268
  standard of care from, 265
American Hospital Association, Patient's Bill of Rights from, 270
American Medical Technologists, code of ethics from, 268. See also *Ethics*.
  examination from, 279
Americans With Disabilities Act of 1990, 251–252
Analgesic, monitoring of, reference values for, 763
Anaphylactic reaction, 365
Anesthesia, billing for, 177
Ankle, radiography of, 478–479
Answering service, for after-hour call, 17
Antepartum, definition of, 466
Antibiotic, candidiasis and, 446
  monitoring of, reference values for, 763
Anticoagulant, definition of, 525
Anticonvulsant, monitoring of, reference values for, 763
Antigen. See also *Reagent; Serology*.
  serology tests and, 639–658
Anus, 557
Apnea, definition of, 313
Apneusis, definition of, 313
Apothecary system, 339t, 340
Appearance, in personnel recruitment, 232
Appointment. See also *Office visit*.
  documentation of, 287
  ethical considerations for, 13
  for clinical test, 13, 15
  for consultation, 13
  for contract patient, 11
  for established patient, 10
  for home visit, 12
  for new patient, 9–10, 10t
  for outpatient surgery, 13, 15
  for physician-referred patient, 9, 10–11
  for problem patient, 11–12
  for Worker's Compensation patient, 11
  general considerations for, 3, 15
  individualized, *6, 7, 7–8*
  late physician and, 12
  legal considerations for, 13
  mission statement and, 3
  nonroutine, 11
  open-slot, 9
  outstanding account and, 12
  system for, 3–15
    category method in, 8–9

Appointment *(Continued)*
  computerized, *5–8*, 13, *14*, 221
  double-book method in, *9*
  factors in, 4
  manual, primary care setting and, 4, *5*, 7
    specialist's office and, 7, 9
  reassessment of, 3, 12–13
  standard, *5*
  stream method in, 8
  time-allotted slot in, 8
  time frame in, 4, 4t, 7
  wave method in, 8
Apron, in specimen collection and processing, 532
Arrhythmia, 509, *511–517*, 512, 515, 517
  aberration as, 515, *515*
  atrial rhythm as, 512, *512*, 513
  atrioventricular block as, 515, *516*, 517, *517*
  electrocardiogram in. See *Electrocardiogram*.
  Holter monitor in, 517
  premature contraction as, 509, *511*, 512
  sinoatrial block as, 517, *517*
  ventricular rhythm as, 512, *514*, 515
Arsenic poisoning, 738t
ASA Relative Value Guide, 177
Ascariasis, 437
Asepsis, 301–306, *304, 305*, 306t. See also *Centers for Disease Control, universal precautions for blood and body fluid from*.
  hand-washing in, 303–304
  sanitation in, 303–304
  sterilization in, *304*, 304–306, *305*, 306t
Aspiration, of fluid, 392–393
Asset, definition of, 123
  in balance sheet, *141*, 142
Astigmatism, definition of, *324*
Atrial fibrillation, 512, *513*
Atrial flutter, 512, *513*
Atrial premature contraction, 509, *511*
Atrial rhythm, 512, *512, 513*
Atrial tachycardia, 512, *512*
Atrioventricular block, 515, *516*, 517, *517*
Attendance record, employee, *130*, 131
Attorney, selection of, 258–259
Attorney General's Office, as information source for federal and state law, 277
Automobile, insurance for, 138–139
  lease *v* purchase of, 56
Autopsy, HIV transmission and, 773

Bacillary dysentry, 435
Bacillus, gram-stain morphology of, 616t, 620
Bacteria, gram-stain morphology of, 616t, 619–620
  in childhood disease, 432–435
  in urinalysis, 570t, *573*, 574
Bacteriostatic preservative, 345
Balance sheet, *141*, 142
Bandage, 394–396. See also *Dressing*.
  cling, 396
  elastic, 394–396
  Gauze roller, 396
Bank statement, 104, *105*, 106
  errors in reconciliation of, 106
  with reconciliation, *107*
Banking, 98–108. See also *Checking account*.
  services included in, 100

Basal body temperature, infertility and, 473–474
Basophils, in electronic blood cell counting, 592
Bathing, of newborn, 406
Battered child syndrome, 438–439
Benefits package, 136, 138, *138*, 239–242
    accounting procedures and, 136, 138, *138*
    changes in, 240
    designing of, 240
    disability insurance and, 138, 241, 253
    general considerations for, 239
    health insurance and, 239–240. See also *Health insurance.*
    legal requirements for, 242, *242*
    life insurance and, 41, 240–241
    miscellaneous, 242
    personal leave and, 241–242
    policy manual and, *247*
    pregnancy and, 241–242
    required costs in, 239
    retirement program and, 239
    sick leave and, 241–242
    wellness program and, 240
Bibliography, in manuscript preparation, 43
Bilirubin, in blood chemistry test, 600t
Bill of Rights, patient's, 269
Billing, 110, 112–122. See also *Fee, collection of.*
    computerization and, 205–206, 207, *215*, 216. See also *Computerization.*
    credit card and, 110
    follow-up for, 114–115, *115–122*, 118–119, 122. See also *Delinquent account, follow-up for.*
    methods for, 112, 114
    procedure for, 114
    sample statement for, 112, *113*
    third-party, computerization in, 205–206. See also *Computerization.*
Bioethics, 270–273. See also *Ethics.*
    abortion and, 271–272
    basic health care and, 270
    euthanasia and, 271
    procreation and, 271
    universal health care and, 270
Biohazard, definition of, 525
Biopsy, needle-guided, ultrasonography in, 522
Biot's respiration, definition of, 313
Birth control. See *Contraception.*
Blade, scalpel, 371, *372*, 377
Bleach(es), poisoning by, 739t
Bleeding, dysfunctional, *668, 669, 670,* 671
    uterine, 451
    oral contraception and, 457
Blind ad, in personnel recruitment, 227
Block letter style, *37*
Blood. See also *Hematology.*
    cell types in, *591*
    chemistry tests for, 597–607. See also *Fecal occult blood test; Hematology.*
        abbreviations in, 598t–600t
        anticoagulants in, 600t
        chemistry analyzers in, 601
        cholesterol level and, 606–607
        common, 597, 598t–600t
        glucose fasting blood sample level and, 602–605, *603–605*
            calibration of glucose meter and, *604,* 604–605, *605*
        glucose tolerance test and, 605–606
        kit methods for, 601

Blood *(Continued)*
        laboratory equipment in, 601
        normal values in, 598t–600t
        preservatives for, 597
        proper specimen handling in, 597, 601
        purpose of, 597, 598t–600t
        quality control in, 601
        reporting procedures in, 601–602
        routine, 597
        specimen integrity in, 597
        terminology in, 597
        tubes for, 597
    collection of, 533–541
        capillary puncture method for, 534–535, *535*
            procedure for, *540,* 540–541
        syringe method in, 534
        vacuum tube system and, 533–534, 534t
            procedure for, 536–539, *536–539*
    diseases and disorders of, diagnosis-related group and, 807
    universal precautions for, 301–303, 768–790. See also *Centers for Disease Control, universal precautions for blood and body fluid from.*
Blood bank, laboratory testing and, 529
Blood pressure, 316–319
    assessment of, 316
        auscultation in, 316–318
        errors in, 316
        guidelines for, 317
        in lower extremities, 319
        in pediatrics, 317, 319, 427, 428t
        medication administration and, 318
        palpation in, 319
        procedure for, 318
    diastolic, 316
    general considerations for, 316
    systolic, 316, 319
Blood smear examination, peripheral. See *Peripheral blood smear examination.*
Blood urea nitrogen, in blood chemistry test, 598t
Blood-forming organ, diseases and disorders of, diagnosis-related group and, 807
Blue Cross/Blue Shield, 158, *159–161,* 160, 161. See also *Health Insurance.*
    central certification plan from, 160, *161*
    claim processing for, *171–172, 174–175*
    Federal Employee Program and, 160, *160*
    permanent reciprocity program from, 161, *161*
    Preadmission Certification for, 158, *159*
    remittance to, 183, *185*
Blue Shield Permanent Reciprocity Program, 161, *161*
Body fluid, universal precautions for, 301–303, 768–790. See also *Centers for Disease Control, universal precautions for blood and body fluid from.*
Body surface area, medication measurement and, 341, *342*
Body weight, 310–311
    desirable, for boys and girls, 752
        for men and women, 751
    in growth and development, 408t, *410,* 410–411, *411.* See also *Growth chart.*
    medication measurement and, 341, *342*
    significance of, 310
Bond, 233
    definition of, 138
Bookkeeping, 77–98. See also *Accounting.*
    accounts payable, 78, 79
    disbursements journal in, 93, *95*

Bookkeeping (Continued)
  accounts receivable, 78, 79, 80
    daily journal in, 78, 80, 84
    monthly analysis in, 122, 122
    patient ledger card in, 82, 83, 84
    trial balance in, 92
  accounts receivable aging record in, 121, 122
  collection ratio in, 121, 122
  disbursements journal in, accounts payable, 93, 95
    pegboard, 94
    single-entry, 93
    trial balance, 94
    year-to-date, 97
  double-entry, 78–79
  pegboard, 79, 81–82, 81–83
    disbursements journal, 94
    posting charges and payments in, 85, 86, 87
  petty cash in, 96, 97–98
  single-entry, 79, 84–85
    disbursements journal, 94
  special accounting entry in, 87, 88–92
    delinquent account as, 87, 88, 89, 90
    insurance nonallowed amount as, 89, 90
    patient refund as, 91, 92
    professional discount as, 90, 90
    returned check as, 91, 91
    reversing entry as, 90
  starting system for, 77–78
  trial balance in, accounts receivable, 92
Boric acid, 531
Bradypnea, definition of, 313
Braxton-Hicks sign, definition of, 466
Breast, abscess of, 452, 453
  cancer of, 454, 454t
    fibrocystic disease and, 452
    self-examination for, 454, 455
  diseases and disorders of, diagnosis-related group and, 804–805
  examination of, ultrasonography in, 522
  fibrocystic disease of, 452
    cancer and, 452
    follow-up for, 454
  self-examination of, 332
Breast milk, universal precautions for, 786
Breast pump, 403, 452
Breastfeeding, flatus and, 408
  nipple care and, 473
Bronchodilator, monitoring of, reference values for, 763
Bruise, child abuse and, 438
Budget, definition of, 123
  monthly, 144, 146
  uses of, 144–145
Bundle branch block, electrocardiogram in detection of, 504, 505
Bunsen burner, in microbiology, 611
  precautions with, 614
Bureau of Workers' Disability, 249
Burn, 671
  child abuse and, 438
  diagnosis-related group and, 808
  ICD-9-CM coding for, 197–198
Burping, newborn, 406
Business letter. See also *Correspondence*.
  parts of, 37, 38, 38–39, 40
  simplified, 40
Calcium, in blood chemistry test, 598t
  in urinalysis, 561t

Calibrated loop method, for urine culture, 634–635, 635, 635t
Calibration, 550–551
  definition of, 525
Camphor poisoning, 739t
Canada, provinces of, abbreviations for, 35, 35t
Cancer. See also *Neoplasm*.
  breast, 454, 454t
    fibrocystic disease and, 452
    self-examination for, 454, 455
  colorectal, test for, 629–631
Candidiasis, 445, 446t, 449
  antibiotics and, 446
  oral contraceptives and, 446
Capillary puncture method, for blood collection, 534–535, 535
  procedure for, 540–541, 541
Capital, definition of, 123
  in balance sheet, 141, 142
  types of, 142
Carbon copy, of correspondence, 39
Carbon dioxide laser unit, 388
Carbon monoxide poisoning, 739t
Carbon tetrachloride poisoning, 740t
Cardiopulmonary resuscitation, 661, 663
  procedure for, 661, 663, 664, 665–667, 666
Cardiovascular drug, monitoring of, reference values for, 763
Cash, petty. See *Petty cash*.
Cash basis accounting, 124. See also *Accounting*.
Cast, urine, 570, 570t, 570–571
Catastrophic Coverage Act of 1988, 187
Catheterization, for urine specimen, 555t, 556–557, 557
  of infant, 556
Cell count, reference values for, 759
Cellophane tape, 620, 621, 622
  examination of, 620, 622
  preparation of, 621
Celsius temperature, conversion to Fahrenheit temperature, 314
Centers for Disease Control, CLIA 1988 Final Rule and, 791
  data from, hepatitis B virus and, 811
    human immunodeficiency virus and, 811
  health care workers and, AIDS-infected, 769, 781
    definition of, 768
    exposure management and, 781–782
    risks to, 769–770
    testing of, 780
  universal precautions for blood and body fluid from, 301–303, 768–790
    applications for, 785–786
    environmental considerations and, 774–776
    for blood and body fluid spills, 776
    for dentistry, 772–773, 786
    for dialysis, 773
    for housekeeping, 776–777
    for infective waste, 777, 788–789
    for invasive procedure, 771–772
    for laboratory, 773–774
    for laundry, 776–777
    for postmortem procedure, 773
    for semen, 785
    for serologic testing, 778–780
    for specimen collection and processing, 532–533
    general considerations for, 768
    implementation of, 777
    update on, 784–790

Centers for Disease Control *(Continued)*
    breast milk and, 786
    dentistry and, 786
    phlebotomy and, 787–788
    protective barriers and, 786–788
    saliva and, 786
    waste management and, 788–789
Centimeter, conversion to inch, 310
Central certification plan, 160, *161*
Centrifuge, microhematocrit, 579, *579*
Cerebrospinal fluid, reference values for, 764
Cerebrovascular accident, 671
Certification, as credential, 279
    education for, *71*
Cervical cap, 465
    efficacy of, 466
Cervical mucus test, 474
Cervical spine, radiography of, 480
Cervix, colposcopy of, 456
Chadwick's sign, definition of, 466
Chain of custody, for specimen, 547–548
    urine, 558, *559*
CHAMPUS. See *Civilian Health and Medical Program of the Uniformed Services.*
Charge slip, 78
Chart of accounts, 124, *125*, 131
Check. See also *Checking Account.*
    acceptance of, 101
    endorsement of, 101, *102*
    returned, bookkeeping for, 91, *91*
    selection of, *98*, *99*, 100
    writing of, *98*, 100–101
Checking account, 98. See also *Check.*
    bank statement and, 104, *105*, 106
        errors in reconciliation of, 106
        with reconciliation, *107*
    business, 98
    deposit to, 101, *103*, 103–104
    individual, 98
    joint, 98
    regular, 98
    special, 98
Chemicals, common, poisoning by, 738t–741t
Chemistry test, 529. See also *Blood, chemistry tests for.*
    panels and profiles in, 529t
Chemotherapy, ICD-9-CM coding for, 201–202
Chemstrip, in urinalysis, 567, 568, *568*, *569*, 626–628
Chest, examination of, radiography in, 481
    ultrasonography in, 522
    growth and development of, 408t, 409–410
Cheyne-Stokes respiration, definition of, 313
Chicken pox, 429
Child abuse, 438–439
Childbirth, diagnosis-related group and, 806–807
    ICD-9-CM coding for, 202–203
Chlamydia, tests for, 544, 545
Chloride, in blood chemistry test, 598t
Cholesterol, in blood chemistry test, 598t
    serum levels of, 606–607
Chronic obstructive pulmonary disease, ICD-9-CM coding for, 203
Cigarette smoking, office policy and, 247, *248*, 251
    oral contraception and, 457
Circular E, Employers' Tax Guide, *135*, 136, *137*
Circulatory system, disorders of, ICD-9-CM coding for, 198
Civil Rights Act, sexual harassment and, 252–253

Civilian Health and Medical Program of the Uniformed Services, 166. See also *Health insurance.*
    Blue Cross/Blue Shield and, 158, 160
    claim form for, 173, *178*, 179
    remittance to, 183, *184*
Classified advertising, for personnel recruitment, 227
CLIA. See *Clinical Laboratory Improvement Amendments of 1988.*
Climacteric, definition of, 441
Clinical Laboratory Improvement Amendments of 1988, 279
    Final Rule, applications of, 791
        copies of, address for, 796
        fees in, 796
        general considerations for, 791
        inspections and, 795–796
        laboratory classification in, 792
        personnel requirements in, 794–795
        proficiency testing in, 792–793
        quality assurance in, 793
        quality control in, 793
        registration certificate from, 791–792
        sanctions in, 796
        test categories in, 792
        timetable for, 791
        waiver certificate from, 791, 792
Clitoris, 557
CO_2 laser unit, 388
Coagulation, laboratory test for, 529. See also *Prothrombin time.*
    reference values for, 759
Cocci, gram reaction of, 616t, 619
Code of ethics, 267–268. See also *Ethics.*
Coding, CPT, 189, 196–197
    computerization and, 221
  digital, terminal, for medical record, 21, *21*, 23
  employee's role in, 195
  ICD, -9-CM, 187–204
    books for, 190–193, *191*, *192*
    computerization and, 207, *214*, 221
    diagnosis-related group and, 203–204
    DRG and, 203–204
    for specific conditions, 197–203
        abortion and, 202
        adverse reaction and, *191*, 199–200
        alcohol abuse and, 197
        burns and, 197
        childbirth and, 202–203
        chronic obstructive pulmonary disease and, 203
        circulatory system disorder and, 198
        complications and, 198
        diabetes mellitus and, 198–199
        dislocation and, 200
        drug abuse and, 197
        drug poisoning and, 199–200
        fracture and, 200
        HIV infection and, 200
        hypertension and, 198
        infectious disease and, 200
        insulin dependency and, 199
        late-effect and, 200
        myocardial infarction and, 198, *199*
        neoplasm and, *200*, 200–202, *201*. See also *Neoplasm.*
        pregnancy and, 202–203
        puerperium and, 202–203
        respiratory system disorder and, 203

Coding *(Continued)*
 future of, 204
 general considerations for, 203
 glossary for, 191, *191*
 guidelines for, 193–195, *194, 195*
  condition appearing under more than one term in, 194
  E codes in, 194
   adverse reaction and, 199–200
  expression of symptoms in, 195
  fifth digit without fourth digit in, 195
  four-digit disease subcategory codes in, 195
  fourth digit in, 189
  instruction to "use an additional code if necessary" in, 195
  NEC (Not Elsewhere Classifiable) in, 195
  nonessential modifiers in, 193, *194*
  NOS (Not Otherwise Specified) in, 195
  See and *See also* instructions in, *194*, 194–195, *195*
  three-digit disease codes in, 195
  two diagnoses or diagnosis with complication in, 195
  two or more codes in, 195
  uncertain diagnosis in, 194
  V codes in, neoplasm and, 202
 history of, 187
 impact of, 187, 189
 medical record as documentation for, 197, 203
 Official Authorized Addendum to, 192–193
 physician education and, 196–197
 prerequisites for, 189
 procedure with, 193
 subscription service for, 192–193
 table of contents in, *188–189*
 terminology in, *192*, 192
 third-party payers' rules for, 195–196
 violations of, 187
 Volume 1, *188–190*, 189–190
 Volume 2, 190, *190, 191*
 Volume 3, 190, *190*
 future of, 204
 procedure for, 193
 third-party payers' rules for, 195–196
Cognition, assessment of, 330, 331t
Coitus, definition of, 441
Cold, application of, 397, 400–401
Colic, 407
Collection agency, 118–119
 accounting and, 129, 131
Collection ratio, *121*, 122
College posting system, 230
Color coding, for medical record, 19, *20*
 in billing follow-up, 114
Color Slide II Mononucleosis Test, 640t, 644–645, *645*
Colposcopy, 456
Coma, diabetic, 672
Combination policy, medical professional liability and, 286
Commission on Office Laboratory Accreditation, address for, 796
 CLIA 1988 Final Rule and, 791, 792, 796. See also *Clinical Laboratory Improvement Amendments of 1988, Final Rule.*
  fees and, 796
  unannounced inspections and, 795–796
  description of, 796
 Community, health and safety of, 549
  relations with, 53

Compensation, overtime. See *Overtime compensation.*
 unemployment, 239
 worker's. See *Worker's compensation.*
Comprehensive Drug Abuse Prevention and Control Act of 1970, 291, *292*, 293, *293*
Computerization, appointment system and, 5–8, 13, *14*, 221
 benefits of, 205–206
 general considerations for, 205
 hardware considerations in, 206
 in record preservation, 24
 literature search with, 42
 precautions for, aged accounts receivable and, 129
  payroll and, 131
 software considerations in, flexibility and, 206
  general considerations for, 207, 222
  HDS Medical Assistance Professional as, 207, *208–221*, 216, 221. See also *HDS Medical Assistance Professional software program.*
 security considerations for, 222
 training and support for, 222–223
 vendor for, 222–223
Concentration, definition of, 597
Condom, 465–466
Condylomata acuminata, 447t
Confidentiality, duty-to-warn rule and, 33
 ethics of, 269
 in research study, 30
 legally required disclosures and, 291
 medical record and, 31–33, *290*, 291
 release of information to government and, 32–33
 state law and, 269
 telephone call and, 16
Connective tissue, diseases and disorders of, diagnosis-related group and, 803–804, 808
Consolidated Omnibus Budget Reconciliation Act of 1985, 253
Constipation, in newborn, 407–408
Construction, of additional space, 47–48, *48*
 of new site, 46–47
Consultant, letter to, 42
 selection of, 258, 259–260
Consultation, appointment system for, 13
Continuing education, 70–71
Contraception, 457
 cervical cap as, 465
  efficacy of, 466
 condom as, 465–466
 diaphragm as, 462, *463–464*, 465, 466. See also *Diaphragm.*
  efficacy of, 466
 general considerations for, 457
 implant as, 458–460
  advantages of, 458
  contraindications for, 458
  efficacy of, 466
  informed consent and, 458
  insertion of, 458–459
  menses and timing of, 458
  removal of, 459–460
  risks of, 458
  side effects of, 458
 intrauterine device as, *460*, 461–462
  efficacy of, 466
 oral, 457
  candidiasis and, 446
  efficacy of, 466

Contraception *(Continued)*
  ovulation method as, 466
  rhythm method as, 466
  vaginal cream as, 465
    efficacy of, 466
  vaginal foam as, 465
    efficacy of, 466
  vaginal sponge as, 465
    efficacy of, 466
  vaginal suppository as, 465
    efficacy of, 466
Contract, medical professional liability and, 280–281, *281, 282*
Contract patient, appointment system for, 11
Controlled substance, 291, *292, 293*
  abuse of. See *Substance abuse.*
  inventory and, 293
  prescription for, 293, *293*
  record-keeping and, 293
  registration and, 291, 293
  uses and effects of, 742–744
Controlled Substances Act, 291, *292, 293*
  drugs and drug products under jurisdiction of, 336, 338t
Conversion formula, 338t, 341
Coombs' test, reference values for, 759
Copayment, collection of, 108
COPD (chronic obstructive pulmonary disease), ICD-9-CM coding for, 203
Coronary artery disease, exercise stress test in, 518
Correspondence, 34–43
  abbreviations for, 35
  carbon copy of, 35, 39
  certified mail as, 36
  classification of, 36
  confidential, 34, 35
  consultant's letter as, 42
  cover letter as, 230
  disability claim form as, 41
  enclosure for, 34, 35, 39
  envelope for, 39–40, *41*
  express mail as, 36
  first-class mail as, 36
  fourth-class mail as, 36
  incoming, 34
  insured mail as, 36–37
  international mail as, 36
  junk mail as, 34
  letter of referral as, 41
  letter-writing format for, *37, 38,* 38–39, *40*
  life insurance company request for, 41
  metered mail as, 35
  military mail as, 36
  outgoing, 34
  postscript to, 39
  registered mail as, 37
  report to patient as, 42
  salutation for, 39
  second-opinion statement as, 41
  signature for, 39
  special delivery as, 37
  special handling items as, 38
  third-class mail as, 36
  written by office personnel for physician, 39
  zip code for, 35
Cost accounting, 144, *145.* See also *Accounting.*
  definition of, 123

Coulter Counter Model T, in electronic blood cell counting, *593,* 593–594
Cover letter, with job application, 230
CPT. See *Current Procedural Terminology.*
Cranial nerve, assessment of, 330, 331t, 332
C-reactive protein, clinical considerations for, 641
  purpose of, 640–641
  test for, 640t, 641–642
Cream, vaginal, 465
  efficacy of, 466
Creatinine, in blood chemistry test, 598t
  in urinalysis, 562t
Credentialing, of personnel, 278–280
Credit, arrangements for, 108
  fee collection and, 108, 110. See also *Fee, collection of.*
Creed, American Association of Medical Assistants Code of Ethics and, 267
Cross-indexing, for medical record, 23
Crying, newborn, 408
Crystal, in urinalysis, 570t, *572*–573, 573–574
Culture. See also *Microbiology, culture techniques in.*
  definition of, 525
  spilled, clean-up for, 614
  stool, 531, 541
  swab for, 531
Current Procedural Terminology, 189, 196–197, 221. See also *Coding.*
  computerization and, 221
Custodial service, 60
Cyanide poisoning, 740t
Cyanmethemoglobin reagent, in hemoglobin concentration, 582–583
Cycle billing, 112
Cyst, ICD-9-CM coding for, 202
Cystitis, screening for, 626–628

DACUM. See *Developing A Curriculum.*
Daily journal, 78, *80*
Day sheet, 124, *126, 126*
D&C (Dilatation and curettage), 441
DEA. See *Drug Enforcement Agency.*
Delinquent account, access to medical record and, 290
  accounting and, 129, 131
  bookkeeping and, 87, *88, 89, 90*
  follow-up for, 114–115, *115–122,* 118–119, 122
    accounts receivable aging record in, *121,* 122
    collection agency in, 118–119
    collection ratio in, *121,* 122
    color-coded system in, 114
    letters in, 114, *115–119*
    monthly analysis in, 122, *122*
    precautions in, 118
    small claims court in, 119, *120,* 122
    telephone collection in, 115, 118
    timetable in, 114, *115*
    undeliverable address and, 114–115
Deltoid muscle, as injection site, *357, 358, 358,* 359
Dentistry, universal precautions for, 772–773, 786. See also *Centers for Disease Control, universal precautions for blood and body fluid from.*
Department of Civil Rights, 252
Deposit, to checking account, 101, *103,* 103–104
Depreciation, of office equipment, 56
Dermal medication, *347,* 348

Design, of additional space, 47–48, *48*
  of new site, 46–47
Developing A Curriculum, 1990 guidelines for, 790–797
  code of ethics and, 268
Diabetes, coma and, 672
  ICD-9-CM coding for, 196
  insulin shock and, 672
Diagnosis, claims processing code for, 177
  computerization and, 207, *213*, *214*
  uncertain, 194, 196
Diagnosis-related group, 203–204. See also *Health insurance*.
  major diagnostic categories for, 800–808
    blood-forming organs and blood diseases and disorders in, 807
    breast diseases and disorders in, 804–805
    burns in, 808
    childbirth, pregnancy, and puerperium in, 806–807
    connective tissue and musculoskeletal diseases and disorders in, 803–804
      addition to, 808
    digestive system diseases and disorders in, 802–803
    ear, nose, and throat diseases and disorders in, 800–801
    endocrine, metabolic, and nutritional diseases and disorders in, 805
    eye diseases and disorders in, 800
    factors in health status and other contacts with health services in, 808
    hepatobiliary system diseases in, 803
    infectious and parasitic diseases in, 807
    injuries, poisonings, and toxic effects of drugs in, 808
    kidney and urinary tract diseases and disorders in, 805–806
    mental diseases and disorders in, 807–808
    metabolic, endocrine, and nutritional diseases and disorders in, 805
    musculoskeletal system and connective tissue diseases and disorders in, 803–804
      addition to, 808
    myeloproliferative disorders in, 807
    nervous system diseases and disorders in, 800
    newborns and other neonates with condition originating in perinatal period in, 807
    nutritional, metabolic, and endocrine diseases and disorders in, 805
    pancreas and hepatobiliary system disorders in, 803
    parasitic and infectious diseases in, 807
    poisonings, injuries, and toxic effects of drugs in, 808
    pregnancy, childbirth, and puerperium in, 806–807
    procedures and disorders not belonging to, 808
    puerperium, pregnancy, and childbirth in, 806–807
    reproductive system diseases and disorders in, 806
    respiratory system diseases and disorders in, 801
    skin and subcutaneous tissue diseases and disorders in, 804–805
    substance use and substance-induced organic mental disorders in, 808
    toxic effects of drugs, poisonings, and injuries in, 808
    urinary tract and kidney diseases and disorders in, 805–806
  reimbursement from, 181
Dialysis, HIV transmission and, 773
Diaper rash, 406, 408
Diaphragm, 462, *463–464*, 465, 466
  efficacy of, 466
  insertion of, 462, *463–464*

Diaphragm *(Continued)*
  removal of, *463–464*
  sizing of, 465
  weight change and, 465
Diarrhea, traveler's, 432
Differential leukocyte count, reference ranges for, 578t
Digestive system diseases and disorders, diagnosis-related group and, 802–803
Digit coding, terminal, for medical record, 21, *21*, 23
Dilatation and curettage, definition of, 441
Diphtheria, pediatric, 432
  skin test for, 745
Dipstick, in urinalysis, 567, 568, *568*, 569
Directigen 123 Testpack Strept A, in group A beta-hemolytic streptococcus, 624–625
Disability, Americans With Disabilities Act of 1990 and, 251–252
  claim form for, 41
  growth and development of child with, 413
  insurance and, 138, 241. See also *Insurance*.
    Medicare, 161, *161*. See also *Medicare*.
  pregnancy and, 253
  pediatric, 413
Disbursement journal, 78
Discharge. See also *Dismissal*.
  by patient, 280, *281*
  by physician, 281, *281*, *282*
  documentation for, 30
  of personnel, 260–261
Discount, professional, bookkeeping for, 90, *90*
Discovery rule, medical professional liability and, 286
Disinfection, HIV transmission and, 774–775
Dislocation, ICD-9-CM coding for, 200
Dismissal, 260–261
  at-will, 246
  just-cause, 246
  office policy and, 245–246
Divorce agreement, minor and, 290
Docking pay, 237
Donor, Uniform Anatomical Gift Act of 1968 and, 294, *294*
Double-book method, for appointment system, 9
Down payment, for office equipment, 55
Draft, of manuscript, 42
Dress, in personnel recruitment, 232
Dressing. See also *Bandage*.
  changing of, 390–391
  draining wound and, 391–392
  of newborn, 406
DRG. See *Diagnosis-related group*.
Drug(s). See *Medication*; named drug.
Drug abuse, 250–251
  equal opportunity practices and, 252
  ICD-9-CM coding for, 197
  medical record release and, 33
  screening for, 250, 293–294
    urine specimen for, 558, *559*
  substance-induced organic mental disorders and, diagnosis-related group and, 808
  toxicology and, reference values for, 764
Drug Enforcement Agency, 291, *292*, 336, 338t
  record-keeping for, 293
  regional offices of, *292*
  registration with, 291, 293
Drug testing, 250, 293–294
  urine specimen for, 559, *559*
Durable power of attorney, 271, 296–297

Duty-to-warn rule, 33
Dysentry, amebic, 436
　bacillary, 435
Dysmenorrhea, definition of, 441
Dyspareunia, definition of, 441

E code, *188*, 194
　adverse reaction and, 199–200
　index for, 190
　table of drugs and chemicals and, *191*
EAP. See *Employee Assistance Program*.
Ear, diseases and disorders of, diagnosis-related group and, 800–801
　medication for, 351–352
　physical examination of, 327, *328*, 329–330
　　foreign body and, 328
　　hearing loss and, 327
　　neurological examination and, 331t
　　precautions in, 329
　　procedure for, 329–330
　　Rinne Test in, 329, 331t
　　screening tests for, 327, 329
　　Weber Test in, 327, 328, 331t
　structure of, *328*
Earnings, retained, definition of, 142
Earnings card, 131, *132*, 135
EBV (Epstein-Barr virus), 643
Echocardiography, 518, 522. See also *Ultrasonography*.
Eclampsia, 471
Ectopic pregnancy, 471–472
　definition of, 466
EDTA. See *Ethylenediaminetetraacetic acid*.
Education, for certificates and licenses, 71
EEOC. See *Equal Employment Opportunity Commission*.
Elbow, radiography of, 482
Elective procedures, fee collection policy for, 108, *108*
Electric loop incinerator, in microbiology, 611
　precautions with, 614
Electrical conduction system and, electrocardiogram, *501*, 501–502, *502*
Electrocardiogram, 499–517
　electrical conduction system and, *501*, 501–502, *502*
　graph paper and measurements for, 502, *503*, 504, *504*
　heart rate in, 502, *503*
　in arrhythmias, 509, *511–517*, 512, 515, 517. See also *Arrhythmia*.
　in bundle branch block, 504, *505*
　in hypertrophy, 506, *508–510*, 509
　in myocardial infarction, 505, 506, *506*, *507*
　normal patterns in, 504
　P wave in, 501, *502*
　PR interval in, 501, *502*
　procedure for, 499–500, *500*
　QRS complex in, 501, *502*
　QRS wave in, 501, *502*
　sinus rhythm in, 502, 504, *504*
　ST segment in, 501, *502*
　T wave in, 502, *502*
　time in, 502, *503*
　voltage in, 502, *503*
　waves and intervals in, 501, *502*
Electronic blood cell counting, 592–594, *593*
　Coulter Counter Model T in, *593*, 593–594
Electrosurgery unit, 389
ELISA. See *Enzyme-linked immunosorbent assay*.

Emergency, office procedures for, 659–675
　airway obstruction and, 667–668, *668–669*
　bleeding and, 668, *669*, *670*, 671
　burns and, 671
　cardiopulmonary resuscitation and, 661, 663, 664, *665–667*, 666
　cerebrovascular accident and, 671
　diabetic coma and, 672
　diabetic insulin shock and, 672
　documentation and, 661, *662*
　emergency cart and, *660*, 661, 663
　epilepsy and, 672–673
　fainting and, 671–672
　fracture and, 673
　general guide for, 661, 663
　hospital admission and, 663
　hypertensive crisis and, 673
　hyperventilation and, 673–674
　medical office emergency chart and, *660*, 661
　myocardial infarction and, 674
　patient assessment and, *663*, 664
　scheduling and, 659–661
　shock and, 674–675
　support systems and, 663
　triage system and, 663–664
　wounds and, 675
Emergency aid, legal considerations for, 286
Emergency chart, *660*, 661
Emotional status, assessment of, 330
Employee Assistance Program, 250
Employee record, retention of, 257
Employer, release of information to, 32
Employment agency, 230
Employment security contribution tax, 136
Endocervical canal, specimen from, 544
Endocrine diseases and disorders, diagnosis-related group and, 805
Endometriosis, 451–452
　definition of, 441
Enema, for newborn, 408
Enterobiasis. See *Pin worm*.
Envelope, address for, 39–40, *41*
Environment, HIV transmission and, 774–776
　medication and, 346–347
Enzyme-linked immunosorbent assay, in HIV screening, *642*, 643
Eosinophils, in electronic blood cell counting, 592
Epilepsy, 672–673
Epithelial cell, gram-stain morphology of, 620
　transitional, 570t, *571*, 571–572, 573
Epstein-Barr virus, in infectious mononucleosis, 643
Equal Employment Opportunity Commission, 252
　guidelines from, 233
Equal opportunity practice, 251–252
Equipment, office. See *Office equipment*.
Erythrocyte sedimentation rate, 584, 759
　reference values for, 578t, 759
Escherichia coli, pediatric, 432
ESR. See *Erythrocyte sedimentation rate*.
Ethical considerations and, appointment system, 13
Ethics, 263–274. See also *Bioethics*.
　American Association of Medical Assistants and, 265, 267–268
　American Medical Technologists and, 268
　conflicts of, 264–265
　DACUM in, 268

Ethics *(Continued)*
    definition of, 263–264
    for medical personnel, 267–268
    general considerations for, 263
    guidelines for, 272–273
    moral principles and, 265–266
    of confidentiality, 269
    of consent, 269
    reasons for, 264
Ethylenediaminetetraacetic acid, in blood chemistry test, 600t
Eupnea, definition of, 313
Euthanasia, 271
Examination room, items needed in, 320
Executive, overtime exemption and, 236–237
Executive, Administrative, Professional and Outside Sales Exemptions Under the Fair Labor Standards Act (Wage and Hour Publication 1363), 236
Exercise stress test, 518
Expected date of confinement, definition of, 467
Expense, definition of, 123
    in accounting, 143
Expiratory grunt, definition of, 313
Eye. See also *Ophthalmology*.
    common defects of, *324*
    common diseases of, *328*
    diseases and disorders of, diagnosis-related group and, 800
    examination of, 324, *324–327*, 327
        equipment for, 324
        external structures in, 327
        extraocular movements in, 327
        neurological examination and, 331t
        ophthalmoscopic examination and, 327
        patient care for, 324
        visual acuity in, 324, *324–327*
        visual field in, 324, 329
    medication for, 349–351

Facilities management, 45–53
    community relations and, 53
    for closing a practice, 48–49
    for new or additional space, 47–48, *48*
    for new practice, 45–47
        design and construction in, 46–47
        renting *v* owning in, 46
        site selection in, 46
        space planning in, 46
        supplies and furniture in, 47
        time frame in, 45–46
    general considerations for, 45
    landlord relations and, 49, *49–52*, 53
    patient survey in, 47
Facsimile machines and services, 65
Fahrenheit temperature, conversion to Celsius temperature, *314*
Fainting, 671–672
Fair Labor Standards Act, 238
Family history, 30
Fasting, definition of, 597
Fax machines and services, 65
Fecal occult blood test, 629–631
Feces, reference values for, 765. See also *Stool*.
Federal Drug Abuse Prevention, Treatment, and Rehabilitation Act (42 U.S.C. Section 290ee-8), 33
Federal Employee Program, 160, *160*
Federal Equal Credit Opportunity Act, 110
Federal Fair Labor Standards Act of 1939, 235–239

Federal government, legislation from. See also names of specific legislation.
    information sources for, 276–277
    laboratory testing and, 279–280
    regulation of medical offices by, 275–276
Federal Insurance Commission Administration, *135*, 136
Federal Register, 279, 280
Federal Tax Deposit Coupon, *147*, 148
Fee, collection of, billing in, 110, 112–122
    credit card, 110
    follow-up for, 114–115, *115–122*, 118–119, 122. See also *Delinquent account, follow-up for*.
    methods for, 112, 114
    procedure for, 114
    sample statement for, 112, *113*
    credit and, 108–122
        arrangements for, 108, 110, *111*, 112
        issues in, 108
        policy for, 108
        staff education and, 108–109
        third-party reimbursement and, 110. See also *Insurance company*.
    policy for, 108
        criteria for, 109
    delinquent. See also *Delinquent account*.
        from insurance company, 183, 186
    discussion of, *108*, 109–110
    for service, 110
Femur, radiography of, 483
FEP *(Federal Employee Program)*, 160, *160*
Fetus, alpha-fetoprotein level and, 472
    monitoring of, 472
    non-stress test and, 472
    oxytocin challenge test and, 472
    ultrasonography for, 472
Fever, pediatric, 435
Fibrillation, atrial, 512, *513*
    ventricular, *514*, 515
Fibrocystic breast disease, 452
Fibula, radiography of, 497–498
FICA. See *Federal Insurance Commission Administration*.
Filing cabinet, *22*, 23
Final Rule, CLIA, 791–796. See also *Clinical Laboratory Improvement Amendments of 1988, Final Rule*.
Financial report. See also *Accounting; Bookkeeping*.
    computerization and, 221
Financial responsibility data, computerization and, 207, *208*
Fire protection, for medical records, 24
    for storage area, 63
First-class mail, 36
First morning specimen, for urinalysis, 555t, 560
Flatus, in newborn, 408
Fluid, aspiration of, ultrasonography in, 522
Fluoride poisoning, 740t
Flutter, atrial, 512, *513*
    ventricular, *514*, 515
Foam, vaginal, 465
    efficacy of, 466
Food and Drug Administration, pregnancy categories for drugs and drug products, 336, 338t
Foot, radiography of, 484–485
Footnote, in manuscript preparation, 43
Forceps, 371, *374*, *375*
    in transferring sterile article, 378–379
Forearm, radiography of, 485–486
Formaldehyde, 531
Formalin, 531

Formula feeding, for infant, 403, 404t–405t
  for newborn, 403, 404t–405t
Fourth-class mail, 36
Fracture, 673
  ICD-9-CM coding for, 200
Fungal infection. See also names of specific fungal infections.
  skin test for, 745
Furniture, for new practice, 47

Gas, in newborn, 408
Genital herpes, 447t
Genital tract, culture techniques for, 636–639, *637*
  oxidase test and, 638–639
  specimen from, 544–545
German measles. See *Rubella*.
Gestation, definition of, 467
Gestational weeks, definition of, 467
Glasses, for specimen collection and processing, 533
Globulin, in blood chemistry test, 599t
Glove, in infection control, 75
  in specimen collection and processing, 532
  in universal precautions, 787–788
Glucose, in blood chemistry tests, 599t
  fasting blood sample level, 599t, 602–605, *603–605*
    calibration of glucose meter and, *604*, 604–605, *605*
    reagent strip insertion and, *603*, 603–604
  glucose tolerance test and, 532, 599t, 605–606
  in urinalysis, 562t
Glucose meter, 602–605, *603–605*
  calibration of, *604*, 604–605, *605*
Goggles, in specimen collection and processing, 533
Gonorrhea, 447t
  clinical considerations for, 628
  tests for, 544–545
    culture techniques in, 636–639, *637*
    direct smear in, 628–629, *629*
Good Samaritan Act, 286, 661
Goodell's sign, definition of, 467
Gown, in specimen collection and processing, 532
Gram stain, 616t, 616–620
  examination of, 619–620
  frequently encountered bacteria and, 616t
  in gonorrhea, 628–629
  purpose of, 616
  smear preparation and, *617*, 617–618
  smear staining and, 618–619
Grammar, common mistakes in, 732–736
Granular cast, in urinalysis, *570*, 570t, *571*
Gravid, definition of, 467
Gravida, 467, 467t
Gross wages, definition of, 147
Grounds, protection of, 59–60
  waste disposal and, 60
Group A beta-hemolytic streptococcus, 623–625
  agar and, 631
  Directigen 123 Testpack Strept A in detection of, 624–625
  serological tests for, 631
  throat culture for, 631–633, *632*
Growth and development, 408t, 409–413, *412–424*, *423*
  chest circumference in, 408t, 409–410
  deviations in, 410
  growth chart for, 413, *415–422*, *423*. See also *Growth chart*.
  head circumference in, 408t, 409
    boys and, *417*

Growth and development *(Continued)*
    girls and, *415*
  height in, 408t, 412–413, *413*, *414*
  of newborn, 408t
  physically handicapped child and, 413
  weight in, 408t, *410*, 410–411, *411*
Growth chart, 413, 415–422, *423*
  for boys, *417*, *418*, *421*, *422*
  for girls, *415*, *416*, *419*, *420*
  materials for, 423
  procedure for, 423
  purpose of, 423
Guaiac, in fecal occult blood test, 629
Gynecology, 441–466. See also *Obstetrics*.
  colposcopy in, 456
  examination in, 442–445, *443*, *444*
    bimanual, *443*, 444
    medical assisting for, 442–443, 444–445
    Pap smear and, 442–443
    physician's implementation of, *443*, 444, *444*
    position for, *321*
    speculum for, 443–445
    spray cytology fixative for, 443
  medical conditions in, 445–456. See also names of specific conditions.
  patient history in, 441
  specimen collection in, 544–545
    vaginal discharge and, 450–451
  terminology in, 441
  ultrasonography in, 522
  wet preparation in. See *KOH preparation*.

Hand, radiography of, 486–487
Hand-washing, 303–304
Handy Reference Guide to the Fair Labor Standards Act, 238
Harassment, sexual, 252–253
Hastings Center Report, 269
Hazard Communication Standard, 549
HCFA. See *Health Care Financing Administration*.
HCG. See *Human chorionic gonadotropin*.
HDS Medical Assistance Professional software program, 207, 208–221, *216*, *221*
  for additional records, 221
  for appointments, 221
  for charge entry, 207, *215*, *216*
  for diagnosis record, 207, *213*, *214*
  for financial responsibility data, 207, *208*
  for ICD-9 menu display, 207, *214*
  for insurance coverage, 207, *209–211*, *216*, *219–221*
  for management reports, 221–222
  for new patient, 207, *208–211*
  for patient information menu, 207, *212*
  for patient list, 207, *208*
  for patient record, 207, *209*
  for payment entry, 207, *215*, *216*, *216*, *218–221*
  for procedure record, 207, *212*, *213*
  for responsible party menu, *216*, *216*, *217*
Head, growth and development of, 408t, 409
  boys and, *415*
  girls and, *415*
Health and welfare agencies and associations, voluntary, 690–692
Health care, quality of. See *Quality of care*.

Health Care Financing Administration, 181
    CLIA 1988 Final Rule from, 791. See also *Clinical Laboratory Improvement Amendments of 1988, Final Rule.*
    HCFA-1500 claim form from, 196
Health care services, telephone numbers for, 693
Health care worker. See also *Personnel.*
    AIDS-infected, 769, 781
    definition of, 768
    hepatitis B virus transmission and, 780. See also *Centers for Disease Control.*
    HIV testing of, 780
    HIV transmission and, 769–770, 781–782. See also *Centers for Disease Control.*
    interaction with Occupational Safety and Health Act guidelines, 830
    job performance of, 71–72
    professional designations for, 726–729
    qualifications of, 70, *71*
Health history, form for, *308*
    medication administration and, 345–346
    prenatal care and, 467, *468–469*, 469
Health insurance, alternatives to, benefits package and, 138
    basic medical, 157–158
    Blue Cross/Blue Shield. See *Blue Cross/Blue Shield.*
    central certification, 160, *161*
    CHAMPUS. See *Civilian Health and Medical Program of the Uniformed Services.*
        claim processing and, 170
            assignment in, 170
            deadline for, *179*
            electronic, 173
            examples of, *182, 183, 184, 185*
            form for, Blue Cross, *171–172, 174–175*
                CHAMPUS, 173, *178*, 179
                equipment and materials for, 173
                Medicaid, *171–172, 176*
                procedural steps for, 173, 175, 177, 179
                standard, *168–169*
            information for, 170
            insurance log for, 179, *180*
            nonparticipating, 170, 173
            participating, 170
            recent legislation for, 170
            with nonallowed adjustment, *89*, 90
        cost containment methods and, 239
        emergency hospital admission and, 158, 175
        Federal Employee Program, 160, *160*
        funding methods for, 240
        general considerations for, 239–240
        health maintenance organization, 166, 186–187, 239–240
            advantages of, 186
            closed, 186
            disadvantages of, 186
            open, 186–187
        hospitalization portion of, 158
        independent practice association, 166, 170
        major medical, 158
        Medicaid. See *Medicaid.*
        Medicare. See *Medicare.*
        payment from, contractual nonalloweds and, 183
            delinquent, 183, 186
            diagnosis-related group and, 181
            explanation of benefit and, 181, *182*, 183
            fee schedule and, 181
            general considerations for, 179, 181
            nonparticipating physician and, 181

Health insurance *(Continued)*
        participating physician and, 181
        resource-based relative value scale and, 181
        usual, customary, and reasonable, 179, 181
    permanent reciprocity program, 161, *161*
    preadmission certification for, 158, *159*
    preferred provider organization, 166, 240
    pregnancy and, 253
    private, 166, *168–169*
    surgical portion of, 158
    types of, 157–158
Health maintenance organization, 166, 186–187, 239–240. See also *Health insurance.*
    advantages of, 186
    closed, 186
    disadvantages of, 186
    open, 186–187
Health services, contact with, health status and, diagnosis-related group and, 808
Hearing, loss of, 327
Heart rate, in electrocardiogram, 502, *503*
Heat, application of, 397–400
    general considerations for, 397
    hot moist pack for, 397–398
    hot water bottle for, 398–400
Heat block, in microbiology, 611
Hegar's sign, definition of, 467
Height, 309–310
    in growth and deevelopment, 408t, 412–413, *413, 414.* See also *Growth chart.*
Heimlich maneuver, 668, *668–669*
Hemacytometer, 585, 586–588, *587, 588*
Hematocrit, 578t, 578–581, *579, 580*
    centrifuge for, 579, *579*, 580
    guidelines for, 578–579
    hemolysis and, 579
    microhematocrit capillary tubes for, 581
    microhematocrit reader for, 579, *580*
    procedure for, 579, *580*, 581
        errors in, 579
    reference values for, 578t, 759
Hematology, 577–597. See also *Blood, chemistry tests for.*
    definition of, 529
    electronic blood cell counting in, 592–594, *593*
        Coulter Counter Model T in, *593*, 593–594
    erythrocyte sedimentation rate in, 584
        reference values for, 578t
    general considerations for, 577–578
    hematocrit in, 578t, 578–581, *579, 580.* See also *Hematocrit.*
    hemoglobin concentration in, 582–583
        cyanmetheglobin reagent in, 582–583
        reference values for, 578t
        turbidity and, 583
    manual leukocyte count in, 585–588, *585–588*
        reference values for, 578t
    peripheral blood smear examination in, 588–592
        blood cell types in, *591*
        guidelines for, 588–589
        preparation for, *590*
        reference values for, 578t
    prothrombin time in, 594–597, *596.* See also *Prothrombin time.*
    reference values for, 578, 578t, 759–762
Hematoma, subdural, 438
Hemoccult II Slide Test, in fecal occult blood, 629–631

Hemoglobin, 582–583
  cyanmethemoglobin reagent and, 582–583
  reference values for, 578t, 579
  turbidity and, 583
Hemolysis, definition of, 597
Heparin, in blood chemistry test, 600t
  subcutaneous injection of, 356
Hepatitis A virus, pediatric, 430
Hepatitis B virus, background of, 811–812
  Occupational Safety and Health Act recommendations for, 809–833. See also *Occupational Safety and Health Act.*
  final standards from, 809–810
  transmission of, health care worker and, 780
    modes of, 812–814
    universal precautions and. See *Centers for Disease Control, universal precautions for blood and body fluid from.*
  vaccine for, 811, 825–831
    Occupational Safety and Health Act and, 809
Hepatobiliary system, diseases of, diagnosis-related group and, 803
Hernia, umbilical, 406
Herpes, genital, 447t
Herpes zoster, pediatric, 431
Hiccoughs, in newborn, 408
Hip, radiography of, 488
Hippocratic oath, 265
Hiring. See *Personnel, recruitment of.*
HIV. See *Human immunodeficiency virus.*
HMO. See *Health maintenance organization.*
Holiday, paid, 237, 238
Holter monitor, 517
Home health care, Medicare coverage for, 164
Home visit, appointment for, 12
  documentation of, 12
Hospital, abbreviations used by, 696–698
  cost containment methods and, 239
  diagnosis-related group effect on, 203–204
  emergency admission to, 663
  fee collection policy for, 108, *108*
  insurance coverage for, 158
  Medicare coverage for, 163–164
Hot moist pack, 397–398
Hot-water bottle, 398–400
Household equivalent, 751
Household measurement, 339t, 340
Housekeeping, 60
  HIV transmission and, 776–777
Human chorionic gonadotropin, clinical considerations for, 646
  definition of, 467
  in ectopic pregnancy, 471
  tests for, 640t, 646–648, *647*
Human immunodeficiency virus. See also *Acquired immune deficiency syndrome.*
  background of, 811–812
  estimated annual number of patients infected with, 778t
  health care workers infected with, 769, 781
    testing of, 780
  ICD-9-CM coding for, 200
  manifestation in female, 447t
  office policy and, 251
  survival of, environment and, 775–776
  tests for, 640t, *642*, 642–643, *643*, 778–780, 779t
    clinical considerations for, 642

Human immunodeficiency virus *(Continued)*
    enzyme-linked immunosorbent assay in, *642*, 643
    health care workers and, 780
    informed consent and, *289*
    patients and, 779–780
    predictive value of, 779t
    sensitivity of, 778
    specificity of, 778–779
    Western Blot test in, *643*, 643
  transmission of, modes of, 812–814
    Occupational Safety and Health Act and, 809–834. See also *Occupational Safety and Health Act.*
    final standards from, 809
    universal precautions for blood and body fluid and, 301–303, 768–790. See also *Centers for Disease Control, universal precautions for blood and body fluid from.*
Humerus, radiography of, 489
Hyaline cast, in urinalysis, *570*, 570t, 570–571
Hydrocarbons, poisoning by, 739t
Hydrochloric acid, 531
  poisoning by, 738t
Hyfrecator, 389
Hygiene, for newborn, 406
Hyperemesis gravidarum, 470
Hypermetropia, definition of, *324*
Hyperpnea, definition of, 313
Hypertension, ICD-9-CM coding for, 198
  pregnancy-induced. See *Preeclampsia.*
Hypertensive crisis, 673
Hypertrophy, electrocardiogram in detection of, 506, *508–510*, 509
Hyperventilation, 673–674
  definition of, 313
Hypotension, supine, *470*, 470–471
Hypoventilation, definition of, 313
Hysterosalpingogram, 474

ICD. See *International Classification of Diseases.*
Ice bag, 400–401
Illustration, in manuscript preparation, 43
Immigration reform, 253, *254–256*, 256–257
Immunization, 424, 424t, 425t
  administration routes for, 425t
  schedule for, 425t
  types of, 425t
Immunology, definition of, 529
Impetigo, pediatric, 432
Inch, conversion to centimeter, 310
Income, net, *142*, 143
Income revenue, definition of, 123
Income statement, *142*, 143
  definition of, 123
Income tax. See *Tax(es).*
Incubator, in microbiology, 609, *610*
Independent practice association, 166, 170
Index, in manuscript preparation, 43
Index Medicus, 42
Indirect immunofluorescence assay, as screening for HIV, *642*, 643
Infant. See also *Newborn.*
  catheterization of, 556
  growth and development of, 408t, 409. See also *Growth and development.*
  stool collection from, 541

Infant *(Continued)*
  urine specimen from, 560
  vital signs, 427, *428*, 428t
Infarction, myocardial. See *Myocardial infarction.*
Infection control, 75
Infectious disease, diagnosis-related group and, 807
  ICD-9-CM coding for, 200
Infertility, 473–474
  definition of, 473
  diagnostic procedures for, 473–474
  etiology of, 473
  general considerations for, 473
Influenza, pediatric, 430
Information, health care, telephone numbers for, 693
Informed consent, ethics of, 269
  for surgery, 287, 287–288, 290
  intrauterine device and, 461
  legal considerations and, 287–288, *287–289*, 290
  levonorgestrel implant and, 458
  minor and, 33
  transparency model for, 269
Injection. See also *Medication, parenteral.*
  advantages of, 352
  adverse effects of, 370
  deltoid muscle as landmark for, 357, 358, *358*, 359
  intradermal, 352, *353*, 353t, *354*, 355
  intramuscular, 353t, 356, *356–358*
    Z-track method of, *365*, 365–366
  legislation regarding, 280
  needle size for, 356, 359, 361
  pain reduction techniques for, 366
  subcutaneous, 353t, *354*, 355, *355*, 358
    heparin and, 356
  syringe for, 361–363
    admixture of two drugs and, 361–362
    air bubbles and, 361
    dead space and, 361
    drawing medication into, 362–363
  vastus lateralis muscle as landmark for, 357, *359*, 359–360
  ventrogluteal site as landmark for, 357, *360*, 360–361
Injury, diagnosis-related group and, 808
  evidence of, 664
Inoculating loop, in microbiology, 611
Instrument, sanitization of, 304
  sterilization of, *304*, 304–306, *305*, 306t
Insulin shock, diabetic, 672
Insurance, automobile, 138
  bond as, 138
  Business Owner's Insurance Package as, 138
  choice of, 138
  commercial, 166, *168–169*
  computerization and, 207, *209–211*, 216, *219–221*
  disability, 138, 161, *161*, 241
    pregnancy and, 253
  discussion of, 109
  fee collection policy and, 108
  for office equipment, 56
  health. See *Health insurance.*
  liability, 139, 286
  life, 138
  new patient information regarding, 28
  renewal of, 138–139
  tickler file for, *138*, 139
  types of, *139*, 139–140
  Worker's Compensation as, 138
Insurance company, as information source for federal and state law, 277

Insurance company *(Continued)*
  information request from, 40–41
  refiles to, 183
  rejections from, 183
  release of information to, 32
Insurance log, 179, *180*
  delinquent unpaid insurance claim and, 183, 186
Insured mail, 36–37
Integrity, definition of, 597
Interlibrary loan, 42
Internal Revenue Code Section 603D, 242
Internal Revenue Service. See *Tax(es).*
International Classification of Diseases, 187–204. See also *Coding, ICD.*
International mail, 36
International Statistical Classification of Diseases and Related Health Problems, 204
International System of Units, 757–758
Interview, exit, 261
  in personnel recruitment, 230–231, *231*
  patient, 306–307, *308*, 309. See also *Patient, new.*
Intrauterine device, *460*, 461–462
  efficacy of, 466
Intrauterine pregnancy, definition of, 467
Inventory, *63*, 63–64
  of controlled substances, 293
Iodine, allergy to, 382
  parenteral medication and, 363
Iodophor, allergy to, parenteral medication and, 363
IPA. See *Independent practice association.*

Jenbec plate, 637, *637*
Job application, *228–229*, 231–232
Job description, 226–227, *227*
Job performance, in quality of care, 71–72
Joint Commission of Health Care Organizations, accreditation from, 67–68
Journal, manuscript preparation for, 42–43
Junctional premature contraction, 509, *511*, 512
Junctional tachycardia, 512, *513*
Junk mail, 34

Kawasaki disease, pediatric, 436
Ketone, in urinalysis, 562t
Kevorkian, Jack, MD, 271
Kidney, diseases and disorders of, diagnosis-related group and, 805–806
  examination of, ultrasonography in, 518, *521*
Knee, radiography of, 490
Knee-chest position, for medical examination, 322
KOH preparation, 544
  for bacterial vaginosis, 446
  for candidiasis, *449*
  for moniliasis, 446
  for trichomonas, *449*
  procedure for, 445–446, 448, 450, *450*
  purpose of, 445
  vaginal swabs for, 545
Korotkoff's sound, 316
Kussmaul's respiration, definition of, 313

Labeling, in specimen collection and processing, 532
  Occupational Safety and Health Act standards for, 809
  of waste, 548, 548t, *549*

Labia majora, 557
Labia minora, 557
Labor law, 131, 135
   drug testing and, 250
   equal opportunity practices and, 251–252
   future trends in, 257–258
   general considerations for, 257–258
   HIV transmission and, 251
   immigration reform and, 253, *254–256*, 256–257
   pregnancy leave and, 253
   retention of employees' records and, 257
   sexual harassment and, 252–253
   smoking and, 251
   substance abuse and, 250–251
   Worker's Compensation and, 248–249. See also *Worker's Compensation.*
Laboratory, CLIA 1988 Final Rule and, 791–796. See also *Clinical Laboratory Improvement Amendments of 1988, Final Rule.*
   HIV transmission and, 773–774
   quality control for, 75
   reference, 526
Laboratory test. See also names of specific laboratory tests.
   abnormal findings in, 34
   authorization to release and assign benefits for, 526, *528*
   categories of, 529
   legislation regarding, 279
   panels and profiles in, 529t, 529–530
   patient instruction for, 530
   reference values for, 757–765
      for cerebrospinal fluid, 764
      for feces, 765
      for semen, 764
      for urine, 762–763
      in hematology, 759–762
      in therapeutic drug monitoring, 753–754
      in toxicology, 764
      International System of Units and, 757–758
   request form for, 526, *527*, *528*
Lactic acid, in blood chemistry test, 599t
Landlord, relations with, 49, *49–52*, 53
Laser surgery, 388
Latex agglutination test, for C-reactive protein, 640t, 641–642
Laundry, HIV transmission and, 776–777
   Occupational Safety and Health Act guidelines for, 829
Lead, in urinalysis, 562t
Lease, 49, *49–52*, 53
   automobile, 56
   office equipment. See also *Office equipment, lease and purchase of.*
      legal counsel in, 57–58
      purchase *v*, 55–56
Leave of absence, 241–242
Ledger card, 78
Legal consideration. See also *Legislation.*
   appointment system and, 13
   office equipment lease and, 58
   personnel recruitment and, *228–229*, 232–233
   policy manual and, 245–246
Legislation. See also names of specific legislation.
   abortion and, 271–272
   basic health care and, 270
   branches of, *276*, 277–278
   death and dying and, 294, *295–297*, 297
   drug screening and, 293–294
   durable power of attorney and, 271

Legislation *(Continued)*
   federal, information sources for, 276–277
      laboratory testing and, 279–280
      regulation of medical offices by, 275–276
   information sources for, 276–277
   injections and, 280
   laboratory testing and, 279–280
   liability and, 280–286. See also *Liability.*
   living will and, 271
   medical assisting practice and, 279–280
   medical records and, *290*, 290–291
   monitoring of, 298
   patient care and, 286–290, *287–290*
      appointments in, 287
      emergency aid in, 286
      informed consent in, 287–288, *287–289*, 290
      minors and, 288, 290
   patients' rights and, 270–272
   personnel credentialing and, 278–280
   public health reporting and, 291, *293*
   radiography and, 280
   regulation of medical offices by, 275–278, *277–278*
   state, in death and dying, 294, *295–297*, 297
      injections and, 280
      medical assisting practice and, 279–280
      medical practice act from, 278–279
      minors and, 290
      radiography and, 280
      regulation of medical offices by, 275–276, *278*
      statute of limitations and, 282, *283–286*, 286
      venipuncture and, 280
   venipuncture and, 280
Letter. See also *Correspondence.*
   business, parts of, *37*, *38*, 38–39, *40*
      simplified, *40*
   collection, 114, *115–119*
   of reference, in personnel recruitment, 232
   of referral, 41
Leukocyte count, manual, 585–588, *585–588*
   reference values for, 578t
   reference values for, 759
Leukocyte esterase, 627–628
Levonorgestrel implant, 458–460, 466. See also *Contraception, implant as.*
Liability, contract and, 280–281, *281*
   definition of, 123
   in balance sheet, *141*, 142
   in discharge by patient, 280, *281*
   in withdrawal by physician, 281, *281*, *282*
   insurance for, 139, 286
   malpractice and, 281
   standard of care and, 281–282, *282*
   statute of limitations and, 282, *283–286*, 286
License. See also *Credentialing, of personnel.*
   education for, 71
Licensure, 278–279
Life insurance, 138, 240–241. See also *Insurance.*
   request for information, 41
   term, 240–241
Life support, withdrawal of, 297
   legal considerations in, 297
Lipemia, definition of, 597
Lipid, serum level of, 606–607
Lithotomy position, for medical examination, *321*
Litigation, medical record and, 24
Liver, examination of, ultrasonography in, 518, *521*
Living will, 271, 294, *295*, 297

Logbook, quality control, 551, 551t
Loop holder, in microbiology, 611
Lumbar spine, radiography of, 491
Lyme disease, pediatric, 436
Lymphocyte, in electronic blood cell counting, 592

Mail. See *Correspondence*.
Mail service, for specimen transport, 547
Maintenance, for office equipment, 58
   for photocopy machine, 64–65
Malfeasance, definition of, 281
Malpractice. See also *Liability*.
   definition of, 281
Mantoux test, 366–367
Manuscript, preparation of, 42–43
Married, semimonthly table for payroll, 136, *137*
Mask, in specimen collection and processing, 533
Mastitis, 452, *453*
Meal period, 237–238
Measure. See *Weights and measures*.
Media, in microbiology, 611–612, *612*, 613t
Medicaid, 33, 164, 166, *167*. See also *Health insurance*.
   Blue Cross/Blue Shield and, 158, 160
   claims processing for, *171–172*, 173, 175, *176*, 177, 179
   limitations of, 166
   refiling claim to, 183
   remittance from, 183
   XIX-TPD-76 form for, 175, *176*
Medical Assistant Society, as information source for federal and state law, 277
Medical ethics. See *Ethics*.
Medical history, 30
Medical practice act, state, 278–279
Medical record, 19–34
   access to, 290
   as validation of coding, 197
   confidentiality and, *290*, 291
   conversion of, 23
   data collection and, 27–28, *29*, 30
   discharge and, 30
   disposal of, 24–25, 291
   documentation in, 72
   employer request for, 32
   faxing of, 31
   filing and identification system for, 19–23
      alphabetic coding in, 20
      color coding in, 19, *20*
      cross-indexing in, 23
      numeric coding in, 20–21
      special indexing in, 25, *25*
      terminal digit coding in, 21, *21*, 23
   filing cabinet for, *22*, 23
   fire protection for, 24
   government request for, 32–33
   ICD-9-CM coding and, 197, 203
   insurance company request for, 32
   legal considerations for, 290–291, *291*
   litigation protection for, 24
   mailed request for, 31
   of minor, 33
   out guide for, 24
   ownership of, 290
   phone request for, 31
   policies for, 72

Medical record *(Continued)*
   preservation of, 23–24
   problem-oriented, 26–27, *27*, *28*
   record retention schedule for, 24–25
   release of, *290*, 291
   research agency request for, 33
   research registry and, 30
   retention of, 290–291
   return visit and, 30
   search warrant for, 34
   SOAP format for, 27
   source-oriented, 25–26, *26*
   specialized terms used in, 730
   subpoena of, 33, 34
   system for, 72
   transfer of, 24
   urinalysis and, *554*, 554
Medicare, 33, 161, *161*. See also *Health insurance*.
   Blue Cross/Blue Shield and, 158, 160
   card for, *161*, 163
   coverage under, 163–164
   deductible for, 164, *166*
   extended patient authorization for, 164, *165*
   fee schedule from, 181
   part A, 163–164
   part B, 164, *165*, 175
   participating *v* nonparticipating, 170, 173
   physician payment reform from, 713–717
      additional amount for supplies in facility-based procedures in, 720
      balance billing limits in, 717
      evaluation and management codes in, 721–725
      evaluation and management service descriptors in, 716
      fee schedule computation in, 714
      new evaluation and management codes in, 715
      new physician payment in, 717
      non-incisional procedures in, 716
      procedure codes subject to outpatient limit in, 718–719
      surgical global package in, 716
      surgical modifier codes in, 717
   refiling claim to, 183
   remittance from, *182*, 183
   resource-based relative scale for, 181
   social security tax and, 136
   suffix codes for, *162–163*, 163
   Travelers, 163, *164*
   United Mine Workers of America and, 163, *164*
Medication. See also names of specific drugs.
   absorption of, *344*, 345
   administration of, 335–370
      environment and, 346–347
      injection for. See *Injection*.
      legal considerations in, 336
      office policy for, 336
      responsibilities in, 335–336
      route and site for, *347*, 347–352
         ear, 351–352
         eye, 349–351
         injection and. See *Injection*.
         mucous membrane, *347*, 347–348
         oral, *347*, *347*
         parenteral, *347*, 348. See also *Medication, parenteral*.
         rectal, 348–349
         topical, *347*, 348, 349–352
   bacteriostatic preservatives in, 345
   cardiovascular, monitoring of, reference values for, 763

Medication *(Continued)*
  checklist for, 346
  delivery of, *344*, 345
  dosage for, 341, *341*, 341t, *342*
    Mg/kg/day formula and, 341, *342*
  drug assessment and, 346
  ear, 351–352
  excretion of, *344*, 345
  eye, 349–351
  factors influencing effects of, 345
  laboratory tests and, 530, 532
  measuring of, 340–341, *340–344*, 345
    conversion formula and, 340, *341*
    oral medication and, *340*, 340–341
    unit dose, 340
  metabolism of, *344*, 345
  mucous membrane, *347*, 347–348
  oral, 347, *347*
    reconstitution of, 341, 341t
    unit dose form of, 340
  parenteral, *347*, 348. See also *Injection*.
    administration of, 363–364
      iodine allergy and, 363
    adverse effects of, 370
    reconstitution of, 341, 341t, 345
    unit dose form of, 340
  patient assessment and, 345–346
  reconstitution of, 341, *343*, 345
    precaution for pediatric and, 345
  rectal, 348–349
  topical, *347*, 348, 349–352
  written and oral orders for, 336, 337t–339t, 340
    abbreviations for, 336, 337t–339t
    controlled substances and, 336, 338t
    measurement systems for, 336, 338t, 339t
    pregnancy and, 336, 338t
Menarche, definition of, 441
Meningitis, pediatric, 433
Menopause, definition of, 441
Menorrhagia, definition of, 441
Menses, cycle for, rhythm method and, 466
  definition of, 441
  "last menstrual period" and, 467
  oral contraception and, 457
  timing of levonorgestrel implant insertion and, 458
Mental disease, diagnosis-related group and, 807–808
Mental status, assessment of, 330
Metabolism, diseases and disorders of, diagnosis-related group and, 805
Metric system, 339t, 340
Metronidazole, 447t
Metrorrhagia, definition of, 441
Mg/kg/day formula, medication measurement and, 341, *342*
MHCRA (Michigan Handicappers' Civil Rights Act), 250, 252
Michigan Handicappers' Civil Rights Act, 250, 252
Microbiology, 609–639
  culture techniques in, 631–639
    genital tract, 636–639, *637*
      oxidase test and, 638–639
    group A beta-hemolytic streptococcus and, 631–633, *632*
    urine, 633–636, *635*, 635t
      calibrated loop method for, 634–636, *635*
      kits for, 634
      pathogens and, 635t, 636
      purpose of, 633
    definition of, 529

Microbiology *(Continued)*
  equipment and supplies in, 609, *610*, 611–612, *613*, 613t, 614t
    Bunsen burner as, 611
      precautions with, 614
    electric loop incinerator as, 611
    heat block as, 611
    incubator as, 609, *610*
    inoculating loops as, 611
    loop holders as, 611
    media as, 611–612, *612*, 613t
    Petri dish holder as, 611
    reagent as, 612, *613*, 614t
    refrigerator as, 611
    stain as, 612, *613*, 614t
    staining rack as, 611
    test kit as, 612
  general considerations for, 609
  microscopic procedures in, cellophane tape and, examination of, 620, 622
    preparation of, 620, *621*
    gram stain and, 616t, 616–620, *617*. See also *Gram stain*.
  safety guidelines in, 614
  screening procedures in, 623–631
    fecal occult blood and, 629–631
    gonorrhea and, 628–629, *629*
    group A beta-hemolytic streptococcus and, 623–625
      Abbott Testpack Strept A in, 624–625
    urine screening tests and, 626–628
  specimen collection and handling in, 615
Microfilm, 23–24
Micronutrient, 754–756
Microorganism, in urinalysis, 570t, *573*, 574
MicroScan ImmunoSCAN RPR Card Test Kit, 651–652, *652*
Minor, definition of, 288
  divorce agreement and, 290
  emancipated, 290
  informed consent and, 33, 288, 290
  mature, 290
  releasing records of, 33
  state legislation and, 290
Misconduct, of personnel, 260–261
Misfeasance, definition of, 281
Mission statement, 3
  appointment system and, 3
MLA Electra 750, 595–597, *596*
Mole, removal of, 389–390
Moniliasis, 446, 446t
Monocyte, in electronic blood cell counting, 592
Mononucleosis, infectious, 643–645, *645*
  Color Slide II Mononucleosis Test for, 640t, 644–645, *645*
  pediatric, 430
Monthly billing, 112
Moral principle, 265–266
Mortician, HIV transmission and, 773
Motor system, assessment of, 330, 331t, 332
Mucocutaneous lymph node syndrome, pediatric, 436
Multigravida, definition of, 467
Multipara, definition of, 467
Mumps, pediatric, 430
Muscle, deltoid, as injection site, *357*, 358, *358*, 359
Musculoskeletal system, diseases and disorders of, diagnosis-related group and, 803–804, 808
Myeloproliferative disorder, diagnosis-related group and, 807

SUBJECT INDEX

Myocardial infarction, 674
    electrocardiogram in detection of, 505, 506, *506*, *507*
    ICD-9-CM coding for, 198, *199*
Myopia, definition of, *324*

Nagele's rule, definition of, 467
National Five-Digit Zip Code and Post Office Directory, 35
Natural Death Act, 294, *295–297*, 297
Near-Vision Acuity Chart, 324, *325*
Needle, precautions with, 533
Needle holder, 371
Needle-guided biopsy, ultrasonography in, 522
Neisseria gonorrhea. See *Gonorrhea.*
Neoplasm. See also *Cancer.*
    coding for, *200*, 200–202, *201*
        alphabetical index in, 190, *190*, 200
        chemotherapy and, 201–202
        classification in, 200–201
        cysts and, 202
        location unknown and, 202
        papilloma and, 202
        possible malignancy and, 202
        radiotherapy and, 201–202
        recurrent malignancy and, 202
        secondary site and, 201
        table of, 200, *200*, *201*
            asterisk in, 202
        V codes and, 202
Nervous system, diseases and disorders of, diagnosis-related group and, 800
Neurological examination, 330, 331t, 332
Neurosonography, 522. See also *Ultrasonography.*
Neutrophil, in electronic blood cell counting, 592
New patient. See *Patient, new.*
New practice. See *Practice, new.*
Newborn, 403, 404t–405t, 406–409, 408t. See also *Infant.*
    and other neonates with condition originating in perinatal period, diagnosis-related group and, 807
    bathing, 406
    breast feeding for, 403
        flatus and, 408
    burping, 406
    circumcised, 406
    common problems of, 407–409
    dressing, 406
    formula feeding for, 403, 404t–405t
    growth and development of, 408t
    hygiene for, 406
    telephone decision guidelines for, 406–407
    umbilical care for, 406
    uncircumcised, 406
Nicotine poisoning, 740t
Nipple, care of, breastfeeding and, 473
    discharge from, 452, *453*
    sore and cracked, 473
Nitric acid, poisoning by, 738t
Nitrite, in urine screening test, 627, 628
Nondiscrimination policy, 251–252
Nonfeasance, definition of, 282
Nonroutine appointment, appointment system for, 11
Non-stress test, fetal heart rate and, 472
Norplant system. See *Contraception, implant as.*
No-show office visit, 11, 13

Nulligravida, definition of, 467
Nullipara, definition of, 467
Numeric coding, for medical record, 20–21
Nutrition, diseases and disorders of, diagnosis-related group and, 805
    medication and, 346
    principal micronutrients and, 754–756
    recommended daily dietary allowances and, 753

OBRA. See *Omnibus Budget Reconciliation Act of 1989.*
Obstetrics, 466–474. See also *Gynecology; Pregnancy.*
    confirmation of pregnancy in, 467
    diagnostic procedures in, 472
        infertility and, 473–474
        ultrasonography in, 522, *522*
    obstetrical disorders and, 469–472. See also names of specific disorders.
    postpartum care in, 473
    routine prenatal care in, 467, *468–469*, 469
        health history and, 467, *468–469*, 469
        physical examination and, 469
    terminology in, 466–467
Occupational Safety and Health Act, bloodborne pathogens
    final standard from, 809–810
    employee records and, 257
    hepatitis B vaccination protection in, 825–831, 829
    Joint Advisory Notice of the Department of Labor and Department of Health and Human Services for protection against HBV and HIV, 811–825
        administrative tasks in, 817
        exposure categories in, 816, 825
        medical provisions in, 820
        national office of, 824
        protective equipment in, 819–820
        recommendations in, 815–816
        record-keeping in, 820
        training and education in, 818
        work practices in, 819
    pathogen exposure control plan in, 825–831
    record-keeping in, 810, 820, 830
    state approval of, 833–834
    waste disposal and, 548–549, *549*
Office equipment, depreciation of, 56
    lease and purchase of, 55–58
        comparison of, 55–57
        coverage in, 56
        depreciation in, 56
        down payment in, 55
        financing in, 56
        legal counsel in, 57–58
        maintenance agreement in, 58
        negotiated terms in, 56
        payment periods in, 56
        policy and procedure development in, 56–58, *57*
        tax advantages in, 56, *57*
    maintenance of, fax machine and, 65
        photocopy machine and, 64–65
    purchase of, fax machine and, 65
        photocopy machine and, 64
    telephone system as, 64
Office manager. See also *Personnel.*
    free-lance, 260
    support and counsel for, 258–260
Office policy, 245–248, *247*, *248*

Office procedure, estimated time requirements for, 4t
Office visit, abbreviations of reasons for, 10t
  fee collection policy for, 108, *108*
  no-show, 11, 13
  outstanding accounts and, 12
  return, 24
  scheduling of, 3–15. See also *Appointment.*
Olfactory system, assessment of, 331t
Oligomenorrhea, definition of, 441
Omnibus Budget Reconciliation Act of 1989, 170, 181, 279
Ophthalmic solution or ointment, 349–351
Ophthalmology. See also *Eye.*
  examination in, 327, 331t
  ultrasonography in, 522. See also *Ultrasonography.*
Oral contraception, 457
  candidiasis and, 446
  efficacy of, 466
OSHA. See *Occupational Safety and Health Act.*
Otitis media, pediatric, 436
Outpatient surgery, appointment system for, 13, 15
Outstanding account, appointment request and, 12
Ova, testing for, 541
Oval fat body, in urinalysis, 570t, *571,* 573
Overtime compensation, 235
  exemptions from, 236–237
  office policy and, 246–247
  registered nurse and, 246–247
  time of payment for, 237
  time off in lieu of, 237, 246–247
  waiving of, 237
Oxidase test, 638–639
Oxytocin challenge test, 472

P wave, in electrocardiogram, 501, *502*
PAC (preadmission certification), for health insurance, 158, *159*
Package, mailing of, 36
Pancreas and hepatobiliary system, disorders of, diagnosis-related group and, 803
Panel, definition of, 597
Pap smear, 442–443
Papilloma, ICD-9-CM coding for, 202
Papillomavirus, 447t
Parasitic disease, diagnosis-related group and, 807
  pediatric, 436
  testing for, 541
Parcel post, 36
Parity, definition of, 467
Parking system, protection for, 59–60
Patient, indigent, 110
  interview with, 306–307, *308, 309*
  new, appointment system for, 9–10, 10t
    clinical information from, 30
    computerization and, 207, *208–211*
    demographic information from, 27–28
    form for, 307, *308*
    insurance information from, 28
    interview with, 307, 309
      chief complaint and, 307, 309
      medical history and, 307, *308*
      personal history and, 307, *308*
      PQRST method and, 309
      SOAP and, 309

Patient *(Continued)*
  referral information from, 28, 30
  noncompliant, appointment request and, 12
  physician-referred, appointment system for, 9, 10–11
  problem, appointment system for, 11–12
  recall letter to, 206
  receipt for, 78
  report to, 42
  rights of, 270–272
  scheduling for, computerization and, 206
  teaching materials for, 679–681
Patient's Bill of Rights, 269
Payroll, attendance record and, *130,* 131
  benefits and, 136, *138,* 138
  docking pay and, 237
  earnings card and, 131, *132,* 135
  estimation of, 131
  gross wages and, 136
  married, semimonthly table for, 136, *137*
  net wages and, 136
  overtime and, 131, 135
  record of, 78, 239
  sample, 136
  state and federal regulations and, 131, 135
  taxes and. See also *Tax(es).*
    Employer's Tax Guide, Circular E and, *135,* 136, *137*
    federal, 147–148, *149*
      year-end report in, *150, 151,* 152
    Medicare, 136
    social security, *135,* 136
    state, 136
  W-4 form and, 131, *133–134*
Pediatrics, 403–439. See also *Infant; Newborn.*
  common problems and communicable diseases in, 429–439. See also names of specific problems and diseases.
  growth and development in, 408t, 409–413, *412–424,* 423. See also *Growth and development.*
  immunizations in, 424, 424t, 425t
  measurement of physically handicapped child in, 413
  stool collection in, 541
Pediculosis pubis, 447t
Pelvic inflammatory disease, 451
Pelvis, examination of, 442–445, *443, 444.* See also *Gynecology, examination in.*
  radiography of, 492
  ultrasonography of, 522
Peripheral blood smear examination, 588–592
  blood cell types in, *591*
  guidelines for, 588–589
  preparation for, *590*
  reference values for, 578t
Personal leave, 241–242
Personnel. See also *Health care worker.*
  benefits package for, 239–242. See also *Benefits package.*
  Clinical Laboratory Improvement Amendments of 1988, Final Rule and, 794–795
  DACUM in evaluation of, 268
  discharge of, 260–261
  ethics and professionalism for, 267–268. See also *Ethics.*
  exit interview for, 261
  management of. See *Office manager.*
  misconduct of, 260–261
  overtime compensation and, registered nurse and, 246–247
    time off in lieu of, 246–247
  part-time, 225–226

Personnel *(Continued)*
    policy manual for, 245–248, *247, 248*
        contents of, 246–247, *247*
        general considerations for, 245
        outline for, 245–246
        updating of, 247–248
        writing of, 247, *248*
    recruitment of, 225–234
        appearance in, 232
        bonding insurance and, 233
        candidate selection in, 234
        checklist for, 225, *226*
        courtesy in, 233
        cover letter in, 230
        immigration reform and, 253, *254–256*, 256–257
        interviewing process in, 230–231, *231*
        job application in, *228–229*, 231–232
        job description in, 226–227, *227*
        legal requirements in, *228–229*, 232–233
        letters of reference in, 232
        planning for, 225–226
        preemployment tests in, 232
        reference checks in, 233
        resume in, 230, 232
            unsolicited, 230
        source for, 227–230
            blind ad as, 227
            classified advertising as, 227
            college posting system as, 230
            direct response as, 227
            employee referral as, 230
            employment agency as, 230
            externship program as, 230
            phone response as, 227–230, *228–229*
            unsolicited, 230
            woman's resource center as, 230
    suspension of, 260
    training and education for, 258
    wage and salary policy for, 234–239, *235*
        confidentiality and, 234–235
        federal wage and hour regulations in, 235–239
            administrative exemption and, 236–237
            executive exemption and, 236
            Fair Labor Standards Act and, 235–239
            holiday and, 237, 238
            monthly salary and, 237
            overtime compensation and, 235
                docking pay and, 237
                exemptions from, 236–237
                penalties and, 238
                record-keeping requirements in, 238–239
                rest periods and, 237–238, 238
                time of payment for, 237
                time off in lieu of, 237
                waiving of payment for, 237
            semimonthly salary and, 237
            time record keeping and, 235–236
            vacation and, 237, 238
            workweek exceeding 40 hours and, 237
        pay scale determination in, 234–235, *235*
    warnings to, 260, 261
Pertussis, pediatric, 434
Petri dish holder, in microbiology, 611
Petroleum distillates, poisoning by, 741t
Petty cash, bookkeeping for, *96*, 97–98
    record of, 78

Pharmaceutical manufacturers, directory of, 682–685
Phenol poisoning, 741t
Phenylketonuria, test for, *423*, 424
    filter-paper blood spot collection and, 426–427, *427*
Phlebotomy, universal precautions for, 787–788
Phosphates, in urinalysis, 570t, *571*, 573
Phosphoric acid, poisoning by, 738t
Phosphorus, in blood chemistry test, 599t
Photocopy machines and services, 64–65
Phrase, commonly misinterpreted, 732–736
Phthirus pubis, 447t
Physical examination, card file for, 319
    complete, 322
    for employment, 333
    for insurance examination, 333
    gynecological. See *Gynecology, examination in.*
    items for, 320
    medical assistant's role in, 333
    of breast, *332*, 333
    of ears, 327, *328*, 329–330. See also *Ear.*
    of eye, 324, *324–328, 327.* See also *Eye.*
    of neurological system, 330, 331t, *332*
    of testis, *333*, 333
    positions for, *320–322*
    proctological, *321*, 322–323
        equipment for, 322
        patient care for, 323
        position for, *321*
        procedure for, 323
Physician-patient contract, 280–281, *281, 282*
Physician sample, 65
Pick-up service, for specimen transport, 547
PID (pelvic inflammatory disease), 451
Pin worm, cellophane tape in detection of, 620, *621*, 622
    examination of, 620, 622
    preparation of, 620, *621*
    clinical considerations for, 620
    in urinalysis, 573
    pediatric, 437
PKU. See *Phenylketonuria.*
Placenta, placenta previa and, 471
    premature separation of, 471
Placenta previa, 471
Plasma, definition of, 525
Platelet, in electronic blood cell counting, 592
    in peripheral blood smear examination, 589–592, *591*
    reference values for, 578t, 759
Poison control centers, directory of, 686–688
Poisoning,
    by common chemicals, 738t–741t
    diagnosis-related group and, 808
    toxicology and, reference values for, 764
    treatment for, 738t–741t
Postage meter, 56
Postcoital test, infertility and, 474
Postmortem procedure, HIV transmission and, 773
Postprandial, definition of, 597
Potassium, in blood chemistry test, 599t
Potassium hydroxide preparation. See *KOH preparation.*
Povidone-iodine, allergy to, parenteral medication and, 363
PPO (preferred provider organization), 166, 240
PQRST method, of interviewing, 309
PR interval, in electrocardiogram, 501, *502*
Practice, closing of, 48–49
    goals of, insurance decisions and, 138

Practice (Continued)
  new, construction and design of, 46–47
    general considerations for, 45
    goal setting in, accounting and, 124, *124*
    renting *v* owning, 46
    site selection for, 46
    space planning for, 46
    supplies and furniture for, 47
    time frame for, 45–46
Preadmission certification, for health insurance, 158, *159*
Preeclampsia, 471
Preferred provider organization, 166, 240
Pregnancy, 467. See also *Obstetrics*.
  complications of, 203
  confirmation of, 467
    test for, 640t, 646–648, *647*
  diagnosis-related group and, 806–807
  drug use during, 336, 338t
  ectopic, 471–472
  employment termination and, 253
  expected date of confinement and, 467
  ICD-9-CM coding for, 202–203
  leave of absence and, 241–242
  legislation and, 253
  medication during, 346
  multiple, 203
  postpartum care and, 473
  prenatal care and, 467, *468–469*, 469
    health history and, 467, *468–469*, 469
    physical examination and, 469
  working and, 241
Prenatal care, 467, *468–469*, 469
  health history and, 467, *468–469*, 469
  physical examination and, 469
Presbyopia, definition of, *324*
Prescription. See *Medication, written and oral orders for*.
  for controlled substance, 293, *293*
Preservative, bacteriostatic, 345
  definition of, 525
  in specimen processing, 531
Primigravida, definition of, 467
Primipara, definition of, 467
Probe, 371, *376*
Problem list, 27, *27*
Problem patient, appointment system for, 11–12
Procreation, technology and, 271
Proctology, examination in, *321*, 322–323
  equipment for, 322
  patient care for, 323
  position for, *321*
  procedure for, 323
Proctosigmoidoscopy, 322
  position for, *321*
Products, health care, telephone numbers for, 693
Professional discount, bookkeeping for, 90, *90*
Professional organizations, 258
Professional Standards Review Organization, 67
Profile, definition of, 597
Profit and loss analysis, *143*, 143–144
Progress note, 26, *26*
Prone position, for medical examination, *321*
Proof, of book or article, 43
Protein, in blood chemistry test, 600t
  in urinalysis, 562t
Prothrombin time, 594–597, *596*
  guidelines for, 594–595

Prothrombin time (Continued)
  MLA Electra 750 in, 595–597, *596*
  procedure for, 595–597, *596*
    errors in, 595
  reference values for, 578t
Pseudomenstruation, newborn, 406
PSRO (Professional Standards Review Organization), 67
Psychopharmacologic drug, monitoring of, reference values for, 763–764
Public health, reporting requirements for, 291
  service agency directory for, 689
Public library, as information source for federal and state law, 276–277
Puerperium, diagnosis-related group and, 806–807
  ICD-9-CM coding for, 202–203
Pulse, *311*, 312–313
  location of, *663*
  pediatric, 427, *428*
  site of, *311*, 312
Purchase order, *140*, 140–141
Purchasing control, 61–62
Pyelonephritis, screening for, 626–628

QRS complex, in electrocardiogram, 501, *502*
QRS wave, in electrocardiogram, 501, *502*
Quality assurance, 67–75
  example of, *70*
  general considerations for, 67–68
  medical records in, 72
  monitoring and evaluation process in, 68–70, *69*
  purpose of, 68
  quality control in, 74–75
  quality of care in, 70–72, *73*, 74
    continuing education and, 70–71
    information vital for, 71–72
    job performance in, 71–72
    personnel qualifications and, 70, *71*
  risk management in, 72, *73*, 74
    report form for, *73*, 74
  terminology in, 68
Quality control, 74–75
  Clinical Laboratory Improvement Amendments of 1988, Final Rule and, 793
  definition of, 525
  for Abbott Testpack Strept A test, 625
  for blood chemistry test, 601
  for Color Slide II Mononucleosis Test, 645
  for microbiology, incubator and, 609, *610*
    media and, *612*, 612
    stains and reagents and, 614t
  for pregnancy test, 648
  for rapid plasma reagin test, 652
  for rheumatoid factor test, 650
  for rubella antibody test, 655
  for specimen collection and processing, 550t, 550–551, 551t
  for streptococcal antibody test, 656
  for urinalysis, 553–554, 628
  in C-reactive protein test, 641
  in fecal occult blood test, 631
Quality of care, 70–72, *73*, 74
  continuing education in, 70–71
  information vital for, 71–72
  job performance in, 71–72
  personnel qualifications in, 70, *71*

Quickening, definition of, 467
Quotation, in manuscript preparation, 42–43

Radiography, 476–499
  general guidelines for, 477
  legislation for, 280
  of abdomen, 478
  of ankle, 478–479
  of cervical spine, 480
  of chest, 481
  of elbow, 482
  of femur, 483
  of fibula, 497–498
  of foot, 484–485
  of forearm, 485–486
  of hand, 486–487
  of hip, 488
  of humerus, 489
  of knee, 490
  of lumbar spine, 491
  of pelvis, 492
  of shoulder, 492–493
  of sinuses, 495–496
  of skull, 493–494
  of thoracic spine, 496–497
  of tibia, 497–498
  of wrist, 498–499
  quality control for, 75
  risks of, 476
  safety in, 476–478
Radiotherapy, ICD-9-CM coding for, 201–202
Rales, definition of, 313
Random, clean-catch specimen, for urinalysis, 560–561
Rapid plasma reagin test, for syphilis, 640t, 650–652, *652*
Rash, diaper, 406, 408
  newborn, 406
RBC cast, in urinalysis, *570*, 570t, 571
RBRVS (resource-based relative value scale payment), 181
RDA, (recommended daily dietary allowances), 753
Reagent. See also *Antigen*.
  cyanmethemoglobin, in hemoglobin concentration, 582–583
  in Abbott Testpack Strept A test, 624–625
  in microbiology, 612, *613*, 614t
Recommended daily dietary allowances, 753
Reconstitution, drug, 341, *343*, 345
  precaution for pediatrics and, 345
Record-keeping. See also *Medical record; Payroll, record of*.
  employee records and, 257
  federal wage and hour regulation requirements for, 238–239
  for controlled substances, 293
  Occupational Safety and Health Act and, 810, 820, 830
  of telephone calls, 16
  time, 235–236
Rectum, examination of, position for, *321*
Recumbent position, for medical examination, *320*
Red blood cell, in peripheral blood smear examination, 589–592, *591*
  in urinalysis, 570t, 571, *571*
  value range for, 578t
Reference laboratory, definition of, 526
Reflex, assessment of, 330, 331t, 332
Refrigeration, for specimen, 531
  urine, 556
  in microbiology, 611

Refund, bookkeeping for, 91, *92*
Registered mail, 37
Registered Medical Assistant, 279
Registration, as credential, 279
Rehabilitative procedure, 397–401
  cold application as, 400–401
  general considerations for, 397
  heat application as, 397–400
    hot water bottle for, 398–400
    moist, 397–398
Reimbursement. See also *Fee*.
  coding for. See *Coding, ICD*.
  computerization and, 207, *215*, 216, *216*, *218–221*
  prospective payment plan for, 203
Renal tubular epithelial cell cast, in urinalysis, *570*, 570t, *571*, 571
Reprint, of journal article, 43
Reproductive system, diseases and disorders of, diagnosis-related group and, 806
Research, medical record release for, 33
  resources for, 42
Research registry, 30
Resource-based relative value scale payment, 181
Respiration, 313
  definition of, 313
  normal, 313
  pediatric, 427, *428*
  terminology in, 313
Respiratory system, diseases and disorders of, diagnosis-related group and, 801
  ICD-9-CM coding for, 203
Rest period, 237–238
Resume, 230, 232
Resuscitation, cardiopulmonary, 661, 663
  procedure for, 661, 663, 664, *665–667*, 666
Retained earnings, definition of, 142
Retirement program, 239
Retractor, 371, *376*
Revenue, in accounting, 123, 124, *125–128*, 131, 143. See also *Accounting, revenue in*.
Rheumatic fever, pediatric, 434
Rheumatoid factor, clinical considerations for, 648–649
  test for, 640t, 649–650
Rheumaton Slide Test Kit, 640t, 649–650
Rhonchi, definition of, 313
Rhythm method, 466
Rights, of patient, 270–271
Rinne test, 329
Roseola, pediatric, 431
Round worm, pediatric, 437
Rubascan card test, 640t, 653–655
Rubella, antibody tests for, 640t, 653–655
  clinical considerations for, 652–653
  pediatric, 431

Safety, 74–75. See also *Occupational Safety and Health Act*.
  asepsis and, 301–306, *304*, *305*, 306t
  employee training in, 249
  in urinalysis, 554
Sales representative, 65–66
  ethics of, 66
  physician samples from, 65
  recourse from, 65–66

Saliva, universal precautions for, 786
Salivary gland, ultrasonography in examination of, 522. See also *Ultrasonography.*
Salmonella, pediatric, 434
Sanitization, 303–304
Scabies, pediatric, 437
Scale, beam balance, 411, *412*
  infant, *411*
Scheduling, in emergency, 659, 661
Scissors, surgical, 371, *373*
Scrotum, ultrasonography in examination of, 523. See also *Ultrasonography.*
Second opinion, 41
Securing Access to Health Care, 270
Security, 74–75
  computerization and, 222
  for grounds and parking systems, 59–60
  for medical practice contents, 58–59
  violation of, 60–61
Seizure, 672–673
Semen, analysis of, 474
  collection of, 542
  reference values for, 764
  universal precautions for, 785
Semi-block letter style, *38*
Sensory system, assessment of, 331t
Serology, 639–658
  C-reactive protein test in, 640t, 641–642
  definition of, 529
  general considerations for, 639–640, 640t
  HIV testing in, 640t, 642, 642–643, *643*, 778–780
    clinical considerations for, 642
    enzyme-linked immunosorbent assay for, *642*, 643
    indirect immunofluorescence assay for, 643
    Western Blot test for, 643, *643*
  in group A beta-hemolytic streptococcus, 631
  infectious mononucleosis antibody test in, 640t, 643–645, *645*
  pregnancy tests in, 640t, 646–648, *647*
  rapid plasma reagin test for syphilis in, 640t, 650–652, *652*
  rheumatoid factor test in, 640t, 648–650
  rubella antibody tests in, 640t, 652–655
  streptococcal antibody test in, 640t, 655–656
Serum, definition of, 526
Serum glutamic-oxaloacetic transaminase, in blood chemistry test, 599t
Serum glutamic-pyruvic transaminase, in blood chemistry test, 599t
Serum lipid study, 607
Sexual harassment, 252–253
Sexually transmitted disease, 446, 447t. See also names of specific sexually transmitted diseases.
  condom in prevention of, 466
SGOT (serum glutamic-oxaloacetic transaminase), 599t
SGPT (serum glutamic-pyruvic transaminase), 599t
Shigellosis, pediatric, 435
Shingles, pediatric, 431
Shock, 674–675
Shoulder, radiography of, 492–493
SI unit (International System of Units) 757–758
Sick leave, 241–242
Sigh, definition of, 313
Sims position, for medical examination, *321*
Sinoatrial block, 517, *517*

Sinus rhythm, in electrocardiogram, 502, 504, *504*
Sinuses, radiography of, 495–496
Site, selection of, for new practice, 46
Sitting position, for medical examination, *320*
Skin and subcutaneous tissue, diseases and disorders of, diagnosis-related group and, 804–805
Skin test, 745
Skip tracing, 114–115
Skull, radiography of, 493–494
Small claims court, for delinquent account, 119, *120*, 122
Snellen eye chart, 324, *326*, *327*
SOAP format, 27, 309
Social Security, as benefit, 239
Social security tax, *135*, 136
Sodium, in blood chemistry test, 600t
  in urinalysis, 562t
Sodium citrate, in blood chemistry test, 600t
Sodium fluoride, in blood chemistry test, 600t
Software. See *Computerization, software considerations in.*
Sonographer, 518
Sonography. See *Ultrasonography.*
Sonologist, 518
Space planning, 46
Special delivery, 37
Specialist, appointment system for, 7, 9. See also *Appointment.*
Specific gravity, of urine, 564, *566*, 567
Specimen. See also names of specific tests.
  collection and processing of, 525–551
    chain of custody in, 547–548, 558, *559*
    culture swab for, 531
    equipment and supplies for, 530–531, 531t
    fasting and, 530, 531–532
    for cellophane tape preparation, 620, *621*
    for Color Slide II Mononucleosis Test, 645
    for C-reactive protein test, 641
    for glucose tolerance test, 605–606
    for Hemoccult II Slide Test, 630
    for pregnancy test, 646
    for rapid plasma reagin test, 651
    for rheumatoid factor test, 649
    for rubella antibody test, 653–654
    for streptococcal antibody test, 656
    in microbiology, 615
    labeling in, 532
    laboratory tests and. See *Laboratory test.*
    medication and, 530
    methods of, 533–545
      for blood, 533–541, 597, 601. See also *Blood, collection of.*
      for genital tract, 544–545
      for semen, 542
      for sputum, 542
      for stool, 541
      for throat, 542, 543
        procedure for, 543–544
      for urine, 615. See also *Urinalysis, specimen collection for.*
    preservatives in, 531
    refrigeration in, 531
    serum lipid studies and, 607
    sterile *v* nonsterile collection cup for, 531
    stool culture and, 531
    terminology in, 525–526
    timing in, 531–532

858 SUBJECT INDEX

Specimen *(Continued)*
  universal precautions and, 532–533
  definition of, 526
  delivery methods for, 381, 547
  disposal of, 548t, 548–549, *549*
  equipment maintenance and, 551
  first morning, 532
  Occupational Safety and Health Act guidelines for, 827
  preparation of, 545, 545t, *546*
  preservation techniques for, 545, 545t, *546*
  quality control for, 550t, 550–551, 551t
  spilled, clean-up for, 614
Speculum, 443–445
  appropriate-size, 445
Sperm, in urinalysis, 570t, *573*, 574
Spina bifida, measurements of child with, 413
Spine, cervical, radiography of, 480
  lumbar, radiography of, 491
  thoracic, radiography of, 496–497
Spirillum, gram-stain morphology of, 620
Spitting up, newborn and, 408
Sponge, vaginal, 465
  efficacy of, 466
Sputum, collection of, 542
Squamous epithelial cell, in urinalysis, 570t, *571*, 573
ST segment, in electrocardiogram, 501, *502*
Stadiometer, 413, *413*, *414*
Stain, in microbiology, 612, *613*, 614t
Staining rack, in microbiology, 611
State, legislation from. See *Legislation, state.*
  medical association of, as information source for federal and state law, 277
  medical practice act from, 278–279
Statement of Claim, 119, *120*, 122
Status epilepticus, 673
Statute of limitations, 282, *283–286*, 286
Sterilization, *304*, 304–306, *305*, 306t
  HIV transmission and, 774–775
  informed consent for, *288*
Stertorous, definition of, 313
Stool, collection of, 541
  culture of, 531
  newborn, 409
Storage space, 62–63
Strabismus, definition of, *324*
Streptococcal infection, clinical considerations for, 623
  pediatric, 435
  screening for, 623–625
    Directigen 123 Testpack Strept A in, 624–625
Streptozyme Test kit, 640t, 655–656
Stridor, definition of, 313
Subcutaneous tissue, diseases and disorders of, 804–805
Subpoena, of drug and alcohol abuse record, 33
  of medical record, 33, 34
Substance abuse, 250–251. See also *Drug abuse.*
  substance-induced organic mental disorders and, diagnosis-related group and, 808
  toxicology and, reference values for, 764
Sulfuric acid, poisoning by, 738t
Supine position, for medical examination, *320*
Supplies, for new practice, 47
Suppository, vaginal, 465
  efficacy of, 466
Surgery, 371–401. See also *Rehabilitative procedure.*
  electrosurgery as, 389–390
  fee collection policy for, 108, *108*

Surgery *(Continued)*
  for incising and draining, 385–387
  for topical and subcutaneous lesion, 383–385
  incising and draining as, 385–387
  indexing by, 25, *25*
  informed consent for, *287*, 287–288, 290
  instruments for, 371, *372–377*, 378. See also names of specific instruments.
    cleaning of, 378
  insurance coverage for, 158
  iodine allergy and, 382
  laser, 388
  minor, preparation for, 382
  opening a sterile package for, 380–381
  outpatient, appointment system for, 13, 15
  precautions for HIV transmission and, 771–772
  transferring sterile articles for, 378–379
Surrogacy, 271
Suspension, of personnel, 260
Suture, 371, *377*
  for simple wound, 383
  removal of, 393–394
Swab-transport media system, 543, *544*
Symbol, in clinical practice, 731
Symptom, date of onset of, 30
Syphilis, 447t
  clinical considerations for, 650
  screening tests for, 640t, 650–652, *652*
Syringe, for blood collection, 534

T wave, in electrocardiogram, 502, *502*
Table, in manuscript preparation, 43
Tachycardia, atrial, 512, *512*
  junctional, 512, *513*
  ventricular, 512, *514*
Tachypnea, definition of, 313
Tandem ICON II HCG Test Kit, 640t, 646–648, *647*
Tax Equity and Fiscal Responsibility Act of 1982, 203
Tax Reform Act of 1986, 242
Taxable and Nontaxable Income, federal publication 525, 138
Tax(es), benefits package and, 242, *242*
  employment security contribution, 136
  federal, 146–155
    Circular E of Employers's Tax Guide and, *135*, 136, *137*
    deposits for, *147*, 148
    forms for, 1096, *152*, 155
      1099, *152*, 155
      W-2, *150*, 152
      W-3, *151*, 152
      W-4, 131, *133–134*
      W-9, *153*, 155
    income, 146–148, *147*, 149–154
      deposits for, *147*, 148
      due date for, 147
      penalties on, 148
      quarterly tax reports and, 148, *149*
      rules for, 147–148
    payroll, 147–148, *149*
    year-end report, *150*, *151*, 152
    penalties on, 148
    quarterly tax reports for, 148, *149*, 152
    social security tax as, *135*, 136
  for equipment purchase or lease, 56, 57
  Internal Revenue Code Section 603D and, 242, *242*

Taxes *(Continued)*
  Medicare, 136
  on employee benefits, 138
  property, 146
  social security, *135*, 136
  state, 136, 146
Telephone call, 15–17
  after-hour, 17
  as follow-up, 16
  collection by, 115, 118
  confidentiality and, 16
  documentation of, 16
  general considerations for, 15
  guidelines for, 16, 406–407
  in personnel recruitment, 227–230, *228–229*
  message flow for, 16
  newborn problem assessment by, 406–407
  screening of, 15–16
  urgency of, 16
Telephone numbers, for health care information, products, and services, 693
Telephone solicitor, 62
Telephone systems and services, 64
Temperature, 313–315, 314t
  Fahrenheit *v* Celsius, *314*
  infertility and, 473–474
  normal, 314–315
  pediatric, 427, 427t
  taking of, *315*, 315–316
  variations in, *314*, 315
Terminal digit coding, for medical record, 21, *21*, 23
Terminology, medical, combining forms in, 703–712
Test kit, in microbiology, 612
Testis, self-examination of, *333*
Thermometer, electronic, 315–316
  types of, 315, *315*
Third-class mail, 36
Third-party payer, coding rules from, 195–196. See also *Coding, ICD.*
Thoracic spine, radiography of, 496–497
Throat, specimen from, *542*, 543
  procedure for, 543–544
Thrush, in newborn, 408
Thyroid, tests for, *423*, 424
  filter-paper blood spot collection and, 426–427, *427*
  ultrasonography in examination of, 523. See also *Ultrasonography.*
Thyroxine T_4, in blood chemistry test, 600t
Tibia, radiography of, 497–498
Timed (24-hour) specimen, for urinalysis, 555t, 561, 561t–562t
  procedure for, 563
Tine test, 366, 368, *369*
Topical medication, *347*, 348, 349–352
Tort action, statute of limitations for, 282, *283–286*, 286
Towel clamp, 371
Toxemia. See *Preeclampsia.*
Toxic screening, in urinalysis, 562t
Toxicology, reference values for, 764
Toxoplasmosis, pediatric, 437
Trade school externship program, 230
Trash, disposal of, 60. See also *Waste, disposal of.*
Trauma, diagnostic-related group and, 808
  evidence of, 664
Traveler's diarrhea, 432
Travelers Medicare, 163, *164*. See also *Medicare.*

Treponema pallidum, infection with. See *Syphilis.*
Triage, in emergency, 663–664
Trichomonas, 445, 446t, 447t, *449*
  in urinalysis, *573*
Triglycerides, in blood chemistry test, 600t
Truth In Lending Act, 108, 110, *111*
Tuberculosis, pediatric, 434
  test for, 366–368, *369*, 745
Turbidity, definition of, 597
Turpentine poisoning, 761t

UCR payment (usual, customary, and reasonable payment), 179, 181
Ultrasonography, 418, *419–422*, 422. See also *Echocardiography; Neurosonography.*
  during pregnancy, 472
  in abdomen examination, 418, *421*, 422
  in breast examination, 522
  in chest examination, 522
  in fluid aspiration, 522
  in gynecology, 522
  in kidney examination, 518, *521*
  in liver examination, 518, *521*
  in male pelvis examination, 522
  in needle-guided biopsy, 522
  in obstetrics, 522, *522*
  in ophthalmology, 522
  in salivary gland examination, 522
  in scrotum examination, 523
  in thyroid examination, 523
  in vascular examination, 523
  intraoperative, 522
  procedure for, 418
  report form for, *520–521*
  requisition form for, *519*
Umbilical care, for newborn, 406
Unemployment, employment security contribution tax for, 136
Unemployment compensation, 239
Uniform Donor Card, 294, *294*
Unit dose medication, 340
United Mine Workers of America, Medicare for, 163, *164*. See also *Medicare.*
United States Department of Labor Publication 1282, 238
United States Immigration and Naturalization Services, handbook from, 253, 254–256, 256–257
Universal health care coverage, 270
Universal precautions for blood and body fluid, 301–303, 768–783. See also *Centers for Disease Control, universal precautions for blood and body fluid from.*
  Occupational Safety and Health Act and, 549, 809–810
Urethra, orifice to, *557*
  specimen from, 544
Urethral syndrome, acute, screening for, 626–628
Urethritis, in gonorrhea, 628
  nongonococcal, 447t
Uric acid, in blood chemistry test, 600t
  in urinalysis, 562t
Urinalysis, 553–575, 626–627
  chemical examination in, *567*, 567–568, *568*
    chemstrip or dipstick in, 567, *568*, 568, *569*
    procedure for, *567*, 567–568
  common pathogens in, 635t
  culture techniques for, 633–636, *635*, 635t

Urinalysis *(Continued)*
    calibrated loop method for, 634–636, *635*
        kits for, 634
        pathogens and, 635t, 636
        purpose of, 633
    definition of, 529
    form for, *554*
    general considerations for, 553
    mailing sample of, 554
    microscopic examination in, 570t, 570–571, *570–573*, 574–575
        casts in, *570*, 570t, 570–571
        cells and particles found in, 570, 570t, 571, *571*, 573
        crystals in, 570t, *572–573*, 573–574
        microorganisms in, 570t, *573*, 574
        procedure for, 574–575
        threads and fibers in, 570t, 574
    physical examination in, 564, 565t, *566*, 566–567
        general appearance in, 564, 565t, 566
        procedure for, *566*, 566–567
        specific gravity in, 564, *566*, 567
        volume in, 564, 567
    quality control for, 553–554
    record-keeping in, *554*, 554
    reference values for, 762–763
    safety considerations for, 554
    specimen collection for, catheterized specimen and, 555t, 556–557, *557*
        container for, 556
        decomposition and, *554*, *555*, 556
        drug screening and, 558, *559*
        first morning specimen and, 555t, 560
        fundamentals of, *554*, 556
        infant specimen and, 556, 560
        procedure for, 556
        random, clean-catch specimen and, 555t, 560–561
        timed (24-hour), 555t, 561, 561t–562t
            procedure for, 563
        two-glass, 563–564
        types of, *554*, 555t
Urinary tract, diseases and disorders of, diagnosis-related group and, 805–806
    infection of, clinical considerations for, 626
        screening for, 626–627. See also *Urinalysis*.
Usual, customary, and reasonable payment, 179, 181
Uterus, dysfunctional bleeding from, 451

V code, *188*, 194
    neoplasm and, 202
Vacation, pay for, 237, 238
Vaccine, 424, 424t, 425t
    administration routes for, 425t
    for hepatitis B virus, 811, 825–831
    schedule for, 425t
    types of, 425t
Vacutainer, 531, 531t
Vacutainer Brand Urine Collection Kit, 615
Vacuum tube system, for blood collection, 533–534, 534t
    procedure for, 536–539, *536–539*
Vagina, cream for, 465
    efficacy of, 466
    discharge from, newborn and, 406
    discharge specimen from, 450–451
    foam for, 465

Vagina *(Continued)*
    efficacy of, 466
    orifice to, *557*
    secretions from, universal precautions for, 785
    specimen from, 544
    sponge for, 465
        efficacy of, 466
    suppository for, 465
        efficacy of, 466
Vaginitis, atrophic, 446t
Vaginosis, bacterial, 445, 446t
Vascular system, ultrasonography in examination of, 523. See also *Ultrasonography*.
Vastus lateralis muscle, as injection site, *357*, *359*, 359–360
VDRL (Venereal Disease Research Laboratory test), 447t
Vena caval syndrome, 470–471, *471*
Vendor, selection of, 61–62
Venereal Disease Research Laboratory test, 447t
Venipuncture, billing for, 177
    legislation for, 280
Ventricular fibrillation, *514*, 515
Ventricular flutter, *514*, 515
Ventricular premature contraction, 512, *512*
Ventricular rhythm, 512, *514*, 515
Ventrogluteal site, *357*, *360*, 360–361
Violation, security, 60–61
Viral condition, pediatric, 429–431
Vital sign, general considerations for, 309
    in emergency procedure, *663*, 664
    infant, 427, *428*, 428t
Vitamin, 754–756
Vocational rehabilitation, Worker's Compensation and, 249
Voice, assessment of, 331t
Voluntary health and welfare agencies and associations, directory of, 690–692
Vulvovaginitis, 445–451, 446t, 447t, *449*, *450*
    atrophic vaginitis as, 446t
    bacterial vaginosis as, 445, 446t
    candidiasis as, 445, 446t, *449*
        antibiotics and, 446
        oral contraceptives and, 446
    moniliasis as, *446*, 446t
    patient education in, 446
    sexually transmitted disease and, 446, 447t
    trichomonas as, 445, 446t, 447t, *449*
    types of, 446t
    vaginal discharge specimen in, 450–451

Wage and Hour Publication 1363, 236
Wart, genital, 447t
    removal of, 389–390
Waste, disposal of, 60
    HIV transmission and, 777
    Occupational Safety and Health Act guidelines for, 829
    universal precautions for, 788–789
Waxy cast, in urinalysis, *570*, 570t, 571
Weber test, 327
Weights and measures, 336, 339t
    comparison of, 339t
    table of, 746–750
        conversion tables in, 748–749
        measures of capacity in, 746
        measures of mass in, 746

Weights and measure *(Continued)*
    metric doses with approximate apothecary equivalents in, 750
    metric measure in, 747
Wellness program, 240
West nomogram, medication measurement and, 341, *342*
Westergren method, for erythrocyte sedimentation rate, 584
    reference values for, 578t
  reference values for, 759
Western Blot test, for HIV, *643*, 643
Wheeze, definition of, 313
White blood cell, gram-stain morphology of, 620
  in peripheral blood smear examination, 589–592, *591*
  in urinalysis, 570t, 571, *571*
  reference ranges for, 578t
  value ranges for, 578t
Whooping cough, pediatric, 434
Wintrobe, reference values for, 759
Woman's resource center, in personnel recruitment, 230
Words, commonly misinterpreted, 732–736
Worker's compensation, appointment system for patient with, 11
  as benefit, 239
  definition of, 138
  fee collection and, 110

Worker's compensation *(Continued)*
  termination of, 249–250
  vocational rehabilitation and, 249
Workweek, over 40 hours, 237
World Health Organization, disease classification from, 187
Wound, 675
  changing sterile dressing for, 390–391
  draining, dressing for, 391–392
Wrist, radiography of, 498–499

Yeast cell, gram-stain morphology of, 620
  in urinalysis, 570t, *573*, 574
  thrush and, 408

Zip code, for correspondence, 35
Z-track technique, *365*, 365–366